Dental Hygiene
in Review

Dental Hygiene in Review

Christina B. DeBiase, BSDH, MA, EdD
Professor and Director
Division of Dental Hygiene
West Virginia University
School of Dentistry
Robert C. Byrd Health Sciences Center
Morgantown, WV

LIPPINCOTT WILLIAMS & WILKINS
A **Wolters Kluwer** Company
Philadelphia · Baltimore · New York · London
Buenos Aires · Hong Kong · Sydney · Tokyo

Acquisitions Editor: John Goucher
Managing Editor: Marette Magargle-Smith
Marketing Manager: Debby Hartman

Copyright © 2002 Lippincott Williams & Wilkins

351 West Camden Street
Baltimore, Maryland 21201-2436 USA

530 Walnut Street
Philadelphia, Pennsylvania 19106 USA

The publisher is not responsible (as a matter of product liability, negligence, or otherwise) for any injury resulting from any material contained herein. This publication contains information relating to general principles of medical care which should not be construed as specific instructions for individual patients. Manufacturers' product information and package inserts should be reviewed for current information, including contraindications, dosages, and precautions.

Printed in the United States of America

Library of Congress Cataloging-in-Publication Data
Dental hygiene board review / Christina B. DeBiase, [editor].
     p.   cm.
   ISBN 0-683-30669-3
    1. Dental hygiene—Examinations, questions, etc. I. DeBiase, Christina B.

RK60.5.D428 2001
617.6'01'076—dc21   2001037618

The publishers have made every effort to trace the copyright holders for borrowed material. If they have inadvertently overlooked any, they will be pleased to make the necessary arrangements at the first opportunity.

We'd like to hear from you! If you have comments or suggestions regarding this Lippincott Williams & Wilkins title, please contact us at the appropriate customer service number listed below, or send correspondence to **book_comments@lww.com**. If possible, please remember to include your mailing address, phone number, and a reference to the book title and author in your message. To purchase additional copies of this book call our customer service department at **(800) 638-3030** or fax orders to **(310) 824-7390**. International customers should call **(301) 714-2324**.

02 03
1 2 3 4 5 6 7 8 9 10

This book is dedicated to Dennis O. Overman, PhD (1943–2000). Dr. Overman dedicated most of his professional life to the teaching of histology to dental and dental hygiene students at West Virginia University. The manner in which he lived his life through community and international service, scholarly excellence, and personal faith is an inspiration to us all.
He is deeply missed.

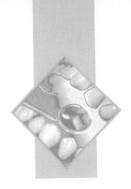

Contributors

Michael Bagby, DDS, PhD
Director
Department of Restorative Dentistry
Division of Dental Materials
West Virginia University
School of Dentistry
Morgantown, West Virginia
Providing Supportive Treatment Services

Peggy W. Coleman, PhD
Professor
Department of Health Sciences and Dental Hygiene
University of Mississippi
School of Health Related Professions
Jackson, Mississippi
Pharmacology

Christina B. DeBiase, BSDH, MA, EdD
Professor and Director
Department of Periodontics
Division of Dental Hygiene
West Virginia University
School of Dentistry
Morgantown, West Virginia
Preparing for the Examination; Taking the Examination; Physiology; Nutrition; Microbiology and Immunology; Assessing Patient Characteristics; Planning and Managing Dental Hygiene Care

Cathryn L. Frere, BSDH, MSEd
Assistant Professor
Department of Periodontics
Division of Dental Hygiene
West Virginia University
School of Dentistry
Morgantown, West Virginia
Performing Periodontal Procedures

Joan Gibson-Howell, RDH, MSEd
Associate Professor
Department of Periodontics
Division of Dental Hygiene
West Virginia University
School of Dentistry
Morgantown, West Virginia
Obtaining and Interpreting Radiographs

Marcia A. Gladwin, RDH, EdD
Professor
Department of Periodontics
Division of Dental Hygiene
West Virginia University
School of Dentistry
Morgantown, West Virginia
Providing Supportive Treatment Services

Joan I. Gluch, RDH, PhD
Director, Health Promotion
Department of Dental Care Systems
University of Pennsylvania
School of Dental Medicine
Philadelphia, Pennsylvania
Analyzing Scientific Information and Applying Research Results

Robert M. Howell, DDS, MSD
Professor
Department of Oral and Maxillofacial Pathology
West Virginia University
School of Dentistry
Morgantown, West Virginia
Pathology

Barbara K. Komives-Norris, RDH, MS
Professor Emeritus
Department of Periodontics
Division of Dental Hygiene
West Virginia University
School of Dentistry
Morgantown, West Virginia
History of Dental Hygiene Board Examinations

Maurice W. Lewis, DDS
Assistant Professor
Department of Diagnostic Services
West Virginia University
School of Dentistry
Morgantown, West Virginia
Anatomic Sciences

Barry T. Linger, EdD
Medical Education Specialist
West Virginia University
School of Medicine
Morgantown, West Virginia
Preparing for the Examination; Taking the Examination

Dennis O. Overman, PhD
Associate Professor
Department of Anatomy
West Virginia University
School of Medicine
Morgantown, West Virginia
Anatomic Sciences

Lauralee Sherwood, DVM
Professor
Department of Physiology
West Virginia University
School of Medicine
Morgantown, West Virginia
Physiology

Margaret Six, BS, MSDH
Assistant Professor
Department of Dental Hygiene
West Liberty State College
West Liberty, West Virginia
**Planning and Managing
Dental Hygiene Care**

Sarah K. Smith, DDS
Owens Community College
Toledo, Ohio
Anatomic Sciences;

Carol Ann Spear, BSDH, MSDH
Professor
Department of Periodontics
Division of Dental Hygiene
West Virginia University
School of Dentistry
Morgantown, West Virginia
**Assessing Patient Characteristics; Planning and
Managing Dental Hygiene Care; Performing Periodontal
Procedures**

Patricia S. Tate, BSDH, MEd
Associate Professor
Department of Dental Hygiene
Raymond Walters College
University of Cincinnati
Cincinnati, Ohio
**Promoting Health and Preventing Disease Within Groups;
Community Health Activities: Participating
in Community Programs**

John G. Thomas, MS, PhD
Professor
Department of Periodontics
Department of Pathology
West Virginia University
Schools of Dentistry and Medicine
Morgantown, West Virginia
Microbiology and Immunology

Dina Agnone Vaughan, BSDH, MS
Member, West Virginia Board of Dental Examiners
Lewisburg, West Virginia
Nutrition

Louise Tupta Veslicky, DDS, MDS, MEd
Senior Associate Dean for Educational Programs
West Virginia University
School of Dentistry
Morgantown, West Virginia
**Assessing Patient Characteristics; Performing Periodontal
Procedures**

Elizabeth R. Walker, PhD
Associate Professor
Department of Anatomy
West Virginia University
School of Medicine
Morgantown, West Virginia
Anatomic Sciences

Jack S. Yorty, DDS
Associate Professor
Department of Restorative Dentistry
West Virginia University
School of Dentistry
Morgantown, West Virginia
Dental Caries/Utilizing Preventive Agents

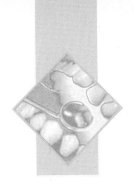

Preface

This textbook has been designed to prepare dental hygiene students to take the National Board Examination by providing them with a comprehensive overview of the basic dental hygiene and dental sciences. Students in the new millenium must be well versed in both question content and format if they hope to be successful in the examination. The text has been divided into four parts and has been organized utilizing the Dental Hygiene Board Examination Specifications. Part I addresses the process of preparing for the Examination, and Parts II, III, and IV represent each of the topic areas covered by the National Board Examination. A separate chapter on dental caries (Chapter 14) has been added rather than as a subtopic area under the "Planning and Managing Dental Hygiene Care" section of the specifications, because the dental hygienist plays a major role in caries assessment and precaution.

Content experts have contributed chapters that thoroughly review the topics with current, accurate information in a relatively concise format. Dental hygiene students may gain some new knowledge, but most of the information presented should serve as a refresher. This textbook may also be a valuable tool to assist dental students with their review for National Board Examinations.

Retrieving previous knowledge learned will assist students in problem-solving the issues of a variety of cases that are representative of the material presented in Chapters 4 to 18. Case-based questions require higher-level learning that essentially involves the integration and application of theory into practice. Cases and related questions are found in the appendix at the end of the text. The majority of the cases involve patients and the provision of clinical dental hygiene services. These patient cases integrate knowledge from the basic and clinical sciences with the application of evidence-based, comprehensive individualized care. The community health cases emphasize the integration of the basic and social sciences with the principles of health education and program planning in the promotion of health for groups of people.

Stand-alone multiple-choice questions appear at the conclusion of each chapter. Photos, radiographs, and illustrations aid in the comprehension of the subject matter and sample questions. In addition, the answers and rationale for selecting them are also provided.

Best of luck to all dental hygiene students taking the National Board Examination. I hope that this review book serves to reduce some of the anxiety associated with preparing to take this examination and is a valuable resource in achieving a successful outcome.

Christina B. DeBiase, BSDH, MA, EdD

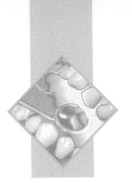

Acknowledgments

I wish to thank all of the contributors to *Dental Hygiene in Review*. A special thank you to those people behind the scenes—to Loreen Hurley for her occasional clerical support when time was of the essence; to Marette Smith and Frank Musick of Lippincott Williams & Wilkins who remained a constant resource throughout this entire process; John Goucher also of Lippincott Williams & Wilkins who recently joined the project as Acquisitions Editor and provided superb guidance and support; West Virginia University School of Dentistry Instructional Technology Department and the Biomedical Communications Department for their assistance with figures; to my loving husband who spent many evenings alone while I sat face-to-face with the computer screen—his love and support are priceless; and to my students who validate my role as an educator every day.

Christina B. DeBiase, BSDH, MA, EdD

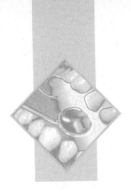

Table of Contents

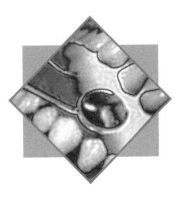

Preparing for Board Examinations

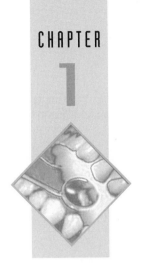

History of Dental Hygiene Board Examinations

BARBARA K. KOMIVES, RDH, MS

 FOUNDATION

Dental hygienists have been interested in creating a dental hygiene national board since the 1950s. At first, the suggestion of a dental hygiene national board received little support from the dental community. Many states had not yet recognized the existing Dental National Board. In states where the Dental National Board had gained acceptance, there was concern about whether enough uniformity existed among dental hygiene education programs to permit national testing. To alleviate this concern, the American Dental Hygienists' Association (ADHA) instituted an achievement testing program in 1959. Concurrently, a liaison committee was established by the ADHA and the American Association of Dental Examiners (AADE) to further enhance support for the dental hygiene national board. The actions of this liaison committee enabled the ADHA to acquire support for a dental hygiene national board from the AADE and the American Dental Association (ADA) Council on Dental Education. (The Council on Dental Education's accreditation authority was transferred to the Commission on Accreditation of Dental and Dental Auxiliary Education Programs in 1975. In 1979, the Commission was renamed the Commission on Dental Accreditation.) In 1960, the ADHA requested that the ADA Board of Trustees consider assigning the development of a dental hygiene national board to an appropriate ADA agency. In 1961, the ADA House of Delegates responded by charging the Council on National Board Examinations with the construction of a written examination program suitable for use by individual state boards of dentistry in the dental hygiene licensure process. A memorandum of agreement was signed by the officers of the ADA and the ADHA, thus establishing a permanent Committee on Dental Hygiene within the Council on National Board Examinations. The committee's composition was designed to ensure continuous ADHA input into the National Board dental hygiene examination program.

 DEVELOPMENT OF THE EXAMINATION

In the summer of 1961, an ADHA education workshop focused on specifications for subject-oriented examinations that were most likely to be accepted by state boards of dentistry. Twelve subjects were identified and grouped in threes to make a four-part examination: Part I = General Anatomy, Dental Anatomy, and Physiology; Part II = Histology, Pathology, and Radiology; Part III = Chemistry, Nutrition, and Microbiology; and Part IV = Pharmacology, Dental Materials, and Preventive Aspects of Dentistry. The Committee on Dental Hygiene adopted examination specifications patterned after those recommended by the 1961 workshop. Each of the four examination parts consisted of 100 multiple-choice test items covering three subjects. In 1962, the first National Board Dental Hygiene Examination was administered. This subject-oriented examination served as the basis for the National Board Dental Hygiene Examination from 1962 to 1972.

 EVOLUTION OF EXAMINATION FORMAT

1969   The Committee on Dental Hygiene recommended replacing the four-part, subject-oriented examination with a comprehensive, function-oriented examination. A steering committee, composed of the four dental hygienists on the Committee on Dental Hygiene plus the ADHA Education Committee, was appointed to develop specifications for a function-oriented examination.

1973   A single, comprehensive dental hygiene examination of approximately 350 test items replaced the four-part, subject-oriented examination. The comprehensive examination was organized around functions that a dental hygienist could be asked to perform. Only functions that may be delegated to a dental hygienist in most states were covered.

1974   The first examination using the new format was administered. The new content outline contained 400 items, including a section on the basic sciences entitled "Scientific Basis for the Practice of Dental Hygiene" and a larger section, "Provision of Clinical Dental Hygiene Services," which focused on clinical care.

1992   The Joint Commission on National Dental Examinations (JCNDE) approved a project to research another change in the structure of the examination. The JCNDE was concerned that some of the test content, particularly the basic science content, was not effectively integrated with the content that addressed the practice of dental hygiene. Some thought that the basic science content bordered on clinical irrelevance. Another concern was that the assessment of the higher levels of knowledge, or the ability to use knowledge in problem solving and critical thinking, was too limited.

1996   A pilot examination was administered to almost all second-year dental hygiene students enrolled in accredited programs. More than 90% of the test items in the case-based component were judged to be appropriate for assessing higher levels of knowledge.

1998   The first examination using a third format was officially administered. This examination is currently in use and focuses a significant portion of its content on criterion-based situations-typical patients with plausible problems. The examination contains a booklet with cases, and the problems are presented as typical sources of information: patient medical and dental history, radiographs, dental chart with periodontal information, clinical photographs, and laboratory reports when applicable. The patient defines the problem, and the multiple-choice test items evaluate the important components of the problem.[5]

◈ CURRENT EXAMINATION FORMAT AND CONTENT

The National Board Dental Hygiene Examination is a comprehensive examination that consists of approximately 350 multiple-choice items. The examination is divided into two components (see Chapters 2 and 3).

The discipline-based Component A includes 200 multiple-choice items or questions (MCQ) that address content in three major areas:

I. **Scientific Basis for Dental Hygiene Practice**
   A. Anatomic Sciences
       1. Anatomy
           a. Head and neck anatomy
           b. Dental anatomy (including tooth morphology, eruption sequence, and occlusion)
               (1) General anatomy
               (2) Root anatomy
       2. Histology and embryology
   B. Physiology
   C. Biochemistry and Nutrition (including nutritional deficiencies)
   D. Microbiology and Immunology
   E. Pathology
       1. General (including inflammation, repair, and neoplasia)
       2. Oral
   F. Pharmacology
II. **Provision of Clinical Dental Hygiene Services**
   A. Assessing Patient Characteristics
       1. Medical and dental history (including vital signs and behavioral factors)
       2. Head and neck examination (including technique and normal and abnormal findings)
       3. Periodontal evaluation (including deposits and stains)
       4. Oral evaluation
       5. Occlusal evaluation
       6. Clinical testing (e.g., thermal, vitalometer, and percussion)
   B. Obtaining and Interpreting Radiographs
       1. Principles of radiophysics and radiobiology
       2. Principles of radiologic health (including radiation protection and measurement)
       3. Technique (including evaluation of quality of radiographs)
       4. Recognition of normalities and abnormalities
   C. Planning and Managing Dental Hygiene Care
       1. Infection control (application)
       2. Recognition of emergency situations and provision of appropriate care
       3. Individualized patient education
           a. Planning of individualized instruction
           b. Provision of instruction for prevention and management of oral diseases
               (1) Dental caries (including dietary counseling)
               (2) Periodontal diseases (including plaque control)
               (3) Oral conditions (including oral cancer, oral habits, tobacco cessation, implants, dental appliance, and exodontia)
       4. Anxiety and pain control
       5. Recognition and management of compromised patients
   D. Performing Periodontal Procedures

1. Etiology and pathogenesis of periodontal diseases
2. Prescribed therapy (including instruments and instrumentation)
   a. Periodontal débridement
   b. Surgical support services (e.g., removing sutures and placing and removing surgical dressings)
   c. Tooth desensitization
3. Reassessment and maintenance (e.g., implant care)
E. Utilizing Preventive Agents
   1. Fluorides-systemic and topical
      a. Mechanisms of action
      b. Toxicology
      c. Methods of administration
         (1) Water fluoridation
         (2) Professionally administered
         (3) Self-administered (including dentifrices, rinses, and tablets)
   2. Pit and fissure sealants
      a. Mechanisms of action
      b. Techniques for application
   3. Other preventive agents
F. Providing Supportive Treatment Services
   1. Properties and manipulation of materials
   2. Polishing natural and restored teeth
   3. Making impressions and preparing study casts
   4. Other supportive services (including placement and removal of temporary restorations, rubber dams, and matrices; and margination and debonding)

III. Community Health Activities
   A. Promoting Health and Preventing Disease within Groups (including media and communication resources)
   B. Participating in Community Programs
      1. Assessing populations and defining objectives
      2. Designing, implementing, and evaluating programs
   C. Analyzing Scientific Information and Applying Research Results

The case-based Component B includes 150 test items that refer to 12 to 15 dental hygiene patient cases.

Adult and child patients are presented in the case format, which includes a patient history, dental/periodontal charting, radiographs, and often intra-oral or extra-oral photographs.

The case-based items address knowledge and skills required in:
   A. Assessing patient characteristics
   B. Obtaining and interpreting radiographs

C. Planning and managing dental hygiene care
D. Performing periodontal procedures
E. Using preventive agents
F. Providing supportive treatment services

RECOGNITION OF NATIONAL BOARD DENTAL HYGIENE EXAMINATION BY STATES

All 53 U.S. licensing jurisdictions accept the National Board Dental Hygiene Examination as fulfilling or partially fulfilling the state written examination requirement. These jurisdictions include all 50 states, the District of Columbia, Puerto Rico, and the U.S. Virgin Islands.

EXAMINATION STATISTICS

More than 4000 individuals take the Dental Hygiene National Board Examination each spring. Since the administration of the current restructured National Board Examination, approximately 92% of first-time candidates have passed. Only 56% of the candidates repeating the examination have passed. This test has a high reliability coefficient of 0.91. The minimum passing raw score is the lowest number of test items that a candidate must answer correctly to pass. This raw score is converted to the reported score of 75%.

Sources

1. American Dental Association: Joint Commission Bylaws. Chicago, ADA, 1990.
2. American Dental Association: Manual for Dental Examiners and Dental Hygiene Educators. Chicago, ADA, 1978.
3. National Board Dental and Dental Hygiene Examinations: 1997 Technical Report: Origins and Purpose of the National Board Dental and Dental Hygiene Examinations. Chicago, ADA, 1997.
4. Joint Commission on National Dental Examinations, Study of the Feasibility of Developing a Case-Based National Board Dental Hygiene Examination. Chicago, ADA, 1994.
5. DeMarais DR: The rationale for patient cases in the national board dental hygiene examinations. J Dent Educ 62:231-234, 1998.
6. Joint Commission on National Boards: History of the National Board Dental Examinations. Chicago, ADA, 1999.
7. American Dental Association: National Board Dental Hygiene Examination Candidate's Guide. Chicago, ADA, 2000.
8. American Dental Association, Department of Testing Services: Report to the National Dental Hygiene Directors' Conference. Chicago, ADA, 1999.

Suggested Sources

http://www.aads.jhu.edu
http://www.ada.org
http://www.adha.org

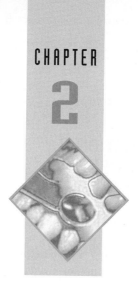

Preparing for the Examination

BARRY T. LINGER, EdD   CHRISTINA B. DeBIASE, EdD

Relax! The hard part is over. You have almost completed your educational program in Dental Hygiene. This chapter is intended to make it easier to prepare for the next step-the dental hygiene licensure examination. It is designed to help you reduce your level of stress and make the most of your study effort by helping you avoid or change poor study habits. Common mistakes made by students when studying for the board examinations include:

- Not knowing the composition of the examination
- Using inefficient or inappropriate study methods
- Not using practice examinations to their maximum benefit
- Starting to study too late
- Not improving their test-taking strategies

 ## YOUR GOAL

Before you start studying for the examination, it is important to remind yourself why you are doing it. You started your educational program because you wanted to become a dental hygienist. Remind yourself of that and focus on it. When it comes time to buckle down and work hard to prepare for the examination, it helps to remember why you are doing it. When you lose sight of your goal, you can get bogged down and overwhelmed.

 ## KNOWING THE EXAMINATION

An important part of preparation for the board examination is knowing the composition of the test. This includes the content areas, the weight of each content area (how many questions are taken from each content area), the format of the questions, and the time allotted to take the examination. The National Board Examination is taken in two sections-a morning (AM) section and an afternoon (PM) section. A total of 350 multiple-choice questions are given. The morning section takes 3½ hours. Approximately 200 "stand-alone" questions are given during this time period. "Stand-alone" means that they do not require information other than that gained from the stem of the question to answer it. These items address all three areas identified on the outline (Scientific Basis for Dental Hygiene Practice, Provision of Clinical Dental Hygiene Services, and Community Health Activities.) Of these items, 5% also address the behavioral sciences, and an additional 5% include ethical and risk management issues.

The remaining 150 questions are case-based items and are given during the afternoon session, which lasts for about 4 hours. These case items are presented in a separate booklet and can only be answered by referring back to descriptions of the patient's history, chartings, photographs, and radiographs. Each case consists of a patient who presents with a problem or a set of circumstances. Questions must address the case and require the selection and use of information from the case components to answer them. There are approximately 12 to 15 cases with 10 to 12 questions accompanying each of them.

The *Candidate's Guide for National Board Dental Hygiene Examinations* includes the specifications for the examination. The specifications are an outline of the topics covered in the examination (see Chapter 1). This outline should be used to guide your study. The number of questions assigned to each topic can help you focus your study on the more heavily weighted areas. Included in the outline are numbers in parentheses that represent the number of items assigned to each topic. For example, there are 60 Anatomic Science items on the National Board. These items are divided into six subject areas.

One of the biggest difficulties that presents to the students with regard to preparing for the examination is knowing what to study. The following excerpt is taken from the Dental Hygiene Examination Specifications:

I. Scientific Basis for Dental Hygiene Practice (60)
   A. Anatomic Sciences (17)
      1. Anatomy(12)
         a. Head and neck anatomy (6)
         b. Dental anatomy (including tooth morphology, eruption sequence, and occlusion) (6)
            (1) General anatomy (3)
            (2) Root anatomy (3)
      2. Histology and embryology (5)
   B. Physiology (5)
   C. Biochemistry and Nutrition (including nutritional deficiencies) (6)
   D. Microbiology and Immunology (10)
   E. Pathology (12)
      1. General (including inflammation and repair, and neoplasia) (5)
      2. Oral (7)
   F. Pharmacology (10)

 ## STUDY METHODS

Few things are more upsetting than to have spent many hours over many weeks faithfully studying, only to find that you remember little of what you have studied. Unfortunately, many students find themselves in this position, not because of insufficient time spent studying but because of the way that they have studied. Memory depends mainly on relating new material to what you have already learned. Doing this allows you to create a chain of inter-related information. Although it is possible to memorize facts in isolation, the information will not stay with you very long. Three strategies for learning that you will help you retain information are mnemonics, linking, and imagery.

Mnemonic Devices

A mnemonic device is a study aid that is often a rhyme or a silly sentence that helps you to recall facts. Mnemonic devices are fun to invent, and they can help you to learn difficult subjects that require extensive memorization. Do-it-yourself mnemonics can be created for any subject. One concern about using mnemonics is that they encourage superficial learning. Learning material for the board examination is more about in-depth learning and critical thinking than quick memorization. Use mnemonics when you think that they are appropriate, but always make meaningful remembering a higher priority. An example of mnemonics involves memorizing the muscles of mastication by the phrase BITEM (**b**uccinator, **i**nternal/medial pterygoid, **t**emporalis, **e**xternal/lateral pterygoid, and **m**asseter). Another example for learning the 12 cranial nerves is memorizing the phrase, "**On** (olfactory) **Old** (optic) **Olympus** (oculomotor) **Towering** (trochlear) **Tops** (trigeminal) **A** (abducens) **Finn** (facial) **And** (accessory) **German** (glossopharyngeal) **Viewed** (vagus) **Various** (vestibulocochlear) **Hops**(Hypoglossal).

Linking

To remember processes or relationships, it is very helpful to find a way to link what you already know to what you are trying to learn. You can then draw a diagram that illustrates

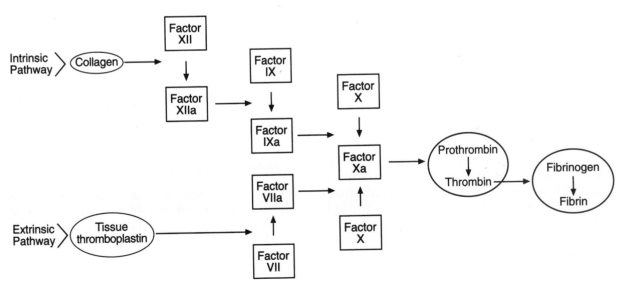

Figure 2-1. The concept of linking used to demonstrate how a clot is formed.

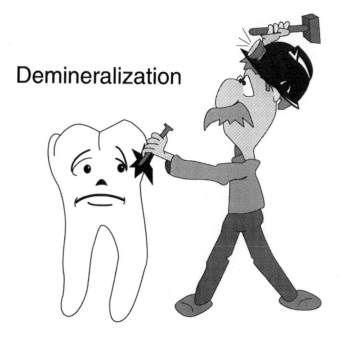

Demineralization

Figure 2-2. Mental pictures such as the miner withdrawing mineral from the tooth to remember the concept of demineralization.

the links. If you are learning a process, the diagram will show the order of actions. If it is a series of relationships, the diagram will show how concepts are related. You must make sure, however, that the linking system accurately depicts the sequence. An example of a link might include a flowchart to depict how a clot is formed (**Figure 2-1**).

Imagery

The use of imagery allows you to use your imagination to build mental pictures to promote active learning. Mental pictures are easy to create and can be a good tool for your memory. When visualizing objects or symbols of concepts, the key is to exaggerate. The more unusual and out of proportion that the images are, the more easily they will be remembered. Once you have created an image, you can expand it to incorporate new material (**Figure 2-2**).

 PRACTICE TESTS

Practice items and tests are some of the most important preparation materials available to you. Practice tests simulate the task that you will be asked to perform, and they provide you with information about your cognitive strengths and weaknesses. Throughout your preparation, you should practice using test items. Make sure that when you are taking practice tests, you approach the items the same way that you will during the real examination. In fact, if at all possible, you should try to visit the actual room where the examination will be administered to familiarize yourself with the

environment. These test-taking preparation strategies will help to improve your overall performance on the testing day. When you sit down to take the real examination, you will not have to think about what you are doing. You will just do it automatically.

 STUDY SCHEDULE

At the start of your preparation for the examination, you should develop a study schedule. Each week you should establish a schedule that takes into account class time, clinic time, meals, and all other obligations. You should decide on a regular time for study and consistently use it for examination preparation only (**Figure 2-3**). During these study periods, study in a quiet place and at the same desk if possible. If you start to daydream or need a break, do it away from your study desk. The desk will become the stimulus for concentration and hard work.

 TIMELINE

3 to 6 Months Before the Examination

At this time, you should start to prepare for the examination. Begin by preparing a study plan, which should include the resources that you are going to use (e.g., create a file by subject that includes your notes, handouts, books, journal articles), the study methods, a weekly study schedule, and an outline of the examination topics.

Before you really begin studying, a good way to determine the strengths and weaknesses in your knowledge base is to take a simulated board examination. This simulated examination should be taken under conditions as close to real examination conditions as possible. This will also help you to evaluate your test-taking abilities.

1 Month Before the Examination

At this point, you should simulate the examination again. You can do this earlier, but do not do it later. If you do it later, there will not be enough time to remedy defects in your knowledge and test-taking strategies.

1 Week Before the Examination

This is the time when you should be reviewing previously learned material. You should not be learning new material during the last week. Focus on reviewing high-yield facts, your notes, and the review chapters of this book.

Try your best to avoid disrupting your routine during the week leading up to the examination. A major disruption can have a negative impact on your mental and physical condition during the examination.

	Monday	Tuesday	Wednesday	Thursday	Friday	Saturday	Sunday
6:00							
7:00							
8:00							
9:00							
10:00							
11:00							
12:00							
1:00							
2:00							
3:00							
4:00							
5:00							
6:00							
7:00							
8:00							
9:00							
10:00							
11:00							
12:00							

Figure 2-3. Weekly schedule to establish study times.

The Day Before the Examination

The night before the examination is the time to rest and relax. Make sure that you have all of the things that you need to take with you to the examination. Do not study any new material. If you feel that you must study, then review very general information. Do not quiz yourself. You may become unnecessarily frustrated. Do not change your daily routine. Go to sleep at your normal time. Students who go to bed much earlier than usual often have difficulty going to sleep.

The Morning of the Examination

Do not do anything different than you do during a normal morning. Wake up at your normal time and eat a normal breakfast. Wear loose comfortable clothing. Arrive at the test site 30 minutes before the time designated for admission. Get to know your testing site before the examination begins (e.g., location of the restroom, water fountain). Each of these things should help you to feel fairly relaxed and comfortable when the examination begins.

After the Examination

Once you leave the examination, do not think about it. There is nothing you can do about it after the test is over. Have fun and relax. Just taking the test is a major achievement. Be proud of your effort and what you have accomplished.

 REVIEW

- Develop and use a study schedule to maximize the efficiency of your preparation for the examination.
- Set up a timeline to follow for the months, weeks, and days leading up to the examination. (Remind yourself of your goal.)
- Begin your preparation 3 to 6 months before the examination.
- Learn as much as you can about the examination.
- Use all of the resources that you have available to you to help you prepare.
- Connect new material to previously learned material by using mnemonic devices, linking, and imagery.
- Use practice tests to determine your strengths and weaknesses and to practice your test-taking strategies.

Suggested Sources

Grant P: Reading and Study Skills. Englewood Cliffs, NJ, Prentice Hall, 1989.

McWhorter KT: Study and Thinking Skills in College. New York, Harper Collins, 1992.

Reynolds JA: Succeeding in College: Study Skills and Strategies. Boston, Allyn & Bacon, 1996.

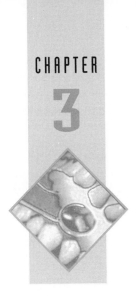

CHAPTER

3

Taking the Examination

BARRY T. LINGER, EDD   CHRISTINA B. DeBIASE, EDD

How you perform on the National Board examination depends on both your fund of knowledge and your test-taking skills. Improving both of these will improve your performance. Chapter 2 addressed how to prepare for the examination by increasing your knowledge and improving your access to the knowledge you have acquired during your professional education. This chapter explains how to improve your test-taking skills and specifically how to deal with case-based questions.

 ## PART 1: GENERAL TEST-TAKING

Attack the Examination

You have studied diligently to prepare for the National Board Examination. Fully learning the material is the most important and obvious variable in your examination performance. Other factors that will affect the outcome of your performance include how you approach the questions. You may consider using the following three-stage strategy. The value of this strategy is that you read every part of the test the first time through to stimulate your memory, and answer the items that you are sure of first. You should not focus on questions that you do not know. Ultimately, if you run out of time and have to guess, you are guessing on only those items that you were uncertain of in the first place.

Stage 1

- Begin with the first item.
- Read the complete question (stem and alternatives or answer choices).
- Answer all of the questions that you immediately know the answer to.
- Make immediate decisions about the remaining questions by marking these questions with either a (+) or a (−).
  - (+) I think that I could answer the question if I had the time to figure it out.

- (−) I don't think that I will ever know the answer to the question even if I have the time to figure it out.
- Do this until you have gone through the test once.

Stage 2

- Go back to the beginning and answer all of the questions marked with a (+).

Stage 3

- Finally, answer all of the questions marked with (−). An example of a three-stage test-taking strategy follows.

  1. Fluoride toxicity manifests in bones as:
     A. rickets
     B. osteoporosis
     C. hypercalcemia
     ○ **D.** osteosclerosis
  2. Which of the following nodes receives lymphatic drainage from maxillary teeth?
     A. Buccal
     + **B.** Submental
     C. Infraorbital
     D. Submandibular
  3. Genetic mutations are likely to result from radiation interaction with which of the following?
     A. Lipids
     − **B.** Proteins
     C. Amino acids
     D. Nucleic acids

Difficult Questions

Questions on the National Board Examination require varying amounts of time to answer and may vary in their level of difficulty. You must not waste time on extremely difficult or time-consuming questions. Mark the question with either a (+)

or a (−) and move on to the next question. Spending excessive time on these questions may prevent you from having adequate time to answer easier questions later in the examination. Remember that this examination is not weighted. Each individual question counts the same as every other question on the test.

As the examination progresses, you will not know the answer to some questions. Do not get discouraged by these questions. A standardized examination is designed to distinguish among all of the individuals taking it. Therefore, you should not expect to know the answer to every question or to answer each question correctly. Do not dwell on these questions. Mark them so that you can come back to them later or make an educated guess. One of the biggest mistakes that examinees often make is that they allow a prior difficult question to have a negative impact on their approach to future questions. When you leave a question, do not think about it again until you see it again.

Another reason to avoid letting a difficult question upset you is that it may not even count toward your final score. On any given test, approximately 15% of the items are included as quality checks.

Guessing

As mentioned earlier, there is no penalty for guessing. An unanswered question counts the same as one that is answered incorrectly. No part of the examination should be left unanswered. When you do not know the answer, make an educated guess. Choose an alternative that you recognize over one that is unfamiliar to you. Choosing the unfamiliar alternative is a common mistake that examinees make. If you studied the subject, nothing should be unfamiliar to you. The unfamiliar alternative is more likely to be a distractor than the correct answer.

Changing Answers

One of the most frustrating things that you can do when taking an examination is to change a correct answer to an incorrect one. You should not change answers that you have already marked unless you have a convincing reason to do so. Many examinees go back at the end of the examination and change their answers-often to wrong answers. Due to fatigue, your performance is much less effective at the end of the examination than when you started it. Unless there is a logical reason to do so, keep your original answer.

Surviving the Examination

Performing your best involves learning how to control your thinking and learning how to stay reasonably relaxed. The ability to control your thinking relates to your attitude. A negative attitude will interfere with your performance during the examination, whereas a positive attitude will enhance your performance. Learning how to relax during the examination is critical to performing well and remaining fresh for the afternoon session.

Throughout the test, it is important that you use "positive self-talk." At the end of each page, say something positive before going on to the next page. For example, say, "Great! I answered most of the items on this page." These positive statements will help to keep you calm and optimistic during the examination.

If you find yourself falling into a pattern of negative thinking, reflect back on your goals. Your goals will help you remember the reason why you are taking the examination, the effort you put in to preparing for it, and the outcome associated with passing the examination. This will also put into perspective the small amount of effort that it will take to focus and concentrate throughout the remainder of the examination.

If you find yourself becoming frustrated or anxious during the examination, try to take a 30-second breather. Close your eyes, breathe deeply, and slowly count to 10. This should help you to continue refreshed. Visualizing a calming place where you would like to be (i.e., island beach) is also effective. This will help to control your anxiety level.

During the lunch break between the examination sections, do something that will give you a mental break from the rigors of the examination. Examples of mental break activities include playing cards with a friend or reading a novel. The only time you should be thinking about the examination is when it is in front of you.

Analysis of Multiple-Choice Questions

A group of 10 to 12 related multiple-choice questions follow the case. Each multiple-choice question has a stem followed by four or five possible answers or alternatives. A multiple-choice item asks for either the **correct** response or the **best** response. Questions asking for the best answer provide alternatives with finer distinctions between correct and incorrect (**Example 1**). The stem may be written in the form of a question or a partial statement (**Examples 2 and 3**). (An asterisk denotes the correct answer.*)

Example 1

Which of the following BEST describes the purpose of potassium sulfate in a mix of irreversible hydrocolloid? **(Stem)**

A. Acts as a filler material
B. Keeps the mix from separating
C. Controls the consistency of the mix
D. Retards the setting of the hydrocolloid
E. Helps produce a hard, dense stone cast surface

Alternatives = one is the correct answer and the remaining are distractors.

Example 2

Which of the following nerves supplies the intrinsic muscles of the tongue?
A. Vagus
B. Facial
C. Lingual
D. Hypoglossal*
E. Glossopharyngeal

Example 3

Radiographic intensifying screens are used for
A. increasing detail.
B. magnifying images.
C. reducing exposure time.*
D. speeding the processing time.
E. decreasing the processing time.

Paired true-false items may also be given. The stem contains two statements. Only four alternatives are given in a question of this type (**Example 4**).

Example 4

One objective of taking medical histories on your patients is to establish baseline information. Another objective is to prevent potential medical emergencies from occurring.
A. Both statements are TRUE.*
B. Both statements are FALSE.
C. The first statement is TRUE; the second statement is FALSE.
D. The first statement is FALSE; the second statement is TRUE.

Cause-and-effect items are also written as two clauses separated by the word, "BECAUSE." The first clause is a statement, followed by the reason that the first statement is factual. Several things must be determined: (1) Is the first statement true or false?; (2) Is the reasoning correct or incorrect?; and (3) Are the statement and the reason related (**Example 5**)?

Example 5

Before undergoing any periodontal surgery, a patient should be controlling the accumulation of plaque, BECAUSE the incidence of disease recurrence increases if a plaque-infected dentition exists after surgery.
A. Both the statement and the reason are correct and related.*
B. Both the statement and the reason are correct, but NOT related.
C. The statement is correct, but the reason is NOT.
D. The statement is NOT correct, but the reason is correct.
E. Neither the statement NOR the reason is correct.

Negative stems are also written in a two-sentence format. One incorrect response must be distinguished from four correct alternatives (**Example 6**).

Example 6

Cyclosporine, an antirejection drug, may produce any of the following conditions, EXCEPT one. Which one is the exception?
A. Candidiasis
B. Xerostomia*
C. Immunosuppression
D. Gingival hyperplasia
E. Hypertension

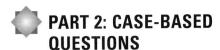

PART 2: CASE-BASED QUESTIONS

Composition of the Examination

As stated in Chapter 2, the National Board Examination is taken in two sections. There is a morning section and an afternoon section, which includes a booklet of cases. A total of 350 multiple-choice questions are given. Approximately 200 questions are referred to as "stand-alone" items. This means that the answer does not require information other than that gained from the stem of the question.

The remaining 150 questions are case-based items, which are presented in a separate booklet and can be answered only by referring back to descriptions of the patient's history, chartings, photographs, and radiographs. Each case consists of a patient who presents with a problem or a set of circumstances. Questions must address the case, and answers require the selection and use of information from the case components. There are approximately 12 to 15 cases with 10 to 12 questions accompanying them. The Joint Commission considers a total score of 75% to be the minimum passing score.

"Stand-alone" questions can be taken from any single topic area identified in the Dental Hygiene Examination Specifications outline. Cases incorporate as many topic areas as possible from the examination specifications outline to present a scenario that integrates basic, dental, and dental hygiene science knowledge to solve patient problems and deliver competent dental hygiene care.

Cases are usually categorized into five areas:

1. Geriatric
2. Adult-periodontal
3. Special needs
4. Medically compromised
5. Pediatric

Some overlap is naturally going to occur, because patients typically present with multiple problems of varying types.

Approximately 80% of the patients identified in the cases are adults and 20% are pediatric patients. Approximately 15% or more of the patients presented in the cases will be medically compromised. Patients with special needs are those with mental or physical conditions, which limit their ability to perform home care or to cooperate with treatment. Examples might include spinal cord injuries, blindness, and cerebral palsy.

Cases also have several components or tools to assist with assessing, planning, and managing the care of the patient presented. Patient history information includes the patient's age, gender, relevant physical characteristics (weight and height), vital signs, medical history, dental history, relevant social history, and chief complaint. Charting is provided and includes periodontal probing depths, furcations, clinically missing teeth, and clinically visible carious lesions. Current oral hygiene status and supplemental oral examination findings are also provided. Each case also contains one or more black and white and/or color photographs of the patient's intraoral findings, radiographs, and study casts. (See the case format in Appendices 1 and 2.)

Approaching Case-Based Questions

Approach one case at a time. First, scan the multiple-choice questions that relate to the case to determine what content areas are being addressed. Then, thoroughly read the case and review each of the assessment tools (i.e., history, charting, radiographs, and photos) and search for the appropriate answer to each question. You will find the answer by integrating information from various sources, much the same way that you do when managing the needs of your "real-life" patients. If you look at the case components or the assessment tools first, you will probably experience information overload, because you do not yet know what you are looking for.

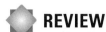 **REVIEW**

- Develop a strategy to attack the examination.
- Use a test-taking strategy that benefits you in some way.
- Do not allow yourself to waste time on difficult questions.
- When you do not know an answer, make an educated guess.
- Do not change your answers unless you find a clue in the test that proves one of your answers to be wrong.
- Whenever you are finished with an item, a section, or the examination itself, do not think about it anymore. Thinking about past items only takes away from your ability to concentrate on what you are currently working on.
- Remain positive throughout the examination.
- Review case multiple-choice items first, then thoroughly read case, and examine assessment tools to locate the correct answer.
- Examine all assessment information (e.g., probing depths, radiographs) before deciding on the correct answer.

Suggested Sources

American Dental Association Joint Commission on National Dental Examinations: Guidelines for the Development of Patient Cases for Dental Hygiene Examinations. Chicago, ADA, 1995.

American Dental Association Joint Commission on National Dental Examinations: Guide for Writing Effective Multiple-Choice Test Stems. Chicago, ADA, 1999.

American Dental Association Joint Commission on National Dental Examinations: National Board Dental Hygiene Examination Candidate Guide. Chicago, ADA, 2001.

McWhorter KT: Study and Thinking Skills in College. New York, Harper Collins, 1992.

Reynolds JA: Succeeding in College: Study Skills and Strategies. Boston, Allyn & Bacon, 1996.

Shain DD: Study Skills and Test-Taking Strategies for Medical Students: Find and Use Your Own Personal Style. New York, Springer-Verlag, 1992.

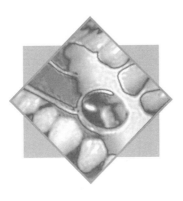

Scientific Basis for Dental Hygiene Practice

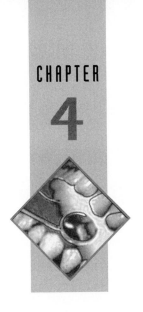

CHAPTER 4

Anatomic Sciences

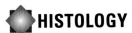 **HISTOLOGY**

DENNIS OVERMAN, PHD
CHRISTINA B. DEBIASE, EDD

Cell Structure

Cells vary considerably in size, shape, and relationship to surrounding structures, but they all have the same basic anatomy. A cell membrane, the **plasmalemma**, surrounds each cell and separates it from its environment. Within the cell, the **nucleus** is the genetic control center. Between the nucleus and the plasmalemma lies the **cytoplasm**, which contains the machinery necessary for cell function and any products being stored by the cell.

Plasmalemma

The plasmalemma is a complex structure that consists of a double layer of lipid molecules plus associated proteins. This layer is remarkable in its property of selective permeability, which is the ability to allow certain materials to enter and leave the cell while preventing other materials from doing the same. Proteins incorporated into the plasmalemma enable cells to recognize each other and allow extracellular materials to recognize specific cells. Many of the cell's organelles have membranes as part of their structure, and these membranes share many structural features with the plasmalemma.

Nucleus

The nucleus is surrounded by a double membrane, the **nuclear envelope,** which separates the nucleus from the cytoplasm. Tiny pores in the nuclear envelope allow for the movement of materials between the cytoplasm and the nucleus. Within the nucleus lies the cell's **chromatin,** which consists of protein and the genetic material responsible for directing the cell's activity. The nucleus also contains a **nucleolus** (or sometimes several nucleoli), consisting of protein and RNA, which helps primarily to produce the **ribosomes** necessary for protein synthesis.

Cytoplasm

Under the direction of the nucleus, the **cytoplasm** performs the various functions of the cell. It surrounds the nucleus and extends to the plasmalemma. Its specific components vary in their presence and relative proportions according to the particular functions of each cell. Specific organelles are responsible for the numerous functions of cells.

Mitochondria have the ability to store energy derived from the metabolism of food in a form that is useful to the cell and then make this energy available to the cell for its various activities.

The **endoplasmic reticulum** is an elaborate network of channels and spaces enclosed within a membrane, and it may be found throughout the cytoplasm. The precise structure of the endoplasmic reticulum varies according to cell activity, and this organelle is involved in the synthesis of cell products and their transportation through the cytoplasm by way of its network arrangement.

The **Golgi complex** is closely related to the endoplasmic reticulum both in structure and function. The final steps in the preparation of a cell's secretory material are undertaken in the Golgi complex; thus, it is described as being a "packaging center" for the cell in preparation for the release of a product.

Lysosomes are membrane-bound structures within the cytoplasm that contain enzymes specifically for the breakdown and destruction of other materials. The enzymes in the lysosomes can degrade and digest foreign materials taken

TABLE 4–1 Classification of Epithelia

TYPE	SHAPE OF SUPERFICIAL CELL LAYER	TYPICAL LOCATIONS
One cell layer		
Simple squamous	Flattened	Endothelium (lining of blood vessels); mesothelium (lining of peritoneum and pleura)
Simple cuboidal	Cuboidal	Lining of distal tubule in the kidney and ducts in some glands; surface of the ovary
Simple columnar	Columnar	Lining of the intestine, stomach, and excretory ducts in some glands
Pseudostratified	All cells rest on basal lamina, but not all reach the lumen; thus, the epithelium appears "falsely stratified"	Lining of the trachea, primary bronchi, nasal cavity, and excretory ducts in parotid gland
More than one cell layer		
Stratified squamous (nonkeratinized)	Flattened (nucleated)	Lining of the esophagus, vagina, mouth, and true vocal cords
Stratified squamous (keratinized)	Flattened (and without nuclei)	Epidermis of skin
Stratified cuboidal	Cuboidal	Lining of ducts in sweat gland
Stratified columnar	Columnar	Lining of large excretory ducts in some glands and the cavernous urethra
Transitional	Dome-shaped (when relaxed); flattened (when) stretched	Lining of the urinary passages from the renal calyces to the urethra

From Gartner LP, Hiatt JL, Strum JM: Cell Biology and Histology. Baltimore, Williams & Wilkins, 1998, p 83.

into the cell, worn-out cell components, and even the entire cell itself in the case of cell death.

The **cytoskeleton** provides supporting elements in the form of tiny **microfilaments** and **microtubules** that maintain a cell's general shape and keep it from collapsing. The microtubules in some cells are involved in the transportation of materials from one part of a cell to another.

Centrioles are organelles that are constructed of microtubules. They form the spindle fibers that are important in the separation of chromosomes during cell division and are required for the formation of **cilia** (i.e., tiny hair-like structures on the surfaces of some cells).

In addition to the various organelles that have specific functional roles in the cell, the cytoplasm may also contain **inclusions,** which are materials that are stored within the cytoplasm but have no independent cellular functions. Fat, glycogen, and pigment granules are examples of inclusions (See Figure 5-1).

Epithelial Tissues

At the microscopic level, everything in the body can be classified into one or a combination of four basic tissue types: epithelial tissues, connective tissues, muscle tissues, or neural tissues. The **epithelial tissues** differ from the other tissue types in their location. All are located at the various surfaces of the body, either internal or external, although some epithelial structures are no longer attached to body surfaces because they have lost their surface connection during development. Epithelial tissues are organized into layers of tightly attached cells resting on a basement membrane, which separates the epithelial tissue from the connective tissue beneath it. Blood supply to the epithelial tissue is by way of blood vessels in the connective tissue, and the blood vessels do not enter the epithelium.

Epithelial tissues may consist of one layer of cells, the **simple epithelial tissues,** or more than one layer or cells, the **stratified epithelial tissues**. Epithelial tissues are further classified depending on the shape of the cells or, if cells with several shapes are present, according to the shape of the cells located at the free surface. Cell shape in epithelial tissue varies from very thin flat cells (**squamous** epithelial cells) to cells shaped like cubes (**cuboidal** epithelial cells) to tall cells shaped like columns (**columnar** epithelial cells) to everything in between. However, only these three shapes (i.e., squamous, cuboidal, and columnar) are used for the purpose of classification (**Table 4-1).**

Epithelial tissues have several functions. Their location at the body surfaces gives them a role in protecting and maintaining homeostasis in the body by regulating the passage of materials into or out of the body. Another important function of epithelial tissues is secretion, and all the glands of the body are epithelial structures. Specialized epithelial tissues function in sensory reception as in, for example, taste buds or the retina of the eye.

Connective Tissues

The connective tissues function to support and connect the numerous structures of the body and enable the body to withstand physical stress. The connective tissues include a group of tissues grouped together under the term **connective tissue proper** plus the more specialized connective tissues of cartilage, bone, blood, bone marrow, adipose, and lymphatic tissue.

All connective tissues consist of **cells** and material located around and between the cells. This material is called the **extracellular matrix.** The composition and arrangement of the extracellular matrix determine the properties of a connective tissue.

Connective tissues are noted for having **relatively few cells.** The cells present in connective tissues are **far apart** and often do not touch each other. The space between the cells is occupied by the extracellular matrix. Connective tissues often **contain many blood vessels,** and in fact the blood vessels use connective tissues as their pathways for travel.

Connective Tissue Components

The connective tissues are made of **cells** and an **extracellular matrix.** The extracellular matrix in turn has two components, both of which are manufactured by the cells. The extracellular matrix consists of three types of **fibers** and a structureless **ground substance.**

Cells

Adult connective tissues are complex and diverse. In very early embryos, only one type of connective tissue and one type of connective tissue cell (i.e., the **mesenchymal cell***)* exist. This cell is famous for its ability to differentiate into all the other connective tissue cells types when required in each different location.

One of the most common, most ubiquitous, and most important types of connective tissue cells is the **fibroblast.** This cell is responsible for the formation of the fibers and the ground substance of the extracellular matrix in the connective tissue proper. **Macrophages** are connective tissue cells that function in defense by using their lysosomal activity to eat and destroy unwanted foreign material and destroy worn-out cells.

Mast cells are characterized by the presence in their cytoplasm of numerous large granules, the contents of which function in mediating immune processes. Their most famous granule contents, **heparin** and **histamine**, play a role in mediating blood vessel function. **Plasma cells** are important connective tissue cells of the immune defense system, because these cells are responsible for the formation of antibodies. Plasma cells are located where they can quickly encounter foreign antigens that enter the body; therefore, the connective tissue just beneath the epithelium of the digestive tract is a common location. All fat in the body is located within **adipose cells.** Within the adipose cell, tiny fat droplets eventually come into contact with each other and begin to coalesce until the cell is entirely filled with a single huge droplet of fat. The nucleus and the cytoplasm, which is stretched to its limits, are forced to occupy the thin outer rim of the cell. They often appear in large clumps where they make up a connective tissue type of their own-adipose tissue. **Leukocytes** (i.e., white blood cells), recently escaped from the circulatory system, are also commonly found in connective tissue **(Figure 4-1)**

Extracellular Matrix

Fibers. The fibers of connective tissue give this tissue its strength and ability to withstand stress. Different types of connective tissue are designed to withstand different types of stress; thus, the fibers vary according to specific needs. **Collagen fibers** are widespread throughout the body and are demonstrated most dramatically in tendons and ligaments, which consist mainly of collagen fibers. The protein of collagen fibers is the most abundant protein in the body, and collagen fibers are an important component of cartilage and bone. **Reticular fibers** are tiny fibers that form a supporting network for cells all over the body. They have been shown to be a type of collagen, but they have retained their own name. **Elastic fibers** are a completely different type of fiber made of a different protein, elastin; these fibers are found in places where resiliency is needed as a property of the connective tissue.

Ground Substance. The ground substance of connective tissues consists of a solution of structural proteoglycans and glycoproteins and varies in consistency from very thin and watery to semigel to gel and even in a few cases to a very stiff gel.

Classification of Connective Tissue Proper

Several different classification schemes for connective tissue are in use. The following method is as good as any and is better than most.

Embryonic Connective Tissues

Two types of connective tissue are found only in the embryo but are important precursors of the adult connective tissue types.

Mesenchyme (mesenchymal connective tissue) is the primitive embryonic connective tissue from which the other types of connective tissue are derived. This primitive type of connective tissue remains almost unchanged in the tooth pulp, but it is not called mesenchyme in adult teeth.

Mucoid (or mucous) connective tissue is an intermediate type of connective tissue through which other connective tissues pass as they differentiate from mesenchyme into something more advanced. This type is most often studied in the umbilical cord, where it never advances beyond this stage of differentiation.

Adult Connective Tissues

The extracellular matrix of adult connective tissue is organized in order to withstand stress. If the tissue is subject to stress from many directions, the fibers will be arranged in many directions. If the stress comes primarily from one direction, the fibers will all be arranged in the same direction. The greater the stress, the larger and stronger and more numerous will be the fibers.

Loose areolar connective tissue (or just plain areolar connective tissue) is found all over the body. This type of

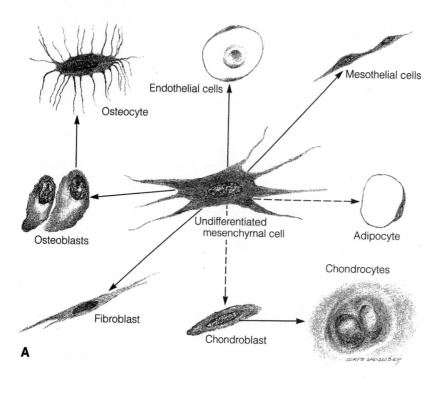

A

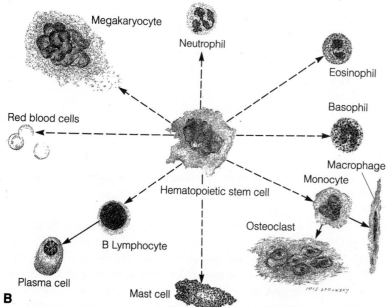

B

Figure 4-1. Diagram showing the origin of connective tissue cells. *A,* Cells arising from undifferentiated mesenchymal cells are formed in connective tissue and remain there. *B,* Cells arising from hematopoietic stem cells are formed in the bone marrow and reside transiently in connective tissue. *Dotted lines* indicate that intermediate cell types occur between those shown. (From Gartner LP, Hiatt JL, Strum JM: Cell Biology and Histology. Baltimore, Williams & Wilkins, 1998, p 83.)

tissue is found beneath the basement membranes of epithelial tissues. It surrounds and supports the blood and lymphatic vessels, bundles of muscle fibers, and the secretory components of glands.

When large clumps of adipose cells occur together, this is referred to as **adipose tissue.** Obviously, the main cell type of adipose tissue consists of adipose cells. Reticular fibers are present in large numbers and form a network to support the adipose cells.

The **dense connective tissues** occur in areas of the body that are subjected to a great deal of stress. If the stress comes primarily from one direction (e.g., in tendons and ligaments), the fibers are arranged in a parallel fashion to withstand this stress. This arrangement is called **dense regular connective tissue.** If the stress in dense connective tissue is applied from various directions, the fibers are arranged in every possible direction to deal with the stress. Such an arrangement is called **dense irregular connective tissue.** The cells of dense irregular connective tissue are mainly fibroblasts. The fibers are usually collagen fibers, such as in the dense irregular connective tissue of the dermis of the skin.

Cartilage

Where there is a need for strong, yet flexible support and the ability to withstand a great deal of pressure, **cartilage** is the type of connective tissue designed to do the job. As a connective tissue, cartilage has the characteristics of all connective tissues, namely relatively few cells surrounded by a great deal of extracellular matrix of fibers and ground substance. Different varieties of cartilage are adapted to accommodate different types of stress, but all have the same basic structural plan.

Cartilage Formation

Cartilage develops from mesenchymal cells that have differentiated to the point of synthesizing extracellular matrix components typical of cartilage. Cells that produce cartilage are no longer mesenchymal cells; instead, they have become **chondroblasts** (i.e., cartilage-forming cells). The extracellular matrix of cartilage consists of fibers and ground substance. The fibers of cartilage consist of a type of collagen fiber, and the ground substance is rich in macromolecules, which give it the consistency of a very stiff gel.

As chondroblasts synthesize the extracellular matrix of cartilage, they become surrounded by this new matrix material and cut off from direct contact with other chondrocytes. Production of additional matrix stops, and the cells no longer form cartilage; from that point on, they are called **chondrocytes.** If the cells were to be removed from the cartilage, the spaces formerly occupied by the cells would remain as little holes in the matrix called **lacunae** (i.e., **little lakes**). Within its lacuna, each chondrocyte is separated from the other chondrocytes by the surrounding matrix. As cartilage grows older, it is common for chondrocytes to divide, with the result that several chondrocytes may occupy the same lacuna. A group of chondrocytes within the same lacuna is called an **isogenous group** (i.e., they have the same beginning). The chondrocytes are separated from each other; however, they are not totally isolated, because they can receive nutrients and eliminate waste products by the slow diffusion of materials through the stiff gel of the matrix. Blood vessels are not usually present in the cartilage tissue; therefore, most of the cells are at some distance from their source of nutrients, resulting in a slow response by the cells when cartilage is damaged by trauma or disease. Healing, therefore, becomes a very slow and difficult process.

Cartilage grows by a combination of two methods. As each chondroblast surrounds itself with cartilage matrix and continues matrix production, the distance between the individual cells increases because more and more matrix is being produced. The cartilage grows by this expansion from within. Growth by expansion from within is called **interstitial growth.** Meanwhile, more mesenchymal cells are being recruited from around the periphery of developing cartilage to become chondroblasts, thus adding more matrix to the surface of the existing cartilage. Growth by the addition of material to the surface of the tissue is called **appositional growth.** Interstitial growth is most important in very early cartilage formation; however, as growth continues, appositional growth takes over and accounts for most of the increase in size.

A layer of dense connective tissue surrounds the cartilage in all except a few locations. Its location (around the cartilage) accounts for the name, the **perichondrium**.

Types of Cartilage

Each type of cartilage has some distinctive differences, but all types show clearly the most important histologic feature of cartilage-the presence of chondrocytes within lacunae.

Hyaline cartilage is the most common and most widespread of the three types of cartilage. It shows all the histologic features described earlier. A perichondrium is present around hyaline cartilage, except where it is attached directly to bone and at the articular surfaces of bones in moveable joints. Hyaline cartilage makes up the fetal skeleton and is found in the nose, larynx, and attachments of the ribs to the sternum. This cartilage provides the slippery surface at the articular ends of the bones and at the same time is able to withstand the great pressure that is often encountered at these locations.

Elastic cartilage consists of everything that hyaline cartilage has plus one more feature-enormous amounts of elastic fibers in the matrix. Elastic cartilage is found in places where very flexible support is required: the external ear, the epiglottis, and a few of the smaller cartilages of the larynx.

Fibrocartilage is found in regions of very great stress and is particularly well adapted to withstand shearing forces in places like the intervertebral disks. It is a composite connective tissue with a combination of properties of hyaline cartilage and dense connective tissue, thus it contains cells located in lacunae within a matrix that looks like dense connective tissue **(Figure 4-2).**

Bone and Osteogenesis

Bone is a specialized connective tissue. It is organized to provide support and accommodate the stress of supporting the whole body in an upright position, protect the delicate organs of the thorax and the brain, and provide a strong and rigid connective tissue as a support for the attachment of the muscles.

As a connective tissue, bone has all the necessary characteristics and components of the connective tissues. Bone has cells and extracellular matrix. The extracellular matrix contains fibers and ground substance. In addition, the ground substance contains inorganic minerals, and as a result bone is hard. Nevertheless, bone is still a living tissue that can grow, change over time, and repair itself. The combination of collagen fibers and inorganic minerals makes bone extremely strong, relatively lightweight, and somewhat resilient; consequently, bone is a remarkable building material.

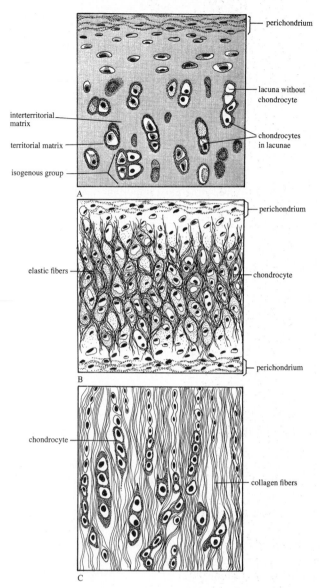

Figure 4-2. The three types of cartilage are shown. *A*, Hyaline cartilage. *B*, Elastic cartilage. *C*, Fibrocartilage. (From Borysenko M, Berringer T: Functional Histology, 2nd ed. Boston, Little, Brown, 1984, p 96.)

Bone Formation

Bone, like cartilage, develops from mesenchyme. However, because bone is hard, the cells cannot receive nutrient materials by diffusion. The individual cells must, therefore, maintain physical contact with each other by means of thin cytoplasmic processes and blood vessels incorporated into bone as it forms.

In areas of mesenchyme where bone is going to form, the mesenchymal cells begin to synthesize extracellular matrix components that are typical of bone. Former mesenchymal cells that now produce bone matrix are called **osteoblasts**. First, the osteoblasts synthesize the organic components of the matrix, then the inorganic minerals are added later. As more bone matrix is produced, the osteoblasts become surrounded and trapped within the matrix, but they remain in

contact with each other by means of cytoplasmic processes. Once surrounded by matrix, the osteoblasts stop forming bone, because there is nowhere to put it; new osteoblasts then differentiate at the surface in order to continue the growth process. The cells that have become trapped in the matrix can no longer be called bone-forming cells, thus from this point on they are called **osteocytes**. As in cartilage, these cells are located within tiny spaces in the matrix called **lacunae**; however, in addition to the lacunae, very tiny tunnels permeate the bone matrix. These tunnels are called **canaliculi** and are occupied by the thin cytoplasmic processes by which the osteocytes remain in contact with each other and with nearby blood vessels.

Mature compact bone consists of cylindrical units of bone called **osteons** or **haversian systems.** The osteons consist of concentric lamellae of bone matrix surrounded by a central **haversian canal**. Lamellar bone is also found at sites other than the osteon. **Volkmann canals** are channels in lamellar bone through which nerves and blood vessels travel from the periosteal and endosteal surfaces to reach the osteon. Volkmann canals do not have concentric lamellae **(Figure 4-3).**

Because bone is hard, it can only grow by the addition of new bone at its surfaces; that is, appositional growth. As bone grows, a layer of dense connective tissue called the **periosteum** forms around its periphery. Most bones, especially the long bones of the body, contain a cavity that is occupied by the bone marrow. This cavity has a lining of connective tissue, the **endosteum,** which consists of a thin layer of rather flat cells and small fibers. The periosteum of bone corresponds to the perichondrium of cartilage, but the endosteum has no counterpart in cartilage because cartilage has no internal cavity.

As bone grows, it must sometimes change its shape in response to varying conditions. Bone is hard and cannot bend or change easily; nevertheless, it does change by the action of cells called **osteoclasts**, which are designed specifically to remove existing bone. These large, multinucleated cells attack the surfaces of bone by enzyme action; as a result of their activity, bone tissue is continuously removed and then replaced by osteoblasts, even as it is being formed. This process is called **remodeling**.

Intramembranous Osteogenesis

Whereas all bone growth is appositional (because bone is hard), there are two different mechanisms of bone formation in different circumstances, both of which involve the same types of cells and fibers and also the same type of ground substance. The mechanism of bone formation already described is called **intramembranous osteogenesis**. In intramembranous osteogenesis, the osteoblasts form new bone matrix at the surfaces of small pieces of bone. These small pieces of bone grow and eventually coalesce into larger and larger pieces of bone until a particular bone is complete.

Endochondral Osteogenesis

Endochondral means "within cartilage," and **endochondral osteogenesis** occurs within a pre-existing cartilage model.

Figure 4-3. A piece of long bone is cut to reveal a cross-section, longitudinal section of the organ, and the wall of the bone marrow cavity. The holes in the marrow cavity wall are openings of canals that carry blood vessels between the bone marrow and bone tissue. On the longitudinal surface of the bone, canals lie longitudinally in the organ and have horizontal branches from one long canal to another and from long canals to the marrow cavity. The cross-cut surface reveals cross-sections of the long canals, each of which is surrounded by several bone lamellae. Each haversian canal and its several lamellae constitute an haversian system. On this surface are also circumferential lamellae, which constitute the outer surface of the organ.

An enlargement of one half of a cross-section of a single haversian system shows the haversian canal surrounded by several haversian lamellae. Between the lamellae are lacunae, which house osteocytes in the living bone. The lacunae are connected to each another and the haversian canal by numerous canaliculi. (From Melfi RC, Alley KE: Permar's Oral Embryology and Microscopic Anatomy. Philadelphia, Lippincott Williams & Wilkins, 2000, p 205.)

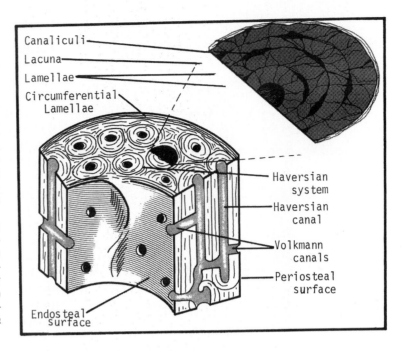

The results of endochondral and intramembranous osteogenesis are the same; the only difference between the two methods is that endochondral osteogenesis involves the formation of bone in an area that originally contained cartilage, which must first be removed. Cartilage does not harden and become bone; rather, it is physically removed and replaced by bone. Removal of the cartilage matrix involves several steps that must occur before bone deposition can begin. In short, the chondrocytes attract inorganic minerals to the cartilage matrix, thus cutting themselves off from their nutrient supply. Starved chondrocytes die and leave behind pieces of calcified cartilage matrix. Cells similar to osteoclasts remove the calcified matrix, while at the same time osteoblasts use the surfaces to begin the deposition of bone matrix. Thus, the cartilage is gradually removed and bone tissue begins to take its place. Bone formation within the former cartilage model barely begins before osteoclasts start to degrade and remove some of the newly formed bone. The result is the formation of a hollow cavity in the shaft of the long bone within which the bone marrow will develop.

The complex steps described in the process of endochondral osteogenesis were to remove the cartilage and deposit bone in its place. The resultant bone tissue is identical to bone formed by the intramembranous method. Both types of osteogenesis are appositional, but in the case of endochondral osteogenesis the original cartilage model had to be removed before bone could be deposited.

Elongation of Long Bones

The long bones of a newborn are not very long. Over a period of years, these bones lengthen dramatically despite the apparent difficulties caused by the hardness of bone. As endochondral osteogenesis begins in the center of the shaft of a long

bone and proceeds toward the ends, and as secondary centers of ossification appear at the ends and grow toward the middle, a band of hyaline cartilage, which is not immediately replaced by bone, remains at each end of the bone. This band of hyaline cartilage is the **epiphyseal plate** or growth plate. Interstitial growth of the cartilage of the epiphyseal plate on the side nearest the end of the bone results in elongation of the bone. Continued growth of the cartilage of the epiphyseal plates is under the control of growth hormone. When growth hormone production stops after puberty, no more cartilage is formed in the epiphyseal plate. Endochondral ossification of the remaining cartilage continues until all the cartilage is replaced by bone and the epiphyseal plates have closed. Thereafter, bones cannot continue to increase in length. Closure of the epiphyseal plates of different bones occurs at predictable ages, and knowledge of the closure times in various bones is useful in the prediction of growth and in forensic determination of the age of bones **(Figure 4-4)**.

Muscle Tissues

The presence of contractile proteins and even the ability to contract to some extent is a property of most cells. **Muscle tissues** contain such high concentrations of contractile proteins that the organization of these proteins may even be visible with the light microscope. The organization of muscle cells in relation to each other is such that their contraction results in coordinated movement.

Three types of muscle exist: (1) **skeletal muscle**, named according to what it is attached to; (2) **smooth muscle**, named according to its appearance; and (3) **cardiac muscle**, named according to its location. Both skeletal muscle and cardiac muscle are **striated;** that is, they show a pattern of stripes or **striations** in their cytoplasm owing to the way that the two types of contractile proteins line up in relation to

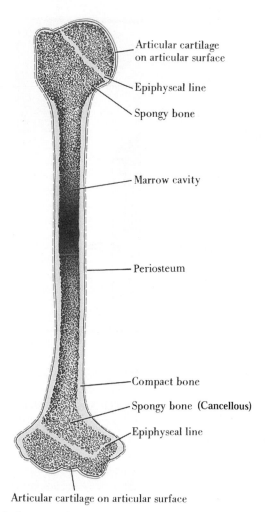

Articular cartilage
on articular surface

Epiphyseal line

Spongy bone

Marrow cavity

Periosteum

Compact bone

Spongy bone (Cancellous)

Epiphyseal line

Articular cartilage on articular surface

Figure 4-4. Structure of a typical long bone. The shaft of the long bone, the diaphysis, contains a large marrow or medullary cavity surrounded by a thick-walled tube of compact bone. A small amount of spongy bone may line the inner surface of the compact bone. The ends of epiphyses of the long bone consist mainly of spongy bone with a thin outer shell of compact bone. An additional term, the metaphysis, refers to the expanded or flared part of the bone at the extremities of the diaphysis. Except for the articular surfaces that are covered by hyaline (articular) cartilage, indicated by the *solid line*, the outer surface of the bone is covered by a fibrous connective tissue capsule called the periosteum, indicated by the *dashed line*. (From Ross MH, Romrell LJ, Kaye GI: Histology: A Text and Atlas. Baltimore, Williams & Wilkins, 1995, p 153.)

each other. Smooth muscle is so-named because it is not striated and, therefore, looks smooth.

Skeletal Muscle

Skeletal muscle gets its name from the fact that it is attached to the skeleton. This type of muscle is under direct voluntary control. Contractions of skeletal muscle are quick and forceful but cannot be easily maintained for a long time. The fibers are long and fairly straight and have a uniform diameter throughout; therefore, skeletal muscle fibers all look basically alike in cross-section.

Cardiac Muscle

Cardiac muscle is named after its location in the heart (Greek **kardia** means **heart**). Cardiac muscle is not under voluntary control, and its contractions are forceful and rhythmic. Contraction of cardiac muscle begins early in embryonic life and can continue uninterrupted for many years.

Cardiac muscle fibers are not multinucleated, although it is not unusual to see cardiac muscle fibers with two nuclei rather than the usual one. The nuclei are centrally located, in contrast to skeletal muscle. The continuous activity of cardiac muscle requires tremendous amounts of energy, thus the fibers contain huge numbers of large mitochondria. Mitochondria are so numerous that the myofibrils cannot get as close to each other as they do in skeletal muscle, with the result that the striations are somewhat less distinct. An extensive blood supply is required, and the large number of capillaries found in cardiac muscle means that the individual fibers are not located as close to each other as were those of skeletal muscle.

At the point where adjacent cardiac muscle fibers make contact with each other end to end, there is an attachment structure called an **intercalated disk**, which functions to attach the fibers to each other and allows direct communication between adjacent fibers.

Organization of Myofibrils

The contractile proteins **actin** and **myosin** are responsible for muscle activity, and their arrangement in skeletal and cardiac muscle creates larger structures called **myofibrils,** many of which form a muscle fiber. The manner in which the actin and myosin myofilaments line up next to each other in the myofibril results in the appearance of striations **(Figure 4-5).**

Smooth Muscle

Smooth muscle contains actin and myosin myofilaments. The myofilaments are not organized into myofibrils and, therefore, the fibers are not striated but instead look smooth compared with the other two types of muscle. The single nucleus of a smooth muscle fiber is centrally located and is famous for its long, narrow, pale appearance. The fibers are fusiform; that is, they are thickest in the middle and taper to a fine point at each end. A cross-section through smooth muscle will cut some of the fibers through the middle and some of them nearer the end, thus the size of the fibers seen in a cross-section will vary, although they will all have approximately the same basically round shape.

Smooth muscle contraction is slow and sustained and is not under voluntary control. The fibers are surrounded by a network of reticular fibers, which unite the individual fibers into layers, sheets, or large bundles. The surrounding reticular fibers help make it possible to coordinate the contractile activity of a whole layer or sheet of smooth muscle.

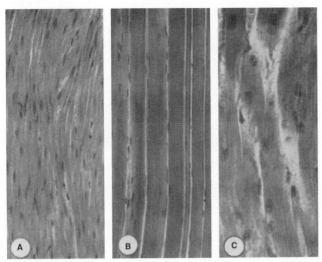

Figure 4-5. Sections of muscle types. *A,* Smooth muscle. *B,* Striated voluntary muscle. *C,* Striated involuntary muscle (cardiac) with intercalated disks. (From Melfi RC, Alley KE: Permar's Oral Embryology and Microscopic Anatomy. Philadelphia, Lippincott Williams & Wilkins, 2000, p 18.)

Neural Tissues

Many different types of cells communicate with each another in various ways; however, this property is extremely well developed in the **neural tissue** (also called nervous tissue). The activities of all body parts are directed and coordinated by means of an extensive network of neural tissue. Cells of the nervous system have the property of **irritability** (i.e., the ability to respond to a stimulus) and **conductivity** (i.e., the ability to transmit information to other cells).

Neurons

Neurons are the communicating cells of the nervous system. In their differentiation, neurons have become very highly specialized for their communicating function. Specialization occurs at the expense of some other cellular functions, namely the ability to replicate by mitosis and the ability to perform some metabolic activities that are carried out routinely in other cells. Because the neurons are so highly specialized, neural tissue also includes cells that function in supporting and nutritive roles.

Because neurons must communicate over long distances, it is not surprising that they are usually large cells with extensive cytoplasmic processes, some of which are extremely long. Most neurons possess a cell body (or **perikaryon**), a number of branching **dendrites**, and a single **axon**. The cell body and the branching dendrites are specialized for receiving nerve impulses from other neurons. The axon is usually specialized for conducting impulses to influence other neurons **(Figure 4-6).**

Supporting Cells

The supporting cells within the central nervous system are called **glia**. Some glia are involved in forming a supportive

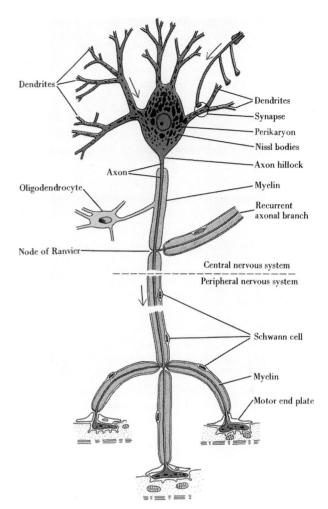

Figure 4-6. Diagram of a motor neuron. The perikaryon, dendrites, and initial part of the axon lie within the central nervous system (CNS). The axon leaves the CNS and, while in the peripheral nervous system (PNS), is part of a nerve (not shown) as it courses to its effectors (striated muscle). In the CNS, the myelin for the axon is produced by and is actually part of an oligodendrocyte; in the PNS, the myelin is produced by and is actually part of a Schwann cell. (From Ross MH, Romrell LJ, Kaye GI: Histology: A Text and Atlas. Baltimore, Williams & Wilkins, 1995, p 258.)

and protective sheath around the axons of neurons. Other glia have different supporting and metabolic functions that aid the neurons.

The supporting cells of the peripheral nervous system are the **Schwann cells** (or neurilemma cells). Schwann cells form a protective covering so that no part of a neuron is exposed to surrounding non-neural tissue.

Nerve Fibers

Axons of neurons and their protective coverings make up **nerve fibers**. The protective covering of a nerve fiber may consist only of supporting cells, or it may include a protein and lipid sheath called **myelin**, which is produced by the supporting cells. As nerve fibers travel throughout the body, they are generally organized into bundles by means of connective tissue coverings. These bundles of nerve fibers make up the nerves seen in gross anatomy.

Blood

Of the four basic tissue types, blood is classified as a connective tissue. Like all connective tissues, it has cell components and an extracellular matrix. The extracellular matrix of blood is a fluid that under normal circumstances does not contain fibers. The fluid component of the blood holds the cells in suspension and maintains various chemicals in solution. Blood has been regarded as essential to life since human life began, and throughout civilization it has been endowed with mysterious and even sacred properties. In an adult, the **5 to 5.5 L** of blood comprise about 8% of the total body weight.

Blood Plasma

Plasma is the fluid component of the blood. When the blood is separated into its various components, plasma comprises approximately 60% of the total volume. Plasma itself is 91.5% water and 7% proteins. The remaining 1.5% consists of nutrients, waste products, enzymes, hormones, and inorganic salts. In addition, the plasma carries heat.

Formed Elements

The cellular components of the blood, considered as a group, are called **formed elements**. This term is used because not all of these components are really cells (see later).

Erythrocytes

The **erythrocytes (red blood cells)** spend their entire functional lifetime inside the circulatory system and are responsible for the transportation and exchange of respiratory gases. Technically speaking, erythrocytes are not true cells because they lack a nucleus, but by virtue of a long and distinguished usage, it is acceptable to refer to them as red blood cells (RBCs).

In males, about 5.5 million erythrocytes per mm^3 of blood are present; in females, approximately 5 million erythrocytes per mm^3 of blood exist. The average functional life span of an erythrocyte is 120 days. The body must produce the amazing number of 2.5 million new erythrocytes every second merely to stay even. During the 120-day life span of an erythrocyte, it travels about 700 miles within the circulatory system. During this time, the erythrocyte is forced through narrow capillaries, gets knocked around in the large vessels, and is pushed into vessel walls at high speeds, while simultaneously being involved in the exchange of gases back and forth across its cell membrane. This continuous activity takes its toll on the membrane. Because erythrocytes lack the necessary cellular machinery to repair or replace the membrane, cells whose membranes begin to wear out are removed from circulation in the spleen, where macrophages degrade them and recycle many of their components.

The red color of erythrocytes is caused by **hemoglobin**. This respiratory pigment has the ability to bind with oxygen or with carbon dioxide and carry it to the lungs (in the case of carbon dioxide) or from the lungs (in the case of oxygen).

Leukocytes

The **leukocytes** [i.e., white blood cells (WBCs)] are true cells that contain nuclei and all other necessary cell machinery. Adults possess about 5,000 to 10,000 leukocytes per mm^3 of blood. Leukocytes do not spend their entire lifetime within the circulatory system, using the circulatory system only for transport from their origin in the bone marrow to their functional location somewhere outside the circulatory system. Leukocytes exit the circulatory system by squeezing between the endothelial cells lining the capillaries. This process is called **diapedesis**. Their travels in the circulatory system may last for only a few hours or as long as a few days. Leukocytes are replaced in the blood at the rate of about 1 million/sec. All the leukocytes are involved in defense against foreign material.

Granular Leukocytes

The **granular leukocytes** are classified on the basis of the staining reaction of granules visible in their cytoplasm with the light microscope.

The **neutrophils** are by far the most numerous of the granular leukocytes, and they account for 60% to 70% of all the leukocytes seen in a blood smear. Granules are present in the cytoplasm of these cells, but it is difficult to determine whether these granules are eosinophilic or basophilic in staining. In fact, there is a mixture of both types, which is what makes a determination difficult. Second, the nucleus of a neutrophil is very dark and segmented into three, four, or even five lobes, which remain attached to each other by thin strands of chromatin. The appearance of the nucleus is responsible for giving neutrophils the names often used clinically: polymorphonuclear leukocytes (**many-shaped nucleus**) or **polymorphs** or simply **PMNs**. Neutrophils can engulf bacteria by phagocytosis and break down the bacteria by means of the granules, some of which are lysosomes.

Eosinophils are granular leukocytes with large red orange granules in the cytoplasm and a nucleus that is typically bilobed and not as dark as that of a neutrophil. Eosinophils defend the body against parasitic infections and function along with mast cells in allergic reactions. They constitute 2% to 4% of the leukocytes in normal blood.

Basophils are the least numerous of all the leukocytes, accounting for only about 0.5% of all the leukocytes in normal blood. The cytoplasm of the basophil is packed with large basophilic granules that are not all the same size. The nucleus is often bilobed, bent into an S shape, and almost to-tally obscured by the granules. Basophils are very closely related to mast cells, both in origin and function. The gran-ules of basophils contain many of the same substances that are found in mast cell granules, and they function along with mast cells in immune reactions.

Agranular Leukocytes

Two types of **agranular leukocytes** exist-monocytes and lymphocytes-neither of which shows cytoplasmic granules with the light microscope.

The **monocytes** are the largest of all the leukocytes, and they make up about 5% of the leukocytes in circulating blood. They are slightly larger than the granular leukocytes, and they may be three times larger than the diameter of an erythrocyte. The nucleus is quite large and horseshoe-shaped and appears to be folded over on itself as if there were not enough room for it in the cell. The cytoplasm is a homogeneous bluish-gray. Like all the other leukocytes, monocytes use the blood for transportation. Once they leave the circulatory system, monocytes differentiate into **macrophages** or into osteoclasts.

The **lymphocytes** are the smallest of the leukocytes (the smallest one being not much larger than an erythrocyte). The nucleus of a lymphocyte is round with a somewhat dark stain. All lymphocytes look the same (except for their size); however, different classes of lymphocytes have different roles in the immune system. **B lymphocytes** (or B cells) are formed in the bone marrow and are the precursors of **plasma cells**, which are the cells responsible for antibody formation. **T lymphocytes** (or T cells) are named after the thymus, on which they depend for their formation. Several different types of T lymphocytes exist, and they play differ-ent roles in the immune defense system. Some are able to destroy foreign cells directly, whereas others play a more peripheral role in stimulating and aiding other cells of the immune system.

Platelets

The **platelets**, or thrombocytes, have an important function in hemostasis, which is to keep the blood in the circulatory sys-tem where it belongs. Platelets accomplish this by promoting blood clotting and helping repair damaged blood vessel walls. Platelets range from 150 to 400 thousand per mm^3 of blood. Platelets are not cells but rather are fragments of cytoplasm broken off from the tips of cytoplasmic processes of large cells of the bone marrow, the **megakaryocytes**. When a blood vessel is injured, platelets aggregate at the site to form a platelet plug. These platelets then release the contents of their granules, which react with proteins of the blood plasma in a complex chemical reaction that leads to the formation of a blood clot (**Tables 4-2 and 4-3**). See also Chapters 7 and 8.

Cardiovascular System

In multicellular organisms, most of the cells are located some distance away from the source of nutrients and the ex-cretory organs; therefore, it becomes necessary to circulate a fluid environment to the cells. The circulatory system is designed to accomplish this function.

The human circulatory system includes a pump, the **heart**, to keep the fluid environment moving; a system of tubes, the **arteries** and **veins**, for transport of the fluid medium; and vast numbers of **capillaries** for the exchange of nutrients and waste products. The cardiovascular system reaches all parts of the body, thus providing a method of communication utilized by the endocrine system.

Capillaries

Capillaries are just large enough in diameter to allow blood cells to pass through in single file. Their structure consists of the very thin simple squamous epithelium, called **en-dothelium**, resting on a basement membrane. This thin en-

TABLE 4–2 Size and Number of Formed Elements in Human Blood

CELL TYPE	DIAMETER (μM)		NO./MM³	% OF LEUKOCYTES
	SMEAR	SECTION		
Erythrocyte	7–8	6–7	5×10^6 (men) 4.5×10^6 (women)	—
Agranulocytes				
Lymphocyte	8–10	7–8	1500–2500	20–25
Monocyte	12–15	10–12	200–800	3–8
Granulocytes				
Neutrophil	9–12	8–9	3500–7000	60–70
Eosinophil	10–14	9–11	150–400	2–4
Basophil	8–10	7–8	50–100	0.5–1
Platelet	2–4	1–3	250,000–400,000	—

From Gartner LP, Hiatt JL: Color Atlas of Histology, 2nd ed. Baltimore, Williams & Wilkins, 1994, p 84.

TABLE 4–3 Selected Characteristics of Granulocytes

CHARACTERISTIC	NEUTROPHILS	EOSINOPHILS	BASOPHILS
Nuclear shape	Lobulated (3 or 4 lobes)	Bilobed	S-shaped
Number of azurophilic granules	Many	Few	Few
Specific granules			
Size	Small	Large	Large
Color*	Light pink	Dark pink	Dark blue to black
Contents	Alkaline phosphatase	Acid phosphatase	Eosinophil chemotactic factor
	Collagenase	Arylsulfatase	(ECF)
	Lactoferrin	β-Glucuronidase	Heparin
	Lysozyme	Cathepsin	Histamine
	Phagocytin	Major basic protein	Peroxidase
		Peroxidase	
		Phospholipase	
		RNase	
Life span	1 week	Few hours in blood; 2 weeks in connective tissue	Very long (1–2 years in mice)
Main functions	Phagocytose, kill, and digest bacteria	Moderate inflammatory reactions by inactivating histamine and leukotriene C	Mediate inflammatory responses in a manner similar to mast cells
Special properties	Form H_2O_2 during phagocytosis	Are decreased in number by corticosteroids	Have receptors for IgE on their plasma membrane

*Cells stained with Giemsa or Wright stain..

dothelium forms a tiny tube; thus, capillaries consist of nothing more than an endothelial tube. Capillaries provide the mechanism of exchange for materials to move between the circulatory system and the surrounding tissues and back again. Their very thin walls and the nature of the cells of their endothelial lining allow for this exchange.

Arteries and Veins

Although arteries and veins appear in many sizes, they are all constructed according to the same basic three-layered plan. The innermost layer is called the **tunica intima** (also called the tunica interna). This layer consists of the endothelium and its basement membrane, plus a thin layer of connective tissue. The middle layer is called the **tunica media**, which is composed mainly of smooth muscle with its fibers arranged circularly. The largest arteries also contain elastic fibers in this layer. The outer coat is the **tunica adventitia** (sometimes called the **tunica externa**). It consists primarily of connective tissue but also has longitudinal smooth muscle in the largest veins. The relative thickness and components of the three layers make it possible to identify the different types of vessels microscopically (**Figure 4-7**).

Heart as a Blood Vessel

Even though the heart is so highly specialized, it is constructed according to the same basic plan as the rest of the blood vessels. The heart consists of three layers, which correspond to the three tunics of the other vessels; however, the names have

been changed. The inner layer of the heart, corresponding to the tunica intima of other vessels, is called the **endocardium** and is similar in anatomy to the tunica intima of large arteries and veins. The middle layer of the heart, corresponding to the tunica media of other vessels, is called the **myocardium.** This layer makes up the bulk of the heart and consists of cardiac muscle rather than smooth muscle. The outer layer of the heart is called the **epicardium** in histology. It consists of connective tissue bounded by a simple squamous epithelium.

Skin

The skin is a complex combination of epithelium, connective tissues, muscle, and neural tissue that together comprises the largest organ in the body. Located at the boundary between the body and the environment, the skin provides protection and sensory interaction between the body and its surroundings, participates in the excretion of waste products, functions in thermoregulation, immune defense, and metabolism of substances applied to its surface.

Anatomy of the Skin

The skin has three main layers. The main connective tissue layer is the **dermis,** named after the Greek word derma, meaning skin (as in dermatology). On top of the dermis lies the epithelial layer of the skin, the **epidermis** (the name means upon the dermis), the outermost boundary of the skin. Under the dermis lies another connective tissue layer, the **hypodermis,** which consists mainly of adipose tissue.

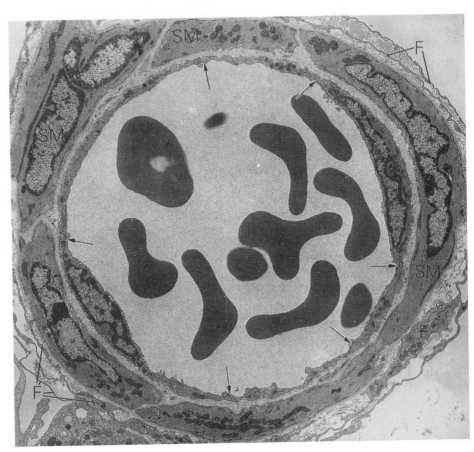

Figure 4-7. Electron micrograph of a relatively small arteriole. The tunica intima of the vessel consists of an endothelium with a very thin layer of subendothelial connective tissue (collagen fibrils and ground substance only). The *arrows* indicate the site of junctions between adjoining endothelial cells. The tunica media consists of a single layer of smooth muscle cells (SM). The tunica adventitia consists of collagen fibrils and several layers of fibroblasts with extremely attenuated processes (F). Several red blood cells are visible in the lumen. (From Ross MH, Romrell LJ, Kaye GI: Histology: A Text and Atlas. Baltimore, Williams & Wilkins, 1995, p 311.)

Epidermis

The epidermis is a keratinized, stratified squamous epithelium resting on a basement membrane that separates it from the underlying dermis. The epidermis contains four layers in all regions of the skin, but the relative thickness of the different layers varies in different parts of the body. The **stratum basale (basal layer)** is in contact with the basement membrane and is the layer responsible for the formation of new cells for the epidermis. As new cells are produced in the stratum basale, older cells are pushed up toward the surface and become part of the next layer of the epidermis, the **stratum spinosum**. The cells of the stratum spinosum are rather polygonal in shape, and they grow flatter as they approach the surface. In the process of becoming keratinized, the cells of the next layer of the epidermis accumulate granules of protein in their cytoplasm. This layer is, therefore, referred to as the **stratum granulosum**. In the surface layer of the epidermis, the **stratum corneum**, the cells have become very flat and completely keratinized. The thickness of this layer varies greatly in different parts of the body and is extremely thick in regions subject to a great deal of abrasion, such as the palms of the hands and soles of the feet. Most of the cells of the epidermis are **keratinocytes**. These cells eventually become keratinized and are gradually lost from the surface of the skin and replaced by new ones. Other cell types in the epidermis are responsible for giving the skin its color, immune function, and special sensory epithelial cells associated with nerve endings.

Dermis

The dermis is the connective tissue portion of the skin, which is located beneath the epidermis and separated from it by the basement membrane. The **papillary layer** of the dermis, which is adjacent to the epidermis, consists of the connective tissue projections (papillae) that extend up to interlock with the downward extensions of epithelium. The remainder of the dermis consists of the **reticular layer**. The name reticular suggests a network arrangement, which refers here to the arrangement of the collagen fibers in this dense, irregular connective tissue. The reticular layer varies considerably in thickness in different locations on the body and in many places is the thickest of all the layers of the skin.

Hypodermis

Adipose tissue forms a layer in connective tissue under the skin called the hypodermis. This layer has an insulating function and is formed primarily under the skin of the abdomen, buttocks, thighs, and upper arms. The non-lactating female breast is also composed of this tissue. When the caloric intake is reduced and adipose tissue elsewhere becomes depleted, the areas noted above remain less affected.

Other Components of the Skin

Hair follicles, sweat glands, and sebaceous glands of the skin are actually extensions of the epidermis but are located in the dermis. Tiny smooth muscles associated with the hair follicles are found in the dermis. In addition, blood vessels and nerves are concentrated in the dermis.

Aging of the Skin

With increasing age, elastic fibers in the connective tissue of the skin begin to deteriorate and at the same time the skin becomes thinner. Sags and wrinkles begin to appear in the skin. The secretory activity of the sweat glands slows down, and the skin becomes drier. Sunlight (or ultraviolet radiation from an artificial source) accelerates and accentuates the normal aging effects on the skin and at the same time impairs the skin's immune properties and promotes the production of skin cancer.

Embryology of the Face

The formation of the human face begins early in embryonic development and continues throughout the lifetime of the individual. The aspects of facial development discussed here occur mainly during the **second month** of prenatal life.

Early Embryology Related to the Face

When the embryo first develops polarity (i.e., a head end and a tail end), it takes the form of a simple flat disk consisting of just two layers of cells: a top layer and a bottom layer. Some of the cells in the top layer begin migrating to a new position between the top and bottom layers of cells, thus establishing a third layer between the other two layers. These three layers of cells in the very early embryo are called the **primary germ layers**. The top layer is the **ectoderm**; the middle layer is the **mesoderm**; and the bottom layer is the **endoderm**. At the anterior end of the flat disk embryo is a region called the **stomodeal plate**, or the **buccopharyngeal plate** in which no mesoderm separates the ectoderm from the endoderm. This region is important in the later development of the face. The flat disk embryo begins to grow rapidly in all directions, but space is limited; as a result, the embryo is forced to change its shape. Lateral growth forces the embryo into a new tubular configuration. Rapid growth in length forces the embryo to assume a C-shaped configuration from front to back. This C-shaped tube consists of ectoderm on the outside of the tube, endoderm lining the inside, and mesoderm in the middle, except at the stomodeal plate and at a similar structure at the tail end of the embryo. The embryo maintains this C shape throughout the rest of its development.

Face at the Start of the Second Month

The face at the beginning of the second month most notably shows a large depression called the **stomodeum**, which is the future site of the mouth. Surrounding the stomodeum are the facial primordia, lumpy-looking structures of various sizes. During the next few weeks, these primordia change their size and shape. Some divide into smaller parts, and others join with each other. As a result of this modeling process, the face begins to appear human.

Above the stomodeum is the largest facial primordium, the **frontonasal process**. It forms the forehead and the middle of the nose, as well as part of the upper lip and dental arch. Below the stomodeum lies the **mandibular arch**, also called the first arch, which eventually forms the mandible and other components of the lower jaw. On either side of the stomodeum are the **maxillary processes**, which originated by pinching off from the mandibular arch. These structures form the maxillary bones, as well as the sides of the nose and the portion of the upper lip that is not formed by the frontonasal process.

Below the mandibular arch lies another complete arch, the **hyoid arch**, which is also referred to by its number; that is, the second arch. Several more arches, which are not complete, lie below the hyoid arch; that is, these arches begin on one side of the face, are interrupted in the middle, then continue on the other side of the face. These arches are not named and are referred to by number only: the third, fourth, and sixth arches. (The fifth arch disappears at an early stage in the human embryo.)

Changes During the Second Month

The first noticeable change in the face occurs at the location of the future nostrils. The epithelium in these areas thickens to form the **nasal placodes**. (**Placode** means an epithelial thickening during development.) Immediately around the future nostrils, the mesenchyme beneath the epithelium begins to thicken above and on either side of each nasal placode, but not below it. This thickening of the mesenchyme leaves the nasal placode sitting at the bottom of the shallow **nasal pit**. The epithelium at the bottom of the nasal pit soon breaks through, opening the nostrils into the oral/nasal cavity. At this stage, only one large cavity exists inside the developing face, with no differentiation between the oral cavity and the nasal cavity. Later, the palate forms to separate the oral cavity from the nasal cavity, and the nasal septum forms, thus dividing the nasal cavity into right and left sides.

Using the newly formed nasal pits as landmarks, the frontonasal process can now be subdivided into some additional parts. The middle part between the two nasal pits forms the right and left **nasomedial processes** (or medial nasal prominence). The structures lateral to the nasal pits are now called the **nasolateral processes** (or lateral nasal prominence). The nasomedial processes extend down farther than the nasolateral processes and form the middle of the nose, the philtrum of the upper lip (the narrow region between the two vertical ridges on the lip), the portion of the dental arch that contains the four upper incisors, and the primary palate. The nasolateral processes do not contribute to the formation of the lip but form the sides of the nose and the **alae** of the nose (the flared "wings" of the nose lateral to the nostrils). The eyes form originally on the sides of the head; however, by the time that the face is completely formed, the eyes are in an anterior position with both eyes facing forward.

The external ears begin to form as a series of small bumps at the boundary between the mandibular arch and the hyoid arch. This location is very low and far forward on the developing face, but like the eyes, differential growth results in proper placement of the ears. Later downward and outward growth of the lower portion of the face at a faster rate than the rest of the face produces an apparent upward and backward relocation of the ears to their final position in the middle of each side of the head.

The maxillary processes, which originally separated from the mandibular arches, now begins to join with the mandibular arch to determine the size of the mouth. In most cases, the extent of union between these structures results in a normal size of mouth. If these structures fail to join, however, the result is **macrostomia** (literally meaning "big mouth"). If the structures join too far, the result is **microstomia** (meaning "small mouth"). Both macrostomia and microstomia, if they appear, may be bilateral or unilateral.

Because the mandibular arch is the only structure located directly below the mouth, it forms the entire lower lip. The upper lip involves both nasomedial processes and both maxillary processes. The nasomedial processes form the middle part of the upper lip, the **philtrum** (intermaxillary segment). The rest of the upper lip is formed by the right and left maxillary processes extending toward the middle of the lip until they make contact with the nasomedial process. If failure of union between any of these structures occurs, the result is a cleft of the lip. Clefts of the lip occur most commonly where the maxillary process joins the nasomedial process and may be either unilateral or bilateral.

Above the upper lip, the maxillary process joins the nasolateral process on each side of the nose. When these two structures first make contact, there is a groove at the point where they meet, the **nasolacrimal groove**, extending from the lower corner of the nose to the inside corner of the eye. In this location, the **nasolacrimal duct** forms for the purpose of draining tears from the eye and transporting them to the nasal cavity **(Figure 4-8)**.

Fate of the Pharyngeal Arches

Collectively, the mandibular, hyoid, third, fourth, and sixth arches are referred to as the **pharyngeal arches**. On both the outside and inside of the developing face, there are grooves at the point where each of the arches meets the arch below it. The grooves on the outside of the embryo are called **pharyngeal clefts**, and those on the inside are called **pharyngeal pouches**.

The external ear develops from lumps and bumps at the location of the first pharyngeal cleft, and the first cleft itself becomes the external auditory meatus. The first pharyngeal pouch develops into the auditory tube, and the very thin membrane where the external auditory meatus meets the auditory tube becomes the **tympanic membrane** (i.e., the eardrum).

The **palatine tonsils** develop in the second pouch. The third pouch, located between the third and fourth arches, forms the thymus and some of the parathyroid glands. The fourth pouch, between the fourth and sixth arches, forms the rest of the parathyroids and some specialized cells of the thyroid gland. The second, third, and fourth pharyngeal clefts disappear without forming anything.

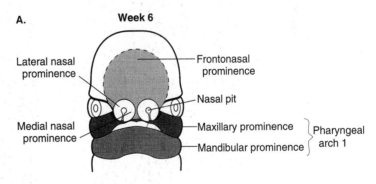

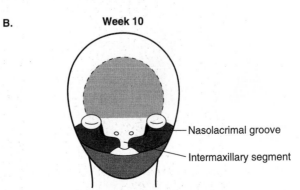

Figure 4-8. Diagram showing the development of the face. Note that pharyngeal arch 1 plays a major role. *A,* At week 6. *B,* At week 10. (From Dudek RW: High-Yield Embryology. Media, Pennsylvania, Williams 7 Wilkins, 2001, p 64.)

Each pharyngeal arch contains a muscular component, a skeletal component, an artery, and a cranial nerve. As the face develops, different parts of the face change position in relation to each other. Any muscles arising from these arches will keep their original innervation from the cranial nerve supplying that arch and blood supply by way of the artery supplying the same arch. This explains why it sometimes seems that certain muscles have an unusual pattern of innervation or blood supply.

Formation of the Palate

The palate develops from the right and left maxillary processes and from the nasomedial process. The portion of the palate that forms from the nasomedial process is the **primary palate**, and the portion forming from the maxillary processes is the **secondary palate**. The first indication of palate formation is the development of the **palatal shelves**, the structures that will form the secondary palate from the maxillary processes. The palate forms a horizontal division between the oral and nasal cavities, but when the palatal shelves form from the maxillary processes they are in a vertical position with the developing tongue between them. In order for these shelves to form the palate, several events must occur on schedule and in the right order. The first event is the **formation of the palatal shelves** in their original vertical orientation. The second event is the **reorientation of the vertical shelves into a horizontal position**, which cannot occur while the tongue is located between the shelves. Growth of the lower part of the face at the same time the palate is forming will result in moving the tongue out of the way. Once the palatal shelves are in a horizontal position, the third important event is **contact between the shelves accompanied by fusion of the epithelium of the two shelves**. Contact occurs first at approximately the middle of the secondary palate, then simultaneously proceeds anteriorly and posteriorly. The final event in palate formation is the **breakdown of the fused epithelium and the establishment of continuity of the mesenchyme from one shelf to the other**. At the same time that the palatal shelves are developing, reorienting, and fusing to form the secondary palate, the primary palate forms as a triangular extension of the nasomedial process and fuses with the two palatal shelves. Meanwhile, the **nasal septum** forms and grows downward to fuse with the palate just as it closes. The original single oral/nasal cavity is now divided into a lower oral cavity and an upper nasal cavity with right and left halves **(Figure 4-9).**

Failure of any one of the several events in palate formation results in a cleft of the palate. A cleft of the palate may involve the primary palate, the secondary palate, or both. It may occur alone or in combination with a cleft of the lip or with other facial malformations. (See Chapter 12.)

Formation of the Tongue

The epithelium and connective tissue of the tongue develop from the pharyngeal arches. Two lateral swellings (i.e., the **lateral lingual swellings)** and a single midline swelling (i.e., the **tuberculum impar),** all of which develop from the first arch, together form the epithelium and connective tissue of the anterior two thirds of the tongue. The posterior third of the tongue is formed by the third arch and also by some of the fourth arches, and the epiglottis develops from the fourth arch. The second pharyngeal arch does not contribute to the formation of the tongue. The muscles of the tongue arise from the back of the head; these muscles migrate to their final location and bring their own original nerve supply with them.

Development of the Teeth

Tooth development **(odontogenesis)** begins approximately 6 weeks in utero or soon after formation of the face begins. Some aspects of tooth development continue throughout the lifetime of the teeth.

Goals of Tooth Development

Before tooth development begins, each future dental arch consists of a single structure with no teeth, lips, or vestibule separating the lips from the teeth. An explanation of the embryology of the teeth must include a description of how the

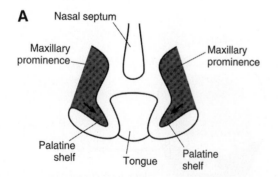 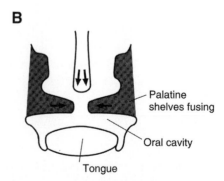

Figure 4-9. Diagram demonstrating the formation of the secondary palate. *A,* At week 6. *B,* At week 8. (From Dudek RW: High-Yield Embryology. Media, Pennsylvania, Williams & Wilkins, 2001, p 65)

dental arch becomes separate from the lips and the cheeks, how the embryonic primordia of the teeth form, and how these primordia form the primary teeth and later the permanent teeth.

Structures Involved in Forming the Teeth

Development of the teeth involves an interaction between epithelial and mesenchymal tissues in which each of these two tissues depends on the other for some direction. Normal teeth are formed as a result of this interaction. The teeth and most of the oral cavity develop in front of the former buccopharyngeal membrane. Thus, the oral cavity, including the dental arches, has an epithelium that is derived from the ectoderm germ layer. Much of the mesenchyme of the head, including that involved in tooth formation, came from the ectoderm by way of the neural crest cells (a byproduct of the formation of neural tissue). Therefore, both tissues involved in tooth development arise from the ectoderm of the very early embryo.

Early Embryogenesis of the Teeth

Formation of the Dental Lamina

The first indication that tooth development is occurring is the formation of an epithelial thickening along a narrow region of the entire upper and lower dental arches. Proliferation of the epithelial cells along the arch causes the cells to invade the underlying mesenchyme, resulting in the formation of the **dental lamina**, which extends along the entire length of each dental arch.

Bud Stage of Tooth Development

At 10 sites along the upper dental lamina and 10 sites along the lower dental lamina, the rapid proliferation of epithelial cells results in the formation of individual swellings or buds. By 8 weeks, these 20 spherical zones of epithelium on the maxillary and mandibular arches delineate the positions of the future primary teeth. These swellings are the **tooth buds**, and this stage is referred to as the **bud stage** of tooth formation. At the same time, the first indication of the involvement of mesenchyme in tooth formation appears as the mesenchyme in the area immediately surrounding the new tooth bud becomes slightly denser than the rest of the mesenchyme.

Cap Stage of Tooth Development

Once again, faster growth of certain cells results in a change of shape leading to the next stage of tooth development. Rapid growth of cells around the equator of the spherical tooth bud causes an indentation to appear. The former bud now resembles a cap, and this stage is known as the **cap stage** (also called the *cup stage*) of tooth development. The **epithelial part** of the future tooth is now called the **enamel organ**. The outer layer of cells in the enamel organ is called the **outer enamel epithelium**, and

the inner layer of cells next to the indentation that appeared when the cap stage formed is called the **inner enamel epithelium**. The enamel organ maintains a basement membrane around itself and separates it from the mesenchyme. The mesenchyme near the tooth during the cap stage of development can be subdivided into the **dental papilla**, which is the connective tissue that actually projects up into the indentation during this stage. The surrounding mesenchyme is called the **dental sac** (also sometimes called the dental **follicle**). Together, the epithelial and mesenchymal components of the developing tooth are called the **odontogenic organ**.

Bell Stage of Tooth Development

The continued growth of cells of the enamel organ results in the enamel organ becoming very highly indented so that it resembles the shape of a bell, hence giving rise to the term **bell stage** of tooth development. The odontogenic organ is a three-dimensional structure with a bell-shaped enamel organ, a papilla of mesenchyme within the bell, and more mesenchyme of the dental sac surrounding it.

At this stage, all the necessary parts and cells types for the formation of the hard tissue, pulp, and periodontal ligament (PDL) of the tooth are present. Some additional structures that were not clearly defined at earlier stages may now be described. The enamel organ, already noted to have an outer enamel epithelium and an inner enamel epithelium, is seen to have additional cells between these two layers. This large region of the enamel organ is called the **stellate reticulum**, a name meaning **star-shaped network**, because the cells in this area have long cytoplasmic branches that form a network with the cytoplasmic processes of adjacent cells and give the individual cells a star-shaped appearance. The stellate reticulum is a rare example of epithelium in which the cells are rather far apart, more like connective tissue. Immediately adjacent to the inner enamel epithelium, between it and the stellate reticulum, lies an intermediate layer of cells, the **stratum intermedium (intermediate layer)**. These cells are close together and appear to be slightly flattened. The cells of the outer enamel epithelium have a rather short columnar shape. Those of the inner enamel epithelium are also columnar, but taller, and eventually they grow very tall. The lip of the bell-shaped enamel organ, where the outer enamel epithelium loops around and becomes the inner enamel epithelium, marks the future anatomic neck of the tooth; therefore, this lip is called the **cervical loop**. A basement membrane still separates the bell stage enamel organ from the mesenchyme of the dental papilla and the dental sac.

A section through the developing tooth at the bell stage shows that the odontogenic organ does not form at the end of the dental lamina but is instead located facially from it. As a direct continuation of the dental lamina, however, the **primordium of the permanent tooth** appears at this time. This is the tooth bud of a permanent tooth, which will not appear in the mouth for quite a few years (**Figure 4-10**).

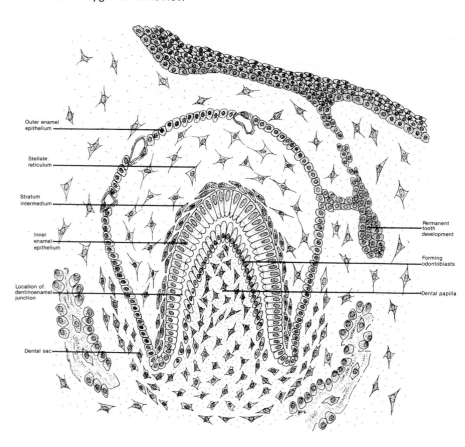

Figure 4-10. Bell stage of odontogenesis, immediately before the onset of dentin and enamel formation. (Original drawing courtesy of D. Overman, PhD, West Virginia University. From DeBiase C: Dental Health Education: Theory and Practice. Philadelphia, Lea & Febiger, 1991, p 51.)

Fate of the Odontogenic Organ

The outermost cells of the dental papilla, which are immediately adjacent to the basement membrane of the enamel organ, soon differentiate into **odontoblasts** and form the **dentin**. The rest of the dental papilla becomes the **pulp**. The cells of the inner enamel epithelium of the enamel organ become **ameloblasts** and produce the **enamel**. Once the root of the tooth has begun to form, some of the cells of the dental sac differentiate into **cementoblasts** and form the **cementum**. The rest of the dental sac contains **fibroblasts,** which form the periodontal ligament (**PDL**).

Formation of the Vestibule

Rapid growth of epithelial cells along the embryonic arch between the dental lamina and the future lips and cheeks results in the formation of another epithelial lamina, the **vestibular lamina**. The vestibular lamina is larger than the dental lamina and begins to form later on. Continued growth of the epithelium in the vestibular lamina causes it to become very large. At about the time of the bell stage, the epithelial cells in the center portion of the vestibular lamina begin to die and break down, thus forming a valley that becomes the vestibule. Epithelial cells are still left on both sides of the valley. The epithelium on the side nearest the lips and cheeks becomes the epithelium of the labial or buccal mucosa. The epithelium on the side nearer to the teeth becomes the epithelium of the alveolar and gingival mucosa.

Formation of Dentin and Enamel

The dentin and enamel start to form at the same place but proceed in opposite directions. Before dentin and enamel start to form, the enamel organ assumes the shape of the future crown of the tooth. Even at this stage, the location of the future cusp tip can be identified, and dentin and enamel formation begins here. Dentin formation starts first with the differentiation of odontoblasts from the outermost cells of the dental papilla. The odontoblasts begin the synthesis of dentin by depositing the organic components first. The inorganic minerals are added later, just as in the formation of bone. Dentin that has just been deposited, but is not yet mineralized, is called **predentin**. Simultaneously, the cells of the inner enamel epithelium differentiate into ameloblasts and begin to synthesize enamel. Both dentin and enamel begin to form at the boundary between the dental papilla and the enamel organ, a region originally marked by the presence of a basement membrane. Once dentin and enamel start to form, the basement membrane is destroyed and the dentin and enamel make contact with each other at the **dentinoenamel junction (DEJ)**. Dentin formation begins at the DEJ and proceeds **inward** toward the pulp. Enamel formation begins at the same place but proceeds **outward**, toward the future surface of the tooth. Both tissues start to form at the cusp tip (or tips, if there are more than one) and spread gradually toward the apex. Once dentin and enamel formation has begun, the configuration of the crown is determined, because the hard tissues cannot be deformed. The shape of the enamel organ, therefore, determines the configuration of the crown.

Because the enamel organ is an epithelial structure, it does not contain blood vessels; however, an abundance of blood vessels exists in the adjacent dental papilla. The onset of mineralization of the dentin and enamel seems to create a problem in that the ameloblasts are now cut off from their blood supply. At this point, an unusual event occurs, namely the **vascularization of an epithelium**. Capillaries invade the outer portion of the enamel organ at the same time that the stellate reticulum begins to collapse. The newly vascularized epithelium ends up adjacent to the ameloblasts, which can now receive their nutrients from a new source. The combination of the now vascularized outer enamel epithelium, the remnants of the collapsed stellate reticulum, and the flattened cells of the previously called stratum intermedium form a new structure-the **reduced enamel epithelium (REE)**-that covers the developing crown. The REE produces a nonmineralized **dental cuticle (secondary enamel cuticle)** over the crown, which will remain in place and isolate the crown from the surrounding connective tissue until the crown appears in the oral cavity. Following eruption, the portion of the REE that remains surrounding the crown is called **junctional or attachment epithelium**. This remnant of the original enamel organ wears away with tooth use. The **primary enamel cuticle** is the last enamel layer produced by ameloblasts and becomes mineralized. The primary and secondary enamel cuticles were once referred to as the **Nasmyth membrane**.

Epithelial-Mesenchymal Interaction in Tooth Development

The shape of the enamel organ determines the configuration of the crown of the tooth. But what determines the shape of the enamel organ? A complex interaction occurs between the epithelium and the mesenchyme in tooth formation, and one outcome of this interaction is the determination of the shape of the enamel organ. By exchanging the mesenchymal and epithelial tissues of developing incisors and molars in organ culture, researchers were able to determine that the mesenchyme of the dental papilla is responsible for determining the original configuration of the enamel organ.

Additional experiments led to the discovery of more interactions between the epithelium and the mesenchyme in developing teeth, the major points of which may be summarized as follows.

The mesenchyme of the dental papilla influences the morphology of the enamel organ by determining its shape and thus also the shape of the crown. Once the enamel organ has formed, the cells of the inner enamel epithelium exert an influence on the outermost cells of the dental papilla. As a result, the mesenchymal cells adjacent to the inner enamel epithelium differentiate into odontoblasts and start to form dentin. Once dentin formation begins, the odontoblasts or the new dentin or perhaps both influence the cells of the inner enamel epithelium to complete their differentiation into ameloblasts. Cells of the

stratum intermedium also have an inductive influence on the new ameloblasts, because enamel formation cannot proceed in the absence of the stratum intermedium.

Root Formation

Root formation begins with the rapid proliferation in cells of the cervical loop of the enamel organ. As newly formed dentin and enamel approach the cervical loop, cell growth beginning at the cervical loop results in the formation of a cylindrical sheath of epithelium outlining the shape of the future root. This sheath is called the **epithelial root sheath**, or the **epithelial root sheath of Hertwig**. The epithelial root sheath includes cells of the inner enamel epithelium and the outer enamel epithelium only, with no stellate reticulum and no stratum intermedium. The inner enamel epithelial cells, which are now part of the root sheath, still induce the differentiation of odontoblasts from the adjacent mesenchymal cells; therefore, as the root sheath elongates, dentin formation proceeds into the root. When the root sheath reaches its full length, it bends sharply to form a diaphragm of epithelium, the **epithelial diaphragm**, at the location of the future apex. An opening in the epithelial diaphragm, called the **apical foramen**, remains for the passage of nerves and blood vessels. If a tooth is to have two roots, the root sheath divides so that its three-dimensional configuration resembles that of a pair of pants, rather than a simple cylinder. In this case, there will be two epithelial diaphragms and two apical foramina. If the tooth is to have three roots, the root sheath assumes the shape of pants with three legs.

One of the roles of the mesenchymal cells of the dental sac is the formation of cementoblasts and the production of cementum. The differentiation of cementoblasts depends on the mesenchymal cells contacting the dentin of the root, but the cells of the dental sac are separated from the root by the root sheath. Therefore, the epithelial root sheath must break down to allow mesenchymal cells of the dental sac to contact the dentin. As the root approaches its full length, the root sheath begins to deteriorate. In three dimensions, the root sheath falls into shreds and the remaining epithelial cells hang together in strings. In a section of a developing tooth, the strings of epithelial cells appear as isolated small clumps of cells called **epithelial rests (or epithelial rests of Malassez)**. Once the root sheath has started to break down, mesenchymal cells of the dental sac are free to contact the dentin. Contact with the dentin causes these cells to differentiate into cementoblasts, and they begin to synthesize cementum. Other mesenchymal cells of the dental sac become fibroblasts and synthesize the strong collagen fibers of the PDL that are incorporated into the cementum as it forms.

Dentin and Pulp

Because the dentin and pulp both develop from the same original population of cells in the dental papilla, they are studied together.

Dentin

The **dentin** makes up the bulk of the tooth and is a mineralized tissue that is slightly harder than bone. The cells that form the dentin, the **odontoblasts**, develop from the cells of the dental papilla closest to the enamel organ. As dentin forms, beginning at the DEJ and progressing inward, the odontoblasts leave behind a slender cytoplasmic process. This **odontoblast process** extends from the odontoblasts at their location in the pulp all the way to the DEJ. Healthy dentin, therefore, is living connective tissue that contains parts of cells (the odontoblast processes) throughout its structure. This gives dentin the ability to react to trauma and disease as described later **(Figure 4-11)**.

The presence of odontoblast processes extending through the dentin means that the hard tissue contains tiny tunnels through which the odontoblast processes pass. These little tunnels are the **dentin tubules**. Each dentin tubule contains an odontoblast process and a small amount of tissue fluid. Over time, some mineralization occurs inside the dentin tubules, causing the tubules to become slightly smaller in di-

ameter. The dentin formed inside the tubules is harder than the rest of the dentin and is properly called **intratubular dentin** but is more commonly called **peritubular dentin**. The rest of the dentin between the tubules is the **intertubular dentin**.

The first dentin deposited immediately adjacent to the DEJ differs from the rest of the dentin only in the orientation of its collagen fibers, a feature that cannot be demonstrated by routine light microscopy. This earliest dentin is the **mantle dentin** and can be identified only by its position. Once mantle dentin formation is complete, the rest of the dentin that is formed until root formation is complete is called **primary dentin**. The dentin tubules follow a gradual S-shaped path through the primary dentin. After the root is anatomically complete, the formation of dentin slows considerably but never stops completely in a healthy tooth. Normal dentin formed after completion of the root is **secondary dentin**. Secondary dentin can be identified by it location next to the pulp chamber and by the fact that the tubules usually make an abrupt change of direction at the boundary between the primary and secondary dentin. Together, the primary and secondary dentin comprise the **circumpulpal dentin**.

Evidence for the regular growth pattern of dentin can be seen in the form of **incremental lines**, but the incremental lines of dentin are not as distinct as those of enamel.

As dentin mineralizes, tiny areas in which the mineralization process is incomplete appear in the tissue. This is known as **interglobular dentin.** It appears as irregularly shaped granules in primary dentin, which occur more commonly in the crown than in the root and usually lie closer to the enamel than to the pulp.

In the mantle dentin of the root, a layer of granular-looking dentin forms near the cementum. At first inspection, it resembles very fine interglobular dentin; however, it consists of the cut ends of twisted and branched dentin tubules. Named after its discoverer, Dr. Tomes, this is the **Tomes' granular layer (Figure 4-12)**.

The histology of the dentin changes as the teeth age and in response to trauma or disease. When odontoblast processes are exposed to the outside environment by wearing away of the tooth surface, dental caries, or injury to the tooth, the result may be the death of the odontoblasts. This leaves a zone of empty dentin tubules that can be seen microscopically as a **dead tract**. When odontoblasts are killed, cells of the pulp may form new odontoblasts. These new cells will form some new dentin at the boundary between the dentin and the pulp in an attempt to protect the pulp. This new dentin is called **tertiary dentin** or **reparative dentin**. Unfortunately, it is also sometimes called irregular secondary dentin, a term that only confuses the situation. Tertiary dentin may also be formed by the original odontoblasts if they are not killed owing to exposure of their odontoblast processes.

The deposition of mineralized dentin inside the dentin tubules sometimes continues until the tubule is totally filled with dentin. When this happens, it is impossible to distin-

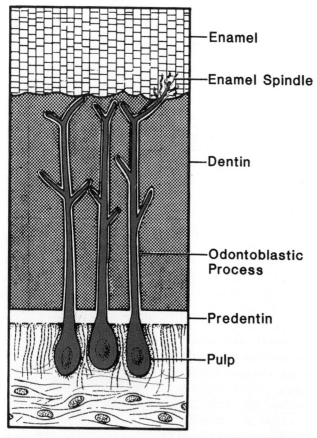

Figure 4-11. A small portion of the crown area shows three odontoblasts. The cell body (nuclear part) of the odontoblast lies in the pulp, and its process extends into the dentinal tubule. Notice the branching of the processes and the entrapped end of a process (an enamel spindle) within the enamel. (From Melfi RC, Alley KE: Permar's Oral Embryology and Microscopic Anatomy. Philadelphia, Lippincott Williams & Wylkins, 2000, p 122.)

Labels in figure:
- Enamel
- Enamel Spindle
- Dentin
- Odontoblastic Process
- Predentin
- Pulp

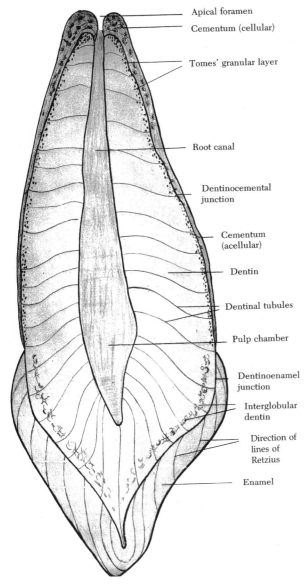

Apical foramen

Cementum (cellular)

Tomes' granular layer

Root canal

Dentinocemental junction

Cementum (acellular)

Dentin

Dentinal tubules

Pulp chamber

Dentinoenamel junction

Interglobular dentin

Direction of lines of Retzius

Enamel

Figure 4-12. The longitudinal faciolingual section of a maxillary canine. (From Melfi RC, Alley KE: Permar's Oral Embryology and Microscopic Anatomy. Philadelphia, Lippincott Williams & Wilkins, 2000, p 82.)

guish between tubules filled with dentin and the rest of the dentin; thus, the dentin looks transparent. For this reason, it is called transparent dentin or **sclerotic dentin**. Formation of transparent dentin is a normal aging process in healthy teeth and occurs more commonly near the apex.

Pulp

The pulp is the soft connective tissue portion of the tooth that is intimately related to the dentin in both structure and function. All the cells of the embryonic dental papilla ultimately result in the pulp. The cell population of the pulp includes the bodies of the odontoblasts, large numbers of fibroblasts, some undifferentiated mesenchymal cells,

cells making up the blood vessels of the pulp, circulating blood cells, and the endings (but not the cell bodies) of neurons.

Each tooth contains both **coronal pulp**, which is located in the crown, and **radicular pulp**, which extends through the root. The coronal pulp includes **pulp horns** that extend toward the cusps. The root may have **accessory root canals** anywhere along its length. Accessory root canals are the result of premature breakdown of the epithelial root sheath. Because the root sheath is required for odontoblast differentiation, its breakdown results in a region in which no dentin forms, thus producing an accessory root canal.

Immediately below the layer of odontoblasts lies an elaborate network of nerve endings, some of which reach between the odontoblasts and travel a short distance up the dentin tubules. This network of nerve endings is called the **subodontoblastic plexus** (of Raschkow). Because the nerve endings are invisible with routine histologic staining, the presence of these apparently invisible nerves creates a region that appears to contain relatively few other types of cells. This region is called the **cell-free zone** (of Weil), also sometimes called the cell-poor zone, and is the zone in which the subodontoblastic plexus is located. Histologists describe a denser cellular region beneath the cell-free zone, which is known as the **cell-rich zone**; however, both the cell-free and cell-rich zones are often difficult to demonstrate.

The pulp is richly supplied with small blood vessels called **arterioles and venules**. As a result of the protected location of the pulp, its blood vessels do not require the usual thickness in their walls; thus, the venules and particularly the arterioles of the pulp are thinner than their counterparts in other locations.

As teeth age, it is common for small concentrations of inorganic material to accumulate in the pulp. These mineralized structures are **denticles** or **pulp stones**. Some denticles are actual bits of dentin formed by real odontoblasts that separated from the rest of the odontoblasts. These are the **true denticles**. Most denticles are merely bits of inorganic material in the pulp and are called **false denticles**. Either type of denticle may be found free in the pulp (**free denticles**), may become attached to the dentin (**attached denticles**), or may become completely embedded in the dentin (**embedded denticles**). Denticles of all types are more common in the coronal pulp chamber than in the radicular pulp (**Figure 4-13**).

Enamel

Enamel is the mineralized tissue that covers the crown of the tooth. Enamel is the hardest tissue in the body and consists of 96% inorganic mineral crystals and 4% organic components and water. Even though enamel is so hard that it seems almost indestructible, the mineral components of enamel are susceptible to the action of acids in the mouth, which can dissolve the mineral and produce dental caries.

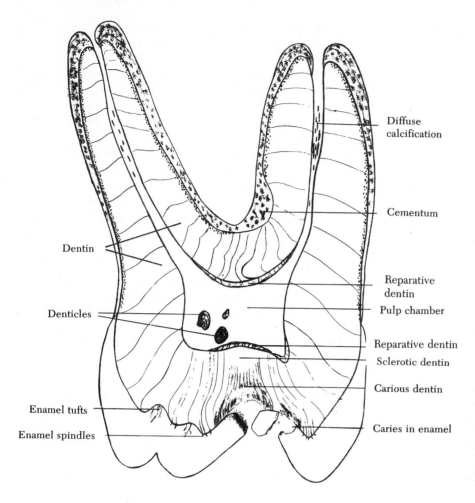

Dentin

Denticles

Enamel tufts

Enamel spindles

Diffuse calcification

Cementum

Reparative dentin

Pulp chamber

Reparative dentin

Sclerotic dentin

Carious dentin

Caries in enamel

Figure 4-13. The longitudinal buccolingual section of a maxillary first molar. Dental caries has destroyed the enamel in the area around a groove on the occlusal surface. The caries has spread horizontally at the dentinoenamel junction and undermined the enamel. Caries has spread pulpward in the dentinal tubules to about two thirds of the thickness of the dentin. The dentin close to the pulp is sclerotic dentin; the tubules are filled with mineral salts. On the pulpal wall beneath the caries lesion, a small amount of reparative dentin has formed. The reparative dentin on the floor of the pulp chamber (next to the root) was not caused by caries; reparative dentin in this location is not unusual. (From Melfi RC, Alley KE: Permar's Oral Embryology and Microscopic Anatomy. Philadelphia, Lippincott Williams & Wilkins, 2000, p 115.)

Amelogenesis

Enamel is formed by cells of the enamel organ, the epithelial component of the odontogenic organ. Under the inductive influence of cells of the dental papilla, the columnar epithelial cells of the inner enamel epithelium begin to differentiate into **ameloblasts**. The presence of the stratum intermedium of the enamel organ is required in order for the ameloblasts to complete their differentiation and begin producing enamel.

Ameloblasts are tall columnar cells that are attached very tightly to each other near the end of the cells closest to the basement membrane. A narrow projection of cytoplasm at the tip of the cell nearest the DEJ is called **Tomes' processes** and is the location where enamel proteins are released from the cell. Soon after dentin formation begins in the area of the dental papilla (immediately adjacent to the enamel organ), the ameloblasts begin to deposit enamel at the former site of the basement membrane. The deposition of enamel continues in an outward direction toward the future surface of the tooth. While enamel is deposited, the ameloblasts move away from the DEJ, but no portion of the ameloblast is left behind in the enamel. Unlike dentin, whose formation continues throughout the lifetime of a tooth (even though very slowly), enamel formation is finished when the crown is completely formed.

Structure and Formation of Enamel Rods

Enamel consists of thousands of elongated structural units called **enamel rods** or **enamel prisms**. Microscopically, each rod has faint cross-striations that make it appear to be constructed of tiny subunits, although the interpretation of this observation is unclear. Individual rods are not straight, but their general orientation is perpendicular to the DEJ and the tooth surface.

The extreme hardness of enamel made it difficult for anatomists to discover the structure of the enamel rods and their relationships to each other. Their shape seems to be determined by the shape of Tomes' processes of the ameloblasts, and the individual ameloblasts appear to overlap in their responsibilities for rod formation. The large head of a rod is formed by one ameloblast, but that same ameloblast contributes a small portion of enamel to the formation of the tails of three surrounding rods.

The outer portion of the enamel of primary teeth and the enamel near the gingiva in permanent teeth lack a rod structure and are called rodless or aprismatic enamel.

Histologic Features

Incremental lines, appearing microscopically as brown bands oriented at approximately right angles to the prisms, are the result of alterations in the availability of nutrients during amelogenesis. These lines provide visual evidence of the gradual increase in enamel during tooth formation. The incremental lines of enamel are often referred to as **lines of Retzius**, in honor of their discoverer.

In the area of the cusp tips of teeth, the enamel rods are often arranged in a very irregular pattern, giving a gnarled appearance to the enamel. **Gnarled enamel** resists splitting in the same way that gnarled firewood resists splitting, thus helping the tooth to withstand heavy occlusal forces.

Changes in the direction of enamel prisms during amelogenesis can sometimes create weakened areas in the mineralized enamel comparable to a geologic fault. These weakened areas accumulate higher concentrations of enamel proteins and consequently have a lower inorganic mineral content. Differences in mineral content make them visible in ground sections of teeth as **enamel tufts**, extending from the DEJ a short distance into the enamel, or **enamel lamellae**, extending from the DEJ all the way to the enamel surface. Tufts and lamellae are both oriented longitudinally in the enamel and, therefore, can be visualized best in cross-sections of teeth. They differ from each other only with regard to whether they extend a short distance from the DEJ or all the way to the tooth surface.

Enamel spindles are the ends of odontoblast processes that crossed the DEJ and extended a short distance into the enamel. Enamel spindles form while the enamel is not yet mineralized; they appear as sharply focused individual projections that are more common near the cusp tip than in other regions of the enamel **(Figure 4-14)**; see also Figures 4-11–4-13).

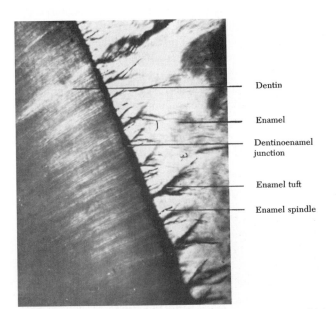

Figure 4-14. Photomicrograph of a small area of tooth crown, which is cut horizontally (low magnification). Among the clearly visible enamel tufts are the much smaller enamel spindles. (From Melfi RC, Alley KE: Permar's Oral Embryology and Microscopic Anatomy. Philadelphia, Lippincott Williams & Wilkins, 2000, p 98.)

The orientation of the enamel rods in this very hard tissue influences the way that light is reflected from the surface of a thin slice of enamel. Light shining on any given region of the surface of a slice of enamel is reflected either toward the viewer's eye or away from it, resulting in a pattern of light and dark bands. These **Hunter-Schreger bands** are visible only by reflected light, and they provide evidence of variation in rod orientation.

Clinical Considerations

The cells that formed the enamel are no longer present in an erupted tooth, consequently enamel has no mechanism for self-repair following damage due to caries or trauma. Fluoride ions from drinking water, toothpastes, or topical fluoride treatments can become incorporated into the enamel and increase its resistance to acids in the mouth, thus helping to protect against caries. Sealants form a physical barrier to the action of acids in locations where topical fluoride is least effective. Even though the dissolving effect of acids is a factor in caries formation, the susceptibility of enamel to acid is taken advantage of in the acid-etching process used in the preparation of the tooth surface for the application of sealants or orthodontic brackets.

Periodontium

The **periodontium (around the teeth)** consists of the tissues that surround and support the teeth and includes the alveolar bone, cementum, PDL, and dentogingival junction.

Alveolar Bone

The **alveolar bone proper** faces the root of the tooth and actually has collagen fibers of the PDL embedded in it. Its dense-looking appearance on radiographs gives it the name **lamina dura (tough layer)**. Its appearance in a dry skull, full of little holes like a sieve, gives it the name **cribriform (sieve-shaped) plate**. Alveolar bone proper is the most precise term.

Alveolar bone that does not actually have fibers of the PDL embedded in it is called **supporting alveolar bone**. The compact bone at the outer surfaces of the mandible or maxilla is called the **cortical plate**. The spongy bone between the cortical plate and the alveolar bone proper is simply called **spongy supporting bone**. The diagram **(Figure 4-15)** uses the bone of mandible as an example; however, the terminology applies in the same way to the maxilla.

Histologically, the alveolar bone appears to be no different from bone in other locations. However, alveolar bone behaves differently when not actually functioning to support the teeth. When the alveolar bone has no teeth to support, it gradually reabsorbs and disappears, thus causing a significant loss of facial height and change of facial profile in edentulous people.

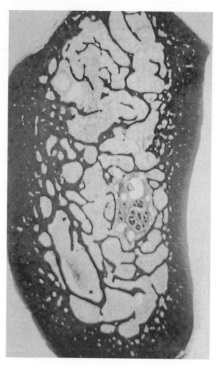

Figure 4-15. The faciolingual histologic section of an edentulous human mandible. The compact bone tissue on the outside is continuous with trabecular (spongy) bone tissue on the inside. The open spaces between the trabecular bone are the sites of the bone marrow tissue. A cross-section of the inferior alveolar canal is surrounded by trabecular bone (*mid-right*). Notice the outline of the inferior alveolar nerve and blood vessels in the canal. (From Melfi RC, Alley KE: Permar's Oral Embryology and Microscopic Anatomy. Philadelphia, Lippincott Williams & Wilkins, 2000, p 198.)

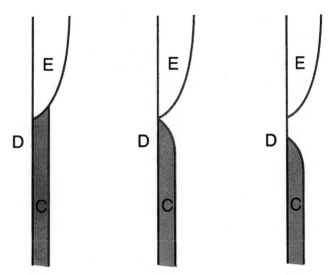

Figure 4-16. Diagrams of the relation of cementum (C) to enamel (E) at the dentinoenamel junction. The most common relation is illustrated at the left, where cementum overlaps the enamel. Illustrated in the center is the next most common relation, where cementum just meets the enamel. The least common relation is illustrated at the right, where cementum does not meet the enamel. Cervical dentin (D) is void of cementum and exposed to the environment. (From Melfi RC, Alley KE: Permar's Oral Embryology and Microscopic Anatomy. Philadelphia, Lippincott Williams & Wilkins, 2000, p 157.)

Cementum

Cementum develops from the dental sac of the odontogenic organ when mesenchymal cells of the dental sac contact the root dentin after the breakdown of the epithelial root sheath. Mesenchymal cells contacting the dentin will differentiate into **cementoblasts** and begin depositing cementum. If mesenchymal cells of the dental sac come into contact with enamel, they also become cementoblasts in that location and deposit cementum on the enamel surface **(Figure 4-16).**

The first cementum, which is called **acellular cementum**, is deposited directly on the dentin of the root and contains no cells. In the cervical one third of the root, the cementum remains thin and acellular. Nearer the apex, the cementum becomes thicker, and cementoblasts become incorporated into the cementum in the same way that osteoblasts become incorporated into developing bone. Trapped cementoblasts become **cementocytes**, and cementum that contains cementocytes is called **cellular cementum** (see Figure 4-12). The terminology used for bone also applies to the cellular cementum. The cementocytes are located in spaces called **lacunae**, and thin cytoplasmic processes from the cementocytes travel in narrow channels in the mineralized cementum called **canaliculi**. Canaliculi in cellular cementum are generally oriented toward the PDL, the source of nutrients for the cementoblasts **(Figure 4-17).**

Although the usual location of cementum deposition is on the root of the tooth, cementoblasts may form occasionally in the PDL or they may separate from the root surface. The result is the formation of a small drop of cementum out in the PDL, a **cementicle**. Cementicles may remain **free** in the PDL, or they may become **attached** to the root surface or completely **embedded** in the cementum covering the root. Overproduction of cementum on the root, **hypercementosis**, may result in the fusion of the roots of a multirooted tooth, the formation of cementum spurs, or ankylosis of the tooth. Hypercementosis may be limited to one or a few teeth. In the case of Paget disease, hypercementosis may involve the entire dentition **(Figure 4-18).**

Periodontal Ligament

The **PDL** is the connective tissue structure responsible for anchoring the tooth to the alveolar bone. The PDL develops from the cells of the dental sac surrounding the enamel organ.

The PDL includes:

1. Type I collagen fibers (**Sharpey fibers**, because they are embedded in a hard tissue) that attach the cementum to the alveolar bone
2. Collagen fibers attaching the surrounding soft tissues to the tooth

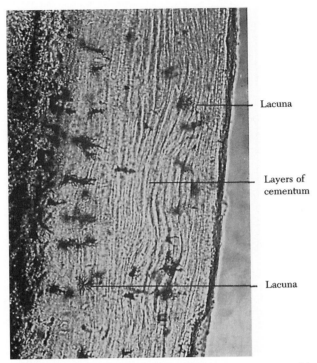

Figure 4-17. Photomicrograph of an area of cementum seen with a higher-power objective. Notice the canaliculi leading from the lacunae; they are often directed chiefly toward the outside surface of the root (to the right). The layer-upon-layer formation of cementum is clear. (From Melfi RC, Alley KE: Permar's Oral Embryology and Microscopic Anatomy. Philadelphia, Lippincott Williams & Wilkins, 2000, p 165.)

3. Fibroblasts responsible for the formation of the fibers
4. Blood vessels and nerves supplying the region
5. Cells of the immune system

This structure is called a ligament, because it functions by joining two hard tissues-bone and cementum-like ligaments elsewhere that join bones to one another. However, in almost all other respects it differs from other ligaments, most notably because the PDL contains large numbers of cells and is highly vascular.

Fibers of the PDL that are embedded in cementum at one end and bone at the other end are called principal fibers and are organized into groups called the **principal fiber groups.** The names of the fiber groups are indicated in **Figure 4-19.**

Other groups of fibers are embedded in bone or cementum at one end and soft tissue at the other end or (in the case of the circular fiber group) are not embedded into either bone or cementum. These **gingival fiber groups** and are seen in **Figure 4-20.**

The **oblique fiber group** is the largest of the fiber groups, and is functionally significant because these fibers receive the majority of the masticatory stress. Their orientation, however, converts pressure on the tooth to tension on the alveolar bone by hanging the tooth in a sling, thus preventing bone reabsorption that would normally result if the tooth put pressure on the bone.

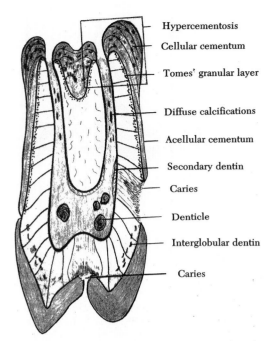

Figure 4-18. Drawing of a longitudinal faciolingual section of a maxillary first premolar. The tip of the lingual root shows a large amount of cementum, which is sometimes referred to as hypercementosis. (From Melfi RC, Alley KE: Permar's Oral Embryology and Microscopic Anatomy. Philadelphia, Lippincott Williams & Wilkins, 2000, p 156.)

The collagen fibers of the PDL, like those of all connective tissues, align themselves to accommodate stress. In the absence of occlusal stress (e.g., in the case of a nonfunctional tooth), the PDL fibers lose their orientation and become disorganized. At the same time, the entire PDL becomes thinner.

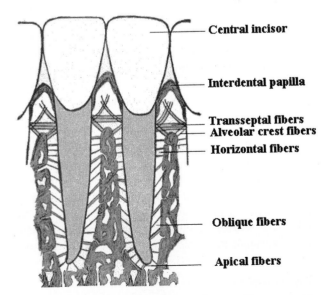

Figure 4-19. Arrangement of periodontal ligament fibers around the tooth roots of mandibular incisors. (From Melfi RC, Alley KE: Permar's Oral Embryology and Microscopic Anatomy. Philadelphia, Lippincott Williams & Wilkins, 2000, p 174.)

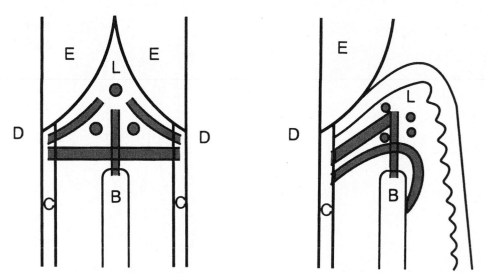

Figure 4-20. Diagram of the functionally arranged fibers within the lamina propria (L) of the free gingiva. The interdental papilla fibers are illustrated (left); dentinogingival fibers extend from the cementum (C) of adjacent teeth and pass into the lamina propria; transseptal fibers extend from the cementum of one tooth, pass over the crest of the interdental bone (B), and continue to the cementum of the other tooth; alveologingival fibers pass from the crest of the alveolar bone to the lamina propria; and circular fibers lie free in the lamina propria. The arrangement of the gingival fibers (right) as seen on the facial or lingual side of a tooth are also illustrated (right); dentinogingival fibers pass from the cementum (C) to the lamina propria; dentinoperiosteal fibers extend from the cementum and pass over the alveolar bone (B) crest to the cortical plate; alveologingival fibers pass from the bone crest to the lamina propria; and circular fibers are free in the lamina propria. (E, enamel; D, dentin.) (From Melfi RC, Alley KE: Permar's Oral Embryology and Microscopic Anatomy. Philadelphia, Lippincott Williams & Wilkins, 2000, p 244.)

Dentogingival Junction

The **dentogingival junction** is the combination of epithelium and connective tissue that attaches the gingiva to the tooth surface. It forms the barrier between the oral environment and the PDL, and loss of integrity in this area can lead to gingivitis and periodontal disease.

The epithelium facing the tooth is called the **attachment epithelium** and consists of two parts: the **sulcular epithelium**, which lines the sulcus, and the **junctional epithelium** directly attached to the tooth. The junctional epithelium is functionally very important in maintaining the gingival attachment, and it differs from the rest of the oral epithelium in several respects. The junctional epithelium is separated from the connective tissue of the gingiva by an external basement membrane, like that found in all epithelial tissues. This basement membrane is formed by the cooperative efforts of both the epithelium and the connective tissue. In addition, it has an internal basement at the tooth surface, and this basement membrane is produced by the junctional epithelium alone. The cell turnover rate in the junctional epithelium is 3 to 6 days, and cell division is not limited to the basal cells at the external basement membrane. Cells directly attached to the tooth at the internal basement membrane are also dividing while maintaining their attachment to the tooth (**Figure 4-21**).

Oral Mucosa

A mucosa always consists of an epithelium and a layer of connective tissue beneath it, which is known as a **lamina propria**. The type of epithelium and the nature of the lamina propria vary according to their location and also depending on the particular combination of the two tissues that best fits the function of the mucosa in that location. The mucosa of the oral cavity shows numerous variations in its different regions, reflecting the many different functions of the oral cavity. If the function of the mucosa in a particular location is to participate in mastication, the epithelium in that area will be keratinized to offer the greatest protection and the mucosa will be tightly attached to the underlying hard tissues. The mucosa in such areas is known as **masticatory mucosa**. In other areas of the oral cavity, the mucosa functions simply to form an internal lining. The epithelium in these areas is nonkeratinized, and the mucosa is loosely attached to the underlying structures. Mucosa in these areas is called **lining mucosa**.

Lip

Histologically, the lip has three different regions: skin on the outside, a red border at the transition from skin to mucosa, and the actual labial mucosa on the inside. The skin of the lip is typical thin skin with hair follicles, sebaceous glands, sweat glands, and a keratinized stratified squamous epithelium. The **red border** (or **vermillion border**) maintains a keratinized stratified squamous epithelium but lacks the other features of skin. Connective tissue papillae that extend into the epithelium and reach rather near the surface give this portion of the lip its characteristic red color. The absence of glands makes the red border susceptible to drying.

The **labial mucosa** begins with an abrupt transition to a thick but nonkeratinized stratified squamous epithelium. A connective tissue lamina propria lies beneath the epithelium;

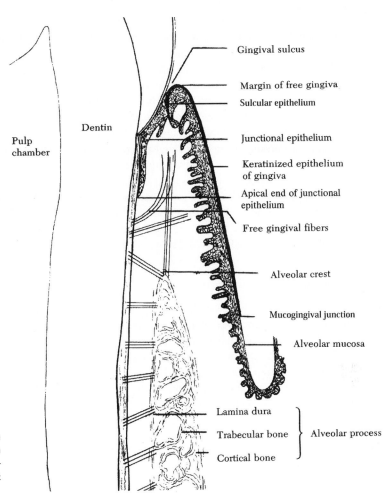

Pulp chamber

Dentin

Gingival sulcus

Margin of free gingiva

Sulcular epithelium

Junctional epithelium

Keratinized epithelium of gingiva

Apical end of junctional epithelium

Free gingival fibers

Alveolar crest

Mucogingival junction

Alveolar mucosa

Lamina dura

Trabecular bone

Cortical bone

Alveolar process

Figure 4-21. A section of the buccal cervical area of a mandibular molar, which is cut buccolingually. (From Melfi RC, Alley KE: Permar's Oral Embryology and Microscopic Anatomy. Philadelphia, Lippincott Williams & Wilkins, 2000, p 243.)

beneath the lamina propria (but not clearly demarcated from it) lies additional connective tissue called the **submucosa**. The connective tissue of the submucosa contains numerous tiny salivary glands, the **labial salivary glands**, which continuously empty their secretion onto the epithelial surface. This region also contains some adipose tissue, blood vessels, and nerves. Deep to the submucosa, the lip contains skeletal muscle, primarily that of the **orbicularis oris muscle**.

Alveolar Mucosa

The space between the lip and the dental arch is called the **vestibule**. The bottom of the vestibule (or the top, in the case of the maxillary arch) is called the **fornix**, and it marks the point of transition between the mucosa of the lip and the **alveolar mucosa**. Beneath the alveolar mucosa lies a submucosa attached to the alveolar bone. The presence of a submucosa here means that the alveolar mucosa itself is not very firmly attached to the alveolar bone and is thus rather mobile.

Gingival Mucosa

The alveolar mucosa is continuous with the **gingival mucosa**, but differences exist between the two. The gingival

mucosa is involved in mastication and requires protection from the masticatory forces. The result is an epithelial transition from nonkeratinized to keratinized stratified squamous epithelium. The epithelial transition at this point is marked by a slight indentation known as the **mucogingival junction**. This junction separates the lining type of alveolar mucosa from the masticatory gingival mucosa. No submucosa is present in the gingival mucosa, and the lamina propria is tightly attached to alveolar bone or to the tooth.

A portion of the gingiva is not attached directly to the tooth surface and is known as the **free gingiva**, whereas the tightly attached gingiva is called the **attached gingiva**. The free gingiva ends at the bottom of the gingival sulcus, and a small groove, the free gingival groove, marks the boundary between free and attached gingiva on the gingiva's outer surface. At points in the gingival mucosa where the epithelium extends deeply into the connective tissue, dimples appear at the epithelial surface, producing the **stippling** of the gingiva that is visible with the naked eye (see Figure 4-21).

Palatal Mucosa

The mucosa of the hard palate is of the masticatory type, and that of the soft palate is typical of lining mucosa. The anterior portion of the **palatal mucosa** is attached very tightly to the bone along the **midline raphe**. The mucosa is less tightly attached on either side of the raphe, and adipose tissue is found between the epithelium and the bone. Posteriorly, palatal glands gradually replace the adipose tissue. These glands spread toward the midline so that in the most posterior part of the palate there are glands beneath the epithelium even at the midline raphe. Transverse ridges, the **palatal rugae**, are prominent in the palatal mucosa anteriorly and become less distinct with advancing age. The lining mucosa of the soft palate continues until it terminates in the **uvula**. After rounding the corner into the nasopharynx, the epithelium changes to the pseudostratified epithelium of the respiratory passages. The pseudostratified epithelium is not part of the oral mucosa **(Figure 4-22)**.

Dorsal Surface of the Tongue

The mucosa of the dorsal surface of the tongue is so different from any mucosa anywhere else that it is referred to simply as a **specialized mucosa**. The epithelium is keratinized, and the surface of the tongue is fuzzy with tiny projections, called **lingual papillae**. Several types of lingual papillae exist; however, only three types are found on the adult human tongue.

The most numerous papillae are the **filiform papillae**, which are found all over the dorsal surface of the tongue. The name means "file-shaped," because these papillae are sharp and pointed like the teeth on a file. They are very highly keratinized and are responsible for the rough texture of the tongues of animals (e.g., cats). Filiform papillae lack taste buds.

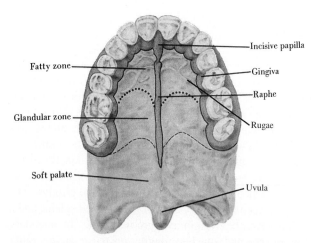

Figure 4-22. Roof of the oral cavity proper. The hard palate, containing bone, is bisected into right and left halves by a raphe. Anteriorly, the hard palate contains fatty tissue in the submucosa; posteriorly, mucous glands lie within the submucosa. Neither the raphe nor the gingiva contains a submucosa; rather, the mucosa is attached directly to the bone. The soft palate has muscle instead of bone in its substance and has glands continuous with those of the hard palate in the submucosa. [Based on Bhaskar SN (ed): Orban's Oral Histology and Embryology, 11th ed. St Louis, CV Mosby, 1991, p 284. From Ross MH, Romrell LJ, Kaye GI: Histology: A Text and Atlas. Baltimore, Williams & Wilkins, 1995, p 405.]

Scattered throughout the anterior two thirds of the tongue are larger slightly dome-shaped papillae that resemble mushrooms, thus they have been called **fungiform (fungus-shaped) papillae**. They are visible with the naked eye as reddish dots that are a little larger than the fuzzy-looking filiform papillae. Their epithelium is thinner than that of the filiform papillae, allowing blood vessels closer to the surface and giving them their redder color. Taste buds may be associated with the fungiform papillae.

The 8 to 10 **circumvallate papillae** (also sometimes just **vallate** papillae) are extremely large and are located along the V-shaped boundary (sulcus terminalis) between the anterior two thirds and the posterior third of the tongue. As their name suggests, these papillae have a surrounding valley. At the bottom of the valley lie the openings of numerous small ducts of the **lingual salivary glands**, which keep the valley full of saliva at all times. The surface epithelium is thin, and smaller papillae may be present on the surface of these large ones. Taste buds are present on both walls of the surrounding valleys, but especially on the sides of the papillae themselves.

Four types of lingual papillae are often described, the fourth being the elusive **foliate papillae**. Some animals have prominent and distinct foliate papillae, but humans do not. Instead, folds in the mucosa at the sides of the tongue are evident. These folds are apparently remnants of foliate papillae. Taste buds are found along these folds, and in animals with prominent foliate papillae, the papillae are richly supplied with taste buds **(Figure 4-23)**.

Taste Buds

Taste buds are small round or oval-shaped collections of cells associated with the circumvallate papillae and the fungiform papillae. They are epithelial structures with a sensory function, thus the epithelium of taste buds is called a **neuroepithelium**. Two types of cells are present in taste buds-the actual sensory taste cells themselves, and the larger and more numerous supporting cells. The cells of the taste bud are oriented around a small opening, the taste pore. The sensation of taste depends on dissolving some of the food in the mouth in saliva, and then saliva with dissolved food must have access to the taste pore of the taste buds **(Figure 4-24)**.

Undersurface of the Tongue

The mucosa of the ventral surface of the tongue is typical lining mucosa with a nonkeratinized stratified squamous epithelium and a large amount of loose connective tissue.

Mucosa of the Cheek

The mucosa of the cheek, the **buccal mucosa**, is quite similar to that of the lip, although some differences exist. The epithelium of this lining mucosa is nonkeratinized. Skin is

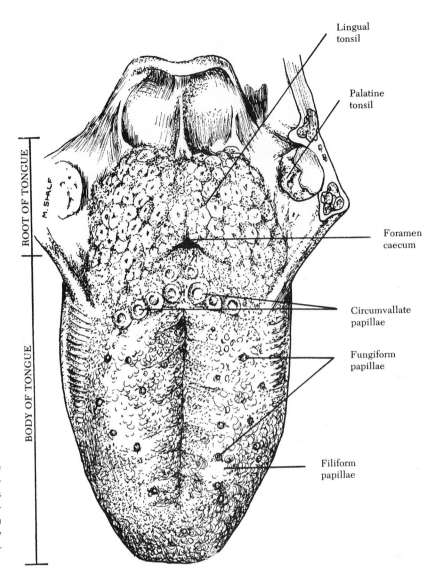

Lingual
tonsil

Palatine
tonsil

Foramen
caecum

Circumvallate
papillae

Fungiform
papillae

Filiform
papillae

ROOT OF TONGUE

BODY OF TONGUE

M. SHALF

Figure 4-23. Diagrammatic drawing of the dorsum of the human tongue. The division between the body and the root is indicated, as are the locations of types of papillae, the foramen cecum, and the lingual tonsil. (From Melfi RC, Alley KE: Permar's Oral Embryology and Microscopic Anatomy. Philadelphia, Lippincott Williams & Wilkins, 2000, p 229.)

present on one side of the cheek and mucosa on the other side, but there is no intermediate zone to compare with the red border of the lip. The connective tissue of the cheek includes large numbers of elastic fibers that help to keep the buccal mucosa pulled away from the teeth during talking and chewing. **Buccal salivary glands** are present, but sometimes they extend deep into the skeletal muscle (unlike those of the lip that are limited to the connective tissue between the epithelium and the muscle).

Salivary Glands

An understanding of the histology of the salivary glands requires a basic understanding of the development and structure of glands in general.

Gland Structure and Development

Glands are epithelial structures. One of the functions of epithelial tissues is secretion, and in many locations groups of epithelial cells are set aside especially for this function. As epithelial structures, they must have a relationship with body surfaces. Most glands are located at body surfaces or are connected to a surface by means of a **duct.**

The development of a gland begins with an epithelium in which some of the cells begin to grow rapidly and invade the connective tissue while still separated from the connective tissue by the basement membrane. These epithelial cells eventually become specialized for their role in secretion. Some glands are so small and simple that they consist only of a few cells growing down into the connective tissue. Salivary glands, however, are larger and more complex and require additional specialization. As a column of epithelial cells for a more complex gland invades the connective tissue, it may branch several times. Each of the new branches will branch again, and probably again and again, until an arrangement like a tree is formed. Finally, at the end of each branch, the epithelial cells become specialized for their secretory function. The cells of the branches themselves form hollow ducts to carry the secretion from the secretory cells

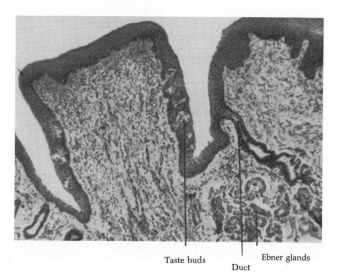

Taste buds   Ebner glands
Duct

Figure 4-24. A vertical section through the dorsum (upper surface) of a human tongue demonstrates a circumvallate papilla. The papillae may be 2 to 3 mm in diameter. Taste buds are located along the side surface; a duct from von Ebner salivary glands empties into the base of the trench around the papilla. This section is cut through the length of the duct, just to one side of the duct opening. Consequently, the exact point at which the duct opens into the trench cannot be seen. (From Melfi RC, Alley KE: Permar's Oral Embryology and Microscopic Anatomy. Philadelphia, Lippincott Williams & Wilkins, 2000, p 232.)

at the ends of the branches, which by this time are far removed from the surface. In some glands, the epithelial cells do not form ducts and lose their connection with the surface epithelium. Glands formed in this way are required to release their secretion into the circulatory system, through which the secretory products are carried to all parts of the body. Such glands are called **endocrine glands**. The glands that maintain their connection to the surface and release their secretions onto a body surface are called **exocrine glands. Salivary glands are all exocrine glands.**

Secretory Units

The little clump of secretory cells at the end of each branch of the duct system is called a **secretory unit**. Each unit consists of a number of secretory epithelial cells grouped around a lumen, which forms the very beginning of the duct system. The salivary glands have two different types of secretory units. The serous type produces a secretion that consists primarily of protein. If a gland contains only serous secretory units, the gland is called a **serous gland**. The other type of secretory unit found in salivary glands is called a mucous secretory unit. The cells of these secretory units produce mucin, a carbohydrate-rich product. If a gland contains only mucous secretory units, it is called a **mucous gland**. Many mucous secretory units possess a little clump of serous cells that form a half-moon-shaped cap structure over the end of the mucous tubule called *a serous demilune*. Glands that contain secretory cells of both types-serous and mucous-are called **mixed glands (Figure 4-25).**

Myoepithelial Cells

Another type of cell is located on the epithelial side of the basement membrane in association with many secretory units. These epithelial cells function in contraction and have been called **myoepithelial cells**. The cells are shaped like an octopus, with a cell body corresponding to the body of an octopus and slender cytoplasmic branches surrounding the secretory unit like the tentacles of an octopus. Contraction of the myoepithelial cells helps to propel the mucous or serous secretion through the duct system.

Major Salivary Glands

The three pairs of major salivary glands each have the same basic structure but differ in the relative proportions of the two types of secretory units. These glands do not secrete continuously but require the stimulation of the presence of food in the mouth (or even the anticipation of food) to release saliva. All are named according to their location.

Parotid Glands

The **parotid glands** are the largest of the salivary glands and are located at the side of the mandible in front of the ear. (Parotid means near the ear.) They are purely serous glands, meaning that they have serous secretory units only.

Submandibular Glands

The **submandibular glands** (sometimes previously called the submaxillary glands) are mixed glands, but most of the

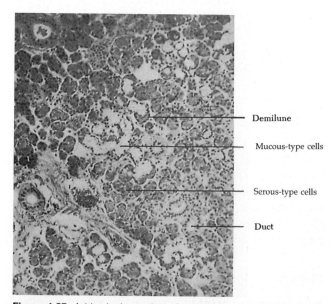

Demilune

Mucous-type cells

Serous-type cells

Duct

Figure 4-25. A histologic section of a human submandibular gland. Both serous and mucous secretory cells are present; the serous type is more numerous. The groups of light-colored mucous cells (center) in some cases are capped on one side by serous cells. In histologic sections, these capping cells have the shape of a "new moon," and some imaginative histologists have called them demilunes (demi = half; lunes = moons). Cross-sections are seen in the section. (From Melfi RC, Alley KE: Permar's Oral Embryology and Microscopic Anatomy. Philadelphia, Lippincott Williams & Wilkins, 2000, p 260.)

secretory units are serous. The submandibular glands are located beneath the base of the tongue. The mucous secretory units have serous demilunes, although they are not necessarily visible on every mucous tubule.

Sublingual Glands

The **sublingual glands** are located under the tongue, where they lie anterior to the submandibular glands. All the secretory units are mucous, but most have serous demilunes, which makes this a mixed gland (**Figure 4-26**).

Minor Salivary Glands

The **minor salivary glands** (intrinsic salivary glands) are characterized by short ducts that empty into the oral cavity close to the gland itself. Unlike the major salivary glands, the minor salivary glands secrete continuously; these glands keep the oral mucosa moist whether or not food is present in the mouth. The glands are all named according to their location in the oral cavity. The minor salivary glands of the lip (**labial glands**), the cheek (**buccal glands**), and the palate (**palatal glands**) are all mucous glands. The tongue contains a number of minor salivary glands (**lingual glands**)-some serous, some mucous, and some mixed.

Biology of Saliva

Saliva is mainly water but also contains the secretions of the salivary glands, cells that have fallen off the lining of the oral mucosa, and calcium and phosphate ions. Saliva has several different functions:

1. **Lubrication** for easy movement of the oral structures

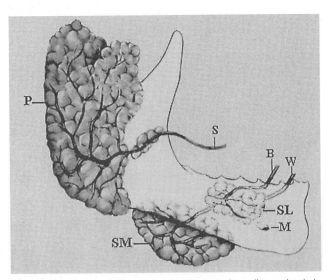

Figure 4-26. Anatomic position of the three major salivary glands in relation to a lateral view of the mandible. (P, parotid gland; S, Stensen duct; SM, submandibular gland; W, Wharton duct; SL, sublingual gland; B, Bartholin duct; M, mental foramen.) (From Melfi RC, Alley KE: Permar's Oral Embryology and Microscopic Anatomy. Philadelphia, Lippincott Williams & Wilkins, 2000, p 257.)

2. **Buffering** to maintain the pH of the oral cavity at a level that is unhealthy for growing bacteria and to protect the enamel from acids formed by the metabolism of sugar
3. **Combating bacteria** with enzymes that actively destroy bacteria (bacteriolytic properties) and via its components, which cause bacteria to clump together and thus prevent their further multiplication (bacteriostatic properties)
4. **Taste**, in that food must be dissolved in saliva in order to come in contact with the sensory cells of the taste buds
5. **Digestion** by way of enzymes that initiate the metabolism of carbohydrates (The actual breakdown, however, is not a major function of the saliva. More important, saliva promotes digestion by preparing food for the more distant parts of the digestive system.)
6. **Protecting** the teeth by cleansing the teeth and other oral structures (The calcium and phosphate ions of saliva play a role in the final mineralization process of the enamel; fluoride-rich saliva has the capacity to remineralize incipient carious lesions.)
7. **Excretion** of excess iron and iodine

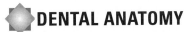 DENTAL ANATOMY

MAURICE W. LEWIS, DDS

In order to be successful in the clinical practice of dental hygiene, a basic knowledge of the anatomic characteristics of the teeth and the surrounding tissues is essential. This knowledge of anatomy is the foundation upon which skills in assessment, planning, implementation, and evaluation of dental hygiene care are developed. A thorough knowledge of crown and root anatomy prepares the dental hygienist to identify teeth present within a patient's dentition, educate the patient in proper oral health maintenance based on the individual's needs, and make decisions regarding the appropriate instruments to use to adapt to the tooth's anatomy. This knowledge of dental anatomy also prepares health care providers to answer any legal or forensic questions that may arise.

This portion of the chapter discusses dental terminology, primary and permanent tooth morphology, eruption and exfoliation, and the intra- and inter-arch relationships.

Trait Categories

A **trait** is a distinguishing characteristic, quality, peculiarity, or attribute that can be quite helpful in describing tooth similarities and differences. **Set traits** (dentition traits) distinguish teeth in the primary (deciduous) dentition from those in permanent (secondary) dentition. Arch traits distinguish maxillary from mandibular teeth. **Class traits** are characteristics that differentiate the four categories or classes of teeth (i.e., incisors, canines, premolars, and molars). **Type traits** differentiate teeth within one class (e.g., differences between central and lateral incisors or between first and second premolars or between first, second, and third molars).

Terminology

The language of the professions of dentistry and dental hygiene is filled with terms and phrases that are foreign to the average person but are the basis of communication within the professional dental community. Familiarity with this terminology is very important.

The common structural parts of all teeth include a **crown,** at least one **root**, and a **pulp cavity**. These structures consist of four types of tissue: enamel, dentin, cementum, and **pulp.**

Enamel is the hard, white, shiny surface of the **anatomic crown**. It is the hardest substance in the human body and consists of 95% calcium hydroxide (inorganic calcified matter); 1% enamel matrix (organic matter); and 4% water. It develops from the enamel organ (ectoderm).

Dentin is the hard yellowish tissue surrounding the pulp and underlying the enamel and cementum, and this tissue makes up the bulk of the tooth. It consists of 70% calcium hydroxide, 18% organic matter (collagen fibers), and 12% water. Dentin develops from the dental papilla (mesoderm).

Cementum is the hard, dull yellow tissue that covers the **anatomic root**. It consists of 65% calcium hydroxide, 23% organic matter (collagen fibers), and 12% water. Cementum develops from the dental sac (mesoderm).

Pulp is the soft (noncalcified) tissue within the **pulp cavity** (the space in the center of the crown and root). It consists of several types of highly differentiated cellular types and substances: loose connective tissue, fibroblasts, blood vessels, lymphatics, nerves, ground substance (water and long carbohydrate chains attached to protein backbones), and undifferentiated mesenchymal cells (which serve to replace injured or destroyed odontoblasts).

The **pulp cavity**, the space within the tooth that contains the pulp, is characterized by three anatomic areas. The **pulp chamber** houses the portion of the pulp within the crown. The **pulp canal**, or **root canal**, contains the portion of the pulp within the root. The **pulp horns** are the most coronal extensions of the pulp chamber. The functions of the dental pulp are:

1. **Formative**: dentin-producing cells (odontoblasts) produce dentin throughout the life of the tooth. This is called **secondary dentin**.
2. **Sensory**: nerve endings permit the sense of pain from heat, cold, drilling, sweet, decay, trauma, or infection.
3. **Nutritive**: nutrient transport from the bloodstream to extensions of the pulp that reach into dentin. Blood in the tooth pulp passed through the heart 6 seconds previously.
4. **Defensive** or **protective**: responds to injury or decay by forming reparative dentin (by the odontoblasts).

Enamel covers the anatomic crown and **cementum covers the anatomic root**. These terms must be differentiated from the **clinical crown** and the **clinical root**. The **clinical crown** is the part of the tooth that is visible in the oral cavity. It may include only part of the anatomic crown if the gingiva still covers part of the cervical portion of the crown, or it may include all of the anatomic crown and part of the anatomic root if the gingiva have receded. The **clinical root** is the part of the tooth that is not visible in the oral cavity. It may include a portion of the anatomic crown if the cervical area of the crown is still covered by the gingiva.

The hard tissues of the tooth meet in three junction areas. The **cementoenamel junction (CEJ)** separates the enamel of the anatomic crown from the cementum of the anatomic root. This area is also known as the **cervical line**. [The part of the root or crown near the CEJ is called the **cervix** (neck).] The **dentinoenamel junction (DEJ)** is the inner surface of the enamel cap and is only visible on cross-section or when preparing a tooth for a restoration. The **cementodentinal junction (CDJ)** is the inner surface of the cementum lining the root and is also only visible on cross-section.

Four of the anatomic characteristics of the root of a tooth should be noted: the **apex, apical foramen, furcation,** and **root** trunk. The **apex** is the end of the root and may be round or pointed. The **apical foramen** is the opening at the apex of the root through which pass blood vessels and nerves. The **furcation** is the area of a multirooted tooth where the root divides. The **root trunk** is the area from the CEJ to the furcation. The **furcation entrance** is the area of opening into the furcation. The **roof of the furcation** is the most coronal part of the furcation. It represents the top, or ceiling, of a mandibular furcation and the bottom, or base, of a maxillary furcation. The **interfurcal** area is the area between the roots of a multirooted tooth **(Figure 4-27)**.

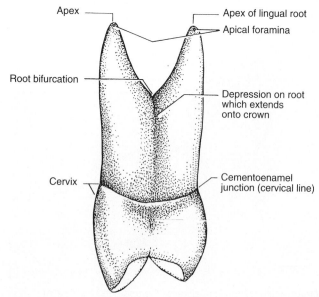

Figure 4-27. Maxillary right first premolar, mesial surface. The space between the two roots is the furcal region, and the root area between the cervical line and the root bifurcation is the root trunk. (From Woelfel JB, Scheid RC: Dental Anatomy: Its Relevance to Dentistry. Baltimore, Williams & Wilkins, 1997, p 99.)

Occasionally, an abnormal tooth will have a crown or root that is twisted (sometimes severely) from the normal linear relationship. This is known as a **dilaceration.**

Several terms are used to identify the surfaces of a tooth. The **facial surface** is the surface that is next to the face; the outer surface of a tooth in the mouth resting against or next to the lips or cheeks. Facial may be used to designate this portion of any tooth, anterior or posterior. When discussing the facial surface of an incisor or canine, the term **labial surface** (i.e., the lip) is commonly used. The same surface on a premolar or a molar is then called the **buccal surface** (i.e., the cheek).

The **proximal surface** is the surface of the tooth that is next to an adjacent tooth. The **mesial surface** is the surface of the tooth nearest the midline of the dental arch. The **distal surface** is the surface of the tooth farthest from the midline of the dental arch. The mesial surface of all teeth approximate (face) the distal surface of the adjacent tooth, except between the central incisors where mesial surface faces another mesial surface. The area of the tooth that touches the adjacent tooth within the same arch is called the **contact area (Figure 4-28).**

The **lingual surface** is the surface toward the tongue and is often referred to as the palatal surface for the maxillary teeth.

The biting surfaces, those surfaces that face each other in the opposing arches, are identified by function in that the anterior teeth are used for gripping, cutting, and tearing, whereas the posterior teeth are used for rending and grinding. The cutting surface of the anterior teeth is called the **incisal edge** or **ridge**.

The **occlusal surface** is the chewing surface of posterior teeth and consists of cusps, ridges, and grooves. This surface is bounded anteroposteriorly by the marginal ridges and faciolingually by the cusp ridges.

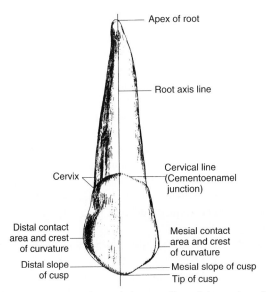

Figure 4-28. Labial surface of the maxillary right canine. (From Woelfel JB, Scheid RC: Dental Anatomy: Its Relevance to Dentistry. Baltimore, Williams & Wilkins, 1997, p 98.)

A **line angle** is the transition area marking the junction of two surfaces (i.e., the mesiobuccal line angle), which designates the transition area of the mesial and buccal surfaces. A **point angle** is the transition point marking the junction of three surfaces of a tooth (i.e., mesioincisolabial point angle).

When reviewing the terms relating to the morphology of the anatomic crown, it is important to note the diversity of bumps, ridges, valleys, crevices and pits. A **cusp** is a point, or peak, on the occlusal surface of molar and premolar teeth and on the incisal edge of canines **(Figure 4-29)**. **Cusp slopes** (also called **cusp ridges** or **cusp arms**) are the inclined surfaces or ridges that form an angle at the cusp tip when viewed from the facial or lingual aspect **(Figure 4-30)**.

Mamelon is one of three tubercles present on permanent incisor teeth that has not been subjected to wear **(Figure 4-31)**. **Cingulum** refers to the large rounded elevation or bulge on the cervical third of the lingual surface of anterior teeth (see Figure 4-31).

Several longitudinal convexities of enamel, identified as ridges, are present on various teeth **(Figure 4-32)**. The **labial ridge** runs incisocervically in the approximate center of the labial surface of canines. Similarly, the **buccal ridge** runs occlusocervically in the approximate center of the buccal surface of premolars (more pronounced on the first premolars than on the second premolars).

The **cervical ridge** runs mesiodistally on the cervical third of the crown of all deciduous teeth and of the permanent molars.

The **marginal ridge** is located on the mesial and distal borders of the lingual surfaces of incisors and canines and on the mesial and distal borders of the occlusal surfaces of premolars and molars.

A **triangular ridge** is on the occlusal surface of a posterior tooth from the cusp tip to the center of the occlusal surface. All posterior tooth cusps have one triangular ridge, except for the mesiolingual cusp of maxillary molars, which has two triangular ridges.

The **oblique ridge** is found only on maxillary molars. It crosses the occlusal surface in an oblique line, connecting the triangular ridges of the mesiolingual and distobuccal cusps.

The **transverse ridge** crosses the occlusal surfaces of most posterior teeth in a buccolingual direction and consists of connecting triangular ridges.

Several concavities are noted in the tooth morphology as well. A **sulcus** is a broad depression or valley on the occlusal surfaces of posterior teeth, the inclines of which meet in a developmental groove and extend outward to the cusp tips.

The **developmental groove** is a sharply defined, narrow, and linear depression, which is short or long, formed during development and usually separating lobes or major portions of teeth **(Figure 4-33)**. This groove is named according to its location **(Figure 4-34)**.

A **fissure** is a narrow channel, cleft, ditch, or crevice, which is sometimes quite deep. It is formed at the depth of a developmental groove during the development of the tooth and extends inward toward the pulp from the groove.

CUSPS

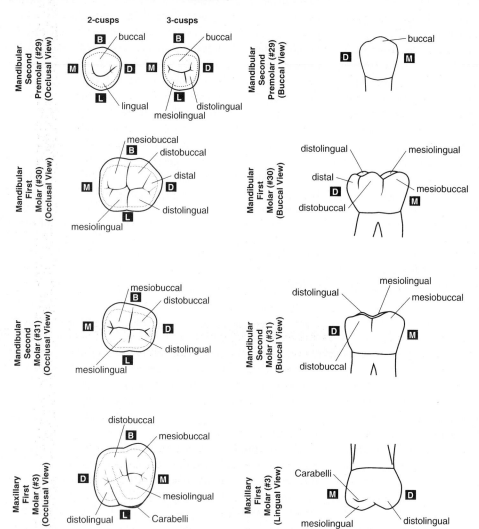

Figure 4-29. Major cusps on various molars and premolars. (From Woelfel JB, Scheid RC: Dental Anatomy: Its Relevance to Dentistry. Baltimore, Williams & Wilkins, 1997, p 103.)

A **fossa** is a depression, or hollow, that is found on the lingual surfaces of some anterior teeth (particularly maxillary incisors) and on the occlusal surfaces of all posterior teeth. **Pits** often occur at the depth of a fossa where two or more grooves join. Like fissures at the depth of grooves, pits are frequently deep and are areas where caries may occur **(Figure 4-35).**

Permanent Dentition

The **permanent dentition** consists of 8 incisors, 4 canines, 8 premolars, and 12 molars. In order to maintain accurate dental records, a uniform code or numbering system must be used for the identification of teeth. Three major systems are used to identify the permanent teeth **(Table 4-4).**

Numbering Systems

The **Universal Numbering System** uses the numbers 1 through 32 to represent the individual teeth. Starting with the maxillary right third molar, which is No. 1, the numbers progress in sequence around the arch to No. 16, which is the maxillary left third molar. The mandibular left third molar is designated as No. 17. The progression is continued as in the maxillary teeth through the arch to the mandibular right third molar (i.e., No. 32).

The **Palmer Notation System** utilizes brackets to represent the four quadrants of the dentition as if facing the patient. The brackets are based on the intersection of a horizontal line, which represents separation of the maxillary and mandibular arches with a vertical line separating the right and left halves of the mouth. The numbers used run from 1 to 8 inches in each quadrant from the central incisor to the third molar.

The **International Numbering System** uses two digits for each tooth. The first digit denotes dentition (permanent or primary), arch, and side, whereas the second digit represents the tooth. As in the Palmer system, the numbers 1 to 8 represent the central incisor to the third molar.

TABLE 4-4 Various Tooth Identification Systems

	TOOTH	UNIVERSAL		PALMER NOTATION		INTERNATIONAL (FDI)	
		RIGHT	LEFT	RIGHT	LEFT	RIGHT	LEFT
DECIDUOUS DENTITION — MAXILLARY TEETH	Central incisor	E	F	A⌐	⌐A	51	61
	Lateral incisor	D	G	B⌐	⌐B	52	62
	Canine	C	H	C⌐	⌐C	53	63
	First molar	B	I	D⌐	⌐D	54	64
	Second molar	A	J	E⌐	⌐E	55	65
DECIDUOUS DENTITION — MANDIBULAR TEETH	Central incisor	P	O	A⌐	⌐A	81	71
	Lateral incisor	Q	N	B⌐	⌐B	82	72
	Canine	R	M	C⌐	⌐C	83	73
	First molar	S	L	D⌐	⌐D	84	74
	Second molar	T	K	E⌐	⌐E	85	75
PERMANENT DENTITION — MAXILLARY TEETH	Central incisor	8	9	1⌐	⌐1	11	21
	Lateral incisor	7	10	2⌐	⌐2	12	22
	Canine	6	11	3⌐	⌐3	13	23
	First premolar	5	12	4⌐	⌐4	14	24
	Second premolar	4	13	5⌐	⌐5	15	25
	First molar	3	14	6⌐	⌐6	16	26
	Second molar	2	15	7⌐	⌐7	17	27
	Third molar	1	16	8⌐	⌐8	18	28
PERMANENT DENTITION — MANDIBULAR TEETH	Central incisor	25	24	1⌐	⌐1	41	31
	Lateral incisor	26	23	2⌐	⌐2	42	32
	Canine	27	22	3⌐	⌐3	43	33
	First premolar	28	21	4⌐	⌐4	44	34
	Second premolar	29	20	5⌐	⌐5	45	35
	First molar	30	19	6⌐	⌐6	46	36
	Second molar	31	18	7⌐	⌐7	47	37
	Third molar	32	17	8⌐	⌐8	48	38

From Woelfel JB, Scheid RC: Dental Anatomy: Its Relevance to Dentistry. Baltimore, Williams & Wilkins, 1997, pp 126 and 134.)

All cusps are basically a gothic pyramid

The cuspal gothic pyramid produces 4 ridges:

1. Mesial cusp ridge
2. Distal cusp ridge
3. Buccal cusp ridge (labial ridge on canines)
4. Triangular ridge on posterior teeth (lingual ridge on canines)

Figure 4-30. Buccal cusps and design with the four cusp ridges numbered 1 to 4 around the cusp tip (X) on a maxillary right first premolar. All cusps have four ridges. The facial ridge (3) is more prominent on some teeth than on others, particularly on maxillary canines and first premolars. Most triangular ridges incline toward the center of the tooth at a slope of approximately 45 degrees. The mesial and distal cusp ridges (1 and 2) form the triangular shape of the cusp when viewed from the facial. (Courtesy of Richard W. Huffman, MD, and Ruth Paulson, MD. From Woelfel JB, Scheid RC: Dental Anatomy: Its Relevance to Dentistry. Baltimore, Williams & Wilkins, 1997, p 100.)

Crown Anatomy

Several characteristics are common to the crowns of all the teeth. All proximal surfaces converge toward the apex from the crests of curvature (see Figure 4-28). Also called the **height of contour**, the **crest of curvature** is the highest point of a curve or the greatest convexity or bulge. Consider the following facts:

1. This convergence allows for the area of interproximal gingiva and bone.
2. The proximal crest of curvature tends to be the contact area in the ideal occlusion and provides stability for adjacent teeth and protection of interproximal gingiva.
3. The proximal heights of contour are located in the incisal/occlusal or middle third of the crown.
4. The mesial crest of curvature tends to be more incisal/occlusal than the distal crest. Mesial outlines are straighter than are distal outlines.

All facial and lingual surfaces converge toward the apex and toward the incisal/occlusal surface from the crest of curvature.

All crowns have convex facial surfaces with the crest of curvature located in the cervical third. Posterior teeth have

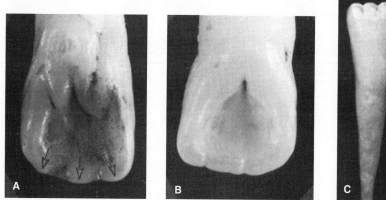

Figure 4-31. Lingual view of the left *(A)* and right *(B)* maxillary central incisors. Both teeth have pronounced lingual marginal ridges and cingula and deeper lingual fossae than normal. They would be called "shovel-shaped" incisors. Both teeth have three rounded protuberances on their incisal edge called mamelons *(arrows)*. The right tooth has a pit on the incisal border of the cingulum-the type of place that caries can penetrate without being easily noticed. Mandibular right central incisor. *C,* Labial surface. The mamelons are unworn. *D,* Lingual surface. The crown surface is concave in the middle and incisal thirds, convex over the cingulum, and nearly smooth. (From Woelfel JB, Scheid RC: Dental Anatomy: Its Relevance to Dentistry. Baltimore, Williams & Wilkins, 1997, pp 122 and 140.)

RIDGES

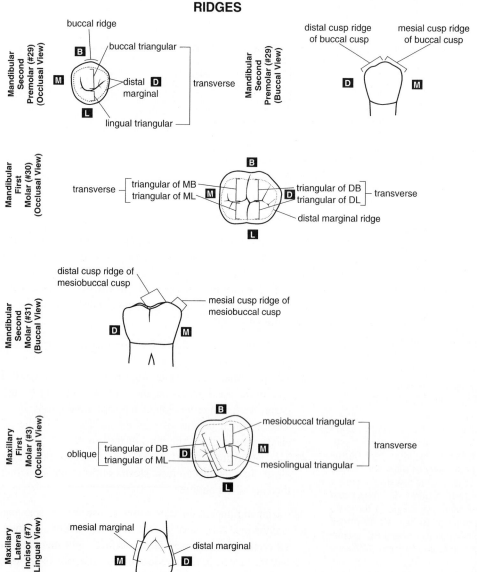

Figure 4-32. Examples of various ridges on molars, premolars, and incisors. (From Woelfel JB, Scheid RC: Dental Anatomy: Its Relevance to Dentistry. Baltimore, Williams & Wilkins, 1997, p 104.)

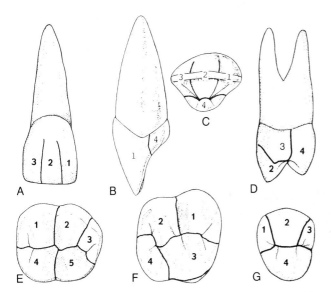

Figure 4-33. Lobes or primary anatomic divisions on teeth. *A*, The maxillary central incisor, like all anterior teeth, has four lobes; the lingual lobe (4) beneath the cingulum is seen in the mesial view (*B*) and incisal view (*C*). *D* and *G*, Maxillary first premolar, mesial, and occlusal views. *E*, The mandibular first molar with three buccal and two lingual lobes. *F*, The maxillary first molar with three large lobes and one small lobe. The Carabelli cusp, when present, is a part of the large mesiolingual lobe. On the posterior teeth, major developmental grooves separate these divisions. Mamelons, when present, are an indication of the three labial lobes on the incisors. (From Woelfel JB, Scheid RC: Dental Anatomy: Its Relevance to Dentistry. Baltimore, Williams & Wilkins, 1997, p 117.)

convex lingual surfaces with crests of curvature in the middle third. Anterior teeth, however, have concave lingual surfaces in the middle third. These contours allow for deflection of food away from the gingiva and facilitate the functions of the teeth.

Proximal cervical lines converge toward incisal/occlusal surfaces and are more prominent on anterior teeth than on posterior teeth. The mesial cervical line curves more than the distal cervical line.

From a proximal view, the long axes of the crown and root are in line, except for the mandibular posterior teeth, which exhibit the long axis of the crown tipping lingual to the long axis of the root. This allows for proper intercuspation of posterior teeth and the distribution of occlusal forces along the long axes.

Proximal surfaces have a lingual convergence (especially on maxillary incisors and canines) on all teeth, except for the mandibular second premolar and the maxillary first molar.

Root Anatomy

The anatomy of the root is less complex than that of the crown, but variations in size, shape, and number often occur. Teeth generally tend to have one, two, or three roots. **One-rooted teeth** include incisors, canines, maxillary second premolars, and mandibular premolars. **Two-rooted teeth** include maxillary first premolars (i.e., buccal and lingual) and mandibular molars (i.e., mesial and distal). The maxillary molars are the **three-rooted teeth** (i.e., mesiobuccal, distobuccal, and lingual). When considering the possible morphologic variations, it must be noted that these numbers can differ in individual cases. Third molars may display multiple roots or rootlets. Mandibular canines sometimes have two roots, whereas maxillary first premolars may develop with only one root.

Multirooted teeth have a root trunk with depressions that deepen until the roots divide at the furcation. Longitudinal depressions are present on some roots. Roots tend to be cone shaped, with their widest point at the CEJ, and then they converge toward the apex.

The cervical cross-section of one-rooted teeth reveals three basic shapes that can be modified by the presence of root concavities.

1. **Triangular**: maxillary incisors
2. **Ovoid**: canines and some mandibular premolars
3. **Elliptical**: maxillary premolars, mandibular incisors, and some mandibular premolars

The lingual surfaces of triangular and ovoid roots tend to be narrower than the facial surfaces. A cervical cross-section of molars follows the form of the crown.

From a facial or lingual view, roots tend to have a **distal inclination** toward the apex of the tooth. (This feature is often used to help differentiate left from right during forensic examinations of individual teeth.) Second and third molars are more likely than first molars to have roots that are closer together (may even be fused) and more distally inclined.

Permanent Incisors

There are four incisors in each arch—two **central incisors** and two **lateral incisors**. Newly erupted incisors have mamelons on the incisal ridge, which are usually worn away shortly after they erupt. Two incisal angles are formed by the proximal surfaces and the incisal ridge.

Central incisal angles are sharper than are the lateral incisal angles. Mesial incisal angles are more acute than distal incisal angles, which are more obtuse.

Lingual outlines are both "S" shaped with a concave lingual fossa and convex cingulum. The **maxillary lateral incisor is the most variable in terms of morphology** and is the second most common congenitally missing tooth (**Figure 4-36**).

Maxillary Incisor Crown

The maxillary central incisor is the largest of the incisors. The lateral incisor is the next largest. When the incisal edges are outlined horizontally, the cingulum of the central appears off-center distally (**Figure 4-37A**), whereas the cingulum of the lateral incisor is centered (see Figure 4-37B).

GROOVES

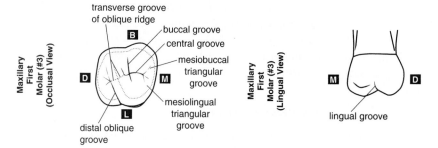

Figure 4-34. Examples of developmental grooves on molars and premolars. (From Woelfel JB, Scheid RC: Dental Anatomy: Its Relevance to Dentistry. Baltimore, Williams & Wilkins, 1997, p 106.)

The mesiodistal dimensions of central incisors are considerably wider than are the faciolingual dimensions. These dimensions are more nearly equal in the lateral incisors.

Lingual anatomy is distinct. The central incisor cingulum is broad, and grooves make it appear scalloped. The lateral incisor cingulum is narrow, and a lingual pit is common.

Maxillary Incisor Root

The central incisor has a short conical root; it is sometimes no longer than the crown. The crown-root ratio is larger in the lateral incisor than in the central incisor.

The cross-sectional appearance is triangular in the central incisor but more ovoid in the lateral incisor. The root of the central incisor is thicker than that of the lateral incisor. The central incisor usually has no prominent root groove, whereas the lateral incisor may have a shallow longitudinal depression on the middle of the mesial surface that extends to about one half of the root. Only one root and one root canal are present.

Mandibular Incisor Crown

The mandibular central incisor is the smallest tooth in the permanent dentition; the lateral incisor is only slightly larger. The faciolingual width is greater than the mesiodistal width. The incisal edges are sharper, and the contact areas are near the incisal ridge. The lingual surface is concave and has indistinct lingual anatomy with no pits. From a facial view, the central incisor appears to be symmetric (**Figure 4-38A**). From lingual and incisal views, the lateral incisor has a distinct skew toward the distal, owing to the cingulum being displaced in that direction (see Figure 4-38B).

Mandibular Incisor Root

Central and lateral incisor roots have similar appearances. Both have a single root with a single root canal. The cross-sectional view shows an elliptical shape with very small facial and lingual surfaces and broad proximal surfaces with root concavities or depressions. The distal depression is

FOSSAE AND PITS

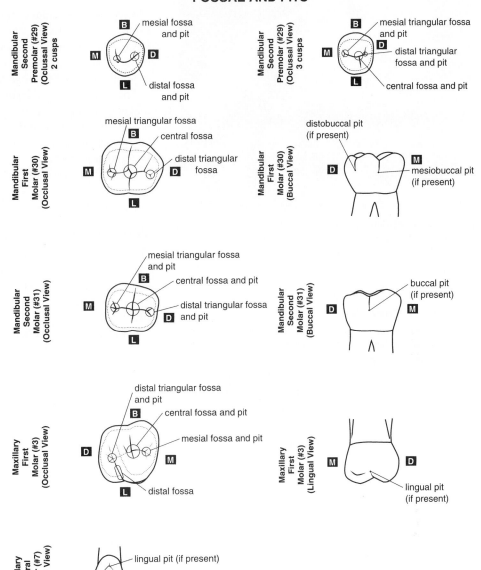

Figure 4-35. Examples of various fossae (often with associated pits) on molars, premolars, and incisors. (From Woelfel JB, Scheid RC: Dental Anatomy: Its Relevance to Dentistry. Baltimore, Williams & Wilkins, 1997, p 105.)

more distinct than the mesial depression. The crown-root ratio strongly favors the root.

Permanent Canines

One canine is found in each quadrant. Canines are the only teeth that have one cusp. They are considered to be the cornerstone teeth because of the long large root externally manifested by the canine eminence of the alveolar bone. They mark the area of transition from cutting activity to grinding activity.

Maxillary Canine Crown (Figure 4-39)

The cusp ridges and tip occupy the incisal third of the crown. Lingual anatomy includes a cingulum, mesial and distal marginal ridges, and a vertical lingual ridge between

two lingual fossae. Lingual pits are rare. In the proximal view, the cusp tip is facial to the long axis of the tooth.

Mandibular Canine Crown (Figure 4-40)

The cusp ridges and tip occupy the incisal fourth of the crown, which appears longer and narrower than the maxillary crown. The lingual anatomy is the same as the maxillary canine but is less prominent. In proximal view, the cusp tip is lingual to the long axis of the tooth.

Canine Root

The root is the longest in the dentition and on average is 1.5 times the length of the crown (the maxillary canine root is usually slightly longer). A cervical cross-section reveals an ovoid shape that is wider labiolingually and has broad facial and proximal surfaces that converge toward the lingual. Proximal longitudinal depressions are present.

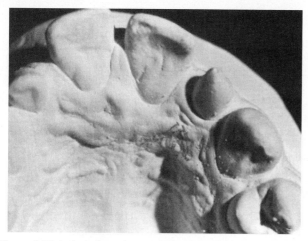

Figure 4-36. Incisal view of a peg-shaped maxillary left lateral incisor. (From Woelfel JB, Scheid RC: Dental Anatomy: Its Relevance to Dentistry. Baltimore, Williams & Wilkins, 1997, p 138.)

Permanent Premolars

The premolars represent characteristics that are common among posterior teeth, such as shorter crowns; less curvature of the CEJ; and occlusal surfaces with marginal ridges, cusps, pits, and grooves. They replace the primary molars. The premolars generally have two cusps and are commonly referred to as bicuspids, even though the mandibular second premolars often manifest a three-cusp, or tricuspate, form. Usually only one root is present, except for the maxillary first premolars, which usually have two roots.

First premolars are often sacrificed for orthodontic purposes. Mandibular second premolars are often congenitally missing.

Mesial marginal ridges are generally more occlusal than distal marginal ridges, which are more cervical. An exception to this rule is on the mandibular first premolars, where distal marginal ridges are in a more occlusal position. Mesial cusp slopes of the buccal cusps are shorter than the distal cusp slopes on all premolars, except the maxillary first premolars that have longer mesial slopes.

Maxillary Premolar Crown (Figure 4-41A and B)

The faciolingual width is greater than the mesiodistal width. From an occlusal view, the outline of the first premolar is hexagonal and angular, whereas the second premolar is rounded and appears more symmetric. There are two cusps of relatively equal size-one facial and one lingual.

The central developmental groove on first premolars is longer (from the mesial to the distal pit) than on the second premolars, where it is only one third or less of the mesiodistal dimension. This groove crosses the mesial marginal ridge on the first premolars.

The first premolar has a distinct concavity in the cervical third of the mesial surface of the crown that extends to the furcation.

Maxillary Premolar Root

The first premolar usually has two roots (i.e., one facial and one lingual) but often has only one root with a prominent mesial root concavity. Occasionally, the premolar has three roots-two facial and one lingual. The second premolar usually has one root.

In cervical cross-section, the roots of both premolars are elliptical and have prominent root concavities.

Mandibular Premolar Crown (Figure 4-42A and B)

Faciolingual and mesiodistal widths are almost equal. The buccal cusp of the first premolar is more pointed than that of the second premolar, which is more obtuse. The first premolar has two cusps-one large facial and one small lingual. The lingual cusp is nonfunctional.

The second premolar is larger and has one large buccal cusp and one (**bicuspate** form) or two (**tricuspate** form) small lingual cusps, all of which are functional cusps. The bicuspate form has a U- or H-shaped groove pattern and two pits. The tricuspate form has a Y-shaped groove pattern and a central pit. Proximal surfaces of this form do not converge toward the lingual. The mandibular second premolar is the third most common congenitally missing tooth.

The first premolar has a strong transverse ridge that separates the mesial and distal triangular fossae, which each have a pit. These pits are often referred to as "snake eyes."

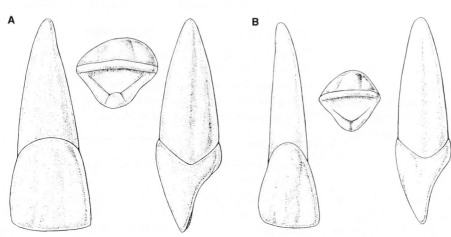

Figure 4-37. *A,* Maxillary right central incisor; labial incisal and mesial views. *B,* Maxillary right lateral incisor; labial, incisal, and mesial views. (From Woelfel JB, Scheid RC: Dental Anatomy: Its Relevance to Dentistry. Baltimore, Williams & Wilkins, 1997, pp 126 and 134.)

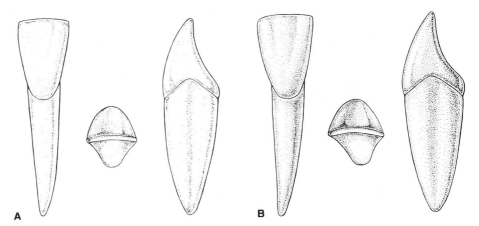

Figure 4-38. *A*, Mandibular right central incisor: labial, incisal, and mesial views. *B*, Mandibular right lateral incisor: labial, incisal, and mesial views. (From Woelfel JB, Scheid RC: Dental Anatomy: Its Relevance to Dentistry. Baltimore, Williams & Wilkins, 1997, p 140.)

Mandibular Premolar Root

In cervical cross-section, these roots are ovoid or elliptical and generally only have one root and one root canal. The first premolar sometimes has a buccolingual apical bifurcation.

Permanent Molars

Permanent molars erupt distal to the primary second molars. The first molars are the largest teeth in the dentition. The second and third molars are progressively smaller. Mandibular molars are the first permanent teeth to erupt.

The presence, size, and shape of third molars can vary greatly. The third molars can resemble either the first or the second molars and are the most commonly missing permanent teeth.

Maxillary Molar Crown

From the occlusal view, the crowns appear to be rhomboid or square. Maxillary molars have pits and grooves on oc-

clusal and lingual surfaces. An oblique ridge runs diagonally from the mesiolingual cusp to the distobuccal cusp.

The first molar has five cusps-four (mesiolingual, mesiobuccal, distobuccal, and distolingual) on the occlusal surface and one on the mesial half of lingual surface called the **cusp of Carabelli (Figure 4-43A).** Each of the four occlusal cusps has a definite triangular ridge. The triangular ridge of the mesiolingual cusp meets the triangular ridge of the mesiobuccal cusp yielding the transverse ridge. The triangular ridges of the mesiolingual and distobuccal cusps form the oblique ridge. The oblique ridge is unique to maxillary molars.

The second molar has four occlusal cusps and resembles the first molar but is smaller. Often the second molar is in tricuspate form with the distolingual cusp missing. Occlusal pits can be noted in mesial, central, and distal fossae.

The outline shape of maxillary molars (with acute mesiobuccal and distolingual angles and obtuse distobuccal and mesiolingual angles) is more twisted on second molars

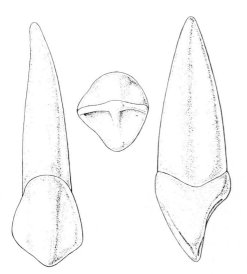

Figure 4-39. A maxillary right canine: labial, incisal, and mesial views. (From Woelfel JB, Scheid RC: Dental Anatomy: Its Relevance to Dentistry. Baltimore, Williams & Wilkins, 1997, p 152.)

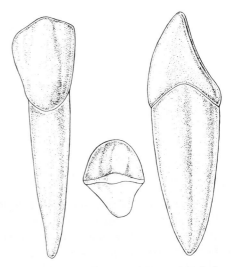

Figure 4-40. A mandibular right canine: labial, incisal, and mesial views. (From Woelfel JB, Scheid RC: Dental Anatomy: Its Relevance to Dentistry. Baltimore, Williams & Wilkins, 1997, p 153.)

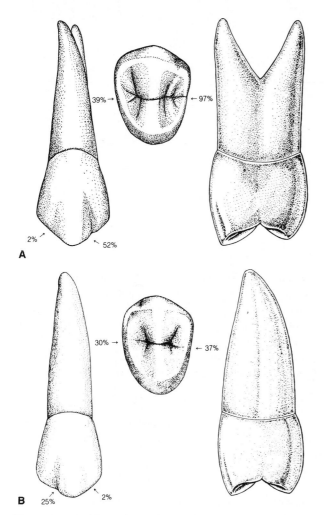

Figure 4-41. *A,* Maxillary right first premolar: buccal, occlusal, and mesial aspects. The percentages by the arrows give the frequency of a deeper depression in the occlusal third or the crown (buccal view) and the frequency of marginal ridge grooves (occlusal view). *B,* Maxillary right second premolar: buccal, occlusal, and mesial aspects. Percentages give frequency of a deeper depression in the occlusal third of the crown (buccal view) and of marginal ridge grooves (occlusal view). (From Woelfel JB, Scheid RC: Dental Anatomy: Its Relevance to Dentistry. Baltimore, Williams & Wilkins, 1997, p 179.)

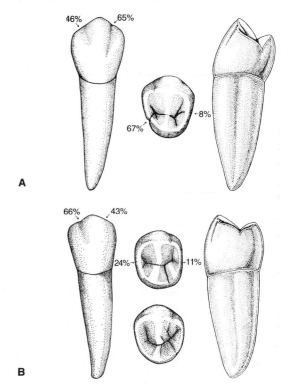

Figure 4-42. *A,* Mandibular right first premolar: buccal, occlusal, and mesial aspects. Percentages (buccal view) give the frequency of notches on the cusp ridges, and in the occlusal view (center), the occurrence of marginal ridge grooves. *B,* Mandibular right second premolar, buccal, and mesial aspects (either type): occlusal aspect, three-cusp type *(above)* occur 54.2% of the time, compared with the two-cusp type *(below center)* and the three-cusp type *(above center)*, the occlusal surface of the three-cusp type is more square or rectangular. (From Woelfel JB, Scheid RC: Dental Anatomy: Its Relevance to Dentistry. Baltimore, Williams & Wilkins, 1997, p 191.)

than on first molars (i.e., acute angles are more acute and obtuse angles are more obtuse) (see Figure 4-43B).

Third molars tend to have large crowns (although still usually smaller than the first or second molars) with short roots. The occlusal surface of a third molar has numerous supplemental grooves and may have extra cusps or tubercles.

Maxillary Molar Root

The three roots found on maxillary molars are mesiobuccal, distobuccal, and lingual (or palatal). The roots are more widely separated on the first molar than on the second molar **(Figure 4-44A and B).** First molar roots are larger and more divergent. The lingual root is the largest and longest and extends beyond the outline of the crown. The roots of the third molar are often fused and pointed.

Furcations are located on the mesial, distal, and buccal surfaces, with the proximal furcation areas located toward the lingual surface. The root trunk of the first molar is shorter than that of the second molar.

Root concavities are found on the mesial surface of the mesiobuccal root, the lingual surface of the lingual root of the first molar, and the furcal surfaces.

Third molars may exhibit accessory roots in excess of the main three.

Mandibular Molar Crown

The mesiodistal width is greater than the buccolingual width, resulting in the rectangular shape of the crown.

The first molar has five cusps-three buccal (mesiobuccal, distobuccal, and distal) and two lingual (mesiolingual and distolingual) **(Figure 4-45)**

Mandibular molars have pits and grooves on the occlusal and buccal surfaces.

First molars have a Y-shaped groove pattern that is formed by the mesiobuccal, distobuccal, and lingual grooves. These grooves are actually connected by the central groove, which separates the buccal cusps from the lin-

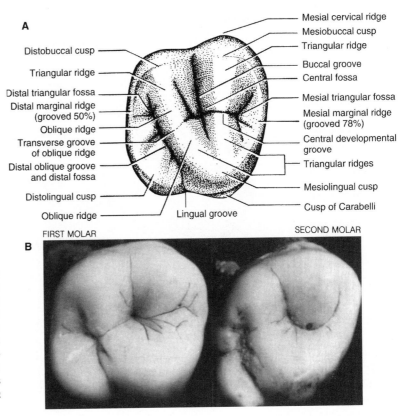

A

Distobuccal cusp
Triangular ridge
Distal triangular fossa
Distal marginal ridge (grooved 50%)
Oblique ridge
Transverse groove of oblique ridge
Distal oblique groove and distal fossa
Distolingual cusp
Oblique ridge

Mesial cervical ridge
Mesiobuccal cusp
Triangular ridge
Buccal groove
Central fossa
Mesial triangular fossa
Mesial marginal ridge (grooved 78%)
Central developmental groove
Triangular ridges
Mesiolingual cusp
Cusp of Carabelli
Lingual groove

FIRST MOLAR   SECOND MOLAR

B

Figure 4-43. *A*, The occlusal surface of a maxillary right first molar with all of the major landmarks named. *B*, *Left*: Maxillary right first molar. *Right*: Maxillary right second molar. Both teeth have all of the morphologic features shown in *A* except for the cusp of Carabelli. Note how the second molar tapers more toward the lingual surface and has a more rounded mesiolingual angle than the first molar. (From Woelfel JB, Scheid RC: Dental Anatomy: Its Relevance to Dentistry. Baltimore, Williams & Wilkins, 1997, p 249.)

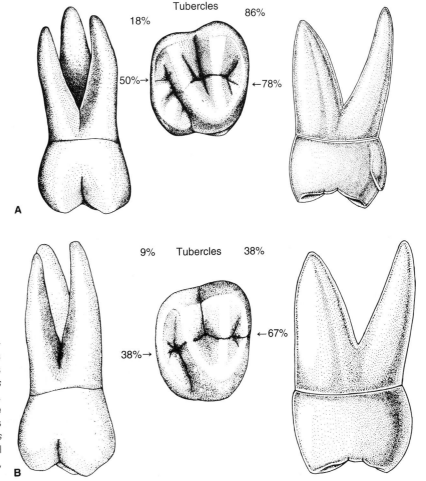

Figure 4-44. *A*, Maxillary right first molar: buccal, occlusal, and mesial views. Percentages give the frequency of marginal ridge tubercles (*above*) and of marginal ridge grooves (*arrows below*). *B*, Maxillary right second molar: buccal, occlusal, and mesial views. Percentages give the frequency of marginal ridge tubercles (*above*) and of marginal ridge grooves (*arrows below*). (From Woelfel JB, Scheid RC: Dental Anatomy: Its Relevance to Dentistry. Baltimore, Williams & Wilkins, 1997, pp 238 and 239.)

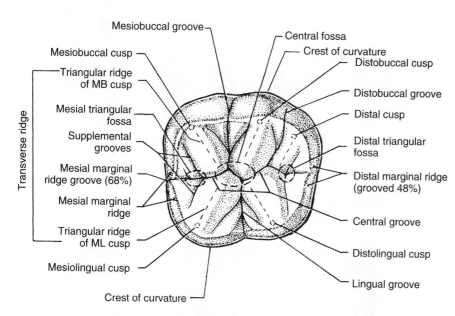

Figure 4-45. Occlusal surface of the mandibular right first molar. After studying these landmarks, cover up the names with a couple of index cards and see how many of the structures at the inner ends of the lines you are able to identify and name. Observe the buccal and lingual crests of curvature. (From Woelfel JB, Scheid RC: Dental Anatomy: Its Relevance to Dentistry. Baltimore, Williams & Wilkins, 1997, p 227.)

gual cusps. The two buccal grooves extend onto the facial surface, and each end in a pit **(Figure 4-46).**

Second molars have four cusps, two buccal and two lingual (the distal cusp is missing), and a +-shaped groove pattern formed by the central, buccal, and lingual grooves. The buccal surface has one groove, which ends in a pit **(Figure 4-47).**

Mandibular molars have a mesial, a distal, and a central pit within the occlusal surface.

As in the maxillary third molars, the mandibular third molars can resemble either first or second molars and may exhibit numerous supplemental grooves, cusps, and tubercles, as well as accessory roots.

When mandibular molars are oriented on a vertical axis, the lingual cusps are longer than the buccal cusps.

Mandibular Molar Root

The roots are the mesial and the distal, with the mesial being the larger root. The mesial root tends to have a distal curvature, whereas the distal root tends to be straighter, especially on mandibular first molars.

First molar roots are larger, longer, and more divergent compared with second molar roots and have a characteristic "plier handle" appearance when viewed from the facial or lingual aspect.

Furcations are located on the buccal and lingual surfaces midway between the proximal surfaces. The first molar has the shortest root trunk of all multirooted teeth and is often the first tooth to manifest furcation involvement when the dentition is periodontally compromised.

Root concavities are found on the mesial surface of the mesial root and on the furcal surface of both mesial and distal roots. The mesial root usually has two canals, whereas the distal root may have one or two canals.

Primary Dentition

The **primary,** or **deciduous dentition** consists of 20 teeth: eight incisors, four canines, and eight molars.

As is utilized with the permanent teeth, three major numbering systems are used to identify the primary teeth (see

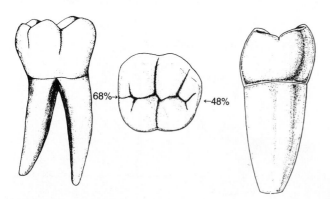

Figure 4-46. Mandibular right first molar: buccal, occlusal, and mesial views. Percentages give the frequency of occurrence of marginal ridge grooves on 215 unrestored first molars examined by Dr. Woelfel. (From Woelfel JB, Scheid RC: Dental Anatomy: Its Relevance to Dentistry. Baltimore, Williams & Wilkins, 1997, p 218.)

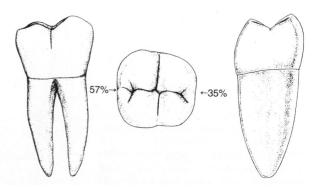

Figure 4-47. Mandibular right second molar: buccal, occlusal, and mesial views. Percentages give the frequency or occurrence or marginal ridge grooves on 233 unrestored teeth examined by Dr. Woelfel. (From Woelfel JB, Scheid RC: Dental Anatomy: Its Relevance to Dentistry. Baltimore, Williams & Wilkins, 1997, p 219.)

Table 4-4). The **Universal Numbering System** utilizes capital letters A through T for the primary teeth, beginning with the maxillary right second molar and ending with the mandibular right second molar.

The **International Numbering System** uses two digits for each tooth as in the permanent dentition. Quadrants are identified by the numbers 5 through 8, designating, in order, the maxillary right and left and the mandibular left and right. The numbers 1 through 5 identify the teeth within that quadrant from the central incisor to the second molar.

The **Palmer Notation System** uses brackets just as in the permanent dentition, but it uses the capital letters A through E to identify the teeth from the midline to the posterior.

Another system is often used by practitioners for record-keeping purposes. This system utilizes the numbers 1 through 20 or the numbers of the corresponding succedaneous teeth to designate the primary teeth in the same manner as the Universal Numbering System. A letter **D** is placed after the number to identify the tooth as part of the deciduous dentition.

The anatomy of the primary teeth is similar to that of the permanent teeth but differs in many ways. Primary teeth are smaller than are their permanent counterparts. The primary molars are larger than the premolars that replace them but are smaller than the permanent molars. Primary teeth are also whiter than permanent teeth.

Primary crowns are shorter than permanent crowns and have pronounced labial and lingual cervical ridges and constricted cervical areas.

The occlusal table is narrower faciolingually, and cuspal anatomy is not as profound.

The enamel depth is more consistent and thinner on the primary teeth.

Relative to the size of the tooth, the pulp chambers of the primary teeth are larger and the pulp chambers extend more occlusally.

Roots are slender and long and approximately twice the length of the crown. Root trunks are shorter, and roots are more divergent in order to accommodate premolar crown development.

Primary teeth have fewer anomalies and variation in tooth form than do permanent teeth. They are less mineralized compared with the analogous permanent teeth, and the attrition rate is rapid. Considerable attrition occurs because of the expanding growth of the jaws and the various positions of occlusion of the teeth before they are shed.

Anatomy of Primary Teeth (Figure 4-48A, B, and C)

Incisors resemble the outline of permanent incisors but have no mamelons on the incisal ridge and no pits on the lingual surface. The mandibular primary central incisors are the only incisors that are wider mesiodistally than they are long incisocervically.

Canines resemble the outlines of permanent canines. The primary maxillary canine cusps have mesial cusp slopes longer than the distal cusp slopes (which differ from the maxillary permanent canines that manifest shorter mesial cusp slopes than the distal cusp slopes).

The primary molars have the same number and position of roots as do the permanent molars. Primary first molars are much smaller than primary second molars (compared with the permanent molars, where the first molars are larger), and they do not resemble any other teeth.

The maxillary primary first molar has an H-shaped groove pattern and usually three cusps with the mesial cusps being largest. The mandibular primary first molar has four or five cusps. The mesial cusps are larger, and the mesiolingual cusp is long, pointed, and angled in on the occlusal surface.

Second primary molars are smaller replicas of the first permanent molars.

Eruption

The process of eruption occurs in two phases. **Phase one** consists of the emergence of the tooth through the gingiva. **Phase two** is the process by which the tooth attains and maintains a relationship with the teeth in the same and the opposing arch. This active process continues throughout the life of the tooth.

Four stages of development relate to the process of eruption **(Table 4-5).**

1. The beginning of hard tissue development
2. Enamel completion, after which the actual tooth movement begins
3. Phase one of eruption
4. Root completion and continuation into phase two (~50% of the root is completed when active eruption begins)

Sequential patterns are reflected throughout the developmental stages, and knowledge of these patterns can be used to predict or approximate the age of one stage, given another.

Generally, mandibular teeth erupt before maxillary teeth. Typically, the first of a particular type of tooth erupts before the second or third of that type. For example, a first premolar is expected to erupt before a second premolar.

The sequential pattern for primary tooth development is central incisor, lateral incisor, first molar, canine, and second molar.

Hard tissue formation begins between 4 and 6 months in utero. Crowns are completed by 1 year of age. Roots are completed between 1.5 and 3 years of age, 6 to 18 months after eruption (see Table 4-5).

By 3 years of age, all of the primary and permanent teeth (except the third molars) are in some stage of development.

Root reabsorption of primary teeth is stimulated by the pressure exerted by the developing permanent teeth and is followed by primary tooth exfoliation in sequential patterns.

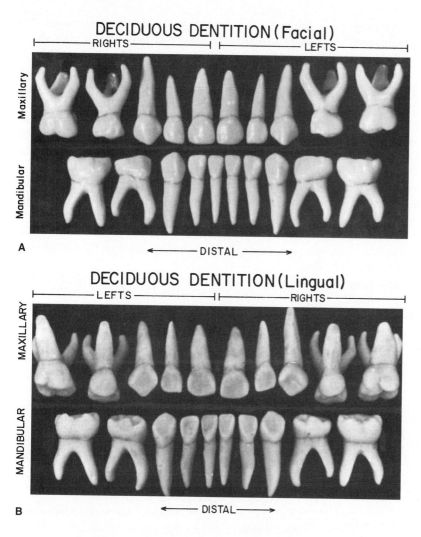

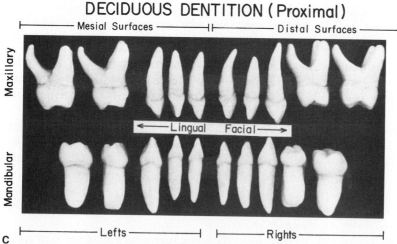

Figure 4-48. *A,* Deciduous dentition (facial view). *B,* Deciduous dentition (lingual view. Notice that the lingual cusps are not as long as the mesiobuccal cusps on the molars. *C,* Deciduous dentition (proximal view). Notice on the molars that more of the occlusal surfaces are visible from the mesial view. Also notice that the roots of anterior teeth bend labially, especially in the maxillary dentition. (From Woelfel JB, Scheid RC: Dental Anatomy: Its Relevance to Dentistry. Baltimore, Williams & Wilkins, 1997, pp 296, 298, and 299.)

The primary dentition ends when the first permanent tooth erupts, marking the beginning of the mixed or transition dentition.

The **transition dentition** (mixed dentition) exists between 6 and 12 years of age with primary tooth exfoliation and permanent tooth eruption. The transition period may actually extend beyond these average times due to various reasons, such as congenitally missing, impacted, or malerupted teeth. This stage of development is called the **"ugly duckling"** stage owing to its characteristic features. These features may include any combination of the following:

TABLE 4–5 Modified from Chronology of the Human Dentition by Logan and Kronfeld (slightly modified by McCall and Schour)

	TOOTH	HARD TISSUE FORMATION BEGINS	CROWN COMPLETED	ERUPTION	ROOT COMPLETED
DECIDUOUS DENTITION — MAXILLARY TEETH	Central incisor	4 mo in utero	4 mo	7½–12 mo	1½ yr
	Lateral incisor	4½ mo in utero	5 mo	9–13 mo	2 yr
	Canine	5 mo in utero	9 mo	16–22 mo	3¼ yr
	First molar	5 mo in utero	6 mo	13–19 mo	2½ yr
	Second molar	6 mo in utero	11 mo	24–33 mo	3 yr
MANDIBULAR TEETH	Central incisor	4½ mo in utero	3½ mo	6–10 mo	1½ yr
	Lateral incisor	4½ mo in utero	4 mo	10–16 mo	1½ yr
	Canine	5 mo in utero	9 mo	17–23 mo	3 yr
	First molar	5 mo in utero	5½ mo	14–18 mo	2¼ yr
	Second molar	6 mo in utero	10 mo	23–31 mo	3 yr
PERMANENT DENTITION — MAXILLARY TEETH	Central incisor	3–4 mo	4–5 yr	7–8 yr	10 yr
	Lateral incisor	10–12 mo	4–5 yr	8–9 yr	11 yr
	Canine	4–5 mo	6–7 yr	11–12 yr	13–15 yr
	First premolar	1½–1¾ yr	5–6 yr	10–11 yr	12–13 yr
	Second premolar	2–2¼ yr	6–7 yr	10–12 yr	12–14 yr
	First molar	birth	2½–3 yr	6–7 yr	9–10 yr
	Second molar	2½–3 yr	7–8 yr	12–15 yr	14–16 yr
	Third molar	7–9 yr	12–16 yr	17–21 yr	18–25 yr
MANDIBULAR TEETH	Central incisor	3–4 mo	4–5 yr	6–7 yr	9 yr
	Lateral incisor	3–4 mo	4–5 yr	7–8 yr	10 yr
	Canine	4–5 mo	6–7 yr	9–10 yr	12–14 yr
	First premolar	1¾–2 yr	5–6 yr	10–12 yr	12–13 yr
	Second premolar	2¼–2½ yr	6–7 yr	11–12 yr	13–14 yr
	First molar	birth	2½–3 yr	6–7 yr	9–10 yr
	Second molar	2½–3 yr	7–8 yr	11–13 yr	14–15 yr
	Third molar	8–10 yr	12–16 yr	17–21 yr	18–25 yr

1. Edentulous areas
2. Disproportionately sized teeth
3. Various clinical crown heights
4. Crowding
5. Enlarged and edematous gingivae
6. Differing shades of tooth coloring

The permanent incisors, canines, and premolars are all called **succedaneous teeth** because they have primary predecessors. The permanent molars are not succedaneous teeth. The primary molars are succeeded by permanent premolars rather than by permanent molars. Furthermore, there are no primary premolars; the premolars exist only in the permanent dentition.

The permanent teeth begin to form between birth and 3 years of age (except for the third molars) (see Table 4-5). The crowns of permanent teeth are completed between 2½ and 8 years of age, at approximately one half the age of eruption. The sequential pattern for the development of permanent teeth is as follows:

MAXILLARY	MANDIBULAR
First molar	First molar
Central incisor	Central incisor
Lateral incisor	Lateral incisor
First premolar	Canine
Second premolar	First premolar
Canine	Second premolar
Second molar	Second molar
Third molar	Third molar

The average age for eruption of the permanent teeth is found in Table 4-5. The roots of the permanent teeth are completed between 9 and 16 years of age, 2 to 3 years after eruption.

Many changes occur in the dentition with age. After the teeth have reached full occlusion, microscopic tooth movements occur to compensate for wear at the contact areas (by mesial drift) and occlusal surfaces (by deposition of cementum at the root apex). (This provides a biologic basis for the cliché, "old and long in the tooth.")

Attrition of incisal ridges and cusp tips may be so severe that the dentin may become exposed and intrinsically stained.

Secondary dentin may be formed in response to dental caries, trauma, and aging and may result in a decrease in size of the pulp cavity and tooth sensitivity.

Occlusal trauma, injury, or even normal use over a long period of time may cause cracks or crazes to appear within the teeth. Some of the cracks may be made more noticeable by staining and may also lead to increased sensitivity of the teeth.

Intra-Arch and Inter-arch Relationships

Each tooth has a relationship with the adjacent teeth in the same and the opposing arch. These relationships are influenced by several factors, including the size and shape of the maxilla, mandible, and teeth and various external factors, such as oral habits and dental disease.

An **intra-arch relationship** indicates the alignment of teeth within an arch and takes into account the position of the teeth in the jaw.

An **inter-arch relationship**, or **jaw relationship**, refers to the position of the mandible relative to the maxillae and should be thought of as a bone-to-bone relationship as well as a tooth-to-tooth relationship.

Vertical Relation or Vertical Dimension

Vertical relation or **vertical dimension** refers to the amount of separation or opening between the mandible and the maxillae. These terms are often used interchangeably.

Vertical relation of occlusion is the amount of separation between the mandible and the maxillae when the teeth are in natural maximum contact (centric occlusion).

Vertical relation of rest position (mandibular physiologic rest position) is the amount of separation of the mandible and the maxillae when the mandible and all of its supporting muscles (eight muscles of mastication plus the suprahyoids and infrahyoids) are in their resting posture. A simple change, such as looking up at the sky, will change the resting position of the jaw, in this case separating the teeth farther due to stretching the skin and underlying fascia on the neck below the mandible **(Figure 4-49)**.

Interocclusal distance or **freeway space** is the normal space of 2 to 6 mm between the incisal and the occlusal surfaces of the maxillary and mandibular teeth with the mandible in physiologic rest position.

Horizontal relations refer to both the anteroposterior and lateral positions of the mandible relative to the maxillae.

The **centric relation** is the most posterior position of the mandible relative to the maxillae at a given vertical dimension. It is really any position with the jaw retruded maximally and rotated open without moving bodily forward **(Figure 4-50)**.

Centric occlusion is the maximum intercuspation or contact attained between the maxillary and mandibular teeth (see Figure 4-50). Several characteristics are noted.

1. **Overjet** is the characteristic of maxillary teeth to overlap the mandibular teeth horizontally.
2. **Overbite** is the characteristic of maxillary teeth to overlap the mandibular teeth vertically.
3. **Intercuspation** is the characteristic of posterior teeth to intermesh in a faciolingual direction. The mandibular facial and the maxillary lingual cusps are centric cusps that make contact interocclusally in the opposing arch.
4. **Interdigitation** is the characteristic of each tooth to articulate with two opposing teeth (except for the mandibular central incisors and the maxillary last molars). A mandibular tooth tends to occlude with its counterpart in the maxillary arch and with the tooth mesial to it. A maxillary tooth tends to occlude with its mandibular counterpart and the tooth distal to it.

Centric relation occlusion (when centric relation and centric occlusion coincide) is the simultaneous even contact between maxillary and mandibular teeth into maximum interdigitation with the mandible in its most retruded position.

Protrusive relation is the position with the mandible moved forward and downward (e.g., when incising food), so that both mandibular condyles and disks are forward in their glenoid, or articular, fossae, functioning against and beneath the articular eminences.

The **lateral relation** is when the mandible is moved to the right or the left side and slightly downward (e.g., when masticating food). The mandible can move almost twice as far sideways as it can forward. The **working side** is the side toward which the mandible moves (i.e., the side where

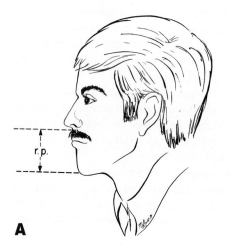
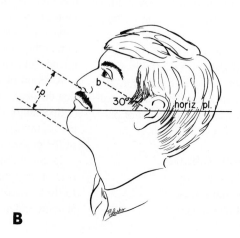

Figure 4-49. *A,* The man assumes a normal posture with his mandible in physiologic rest position and the posterior teeth separated (interocclusal distance). *B,* This man is looking up at an airplane and his mandible is again in physiologic rest position with his posterior teeth separated, more so than in *A,* because of the stretch of fascia, skin, and the suprahyoid and infrahyoid muscles. The resting position of the mandible varies with factors such as body posture, fatigue, and stress. (From Woelfel JB, Scheid RC: Dental Anatomy: Its Relevance to Dentistry. Baltimore, Williams & Wilkins, 1997, p 316.)

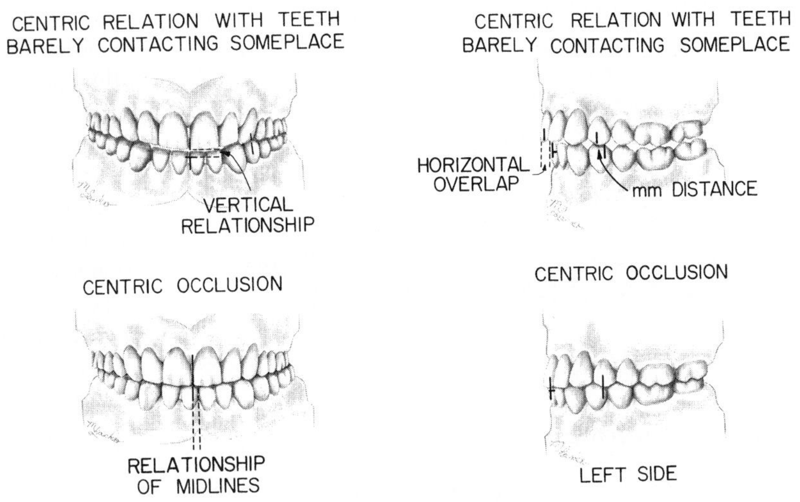

Figure 4-50. *Upper left and upper right:* The mandible has closed in the most retruded position until the first tooth contact between any upper and lower teeth (centric relation, prematurity, or deflective contact). *Lower left and lower right:* The mandible has continued to close from the first tooth contact into maximum intercuspation (centric occlusion) and, as a result, the mandible has deviated forward and to the left. The deviation of the mandible was caused by deflective tooth interferences, which guided the terminal (most upward) portion of jaw closure. Two or more opposing teeth first make contact, and then they all slide into centric occlusion. In the centric occlusion figures, observe the normal anterior and posterior maxillary to mandibular tooth relationships as described in the text. (From Woelfel JB, Scheid RC: Dental Anatomy: Its Relevance to Dentistry. Baltimore, Williams & Wilkins, 1997, p 317.)

chewing or work occurs). The **balancing side** is the side away from which the mandible moves and usually involves no contact with the teeth. Any balancing side contacts are thought to be destructive to the involved teeth and damaging to the craniomandibular (temporomandibular) joint on the opposite side.

Eccentric relations refer to any deviation of the mandible from the centric occlusion position. This includes lateral and protrusive movements and any combination of movements.

In an ideal alignment, teeth contact at their proximal crests of curvature and a continuous arch form is observed from the occlusal view.

Axial positioning is the relationship of the long axes of individual teeth to an imaginary, horizontal or median plane. Ideally, each tooth "sits" at an angle that best withstands the forces placed upon it.

1. Incisors are placed in with their axes at about 60 degrees to the horizontal plane; the more posterior the tooth, the less acute will be the angle.
2. Mandibular posterior teeth tip lingually toward the median plane. The long axes of maxillary posterior teeth are more parallel to the median plane.

Curves of the occlusal plane (a line connecting the cusp tips of the canines, premolars, and molars) are observed from a buccal and a proximal view. The **curve of Spee**, an anteroposterior curve, is convex in mandibular teeth and concave in maxillary teeth. The **curve of Wilson**, a side-to-side curve, is concave for mandibular teeth and convex for maxillary teeth.

Intra-arch contacts do not always exist. Some permanent dentitions have normal spacing. Primary dentitions often have developmental spacing in the anterior area. Some primary dentitions have a pattern of spacing called **primate spaces** (See Figure 10-11).

Disturbances to the intra-arch alignment are often observed. Open contacts or **diastemas** occur because of tooth-jaw size differences, missing teeth, oral habits, dental disease, or overdeveloped frena. **Versions** occur when the position of the tooth or contact with the tooth is at an unexpected area because of developmental disturbances, crowding, oral habits, dental caries, or periodontal disease. Versions are named after their misplaced position: facial, lingual, mesial, distal, supra- (supererupted), infra- (undererupted), and torso (rotated) version.

Classifications of Inter-arch Relationships

Edward H. Angle classified inter-arch relationships using the first permanent molars (See Chapter 10).

Dynamic inter-arch relationships are a result of functional mandibular movements that start and end with centric occlusion during mastication. Five types of mandibular movements are possible.

1. **Elevation** (closing) results from the bilateral contraction of the right and left temporalis, masseter, and medial pterygoid muscles.
2. **Depression** (opening) results from bilateral contraction primarily of both lateral pterygoid muscles but assisted by suprahyoid and infrahyoid muscles.
3. **Retraction** (retruding the jaw) results from the bilateral contractions of the posterior fibers of the temporalis muscles assisted by the suprahyoids.
4. **Protraction** (protrusion of the jaw) results from the simultaneous contractions of the right and left lateral pterygoid muscles.
5. **Lateral excursion** (sideways movement) results from the contraction of one lateral pterygoid muscle on the opposite side.

Mandibular movements from centric occlusion are guided by the maxillary teeth. Protrusion is guided by the incisors and is called **incisal guidance**.

Lateral movements are guided by the canines on the working side in the young, unworn dentitions (**canine pro-**

tected occlusion) and may be guided by incisors and posterior teeth in older worn dentitions.

As mandibular movements commence from centric occlusion, the posterior teeth should disengage in protrusion. The posterior teeth on the balancing side should disengage in lateral movement. If tooth contact occurs where teeth should be disengaged, occlusal interferences or premature contacts exist.

HEAD AND NECK ANATOMY

SARAH K. SMITH, DDS

Skeletal System (Figures 4-51 to 4-53)

Representation of the skeletal system in the head and neck includes the **cranium, mandible**, and **cervical vertebrae**. Each bone consists of a core of spongy, **trabecular,** or **cancellous bone** (loosely packed bony spicules interspersed with marrow or blood-producing tissue) and a hard outer covering of **compact bone**.

The cranium is one of two places in the human body where both types of embryonic bone development occur. The base of the skull develops from a cartilage model (**endochondral development**), and the top plates develop from within a membrane (**membranous development**).

Head and neck bones fit together in **joints,** which are often held together with ligaments. Several types of joints are seen in the head and neck region. **Immobile joints** are found between the plates of the cranium and are called **sutures**. These joints are separated by fibrous tissue; in the developing fetus and infant, the joints are seen as wide membranous gaps called **fontanels**. They allow flexibility during childbirth. These cranial bones come closer with time and may even fuse in old age. **Gliding**, **hinge**, **and rotational joints** are apparent in the joints between the cervical vertebrae, giving the neck a wide range of motion. The **temporomandibular joint (TMJ)** consists of the mandible articulating with the cranium (temporal bone). The TMJ is a unique "dual" joint in the body with two compartments that allow both hinge and gliding motion necessary for mastication (chewing) by the human omnivore.

Terminology associated with bones follows. **Foramina** (**foramen**-singular) are "holes" in bone that allow the passage of nerves, arteries, and veins to the other side of the bone. **Fossae** (*fossa*-singular) are concave areas in bone. **Processes** are convex projections of bone that often serve as attachment sites for muscles, tendons, or ligaments. **Ligaments** are connective tissue straps that hold bones together, whereas **tendons** hold muscle to bone.

Cervical Vertebrae

Seven bones make up the bones of the neck or the **cervical vertebrae**. Each vertebra resembles the other, having a ring shape that consists of a bony articulating body, a dorsal spin-

ous process, and a large central foramen for passage of the spinal cord. Two smaller foramina on the right and left sides allow passage of blood vessels in the neck, thus creating a tunnel when the vertebrae are stacked.

The cervical vertebrae are named **C1, C2, C3, C4, C5, C6,** and **C7** and are stacked upon each other; the body portions articulate with a cartilaginous disk interposed. C1 is also called the **atlas** and is shaped differently; this vertebra lacks a large spinous process and has two large articulating facets on the superior aspect to support the cranium. C2, also called the **axis**, is the only vertebra to have a vertical process that serves as a rotational axis. The atlas supports the cranium, and the axis allows rotational movement of the head. C3 through C7 are similar in appearance. The cervical vertebrae support the head and allow for flexing and rotational movements.

Hyoid Bone

An unusual-shaped bone, the **hyoid bone**, lies in the antero-superior neck alone. This C-shaped bone has four processes or spines on its ends. The hyoid serves as an attachment site for the thin, strap-like muscles of the anterior neck called the hyoid muscles, which make their actions possible. The muscles located above the hyoid bone are called the suprahyoid muscles, and those below it are called the infrahyoid muscles.

Cranial Bones

The skull or head bones consist of the **cranium** and **mandible** or jaw. The cranium consists of 12 bones, some of which are paired whereas others are not. These bones are joined by sutures, which make the cranium resemble one large bone. The particular anatomy of each of the cranial bones is discussed. Different views of the cranium (the head and neck) are used: **frontal view** (from the front), **sagittal** (from the side), **inferior** (underneath), and **interior** (inside). Attention is paid to their foramina and what passes through them and also their processes with attaching structures **(Table 4-6)**.

Frontal Bone

The **frontal bone** is a single bone that makes up the forehead area of the cranium. The inferior edge comprises the brow and extends into the **orbits** (eye sockets). Trace its outline on the figures and also note its extent from the interior view. From the interior view, the frontal bone forms a large concave area, which holds the anterior cerebrum. This area is the **anterior cranial fossa** (the last portion of the fossa is another bone-the sphenoid). A portion of the ethmoid bone is located in the middle of the interior frontal bone.

From the frontal aspect, two **supraorbital foraminae** are located above the orbits; these foraminae allow passage of the supraorbital nerves, arteries, and veins.

With most anatomic names, a foramen will have the same name as the vessels and nerves that pass through it. A nerve, artery, and vein usually accompany each other for distribution (see Table 4-6).

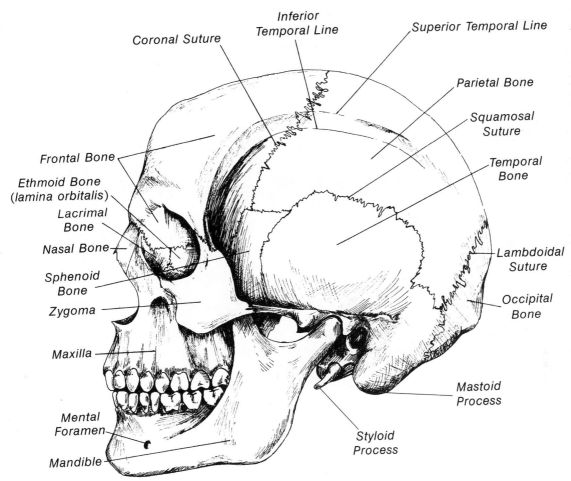

Figure 4-51. A lateral view of the skull. (From Fried LA: *Anatomy of the Head, Neck, Face, and Jaws,* 2nd ed. Philadelphia, Lea & Febiger, 1980.)

Parietal Bones

Two large **parietal bones** make up the top and sides of the cranium. Note their extent from the sagittal and interior view shown. No important foramina exist; however, from the interior, a large concave groove passes between the two bones, along the suture line. This groove is for the superior sagittal sinus, which is the largest vein in the brain and lies between its two hemispheres.

Occipital Bone

The **occipital** bone is a large, thick bone that forms the back of the cranium. The interior view shows that a large foramen, called a **foramen magnum**, is located in the occipital bone. This large opening accommodates the passage of the spinal cord out of the cranium. Above the foramen, this nervous tissue is called the brainstem. A **hypoglossal foramen** lies on either side of the foramen magnum. Each of these allows passage of the hypoglossal nerve as it travels to the tongue. The occipital's interior forms the last concavity, the **posterior cranial fossa,** which holds the cerebellum.

Temporal Bones

The "temples" of the head are formed by the two **temporal bones**. Each bone has a distinctive shape with important processes. From the sagittal view, note the long, thin horizontal process that forms the back of the "cheekbone." The **zygomatic process**, or cheekbone, is actually formed from three bones: the temporal bone, the zygoma bone, and the maxillary bone. Posterior to this lies the opening for the ear called the **external auditory meatus**. The temporal bone houses the entire ear and can be seen by looking at an interior view for a tent-shaped bony area. The middle and inner ear cavities lie below this area. This location is the **middle cranial fossa**, the second concave area of the interior cranium. The middle portion of the cerebrum lies here. An **internal meatus** can also be seen in the temporal bone. A large, ragged foramen can be seen at the border of the temporal and occipital bones. This is the **jugular foramen** for the interior jugular vein, and an S-shaped groove can be seen trailing off from it for the sigmoid sinus.

From the sagittal view, find the **mastoid process,** which is the round process posterior to the external meatus. It

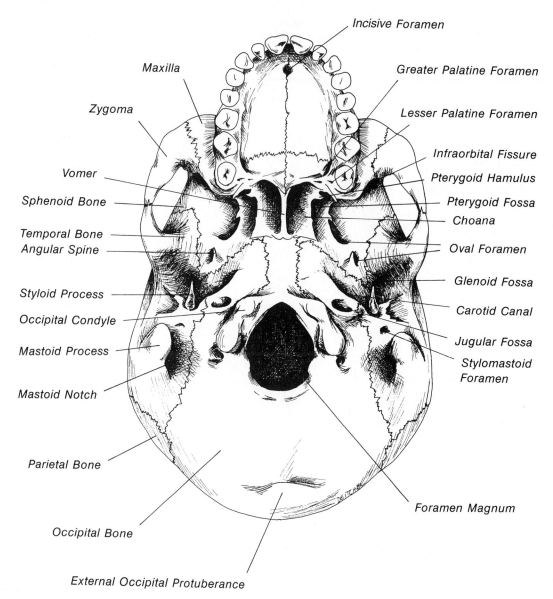

Figure 4-52. Base of the skull. (From Fried LA: *Anatomy of the Head, Neck, Face, and Jaws,* 2nd ed. Philadelphia, Lea & Febiger, 1980.)

serves as a muscle attachment site for the **sternocleidomastoid muscle (SCM)** and also for the digastric muscle. Lateral to the mastoid and slightly anterior is the pencil-shaped **styloid process**, which is necessary for the attachment of two muscles (i.e., the styloglossus and the stylohyoid) and one ligament (i.e., the stylohyoid). These aid in attaching the mandible, tongue, and hyoid bone.

Only from an inferior view can one appreciate the **mandibular fossa** of the temporal bone where the mandible "fits," although its true articulation lies on the **articular eminence** (i.e., a ridge anterior to the fossa).

Sphenoid Bone

The **sphenoid** is a butterfly-shaped bone that can be seen best from an interior view. On the sagittal view, however, the sphenoid lies next to the temporal bone. On either side

of the cranium, these two bones along with parts of the parietal and temporal bones form a shallow concave area called the **temporal fossa**. This area is continuous with and gives rise to the more inferior **infratemporal fossa**, beneath the zygomatic process. Deeper still lies the **pterygopalatine fossa**, which is the entire concavity's endpoint, butting up against the maxillary bone. Several important structures occupy this concavity, including the temporalis muscle, the maxillary artery, the pterygoid plexus and ganglion, and the maxillary division of the trigeminal nerve.

The interior view of the sphenoid shows several paired foramina. Beginning with the most anterior on one side is the **superior orbital fissure**, a large crack formed between the frontal and the sphenoid, which passes into the orbit (see the frontal view). This fissure may continue as the **inferior orbital fissure** of the orbit. Important nerves pass through

TABLE 4–6 Foramina and Their Structures

FORAMEN	PASSAGE
Optic foramen	Optic nerve (CN I)
Supraorbital foramen	Supraorbital nerve (VI), artery, vein
Superior orbital fissure	V1, CN III, IV, VI
Foramen rotundum	Maxillary division (V2)
Foramen ovale	Mandibular division (V3)
Infraorbital foramen	Infraorbital nerve (V2), artery, vein
Mental foramen	Mental nerve (V3), artery, vein
Incisive foramen	Nasopalatine nerve (V2), artery, vein
Greater palatine foramen	Greater palatine nerve (V2), artery, vein
Carotid canal	Internal carotid artery
Jugular foramen	Internal jugular vein, CN IX, X, XI
Foramen magnum	Spinal cord
Hypoglossal foramen	Hypoglossal nerve (CN XII)
Mandibular foramen	Inferior alveolar nerve (V3), artery, vein
Pituitary fossa and area	Pituitary gland, internal carotid arteries, CN V and trigeminal ganglia, CN III, IV, VI, cavernous sinus, optic chiasm (CN II)
Pterygopalatine fossae	Maxillary artery, pterygoid plexus, pterygopalatine ganglion, V2 (PSA nerve)
Sternocleidomastoid border	Internal jugular vein, carotid arteries, CN X, CN XI, cervical lymph nodes

CN, cranial nerve; PSA, posterior superior alveolar nerve.

here to the eye, including cranial nerves III, IV, and VI and the division V1 (ophthalmic). Medial to it lies a rounder foramen, the **optic foramen**, lying on the edge of the anterior fossa. Its openings also pass to the orbit. The optic foramen contains the optic nerve (cranial nerve I), which leads to the eyeball. These nerves cross and connect in the middle of sphenoid in the optic chiasm. Posterior to these two foramina, lies each **foramen rotundum**, which are smaller round openings. The maxillary division of the trigeminal (V2) nerve passes through here on its way to the maxilla. Posterior and lateral to them lie the oval-shaped **foramina ovale**. These foramina contain the mandibular division (V3) of the trigeminal nerve, as they pass to the mandible. Just lateral to the foramina ovale are two very small holes called the **foramina spinosum**, which carry meningeal vessels and have a small spine of bone next to them.

In the center of the sphenoid are two large irregular foramina or "canals." These **carotid canals** carry the internal carotid arteries into the brain in a twisting, curved pathway. Many structures intersect in the middle of sphenoid in the unusual-shaped area known as the **pituitary fossa**. This concave area contains the pituitary gland (hypophysis). Around it are bony processes that form the **sella turcica** or "Turkish saddle." Passing around the area of the pituitary fossa are the carotid arteries and the circle of Willis; the optic chiasm; the cavernous sinus; cranial nerves III, IV, and VI; and the trigeminal nerve.

Finally, from the inferior view, locate the sphenoid bone. On the bottom of the "butterfly," some double wing-shaped processes called the **pterygoid plates** can be seen. These processes serve as attachment sites for the pterygoid muscles and the muscles of the pharynx.

Vomer Bone, Palatine Bone, and Ethmoid Bone

Another cranial bone, the **vomer**, is seen from the inferior view of the cranium. This small plough-shaped bone forms the posterior portion of the nasal septum. The anterior portion belongs to the ethmoid bone, which can be visualized better from other views of the nasal septum.

The top of the **ethmoid** can be seen nestled in the frontal bone in an interior cranial view. The ethmoid appears as a walnut-shaped bone. The horizontal portion is perforated with many small foramina and is called the **cribriform plate** of the ethmoid. The vertical portion is called the **crista galli**. The ethmoid then extends this vertical plate below the surface to become the top of the nasal septum. Other smaller vertical portions of the ethmoid form parts of the **paranasal sinuses**.

The **nasal septum** can be seen from an interior sagittal view of the nose. It consists of bone and cartilage and subdivides the nasal cavity into a right and left nasal fossa. The septum is formed mainly by the vomer and ethmoid, with some contributions from the palatine and maxillary bones.

The sides of the nasal cavity can be seen to have three structures suspended from its walls. These structures are called the superior, middle, and inferior **nasal turbinates (conchae).** Some anatomists consider the inferior turbinate to be a separate bone, whereas others believe that all three turbinates derive from the maxilla. These processes can be found from the frontal view and from the view of the nose without the septum. Passageways from the paranasal sinuses called **meatii** empty out into the nasal cavity under the turbinates. The **paranasal sinuses** are hollowed out areas in the maxillary, sphenoid, ethmoid, and frontal bones that surround the nasal cavity. These sinuses are lined with mucous membranes and drain into the nose. They lighten the cranium with their spaces.

From the inferior view, find the palatine bones, which are a pair of very small bones that form the back of the hard palate. They each have a small hook-like process called a **hamulus** (the plural *is* **hamuli**). The palatine bones also have large and small foramina. The larger foramen is called the **greater palatine foramen**; a nerve, artery, and vein of that name pass through the foramen.

Maxillary Bones

Although they appear to be one bone, the **maxillary bone** actually consists of two bones. The suture between them can be seen in a frontal view at the bottom of the nasal orifice, forming a projection called the **nasal spine**, directly below the septum. The maxilla forms the middle third of the face and contains the maxillary teeth. The bones are particularly convex over the roots of the canine teeth and form the **ca-**

nine **eminences**. Directly below the orbits are two foramina, the **infraorbital foramina**, which pass nerves, arteries, and veins of the same name. The maxilla begins the cheekbone and also forms most of the **hard palate**. The maxilla can be seen on an interior view. Another line called the **midpalatine suture** reveals the joint between the two maxilla, while a horizontal suture joins it to the palatine bones. The hard palate, therefore, consists of four separate bones. On the anterior aspect of the palate is a foramen called the **incisive foramen**, which lies directly behind teeth numbers 8 and 9. The nasopalatine nerve, artery, and vein pass through this foramen en route to the anterior palate (note that these do not have the same names).

Nasal Bones and Lacrimal Bones

A small pair of bones form the bridge of the nose called the **nasal bones**, which can be seen in a frontal view. From the sagittal, another pair, the **lacrimal bones** can be seen within the orbit near its medial rim. The lacrimal or tear duct sits on this bone and drains through foramina into the nasal cavity. The lacrimal bones are the two smallest cranial bones.

The **ossicles** are three pairs of smaller bones within the ear; however, they are studied along with the ear.

Mandible and the Temporomandibular Joint (TMJ)

The **mandible** or lower jaw is a single bone that developed from two processes. The horizontal portion is called the **body**, which contains the mandibular teeth, and the two vertical components are called the **rami (ramus** is the singular). The **angle of the mandible** lies at the junction of the ramus and the body of the mandible. The ramus has two processes: the condyle process and the coronoid process. The **condyle** is an egg-shaped process, which is the articulating portion of the jaw. The **coronoid process** is a flat, pointed process, which exists for the attachment of the temporalis muscle. The **sigmoid notch** lies between the two processes. The ramus ends in two ridges as it joins the body. These ridges are the **superior and inferior oblique lines**, and they show the attachment sites of the buccinator muscle.

On the outer aspect of the mandible, a foramen exists directly below the first and second premolars called the **mental foramen**. A nerve, artery, and vein of the same name exit here. Fossae, called the **mental fossae**, are also present in the region of the chin, on the right and left sides. The mentalis muscles are located within them.

On the inner aspect of the mandible, the **mandibular foramen** is located on the ramus below its processes. This foramen becomes the **mandibular canal** as it travels inside the body of the mandible. It contains the inferior alveolar nerve, artery, and vein (which do not have the same names). The **submandibular fossa**, which contains the submandibular salivary gland, lies below the mandibular foramen. Anterior to this is a horizontal ridge on the inside of the body

called the mylohyoid line, which is the attachment site for the mylohyoid muscle.

Two "bumps" or **genial tubercles** are located on the inner aspect of the "chin." These processes provide attachment for the geniohyoid and genioglossus muscles. Inferior and lateral to these processes lie the **digastric fossae**, which are two concave areas where the digastric muscle bellies attach.

The **TMJ**, as mentioned earlier, is a unique joint that consists of the condyle of the mandible, the mandibular fossa, the articular eminence, the temporomandibular (TM) capsule and ligaments, the TM disk, and two accessory ligaments. The lateral pterygoid muscle inserts into the joint and condyle. Histologically, it is different, because its bony coverings on the condyle and eminence are fibrous instead of cartilaginous. Furthermore, a fibrous disk is interposed between the articulating surfaces. This disk divides the joint into two compartments, allowing a gliding motion in the superior joint compartment and a hinge action in the lower joint compartment. Thus, the TMJ can act like a "dual joint." Synovial fluid fills both compartments for lubrication.

Look at the outer aspect of the TMJ. The **TM ligament** surrounds the joint and is divided into an outer vertical fibrous layer and two horizontal **lateral ligaments**. Both help to suspend the mandible in the fossa while holding it up to the articulating eminence. The **TM capsule** is continuous with the ligament and contains the synovial membrane that creates its fluid. The **TM disk**, which is oval and biconcave, splits the joint into two compartments (i.e., the **superior and inferior joint cavities**) and provides a cushion between the condyle and its eminence. The disk is held in position by the lateral pterygoid muscle during jaw excursions (movements). If the disk is displaced, popping or crepitus sounds signal a dysfunction. Two other **accessory ligaments** (the **sphenomandibular** and **stylomandibular**) help to suspend the mandible in place.

The mandible is capable of basic movements or **excursions** owing to its joints and musculature. The shape of the teeth also helps to guide jaw movements. **Opening** and **closing** are simple hinge motions using the lower joint compartment along with the elevator and depressor muscles. **Lateral movements** are gliding movements that utilize the superior compartment and one side lateral pterygoid muscles. **Protrusion** is a gliding motion that uses both lateral pterygoids, whereas its opposite **retrusion** uses elevator muscles.

Muscular System (Figures 4-54 to 4-56)

The named muscles of the head and neck that are reviewed are mainly **skeletal-type muscles**, which consist of striated multinucleated fibers bundled together as a voluntary unit. A muscle does its work by **contraction**: It grows shorter upon receiving a neuronal signal by sliding filaments, and it moves a bone or skin. Muscles usually have two attachments: one attachment is to a stationary structure called its origin, and the other attachment is to a moving structure called its **insertion**. The work that a muscle does is its **action**. The nerve that causes its contraction is its **innervation**. All major muscles have an origin, insertion, action, and innervation.

The muscles of the head and neck are grouped by their similar actions and innervations. Each major group and its members are described and identified. To better understand

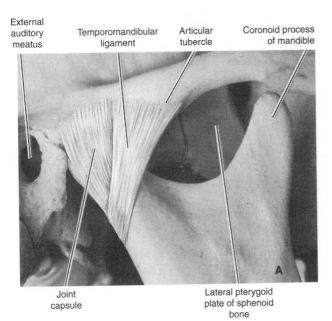

External auditory meatus | Temporomandibular ligament | Articular tubercle | Coronoid process of mandible

Joint capsule | Lateral pterygoid plate of sphenoid bone

Joint capsule | Superior synovial compartment | Articular disk | Temporomandibular ligament

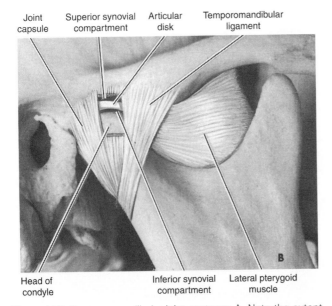

Head of condyle | Inferior synovial compartment | Lateral pterygoid muscle

Figure 4-53. Temporomandibular joint anatomy. A. Note the extent of the capsule model and the differentiated lateral ligament (temporomandibular ligament). B. Observe that the capsule model has been cut away to reveal the disk and its relationship to the articulating surfaces of the joint. (From Hiatt JL, Gartner LP: *Textbook of Head and Neck Anatomy*, 3rd ed. Philadelphia, Lippincott, Williams & Wilkins, 2001.)

their actions, one should imagine what would occur in the picture if the muscle were shorter (contracted). Origins and insertions can be seen on the drawings by locating the structures that each end attaches to.

Muscles of Facial Expression

The **muscles of facial expression** are superficial; that is, they are located directly beneath the skin. These muscles insert into the skin of the face and make possible a wide variety of communicative facial expressions. This group of muscles is innervated by cranial nerve VII, the facial nerve, which emerges from the cranium behind the ear. This nerve passes over and through the parotid gland to spread across the face below the skin, branching to each facial expression muscle. The facial nerve is, therefore, very susceptible to injury. Damage to the facial nerve leads to a condition called **Bell palsy** (i.e., hemifacial paralysis).

The muscles of facial expression follow. (Innervation is from cranial nerve VII; origins are on the areas of the face pictured on bone; insertions are into overlying skin; and actions are included with the muscle.)

Platysma: grimace
Frontalis (pair): wrinkle the brow
Orbicularis oculi (pair): close the eye
Orbicularis oris: pucker the mouth
Nasalis (pair): flare the nostrils
Levators (group): raise the mouth
Depressors (group): lower the mouth
Mentalis: pout
Buccinator: position a food bolus

One oral muscle occurs in this group-the **buccinator** muscle, whose horizontal fibers line the cheek. This muscle originates on the oblique lines and raphe and inserts into the orbicularis oris. The buccinator muscle acts to center food on the tongue during mastication (chewing) and deglutition (swallowing), and this muscle is pierced by the duct of the parotid gland (**Stensen duct**) as it enters the oral cavity.

Muscles of Mastication

The **muscles of mastication** function during chewing (mastication), although they also contract during all jaw movements, including swallowing and speech. The four pairs of masticatory muscles are all innervated by cranial nerve V3 (i.e., the trigeminal, mandibular division, motor branch). All four pairs insert onto the mandible and originate in the cranium. Three of these pairs of muscle elevate the mandible, which means that when they contract they raise or close the jaw. Review their origins (o), insertions (i), innervations (inv), and actions (a).

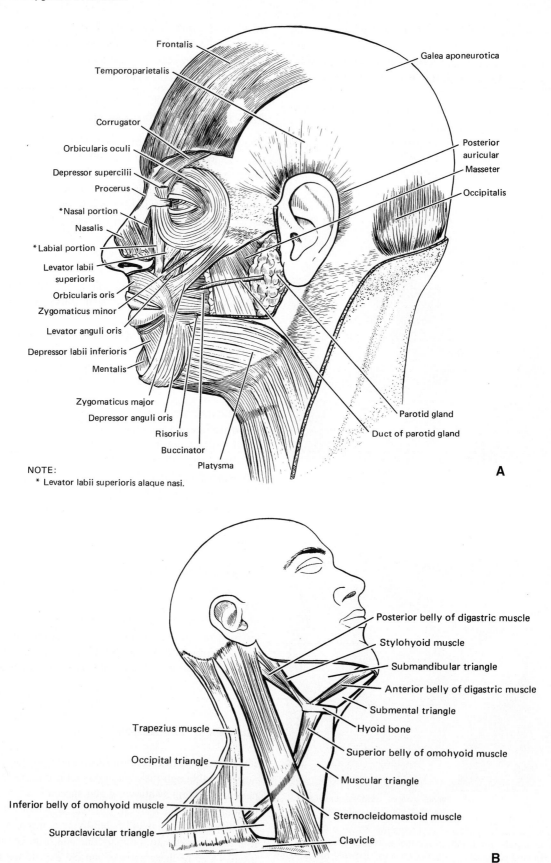

Figure 4-54. *A.* Muscles of facial expression. *B.* Triangles of the neck. (From Hiatt JL, Gartner LP: *Textbook of Head and Neck Anatomy,* 3rd ed. Philadelphia, Lippincott, Williams & Wilkins, 2001.)

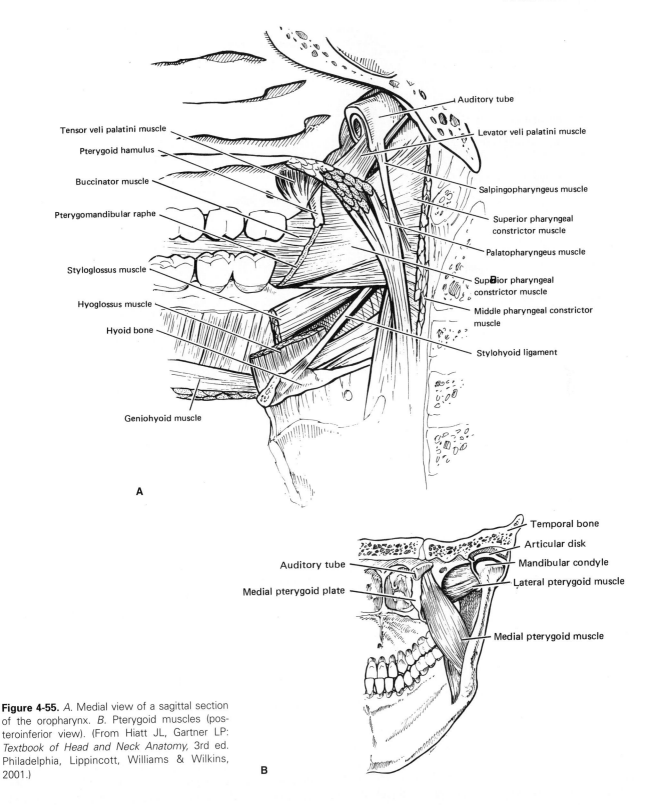

Tensor veli palatini muscle

Pterygoid hamulus

Buccinator muscle

Pterygomandibular raphe

Styloglossus muscle

Hyoglossus muscle

Hyoid bone

Geniohyoid muscle

Auditory tube

Levator veli palatini muscle

Salpingopharyngeus muscle

Superior pharyngeal constrictor muscle

Palatopharyngeus muscle

Superior pharyngeal constrictor muscle

Middle pharyngeal constrictor muscle

Stylohyoid ligament

A

Auditory tube

Medial pterygoid plate

Temporal bone

Articular disk

Mandibular condyle

Lateral pterygoid muscle

Medial pterygoid muscle

B

Figure 4-55. *A.* Medial view of a sagittal section of the oropharynx. *B.* Pterygoid muscles (posteroinferior view). (From Hiatt JL, Gartner LP: *Textbook of Head and Neck Anatomy,* 3rd ed. Philadelphia, Lippincott, Williams & Wilkins, 2001.)

Temporalis
  o- temporal fossa | i- coronoid process | a- elevates the mandible | inv- CN V3

Masseter
  o- zygomatic arch | i- angle of the mandible | a- elevates the mandible | inv- CN V3

Medial pterygoid
  o- pterygoid plate | i- angle of the mandible | a- elevates the mandible | inv- CN V3

Lateral pterygoid
  o- pterygoid plate | i- condyle, TM disk/ capsule | a- (one) lateral move | inv- CN V3 (both) protrusion

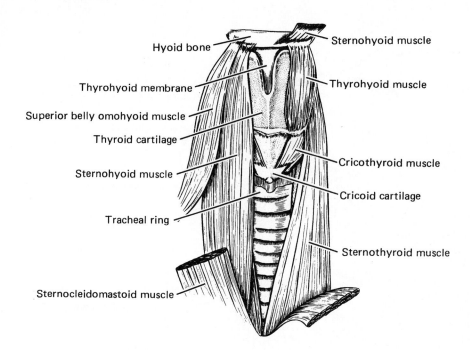

Hyoid bone

Sternohyoid muscle

Thyrohyoid membrane

Thyrohyoid muscle

Superior belly omohyoid muscle

Thyroid cartilage

Sternohyoid muscle

Cricothyroid muscle

Cricoid cartilage

Tracheal ring

Sternothyroid muscle

Sternocleidomastoid muscle

Figure 4-56. *A.* Infrahyoid muscles. The thyroid gland has been removed. (From Hiatt JL, Gartner LP: *Textbook of Head and Neck Anatomy,* 3rd ed. Philadelphia, Lippincott, Williams & Wilkins, 2001.)

Which three of the muscles of mastication are elevators? The lateral pterygoids constitute the only pair that has horizontally directed fibers, thus its main actions are different. If one lateral pterygoid contracts, the pair pulls the mandible to one side (lateral movement). If both pterygoids contract, protrusion of the mandible occurs.

Posterior Neck

The muscles of the **posterior neck** are thick muscles-the muscles that support the head on the neck and move it. Most of these muscles insert into the occipital bone. The largest of this group is the **trapezius**, a huge quadrilateral muscle, which connects the shoulders and head. The trapezius also runs down the length of the back and inserts into the spine. The trapezius is innervated by cranial nerve XI (spinal accessory nerve). Three more layers of muscle lie under the trapezius, but they are not described here. They are similar in shape and function but are innervated by cervical nerves. They create a thick support of musculature for the posterior neck.

Another pair of strong muscles, the **sternocleidomastoid SCM** muscles, lie on the right and left sides, running posterior to the anterior. Find them and note that as the name indicates, they have three attachments: The SCM originates on the mastoid process and runs obliquely down to attach on both the sternum and the clavicle. This muscle can flex the head when both contract and turn the head when each contract. The SCM is also innervated by cranial nerve XI and is often used in anatomy as a **"landmark"** to locate other structures that lie beside it. It can also be seen to divide the neck region into a **posterior triangle** and an **anterior triangle**.

Anterior Neck

All hyoid muscles are thin, paired, strap-like muscles that are small compared with those of the posterior neck. Most of these muscles are innervated by the cervical nerves. They are important in the functions of mastication and deglutition. Most hyoid muscles are named after their origins and insertions.

Suprahyoid Muscles

The anterior neck muscles located above the hyoid bone are called the **suprahyoid muscles**. These muscles are found in four pairs and are located in the diagrams on the sagittal and frontal neck. The main function of the suprahyoids is to depress the mandible (the opposite of the elevators). They also help to create a strong base for the tongue during swallowing.

Digastric	o- mastoid process	i- digastric fossa
Stylohyoid	o- styloid process	i- hyoid
Mylohyoid	o- hyoid bone	i- mylohyoid line mandible
Geniohyoid	o- hyoid bone	i- genial tubercles

Note that the digastric is a "two-belly" muscle that acts as a pulley. The middle portion slips through a "strap" of tissue on the hyoid bone before passing up to the mandible. This muscle is the main depressor of the mandible. The mylohyoid forms the "floor of the mouth" and thus supports the tongue. It is innervated by cranial nerve V3, as is the anterior belly of the digastric.

Infrahyoid Muscles

The muscles that lie below the hyoid bone are the **infrahyoids**. They act together with the suprahyoids to stabilize the hyoid bone as a base for other actions, such as deglutition and mastication. The infrahyoid muscles, which consist of four pairs, are innervated by the cervical nerves.

Sternohyoid	o- sternum	i- hyoid
Sternothyroid	o- sternum	i- thyroid cartilage
Thyrohyoid	o- thyroid cartilage	i- hyoid bone
Omohyoid	o- clavicle	i- hyoid bone

The omohyoid is also a two-belly muscle like the digastric. The middle of the muscle goes through a tendinous slip, giving the action of a pulley. The thyroid gland lies on top of the infrahyoids and thyroid cartilage of the larynx, giving it its name.

Tongue

The structure that fills the oral cavity is actually a membrane-bound "sac" of muscles-the **tongue**. The body and root of the tongue is filled with small groups of muscle fibers that run in three directions: vertical, horizontal, and transverse. These muscle fibers are collectively called the **intrinsic muscles of the tongue**. They are capable of the many fine movements of the tongue that are necessary for the initiation of swallowing and speech. Intrinsic muscles are innervated by the hypoglossal nerve.

The gross motor movements of the tongue are done by the **extrinsic muscles** of the tongue and consist of any muscle name containing the word "glossus," which means tongue. All glossal muscles insert into the base of the tongue; they are paired; and all are innervated by cranial nerve XII, the hypoglossal nerve. Find them in the sagittal section.

Hyoglossus	o- hyoid	i- tongue
Styloglossus	o- styloid process	i- tongue
Genioglossus	o- genial tubercles	i- tongue

Palate/Pharynx

The **pharynx** is the beginning of the digestive "tube." It begins where the oral cavity ends and is a mucosa-lined muscular tube that is designed to produce a squeezing action. Food that is passed down the pharynx to the esophagus and then to the stomach assumes the form of a soft, moistened ball called a **bolus**. The passage of a bolus from the oral cavity into the pharynx is called **deglutition** (swallowing), which begins as a voluntary action and ends as a reflex or involuntary action of the musculature.

The **constrictor muscles** of the pharynx wrap around the mucosal tube in three groups to provide a squeezing action. Locate the **superior, middle, and inferior constrictors** on the drawings. The superior constrictor originates at the base of the skull and inserts on both sides into the mandible and raphe. The **pterygomandibular raphe** is the tendinous junction where the superior constrictor and buccinator muscles meet. It can be seen as a mucosal landmark in the opened mouth, forming a vertical cord of tissue.

All constrictor muscles are innervated by cranial nerve X (i.e., the vagus nerve). This nerve is the main parasympathetic nerve to the digestive system. The constrictors are unique in that they consist of a blend of skeletal and smooth muscle fibers and show the transition from voluntary to involuntary function. The superior constrictor has the greatest proportion of skeletal fibers, whereas the distal end of the inferior constrictor contains the smoothest fibers. By the level of the esophagus, the muscular layers are completely smooth muscle.

The palate (**soft palate**) contains the insertions of four different muscle pairs that allow it to function. The soft palate is raised and stretched up against the posterior wall of the pharynx during each swallow, in order to seal off the nasopharynx from the passage of food. The palate also functions during speech in more subtle actions. Find the palatal muscles in the drawings. Innervation is mixed.

Tensor veli palatini (TVP)
o- base of skull	i- soft palate	inv- CN V

Levator veli palatine (LVP)
o- base of skull	i- soft palate	inv- CN VII

Palatoglossus
o- tongue	i- soft palate	inv- CN XII

Palatopharyngeus
o- pharyngeal wall	i- soft palate	inv- CN X

The TVP is an interesting muscle. This two-belly muscle has a tendinous center that wraps around the **hamular process** before inserting into the palate. Its acts on the palate like a pulley, causing the soft palate to stretch or tense. A separate portion of the superior belly inserts into the **tympanic** or **eustachian tube**, causing it to open or dilate each time a swallow occurs. The tympanic tube provides the middle ear with a way of equalizing its internal pressure.

Other Muscles

Other small muscles present in the head and neck are not illustrated. Two small muscles in the ear called the **stapedius** (cranial nerve VII) and the **tensor tympani** (cranial nerve V) function on the ossicles. Several **laryngeal muscles** regulate speech and also lift the larynx up against the epiglottis during a swallow.

Nervous System (Figures 4-57 to 4-68)

Systems and Pathways

Representation of the nervous system is great in the head and neck, including the **brain, cervical spinal cord**, and **cranial and cervical nerve pairs**. A short review of the system and its terminology follows.

Neurons are the building blocks of the nervous system. In general, neurons consist of receiving processes called **dendrites**, a **cell body**, and a sending process called an *axon*. The information or signal travels in one direction down the neuron from the dendrite to the axon and then connects to another neuron by chemically jumping the gap or **synapse**. Combinations of neurons create **pathways**, which may be as simple as two neurons. **Sensory neurons (affectors)** are used to sense the environment, and **motor neurons (effec-**

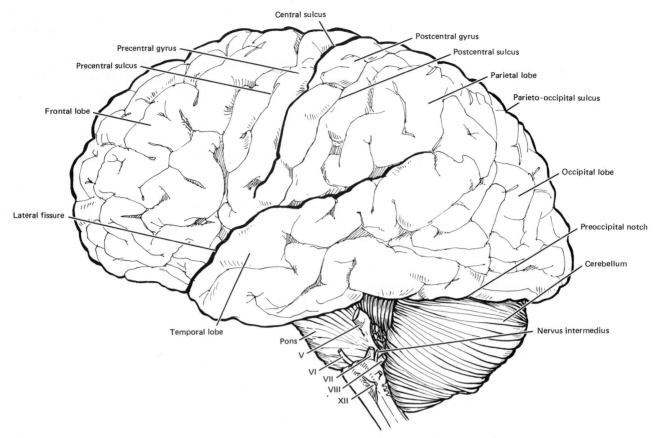

Figure 4-57. Lateral view of the whole brain. (From Hiatt JL, Gartner LP: *Textbook of Head and Neck Anatomy,* 3rd ed. Philadelphia, Lippincott, Williams & Wilkins, 2001.)

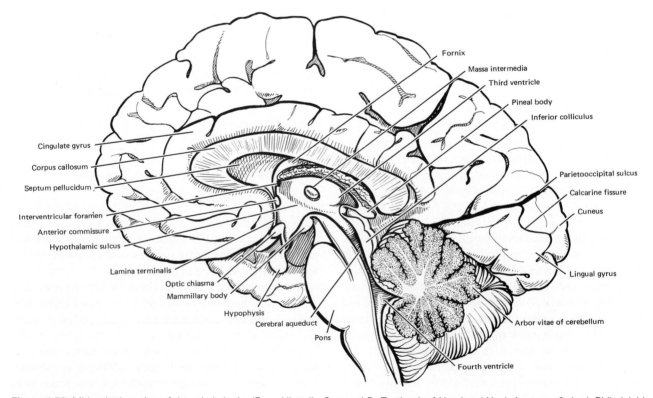

Figure 4-58. Midsagittal section of the whole brain. (From Hiatt JL, Gartner LP: *Textbook of Head and Neck Anatomy,* 3rd ed. Philadelphia, Lippincott, Williams & Wilkins, 2001.)

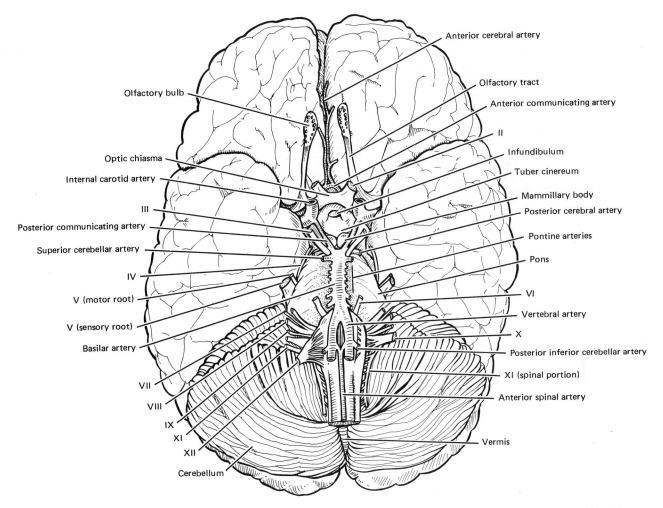

Figure 4-59. Ventral view of the whole brain and its major arterial supply. (From Hiatt JL, Gartner LP: *Textbook of Head and Neck Anatomy*, 3rd ed. Philadelphia, Lippincott, Williams & Wilkins, 2001.)

tors) cause either a muscle to contract or a gland to secrete. Sensory neurons bring information into the central nervous system (CNS), and motor neurons take the action out to the body. Several neuron processes that combine together travel in bundles called **nerves**. Their cell bodies either lie in lumps attached to the nerves (called **ganglia**) or in clumps (called **nuclei**) within the CNS.

The nervous system is divided anatomically into the **CNS** and the **peripheral nervous system (PNS).** The CNS consists of the brain and spinal cord, and the PNS includes all other nerves outside of the CNS. Functionally, the nervous system is divided into the **somatic nervous system** (voluntary) and the **autonomic nervous system** (involuntary). The autonomic system is subdivided into the sympathetic and parasympathetic systems. **Sympathetic** pathways are concerned with "fright or flight" responses of the organism to its environment, whereas **parasympathetic** pathways deal with daily maintenance functions, such as heartbeat, respiration, and digestion.

The brain is divided into functional and anatomic areas. The **cerebrum** is the largest area and is considered to be the seat of all conscious activity. Below the cerebrum lies the **cerebellum**, a center for motor coordination. Below that lies the **brainstem,** which is a collection of nuclei and pathways associated with regulation of vital body functions such as heartbeat and respiration. The spinal nerves are paired nerves that leave and enter the spinal cord. The **cervical nerves** are the seven pairs of spinal nerves found in the neck and are labeled C1 through C7 as the vertebrae. The **cranial nerves** are paired nerves that come off of the brainstem and cerebrum.

Neuronal pathways to and from the body connect at the spinal cord (or brainstem). **Sensory pathways** involve reception of sensation by receptor neurons (which may be highly specialized) and the passing of this information towards the CNS. The **ganglia** of sensory neurons form paired lumps on either side of the spinal cord or, for cranial nerves, near their brainstem exit. **Motor pathways** leave the CNS and travel to innervate muscles or glands of the body, leaving their cell bodies in the cord or stem as **nuclei**. The two pathways connect within the CNS, either directly

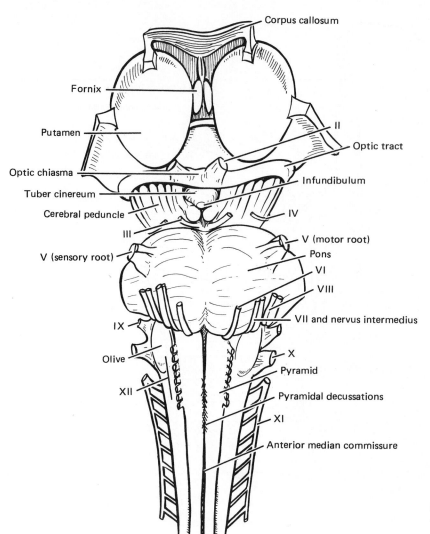

Figure 4-60. Ventral view of the brainstem. (From Hiatt JL, Gartner LP: *Textbook of Head and Neck Anatomy*, 3rd ed. Philadelphia, Lippincott, Williams & Wilkins, 2001.)

or by **interneurons**. Additional pathways may run up the spinal cord or brainstem to higher connecting centers in the brain. The simplest pathway involves only two neurons connecting in the spinal cord, called a **reflex pathway**. **Sympathetic pathways** involve at least three neurons, with an extra cell body lying within the sympathetic chain ganglia, a chain lying next to the spinal column. **Parasympathetic pathways** also involve three neurons, and the extra ganglion lies within the organ innervated.

Cranial Nerves

A brief description of each of the 12 pairs of cranial nerves is given in **(Table 4-7)**. Attention is directed to the name and number (Roman numeral) of each nerve and also to the names of its branches or divisions, the pathways to the nerve and the structure that it innervates, the type of innervation (i.e., sensory, motor, or mixed), and the skeletal foramina through which it passes.

Find the drawing of the brainstem, and locate these 12 pairs of nerves as they leave this area (except for cranial nerve I). Separate drawings of cranial nerves V, VII, IX, X, XII and their pathways are included. The trigeminal nerve is reviewed last, because this nerve is the most complex and relates greatly to the oral cavity.

Cranial Nerve I: Olfactory Nerve

The **olfactory** pair of nerves is responsible for the sense of smell and connects directly to the cerebrum rather than the brainstem. They appear as two "antennae" projecting out from the inferior cerebrum, lying on top of the cribriform plate. Smell sensory neurons of the nasal mucosa receive chemical stimulation and convert the neuronal signal to pass to neurons in the **olfactory bulb** (the end of the "antennae") through the foraminae of the cribriform plate. From this point, neurons connect with the cerebrum in a primitive area that is linked closely to memory. Cranial nerve I is a sensory nerve.

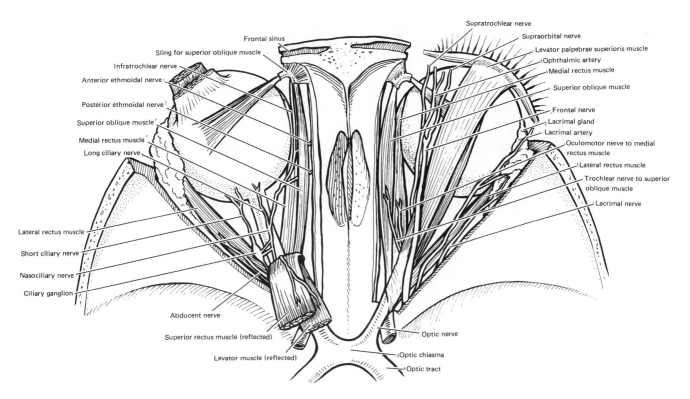

Figure 4-61. Structures within the orbit. Observe that the orbital plate of the frontal bone has been removed, as has the periorbital fascia and fat. The right side represents a superficial dissection and the left side is a deeper view. (From Hiatt JL, Gartner LP: *Textbook of Head and Neck Anatomy,* 3rd ed. Philadelphia, Lippincott, Williams & Wilkins, 2001.)

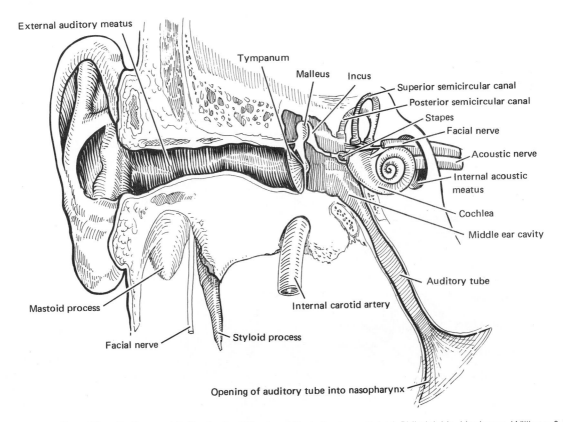

Figure 4-62. The ear. (From Hiatt JL, Gartner LP: *Textbook of Head and Neck Anatomy,* 3rd ed. Philadelphia, Lippincott, Williams & Wilkins, 2001.)

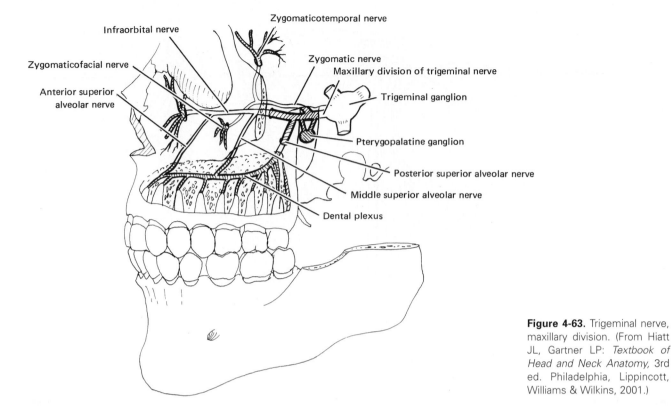

Figure 4-63. Trigeminal nerve, maxillary division. (From Hiatt JL, Gartner LP: *Textbook of Head and Neck Anatomy*, 3rd ed. Philadelphia, Lippincott, Williams & Wilkins, 2001.)

Cranial Nerve II: Optic Nerve

The **optic nerves** are sensory nerves that are responsible for delivering the sense of sight to the cerebrum for interpretation. They begin at the posterior aspect of each eyeball and exit through the optic foramina into the interior cranium where they immediately cross and connect at the **optic chi-** asm, which lies near the pituitary fossa. Upon entering the brain, these neurons connect with the **lateral geniculate bodies** and other nuclei that eventually take information to the **visual cortex**, which is located in the occipital lobes along the calcarine fissure. Visual information from the right and left eyes is shared by both sides of the brain, owing to the chiasm.

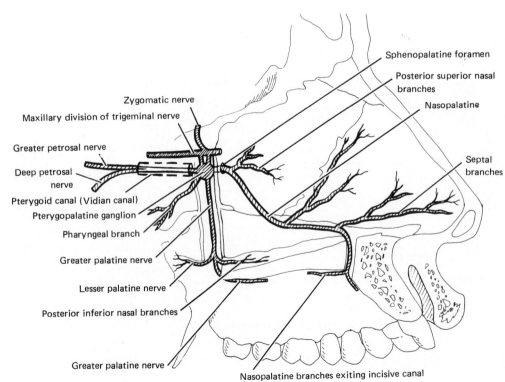

Figure 4-64. Pterygopalatine ganglion and connections. (From Hiatt JL, Gartner LP: *Textbook of Head and Neck Anatomy*, 3rd ed. Philadelphia, Lippincott, Williams & Wilkins, 2001.)

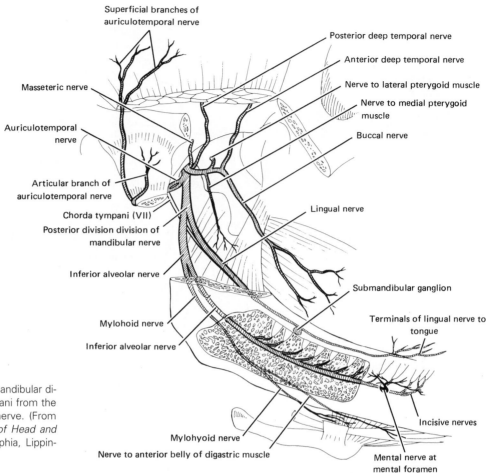

Figure 4-65. Trigeminal nerve, mandibular division. Observe the chorda tympani from the facial nerve joining the lingual nerve. (From Hiatt JL, Gartner LP: *Textbook of Head and Neck Anatomy,* 3rd ed. Philadelphia, Lippincott, Williams & Wilkins, 2001.)

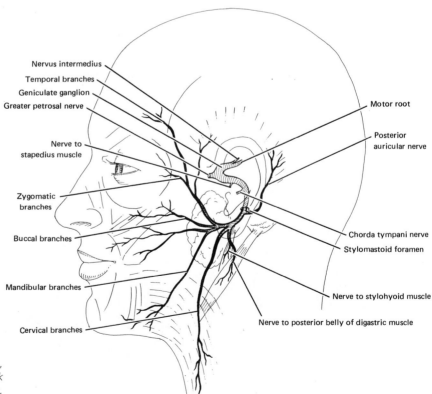

Figure 4-66. VII. Facial nerve. (From Hiatt JL, Gartner LP: *Textbook of Head and Neck Anatomy,* 3rd ed. Philadelphia, Lippincott, Williams & Wilkins, 2001.)

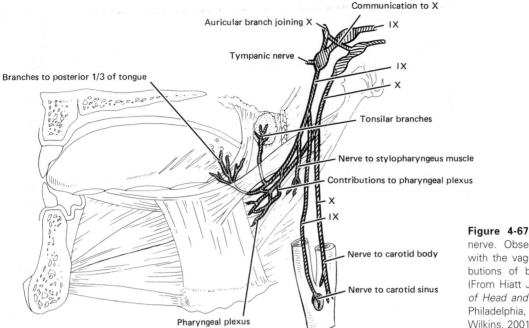

Figure 4-67. IX. Glossopharyngeal nerve. Observe the communication with the vagus nerve and the contributions of both to the pharyngeal. (From Hiatt JL, Gartner LP: *Textbook of Head and Neck Anatomy*, 3rd ed. Philadelphia, Lippincott, Williams & Wilkins, 2001.)

Cranial Nerve III (the Oculomotor Nerve), Cranial Nerve IV (the Trochlear Nerve), and Cranial Nerve VI (the Abducens Nerve)

These three pairs of motor nerves-the **oculomotor (III)**, **trochlear (IV),** and **abducens (VI)**-have similar functions and are reviewed together. They travel through the superior orbital fissure to innervate the small muscles that move the eyeball and its lids. A small branch of cranial nerve III provides parasympathetic function to the iris and lens.

Cranial Nerve VII: Facial Nerve

The **facial nerve (CN VII)** is a large mixed nerve with several branches. A large branch rides with cranial nerve V3 through the foramen ovale down to the mandible, giving a branch for taste to the anterior tongue called the **chorda**

tympani. The sensory ganglion is the **geniculate ganglion,** the brainstem connection in the **gustatory portion of the solitarius.**

A second portion (parasympathetic) travels to submandibular and sublingual salivary glands to innervate their secretion. Another small parasympathetic branch passes through superior orbital fissure to the lacrimal gland and nasal mucosa for secretion. Parasympathetic ganglia are the **submandibular** and **pterygopalatine ganglia.** CNS connection is to the **superior salivatory nucleus.**

The largest portion of facial nerve is its motor branch, which exits through stylomastoid foramen, behind the ear, to spread across the superficial face, innervating the muscles of facial expression. Central connections are with the **facial motor nucleus.**

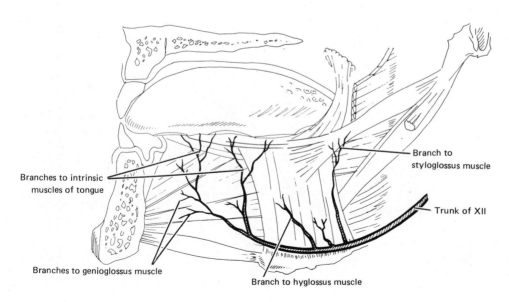

Figure 4-68. XII. Hypoglossal nerve. (From Hiatt JL, Gartner LP: *Textbook of Head and Neck Anatomy,* 3rd ed. Philadelphia, Lippincott, Williams & Wilkins, 2001.)

TABLE 4–7 Cranial Nerves

CRANIAL NERVE	TYPE	FORAMEN	GANGLIA/NUCLEI	INNERVATION
I Olfactory	Sensory	Cribriform plate	Olfactory bulb	Nasal mucosa to the cerebrum—smell
II Optic	Sensory	Optic foramen	Lateral geniculate bodies	Eyeball to the visual cortex—sight
III Oculomotor	Motor	Superior orbital fissure	Ciliary ganglia/motor nuclei	Muscles of the eye—movement/iris lens—opening (para)
IV Trochlear	Motor	Superior orbital fissure	Motor nuclei	Brainstem to muscles of the eye—movement of the eye
VI Abducens	Motor	Superior orbital fissure	Motor nuclei	Brainstem to muscles of the eye—movement of the eye
V Trigeminal	Mixed			
VI Ophthalmic	Sensory	Superior orbital fissure	Trigeminal ganglion/sensory nucleus V	Orbital area and forehead to the pons
Frontal Supraorbital Nasociliary Lacrimal		Supraorbital foramen		Skin of the forehead—general sensation
V2 Maxillary	Sensory	Foramen rotundum	Trigeminal ganglion/sensory nucleus V	Maxilla to the pons
Infraorbital		Infraorbital foramen		Skin of the maxillae—general sensation
Superior alveolar PSA, MSA, ASA				Maxilla and facial teeth—general sensation
Nasopalatine		Incisive foramen		Anterior palate, lingual teeth—general sensation
Greater palatine		Greater palatine foramina		Posterior palate, lingual teeth—general sensation
V3 Mandibular	Mixed	Foramen ovale	Trigeminal ganglion/V sensory nucleus	Mandible to the pons
Auriculotemporal				TMJ—general sensation
Lingual				Anterior tongue—general sensation
Buccal				Cheek—general sensation
Inferior alveolar		Mandibular foramen		Mandible and teeth—general sensation
Mental		Mental foramen		Skin of the chin—general sensation
Motor			Motor nucleus V	Pons to the muscles of mastication—mastication and mylohyoid/anterior digastric
VII Facial	Mixed			
Chorda tympani		Foramen ovale	Geniculate ganglion/gustatory of nucleus solitarius	Palate and ant. tongue—taste (on lingual n. V3) to the brainstem
		Internal meatus, stylomastoid foramen	Motor nucleus VII	Brainstem to the muscles of facial expression—fac. expression
		Superior orbital fissure, foramen ovale, internal meatus	Ciliary, pterygopalatine, submandibular ganglia/ superior salivatory nucleus	Brainstem to the lacrimal, palatal salivary glands (on CNV) Submandibular, sublingual salivary glands (on CNV)—secretions
VIII Vestibulocochlear	Sensory	Internal meatus		
Vestibular nerve			Vestibular ganglia/vestibular nuclei	Vestibular hair cells to the cerebellum—balance
Cochlear nerve			Spiral ganglia/cochlear nuclei Medial geniculate bodies	Hair cells of cochlea to the auditory cortex—hearing
IX Glossopharyngeal	Most sensory	Jugular foramen	Superior and inferior petrosal ganglia/nucleus solitarius	Skin of the ear, mucosa of the palate, pharynx Post. tongue to the brainstem—general sensation Carotid bodies and sinus—baro/chemoreception
			Gustatory of nucleus solitarius	Posterior tongue to the brainstem—taste
			Nucleus ambiguus/otic ganglia/ inferior salivatory nucleus	Brainstem to the stylopharyng./sup. constr.—motor Brainstem to the parotid gland—secretion (para)
X Vagus	Most motor (para)	Jugular foramen	Superior and inferior petrosal/nucleus solitarius	Skin of the ear—general sensation Pharynx, larynx, GI—visceral sensation
			Nucleus ambiguus	Brainstem to the musc. pharynx/larynx
			Dorsal motor nucleus X	Stem to GI/heart/lungs—(parasym. control)
XI Spinal accessory	Motor	Jugular foramen	Nucleus ambiguus	Cerebrum/stem to the sternocleidomastoid, trapezius muscles—motor
XII Hypoglossal	Motor	Hypoglossal foramina	Hypoglossal nucleus	Cerebrum/stem to the tongue muscles—motor

ASA, anterior superior alveolar; MSA, middle superior alveolar; PSA, posterior superior alveolar; TMJ, temporomandibular joint.

Cranial Nerve VIII: Vestibulocochlear Nerve

The **vestibulocochlear** is a sensory nerve passes on right and left sides through the internal meatus to the inner ear. It has two portions-the **vestibular nerve** and the **cochlear nerve**-each with a sensory ganglion located near the foramen (i.e., the **spiral and vestibular ganglia**). The vestibular nerve carries information from the hair cells of the vestibule and semicircular ampullae for positional sense or for balance. This information travels first to the **vestibular nuclei** and then to the cerebellum, brainstem, and cerebrum. It is important for muscle movement and coordination.

The cochlear branch carries information from the **hair cells** of the cochlea, responsible for the sense of hearing. Receptors of the inner ear (cochlea) sense differences in sound and transmit them through cranial nerve VIII to the cochlear nuclei, then to the **medial geniculate** bodies of the cerebrum, and finally to the auditory cortex for interpretation. The **auditory cortex** lies in the temporal lobes along the lateral sulcus.

Cranial Nerve IX: Glossopharyngeal Nerve

As the name suggests, the **glossopharyngeal nerve** is important for innervating the pharynx and the tongue. This mixed nerve has several branches. The glossopharyngeal branches pass through the jugular foramen to exit the cranium. The sensory ones are as follows: A small branch goes to the ear. A larger branch innervates general sensation to the posterior tongue, and pharynx, helping regulate the swallow (or gag) reflex. Taste to the posterior tongue and palate is carried on this branch also. A third branch is to the **carotid bodies and sinus** of that artery and is important in the regulation of blood flow by baroreceptor and chemoreceptor information. Sensory ganglia associated with these nerves are the **superior and inferior petrosal ganglia**. Brainstem nucleus connection to the carotid information is the **nucleus solitarius** and for taste to its **gustatory portion.**

Motor branches of cranial nerve IX include a few fibers to the stylopharyngeus and superior constrictor muscles. Parasympathetic fibers that regulate the parotid gland begin in the **inferior salivatory nucleus** of the brainstem. The parasympathetic ganglion of the parotid is the **otic ganglion**.

Cranial Nerve X: Vagus Nerve

The name "vagus" means "the wanderer," which is appropriate for this large, mixed nerve pair, because it travels out of the head and neck region to the trunk of the body. The **vagus** is the main source of parasympathetic innervation to the viscera.

The smaller sensory branches begin at the ear and give general sensation there. More branches give visceral sensation to the pharynx, larynx, esophagus, stomach, small intestine, part of the large intestine, the heart, and the lungs. The **superior and inferior petrosal ganglia** are associated sensory ganglia. Visceral sensation also connects with the **nucleus solitarius** of the brainstem.

The motor component of the vagus is large, and it sends parasympathetic fibers to the entire respiratory system, most of the digestive system, and the heart. It begins with innervation of the muscles of the pharynx and larynx, connecting with the **nucleus ambiguus**. It is important for deglutition and the gag reflex.

Regulation of respiration, digestion, and heartbeat falls in the domain of the vagus nerve. Parasympathetic ganglia are located within the organ walls, and the brainstem connection is through the **dorsal motor nucleus** of the brainstem.

Companion sympathetic fibers travel with all the parasympathetic nerves, but their source is the sympathetic chain ganglia near the spinal column.

The large vagus nerve exits the cranium through the jugular foramina and travels down the neck near the SCMs, along their borders.

Cranial Nerve XI: Spinal Accessory Nerve

The 11th cranial nerve is named **spinal accessory**, because a portion of its fibers arise from the cervical nerves below. This motor nerve carries innervation to the SCMs and the trapezius muscle. Cranial nerve XI exits the cranium by the jugular foramen and has connections to the **nucleus ambiguus.**

Cranial Nerve XII: Hypoglossal Nerve

The **hypoglossal** is the motor nerve that passes out of the hypoglossal foramina, swings down and forward to go under the base of the tongue, and then spreads to all "glossal" muscles. All muscles of the tongue are innervated by cranial nerve XII, which is connected to the **hypoglossal motor nucleus** of the brainstem.

Cranial Nerve V: Trigeminal Nerve

Perhaps the most complex and important to dentistry is the **trigeminal nerve**, so-named for its three divisions: **V1-ophthalmic division**, **V2-maxillary division**, and **V3-mandibular division**. Each division and its branches will be traced. Find the diagram of cranial nerve V both in place in the cranium and separated from it. V1 and V2 are sensory nerves, and V3 is mixed.

The trigeminal begins exiting an area of the brainstem known as the **pons**, on its right and left sides. A large ganglion, called the **trigeminal ganglia**, is attached to the root of each nerve. Each trigeminal ganglion lies in a small fossa on either side of the pituitary fossa. The trigeminal immediately branches into its three divisions, and each division exits the cranium as follows: V1 exits through the superior orbital fissure toward the orbit; V2 exits through the foramen rotundum toward the maxilla; and V3 exits through the foramen ovale toward the mandible.

Divisions. Ophthalmic Division: VI. Look at each division of the trigeminal as its branches are described. Only major branches and their innervations are reviewed. Begin with the **V1, ophthalmic division** as it heads toward the orbit. Branches are as follows:

Frontal nerve: passes superiorly and a portion exits as the supraorbital nerve-the sensory nerve to the skin of the forehead and orbit

Nasociliary nerve: part to the eye (ciliary gland-parasympathetic, and orbital skin-sensory), part to the nasal sinus, connected to the ciliary ganglion and cranial nerve III.

Lacrimal nerve: passes to the lacrimal gland, with cranial nerve VII.

Maxillary Division: V2. The **maxillary division, V2,** branches immediately upon entering the posterior of the maxillary bone. Its branches are connected in a large loop and are:

Nasopalatine nerve: connected to pterygopalatine ganglion (cranial nerve VII), sends nasal branches to the mucosa (parasympathetic) and sensory branches to the anterior palate, the lingual side of its teeth (i.e., centrals, laterals, mesial canines), and its periodontium. It passes through the incisive foramen.

Greater palatine nerve: branching from the same point as the nasopalatine, goes to the posterior palate and the lingual of its teeth (i.e., molars, premolars, distal canines) and their periodontium.

Superior alveolar nerve: sensory to the facial side of the maxillary teeth and periodontium, three loops (sub-branches):
1. **Posterior superior alveolar (PSA) nerve**: innervates the facial molars (i.e., the second and third molars and the distal first molars).
2. **Middle superior alveolar (MSA) nerve**: innervates the facial premolars (i.e., the mesial first molars, premolars, and distal canines).
3. **Anterior superior alveolar (ASA) nerve**: innervates facial anteriors (i.e., centrals, laterals, mesial canines).

Infraorbital nerve: the anterior portion of the superior alveolar/nasopalatine loop that exits the infraorbital foramen, giving sensation to the skin on the midface.

Mandibular Division: V3. The **mandibular division, V3,** passes behind the condyle of the mandible, giving some branches before entering the mandibular foramen into the mandibular canal. Its branches are as follows:

Auriculotemporal nerve: a small branch around and to the TMJ and outer ear.

Motor branch V: four motor nerves to each of the muscles of mastication.

Buccal nerve: sensation to the cheek and the facial side of mandibular molars.

Lingual nerve: general sensation to the anterior two thirds of the tongue; branches of cranial nerve VII ride on it (one to "sub" salivary glands, and chorda tympani for taste to the anterior two thirds of the tongue).

Mylohyoid nerve: motor to the mylohyoid muscle.(All of the above branch before the mandibular foramen.)

Inferior alveolar nerve: the large nerve traveling in the mandibular canal, sensory to all mandibular teeth and their periodontium.

Mental nerve: the small sub-branch of the inferior alveolar that exits the mental foramen and is sensory to the skin on the chin.

Branches. The locations of the branches of the trigeminal nerve are important to anesthetize teeth. The following list denotes the branches that must be anesthetized to fully numb each tooth type.

Maxillary
Third molar, second molar: PSA, greater palatine
First molar: PSA, MSA, greater palatine
Premolars: MSA, greater palatine
Canines: MSA, ASA, greater palatine, nasopalatine
Incisors: ASA, nasopalatine

Mandibular
Molars: inferior alveolar, buccal
All others: inferior alveolar only

Review the sensory innervation of the face (in thirds) as it relates to the three divisions of the trigeminal nerve. Also note the three paired foramina of the face through which these nerves exit (see Table 4-6).

The central connections of the trigeminal nerve are as follows. We have already seen the large sensory ganglion on the exterior nerve trunk, the **trigeminal ganglion**. Former names for this ganglion are the gasserian or semilunar ganglion. A large sensory nucleus, which also has three centers, is found in the pons. The **mesencephalic nucleus** is the topmost portion, which receives mainly proprioception. The **chief sensory nucleus** lies in the middle and handles signals for general sensation such as touch, whereas the **spinal nucleus** lies at the bottom deals mainly with pain signals. Many connections exist between the sensory input of cranial nerve V and the CNS. Sensation is largely relayed to the **VPM nucleus of the thalamus** and then to sensory areas of the cortex. Medial to the sensory nuclei, lie the **motor nuclei of V**, which are the cell bodies of the nerves to the muscles of mastication. The motor nuclei have connections to other centers of the brainstem, including the **masticatory center**.

Summary of Sensory Organs

General sensation includes touch, pressure, temperature, and pain. Specialized sensation (e.g., smell, taste, vision, and hearing/balance) requires separate organs, and specialized receptor neurons have developed for this purpose.

Smell

The special sensory **receptors for smell** are stimulated chemically by airborne particles and are located in the superior nasal mucosa. Neuronal pathways include those of cranial nerve I (i.e., the **olfactory nerve**) and its **olfactory bulbs**. Their connection is directly to the **cerebrum** for the purpose of interpretation, and this information blends with taste data as well as emotion and memory.

Taste

The special sensory receptors called **taste cells** are found mainly on the dorsal tongue, although they are scattered throughout the oral mucosa. Most of these receptors lie in the circumvallate papillae and are stimulated chemically, being first presented in a liquid form by saliva. Only four basic taste sensations exist (i.e., salty, sweet, bitter, and sour), but the wide variety of tastes are enhanced by the sense of smell. Innervation of the anterior tongue for taste is by achieved by cranial nerve VII (chorda tympani) and the posterior third by cranial nerve IX. Pathways are directed into the **gustatory portion of the solitarius nuclei** in the brainstem and then to the cerebrum. General sensation to the tongue travels on cranial nerve V (lingual) for the anterior region and on cranial nerve IX for the posterior region.

Vision

The eyeball is said to work like a camera, with light focusing through a small hole (the **pupil**) and **lens**, onto the back of the ball on a layer called the **retina**. The retina contains its receptor neurons (the **rods and cones**) in a small area called the **fovea**. These receptors are stimulated by light and dark, and color begins a pathway from cranial nerve II (**optic nerve**) to the occipital lobe (visual cortex), which crosses information from each eye at the chiasm. This information goes through other nuclei of the brain called the **lateral geniculate bodies.**

Hearing/Balance

Hearing is the perception of vibrating air waves and begins with that vibration being translated into mechanical motion by the **tympanic membrane** of the outer ear. That mechanical vibration passes through the ossicles (i.e., the **malleus, incus, and stapes**) of the middle ear to the membranous, fluid-filled inner ear. The portion of the inner ear known as the **cochlea** contains **hair cells,** which are the specialized receptors for hearing. Each hair cell is tuned to a particular pitch. Pathways to the **auditory cortex** of the temporal lobe begin at the **cochlear nerve (cranial nerve VIII) and its ganglion** and go through other nuclei of the brainstem and cerebrum as the **medial geniculate bodies.**

Balance is sensed by the other portion of the inner ear, the **vestibule** and **semicircular canals**, whose hair cells are triggered by fluid motion much as that of a carpenter's level. Information on the position of the head is taken down the **vestibular nerve (cranial nerve VIII)** and the **ganglion** to make multiple connections with the brainstem and **cerebellum**, which aids in muscle control of the body.

Circulatory System (Figures 4–69 to 4–71)

Circulation implies the circular travel of substances. In this case, blood and lymph travel in circular routes around the body to deliver nutrients and oxygen to the cells and to rid the body of wastes and CO_2. The **vascular system** consists of the blood vessels, heart, and blood. It is a closed system of tubes. Leading away from the pump (i.e., the heart) are the thick-walled **arteries** that supply the body with blood. They branch into smaller and smaller vessels, until the cellular level is reached by the **capillaries**. Nutrients and oxygen are delivered at the capillary level, and waste products picked up. The vessels then enlarge and create the veins or venous side of the circle. **Veins** lead toward the heart and are thin-walled vessels. Only the major arteries and veins have anatomic names.

The **lymphatic system** is an open system, consisting of vessels, nodes, lymph fluid, and lymphocytes. The system begins at the cellular level with the fluid that bathes the cells. This fluid drains into the **lymph vessels**, along which lie **lymph nodes** that act as filters of the fluid; furthermore, they increase the lymphocytes. Lymph vessels branch into larger vessels, which eventually empty into the venous system via the **thoracic duct**. Fluid will leak back out to the cells through the capillaries and some veins.

Vascular System

The major arteries and veins of the head and neck are identified, and their distribution is shown on the diagrams. Most vessels are paired, right and left.

Arteries of the Head and Neck

The major arterial supply to the head and neck is by way of the **carotid arteries**, which branch off of the large vessels of the heart. The largest branches that travel up the neck from the chest are the common carotid arteries, which are located below the borders of the SCM. The **common carotid** branches below the mandible into two major arteries: the **internal carotid** (which supplies the brain) and the **external carotid** (which supplies all external structures). A third pair of smaller vessel, the **vertebral arteries**, are separate from the carotids and ascend the neck within a foraminal "tunnel" created by the cervical vertebrae on the right and left sides. They also enter the brain. The smaller branches of the external and internal carotid and their distribution are listed. Find each branch on the diagram.

The branches of the external carotid artery include:

Thyroid arteries: supply the thyroid gland.
Lingual arteries: supply the tongue from below.
Facial arteries: run over the mandibular body to the superficial face to supply it.
Occipital arteries, retroauricular arteries: supply the back of the head.
Superficial temporal arteries: spread over the surface of the sides and top of the head.
Maxillary arteries: supply the maxilla and mandible and its structures.

The **maxillary artery** is important to the study of the oral cavity because it supplies the cavity with its branches. This large artery passes behind the condyle of the mandible and then gives off several branches. Note also the foramina that

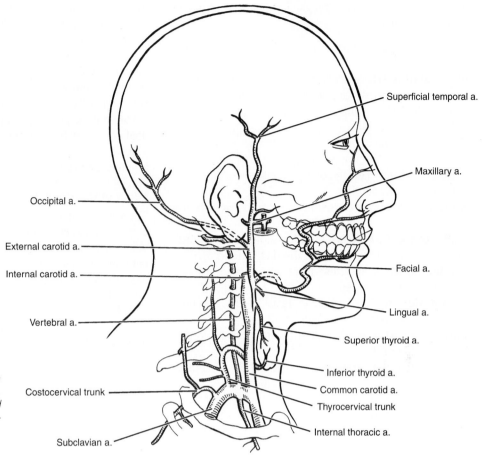

Figure 4-69. Major arteries of the head and neck. (From Hiatt JL, Gartner LP: *Textbook of Head and Neck Anatomy,* 3rd ed. Philadelphia, Lippincott, Williams & Wilkins, 2001.)

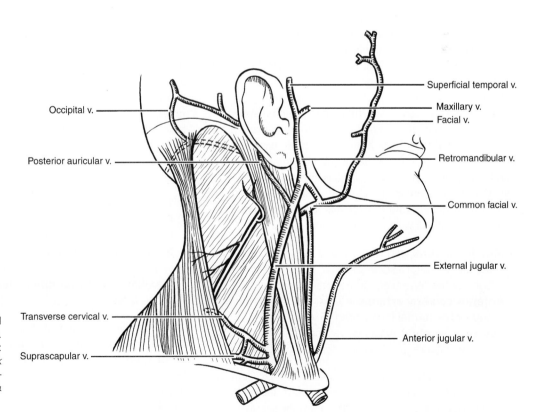

Figure 4-70. Superficial veins of the face and neck. (From Hiatt JL, Gartner LP: *Textbook of Head and Neck Anatomy,* 3rd ed. Philadelphia, Lippincott, Williams & Wilkins, 2001.)

some of these vessels pass through. The branches of maxillary artery include:

Sphenopalatine artery: to the palate, further sub-branches.

Nasopalatine artery (through the incisive foramen): to the anterior palate and lingual of the anterior teeth (i.e., the incisors and mesial canines) and periodontium.

Greater palatine arteries (through the greater palatine foramina): to the posterior palate and lingual to the posterior teeth (i.e., the distal canine, premolars, molars) and periodontium.

Superior alveolar arteries: to the maxilla, facial of the maxillary teeth and periodontium.

(Posterior) PSA arteries: to facial of posterior teeth (second and third molars, the distal first molar).

(Middle) MSA arteries: to facial of the premolars and mesial canines.

(Anterior) ASA arteries: to facial of the anteriors (i.e., the distal canine, incisors)

Infraorbital arteries (through the infraorbital foramen): to the skin of the maxilla

Inferior alveolar arteries (through the mandibular foramen): to the mandible and its teeth

Mental arteries (through the mental foramina): to the skin of the chin.

Buccal arteries: to the cheek and facial of the mandibular molars.

Note that the arterial supply of the oral cavity mirrors the nervous supply by V2 and V3, with all of the same branch names and distribution. The veins are the same, because an artery, vein, and nerve of the same name travel together for a distribution site. The foramina also usually go by the name of the vessels and nerves that pass through them. The only difference is that the superior and inferior alveolar arteries (and veins) are both branches of the maxillary vessel, whereas there are separate maxillary and mandibular nerves.

The branches of the internal carotid artery consist of the **internal carotids,** which branch off from the common carotid at a level just below the mandibular angle. They pass into the cranium through the tortuous **carotid canals** on either side of the pituitary fossa. These curved, large vessels branch immediately into vessels that supply the cerebrum. Find them on the drawing. They are also paired.

Middle cerebral arteries: largest of the three; they supply the outer aspect of most of the cerebrum, especially the temporal and parietal lobes.

Anterior cerebral arteries: a small pair run anterior to supply the frontal lobe from the inner aspect.

Posterior cerebral arteries: run posteriorly to supply the occipital region from the inner aspect.

The brain demands a rich and rapid supply of oxygenated, nutrient-rich blood in order to function. Thus, the brain has a second supply of arterial blood that joins the supply of the internal carotids. The **vertebral arteries** that ascend the cervical spinal column enter through the foramen magnum on the base of the brainstem, where they fuse to become the **basilar artery.** This single vessel then gives paired branches to the brainstem and cerebellum, before joining the internal carotid circulation. This happens through small vessels, called the **circle of Willis,** which are arranged in a circle around the pituitary gland. In addition to connecting the dual source of blood to the brain, the circle of Willis provides a safety mechanism; in case of damage to a vessel, blood can be re-routed around the brain.

Veins of the Head and Neck

The veins begin as smaller vessels (capillaries) and then coalesce into larger ones (veins). Blood flow (drainage) of the veins is toward the heart. For the most part, veins accompany arteries and have similar distributions and names. A few differences are pointed out. For example, the large veins of the brain are called **sinuses,** and a network of veins is called a **plexus.**

The major veins that drain the head and neck are the jugular veins. They go downward into the superior vena cava in the chest and then into the heart. The major veins consist of three pairs of jugular veins and one pair of vertebral veins. Their branches are discussed.

Anterior jugular veins are the anterior-most pair; these veins join together in the front of the superficial neck. They are small and irregular, and they drain this area.

Unlike the accompanying vertebral arteries, the **vertebral veins** do not originate in the brain but rather drain the occipital region. They travel with the arteries in the "tunnel" created by the cervical vertebral foramina

The **external jugular veins** are the large vessels that drain the external face, head, and neck. There is no common jugular, as is found with the arterial supply; instead, the internal and external jugular veins connect directly to the brachiocephalic veins in the chest. The internal and external jugular veins, however, are connected at a higher level, behind the angle of the mandible by way of the **retromandibular vein.** The remaining branches of the external jugular are very similar to the arteries that supply the same areas. They are paired.

Thyroid veins: drain the thyroid glands.
Facial veins: drains the superficial face.
Lingual veins: drain the tongue from below.
Superficial temporal veins: drain the sides and top of the head.
Maxillary vein/Pterygoid plexus: drain the maxilla and mandible.

Only a short segment of the maxillary vein is present. Instead, the maxillary vein spreads out into a network of small veins called the **pterygoid plexus.** Both the maxillary artery and the pterygoid plexus lie in the bottom of the infratemporal fossa, in a portion called the **pterygopalatine fossa.** Also present in this fossa is V2 (maxillary divi-

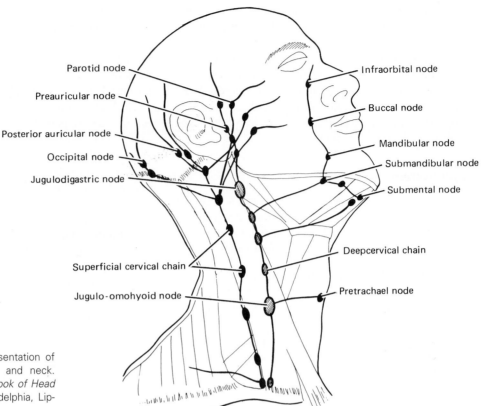

Parotid node
Preauricular node
Posterior auricular node
Occipital node
Jugulodigastric node
Superficial cervical chain
Jugulo-omohyoid node

Infraorbital node
Buccal node
Mandibular node
Submandibular node
Submental node
Deepcervical chain
Pretrachael node

Figure 4-71. Diagrammatic representation of lymphatic drainage of the head and neck. (From Hiatt JL, Gartner LP: *Textbook of Head and Neck Anatomy*, 3rd ed. Philadelphia, Lippincott, Williams & Wilkins, 2001.)

sion of the trigeminal) and its pterygopalatine ganglion. This is interesting, because this is the site of a frequent dental anesthetic injection-the PSA block. Care must be taken while injecting into this space not to damage the vessels, thus causing a hematoma. This situation is avoided by using an aspirating technique.

The branches of the **maxillary vein/pterygoid plexus** are the same as those of the arterial supply. They accompany the arteries through the same foramina.

Nasopalatine vein (through the incisive foramen): from the anterior palate and the lingual anterior teeth.

Greater palatine veins (through the greater palatine foramina): from the posterior palate and the lingual posterior teeth.

Infraorbital veins (through the infraorbital foramina): from the maxillary skin

Superior alveolar veins: from the maxilla, the facial of its teeth and the periodontium

PSA veins: from the facial second molars, third molars, and distal first molars

MSA veins: from the mesial first molar, premolars, and distal canines

ASA veins: from the mesial canines and incisors

Inferior alveolar veins (through the mandibular foramen into the mandibular canal): from the mandible and the teeth

Mental veins (through the mental foramina); from the skin on the chin

Buccal veins: to the cheek and facial of mandibular molars

The internal jugular vein is the largest of the jugulars and drains the interior cranium or brain. The large veins of the brain are called sinuses. The internal jugular passes through the jugular foramen on its way out of the cranium. Some of the larger venous sinuses "carve out" grooves in the cranial bone where they lie between the bone and the surface of the brain. Identify the following branches.

Superior sagittal sinus: This large, midline vein lies between the cerebral hemispheres and drains this region. Cerebrospinal fluid also arises from this area.

Inferior sagittal sinus: a single vessel directly below the superior, drains the interior cerebrum

Transverse sinuses: diverging from the sagittal sinuses right and left, across the cerebellum

Sigmoid sinuses: S-shaped curves that connect the sinuses to the internal jugular veins

Cavernous sinus: plexus-like sinus that drains the base of the brain and connects to the face and pterygoid plexus

The most interesting of the venous sinuses is the **cavernous sinus**. Anatomically, it resembles a sponge that is full of different pathways and spaces. It lies around and on top of the pituitary fossa, and several structures in that area actually pass through it (i.e., the internal carotids and branches of cranial nerves V, III, IV, and VI). This thin-walled fragile structure is susceptible to pooling of blood and thus presents a hazard for infection and for damage to the material that passes through it. For example, if an infected needle penetrates the pterygoid plexus, the needle would pass infection directly to this area of the brain. Passage of infection is also possible from the facial/nasal area.

Lymph System

Several groups of **lymph nodes** and their vessels drain the head and neck (in that direction) down toward thoracic duct in the chest. These groups are identified, and their drainage sites are named. The groups are paired, right and left.

Occipital, postauricular nodes: drain the back of the head and ear

Parotid, preauricular nodes: drain the front of the ear and parotid region

Facial nodes: drain the anterior superficial face

Submental nodes: drain the mandibular anterior teeth and the chin

Submandibular nodes: located near the submandibular salivary glands, they drain most of the teeth, maxilla, and mandible.

Cervical nodes: all of the above groups of nodes drain into the cervical chain of nodes, down the neck (i.e., the superficial and deep groups).

The cervical nodes and their vessels from a chain of drainage points that descend the neck along the border of the SCM. The largest node of the chain is the **jugulodigastric node**, which lies at the level of the angle of the mandible in the neck. Nodes are important diagnostic indicators of pathology. They become swollen and tender when infection and subsequent drainage is present. They may be hard and "rubbery" to palpation when cancerous processes are present.

List the structures that we can find along the borders of the SCM-the landmark muscle:

1. The carotid vessels (A good place to find the carotid pulse is along the SCM, near the jaw.)
2. Internal jugulars
3. Cranial nerves X and XI
4. Cervical lymph nodes

Other Systems (Figures 4-72 to 4-73)

Digestive System

Oral Cavity

Refer to the complete sagittal section of the head and neck to find the parts of the digestive system represented in the area. The beginning of the system is the **oral cavity**, which begins at the lips and encompasses the space that contains the maxillary and mandibular arches, their periodontium and teeth, the **hard and soft palate,** and the anterior tongue (the body). The function of the oral cavity in digestion is the breakdown of food substances by the teeth (mastication) and the addition of saliva to moisten the resultant bolus. This begins mechanical and chemical digestion.

The major salivary glands empty into the oral cavity as follows (all are paired): The **parotid gland** lies superficial to the skin, just anterior to the TMJ and ear on right and left sides. Its major duct, the **Stensen duct**, pierces the buccinator muscle to enter at the level of the maxillary second molar into the oral cavity through the **parotid papilla**. This is a mainly serous gland (which produces protein and water) that is innervated by cranial nerve IX. The **submandibular glands** are located in the submandibular fossae of the mandible, which are in between the skin of the chin (near the angle) and the mylohyoid muscle. Their ducts (**Wharton ducts**) travel forward in the floor of the mouth to empty under the tongue into the oral cavity into the **sublingual caruncles**. The **sublingual glands** are located in the floor of the mouth, directly under the mucosa below two folds called the **sublingual plicae**. Multiple small ducts (the **ducts of Rivinus**) are associated with the sublingual, which empty into the oral cavity through the plicae.

Landmarks of the oral cavity are shown in a diagram to be reviewed. All of these structures are covered with **oral mucosa**, underneath which is muscle, some glands, and other bone or connective tissue. Locate the **buccal mucosa** (over the buccinator), the **raphe** (joining of the superior constrictor and buccinator), the **soft palate** and **uvula,** the **tonsillar pillars** (over the palatoglossus and palatopharyngeus), and the **palatine tonsil** between them.

The **pharynx** begins where the oral cavity ends, at the tonsillar pillars and at the end of the soft palate and posterior tongue. The pharynx is a muscular tube, lined with mucosa, which is divided into three regions: the nasopharynx, the oropharynx, and the pharynx proper. Find these regions on the drawing. The **nasopharynx** lies above the soft palate and is not part of the digestive system but contains the **tympanic tubes** and **pharyngeal tonsils**. The nasopharynx is sealed off from the oropharynx during swallowing by the soft palate. The **oropharynx** (or "back of the throat") begins the deglutition process by sending boluses downward into the pharynx proper and thence into the esophagus. The muscles of the pharynx are the constrictors and are innervated by cranial nerve X, whereas the mucosa's sensory innervation is by cranial nerve IX. The **epiglottis** is present at the base of the tongue in the **pharynx proper**, to seal off the respiratory tract from the passage of food.

Esophagus

A small portion of the **esophagus** is present in the neck. This smooth muscular tube propels the bolus downward by peristalsis into the stomach. The esophagus is innervated by cranial nerve X. No digestive glands are present.

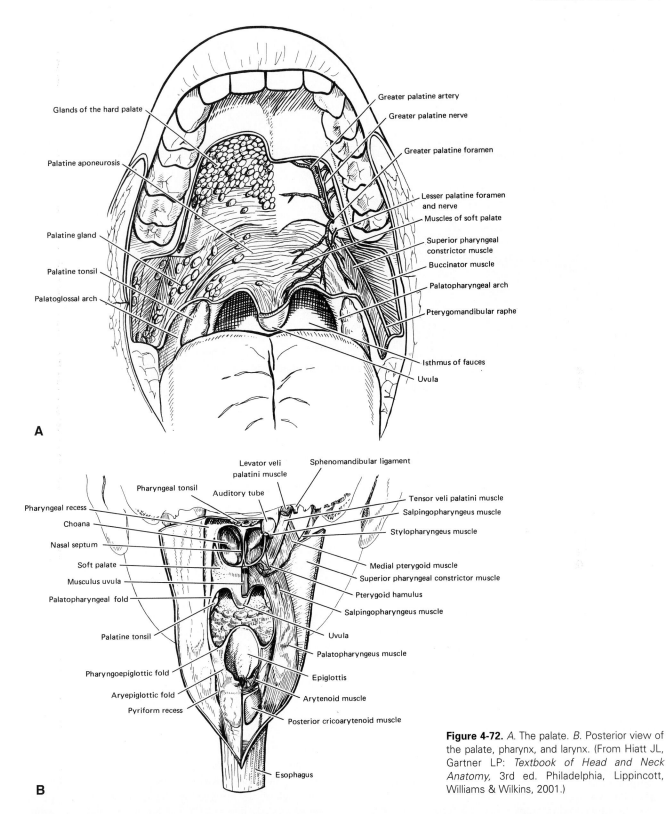

Figure 4-72. *A.* The palate. *B.* Posterior view of the palate, pharynx, and larynx. (From Hiatt JL, Gartner LP: *Textbook of Head and Neck Anatomy,* 3rd ed. Philadelphia, Lippincott, Williams & Wilkins, 2001.)

Mastication is the breakdown of large food substances by the teeth into a package (i.e., the bolus) that is small enough to be sent down the pharynx. Mastication is accomplished by the mandibular excursions (the mandible and its musculature in function) and the occlusion of the dentition during mandibular movement.

The human **dentition** is designed to handle an omnivore diet (i.e., meat and vegetable) and thus has a double-cusped occlusion. Each group of teeth is built to do a job. The anterior teeth incise (incisors), pierce, and hold food (canines); these teeth then pass the food to the posterior oral cavity and the teeth. **Trituration**, the grinding of food into smaller par-

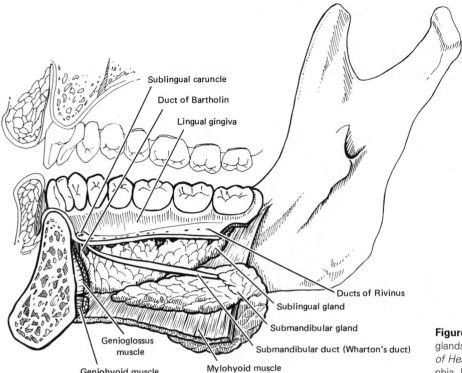

Figure 4-73. Submandibular and sublingual glands. (From Hiatt JL, Gartner LP: *Textbook of Head and Neck Anatomy*, 3rd ed. Philadelphia, Lippincott, Williams & Wilkins, 2001.)

ticles, is accomplished by the premolars and molars in the fashion of a mortar and pestle. Elevations of enamel called cusps fit into concave areas of the opposing molars, thus allowing grinding to occur. The set of cusps that do this work are called the **working or centric cusps**. These cusps are rounded and strong. The second set of cusps allows the dentition to unlock from its grinding function; these cusps are called the **balancing cusps**. They are pointed and slim.

The **mandibular excursions** or movements are combined in mastication. They include opening and closing, lateral movement, and protrusion and retrusion. The structure of the TMJ and teeth is important to allow these movements. Its dual joint cavities allow for a hinge-type movement in the lower portion and a gliding type of motion in the superior portion. The combination of excursions produces an **elliptical pattern of mastication** that is typical for omnivores. The main muscles that cause the different mandibular movements are summarized along with their innervations.

Opening (elevation)
temporalis, medial pterygoid,   (cranial nerve V3)
    masseter
Closing (depression)
suprahyoids   (cranial nerve V3)
Lateral movement
lateral pterygoid (single)   (cranial nerve V3)
Protrusion
lateral pterygoid (both)   (cranial nerve V3)
Retrusion
temporalis   (cranial nerve V3)

As can be seen, the **muscles of mastication** are the major group involved as well as the motor branch of the trigeminal nerve (the mandibular division). Nerve pathways to and from the muscles

involve sensation from the oral cavity, which is delivered on trigeminal branches and motor pathways that begin in the brainstem in the trigeminal motor nucleus. Some cerebral connections are wired into these pathways, but a great deal of mastication relies on involuntary, unconscious centers. The **masticatory center** in the brainstem is associated with the rhythmic, unconscious activity of mastication. Also, some mandibular reflex actions occur during sensory stimulation, such as when an unwanted hard object between the teeth causes the jaw to open. Stimulation from the proprioceptors of the periodontal ligaments and the TMJ is important for knowing where the mandible (and teeth) is in space during mastication. This information also travels into the CNS by way of the trigeminal nerve and the **mesencephalic nucleus** in the brainstem.

Deglutition

By this time, the food bolus has been finished by mastication and moistened by the addition of saliva by the major and minor salivary glands. It is ready for **deglutition** or swallowing to occur. Deglutition is usually divided into three phases: oral, pharyngeal, and esophageal.

During the **oral phase**, the bolus is positioned on the posterior end of the tongue by the intrinsic muscles of the tongue (cranial nerve XII) and buccinator muscle (cranial nerve VII). The glossopharyngeal nerve (cranial nerve IX) picks up the sensation of the presence of the bolus and triggers the muscular action of the pharynx via cranial nerve X (the vagus). If cranial nerve IX detects an unwanted object in the posterior oral cavity, it may trigger a reverse contraction of cranial nerve X, thus causing expulsion of the object (which is called the **gag reflex**).

During the **pharyngeal phase**, the soft palate rises and stretches the TVP, LVP, palatoglossus, palatopharyngeus-cranial nerves V, VII, XII, and X-to seal off the nasopharynx from the passage of food. This also occurs with liquids. The bolus is forced downward into the pharynx. Meanwhile, the TVP also opens the tympanic tube. The superior constrictor first squeezes the bolus downward, followed by the middle constrictors and then by the inferior constrictors (cranial nerve X).

The **esophageal phase** indicates the passage of the bolus from the pharynx into the esophagus by constrictor action (cranial nerve X). At the top of the pharyngeal tube, we began with skeletal muscle and voluntary control; by the time the bolus arrives at the bottom, smooth muscle and involuntary control have taken over. The squeezing motion of the digestive tube is now called **peristalsis,** which is caused by the action of the three layers of smooth muscle around the tube. Before the bolus passes into the esophagus, it is directed away from the respiratory tube, the larynx, by the epiglottis. The epiglottis is a large cartilaginous flap, against which the larynx is raised during deglutition. If the respiratory tract is not sealed off during deglutition, objects may get into the airway. This is called **aspiration.**

Deglutition begins as a conscious action but is then governed by involuntary brainstem controls. As well as a masticatory center, a swallowing center can be found in the brainstem; this center coordinates the information and action of several cranial nerves. Information sent from taste receptors in the mouth (and especially the tongue) are important regarding the decision to swallow. This information travels on cranial nerves VII and IX.

Respiratory System

Larynx

Respiration is the inhalation and exhalation of air into the body. Air is brought into the body through the nasal and oral cavities and sent down into the **larynx.** Find this second "tube" under the epiglottis and anterior to the pharyngeal tube. The larynx and the trachea (which lies below the larynx) are rigid tubes that are maintained in a constantly open state (a patent airway). The trachea divides into two bronchi in the thorax and then into smaller and smaller passageways in the lungs, which provide a surface area for body gas exchange. Oxygen is taken in and loaded on the erythrocytes as carbon dioxide (CO_2) is unloaded for removal by exhalation.

The **nasal cavity** is divided by the **nasal septum** and has three pairs of lateral processes, the **turbinates,** extending into them. The entire cavity is lined with respiratory mucosa (pseudostratified, ciliated epithelium with mucous cells). The **paranasal sinuses** and the lacrimal gland drain into the nasal cavity via the **meatii.** The nasal cavity acts as a filter of incoming air and also warms and moistens it. It joins the nasopharynx at its posterior aspect and sends air downward. The **nasopharynx** contains the tympanic tube orifices for ventilation of the middle ears.

Air continues down the pharynx until it meets the larynx below the root of the tongue. The epiglottis is a mucosa-covered cartilaginous flap that is used to seal off the larynx during deglutition. The **larynx** is called the "voice box" because it contains the **vocal folds or cords** (two cords of connective tissue that vibrate when air passes over them) that produce sound. This area is innervated by cranial nerve X and is responsible for vocalization (speech). The larynx is protected on the outside by a large cartilage shield, the **thyroid cartilage,** thus named for the thyroid gland that rests on it.

Below the larynx, the airway continues with the **trachea.** This tube consists of a series of cartilaginous **rings** that is connected by connective tissue and lined with respiratory mucosa. A patent airway is provided down the neck, anterior to the esophagus into the thorax.

Endocrine System

Pituitary Gland

Several glands of the endocrine system are present in the head and neck. This system is one that regulates other body systems by way of blood-borne chemicals (i.e., the **hormones**). The so-called master gland, the **pituitary or hypophysis**, lies in the pituitary fossa at the base of the brain. The pituitary gland is actually two glands: the adenohypophysis and the neurohypophysis. The **neurohypophysis** is a collection of nerve endings of the brain. Its hormones have influence over the kidneys and uterus.

The **adenohypohysis** secretes five different hormones from its glandular cells, which range in effect from the regulation of growth to sexual regulation to thyroid and adrenal regulation.

Thyroid Gland

The **thyroid gland** regulates the metabolism of ingested food substances. Its hormone is **thyroxine.** Located superficial to the skin of the anterior neck, the thyroid gland lies on top of the thyroid cartilage of the larynx; it is a bilobed gland with a rich blood supply. **C cells** are located within the substance of the main gland, which secretes **calcitonin.** These cells help to regulate calcium metabolism, which is important for maintaining health bone structure and muscle function.

Parathyroid Glands

The **parathyroids** are four small round glands found within the substance of the thyroid gland. They are also important for calcium metabolism, and they secrete **parathormone.**

Other Anatomic Features

Pineal Gland (Epiphysis)

The **pineal gland** is actually part of the brain but has a unique histology. Its function is still unclear, but it appears to be important for the regulation of the biorhythms of the body. The pineal gland secretes **melatonin.**

Lymphoid Tissue

Although the **thymus** appears to be a gland, it consists of lymphoid tissue that resembles nodes. The thymus is only present during childhood and involutes at approximately 12 years of age. The thymus is the source of T cell lymphocytes for the body. It is located in the anterior neck, behind the sternum.

Lymphoid tissue that remains in the adult is present in three places in the head and neck and is called the **tonsils**. The tonsils all lie about the end of the oral cavity and beginning of the pharynx. Collectively, they are called the **Waldeyer ring** and are thought to provide a protective shield against foreign substances that enter the respiratory and digestive systems.

The first pair is the **palatine tonsils**, located between the tonsillar pillars of the oropharynx. The **lingual tonsils** are one mass, located on the dorsum of the posterior tongue, or root. They are not usually visible from the oral cavity, and they lie just above the epiglottis. The third pair consists of the **pharyngeal tonsils**. They lie in the nasopharynx, close to the orifices of the tympanic tubes.

Fascia and Spaces (Figures 4-74 to 4-75)

Up to this point the separate organs and muscles of the head and neck have been discussed. Each of these structures is wrapped in a sleeve of connective tissue called **fascia** and separated from each other by **spaces**. Tissue fluid and fat (adipose tissue) in the spaces allows lubrication, so that the various parts can glide past each other.

A few of the major fascias and spaces have been shown in sectional views. They are as follows:

Fascia of the trapezius, SCM, temporal muscles: envelopes these muscles
Middle cervical fascia: envelopes the hyoid muscles
Vertebral fascia: envelopes the cervical vertebrae and its small muscles
Visceral fascia: envelopes the trachea and esophagus/pharynx

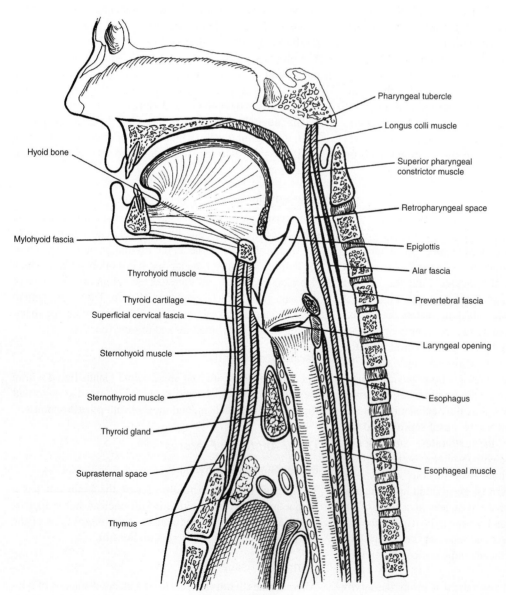

Figure 4-74. SCervical fascia in midsagittal view. (From Hiatt JL, Gartner LP: *Textbook of Head and Neck Anatomy,* 3rd ed. Philadelphia, Lippincott, Williams & Wilkins, 2001.)

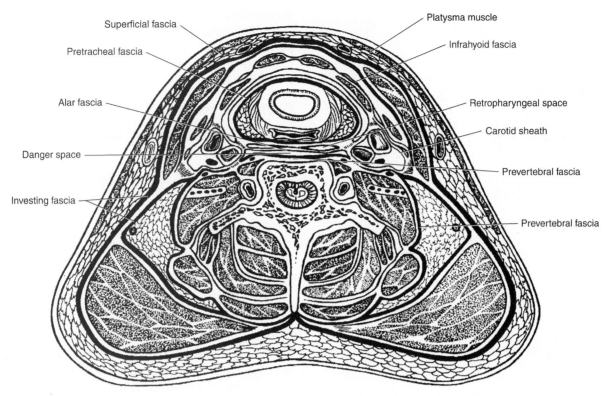

Superficial fascia
Pretracheal fascia
Alar fascia
Danger space
Investing fascia

Platysma muscle
Infrahyoid fascia
Retropharyngeal space
Carotid sheath
Prevertebral fascia
Prevertebral fascia

Figure 4-75. Cervical fascia and spaces. The view is approximately at the level of the seventh cervical vertebra. (From Hiatt JL, Gartner LP: *Textbook of Head and Neck Anatomy,* 3rd ed. Philadelphia, Lippincott, Williams & Wilkins, 2001.)

Parotid, parotideomasseteric fascia: envelopes the parotid gland continuous with the masseteric fascia around the masseter, mandible, and medial pterygoid.

Carotid sheath: envelopes the carotids and internal jugulars, cranial nerves X and XI

Alar fascia: connects the vertebral and visceral fascias

Pterygoid fascia: envelopes medial and lateral pterygoid muscles, attaching to the mandibular border.

The **spaces** created between these fascia are important in the diagnosis, because they become pockets where fluid or exudate may accumulate and swell during the infection and healing process. They may point to the source of the infection or disease process. The major spaces are as follows:

Retropharyngeal space: between the vertebral, alar, and visceral fascias

Temporal space: contains the temporalis muscle

Carotid space: contains major neck vessels

Parotid space: contains the parotid gland, continuous with the masticator space

Buccal space and fat pad: anterior to the parotid gland, a large sac of adipose tissue

Masticator space: contains the masseter, mandible, and medial and lateral pterygoid muscles

Pterygomandibular space: the triangular space around the mandibular foramen and the inferior alveolar nerve between the pterygoids and the sphenomandibular ligament

Submandibular space: below the mylohyoid and above the deep fascia of the skin, contains submandibular salivary glands and nodes

Submental space: the small space under the chin, bordered by the digastrics and the mandible, contains submental lymph nodes

 GENERAL ANATOMY

ELIZABETH WALKER, PhD

Descriptive Terms

The subject is in the **anatomic position**-an erect body position with the arms at the sides and the forearms supinated (palms facing toward the front of the body), except for the pronated right forearm (**Figure 4-76**) Using Figure 4-76, the position of one structure with respect to another in the body can be described. **Superior** (cranial) refers to a structure nearer to the head; **posterior** (synonymous with the term **dorsal**) refers to the back of the body. **Anterior** (synonymous with the term **ventral**) means nearer the front of the body. Note that when the body is in the anatomic position, the **palmar** surface of the hand is anterior to the **dorsal** surface (the back) of the hand. **Inferior (caudal)** means nearer to the feet. Note that the **plantar** surface (i.e., the sole of the foot) is inferior to the **dorsum** (i.e., the top of the foot).

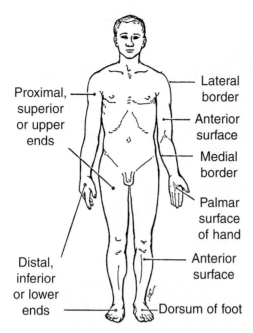

Proximal, superior or upper ends

Lateral border

Anterior surface

Medial border

Palmar surface of hand

Distal, inferior or lower ends

Anterior surface

Dorsum of foot

Figure 4-76. The subject in the anatomic position-except for the right forearm, which is pronated. (From Basmajian JV: Grant's Method of Anatomy, 9th ed. Baltimore, Williams & Wilkins, 1975, xiii.)

Relative positions of structures in the body illustrated in Figure 4-76 are:

superficial: nearer to the surface
deep: farther from the surface
medial: near to the median plane
lateral: farther away from the median plane
proximal: near the trunk or point of origin
distal: farther from the trunk or point of origin

For the purpose of study, the body is shown in a plane or section, which is an imaginary cut through the entire body. The **median plane** is a vertical plane that divides a body into right and left halves **(Figure 4-77)**. A **coronal or frontal plane** is a vertical plane that forms at right angles to the sagittal plane and divides the body into anterior and posterior sections.

Body Cavities

A **sagittal view** is a vertical plane that divides a body into right and left halves. The midsagittal section of the body shows the dorsal cavity, which contains the **central nervous system (CNS)-brain and spinal cord.** These are contained in the **cranial cavity**, which is formed by bones of the skull, and the **vertebral canal**, which is formed by the vertebral column. A ventral cavity has two major spaces-the **thorax** and the **abdominopelvic cavity)**-separated by a large dome-shaped skeletal muscle, the **diaphragm.** The frontal section gives an **anterior view** and shows the thorax divided into the **pericardial cavity**, which surrounds the heart, and two **pleural cavities,** which enclose the lungs. The double line surrounding these cavities indicates that each cavity has a thin lining separating it from the surrounding structures.

Pericardium surrounds the heart; **pleura** surround the lungs. In the abdominopelvic cavity, the lining is called the **peritoneum.** The **abdominopelvic cavity** contains the major part of the **digestive system, urinary system, and reproductive system** (see Figure 4-77).

Skeletal System

Axial Skeleton-Thorax and Vertebral Column

Ribs (12 pairs)

Posteriorly, the ribs articulate with the **bodies** and the **transverse processes** of its corresponding thoracic vertebrae. Anteriorly, the **true ribs** (pairs 1-7) articulate directly with the sternum through the costal cartilages. The **false ribs** (pairs 8-12) attach anteriorly to **costal cartilages** of higher ribs (pairs 8, 9, and 10) or float (pairs 11 and 12). The floating ribs attach only to the vertebral column with no anterior attachment. The ribs curve outward, forward, and then downward to attach to the sternum.

Sternum

The sternum consists of three parts-the **manubrium, body,** and **xiphoid process.** The clavicles of the appendicular skeleton articulate with the upper part of the **manubrium.** The first ribs also articulate with the manubrium. The second ribs articulate with the sternum at the **sternal angle**, the junction between the manubrium and the body of the sternum. Ribs 3 to 7 attach anteriorly to the sternum through the costal cartilages.

Vertebral Column

Developments of the Curvatures of the Vertebral Column. The thoracic and sacral curvatures are primary, and the cervical and lumbar curvatures are secondary **(Figure 4-78)**

Axial Skeleton. Observe the five regions of the vertebral column. Notice the 24 separate vertebrae (cervical, thoracic, lumbar); the sacral segments are fused to form the sacrum. The four coccygeal segments fuse to form the coccyx **(Figure 4-79)**

The vertebral column is part of the axial skeleton. It forms a strong, flexible structure that supports the head, encloses the spinal cord, and in the thorax region provides a posterior articulation for the ribs. Figure 4-79 illustrates the 33 individual vertebrae that make up the spinal column: 7 **cervical**, 12 **thoracic**, 5 **lumbar**, 5 **sacral**, and 4 **coccygeal**. In the sacral region, five fused vertebrae, the **sacrum**, which form a triangular shape that fits between the pelvic bones. The coccygeal vertebrae (i.e., the **coccyx**) consist of four pieces fused together that laymen call the "tail bone."

From a lateral view (see Figure 4-79), four curves are present in the adult. The **two primary concave curves** (i.e., the thoracic and sacral) are present from birth (see Figure 4-78). **Two secondary curves** are present. The cervical curve appears when the baby holds up the head, and the lumbar curve develops when the baby walks at approximately 1 year of age (see Figure 4-78). Defects of the cur-

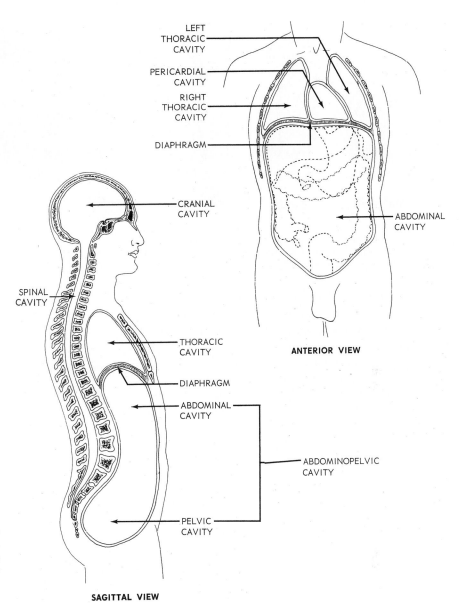

Figure 4-77. A median plane-a vertical plane that divides a body into right and left halves. The midsagittal section of the body shows the *dorsal cavity*-*cranial cavity* and *vertebral canal* and the *ventral cavities*-the *thorax* and the *abdominopelvic cavity*. (From Butterworth BB: Laboratory Anatomy of the Human Body, 4th ed. Dubuque, IA, WB Brown, 1992, p 7.)

vatures fall into three categories: (1) **lordosis** (i.e., an exaggerated lumbar concavity), (2) **scoliosis** (i.e., a lateral curvature of any region, and (3) **kyphosis** (i.e., and exaggerated convexity in the thoracic region).

Nervous System

The **CNS** refers to the brain and spinal cord. The **peripheral nervous system (PNS)** consists of cranial nerves, which originate from the brain (12 pairs), and **spinal nerves** (31 pairs), which originate from the spinal cord. The 31 pairs of spinal nerves consist of 8 pairs of cervical nerves, 12 pairs of thoracic nerves, 5 pairs of lumbar nerves, 5 pairs of sacral nerves, and 1 pair of coccygeal nerves **(Figure 4-80)**.

In addition to the CNS and PNS, the **autonomic nervous system (ANS)** is an efferent system that utilizes both the CNS and the PNS to reach target tissues (i.e. cardiac muscle, smooth muscle, and glands). The two divisions of ANS

are the parasympathetic and the sympathetic. The **parasympathetic** conserves and restores the body's energy in daily activities. An example of parasympathetic innervation is stimulation to the gastrointestinal (GI) tract for digestion. Another example is the stimulation to the heart to maintain a slow rhythm. The **sympathetic** division of the ANS is responsible for expenditure of energy during high-demand "stressful" situations. An example is stimulation to increase the heart rate with exercise or stimulation to open airways with hypoxia. Terminology describing the nervous system follows in **Table 4-8**.

Vertebral Column/Spinal Cord Relationships

The **spinal cord** extends from the **foramen magnum** to the level of the L1 or L2 vertebrae. The 31 pairs of spinal nerves arise from the spinal cord in a segmental manner and exit through the appropriate **intervertebral foramina** (lat-

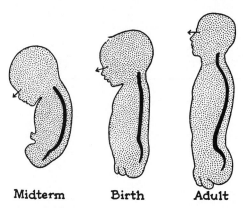

Midterm   Birth   Adult

Figure 4-78. Developments of the curvatures of the vertebral column. The thoracic and sacral curvatures are primary, and the cervical and lumbar are secondary. (From Basmajian JV: Grant's Method of Anatomy, 9th ed. Baltimore, Williams & Wilkins, 1975, p 15.)

eral spaces between the vertebrae). Inferior to the spinal cord at the L1 or L2 vertebral level, the **lumbar and sacral spinal nerve roots** float in the **cerebrospinal fluid (CSF)** of the **subarachnoid space** before exiting through their appropriate intervertebral foramen in the lumbar and sacral region. These nerve roots are called **cauda equina** because they resemble a horse's tail. This area inferior to the spinal cord provides the clinician with a pool of accessible CSF that can be withdrawn without damaging the spinal cord. Only the **cauda equina**, the bundle of spinal nerve roots, are located in this cistern of CSF extending inferiorly into the sacral region. These move away from an aspiration needle without being harmed. This procedure is called a spinal tap, lumbar tap, or lumbar puncture.

Spinal nerves exit from the spinal cord through spaces between the vertebrae, the **intervertebral foramina.** After exiting the intervertebral foramina, the spinal nerves send one branch, the dorsal ramus, to the posterior part of the body (i.e., the area behind the transverse processes of the vertebral column) and one larger branch to the anterolateral part of the body. This is called the ventral ramus or branch and serves a much larger area of the body than the dorsal ramus.

The ventral rami of the spinal nerves form plexuses that serve the neck and the upper and lower extremities. In addition, the ventral rami serve the anterolateral walls of the trunk. In the thoracic region, each ventral ramus (branch) travels along the lower border of the rib with an intercostal artery and vein to form the neurovascular bundle to that rib space. A similar segmental arrangement is present in the abdominal body wall.

Eight pairs of **cervical nerves** exist. Ventral rami of C1 through C4 form the cervical plexus. The phrenic nerves, which are important nerves of the cervical plexus and originate from spinal cord segments C3, C4, and C5, travel through the thorax and pass along the sides of the pericardial sac to innervate the diaphragm. Damage to the cervical spinal cord at the C3 to C5 level can be life threatening, because phrenic nerve supply to the skeletal muscle of the diaphragm is an important part of normal respiration.

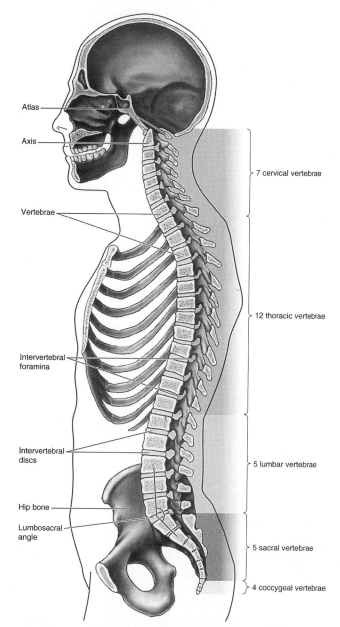

Atlas

Axis

Vertebrae

Intervertebral foramina

Intervertebral discs

Hip bone

Lumbosacral angle

7 cervical vertebrae

12 thoracic vertebrae

5 lumbar vertebrae

5 sacral vertebrae

4 coccygeal vertebrae

Figure 4-79. The axial skeleton. Observe the five regions of the vertebral column. Notice also the 24 separate vertebrae (cervical, thoracic, lumbar) and the fact that the sacral segments are fused to form the sacrum. The four coccygeal segments fuse to form the coccyx. (From Moore KL, Dalley AF: Clinically Oriented Anatomy, 4th ed. Philadelphia, Lippincott Williams & Wilkins, 1999, p 433.)

The spinal cord has enlargements in the cervical and lumbar regions to accommodate the increased number of nerve cell bodies serving the nerves of the **brachial plexus (C5 through T1)** to the upper limb and the nerves of the **lumbosacral plexus (L4-S3)** to the lower limb. The ventral rami of T1 through L5 also innervate the body walls in a segmental pattern (see Figure 4-80).

The strips of skin supplied by the various levels or segments of the spinal cord are called **dermatomes.** In each segment, the **myotome** (the skeletal muscle underlying the dermatome) and the **sclerotome** (bone) are also innervated

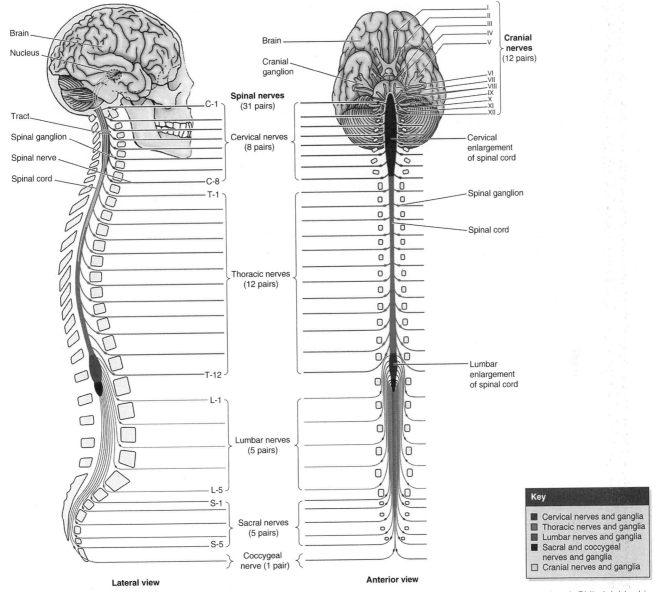

Figure 4-80. Basic organization of the nervous system. (From Moore KL, Dalley AF: Clinically Oriented Anatomy, 4th ed. Philadelphia, Lippincott Williams & Wilkins, 1999, p 40.)

by the same spinal nerve. This permanent relationship between the spinal nerve and the segment is established early in development even when the segment migrates, which occurs in the upper and lower limbs **(Figure 4-81).**

Coverings or **meninges** of the spinal cord inside the vertebral canal are continuous with the coverings of the brain **(Figure 4-82).** The brain and the spinal cord are surrounded by three **meningeal layers.** The **dura mater** is the tough fibrous outermost layer of connective tissue. The two layers of the dura separate to form the **dural venous sinuses,** such as the **superior sagittal sinus.** The **arachnoid,** the delicate web-like meningeal layer, underlies the dura mater. These two layers extend from the superior aspect of the brain inferiorly into the sacral region of the vertebral canal. A space deep to the arachnoid membrane, the **subarachnoid space** contains **CSF.** The CSF surrounds the **brain** and **spinal cord** and provides nourishment and

protection to the **CNS.** The **pia mater,** a delicate vascular membrane, adheres to the surface of brain and spinal cord. The CSF is produced by **choroid plexuses (capillaries)** located in the **ventricle system of the brain.** The CSF passes from the lateral ventricles to the third ventricle to the fourth ventricle and passes out through three small apertures in the fourth ventricle into the **subarachnoid space,** which is located on the outside of the brain and spinal cord. The CSF is returned to the general venous system through **arachnoid granulations** projecting into the **dural venous sinuses.** The **superior sagittal sinus** on the superior aspect of the brain receives most of the CSF.

Brain

In a midsagittal section, the **ventricles** of the brain (lateral, third, and fourth) are observed. The major areas shown are: the

TABLE 4–8 Nervous System Terminology

Afferent	Nerve fiber that carries impulses toward the central nervous system (CNS)
Autonomic Nervous System (ANS)	Sensory neurons that convey information primarily from the viscera and motor neurons that involuntarily influence glands, smooth muscle, and cardiac muscle
Arachnoid	Middle layer of the CNS coverings (attached to the dura mater)
Choroid Plexus	Vascular structures located in the roof of the brain ventricles, which produce cerebrospinal fluid (CSF)
CNS	Overall nervous control center consisting of the brain and spinal cord
Columns	Principal regions of white matter in the spinal cord
Contralateral	On the opposite side
Cranial Nerves	12 pairs of nerves leaving the brain that supply the head and neck and part of the trunk
CSF	Fluid that circulates in the ventricles and the subarachnoid space around the brain and spinal cord
Dura Mater	Tough outermost covering of the brain and spinal cord
Dural Venous Sinuses	Openings within the two layers of the dura mater into which the venous blood of the brain drains, leading to the internal jugular vein
Efferent	Nerve fiber that carries impulses away from the CNS
Ganglia	A group of neuron cell bodies in the peripheral nervous system (PNS)
Glial Cells	Cells in the nervous tissue that function primarily to support and protect neurons
Gray Matter	Region of nonmyelinated nervous tissue
Horns	Principal regions of neuron cell bodies (nuclei) in the spinal cord
Ipsilateral	On the same side of the body
Meninges	Connective tissue coverings that run continuously around the brain and spinal cord
Nerve	A bundle of axons or dendrites with their associated connective tissue in the PNS
Neurons	Cells in nervous tissue that function primarily to conduct electrical impulses
Nucleus	A group of neuron cell bodies in the CNS
Parasympathetic	Relates to the part of the ANS that maintains the normal function of organs
Pia Mater	Thin innermost covering of the brain and spinal cord
PNS	The nerves that carry impulses to and away from the CNS
Somatic Nervous System (SNS)	Motor neurons that voluntarily control skeletal muscle and the sensory neurons that convey information from skeletal muscle in the head, body wall, and extremities.
Sympathetic	The part of the ANS that stimulates organs during stress
Tract	A bundle of nerve fibers (axons or dendrites) in the CNS
Visceral	Pertaining to the organs or their coverings
White Matter	Region of nervous tissue rich in myelinated nerve fibers

cerebrum, midbrain, pons, medulla oblongata, and cerebellum. The **diencephalon** located on both sides of the third ventricle is not shown in this midsagittal section **(Figure 4-83).** (see also Figures 4-57 to 4-60.)

Cerebrum

The cerebrum occupies most of the cranium and is composed of two hemispheres that are separated by the longitudinal fissure. The **cerebral cortex** consists of gray matter (mainly cell bodies and supporting tissue) near the surface of the cerebrum. This mantle of gray matter is organized into **gyri** (folds) and **sulci** (grooves). **White matter of the cerebrum** is found underlying the cerebral cortex. It appears white because of the **myelination** of the nerve fibers. The fibers located in the cerebrum have different destinations: **association fibers** transmit impulses between gyri in same hemisphere; **commissural fibers** transmit impulses to gyri in the other hemisphere; the **corpus callosum** is the major group of commissural fibers between hemispheres; **projection fibers** transmit impulses from the cerebrum to other brain and spinal cord regions.

Functional areas of the cerebral cortex are: **occipital lobes** (primary visual area), **temporal lobes** (primary auditory area), **parietal lobes** (language and association), **postcentral gyri in the parietal lobes** (general sensory area), **precentral gyri in the frontal lobes** (general motor area), and the **frontal lobes** (personality).

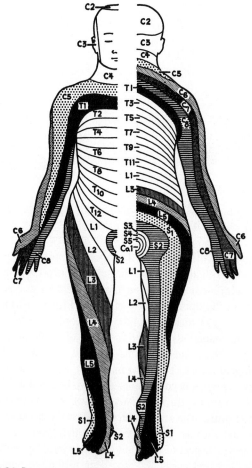

Figure 4-81. Dermatomes. The sensory pattern of the skin reveals the segmental innervation of body. (From Basmajian JV: Grant's Method of Anatomy, 9th ed. Baltimore, Williams & Wilkins, 1975, p 44.)

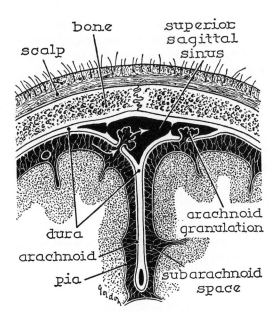

Figure 4-82. The meninges and their relationship to the calvaria (skullcap), brain. (From Basmajian JV: Primary Anatomy, 5th ed. Baltimore, Williams & Wilkins, 1964, p 307.)

Diencephalon

The diencephalon is located in the center of the brain, lateral to the midline third ventricle. It consists of several subdivisions of which the thalamus and hypothalamus are most important. The **thalamus** contains groups of nuclei above the midbrain that relay or interpret sensory impulses ascending from the spinal cord. The **hypothalamus**, which lies between the thalamus and the pituitary gland, controls and integrates the ANS and also connects the CNS with the endocrine system. The hypothalamus controls body temperature, hunger, and thirst.

The **limbic system** refers to a group of structures in the deep part of the cerebrum and diencephalon with primary function in emotions such as pain, pleasure, anger, rage, fear, sorrow, sexual feelings, docility, and affection. This system is also involved in memory formation.

Brain Stem

The parts of the brain stem are the **medulla oblongata,** the **pons,** and the **midbrain.** This area of the brain regulates visceral activity of the body. One of its most important functions is that it houses the reticular activating system (RAS), which is involved in maintaining consciousness and the sleep cycle.

Midbrain

The **midbrain** extends from the base of the diencephalon to the pons. The **cerebral peduncles** contain motor fibers that connect the cerebral cortex to the pons and spinal cord as well as sensory fibers, which connect the spinal cord to the thalamus. The **colliculi,** reflex centers for the eye, head, and trunk movements in response to visual and auditory stimuli, are located on the dorsal aspect of the midbrain.

Pons

The **pons** is located above the medulla and in front of the cerebellum. The name pons means bridge, and it serves to

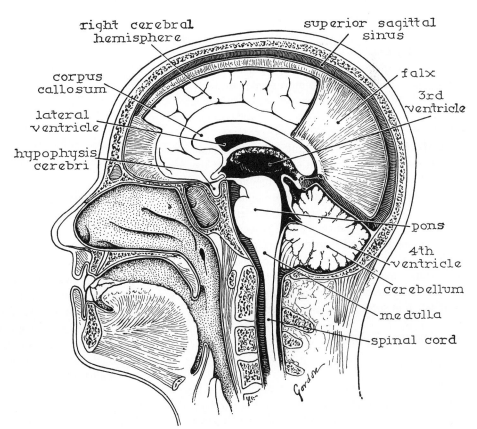

Figure 4-83. Midsagittal section of the brain. (From Basmajian JV: Primary Anatomy, 5th ed. Baltimore, Williams & Wilkins, 1964.)

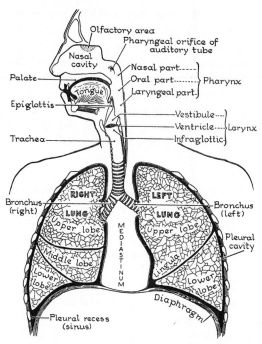

Figure 4-84. Diagram of the respiratory system. (From Basmajian JV: Grant's Method of Anatomy, 9th ed. Baltimore, Williams & Wilkins, 1975, p 297.)

send relay to nerve fibers to the cerebellum, as well as CNS structures superior and inferior to the pons. It also contains the part of the respiratory center that controls breathing.

Medulla Oblongata

The **medulla oblongata** is continuous with the spinal cord. The pyramids, which constitute a prominent feature of the medulla, are located on the ventral surface near the midline. They represent the decussation (crossing over) of the motor pathway that controls voluntary movement in the body. This tract is called the lateral corticospinal or pyramidal tract.

Cerebellum

The **cerebellum** is sometimes called the "little brain," because it shows an organization similar to that of the cerebrum. The gray matter is situated on the outside; the **cerebellar cortex** with the white matter underlies the gray matter. As in the cerebrum, cerebellar nuclei are embedded in this white matter. The cerebellum is located behind the **pons and medulla** and below the **occipital lobes** of the **cerebrum.** It is concerned with subconscious skeletal movements required for coordination, balance, and posture maintenance. Cerebellar damage manifests itself as loss of coordination in speech, gait, and movement.

Respiratory System

Bronchial Tree

The **trachea** is approximately 12 cm long, located in front of the esophagus, and contains C-shaped hyaline cartilage rings that prevent its collapse. At the level of the T4 vertebra, the trachea divides into left and right primary bronchi; these

bronchi enter the left and right lung at the **hilus** or root of the lung. The right primary bronchus has a larger diameter compared with the left primary bronchus and comes off almost in a straight line from the trachea. The clinical significance of this is that any small object that enters the bronchial tree will probably enter the right bronchus instead of the left bronchus. Inside the lungs, the two main bronchi branch into secondary (lobar) bronchi to the lobes. The right lung has three lobes: superior, middle, and inferior. The left lung has two lobes: superior and inferior (**Figure 4-84**).

Pleurae and Lungs

Each lung is invested by a serous membrane, which is arranged like a closed sac called the **pleura** and which is invaginated by the lung like a fist invaginating an underinflated balloon. The visceral pleura adhere to the surface of the lung, whereas the parietal pleura attach to the thoracic wall. Normally, the lung is inflated, filling the entire thoracic space; the parietal and visceral layers of pleura are separated only by the pleural cavity. This cavity is a potential space, which is only large when the lung has collapsed. The visceral pleura reflect off the lung onto the thoracic wall at the hilus. In this area, the main bronchi, the pulmonary arteries, and pulmonary veins enter the lung.

Pulmonary Circulation

The pulmonary trunk from the right ventricle of the heart divides into right and left pulmonary arteries, which transport poorly oxygenated blood to the lungs. The pulmonary arteries subdivide into lobar and segmental arteries within the lungs. After passing through the pulmonary capillaries where gas exchange (O_2 and CO_2) occurs, the blood drains into the pulmonary veins, which return the well-oxygenated blood to the left atrium of the heart. These vessels of the root of the lung enter and leave the lung at the hilum. An artery is defined as a blood vessel that carries blood away from the heart, whereas a vein carries blood back to the heart. The pulmonary circulation is one of the few cases in which the artery contains deoxygenated blood and the vein contains oxygenated blood.

Circulatory System

Heart

The heart, which is located behind the sternum, is enclosed in the **pericardial sac** and is the size of a human fist. The **apex of the heart** points down and to the left and is located in a space between the lungs in the thoracic cavity known as the **mediastinum.** The heart consists of four chambers: two **atria** and two **ventricles.** The atria are the receiving chambers and have a thinner wall, whereas the ventricles are the pumping chambers and have thick walls. The heart serves as a double pump that moves blood to the lungs from the right ventricle (pulmonary circulation) or to the body from the left ventricle (systemic circulation).

After the pericardial sac is opened, the great vessels of the heart can be observed. From right to left, they are: the **supe-**

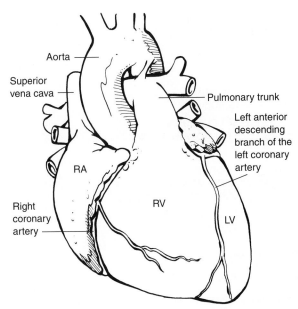

Figure 4-85. Anterior view of the heart showing the chambers, the great vessels, and the coronary arteries. (From Abeloff D: Medical ARt Graphics for Use. Baltimore, Williams & Wilkins, 1982, p 4.5.)

rior vena cava (returns venous blood from the body above the diaphragm to the right atrium), the **aorta** (arising from the left ventricle), and the **pulmonary trunk** (arising from the right ventricle). The left anterior descending (LAD) branch of the **left coronary artery** lies on the anterior interventricular wall (between the right and left ventricle). The **right coronary artery** is located in a groove between the right atrium and the right ventricle. These arteries supply oxygenated blood to the myocardium (heart muscle). Occlusion of these arteries is clinically associated with heart disease, such as myocardial infarction (heart attack). Anastomoses of branches of the coronary arteries provide collateral circulation to the heart wall in case of blockage of one vessel **(Figure 4-85)**.

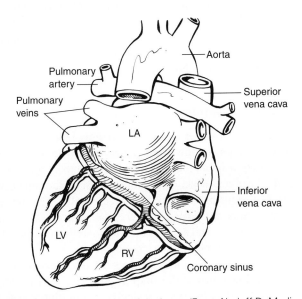

Figure 4-86. Posterior aspect of the heart. (From Abeloff D: Medical ARt Graphics for Use. Baltimore, Williams & Wilkins, 1982, p 4.5.)

The **left atrium** is the thin-walled chamber that lies completely on the posterior aspect of the heart. It can be recognized by the four **pulmonary veins** that enter it (two from the right lung and two from the left lung). Separating the left atrium from the left ventricle is the **coronary sulcus (groove)**, which contains a large vein that drains venous blood away from the heart. This vein, the **coronary sinus**, opens into the right atrium; so too does the **superior vena cava**, which returns venous blood from the upper part of the body (above the diaphragm), and the **inferior vena cava**, which returns venous blood from the lower part of the body (below the diaphragm) **(Figure 4-86)**.

The heart wall consists of three layers from superficial to deep-**epicardium, myocardium** (cardiac muscle), and **endocardium**, a smooth continuous covering lining the valves and chambers. Valves of the heart are unique. **Atrioventricular (AV) valves** are composed of tough, fibrous tissue; these valves remain open except when the ventricles contract. The AV valves hang into the ventricles like leaves and are held in place by **chordae tendineae** at the edge of the valves, which are attached to **papillary muscles**-extensions from the ventricle walls. The **tricuspid AV valve** on the right side has three flaps. The **bicuspid AV valve (mitral valve)** has two flaps. The **semilunar (SL) valves**, which are located at the point where the **great arteries, pulmonary trunk, and aorta** exit from the ventricles, remain closed until the ventricles contract. The **pulmonary SL valve** is located on the right, and the **aortic SL valve** is located on the left **(Figure 4-87)**.

Circulation Through The Heart

The left side of the heart serves the body. The left ventricle (part of the systemic circulation) pumps oxygenated blood to the body through the aorta, the largest artery in the body. Use Figure 4-96 to review the circulation of blood through the pulmonary circulation and the heart to the aorta. Use blue arrows to indicate the path of deoxygenated blood and the color red to indicate oxygenated blood in Figure 4-87.

Systemic Circulation

The **aorta** arises from the left ventricle and is considered in three parts: the ascending, the arch of the aorta, and the descending aorta in the thorax and abdomen. The **aorta** ends by bifurcating at the vertebral level L4 into the **common iliac arteries**. The **venae cavae** enter the right atrium. The **superior vena cava** receives venous blood from the entire body above the diaphragm. The **inferior vena cava** receives all the venous blood from the body below the diaphragm **(Figure 4-88)**.

Arterial Circulation
Ascending Aorta

The ascending aorta arises from the left ventricle. Immediately distal to the aortic valves, the coronary arteries are given off to the walls of the heart.

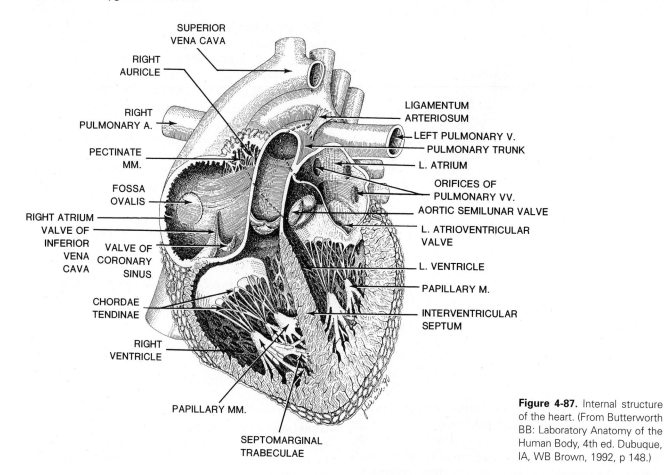

Figure 4-87. Internal structure of the heart. (From Butterworth BB: Laboratory Anatomy of the Human Body, 4th ed. Dubuque, IA, WB Brown, 1992, p 148.)

Arch of the Aorta

The aorta arches to the left and gives rise to three major trunks in this order: (1) the **brachiocephalic artery**, which provides arterial blood to the right head and neck via the right common carotid artery and the right upper limb via the right subclavian artery; (2) the **left common carotid artery**, which distributes blood to the left side of the head and neck; and (3) the **left subclavian artery** to the left upper limb.

Descending Aorta

This portion of the aorta extends through the **posterior mediastinum** of the thorax. The **thoracic branches** are **posterior intercostal arteries** that supply the rib spaces; **bronchial arteries** that travel along the outside of the bronchial tree, carrying oxygenated blood to the lungs; and **esophageal arteries** that supply the esophagus.

Abdominal Branches of the Aorta

The aorta has three types of abdominal branches: (1) paired arteries (to the body wall), (2) unpaired arteries (to the GI tract), and (3) paired arteries (to the glands).

The paired arteries (to the body wall) are: the inferior **phrenic arteries** to the diaphragm and the **lumbar arteries** to the body wall, which are arranged in a segmental pattern.

The unpaired arteries (to the GI tract) are: the **celiac artery**, which supplies the upper one third of the GI tract (i.e., the stomach, liver, and half of the duodenum) and the spleen (which is a lymphoid organ that develops in this area of the

abdomen on the left side behind the stomach); the **superior mesenteric artery**, which distributes to the middle third of the GI tract (i.e., half of the duodenum, jejunum, and ileum of the small intestines), pancreas, and part of the large intestine (i.e., the ascending colon and two thirds of the transverse colon); and the **inferior mesenteric artery**, which supplies arterial blood to the rest of the large intestines (e.g., the distal third of the transverse colon, the descending colon, the sigmoid colon, and the upper rectum) **(Figure 4-89)**.

Paired arteries (to the glands) are: the **renal arteries** to the kidneys arising from the sides of the aorta at vertebral level L2, the **middle suprarenal arteries** to the suprarenal glands, and the **gonadal arteries** to the testes and ovaries.

Venous Circulation

The superior vena cava receives venous blood from the entire body above the diaphragm. Its tributaries are the **left and right brachiocephalic veins** from the upper limbs and the head and neck. In addition, the superior vena cava receives venous blood from the thoracic walls. The **azygos system** drains the posterior intercostal veins of the body wall in the thorax and empties into the superior vena cava by arching over the root of the right lung.

The inferior vena cava receives all the venous blood from the body below the diaphragm. The inferior vena cava is formed by the right and left **common iliac veins.** It ascends on the right side of the vertebral body, posterior to

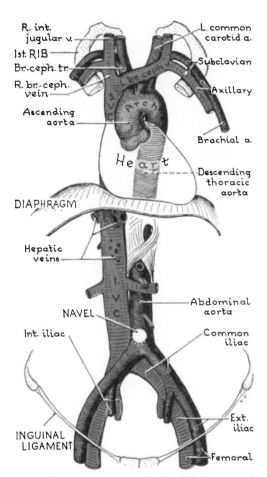

Figure 4-88. The great arteries and veins of the systemic circuit. (From Basmajian JV: Grant's Method of Anatomy, 9th ed. Baltimore, Williams & Wilkins, 1975, p 32.)

the liver, and passes through an opening in the diaphragm to empty into the right atrium. The inferior vena cava receives numerous tributaries along its pathway: **gonadal veins** (from the testes and ovaries), **renal veins** (from the kidneys), **posterior abdominal veins** (from the posterior abdominal wall), **suprarenal veins** (from the suprarenal or adrenal glands), and **phrenic veins** (from the diaphragm) and the **hepatic portal system**.

Hepatic Portal System

The **portal vein** is formed by the union of the **splenic vein** with the **superior mesenteric vein** and the **inferior mesenteric vein**.

This venous system is responsible for draining blood from the GI tract and the spleen, through the liver sinusoids for the purpose of depositing nutrients and cleaning the blood before it enters the inferior vena cava on the posterior surface of the liver. The **superior mesenteric vein** drains venous blood from the stomach, small intestines, and ascending colon. The **inferior mesenteric vein** drains venous blood from the descending colon and the upper rectum. The **splenic vein** drains blood from the spleen **(Figure 4-90)**.

Portal Hypertension

When the portal circulation becomes obstructed (e.g., liver disease), blood from the GI tract is diverted away from the portal venous system to the inferior vena cava through the collateral venous circulation. Clinical manifestations such as bleeding and enlarged veins are seen in areas where there are portocaval anastomoses, such as the esophagus (esophageal bleeding), the paraumbilical veins (enlarged superficial veins around the umbilicus), and the anorectal area (hemorrhoids).

Lymphatic System

The lymphatic system consists of lymphatic vessels and lymph nodes. It functions to return tissue fluid to the venous system and to help protect the body from disease. The lymphatic system is closely related to the circulatory system because the small fragile lymphatic vessels and lymph nodes lie on the outside of veins. The main differences in the lymphatic system compared with the circulatory system are that the flow of lymph is only in one direction (back toward the heart) and the lymphatic system is open to the interstitial spaces of the body. The lymphatic capillaries are open on one end where they collect excess interstitial (tissue) fluid from the periphery of the body. The possibility then arises of aberrant (e.g., cancer) cells entering the lymphatic system from the interstitial spaces of the body. Lymph is filtered through

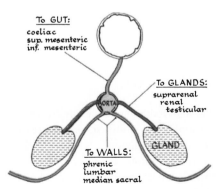

Figure 4-89. Abdominal aorta: Three types of branches.(From Anderson JE: Grant's Atlas of Anatomy, 8th ed. Baltimore, Williams & Wilkins, 1983.)

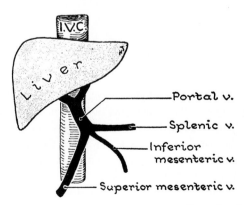

Figure 4-90. The hepatic portal system. (From Basmajian JV: Grant's Method of Anatomy, 9th ed. Baltimore, Williams & Wilkins, 1975, p 208.)

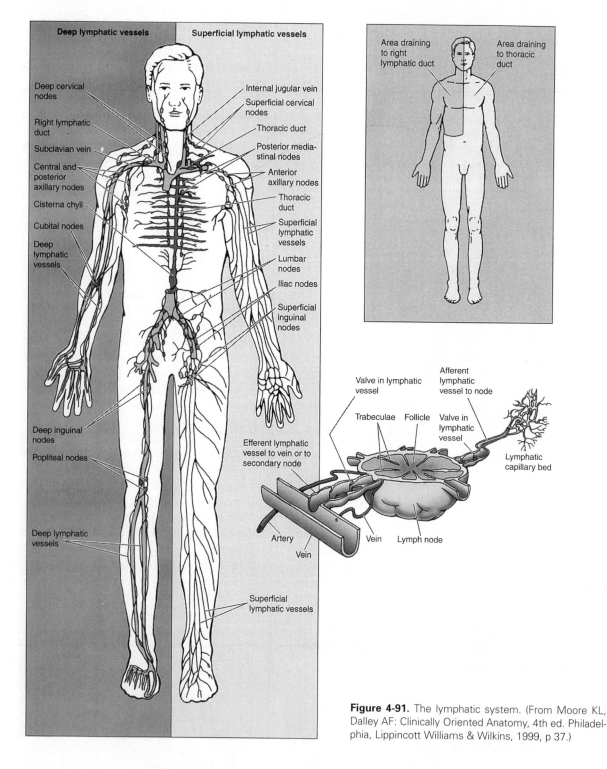

Figure 4-91. The lymphatic system. (From Moore KL, Dalley AF: Clinically Oriented Anatomy, 4th ed. Philadelphia, Lippincott Williams & Wilkins, 1999, p 37.)

lymph nodes, which are kidney-shaped structures along the lymphatic vessels that contain the body's defensive cells located in lymphoid follicles (i.e., spherical masses of lymphoid cells in the lymph nodes). Near the heart, the largest lymphatic vessels drain into the subclavian veins. The **right lymphatic duct** drains lymph from the right side of the head and neck, the right upper limb and the pectoral region, and the right half of the thorax. The **thoracic duct** drains lymph from the remainder of the body (**Figure 4-91**).

Digestive System

In the thorax and abdominopelvic cavity, the gut tube consists of the **esophagus, stomach, small intestines** (i.e., the **duodenum, jejunum, ileum**), **large intestines** (i.e., the **cecum, ascending colon, transverse colon, descending colon, sigmoid colon**) the **rectum,** and the **anus.** Accessory organs have ducts that secrete into the gut tube. The liver produces **bile** (for fat digestion), which is stored in the

gallbladder and secreted to the duodenum through the **common bile duct**. The pancreas secretes pancreatic juice through the **main and accessory pancreatic ducts**, which also enter the duodenum. Although the spleen is shown with the digestive system, it is a lymphoid organ and is not part of the digestive system (**Figure 4-92**).

Figure 4-93 illustrates the major features of the developing gut tube. The **peritoneum** is the serosal membrane of the abdominal cavity. The disposition of the peritoneum is similar to that of the serosal layers around the heart (i.e., the pericardium) and lungs (pleura). Peritoneum attached to the body wall is parietal. It reflects on to the outer wall of the viscera to become visceral peritoneum. The larger part of the gut tube is suspended in the peritoneal cavity. Peritoneal layers that suspend organs are called **mesenteries**. Vessels and nerves to the intestines and stomach travel in the mesenteries. The source vessels such as the abdominal aorta are **retroperitoneal**.

Structures behind the parietal peritoneum are retroperitoneal (still in the abdominal cavity but not suspended in the peritoneal cavity). The retroperitoneal organs of the posterior abdominal wall are the aorta (left), the inferior vena cava (right), the kidneys, and the suprarenal gland. Other retroperitoneal organs not shown are part of the duodenum, the pancreas, and the ascending and descending colon (**Figure 4-94**).

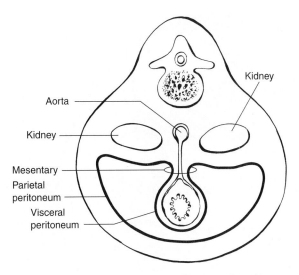

Figure 4-93. Cross-section of the developing digestive system. (From Tweiltmeyer A, McCracken T: Coloring Guide to Regional Human Anatomy, 2nd ed. Lea & Febiger, 1992, p 89.)

The gut tube usually has four layers, although each region has some specializations that reflect function. The **mucous coat** consists of the epithelial lining, underlying connective tissue called lamina propria, and a thin layer of smooth muscle, the muscularis mucosae. Lymphoid nodules may be located in the lamina propria and the submucosa. The **submucosal coat** underlying the mucosa contains glands and the **Meissner plexus**, which consists of autonomic nerves and cell bodies (sympathetic and parasympathetic) that reg-

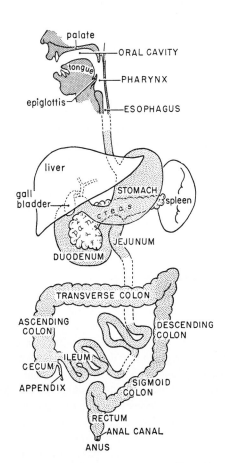

Figure 4-92. Diagram of the Digestive System. (From Basmajian JV: Grant's Method of Anatomy, 9th ed. Baltimore, Williams & Wilkins, 1975, p 53.)

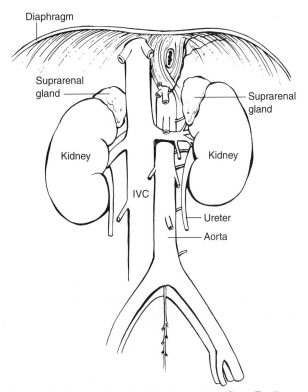

Figure 4-94. Retroperitoneal abdominal organs. (From Tweiltmeyer A, McCracken T: Coloring Guide to Regional Human Anatomy, 2nd ed. Lea & Febiger, 1992, p 89.)

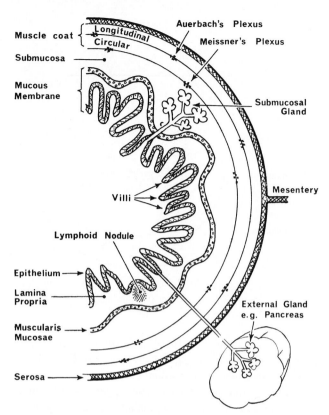

Figure 4-95. Basic histologic plan of the gut tube. (From Cruickshank B, Dodds TC, Gardner DL: Human Histology, 2nd ed. Baltimore, Williams & Wilkins, 1969, p 95.)

ulate secretion from the submucosal glands. The **muscular coat** usually consists of two layers of smooth muscle. The **Auerbach plexus** (autonomic nerve and cell bodies) is located between the layers of smooth muscle for regulation of smooth muscle contraction (peristalsis). In most parts of the digestive system, the inner layer is circular and the outer layer is longitudinal in orientation. The stomach, however, has an extra oblique layer to aid the mechanical breakdown of the food, and the large intestine has an incomplete longitudinal layer. The **serous coat,** which is also the visceral peritoneum, is continuous with the mesentery.

The muscular layer in the esophagus moves the bolus along to the stomach by peristaltic contractions. In the stomach, the bolus is treated by mechanical and chemical digestion, then it is passed into the highly coiled small intestines for more enzymatic and mechanical digestive processes. Small molecular nutrients are extracted, absorbed by lining cells, and transferred to capillaries. Liver-produced bile stored in the gallbladder is discharged into the duodenum by bile ducts. Digestive enzymes from the pancreas enter the duodenum as well. The large intestine is mainly concerned with the absorption of water, minerals, and certain vitamins. The residue of the ingested bolus is moved through the rectum and anal canal to the outside. Nutrients absorbed through the tract are transported to the liver by the hepatic portal system for processing and distribution to the body's cells **(Figure 4-95)**.

Urinary System

The paired **kidneys** and **ureters** lie posterior to the parietal peritoneum (retroperitoneal) of the abdominal cavity on either side of the vertebral column (see Figure 4-103). The kidneys are encased in pararenal fat, secured by an outer, stronger layer (renal fascia), and then packed in pararenal fat. These layers of fat, fascia, and fat provide protection for the kidneys and secure them against vibration or injury from impact.

The renal artery and vein and the ureter enter the kidney at the **hilus.** Renal circulation is the renal artery to the interlobar artery to the arcuate artery to the afferent arteriole to the **glomerulus** to the efferent arterioles to the secondary capillary network to the interlobular vein to the arcuate vein to the interlobar vein to the renal vein. The **glomerulus**, in association with the **Bowman (glomerular) capsule** of a nephron, forms the filtering apparatus of the kidney-the **renal corpuscle.** The **nephron** is the functional unit of the kidney, which consists of the filtering apparatus and tubules. The kidney contains approximately 1 million nephrons. Renal corpuscles are located in the outer part of the kidney, the **cortex.** The kidney tubules are found in the cortex and in the inner part of the kidney, called the **medulla.** The medulla is organized into pyramids. The apex of each pyramid projects into a **minor calyx,** which is a cup-shaped funnel that receives the concentrated urine. These funnels, which number 8 to 18, open into three much larger **major calyces**-all of which open into the renal pelvis. At the hilus of the kidney, the renal pelvis narrows to form the ureter, which travels retroperitineally to the urinary **bladder (Figure 4-96).**

The urinary bladder lies behind the symphysis pubis in the true pelvis. It serves as a reservoir for urine and can hold as much as 1 L. The urinary bladder is lined by transitional epithelium, which allows distention of the organ without injury. The mucosal area between the two urethral openings and the urethra is called the **trigone.** The smooth muscle in this area, the detrusor muscle, controls the amount of urine in the bladder. The male urethra consists of three parts (i.e., **prostatic, membranous,** and **spongy)** and is longer (~20 cm) than the female urethra (~4 cm) **(Figure 4-97).**

Reproductive System

In the male, the prostate gland and the penis are used both by the urinary system and the reproductive system. The **prostatic urethra** receives urine from the urinary bladder, sperm from the ejaculatory ducts, seminal fluid from the **seminal vesicles,** and secretion from the prostate via several ducts. Reflex contraction of the bladder neck muscles prevent contraction and prevent voiding of urine during the expulsion of semen. The urethra continues through the prostate gland, the urogenital diaphragm (membranous urethra), and the penis (penile or spongy urethra). The penis consists of three bodies of erectile tissue. The two dorsal bodies, the **corpora cavernosa,** are anchored to the pubic rami. The ventral **corpus spongiosum** widens out posteri-

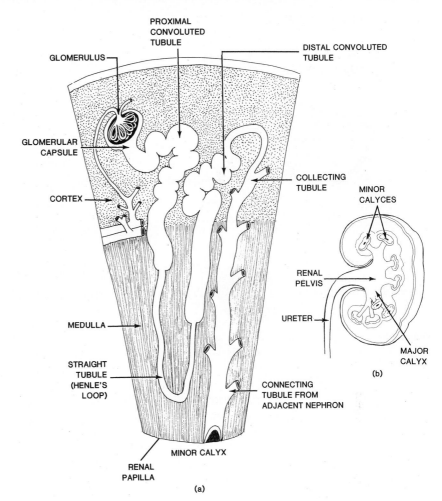

Figure 4-96. A nephron and its relationship to cortex and the medulla. The left kidney is sectioned. (From Butterworth BB: Laboratory Anatomy of the Human Body, 4th ed. Dubuque, IA, WB Brown, 1992, p 168.)

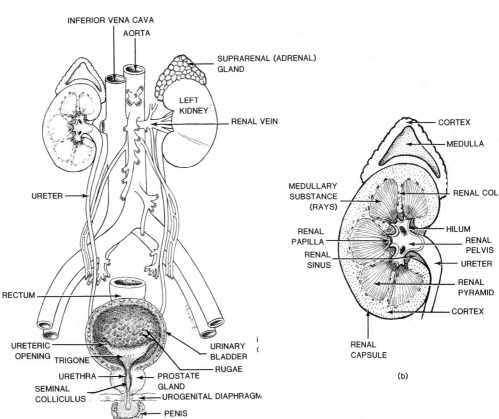

Figure 4-97. The urinary organs and the right kidney (midsagittal section). (From Butterworth BB: Laboratory Anatomy of the Human Body, 4th ed. Dubuque, IA, WB Brown, 1992, p 167.)

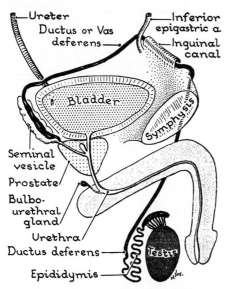

Figure 4-98. Diagram of the male pelvis and perineum. (From Basmajian JV: Grant's Method of Anatomy, 9th ed. Baltimore, Williams & Wilkins, 1975, p 186.)

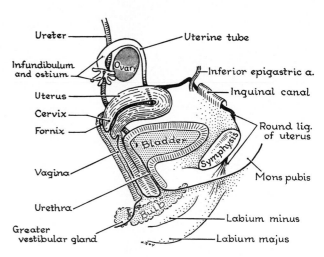

Figure 4-99. Female reproductive system shown in the median section of the pelvis and perineum. (From Basmajian JV: Grant's Method of Anatomy, 9th ed. Baltimore, Williams & Wilkins, 1975, p 66.)

orly into the bulb of the penis and anteriorly into the glans penis. The penile urethra is located in the corpus spongiosum. The testes are located in the scrotal sacs outside the body cavity in order to maintain the optimal temperature (lower than body temperature) for sperm production. Spermatozoa are produced in the **seminiferous tubules** of the testes; stored in the **epididymis**; and transported through the ductus (vas) deferens to the posterior wall of the prostate gland, where sperm enters the ejaculatory duct that leads to the prostatic urethra. **Figure 4-98** is a schematic diagram that shows all structures of the male reproductive system. The bladder, prostate gland, and penis are accurately shown and described as midline structures. However, only one testis, the ductus deferens, seminal vesicle, and ejaculatory duct are shown, although these bilateral structures are present on both the left and right sides of the body.

The female reproductive organs consist of paired ovaries and uterine tubes, an unpaired uterus, and a vagina. The primary organ of the female reproductive system is the **ovary,** which produces the female germ cell (ova). Each month during the time of ovulation, an ovum ruptures through the surface of the ovary. This ovum is picked up by the fimbriae of the uterine tube and is transported to the cavity of the uterus for implantation (if fertilized) or for passing out of the body through the vagina (if not fertilized). The uterus is normally tipped forward at right angles to the vagina and lies over the superior aspect of the urinary bladder.

The external genitalia are located in the **perineum.** The labia majora are fat filled folds of skin surrounding the space called the vestibule, which contains urethral and vaginal openings. Inside the labia majora, the labia minora (smaller folds) run anteriorly to the clitoris. The **clitoris** has an erectile structure homologous to the penis. The two crura are anchored onto the ischiopubic rami and anteriorly form the body of the clitoris. The **glans** caps the body of the clitoris. The vestibu-

lar bulbs lateral to the labia minora are homologous to the bulb of the penis. The main difference is that in the female there are two midline openings-the urethra and the vagina. In the male, the urethra, which serves both the urinary and reproductive systems, is enclosed in the corpus spongiosum and opens through the glans penis to the outside (**Figure 4-99**).

Suggested Sources

Histology

Avery JK: Oral Development and Histology. New York, Thieme Medical Publishers, 1994.

Bath-Balogh M, Fehrenbach MJ: Illustrated Dental Embryology, Histology, and Anatomy. Philadelphia, WB Saunders, 1997.

Dudek RW, Fix JD: Embryology. Baltimore, Williams & Wilkins, 1998.

Gartner LP, Hiatt JL, Strum JM: Cell Biology and Histology. Baltimore, Williams & Wilkins, 1998.

http://wberesford.hsc.wvu.edu

http://histologyatlas.com

Melfi RC, Alley KE: Permar's Oral Embryology and Microscopic Anatomy. Philadelphia, Lippincott Williams & Wilkins, 2000.

Riviere HL: Normal Oral Histology. Chicago, Quintessence Publishing Co., 2000.

Ross MH, Romrell LJ, Kaye GI: Histology: A Text and Atlas. Baltimore, Williams & Wilkins, 1995.

Smith SK, Karst NS: Head and Neck Histology and Anatomy. East Norwalk, CT, Appleton & Lange, 1999.

Dental Anatomy

Bath-Balogh M, Fehrenbach MJ: Illustrated Dental Embryology, Histology, and Anatomy. Philadelphia, WB Saunders, 1997.

Karst NS, Smith SK: Dental Anatomy: A Self-Instructional Program. East Norwalk, CT, Appleton & Lange, 1998.

Woelfel JB, Scheid RC: Dental Anatomy: Its Relevance to Dentistry. Baltimore, Williams & Wilkins, 1997.

Head and Neck Anatomy

Fehrenbach MJ, Herring SW: Illustrated Anatomy of the Head and Neck. Philadelphia, WB Saunders, 1996.

Hiatt JL, Gartner LP: Textbook of Head and Neck Anatomy, 3rd ed. Philadelphia, Lippincott Williams & Wilkins, 2001.

Smith SK, Karst NS: Head and Neck Histology and Anatomy. East Norwalk, CT, Appleton & Lange, 1999.

General Anatomy

Abeloff D: Medical Art Graphics for Use. Baltimore, Williams & Wilkins, 1982.

Anderson JE: Grant's Atlas of Anatomy, 8th ed. Baltimore, Williams & Wilkins, 1983.

Basmajian JV: Grant's Method of Anatomy, 9th ed. Baltimore, Williams & Wilkiins, 1975.

Basmajian JV: Primary Anatomy, 5th ed. Baltimore, Williams & Wilkins, 1964.

Butterworth BB: Laboratory Anatomy of the Human Body, 4th ed. Dubuque, IA, WB Brown, 1992.

Guy J: Learning Human Anatomy. East Norwalk, CT, Appleton & Lange, 1998.

Mathers LH, Chase RA, Dolph J, et al: Clinical Anatomy Principles. St. Louis, CV Mosby, 1996.

Moore KL, Dalley AF: Clinically Oriented Anatomy, 4th ed. Philadelphia, Lippincott Williams & Wilkins, 1999.

Olson TR: A.D.A.M. Student Atlas of Anatomy. Baltimore, Williams & Wilkins, 1996.

The Anatomy Lab-Human Anatomy Laboratory and Tutorial CD-ROM. (614) 470-3123

Tweiltmeyer A, McCracken T: Coloring Guide to Regional Human Anatomy, 2nd ed. Baltimore, Lea & Febiger, 1992.

Questions and Answers

Questions

Histology

1. Odontoblasts are responsible for the formation of which one of the following structures?
   A. Cementum
   B. Enamel
   C. Dentin
   D. Periodontal ligament

2. The type of epithelium associated with the vermillion border of the lip is:
   A. stratified squamous nonkeratinized.
   B. pseudostratified ciliated columnar.
   C. stratified squamous keratinized.
   D. stratified cuboidal.

3. Which of the following statements concerning the principal bundles of the periodontal ligament is true?
   A. They are composed of elastin.
   B. They consist of collagen.
   C. They extend from the cementum to the enamel.
   D. They extend from one tooth to the next tooth.

4. Which of the following statements regarding osteoclasts is true?
   A. They are enucleated cells.
   B. They produce collagen.
   C. They occupy Howship lacunae.
   D. They are derived from osteoprogenitor cells.

5. Which of the following cells arise from monocytes?
   A. Plasma cells
   B. Fibroblasts
   C. Lymphocytes
   D. Macrophages

6. Which of the following cells is under voluntary control?
   A. Skeletal muscle cells
   B. Smooth muscle cells
   C. Cardiac muscle cells
   D. Myoepithelial cells

7. Myelination of peripheral nerves is accomplished by:
   A. astrocytes.
   B. oligodendrocytes.
   C. Schwann cells.
   D. neural crest cells.
   E. basket cells.

8. Which of the following cells possess specific granules?
   A. Monocytes
   B. Lymphocytes
   C. Thrombocytes
   D. Basophils

9. The intermaxillary segment forms by the fusion of the:
   A. maxillary prominences.
   B. mandibular prominences.
   C. palatine shelves.
   D. lateral nasal prominences.
   E. medial nasal prominences.

10. The number of roots that a tooth will possess is determined by:
    A. junctional epithelium.
    B. epithelial rests of Malassez.
    C. Tomes granular layer.
    D. Hertwig root sheath.

11. The last enamel layer that becomes mineralized and is produced by ameloblasts is the:
    A. primary enamel cuticle.
    B. secondary enamel cuticle.
    C. outer enamel epithelium.
    D. inner enamel epithelium.

12. Weakened areas of mineralized enamel that extend from the DEJ a short distance into the enamel are referred to as enamel
    A. spindles.
    B. tufts.
    C. lamellae.
    D. prisms.

13. Acellular cementum is found at which of the following root locations?
    A. Cervical third
    B. Middle third
    C. Apical third

14. The most common relationship of cementum to enamel is:
    A. cementum does not meet enamel.
    B. cementum just meets enamel.
    C. cementum overlaps enamel.
    D. enamel overlaps cementum.

15. Which of the principal fibers of the periodontal ligament receive the majority of masticatory stress?
    A. Transseptal
    B. Oblique
    C. Horizontal
    D. Apical
    E. Alveolar crestal

16. The gingival attachment epithelium consists of the:
    A. sulcular epithelium and the basement membrane.
    B. sulcular epithelium and junctional epithelium.
    C. free gingival fibers and the lamina propria.
    D. lamina dura and the alveolar mucosa.

17. The epithelial transition separating the lining type of alveolar mucosa from the masticatory gingival mucosa is known as the:
    A. vestibule.
    B. zone of attached gingiva.
    C. submucosal plexus.
    D. mucogingival junction.

18. The most numerous papillae on the tongue are the:
    A. lingual.   D. fungiform.
    B. folate.   E. circumvallate.
    C. filiform.

19. The parotid gland consists of which of the following secretory units?
    A. Mucous
    B. Serous
    C. Mixed

20. Odontogenesis begins at approximately _____ weeks in utero.
    A. 3   C. 9
    B. 6   D. 12

Dental Anatomy

21. What name is given to the enamel elevations that form the mesial and distal borders of the occlusal surface of a tooth?
    A. Oblique ridge
    B. Transverse ridge
    C. Marginal ridge
    D. Triangular ridge

22. Which of the following teeth guide protrusive mandibular movement?
    A. Working cusps of molars
    B. Buccal cusps of premolars
    C. Canines
    D. Incisors

23. What name is given to the disturbance to intra-arch alignment in which a tooth is rotated from its usual position?
    A. Torsoversion
    B. Supraversion
    C. Facial version
    D. Mesial version

24. In centric occlusion, the mesiobuccal cusp of tooth No. 3 is in the facial embrasure between tooth No. 30 and tooth No. 31. What is the classification for this malocclusion?
    A. Normal   C. II
    B. I   D. III

25. Which of the following is normally observed in lateral mandibular movement in a young unworn dentition?
    A. Incisors guide the movement.
    B. Posterior teeth on the balancing side guide the movement.
    C. Canines on the working side guide the movement.
    D. There is bilateral contact of maxillary and mandibular posterior teeth.

26. Which of the following cannot be observed during a routine oral examination?
    A. Clinical crown
    B. Anatomic root
    C. Anatomic crown
    D. Clinical root

27. Which is the largest and longest root of the maxillary molars?
    A. Mesiobuccal
    B. Lingual
    C. Distobuccal
    D. None of the above, because all roots are equal in size and length

28. What is the most probable effect on the position of the maxillary molars if their mandibular antagonists are lost and not replaced?
    A. Supereruption
    B. Mesial drift
    C. No effect
    D. Undereruption or even impaction

29. What is the most likely relationship between tooth No. 14 and tooth No. 19 if tooth No. 14 is in a normal axial position and tooth No. 19 is in buccal version?
    A. Excessive overjet
    B. Openbite
    C. Crossbite
    D. Excessive overbite

30. Which of the following could most likely result in reddened, enlarged gingiva lingual to the maxillary incisors?
    A. Anterior crossbite
    B. Excessive overbite
    C. Excessive overjet
    D. Anterior open bite

31. What identification is given in the International Numbering System for the tooth that is identified as No. 19 in the Universal Numbering System?
    A. 19   C. 46
    B. 36   D. L

32. Which of the following is found only on anterior teeth?
    A. Cingulum
    B. Marginal ridges
    C. Fossa
    D. Pits

33. What are the last succedaneous teeth to erupt?
    A. Third molars
    B. Maxillary second molars
    C. Maxillary canines
    D. Maxillary first premolars

34. Which of the following would be used to differentiate central and lateral incisors?
    A. Set traits   C. Class traits
    B. Arch traits   D. Type traits

35. The cervical cross-section of one-rooted teeth reveals all of the following basic shapes EXCEPT one. The exception is
    A. triangular.   C. elliptical.
    B. ovoid.   D. rhomboidal.

36. Approximately when is root formation completed in the permanent teeth?

A. 2 to 6 months before eruption
B. 6 months after eruption
C. 1 year after eruption
D. 2 to 3 years after eruption

37. What horizontal relationship exists when there is simultaneous even contact between maxillary and mandibular teeth into maximum interdigitation with the mandible in its most retruded position?
    A. Centric occlusion
    B. Centric relation
    C. Centric relation occlusion
    D. Lateral relation

38. Which of the following is not a characteristic of the "ugly duckling" stage of development of the dentition?
    A. Disproportionately sized teeth
    B. Enlarged and edematous gingivae
    C. Carious first molars
    D. Differing shades of tooth color

39. Which of the following is characterized by a strong transverse ridge separating the mesial and distal triangular fossae?
    A. Maxillary first premolar
    B. Maxillary second premolar
    C. Mandibular first premolar
    D. Mandibular second premolar

40. All of the following locations normally have a groove that extends from the occlusal surface EXCEPT one. The exception is:
    A. facial surface of the mandibular first molars.
    B. facial surface of the maxillary second molars.
    C. lingual surface of the maxillary first molars.
    D. mesial surface of the maxillary first premolars.

Head and Neck Anatomy

41. Which of the following structure(s) pass around the pituitary fossa?
    A. carotid arteries
    B. cavernous sinus
    C. cranial nerve I
    D. cranial nerve V
    E. all of the above.

42. All of the following are structures found in the pterygopalatine fossa EXCEPT one. The exception is:
    A. Maxillary artery
    B. Cranial nerve III
    C. Cranial nerve V2
    D. Pterygoid plexus
    E. Temporalis

43. All of the following muscles are infrahyoid muscles EXCEPT one. The exception is:
    A. Sternohyoid   C. Omohyoid
    B. Sternothyroid   D. Mylohyoid

44. All of the following structures are part of the visual pathway EXCEPT one. The exception is:
    A. Optic nerve
    B. Optic chiasm
    C. Medial geniculate bodies
    D. Visual cortex

45. All of the following nerves are branches of the trigeminal, mandibular division (V3) EXCEPT one. The exception is:
    A. Lingual
    B. Inferior alveolar
    C. Mental
    D. Buccal
    E. Nasopalatine

46. Which of the following structures is not considered to be a head and neck space?
    A. Retropharyngeal
    B. Alar
    C. Submandibular
    D. Buccal
    E Terygomandibular

47. The cranium is composed of how many different bones?
    A. 10   C. 12
    B. 11   D. 13

48. A large opening for passage of the spinal cord through the occipital bone is called the ____.
    A. foramen ovale.
    B. foramen rotundum.
    C. foramen spinosum.
    D. foramen magnum.

49. The _____ process consists of the zygoma, maxillary, and temporal bones.
    A. zygomatic.   C. styloid.
    B. mastoid.   D. coronoid.

50. The coronoid process exists for the attachment of the _____ muscle.
    A. masseter.
    B. medial pterygoid.
    C. lateral pterygoid.
    D. temporalis.

51. The TMJ is a unique _____ joint, because it allows gliding and hinge movements.
    A. cartilagenous.
    B. dual.
    C. single.

52. Which muscle group is innervated by cranial nerve VII, the facial nerve?
    A. Muscles of mastication
    B. Muscles of anterior neck
    C. Muscles of facial expression
    D. Sternocleidomastoid

53. Which muscle: 1. originates on the pterygomandibular raphe, 2. is pierced by Stensen duct, 3. inserts into the orbicularis oris?
    A. Buccinator
    B. Masseter
    C. Superior constrictor

54. Which muscle serves as a landmark to locate the carotids, internal jugular, and the cervical nodes?
    A. Sternohyoid
    B. Sternothyroid
    C. Sternocleidomastoid

55. The soft palate is a muscular flap that acts to seal off the oropharynx from the _____.
    A. pharynx proper.
    B. trachea.

C. nasal cavity.

56. Taste sensation to the anterior tongue travels on the _____ branch of CN VII (facial nerve).
    A. lingual.
    B. motor.
    C. chorda tympani.
    D. submandibular.

57. Two cranial nerves serve the pharynx (sensory and motor). Which are they?
    A. V and VII
    B. VII and IX
    C. IX and VIII
    D. IX and X

58. The trigeminal is mainly a sensory type of nerve. Which division of the trigeminal nerve carries motor fibers and to which muscles does it innervate?
    A. V1-muscles of tongue
    B. V2-muscles of facial expression
    C. V3-muscles of mastication

59. The brain has a dual source of arterial blood by way of the _____ arteries and the _____ arteries.
    A. carotid, jugular.
    B. internal carotid, external carotid.
    C. internal carotid, vertebral.
    D. vertebral, basilar.

60. A network of veins accompanies the maxillary artery in the pterygopalatine fossa called the _____. It poses a risk when performing PSA dental block injections.
    A. maxillary.
    B. cavernous sinus.
    C. pterygoid plexus.

General Anatomy

Nervous System

61. The central nervous system, CNS, consists of the:
    A. brain, spinal cord, and cranial nerves.
    B. brain, cranial nerves, and autonomic nervous system.
    C. brain and spinal cord only.
    D. brain, cranial nerves, spinal nerves, and sympathetic ganglia.

62. Gray matter primarily contains:
    A. blood vessels.
    B. myelinated nerve fibers.
    C. neuron cell bodies and synapses.
    D. cerebrospinal fluid.

63. A stroke can result from a cerebral vessel
    A. blockage (e.g., a clot).
    B. narrowing (e.g., atherosclerosis).
    C. weakening (e.g., aneurysm).
    D. all of the above.

64. Pain from the teeth is associated with which nerve?
    A. Trigeminal nerve
    B. Facial nerve
    C. Glossopharyngeal nerve
    D. Vagus nerve

65. In diagnostic lumbar puncture, a sample of cerebrospinal fluid is obtained from the:
    A. subdural space.
    B. subarachnoid space.
    C. epidural space.
    D. central canal of the spinal cord.

Circulatory System

66. All arteries of systemic circulation branch from the:
    A. aorta.
    B. pulmonary artery.
    C. superior vena cava.
    D. circle of Willis.

67. A thrombus in the first branch of the arch of the aorta would effect the flow of blood to the:
    A. left side of the head and neck.
    B. myocardium of the heart.
    C. right side of the head and neck and right upper extremity.
    D. left upper extremity.

68. An obstruction in the inferior vena cava would hinder the return of blood from the:
    A. head and neck.
    B. upper limbs.
    C. abdomen and pelvis.
    D. thorax.

69. Which of the following are involved in pulmonary circulation?
    A. Superior vena cava, right atrium, and left ventricle
    B. Inferior vena cava, right atrium, and left ventricle
    C. Right ventricle, pulmonary artery, and left atrium
    D. Left ventricle, aorta, and inferior vena cava

70. If a thrombus in the left common carotid artery broke free, into which area of the body might it first find its way?
    A. Brain
    B. Kidneys
    C. Lungs
    D. Left arm

71. The thoracic duct receives lymph from the:
    A. lower limbs.
    B. abdomen.
    C. pelvis.
    D. left side of the thorax.
    E. all of the above.

72. Both the thoracic duct and the right lymphatic duct empty directly into the:
    A. superior vena cava.
    B. inferior vena cava.
    C. subclavian arteries.
    D. subclavian veins.

Urinary System

73. In the kidney, filtration occurs in the:
    A. proximal convoluted tubules.
    B. distal convoluted tubule.
    C. renal corpuscle.
    D. loop of Henle.

74. Which of the following is *not* part of the nephron of the kidney?
    A. Glomerulus
    B. Bowman capsule
    C. Proximal convoluted tubule
    D. Distal convoluted tubule

Miscellaneous

75. Microvilli are prominent and abundant on the free surfaces of cells of each of the following except the:
    A. mucosa of the small intestines.
    B. lining of the urinary bladder.
    C. endothelium of blood vessels.
    D. lining of the trachea.

76. Which of the terms for muscular layer is incorrectly matched with the organ?
    A. Myocardium-heart
    B. Myometrium-stomach
    C. Tunica media-blood vessel
    D. Muscularis-intestines

77. Which of the following terms does not refer to the outer layer of an organ wall?
    A. Epicardium
    B. Tunica adventitia
    C. Endometrium
    D. Serosa

78. All of the following terms refer to linings except one. The EXCEPTION is:
    A. pericardium.   C. pleura.
    B. perineum.   D. peritoneum.

79. Bowman glands are found in the:
    A. kidney.   C. liver.
    B. pancreas.   D. nasal cavity.

80. The macula lutea is found in the:
    A. kidney.   C. eye.
    B. ovary.   D. ear.

ANSWERS

Histology

1. **C.** Dentin is manufactured by odontoblasts. Ameloblasts form enamel; cementoblasts form cementum; and fibroblasts produce periodontal ligament.

2. **C.** The external aspect (vermillion zone) of the lip is comprised of stratified squamous keratinized epithelium. The inside of the lips is lining mucosa; a wet mucosa containing a stratified squamous nonkeratinized epithelium.

3. **B.** The principal fiber bundles of the periodontal ligament consist of collagen fibers. They suspend a tooth in its alveolus, extending from the cribiform plate of the alveolar bone to the cementum on the root of the tooth. The fibers that extend from one tooth to the next are the transseptal gingival fibers.

4. **C.** Osteoclasts are multinucleated cells that produce proteolytic enzymes and occupy Howship lacunae. They are not derived from osteoprogenitor cells but from monocyte precursors.

5. **D.** Monocytes leave the bloodstream and migrate into the connective tissue where they mature into functional macrophages.

6. **A.** Skeletal muscle cells are under voluntary control. All the other cells listed are controlled by the autonomic nervous system.

7. **C.** Schwann cells produce myelin in the PNS; oligodendrocytes produce myelin in the CNS. Astrocytes, neural crest cells, and basket cells do not produce myelin.

8. **D.** Granulocytes are leukocytes that possess specific granules with type-specific contents. They are basophils, eosinophils, and neutrophils. Thrombocytes are platelets, and lymphocytes and monocytes are agranulocytes.

9. **E.** The intermaxillary segment forms when the two medial nasal prominences fuse in the midline.

10. **D.** Hertwig root sheath determines the outline of the root dentin before cementum formation begins and also the number of roots that a tooth will have.

11. **A.** Primary enamel cuticle is the last product of enamel-forming ameloblasts and becomes mineralized. The secondary enamel cuticle is a product of REE and is not mineralized. It is the outermost layer and will wear away after tooth use.

12. **B.** Enamel tufts resemble small paintbrushes that extend beyond the DEJ. Enamel spindles also extend across the DEJ, but they are the peripheral ends of odontoblasts.

13. **A.** Cementocytes are not usually found throughout the cementum. The thin cementum on the cervical portion of the root is acellular, whereas the apex of the root is thick and cellular. Cementum close to the dentin may have few cementocytes, and the outer layers may contain many irregularly distributed cells.

14. **C.** Cementum most often overlaps enamel. The next most common occurrence is cementum meeting enamel, and the third most frequent scenario is that enamel and cementum do not meet. Enamel never overlaps cementum.

15. **B.** The oblique fibers of the periodontal ligament are extremely strong and prevent the apex of the tooth from being jammed against the bottom of the socket during clenching, mastication, and so forth.

16. **B.** The junctional epithelium or attachment epithelium consists of stratified squamous epithelium that is attached to the tooth surface at the cervical portion of all teeth. It continues coronally with the sulcular epithelium and over the gingival margin with the epithelium on the outer surface of the gingiva.

17. **D.** The mucogingival junction is the junction where the gingiva and the alveolar mucosa meet. This transitional zone changes from keratinized to nonkeratinized epithelium.

18. **C.** Although the filiform papillae are the most numerous, they lack taste buds.

19. **B.** The largest salivary glands are the parotids. They produce serous saliva. The main duct (Stensen duct) opens into the oral cavity on the wall of the buccal mucosa opposite the maxillary second molar. The other salivary glands are mixed.

20. **B.** Odontogenesis refers to the origin of tooth formation. The earliest sign of tooth development is found in the mandibular anterior region when the embryo is 5 to 6 weeks old.

Dental Anatomy

21. **C.** The triangular ridge runs from the cusp tip toward the center of the tooth. Both the oblique ridge and the transverse range are made up of connecting triangular ridges. Only marginal ridges are on the mesial and distal borders of the occlusal surface.

22. **D.** The incisors guide protrusive mandibular movement in the normal dentition. Canines, premolars, and molars usually disocclude during protrusive movement.

23. **A.** Versions occur where contact or the position of the tooth is at an unexpected area and are named after their misplaced positions. The prefix *torso-* indicates rotation, whereas the term *supraversion* indicates supereruption.

24. **D.** Occlusion is classified by the relationship of the mesiobuccal cusp of the maxillary permanent first molar with the mesiobuccal groove of the mandibular first permanent first molar. In class I occlusion and malocclusion, the groove and cusp are aligned. In class II malocclusion, the groove is distal to the cusp. The groove is mesial to the cusp in class III malocclusion.

25. **C.** Lateral movements are guided by the canines on the working side in young, unworn dentitions and may be guided by incisors and posterior teeth in older, worn dentitions. Posterior teeth on the balancing side should disengage in lateral movement.

26. **D.** By its definition, the clinical root is the part of the tooth that is not visible in the oral cavity.

27. **B.** The lingual root is the largest and longest root of the maxillary molars.

28. **A.** If the antagonist tooth is lost and not replaced, the same process that compensates for occlusal wear will take place. Cementum will be deposited at the root apex and will result in the supereruption of the counterpart tooth. This process will continue actively until occlusal contact is re-established.

29. **C.** The terms overjet and overbite refer to the characteristics of maxillary teeth to overlap the mandibular teeth in horizontal and vertical relations, respectively. Crossbite occurs when the mandibular tooth occludes facially to its maxillary counterpart(s).

30. **B.** Excessive overbite could result in trauma to the soft tissue lingual to the maxillary incisors from the incisal edges of the mandibular incisors.

31. **B.** The International Numbering System uses two digits to identify each tooth. The first digit denotes dentition, arch, and side (1 to 4 for the permanent quadrants and 5 to 8 for the deciduous quadrants), whereas the second digit represents the tooth (1 to 8 for the central incisor to the third molar).

32. **A.** The cingulum is the large, rounded elevation, or bulge, on the cervical third of the lingual surface of an anterior tooth.

33. **C.** Maxillary canines are usually the last succedaneous teeth to erupt. Molars are not succedaneous teeth.

34. **D.** Set traits differentiate permanent and deciduous teeth. Arch traits distinguish maxillary from mandibular teeth. Class traits differentiate the four categories of teeth. Type traits differentiate teeth within one class.

35. **D.** The cervical cross-section of one-rooted teeth yields three basic shapes that can be modified by the presence of root concavities: triangular, ovoid, and elliptical.

36. **D.** The roots of deciduous teeth are completed 6 to 18 months after eruption. Roots of the permanent teeth are completed 2 to 3 years after eruption.

37. **C.** Centric occlusion is the maximum intercuspation or contact attained between maxillary and mandibular teeth. Centric relation is the most posterior position of the mandible relative to the maxillae at a given vertical dimension. Centric relation occlusion refers to the coincidental occurrence of centric relation and centric occlusion. Lateral relation refers to right and left movement of the mandible.

38. **C.** Even though they may be ugly and may be observed in many young patients during the "ugly duckling" stage of development, carious first molars are not a defining characteristic. Many parents misidentify the permanent first molars as "baby teeth" and allow them to decay, because they think they are going to fall out soon anyway.

39. **C.** This is a strong identifying trait of the mandibular first premolar, especially when the pits ("snake-eyes") are prominent.

40. **B.** The facial surface of the mandibular first molars will have one or two grooves that extend from the occlusal surface. The mesial marginal ridge of the first premolar is crossed by a groove that extends from the central developmental groove. The facial surfaces of maxillary second molars normally have no grooves.

Head and Neck Anatomy

41. **E.** The carotid arteries and cavernous fossa are lateral to the pituitary fossa, and cranial nerves I and V are located around the pituitary fossa.

42. **B.** All of the structures, with the exception of cranial nerve III, are found in the pterygopalatine fossa. Cranial nerve III is located in the orbit of the eye.

43. **D.** The mylohyoid is a suprahyoid muscle.

44. **C.** The medial geniculate bodies are part of the auditory pathway. The optic chiasm is a crossover of cranial nerve VIII.

45. **E.** The nasopalatine nerve is not a branch of the mandibular division of the trigeminal nerve. The nasopalatine nerve innervates the anterior palate.

46. **B.** The alar is fascia and is not a space.

47. **C.** The cranium contains 12 different bones.

48. **D.** V3 passes through the foreman ovale; V2 passes through the foramen rotundum; the meningeal vessel passes through the foramen spinosum.

49. **A.** The mastoid and styloid are posterior to the ear. The coronoid process is the anterior notch, which is located on the ramus of the mandible.

50. **D.** The temporalis attaches to the coronoid process to permit elevation and rapid movement of the mandible.

51. **B.** The TMJ has fibrous articular surfaces and acts as a dual joint to permit gliding and hinge movements.

52. **C.** The muscles of mastication are innervated by V3. The muscles of the anterior neck are innervated by the cervical nerves. The sternocleidomastoid muscle is innervated by cranial nerve XI.

53. **A.** The masseter is more superficial, and the superior constrictor muscle attaches posterior to the buccinator.

54. **C.** The sternohyoid muscle is anterior to the sternocleidomastoid muscle and would be located too far anteriorly to serve as a landmark. The sternothyroid muscle is medial and deep to the sternohyoid and inserts on the thyroid cartilage.

55. **C.** The pharynx proper is below the palate, and the trachea is located even further below the palate.

56. **C.** The lingual nerve is a branch of cranial nerve V; the motor nerve is a sensory nerve; and the submandibular branch does not exist.

57. **D.** Cranial nerves V and VII provide sensation and movement to the tongue. Cranial nerves VII and IX supply the salivary glands, and cranial nerve VIII innervates the ear.

58. **C.** Cranial nerve V1 is sensory to the upper part of the face, and V2 is sensory to the middle part of the face.

59. **C.** The jugular is a vein; the external carotid goes to the face; and the basilar artery consists of both vertebral arteries fused.

60. **C.** The maxillary sinus does not specify an artery or vein, and the cavernous sinus is within the brain.

General Anatomy

61. **C.** The CNS refers to the brain and spinal cord. The PNS refers to the cranial nerves and the spinal nerves.

62. **C.** Gray matter refers to the color of areas containing cell bodies, synapses, and unmyelinated nerve fibers.

63. **D.** A stroke is a general term for a cerebral vascular accident (CVA).

64. **A.** The trigeminal nerve provides all sensory innervation to the teeth.

65. **B.** CSF is produced in the ventricles of the brain continuously; it moves to the outside of the CNS from the fourth ventricle to circulate in the subarachnoid space. The fluid returns to the venous bloodstream through arachnoid granulations that protrude into the superior sagittal sinus and other dural venous sinuses.

66. **A.** The aorta arises from the left ventricle, arches posteriorly and to the left, descends through the thorax and abdominal region, and divides into the common iliac arteries in the pelvic area.

67. **C.** The first branch from the arch of the aorta, the brachiocephalic artery, divides into the right subclavian artery to the right upper limb and the right common carotid artery, which serves the right side of the head and neck.

68. **C.** The IVC collects venous blood from the body below the diaphragm and returns it to the right atrium of the heart.

69. **C.** The pulmonary circulation carries deoxygenated blood from the heart to the lungs through the pulmonary arteries and returns oxygenated blood from the lungs to the heart through the pulmonary veins. By definition, an artery always goes away from the heart and a vein always returns to the heart. This is one of the few cases in which the artery contains deoxygenated blood and the vein contains oxygenated blood.

70. **A.** The left common carotid divides into the internal carotid artery, which serves the brain by entering the circle of Willis and the external carotid artery serves the left side of the head and neck. Either area could be compromised by a blockage in a branch of the left common carotid artery.

71. **E.** The thoracic duct, the largest lymphatic vessel in the body, originates in the upper abdomen under the diaphragm. It receives smaller lymphatics from lower limbs and the abdomen, travels through the thorax, and enters the left subclavian vein. Lymphatics from the left side of the thorax, head, and neck enter the thoracic duct immediately before it drains into the left subclavian vein.

72. **D.** The thoracic duct empties into the left subclavian vein; the right lymphatic duct empties into the right subclavian vein. On both sides, this occurs at the junction where the subclavian vein meets the internal jugular vein to form the brachiocephalic vein.

73. **C.** In the kidney, filtration of the blood occurs in the renal corpuscle, which consists of a blood capillary arranged in a ball enclosed in the beginning part of the nephron called the Bowman capsule.

74. **A.** The glomerulus is a blood capillary that retains large molecules with a molecular weight of less than 10,000, while allowing smaller molecules to pass into the urinary space of the Bowman capsule, the beginning of the nephron.

75. **C.** Microvilli increase the surface area of the epithelial surface. They are found where exchange of materials across the epithelial layer to the underlying blood and lymph capillaries is needed.

76. **B.** The smooth muscle layer of the gut tube, including the stomach, is called a muscularis, and the thick smooth muscle layer of the uterus is the myometrium.

77. **C.** The inner layer of the uterus is the endometrium. The outer layer of the heart is called the epicardium; the outer layer of a blood vessel is called the tunica adventitia; and the outer layer of the organs is the serosa.

78. **B.** The perineum is the region below the pelvis that contains the genitalia. Pericardium lines the heart; pleura line the lungs; peritoneum lines the abdominal viscera.

79. **D.** Bowman glands, also called olfactory glands, are found in the nasal cavity. Dr. Bowman also has a kidney structure named after him. What is it?

80. **C.** The macula lutea is a yellow pigmented area that surrounds the fovea centralis, the area of greatest visual acuity in the retina of the eye.

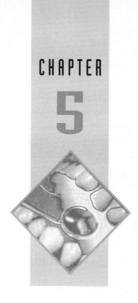

5

Physiology

LAURALEE SHERWOOD, DVM   CHRISTINA B. DeBIASE, EdD

Physiology is the study of how the body functions. It is closely related to anatomy because structure and function are inseparable. The basic unit of structure and function is the **cell**.

 ## HOMEOSTASIS

Homeostasis is the maintenance of a stable internal environment (i.e., the concentration of O_2, CO_2, nutrients, wastes, pH, salt and other electrolytes, temperature, and volume and pressure) in the **extracellular fluid (ECF)** bathing the cells. Homeostasis is essential for the survival of cells. Cells are organized into functional groupings, with cells of similar structure and specialized activity organized into tissues. Tissues are further organized into organs, which are structures composed of several types of primary tissue that work together to perform particular functions. Body systems are collections of organs that perform similar functions and interact to accomplish a common activity essential for survival of the body. Body systems maintain homeostasis. Components of body systems can be found in **Table 5-1**.

 ## CELLULAR PHYSIOLOGY

Most cells have three major subdivisions (**Figure 5-1**). The **nucleus** contains DNA, the genetic blueprint for protein synthesis and cell replication. **Cytoplasm** is made up of a gelatin-like mass called **cytosol**. Cytoplasm surrounds the nucleus and contains six highly organized membrane structures known as **organelles**:

1. **Endoplasmic reticulum**: synthesizes proteins for export out of the cell (secretory products)
2. **Golgi complex**: modification, packaging, and distribution center for newly synthesized proteins

3. **Lysosomes:** intracellular digestive system of the cell
4. **Peroxisomes:** detoxifies intracellular wastes
5. **Mitochondria:** energy source of the cell; generates adenosine triphosphate (ATP)
6. **Vaults:** cellular vehicles for transporting messenger RNA

The **plasma membrane** is a selectively permeable membrane that surrounds each cell and **separates the intracellular fluid (ICF)** from the ECF.

 ## MEMBRANE PHYSIOLOGY

The survival of cells depends on the maintenance of intracellular contents unique to that cell type despite the different composition of ECF surrounding it. This difference in fluid composition inside and outside the cell is maintained by the **plasma membrane**, which is a very thin layer of lipids and proteins that forms the outer boundary of every cell and encloses the intracellular contents. In addition to serving as a mechanical barrier that traps necessary molecules within the cell, the plasma membrane plays an active role in determining the composition of the cell by selectively permitting passage of specific substances between the cell and its environment.

Cell-to-Cell Adhesions

Desmosomes serve as adhering junctions to mechanically hold cells together and are especially important in tissues subject to a lot of stretching. **Tight junctions** actually fuse cells together to seal off passage between cells, thus permitting only regulated passage of materials through the cells. These impermeable junctions are found in the epithelial sheets that separate compartments with very different chemical compositions. Cells joined by **gap junctions** are con-

118

TABLE 5–1 Components of Body Systems

SYSTEM	COMPONENTS	FUNCTION
Circulatory system	Heart, blood vessels, blood	Transports nutrients, O_2, CO_2, wastes, electrolytes, and hormones
Digestive system	Mouth, pharynx, esophagus, small intestine, large intestine, salivary glands, exocrine pancreas, liver, gallbladder	Degrades dietary food into nutrients Transfers water and electrolytes from the external to internal environment Eliminates undigested food
Respiratory system	Nose, pharynx, larynx, trachea, bronchi, lungs	Obtains O_2 and eliminates CO_2 Helps to regulate pH by adjusting the rate of removal of acid-forming CO_2
Urinary system	Kidneys, ureters, urinary bladder, urethra	Removes waste products from plasma and removes excess water, salt, and electrolytes and eliminates them in urine Regulates volume, electrolyte composition, and acidity of extracellular fluid
Skeletal system	Bones, cartilage, joints	Support and protect body parts and allow body movement; heat-generating muscle contractions important in temperature regulation; calcium stored in bone
Muscular system	Skeletal muscles	
Integumentary system	Skin, hair, nails	Serves as protective barrier between the external environment and the remainder of the body; sweat glands and adjustments in the blood flow in the skin are important in temperature regulation
Immune system	White blood cells, thymus, bone marrow, tonsils, adenoids, lymph nodes, spleen, appendix, gut-associated lymphoid tissue, skin-associated lymphoid tissue	Defends against foreign invaders and cancer cells; paves way for tissue repair
Nervous system	Brain, spinal cord, peripheral nerves, special sense organs	Acts through electrical signals to control rapid responses of the body; also responsible for higher functions (e.g., consciousness, memory, and creativity)
Endocrine system	All hormone-secreting tissues, including the hypothalamus, pituitary, thyroid, adrenals, endocrine pancreas, parathyroids, gonads, kidneys, intestine, heart, thymus, pineal, and skin	Secretes hormones into the blood, which control metabolic activities, water and electrolyte balance, and other processes that require duration rather than speed
Reproductive system	Male: testes, penis, prostate gland, seminal vesicles, bulbourethral glands, and associated ducts Female: ovaries, oviducts, uterus, vagina, and breasts	Not essential for homeostasis, but essential for perpetuation of the species

nected by small tunnels that permit exchange of ions and small molecules between the cells. Such movement of ions plays a key role in the spread of electrical activity to synchronize contraction in heart and smooth muscle.

Membrane Transport

Materials can pass between the ECF and ICF across the plasma membrane by the following pathways. Nonpolar (lipid-soluble) molecules of any size can dissolve in and pass through the lipid bilayer. Small ions traverse through protein channels specific for them. Movement of particles through these pathways occurs passively down electrochemical gradients. **Osmosis** is a special case of water moving down its own concentration gradient.

Other substances can be selectively transferred across the membrane by specific carrier proteins, being moved either down a concentration gradient without energy expenditure (**facilitated diffusion**) or against a concentration gradient at the expense of cellular energy (**active transport**). Carrier mechanisms are important for transfer of small polar molecules and for selected movement of ions.

Large polar molecules and multimolecular particles can leave or enter the cell by being wrapped in a piece of membrane to form vesicles that can be internalized (**endocytosis**) or externalized (**exocytosis**). This is referred to as vesicular transport.

Membrane Potential

The plasma membrane is polarized electrically, with excess negative charges lined up along the inside of the membrane and excess positive charges along the outside. The membrane-bound Na^+-K^+ pump actively transports Na^+ out of and K^+ into the cells, leading to a high concentration of Na^+ in the ECF and high concentration of K^+ in the ICF. Because the resting membrane is considerably more permeable to K^+ than to Na^+, more K^+ exits the cell than Na^+ enters down

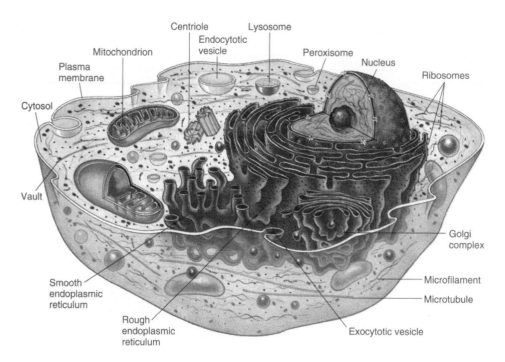

Figure 5-1. Schematic three-dimensional illustration of cell structures visible under an electron microscope. (From Sherwood L: Human Physiology: From Cells to Systems, 4th ed. Pacific Grove, CA, Brooks/Cole, 2001, p 19.)

their respective concentration gradients. Because more positive charges leave than enter, excess positive charges accumulate on the outside, leaving behind unbalanced negative charges on the inside. The result is a resting membrane potential of −70 mV.

When appropriately triggered, nerve and muscle cell membranes undergo brief, rapid reversals of membrane potential; these reversals serve as electrical signals known as **action potentials**, and they are able to spread throughout the membrane in nondecremental fashion. To understand the processes that occur during an action potential, it is necessary to be familiar with the following terms (**Figure 5-2**).

1. **Polarization:** the membrane has potential; there is a separation of opposite charges.
2. **Depolarization:** the membrane potential is reduced from resting potential; it has decreased or moved toward 0 mV; fewer charges are separated than at resting potential.
3. **Hyperpolarization:** the potential is greater than resting potential; it has increased or become even more negative; more charges are separated than at resting potential.
4. **Repolarization:** return to resting potential after having been depolarized.

One possibly confusing point should be clarified. On the device used for recording rapid changes in potential, a decrease in potential is represented as an upward deflection whereas an increase is potential is represented as a downward deflection.

Consider the changes that occur in the membrane potential during an action potential (**Figure 5-3**). To initiate an action potential, a triggering event causes the membrane to de-

polarize from the resting potential of −70 mV. Depolarization proceeds slowly at first until it reaches a critical level known as **threshold potential**, which is typically between −50 and −55 mV. At threshold potential, an explosive depolarization takes place. A recording of the potential at this time shows a sharp upward deflection to +30 mV as the potential rapidly decreases toward 0 mV, then reverses itself so that the inside of the cell becomes positive compared with the outside. Just as rapidly, the potential drops back to resting potential as the membrane repolarizes. The entire rapid change in potential from threshold to peak reversal and then back to resting is called the **action potential**.

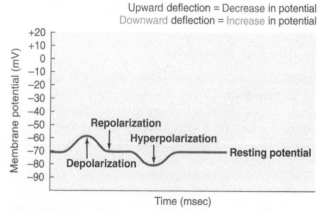

Figure 5-2. Types of changes in membrane potential. (From Sherwin L: Human Physiology: From Cells to Systems, 4th ed. Pacific Grove, CA, Brooks/Cole, 2001, p 89.)

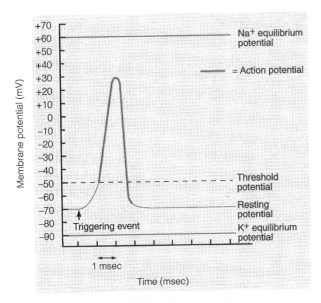

Figure 5-3. Changes in membrane potential during an action potential. (From Sherwin L: Fundamentals of Physiology, 2nd ed. Minnesota, West Publishing, 1995, p 61.)

K^+ makes the greatest contribution to the establishment of the resting potential, because the membrane when at rest is considerably more permeable to K^+ than to Na^+. During an action potential, marked changes in membrane permeability to Na^+ and K^+ occur, thus permitting rapid fluxes of these ions down their electrochemical gradients. These ion movements carry the current responsible for the potential changes that occur during an action potential. At threshold potential, membrane permeability to Na^+ greatly increases. The resultant inward movement of positively charged Na^+ is responsible for the rising phase of the action potential. At the peak of the action potential, membrane permeability to Na^+ falls to its low resting value whereas permeability to K^+ greatly increases. The resultant outward movement of positively charged K^+ is responsible for the falling phase of the action potential, returning the membrane to resting potential.

Synapses

The primary method by which one neuron directly interacts with another neuron is through a **synapse.** An action potential in the presynaptic neuron triggers the release of a **neurotransmitter**, which combines with receptor sites on the postsynaptic neuron. This combination brings about opening of chemical messenger-gated channels. The resultant changes in ionic movement lead to excitatory (depolarizing) or inhibitory (hyperpolarizing) fluctuations in potential of the postsynaptic cell, depending on the permeability changes induced by neurotransmitter binding.

 NERVOUS SYSTEM

The nervous system is one of the two control systems of the body, the other being the endocrine system. In general, the nervous system coordinates rapid responses, whereas the endocrine system regulates activities that require duration rather than speed.

The nervous system consists of the **central nervous system (CNS),** which includes the brain and spinal cord, and the **peripheral nervous system,** which includes the nerve fibers carrying information to **(afferent division)** and from **(efferent division)** the CNS. Three classes of neurons-afferent neurons, efferent neurons, and interneurons-compose the **excitable cells** of the nervous system. Afferent neurons apprise the CNS of conditions in both the external and internal environment. Efferent neurons carry instructions from the CNS to effector organs, namely muscles and glands. **Interneurons** are responsible for integrating afferent information and formulating an efferent response, as well as for all higher mental functions associated with the "mind."

Protection and Nourishment of the Brain

Glial cells form the connective tissue within the CNS and physically and metabolically support the neurons. The brain is provided with several protective devices, which is important because neurons cannot divide to replace damaged cells. The brain is wrapped in three layers of protective membranes-**the meninges**-and is further surrounded by a hard bony covering. **Cerebrospinal fluid (CSF)** flows within and around the brain to cushion it against physical jarring. Protection against chemical injury is conferred by a **blood-brain barrier** that limits access of blood-borne substances to the brain.

The brain depends on a constant blood supply for delivery of O_2 and glucose, because it is unable to generate ATP in the absence of either of these substances.

Cerebral Cortex

The **cerebral cortex** is the outer shell of **gray matter** that caps an underlying core of white matter; the **white matter** consists of bundles of nerve fibers that interconnect various cortical regions with other areas. The cortex itself consists primarily of neuronal cell bodies and dendrites.

Ultimate responsibility for many discrete functions is known to be localized in particular regions of the cortex as follows: (1) the occipital lobes house the visual cortex; (2) the auditory cortex is found in the temporal lobes; (3) the parietal lobes are responsible for reception and perceptual processing of somatosensory input; and (4) voluntary motor movement is set into motion by frontal lobe activity. Language ability depends on the integrated activity of two primary language areas located in the left hemisphere only.

The association areas are areas of the cortex that are not specifically assigned to process sensory input or command motor output or language ability. These areas provide an integrative link between diverse sensory information and purposeful action; they also play a key role in higher brain functions such as memory and decision-making.

Subcortical Structures and Their Relationship with the Cortex in Higher Brain Functions

The **subcortical brain structures**, which include the basal nuclei, thalamus, and hypothalamus, interact extensively with the cortex in the performance of their functions. The **basal nuclei** inhibit muscle tone; coordinate slow, sustained postural contractions; and suppress useless patterns of movement. The **thalamus** serves as a relay station for preliminary processing of sensory input on its way to the cortex. It also accomplishes a crude awareness of sensation and some degree of consciousness. The **hypothalamus** regulates many homeostatically directed activities, such as maintenance of body temperature, thirst, and urine output, in part through its extensive control of the autonomic nervous system and endocrine system. The **limbic system,** which includes portions of the hypothalamus and other forebrain structures, is responsible for emotion as well as basic, inborn behavior patterns related to survival. It also plays an important role in motivation and learning.

Memory is broken down into two types: (1) short-term memory with limited capacity and brief retention, coded at least in part by temporary modifications in transmitter release; and (2) long-term memory with large storage capacity and enduring memory traces, presumably involving relatively permanent structural or functional changes between already existing neurons.

Cerebellum and Brainstem

The **cerebellum** helps to maintain balance, enhances muscle tone, and helps coordinate voluntary movement. It is especially important in smoothing out fast, phasic motor activities.

The **brainstem** is an important link between the spinal cord and higher brain levels and is the origin of the cranial nerves. The brainstem contains centers that control cardiovascular, respiratory, and digestive function; it regulates postural muscle reflexes; it controls the overall degree of cortical alertness; and it establishes the sleep-wake cycle. The prevailing state of consciousness depends on the cyclical interplay between an arousal system (the reticular-activating system), a slow-wave sleep center, and a paradoxical sleep center, which are all located in the brainstem.

Spinal Cord

The **spinal cord** has two vital functions. First, it serves as the neuronal link between the brain and the peripheral nervous system. All communication up and down the spinal cord is located in well-defined, independent ascending and descending tracts in the cord's outer white matter. Second, the spinal cord is the integrating center for spinal reflexes, including some of the basic protective and postural reflexes and those involved with the emptying of the pelvic organs. The components of a basic **reflex arc** include a receptor, an afferent pathway, an integrating center, an efferent pathway, and an effector. The centrally located gray matter of the spinal cord contains the interneurons interposed between the afferent input and efferent output as well as the cell bodies of efferent neurons. The afferent and efferent fibers, which carry signals to and from the spinal cord, respectively, are bundled together into **spinal nerves**. These nerves are attached to the spinal cord in paired fashion throughout its length. They supply specific regions of the body.

AFFERENT INPUT: SPECIAL SENSES

Receptors are specialized peripheral endings of afferent neurons; they respond to particular stimuli, translating the energy forms of the stimuli into electrical signals, the language of the nervous system. There are discrete labeled-line pathways from the receptors to the CNS so that information about the type and location of the stimuli can be deciphered by the CNS, even though all the information arrives in the form of action potentials. Information that reaches the conscious level is called **sensory information,** which includes **somatic sensation (body awareness)** and the **special senses** (i.e., **seeing, hearing, tasting,** and **smelling**). Afferent input is necessary for arousal, perception, and determination of efferent output.

Pain

Painful experiences are elicited by noxious mechanical, thermal, or chemical stimuli and consist of two components: the perception of pain combined with emotional and behavioral responses to it. Transmission of pain signals takes place over two afferent pathways: (1) a fast pathway that carries sharp prickling pain signals; and (2) a slow pathway that carries dull aching, persistent pain signals. Afferent pain fibers terminate in the spinal cord on ascending pathways that transmit the signals to the brain for processing. Descending pathways from the brain use endogenous opiates to suppress the release of substance P, the neurotransmitter from the afferent pain fiber terminal, thus blocking further transmission of the pain signal and serving as a built-in analgesic system.

Eye: Vision

The eye is a specialized structure that contains the light-sensitive receptors that are essential for vision perception-namely, the rods and cones found in its **retinal layer**. The **iris** controls the size of the pupil, thus adjusting the amount of light permitted to enter the eye. The **cornea** and lens are the primary refractive structures that bend the incoming light rays to focus the image on the retina. The cornea contributes most to the total refractive ability of the eye. The strength of the lens can be adjusted through action of the ciliary muscle to accommodate for differences in near and far vision.

Rods and cones are activated when the photopigments that they contain differentially absorb various wavelengths of light, causing a biochemical charge in the photopigment that is ultimately converted into a change in the rate of action potential propagation in the visual pathway leaving the retina. The visual message is transmitted to the visual cortex in the brain for perceptual processing.

Cones display high acuity but can be used only for day vision because of their low sensitivity to light. Different ratios of stimulation of three cone types by varying wavelengths of light lead to color vision. Rods provide only indistinct vision in shades of gray; however, because they are very sensitive to light, they can be used for night vision.

Ear: Hearing and Equilibrium

The ear performs two unrelated functions: (1) **hearing**, which involves the external ear, middle ear, and cochlea of the inner ear; and (2) sense of **equilibrium**, which involves the vestibular apparatus of the inner ear. Hearing depends on the ear's ability to convert airborne sound waves into mechanical deformations of receptive hair cells, thus initiating neural signals. Sound waves consist of high-pressure regions of compression alternating with low-pressure regions of rarefaction of air molecules. The **pitch (tone)** of a sound is determined by the frequency of its waves and the **loudness (intensity)** by the amplitude of the waves. Sound waves are funneled through the external ear canal to the **tympanic membrane**, which vibrates in synchrony with the waves. Middle-ear bones that bridge the gap between the tympanic membrane and the inner ear amplify the tympanic movements and transmit them to the oval window, whose movement sets up traveling waves in the cochlear fluid. These waves, which are at the same frequency as the original sound waves, set the **basilar membrane** in motion. Various regions of this membrane selectively vibrate more vigorously in response to different frequencies of sound. On top of the basilar membrane are the receptive hair cells of the **organ of Corti**, whose hairs are bent as the basilar membrane is deflected up and down in relation to the overhanging stationary tectorial membrane in which the hairs are embedded. This mechanical deformation of specific hair cells in the region of maximal basilar membrane vibration is transduced into neural signals that are transmitted to the auditory cortex in the brain for sound perception.

The **vestibular apparatus** in the inner ear consists of: (1) the **semicircular canals**, which detect rotational acceleration or deceleration in any direction, and (2) the **utricle** and **saccule**, which detect changes in the rate of linear movement in any direction and provide information important for determining head position in relationship to gravity. Neural signals are generated in response to mechanical deformation of hair cells caused by specific movement of fluid and related structures within these sense organs.

Chemical Senses: Taste and Smell

Taste and smell are chemical senses. In both cases, attachment of specific dissolved molecules to binding sites on the receptor membrane causes receptor potentials that, in turn, set up neural impulses that signal the presence of the chemical. **Taste receptors** are housed in taste buds on the tongue; **olfactory receptors** are located in the mucosa in the upper part of the nasal cavity. Both sensory pathways include two routes: one to the limbic system for emotional and behavioral processing, and one through the thalamus to the cortex for conscious perception and fine discrimination.

 EFFERENT OUTPUT

The efferent division of the peripheral nervous system carries directives from the CNS to the effector organs. Cardiac muscle, smooth muscle, and exocrine glands are innervated by the autonomic nervous system, which is considered to be the involuntary branch of the peripheral efferent division. Skeletal muscle is innervated by the somatic nervous system, which is the voluntary branch of the efferent division.

The **autonomic nervous system** consists of two subdivisions-the **sympathetic** and **parasympathetic** nervous systems. An autonomic nerve pathway consists of a two-neuron chain. The preganglionic fiber originates in the CNS and synapses with the cell body of the postganglionic fiber in a ganglion outside the CNS. The postganglionic fiber terminates on the effector organ. All preganglionic fibers and parasympathetic postganglionic fibers release **acetylcholine (ACh)**. Sympathetic postganglionic fibers release **norepinephrine.**

A given autonomic fiber either excites or inhibits activity in the organ that it innervates. Most visceral organs are innervated by both sympathetic and parasympathetic nerve fibers, which generally produce opposite effects in a particular organ. Dual innervation of visceral organs by both branches of the autonomic nervous system permits precise control over an organ's activity. The sympathetic system dominates in emergency or stressful situations and promotes

TABLE 5–2 Effects of the Autonomic Nervous System on Various Organs

ORGAN	EFFECT OF SYMPATHETIC STIMULATION	EFFECT OF PARASYMPATHETIC STIMULATION
Heart	Increased rate, increased force of contraction (of the whole heart)	Decreased rate, decreased force of contraction (of the atria only)
Blood vessels	Constriction (most organs)	Dilation of vessels supplying the penis and clitoris only
Lungs	Dilation of bronchioles (airways)	Constriction of bronchioles
	Inhibition of mucus secretion (?)	Stimulation of mucus secretion
Digestive tract	Decreased motility (movement)	Increased motility
	Contraction of sphincters (to prevent forward movement of contents)	Relaxation of sphincters (to permit forward movement of contents)
	Inhibition of digestive secretions (?)	Stimulation of digestive secretions
Urinary bladder	Relaxation	Contraction (emptying)
Eye	Dilation of the pupil	Constriction of the pupil
	Adjustment of the eye for far vision	Adjustment of the eye for near vision
Liver (glycogen stores)	Glycogenolysis (glucose released)	None
Adipose cells (fat stores)	Lipolysis (fatty acids released)	None
Exocrine glands	Inhibition of pancreatic exocrine secretion	Stimulation of pancreatic exocrine secretion (important for digestion)
	Stimulation of secretion by most sweat glands	Stimulation of secretion by some sweat glands
	Stimulation of small volume of thick saliva rich in mucus	Stimulation of large volume of watery saliva rich in enzymes
Adrenal medulla	Stimulation of secretion of epinephrine and norepinephrine	None
Genitals	Ejaculation and orgasmic contractions (males); orgasmic contractions (females)	Erection [caused by dilation of blood vessels in the penis (male) and clitoris (female)]
Brain activity	Increased alertness	

responses that prepare the body for strenuous physical activity. The parasympathetic system dominates in quiet, relaxed situations and promotes body maintenance activities such as digestion (**Table 5-2**).

The **somatic** nervous system consists of the axons of motor neurons, which originate in the spinal cord and terminate on skeletal muscle. ACh, the neurotransmitter released from a motor neuron, stimulates muscle contraction. Motor neurons are the final common pathway by which various regions of the CNS exert control over skeletal muscle activity.

Each axon terminal of a motor neuron forms a **neuromuscular junction** with a single muscle cell (fiber). Because these structures do not make direct contact, signals are passed between the nerve terminal and muscle fiber by means of the chemical messenger ACh. An action potential in the axon terminal causes the release of ACh from its storage vesicles. The released ACh diffuses across the space separating the nerve and muscle cell and binds to special receptor sites on the underlying motor end-plate of the muscle cell membrane. This combination of ACh with the receptor sites triggers the opening of specific channels in the motor end-plate. The subsequent ion movements depolarize the motor end-plate, producing the end-plate potential (EPP). Local current flow between the depolarized end-plate and adjacent muscle cell membrane brings these adjacent areas to threshold, initiating an action potential that is propagated throughout the muscle fiber. This muscle action potential triggers muscle contraction. Acetylcholinesterase inactivates ACh, terminating the EPP and, subsequently, the action potential (**Figure 5-4**).

MUSCULOSKELETAL SYSTEM

Muscle cells are specialized for contraction. The contractile units in muscle, **sarcomeres,** are made up of alternating, slightly overlapping stacked sets of **myosin**-containing **thick filaments** and **actin**-containing **thin filaments** (see Chapter 4).

During muscle contraction, **cross-bridges** extending from the thick filament bind to the thin filament, then bend to pull the thin filaments closer together between the thick filaments. This **sliding-filament mechanism of muscle contraction** results in shortening and tension development (i.e., contraction) of the muscle fiber. The energy-consuming cross-bridge power stroke that results in contraction is switched on by a rise in cytosolic Ca^{2+} brought about in response to an action potential (**excitation-contraction coupling**). Depending on the type of muscle, Ca^{2+} may be released from an intracellular store, the **sarcoplasmic reticulum,** or enter through opened Ca^{2+} channels from the ECF. The means by which Ca^{2+} turns on cross-bridge stroking also varies with muscle type (**Table 5-3**).

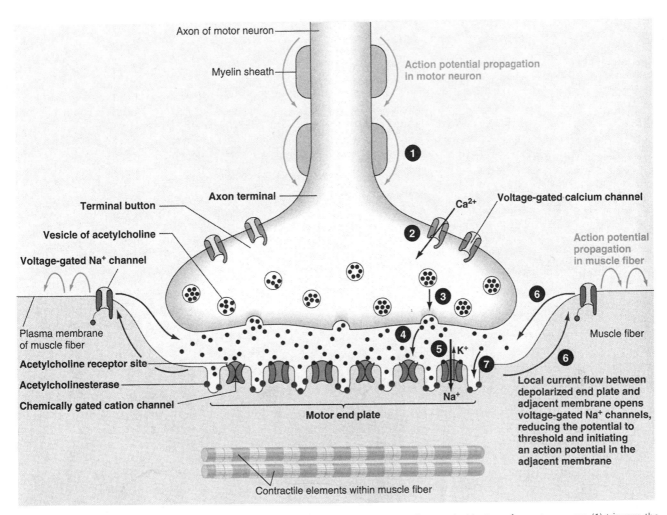

Figure 5-4. Events at a neuromuscular junction. Propagation of an action potential to the terminal button of a motor neuron (1) triggers the opening of voltage-gated Ca^{2+} into the terminal button (2). Ca^{2+} triggers the release of acetylcholine by exocytosis from a portion of the vesicles (3). Acetylcholine diffuses across the space separating the nerve and muscle cells and binds with receptor sites specific for it on the motor end-plate of the muscle cell membrane (4). This binding brings about the opening of cation channels, leading to a relatively large movement of Na^+ into the cell compared with a smaller movement of K^+ outward (5). The result is an end-plate potential. Local current flow between the depolarized end-plate and adjacent membrane initiates an action potential, which is propagated throughout the muscle fiber (6). Acetylcholine is subsequently destroyed by acetylcholinesterase, an enzyme located in the muscle cell membrane, terminating the muscle cell's response. (From Sherwin L: Human Physiology: From Cells to Systems, 4th ed. Pacific Grove, CA, Brooks/Cole, 2001.)

The three types of muscle are: **skeletal, smooth,** and **cardiac.** Skeletal muscle is striated and voluntary, and it attaches to bones. The two types of skeletal muscle contraction are-**isometric** (constant length) and **isotonic** (constant tension)-depending on the relationship between muscle tension and the load. If tension is less than the load, the muscle cannot shorten and lift the object but remains at constant length, producing an isometric contraction. In an isotonic contraction, the tension exceeds the load thus the muscle can shorten and lift the object, maintaining constant tension throughout the period of shortening.

Smooth muscle is unstriated, involuntary and forms the walls of hollow organs. Smooth muscle can be divided into two types: (1) **multiunit smooth** muscle is neurogenic and requires stimulation of individual muscle fibers by its autonomic nerve supply to trigger a contraction, and (2) **single-unit smooth** muscle is myogenic and initiates its own contraction without any external influence as a result of spontaneous depolarizations to threshold potential, which are brought about by automatic shifts in ionic fluxes. The autonomic nervous system as well as hormones and local metabolites can modify the rate and strength of the self-induced contractions. Smooth muscle contractions are energy efficient, thus enabling this type of muscle to economically sustain long-term contractions without fatigue. This economy, combined with the fact that single-unit smooth muscle is able to exist at various lengths with little change in tension, makes single-unit smooth muscle ideally suited for its task of forming the walls of distensible hollow organs. Cardiac muscle is striated, involuntary and myogenic and is found only in the heart.

TABLE 5–3 Comparison of Muscle Types

CHARACTERISTIC	SKELETAL	MULTI-UNIT SMOOTH	SINGLE-UNIT SMOOTH	CARDIAC
Location	Attached to the skeleton	Large blood vessels, eye, and hair follicles	Walls of hollow organs in the digestive, reproductive, and urinary tracts and in small blood vessels	Heart only
Function	Movement of the body in relation to the external environment	Varies with the structure involved	Movement of the contents within hollow organs	Pumps blood out of heart
Mechanism of contraction	Sliding-filament mechanism	Sliding-filament mechanism	Sliding-filament mechanism	Sliding-filament mechanism
Innervation	Somatic nervous system (motor neurons)	Autonomic nervous system	Autonomic nervous system	Autonomic nervous system
Level of control	Under voluntary control; also control subject to subconscious regulation	Under involuntary control	Under involuntary control	Under involuntary control
Initiation of contraction	Neurogenic	Neurogenic	Myogenic	Myogenic
Role of nervous stimulation	Initiates contraction	Initiates contraction	Modifies contraction	Modifies contraction
Modifying effect of hormones	No	Yes	Yes	Yes
Presence of thick myosin and thin actin filaments	Yes	Yes	Yes	Yes
Striated due to orderly arrangement of filaments	Yes	No	No	Yes
Cross Bridges Turned on by Ca^{2+}	Yes	Yes	Yes	Yes
Source of increased cytosolic Ca^{2+}	Sarcoplasmic reticulum	Extracellular fluid and sarcoplasmic reticulum	Extracellular fluid and sarcoplasmic reticulum	Extracellular fluid and sarcoplasmic reticulum
Site of Ca^{2+} regulation	Troponin in thin filaments	Myosin in thick filaments	Myosin in thick filaments	Troponin in thin filaments
Mechanism of Ca^{2+} action	Physically repositions the blocking troponin-tropomyosin complex to uncover actin cross-bridge	Chemically brings about phosphorylation of myosin cross-bridges so that they can bind with actin	Chemically brings about phosphorylation of myosin cross-bridges so that they can bind with actin	Physically repositions the sarcoplasmic reticulum blocking troponin-tropomyosin complex

CIRCULATORY SYSTEM

The Heart

Anatomic Considerations

The **heart** is basically a dual pump that provides the driving pressure for blood flow through the pulmonary and systemic circulations. The heart has four chambers; there is an **atrium**, or venous input chamber, and a **ventricle**, or arterial output chamber, in each half of the heart. Four heart valves direct the blood in the proper direction and prevent its flow in the reverse direction (**Figure 5-5**). The heart is self-excitable and initiates its own rhythmic contractions. Contraction of the spirally arranged cardiac muscle fibers produces a wringing effect that is important for efficient pumping. Also important for efficient pumping is the fact that the muscle fibers in each chamber act as a functional syncytium; they contract as a coordinated unit.

Electrical Activity of the Heart

The cardiac impulse originates at the **sinoatrial (SA) node,** the pacemaker of the heart, which has the fastest rate of spontaneous depolarization to threshold. Once initiated, the action potential spreads throughout the right and left atria, partially facilitated by specialized conduction pathways, but mainly by cell-to-cell spread of the impulse through gap junctions. The impulse passes from the atria into the ventricles through the **atrioventricular (AV) node,** the only point of electrical contact between these chambers. The action potential is delayed briefly at the AV node, ensuring that atrial excitation and subsequent contraction precedes ventricular excitation and contraction to allow complete ventricular filling. The impulse then rapidly travels down the interventricular septum via the **bundle of His** and is rapidly dispersed throughout the myocardium by means of the **Purkinje fibers.** The remainder of the ventricular cells are activated by cell-to-cell spread of the impulse through

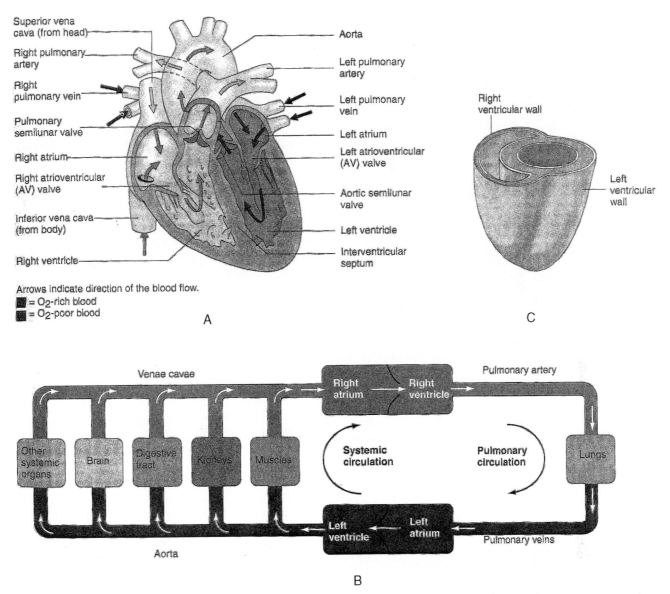

Arrows indicate direction of the blood flow.
■ = O₂-rich blood
■ = O₂-poor blood

A

C

B

Figure 5-5. Blood flow through and pump action of the heart. *A,* Blood flow through the heart. *B,* Dual pump action of the heart. The right side of the heart receives O₂-rich blood from the systemic circulation and pumps it into the pulmonary circulation. The left side of the heart receives O₂-rich blood from the pulmonary circulation and pumps it into the systemic circulation. *C,* Comparison of the thickness of the right and left ventricular walls. Note that the left ventricular wall is much thicker than the right wall. (The relative volume of blood flowing through each organ is not drawn to scale.) (From Sherwin L: Human Physiology: From Cells to Systems, 4th ed. Pacific Grove, CA, Brooks/Cole, 2001, p 285.)

gap junctions. Thus, the atria contract as a single unit, followed after a brief delay by a synchronized ventricular contraction.

The action potentials of contractile cardiac muscle fibers exhibit a prolonged positive phase, or plateau, accompanied by a prolonged period of contraction, which ensures adequate ejection time. This plateau is primarily due to activation of slow Ca²⁺ channels. Because a long refractory period occurs in conjunction with this prolonged plateau phase, summation and tetanus of cardiac muscle are impossible, thus ensuring the alternate periods of contraction and relaxation that are essential for pumping blood.

The spread of electrical activity throughout the heart can be recorded from the surface of the body. This record, the electrocardiogram (ECG), can provide useful information about the status of the heart **(Figure 5-6).**

Mechanical Events of the Cardiac Cycle

The cardiac cycle consists of three important events: (1) the generation of electrical activity as the heart autorhythmically depolarizes and repolarizes; (2) mechanical activity consisting of alternate periods of systole (contraction and emptying) and diastole (relaxation and filling), which are

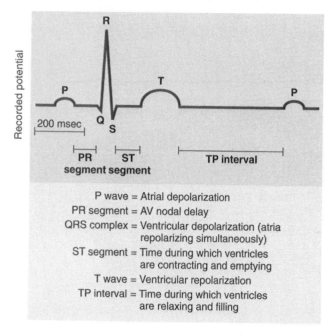

P wave = Atrial depolarization
PR segment = AV nodal delay
QRS complex = Ventricular depolarization (atria
                    repolarizing simultaneously)
ST segment = Time during which ventricles
                    are contracting and emptying
T wave = Ventricular repolarization
TP interval = Time during which ventricles
                    are relaxing and filling

Figure 5-6. Electrocardiogram waveforms in lead II. (From Sherwin L: Human Physiology: From Cells to Systems, 4th ed. Pacific Grove, CA, Brooks/Cole, 2001, p 300.)

initiated by the rhythmical electrical cycle; and (3) directional flow of blood through the heart chambers, guided by valvular opening and closing induced by pressure changes that are generated by mechanical activity. Closure of the valve gives rise to two normal heart sounds. The first heart sound is caused by closure of the AV valves and signals the onset of **ventricular systole**. The second heart sound is caused by closure of the aortic and pulmonary valves at the onset of **diastole**.

Defective valve function produces turbulent blood flow, which is audible as a heart murmur. Abnormal valves may be either stenotic (and not open completely) or insufficient (and not close completely).

Cardiac Output and Its Control

Cardiac output, the volume of blood ejected by each ventricle each minute, is determined by the heart rate times the stroke volume. **Heart rate** is varied by altering the balance of parasympathetic and sympathetic influence on the SA node, with parasympathetic stimulation slowing the heart rate and sympathetic stimulation speeding it up **(Table 5-4)**.

Stroke volume depends on: (1) the extent of ventricular filling, with an increased end-diastolic volume resulting in a larger stroke volume by means of the length-tension relationship (intrinsic control), and (2) the extent of sympathetic stimulation, with increased sympathetic stimulation resulting in increased contractility of the heart; that is, increased strength of contraction and increased stroke volume at a given end-diastolic volume (extrinsic control).

Nourishing the Heart Muscle

Cardiac muscle is supplied with oxygen and nutrients by blood delivered to it by the coronary circulation, not by blood within the heart chambers. Most coronary blood flow occurs during diastole, because the coronary vessels are compressed by the contracting heart muscle during systole. Coronary blood flow is normally varied to keep pace with cardiac oxygen needs.

Coronary blood flow may be compromised by the development of **atherosclerotic plaques**. These plaques can lead to ischemic heart disease, ranging in severity from mild chest pain on exertion to fatal heart attacks. The exact cause of atherosclerosis is unclear, but apparently the ratio of cholesterol carried in the plasma in conjunction with high-density lipoproteins (HDLs) compared to low-density lipoproteins (LDLs) is an important factor. Evidence is also rapidly accumulating to support the notion that an infectious agent may be the underlying culprit in a significant number of atherosclerotic cases. Among the leading suspects are gum disease-causing bacteria. Perhaps the infectious oral bacteria responsible for chronic gum disease, or gingivitis, may become blood-borne and injure the blood vessels, thus setting the stage for the buildup of cholesterol-containing plaque.

BLOOD VESSELS AND BLOOD PRESSURE

The blood vessel network connects various parts of the body with each other and with the external environment in order

---

TABLE 5–4 Effects of the Autonomic Nervous System on the Heart

PARASYMPATHETIC STIMULATION	SYMPATHETIC STIMULATION
Decreases the heart rate	Increases excitability of all areas of the heart, decreasing AV nodal delay and speeding up conduction of the impulse through the heart
Increases AV nodal delay	Increases contractility (strength of contraction) of the atria and ventricles
Weakens atrial contraction	Promotes secretion of epinephrine, which augments the sympathetic nervous system
Increases the heart rate	Increases venous return, which increases stroke volume through the Frank-Starling mechanism

to exchange materials. Organs that replenish nutrient supplies and remove metabolic wastes from the blood receive a greater percentage of the cardiac output than is warranted by their metabolic needs. These "reconditioning" organs can better tolerate reductions in blood supply than can organs that receive blood solely for the purpose of meeting their own metabolic needs. The brain is especially vulnerable to reductions in its blood supply. Therefore, the maintenance of adequate flow to this vulnerable organ is a high priority in circulatory function.

Blood flows in a closed loop between the heart and the tissues. The **arteries** transport blood from the heart throughout the body. The **arterioles** regulate the amount of blood that flows through each organ. The **capillaries** are the actual site of exchange of materials between the blood and the surrounding tissue. The **veins** return the blood from the tissues to the heart.

The **flow rate** of blood through a vessel is directly proportional to the pressure gradient and inversely proportional to the resistance. The higher pressure at the beginning of a vessel is established by the pressure imparted to the blood by cardiac contraction. The lower pressure at the end is caused by frictional losses as flowing blood rubs against the vessel wall. **Resistance**, the hindrance to blood flow through a vessel, is influenced most extensively by the vessel's radius. Resistance is inversely proportional to the fourth power of the radius, thus small changes in radius greatly influence flow. As the radius increases, resistance decreases and flow increases.

Arteries

Arteries are large-radius, low-resistance passageways from the heart to the tissues and also serve as a pressure reservoir. Because of their elasticity, arteries expand to accommodate the extra volume of blood pumped into them by cardiac contraction and then recoil to continue driving the blood forward when the heart is relaxing.

Systolic pressure is the peak pressure exerted by the ejected blood against the vessel walls during cardiac systole. **Diastolic pressure** is the minimum pressure in the arteries when blood is draining off into the vessels downstream during cardiac diastole.

Arterioles

Arterioles are the major resistance vessels. Their high resistance produces a large drop in mean pressure between the arteries and capillaries. This decline enhances blood flow by contributing to the pressure differential between the heart and the tissues. **Tone**, a baseline of contractile activity, is maintained in arterioles at all times. **Arteriolar vasodilation**, an expansion of arteriolar caliber above tonic level, decreases resistance and increases blood flow through the vessel, whereas **vasoconstriction**, a narrowing of the vessel, increases resistance and decreases flow.

Arteriolar caliber is subject to two types of control mechanisms: local controls and extrinsic controls. Local controls involve local chemical changes associated with changes in the level of metabolic activity in a tissue; these controls act directly on the arteriolar smooth muscle in the vicinity to induce changes in the caliber of the arterioles that supply the tissue. By adjusting the resistance to blood flow in this manner, the local control mechanism adjusts blood flow to the tissue to match the momentary metabolic needs of the tissue. Adjustments in arteriolar caliber can be accomplished independently in different tissues by local control factors. Such adjustments are important in determining the distribution of cardiac output.

Extrinsic control is accomplished primarily by sympathetic nerve influence and to a lesser extent by hormonal influence over arteriolar smooth muscle. Extrinsic controls are important in maintaining mean arterial blood pressure. Arterioles are richly supplied with sympathetic nerve fibers, whose increased activity produces generalized vasoconstriction and a subsequent increase in mean arterial pressure. Decreased sympathetic activity produces generalized arteriolar vasodilation, which lowers mean arterial pressure. These extrinsically controlled adjustments of arteriolar caliber help maintain the appropriate pressure head for driving blood forward to the tissues.

Capillaries

The thin-walled, small-radius, extensively branched **capillaries** are ideally suited to serve as sites of exchange between the blood and surrounding tissues. Anatomically, the surface area for exchange is maximized and diffusion distance is minimized in the capillaries. Furthermore, because of the capillaries' large total cross-sectional area, the velocity of blood flow through them is relatively slow, providing adequate time for exchanges to take place.

Two types of passive exchanges-**diffusion** and **bulk flow** - take place across capillary walls. Individual solutes are exchanged primarily by diffusion down concentration gradients. Lipid-soluble substances pass directly through the single layer of endothelial cells lining a capillary, whereas water-soluble substances pass through water-filled pores between the endothelial cells. Plasma proteins generally do not escape.

Imbalances in physical pressures acting across capillary walls are responsible for bulk flow of fluid through the pores back and forth between the plasma and the interstitial fluid. Fluid is forced out of the first portion of the capillary (ultrafiltration) where outward pressures (mainly capillary blood pressure) exceed inward pressures (mainly blood-colloid osmotic pressure). Fluid is returned to the capillary along its last half when outward pressures fall below inward pressures. The reason for the shift in balance down the length of the capillary is the continuous decline in capillary blood pressure, whereas the blood-colloid osmotic pressure remains constant. Bulk flow is responsible for the distribution of ECF between the plasma and interstitial fluid.

Normally, slightly more fluid is filtered than is reabsorbed. The extra fluid, any leaked proteins, and tissue contaminants such as bacteria are picked up by the lymphatic system. Bacteria are destroyed as lymph passes through the lymph nodes en route to being returned to the venous system.

Veins

Veins are large-radius, low-resistance passageways for return of blood from the tissues to the heart. Additionally, they can accommodate variable volumes of blood, thus acting as a blood reservoir. The capacity of veins to hold blood can change greatly with little change in venous pressure. Veins are thin-walled, highly distensible vessels that can passively stretch to store a larger volume of blood.

The primary force responsible for venous flow is the pressure gradient between the veins and the atrium (i.e., what remains of the driving pressure imparted to the blood by cardiac contraction.) **Venous return** is enhanced by sympathetically induced venous vasoconstriction and by external compression of the veins resulting from contraction of surrounding skeletal muscles, both of which drive blood out of the veins. One-way venous valves ensure that blood is driven toward the heart and prevented from flowing back toward the tissues. Venous return is also enhanced by the respiratory pump and the cardiac-suction effect. Respiratory activity produces a less-than-atmospheric pressure in the chest cavity, thus establishing an external pressure gradient that encourages flow from the lower veins that are exposed to atmospheric pressure to the chest veins that empty into the heart. In addition, slightly negative pressures created within the atria during ventricular systole and within the ventricles during ventricular diastole exert a suctioning effect that further enhances venous return and facilitates cardiac filling.

Blood Pressure

Regulation of mean arterial pressure depends on control of its two main determinants: cardiac output and total peripheral resistance. Control of **cardiac output**, in turn, depends on regulation of heart rate and stroke volume, whereas **total peripheral resistance** is determined primarily by the degree of arteriolar vasoconstriction. Short-term regulation of blood pressure is accomplished primarily by the baroreceptor reflex. Carotid-sinus and aortic-arch baroreceptors continuously monitor mean arterial pressure. When they detect a deviation from normal, they signal the medullary cardiovascular center, which responds by adjusting autonomic output to the heart and blood vessels to restore the blood pressure to normal. Long-term control of blood pressure involves maintenance of proper plasma volume through the kidneys' control of salt and water balance.

Blood pressure can be abnormally high (**hypertension**) or abnormally low (**hypotension**). Severe sustained hypotension resulting in generalized inadequate blood delivery to the tissues is known as circulatory shock.

BLOOD AND BODY DEFENSES

Plasma

The 5- to 5.5-L volume of blood in an adult consists of 42% to 45% erythrocytes, less than 1% leukocytes and platelets, and 55% to 58% plasma. The percentage of whole blood volume occupied by erythrocytes is known as the **hematocrit**.

Plasma is a complex liquid that serves as a transport medium for substances being carried in the blood. All plasma constituents are freely diffusible across the capillary walls except the plasma proteins, which remain in the plasma and perform various functions.

Erythrocytes

Erythrocytes (red blood cells) are specialized for their primary function of O_2 transport in the blood. They do not contain a nucleus, organelles, or ribosomes but instead are packed full of **hemoglobin**, which is an iron-containing molecule that can loosely, reversibly bind with O_2. Because O_2 is poorly soluble in blood, hemoglobin is indispensable for O_2 transport. Hemoglobin also contributes to CO_2 transport and buffering of blood by reversibly binding with CO_2 and H^+.

Because erythrocytes are unable to replace cell components, they are destined to a short life span of about 120 days. Undifferentiated stem cells in the red bone marrow give rise to all cellular elements of the blood. Erythrocyte production (**erythropoiesis**) by the marrow normally keeps pace with the rate of erythrocyte loss to keep the red blood cell count constant. Erythropoiesis is stimulated by erythropoietin, a hormone secreted by the kidneys in response to reduced O_2 delivery.

Platelets and Hemostasis

Platelets are cell fragments derived from large megakaryocytes in the bone marrow. Platelets play an important role in hemostasis, which is the arrest of bleeding from an injured vessel. The three main steps in hemostasis are: (1) vascular spasm, (2) platelet plugging, and (3) clot formation. **Vascular spasm** reduces blood flow through an injured vessel, whereas **aggregation of platelets** at the site of vessel injury quickly plugs the defect. Platelets start to aggregate upon contact with exposed collagen in the damaged vessel wall.

Clot formation (blood coagulation) reinforces the platelet plug and converts blood in the vicinity of a vessel injury into a nonflowing gel. Most factors necessary for clotting are always present in the plasma in inactive precursor form. When a vessel is damaged, exposed collagen initiates a cascade of reactions involving successive activation of these clotting factors, ultimately converting fibrinogen into fibrin. **Fibrin,** an insoluble thread-like molecule, is laid down as the meshwork of the clot, entangling blood cells to complete clot formation. Blood that has escaped into the tissues is also coagulated upon exposure to **tissue thromboplastin,** which likewise sets the clotting process into motion. When no longer needed, clots are dissolved by **plasmin,** a fibrinolytic factor also activated by exposed collagen.

    Leukocytes (white blood cells) are the defense corps of the body. They attack foreign invaders, destroy abnormal cells that arise in the body, and clean up cellular debris. There are five types of leukocytes, each with a different task:

1. **Neutrophils,** the phagocytic specialists, are important in engulfing bacteria and debris.
2. **Eosinophils** specialize in attacking parasitic worms and play a key role in allergic responses.
3. **Basophils** release two chemicals: histamine, which is also important in allergic responses, and heparin, which helps clear fat particles from the blood.
4. **Monocytes,** upon leaving the blood, set up residence in the tissues and greatly enlarge to become the large tissue phagocytes known as **macrophages.**
5. **Lymphocytes** are primarily responsible for the acquired immune defenses that occur against a specific foreign invader to which the body has been exposed.

Leukocytes are present in the blood only while in transit from their site of production and storage in the bone marrow (and also in the lymphoid organs in the case of the lymphocytes) to their site of action in the tissues. At any given time, most leukocytes are out in the tissues on surveillance missions or performing actual combative activities. All leukocytes have a limited life span and must be replenished by ongoing differentiation and proliferation of precursor cells. The total number and percentage of each of the different types of leukocytes produced varies depending on the momentary defense needs of the body.

Innate Immune Responses

Immunity, the body's ability to resist or eliminate potentially harmful foreign invaders and newly arisen cancer cells, includes both innate and acquired immune responses. **Innate** responses nonselectively defend against foreign material even upon initial exposure to it, whereas **acquired** responses are specifically aimed at the destruction of particular invaders to which the body has had prior exposure and is specially prepared for selective attack. Innate, nonspecific immune defenses include inflammation, interferon, natural killer cells, and the complement system (see Chapter 7).

    Inflammation is a nonspecific response to foreign invasion or tissue damage mediated mainly by the professional **phagocytes** (neutrophils and monocytes/ macrophages) and

their secretions. The phagocytic cells destroy foreign and damaged cells both by phagocytosis and by the release of lethal chemicals. Histamine-induced vasodilation and increased permeability of local vessels at the site of invasion or injury permit enhanced delivery of more phagocytic leukocytes and inactive plasma protein precursors crucial to the inflammatory process, such as clotting factors and components of the complement system. These vascular changes are also largely responsible for the observable local manifestations of inflammation-swelling, redness, heat, and pain (see Chapter 8).

    Interferon is nonspecifically released by virus-infected cells and transiently inhibits viral multiplication in other cells to which it binds. Interferon further exerts anticancer effects by slowing division and growth of tumor cells as well as by enhancing the power of killer cells.

    Natural killer cells nonspecifically lyse and destroy virus-infected cells and cancer cells on first exposure to them.

    Upon being activated by locally released factors or microbes themselves at the site of invasion, the **complement system** directly destroys the foreign invaders by lysing their membranes and furthermore augments other aspects of the inflammatory process.

Acquired Immune Responses

After the initial exposure to a microbial invader, specific components of the immune system become especially prepared to selectively attack the particular foreigner. The immune system is able not only to recognize foreign molecules as different from self-molecules-so that destructive immune reactions are not unleashed against the body itself-but it can also specifically distinguish between millions of different foreign molecules. The cells of the acquired immune system, the lymphocytes, are each uniquely equipped with surface membrane receptors that are able to bind lock-and-key fashion with only one specific, complex foreign molecule, which is known as an **antigen** (see Chapter 7).

 # RESPIRATORY SYSTEM

Internal respiration refers to the intracellular metabolic reactions that utilize O_2 and produce CO_2 during energy-yielding oxidation of nutrient molecules. **External respiration** encompasses the various steps involved in the transfer of O_2 and CO_2 between the external environment and tissue cells. The respiratory and circulatory systems function together to accomplish external respiration.

    The **respiratory system** accomplishes exchange of air between the atmosphere and the lungs through the process of ventilation. Exchange of O_2 and CO_2 between the air in the lungs and the blood in the pulmonary capillaries takes place across the extremely thin walls of the air sacs, or **alveoli. Respiratory airways** conduct air from the atmosphere to this gas-exchanging portion of the lungs. The lungs are housed within the closed compartment of the thorax or chest, the volume of which can be changed by contractile activity of surrounding respiratory muscles.

Respiratory Mechanics

Ventilation, or breathing, is the process of cyclically moving air in and out of the lungs so that old alveolar air that has already participated in exchange of O_2 and CO_2 with the pulmonary capillary blood can be exchanged for fresh atmospheric air. Ventilation is mechanically accomplished by alternately shifting the direction of the pressure gradient for airflow between the atmosphere and alveoli through cyclical expansion and recoil of the lungs. Alternate contraction and relaxation of the inspiratory muscles (primarily the diaphragm) indirectly produces periodic inflation and deflation of the lungs by cyclically expanding and compressing the thoracic cavity, with the lungs passively following its movements.

Inspiration and Expiration

Because energy is required for contraction of the inspiratory muscles, **inspiration** (breathing air in) is an active process, but **expiration** (breathing air out) is passive during quiet breathing because it is accomplished by elastic recoil of the lungs on relaxation of inspiratory muscles at no energy expense. For more forceful active expiration, contraction of the expiratory muscles (i.e., the abdominal muscles) further decreases the size of the thoracic cavity and lungs, which further increases the intra-alveolar-to-atmospheric pressure gradient. The larger the gradient between the alveoli and the atmosphere in either direction, the larger will be the airflow rate, because air continues to flow until the intra-alveolar pressure equilibrates with atmospheric pressure.

Besides being directly proportional to the pressure gradient, airflow rate is also inversely proportional to **airway resistance**. Because airway resistance, which depends on the caliber of the conducting airways, is normally very low, airflow rate usually depends primarily on the pressure gradient established between the alveoli and the atmosphere. If airway resistance is pathologically increased by chronic obstructive pulmonary disease, the pressure gradient must be correspondingly increased by more vigorous respiratory muscle activity to maintain a normal airflow rate.

The lungs are able to be stretched to varying degrees during inspiration and then to recoil to their preinspiratory size during expiration because of their elastic behavior. **Pulmonary compliance** refers to the distensibility of the lungs-how much they stretch in response to a given change in the transmural pressure gradient, the stretching force exerted across the lung wall. **Elastic recoil** refers to the phenomenon of the lungs returning to their resting position during expiration. Pulmonary elastic behavior depends on the elastic connective tissue meshwork within the lungs and on alveo-

lar surface tension/pulmonary surfactant interaction. Alveolar surface tension, which is due to the attractive forces between the surface water molecules in the liquid film lining each alveolus, tends to resist the alveolus being stretched upon inflation (decreases compliance) and tends to return it back to a smaller surface area during deflation (increases lung rebound). If the alveoli were lined by water alone, the surface tension would be so great that the lungs would be poorly compliant and would tend to collapse. Type II alveolar cells secrete **pulmonary surfactant**, a phospholipoprotein that intersperses between the water molecules and lowers the alveolar surface tension, thus increasing the compliance of the lungs and counteracting the tendency for alveoli to collapse.

Normally, the lungs operate at "half-full." The lung volume typically varies from about 2 to 2½ L as an average **tidal volume** of 500 ml of air is moved in and out with each breath. The lungs can be filled an additional 3 L upon maximal inspiratory effort or emptied to about 1 L upon maximal expiratory effort.

The amount of air moved in and out of the lungs in one minute, the **pulmonary ventilation**, is equal to the tidal volume multiplied by the respiratory rate. However, not all of the air moved in and out is available for O_2 and CO_2 exchange with the blood because part of it occupies the conducting airways, known as the **anatomic dead space**. **Alveolar ventilation,** the volume of air exchanged between the atmosphere and alveoli in 1 minute, is a measure of the air that is actually available for gas exchange with the blood.

$$\text{Alveolar ventilation} = (\text{tidal volume - the dead space volume}) \times \text{respiratory rate}$$

Gas Exchange

Oxygen and CO_2 move across body membranes by passive diffusion down partial pressure gradients. Net diffusion of O_2 occurs first between the alveoli and the blood and then between the blood and the tissues as a result of the O_2 partial pressure gradients created by continuous utilization of O_2 in the cells and continuous replenishment of fresh alveolar O_2 provided by ventilation. Net diffusion of CO_2 occurs in the reverse direction, first between the tissues and the blood and then between the blood and the alveoli, as a result of the CO_2 partial pressure gradients created by continuous production of CO_2 in the cells and continuous removal of alveolar CO_2 through the process of ventilation.

Gas Transport

Because O_2 and CO_2 are not very soluble in the blood, they must be transported primarily by mechanisms other than simply being physically dissolved. Only 1.5% of the O_2 is physically dissolved in the blood; 98.5% is chemically bound to hemoglobin (Hb). The primary factor that determines the extent to which Hb and O_2 are combined (the percentage of Hb saturation) is the PO_2 of the blood. The relationship between blood PO_2 and the percentage of Hb saturation is such that in the PO_2 range found in the pulmonary capillaries, Hb is still almost fully saturated even if the blood PO_2 falls as much as 40%, thus providing a margin of safety in ensuring near-normal O_2 delivery to the tissues despite a substantial reduction in arterial PO_2. On the other hand, in the PO_2 range found in the systemic capillaries, large increases in Hb unloading occur in response to a small local decline in blood PO_2 associated with increased cellular metabolism, thus providing more O_2 to match the increased tissue needs.

Carbon dioxide picked up at the systemic capillaries is transported in the blood by three methods: (1) 10% is physically dissolved, (2) 30% is bound to Hb, and (3) 60% is in the form of bicarbonate (HCO_3^-). The erythrocytic enzyme **carbonic anhydrase** catalyzes the conversion of CO_2 to HCO_3^- according to the reaction:

$$CO_2 + H_2O \equiv H_2CO_3 \equiv H^+ + HCO_3^-$$

The generated H^+ binds to Hb. These reactions are all reversed in the lungs as CO_2 is eliminated to the alveoli.

Control of Respiration

The two distinct aspects of ventilation, both of which are subject to neural control, are: (1) rhythmic cycling between inspiration and expiration and (2) regulation of the magnitude of ventilation, which in turn depends on control of respiratory rate and depth of tidal volume. Respiratory rhythm is established by rhythmic firing of inspiratory neurons located in the respiratory control center in the medulla of the brainstem. When these inspiratory neurons fire, impulses ultimately reach the inspiratory muscles to bring about inspiration. When the inspiratory neurons cease firing, the inspiratory muscles relax and expiration takes place. If active expiration is to occur, the expiratory muscles are activated by output from the medullary expiratory neurons at this time. This basic rhythm is smoothed out by a balance of activity in the apneustic and pneumotaxic centers located higher in the brainstem in the pons. The apneustic center prolongs inspiration, whereas the more powerful pneumotaxic center limits inspiration.

Three chemical factors play a role in determining the magnitude of ventilation: the **PCO_2**, **PO_2**, and **H^+** concentration of the arterial blood. The dominant factor in the minute-to-minute regulation of ventilation is the arterial PCO_2. An increase in arterial PCO_2 is the most potent chemical stimulus for increasing ventilation. Changes in arterial PCO_2 alter ventilation primarily by bringing about corresponding changes in the brain ECF H^+ concentration, to which the central chemoreceptors are exquisitely sensitive. The peripheral chemoreceptors respond to an increase in arterial H^+ concentration, which likewise reflexly brings about increased ventilation. The resultant adjustment in arterial H^+-generating CO_2 is important in maintaining the acid-base balance of the body. The peripheral chemoreceptors also reflexly stimulate the respiratory center in response to a marked reduction in arterial PO_2

RENAL PHYSIOLOGY

The **kidneys** eliminate unwanted plasma constituents into the urine while conserving materials of value to the body. The urine-forming functional unit of the kidneys is the **nephron**, which consists of interrelated vascular and tubular components. The vascular component consists of two capillary networks in series, the first being the **glomerulus**, a tuft of capillaries that filters large volumes of protein-free plasma into the tubular component. The second capillary network consists of the **peritubular capillaries**, which wind around the tubular component. The peritubular capillaries nourish the renal tissue and participate in exchanges between the tubular fluid and the plasma. The tubular component begins with the **Bowman capsule**, which cups around the glomerulus to catch the filtrate, then continues a specific tortuous course to ultimately empty into the **renal pelvis**. As the filtrate passes through the various regions of the tubule, it is modified by the cells lining the tubules to return to the plasma only those materials necessary for maintaining the proper ECF composition and volume. The filtrate that is left behind in the tubules is excreted as **urine**.

The kidneys perform three basic processes when carrying out their regulatory and excretory functions: (1) **glomerular filtration**, the nondiscriminating movement of protein-free plasma from the blood into the tubules; (2) **tubular reabsorption,** the selective transfer of specific constituents in the filtrate back into the blood of the peritubular capillaries; and (3) **tubular secretion,** the highly specific movement of selected substances from the peritubular capillary blood into the tubular fluid. Everything that is filtered or secreted but not reabsorbed is excreted as urine.

Glomerular Filtration

Glomerular filtrate is produced as a portion of the plasma flowing through each glomerulus is passively forced under pressure through the glomerular membrane into the lumen of the underlying Bowman capsule. The net filtration pressure that induces filtration is caused by an imbalance in the physical forces acting across the glomerular membrane. A high glomerular-capillary blood pressure favoring filtration outweighs the combined opposing forces of blood-colloid osmotic pressure and the hydrostatic pressure of the Bowman capsule.

Typically, 20% to 25% of the cardiac output is delivered to the kidneys for the purpose of being acted on by renal regulatory and excretory processes. Of the plasma flowing through the kidneys, normally 20% is filtered through the glomeruli, producing an average **glomerular filtration rate (GFR)** of 125 ml/min. This filtrate is identical in composition to plasma, except for the plasma proteins that are held back by the glomerular membrane.

The GFR can be deliberately altered by changing the glomerular capillary blood pressure as a result of sympathetic influence on the afferent arterioles, the vessels that deliver blood to the glomeruli. Afferent arteriolar vasoconstriction decreases the flow of blood into the glomerulus, resulting in a reduction in glomerular blood pressure and a fall in the GFR. Conversely, afferent arteriolar vasodilation leads to increased glomerular blood flow and a rise in the GFR. Sympathetic control of the GFR is part of the baroreceptor reflex response to compensate for a change in arterial blood pressure. As the GFR is altered, the amount of fluid lost in the urine is changed correspondingly, providing a mechanism to adjust plasma volume as needed to help restore blood pressure to normal on a long-term basis.

Tubular Reabsorption

After a protein-free plasma is filtered through the glomerulus, each substance is handled discretely by the tubules, so that even though the concentrations of all constituents in the initial glomerular filtrate are identical to their concentrations in the plasma (with the exception of plasma proteins), the concentrations of different constituents are variously altered as the filtered fluid flows through the tubular system. The reabsorptive capacity of the tubular system is tremendous. **More than 99% of the filtered plasma is returned to the blood through tubular reabsorption.** The major substances actively reabsorbed are Na^+ (the principal cation in the ECF), most other electrolytes, and organic nutrients such as glucose and amino acids. The most important passively reabsorbed substances are Cl^-, H_2O, and urea.

Tubular Secretion

The kidney tubules are able to selectively add some substances to the quantity already filtered by means of the process of tubular secretion. Secretion of substances hastens their excretion in the urine. The most important secretory systems are for: (1) H^+, which is important in the regulation of acid-base balance; (2) K^+, which keeps the plasma K^+ concentration at an appropriate level to maintain normal membrane excitability in muscles and nerves, and (3) organic anions and cations, which accomplish more efficient elimination of foreign organic compounds from the body.

Urine Excretion and Plasma Clearance

Of the 125 ml/min filtered in the glomeruli, normally only 1 ml/min remains in the tubules to be excreted as **urine**. Only wastes and excess electrolytes that are not wanted by the body are left behind, dissolved in a given volume of H_2O, and eliminated in the urine. Because the excreted material is removed or "cleared" from the plasma, the term **plasma**

clearance refers to the volume of plasma being cleared of a particular substance each minute by means of renal activity.

The kidneys are able to excrete urine of varying volumes and concentrations to either conserve or eliminate H_2O, depending respectively on whether the body has an H_2O deficiency or excess. The kidneys are able to produce urine ranging from 0.3 ml/min at 1200 mOsm/L to 25 ml/min at 100 mOsm/L by reabsorbing variable amounts of H_2O from the distal portions of the nephron.

Once formed, urine is propelled by peristaltic contractions through the **ureters** from the kidneys to the **urinary bladder** for temporary storage. The bladder can accommodate up to 250 to 400 ml urine before stretch receptors within its wall initiate the **micturition reflex**. This reflex causes involuntary emptying of the bladder by simultaneous bladder contraction and opening of both the internal and external urethral sphincters. Micturition can transiently be voluntarily prevented until a more opportune time for evacuation by deliberately tightening the external sphincter and surrounding pelvic diaphragm.

Fluid Balance

On average, the body fluids compose 60% of total body weight. This figure varies among individuals, depending on how much fat (low H_2O content in the tissue) they possess. Two thirds of the H_2O in the body is found in the **ICF**. The remaining one third in the **ECF** is distributed between the plasma (20% of the ECF) and the **interstitial fluid** (80% of the ECF).

The essential components of fluid balance are: (1) **control of ECF volume** by maintaining **salt balance,** and (2) **control of ECF osmolarity** by maintaining **water balance**. Because of the osmotic holding power of Na^+, the major ECF cation, a change in the body's total Na^+ content brings about a corresponding change in ECF volume, including plasma volume, which in turn, alters the arterial blood pressure in the same direction. Appropriately, changes in ECF volume and arterial blood pressure are compensated for in the long term by Na^+-regulating mechanisms. Salt intake is not controlled in humans, but control of salt output in the urine is closely regulated. Blood pressure-regulating mechanisms can vary the GFR, and accordingly the amount of Na^+ filtered, by adjusting the caliber of the afferent arterioles supplying the glomeruli. Simultaneously, blood pressure-regulating mechanisms can vary the secretion of **aldosterone**, which is the hormone that promotes Na^+ reabsorption by the renal tubules. By varying Na^+ filtration and reabsorption, the extent of Na^+ excretion in the urine can be adjusted to regulate the plasma volume and subsequently the arterial blood pressure in the long term.

Changes in the osmolarity of the ECF are primarily detected and corrected by systems responsible for maintaining H_2O balance. The osmolarity of the ECF must be closely regulated to prevent osmotic shifts of H_2O between the ECF and the ICF, because cell swelling or shrinking is deleterious, especially to brain neurons. Excess free H_2O in the ECF dilutes the ECF solutes, with the result that ECF hypotonicity drives H_2O into the cells. An ECF-free H_2O deficit, on the other hand, concentrates the ECF solutes, and consequently H_2O leaves the cells to enter the hypertonic ECF. To prevent these detrimental fluxes, regulation of free H_2O balance is accomplished mainly by **vasopressin** and, to a lesser degree, by **thirst**. Changes in vasopressin secretion and thirst are both governed primarily by hypothalamic osmoreceptors, which monitor ECF osmolarity. The amount of vasopressin secreted determines the extent of free H_2O reabsorption by the distal portions of the nephrons, thus determining the volume of urinary output. Simultaneously, the intensity of thirst controls the volume of fluid intake. However, because the volume of fluid drunk is often not directly correlated with the intensity of thirst, control of urinary output by vasopressin is the most important regulatory mechanism for maintaining H_2O balance.

Acid-Base Balance

Acids liberate free hydrogen ions (H^+) into solution; **bases** bind with free hydrogen ions and remove them from solution. **Acid-base balance** refers to the regulation of H^+ concentration ($[H^+]$) in the body fluids. To precisely maintain $[H^+]$, input of H^+ by means of metabolic production of acids within the body must continually be matched with H^+ output by way of urinary excretion of H^+ and by respiratory removal of H^+-generating CO_2. Furthermore, between the time of its generation and elimination, H^+ must be buffered within the body to prevent marked fluctuations in $[H^+]$.

Hydrogen ion concentration is often expressed in terms of the pH, which is the logarithm of $1/[H^+]$. The normal pH of the plasma is 7.4, which is slightly alkaline compared with neutral H_2O, which has a pH of 7.0. A pH lower than normal (higher $[H^+]$ than normal) is indicative of a state of **acidosis**. A pH higher than normal (lower $[H^+]$ than normal) characterizes a state of **alkalosis**. Fluctuations in $[H^+]$ have profound effects on body chemistry, most notably: (1) changes in neuromuscular excitability, with acidosis depressing excitability, especially of the CNS, and alkalosis producing overexcitability of both the peripheral nervous system and the CNS; (2) disruption of normal metabolic reactions by altering the structure and function of all enzymes; and (3) alterations in plasma $[K^+]$ brought about by H^+-induced changes in the rate of elimination of K^+ by the kidneys.

The primary challenge in controlling acid-base balance is the maintenance of normal plasma alkalinity in the face of continual addition of H^+ to the plasma from ongoing metabolic activity. The three lines of defense for resisting changes in $[H^+]$ are: (1) the chemical buffer systems, (2) respiratory control of pH, and (3) renal control of pH.

Chemical buffer systems, the first line of defense, each consist of a pair of chemicals involved in a reversible reaction, one that can liberate H^+ and the other that can bind H^+.

A buffer pair acts to minimize any changes in pH that occur by acting according to the law of mass action, either liberating or binding H^+ as needed.

The **respiratory system**, constituting the second line of defense, normally eliminates the metabolically produced CO_2 so that H_2CO_3 does not accumulate in the body fluids. When the chemical buffers alone have been unable to immediately minimize a pH change, the respiratory system responds within a few minutes by altering its rate of CO_2 removal. An increase in $[H^+]$ arising from noncarbonic acid sources stimulates respiration so that more H_2CO_3-forming CO_2 is blown off, compensating for the acidosis by reducing the generation of H^+ from H_2CO_3. Conversely, a fall in $[H^+]$ depresses respiratory activity so that CO_2 and thus H^+-generating H_2CO_3 can accumulate in the body fluids to compensate for the alkalosis.

The **kidneys** are the third and most powerful defense mechanism. They require hours to days to compensate for a deviation in body fluid pH. The kidneys vary their rate of H^+ excretion in the urine, depending on the H^+ concentration in the body fluids. Furthermore, the kidneys vary their rate of excretion of HCO_3 in the urine in response to changes in H^+ concentration in the body fluids, thus adjusting the ECF concentration of this important buffer as needed.

The four types of acid-base imbalance are: (1) respiratory acidosis, (2) respiratory alkalosis, (3) metabolic acidosis, and (4) metabolic alkalosis. Respiratory acid-base disorders originate with deviations from normal $[CO_2]$, whereas metabolic acid-base imbalances encompass all deviations in pH other than those caused by abnormal $[CO_2]$.

 # DIGESTIVE SYSTEM

The four basic digestive processes are **motility, secretion, digestion,** and **absorption**. Digestive activities are carefully regulated by synergistic autonomous, neural (both intrinsic and extrinsic), and hormonal mechanisms to ensure that the ingested food is maximally made available to the body for energy production and as synthetic raw materials.

Digestive Tract

The **digestive tract** consists of a continuous tube that runs from the mouth to the anus, with local modifications that reflect regional specializations for carrying out digestive functions. The lumen of the digestive tract is continuous with the external environment, thus its contents are technically outside of the body; this arrangement permits digestion of food without allowing self-digestion in the process.

Mouth, Pharynx, and Esophagus

Food enters the digestive system through the mouth, where it is chewed and mixed with **saliva** to facilitate swallowing.

The salivary enzyme, **amylase**, begins the digestion of polysaccharides (complex carbohydrates), a process that continues in the stomach after the food has been swallowed until amylase is eventually inactivated by the acidic gastric juice. More important than its minor digestive function, saliva is essential for articulate speech and plays an important role in dental health. Salivary secretion is controlled by a salivary center in the medulla, mediated by autonomic innervation of the salivary glands.

Following chewing, the tongue propels the bolus of food to the rear of the throat, which initiates the **swallowing reflex**. The swallowing center in the medulla coordinates a complex group of activities that result in closure of the respiratory passages and propulsion of the food through the pharynx and esophagus into the stomach.

The esophageal secretion, mucus, is protective in nature. No nutrient absorption occurs in the mouth, pharynx, or esophagus.

Stomach

The **stomach,** a sac-like structure located between the esophagus and the small intestine, stores ingested food for variable periods until the small intestine is ready to further process it for final absorption. The four aspects encompassing **gastric motility** are gastric filling, storage, mixing, and emptying. **Gastric filling** is facilitated by vagally mediated receptive relaxation of the stomach musculature. **Gastric storage** takes place in the body of the stomach, where peristaltic contractions of the thin muscular walls are too weak to mix the contents. **Gastric mixing** takes place in the thick-muscled antrum as a result of vigorous peristaltic contractions. **Gastric emptying** is influenced by factors both in the stomach and duodenum. The volume and fluidity of **chyme** (a mixture of food and gastric secretions) in the stomach tend to promote emptying of the stomach contents. The duo-denal factors, which are the dominant factors controlling gastric emptying, tend to delay gastric emptying until the duodenum is ready to receive and process more chyme. The specific factors in the duodenum that delay gastric emptying by inhibiting stomach peristaltic activity are fat, acid, hypertonicity, or distention.

Carbohydrate digestion continues in the body of the stomach under the influence of the swallowed salivary amylase; protein digestion is initiated in the antrum of the stomach, where vigorous peristaltic contractions mix the food with gastric secretions, converting it to a thick liquid mixture known as chyme. **Gastric secretions** in the stomach lumen include: (1) **HCl**, which activates pepsinogen, denatures protein, and kills bacteria; (2) **pepsinogen**, which, once activated, initiates the digestion of protein; (3) **mucus**, which provides a protective coating to supplement the gastric mucosal barrier, thus enabling the stomach to contain the harsh luminal contents without self-digestion; and (4) **intrinsic factor**, which plays a vital role in vitamin B_{12} absorption, a constituent essential for normal red blood cell production. The stomach also secretes into the blood the hormone **gastrin**, which plays a dominant role in regulating gastric secretion. **Histamine**, a potent gastric stimulant that is not normally secreted, is released into the stomach lumen with devastating effects during ulcer formation.

Both gastric motility and gastric secretion are under complex control mechanisms; they involve not only gastrin but also vagal and intrinsic nerve responses and enterogastrone hormones (**secretin, cholecystokinin,** and **gastric inhibitory peptide**) secreted from the mucosa of the small intestine. Regulation of the stomach is aimed at balancing the rate of gastric activity with the ability of the small intestine to handle the arrival of acidic, fat-laden contents from the stomach.

No nutrients are absorbed from the stomach (**Table 5-5**).

TABLE 5–5 Factors Regulating Gastric Motility and Emptying

FACTORS	MODE OF REGULATION	EFFECTS ON GASTRIC MOTILITY AND EMPTYING
Within the Stomach		
Volume of chyme	Distention has a direct effect on gastric smooth-muscle excitability, as well as acting through intrinsic plexuses, vagus nerve, and gastrin	Increased volume stimulates motility and emptying
Degree of fluidity	Direct effect; contents must be in fluid form to be evacuated	Increased fluidity allows more rapid emptying
Within the Duodenum		
Presence of fat, acid, hypertonicity, or distention	Initiates enterogastric reflex or triggers release of enterogastrones (cholecystokinin, secretin, gastric inhibitory peptide)	These factors in the duodenum inhibit further gastric motility and emptying until the duodenum has coped with factors already present
Outside the Digestive System		
Emotion	Alters autonomic balance	Stimulates or inhibits motility and emptying
Intense pain	Increases sympathetic activity	Inhibits motility and emptying

Pancreatic and Biliary Secretions

Pancreatic exocrine secretions and bile from the liver both enter the duodenal lumen. **Pancreatic secretions** include: (1) potent digestive enzymes from the pancreatic acinar cells that digest all three categories of foodstuff (i.e., **pancreatic amylase** for carbohydrates; **lipase** for fats; and **trypsin, chymotrypsin,** and **carboxypeptidase** for proteins), and (2) an aqueous $NaHCO_3$ solution from the cells of the pancreatic duct, which neutralizes the acidic contents emptied into the duodenum from the stomach. This neutralization is important to protect the duodenum from acid injury and to allow the pancreatic enzymes, which are inactivated by acid, to perform their important digestive functions. Pancreatic secretion is primarily under hormonal control, which matches the composition of the pancreatic juice with the needs in the duodenal lumen.

The **liver**, the body's largest and most important metabolic organ, performs many varied functions. Its contribution to digestion is the secretion of **bile**, which contains bile salts. **Bile salts** aid fat digestion through their detergent action and facilitate fat absorption through formation of water-soluble micelles that can carry the products of fat digestion to their absorptive site. Between meals, bile is stored and concentrated in the **gallbladder**, which is hormonally stimulated to contract and empty the bile into the duodenum during digestion of a meal. After participating in fat digestion and absorption, bile salts are reabsorbed and returned via the hepatic portal system to the liver, where they are not only resecreted but act as a potent **choleretic** to stimulate the secretion of even more bile. Bile also contains **bilirubin**, a derivative of degraded hemoglobin, which is the major excretory product in the feces and is responsible for the color of feces.

Small Intestine

The **small intestine** is the main site for digestion and absorption. **Segmentation,** its primary motility, thoroughly mixes the food with pancreatic, biliary, and small intestinal juices to facilitate digestion; it also exposes the products of digestion to the absorptive surfaces. Between meals, the **migrating motility complex** sweeps the lumen clean. The juice secreted by the small intestine does not contain any digestive enzymes. The enzymes synthesized by the small intestine act intracellularly within the brush border membranes of the epithelial cells. These enzymes complete the digestion of carbohydrates (**maltase, sucrase,** and **lactase**) and protein (**aminopeptidases**) before these nutrients enter the blood. The energy-dependent process of Na^+ absorption provides the driving force for Cl^-, water, glucose, and amino acid absorption. Fat digestion is accomplished entirely in the lumen of the small intestine by pancreatic lipase (**Table 5-6**). Because of their water insolubility, the products of fat digestion must undergo a series of transformations that enable them to be passively absorbed and eventually enter the lymph. The small intestine absorbs almost everything presented to it, from ingested food to digestive secretions to sloughed epithelial cells. Only a small amount of fluid and nondigestible food residue passes on to the large intestine.

The lining of the small intestine is remarkably adapted to its digestive and absorptive function. It is thrown into folds that bear a rich array of finger-like projections, the **villi,** which are furnished with a multitude of even smaller hair-like protrusions, the **microvilli**. Altogether, these surface modifications greatly increase the area available to house the membrane-bound enzymes and to accomplish both active and passive absorption. This impressive lining is replaced approximately every 3 days to ensure an optimally healthy and functional presence of epithelial cells despite the harsh luminal conditions.

Large Intestine

The **colon** serves primarily to concentrate and store undigested food residues and biliary waste products until they can be eliminated from the body as feces. No secretion of digestive enzymes or absorption of nutrients takes place in the colon. All nutrient digestion and absorption is completed in the small intestine. **Haustral contractions** slowly shuffle the colonic contents back and forth to accomplish absorption of most of the remaining fluid and electrolytes. **Mass movements** occur several times a day, usually after meals, propelling the feces long distances. Movement of feces into the rectum triggers the **defecation reflex**, which can be voluntarily prevented by contraction of the external anal sphincter if the time is inopportune for elimination. The alkaline mucus secretion of the large intestine is primarily protective in nature.

ENERGY BALANCE AND TEMPERATURE REGULATION

Energy Balance

Energy input to the body in the form of food energy must equal energy output, because energy cannot be created or destroyed. **Energy output** or expenditure includes: (1) **external work**, performed by skeletal muscles to accomplish movement of an external object or movement of the body through the external environment; and (2) **internal work**, which consists of all other energy-dependent activities that do not accomplish external work, including active transport, smooth and cardiac muscle contraction, glandular secretion, and protein synthesis. Only about 25% of the chemical energy in food is harnessed to do biologic work. The rest is converted immediately to heat. Furthermore, all of the energy expended to accomplish internal work is eventually converted into heat, and 75% of the energy expended by working skeletal muscles is lost as heat. Therefore, most of the energy in food ultimately appears as body heat. The **metabolic rate**, which is energy expenditure per

TABLE 5–6   Digestive Processes for the Three Major Categories of Nutrients

NUTRIENTS	ENZYMES FOR DIGESTING NUTRIENT	SOURCE OF ENZYMES	SITE OF ACTION OF ENZYMES	ACTION OF ENZYMES	ABSORBABLE UNITS OF NUTRIENTS
Carbohydrate	Amylase	Salivary glands Exocrine pancreas	Mouth and body of the stomach Small intestine lumen	Hydrolyzes to polysaccharides to disaccharides	Monosaccharides, especially glucose
	Disaccharidases (maltase, sucrase, lactase)	Small intestine epithelial cells	Small intestine brush border	Hydrolyzes to disaccharides to monosaccharides	
Protein	Pepsin	Stomach chief cells	Stomach antrum	Hydrolyzes protein to peptide fragments	
	Trypsin, chymotrypsin, carboxypeptidase	Exocrine pancreas	Small intestine lumen	Attack different peptide fragments	
	Aminopeptidases	Small intestine epithelial cells	Small intestine brush border	Hydrolyze peptide fragments to amino acids	Amino acids and a few small peptides
Fat	Lipase	Exocrine pancreas	Small intestine lumen	Hydrolyzes triglycerides to fatty acids and monoglycerides	
	Bile salts (not an enzyme)	Liver	Small intestine lumen	Emulsify large fat globules for attack	

unit of time, is measured in kilocalories of heat produced per hour.

For a neutral energy balance, the energy in ingested food must equal the energy expended in performing work. If more food is consumed than energy expended, the extra energy is stored in the body, primarily as adipose tissue, thus body weight increases. On the other hand, if more energy is burned than is available in the food, body energy stores are used to support energy expenditure, therefore body weight decreases. Usually, body weight remains fairly constant over a prolonged period (except during growth), because food intake is adjusted to match energy expenditure on a long-term basis. Food intake is controlled primarily by the hypothalamus by means of complex, poorly understood regulatory mechanisms in which **hunger** and **satiety** (fullness) are important components.

Temperature Regulation

The body can be thought of as a heat-generating core (internal organs, CNS, and skeletal muscles) surrounded by a shell of variable insulating capacity (the skin). The skin exchanges heat energy with the external environment, with the direction and amount of heat transfer depending on the environmental temperature and the momentary insulating capacity of the shell. The four physical methods by which heat is exchanged between the body and the external environment are: (1) **radiation** (net movement of heat energy via electromagnetic waves); (2) **conduction** (exchange of heat energy by direct contact); (3) **convection** (transfer of heat energy by means of air currents); and (4) **evaporation** (extraction of heat energy from the body by the heat-requiring conversion of liquid H_2O to H_2O vapor).

To prevent serious cellular malfunction, the *core* **temperature** must be held constant at about 100°F (equivalent to an average oral temperature of 98.2°F) by continuously balancing heat gain and heat loss despite changes in environmental temperature and variation in internal heat production. This thermoregulatory balance is controlled by the hypothalamus. The primary method of heat gain is heat production by metabolic activity, the biggest contributor being skeletal muscle contraction. On cold exposure, the hypothalamus triggers heat-generating **shivering**; in response to excessive heat, it reduces muscle tone. Heat loss is adjusted by **sweating** and by controlling to the greatest extent possible the temperature gradient between the skin and the surrounding environment. The latter is accomplished by hypothalamic regulation of the caliber of the skin's blood vessels. **Vasoconstriction of the skin vessels** in response to cold exposure reduces the flow of warmed blood through the skin so that skin temperature falls. The layer of cool skin between the core and the environment increases the insulating barrier between the warm core and the external air. Conversely, **skin vasodilation** in the face of excessive heat exposure brings more warmed blood through the skin so that skin temperature approaches the core temperature, thus reducing the insulative capacity of the skin.

A **fever** occurs when **endogenous pyrogen** released from white blood cells in response to infection raises the hypothalamic set point. An elevated core temperature develops as the hypothalamus initiates cold-response mechanisms to raise the core temperature to the new set point.

ENDOCRINE SYSTEM

General Principles of Endocrinology

Hormones are long-distance chemical messengers secreted by the ductless **endocrine glands** into the blood, which transports them to specific target sites where they regulate or direct a particular function by altering protein activity within the target cells. Even though hormones are able to reach all tissues via the blood, they exert their effects only at their target cells because of target-cell specificity. Through its slowly acting hormonal messengers, the endocrine system controls activities that require duration rather than speed. It is especially important in regulating fuel metabolism, H_2O and electrolyte balance, growth, and reproduction.

The three chemical classes of hormones are **peptides, steroids,** and **amines**, the latter including thyroid hormones and adrenomedullary catecholamines. Peptides and catecholamines are hydrophilic; steroid and thyroid hormones are lipophilic. **Hydrophilic hormones** are synthesized and packaged for export by the endoplasmic reticulum/Golgi apparatus route, stored in secretory vesicles, and released by exocytosis upon appropriate stimulation. They dissolve freely in the blood for transport to their target cells where they bind with surface membrane receptors. Upon binding, a hydrophilic hormone triggers a chain of intracellular events by means of a second messenger system that ultimately alters pre-existing cellular proteins, usually enzymes, which exert the effect leading to the target cell's response to the hormone.

Steroids are synthesized by modifications of stored cholesterol by means of enzymes specific for each steroidogenic tissue. Steroids are not stored in the endocrine cells. Being lipophilic, they diffuse out through the lipid membrane barrier as soon as they are synthesized. Control of steroids is directed at their synthesis. Thyroid hormone is synthesized and stored in large amounts within extracellular storage pools sequestered "inland" in the thyroid gland. Lipophilic steroids and thyroid hormone are both transported in the blood mainly bound to carrier plasma proteins, with only free, unbound hormone being biologically active. **Lipophilic hormones** readily enter through the lipid membrane barriers of their target cells and bind with intracellular receptors. Hormonal binding activates the synthesis of new intracellular proteins that carry out the hormone's effect on the target cell.

Hypothalamus and Pituitary

The **pituitary gland** consists of two distinct lobes, the **posterior pituitary** and the **anterior pituitary**. The posterior pituitary is essentially a neural extension of the **hypothalamus**. Two small peptide hormones, **vasopressin** and **oxytocin**, are synthesized within the cell bodies of neurosecretory neurons located in the hypothalamus, from which they pass down the axon to be stored in nerve terminals within the posterior pituitary. These hormones are independently released from the posterior pituitary into the blood in response to action potentials originating in the hypothalamus.

The anterior pituitary secretes six different peptide hormones that it produces itself: **growth hormone, thyroid-stimulating hormone (TSH), adrenocorticotropic hormone (ACTH), follicle-stimulating hormone (FSH), luteinizing hormone (LH),** and **prolactin**. Most of these hormones are **tropic**; that is, they stimulate hormone secretion by other endocrine glands.

The anterior pituitary releases its hormones into the blood at the bidding of releasing and inhibiting hormones from the hypothalamus. The hypothalamus, in turn, is influenced by various neural and hormonal controlling inputs. Both the hypothalamus and the anterior pituitary are inhibited in negative-feedback fashion by the product of the target organ in the hypothalamus/anterior pituitary/target organ axis.

Hormonal Control of Growth

Growth hormone promotes growth by stimulating cellular protein synthesis, cell division, and lengthening and thickening of bones. It also exerts metabolic actions unrelated to growth, such as enhancing mobilization of fat and conservation of glucose.

Growth hormone secretion by the anterior pituitary is regulated in negative-feedback fashion by two hypothalamic hormones, **growth hormone-releasing hormone** and **growth-hormone-inhibiting hormone**. Growth hormone levels are not highly correlated with periods of rapid growth. The primary signals for increased growth hormone secretion are related to metabolic needs rather than growth, namely, deep sleep, stress, exercise, and low blood glucose levels.

Thyroid Gland

The **thyroid gland** contains two types of endocrine secretory cells: (1) **follicular cells**, which produce the iodine-containing hormones, T_4 (**thyroxine** or **tetraiodothyronine**) and T_3 (**triidothyronine**), collectively known as **thyroid hormone**, and (2) **C cells**, which synthesize a Ca^{2+}-regulating hormone, **calcitonin**.

Thyroid hormone is the primary determinant of the overall metabolic rate of the body. By accelerating the metabolic rate of most tissues, it increases heat production. Thyroid hormone also enhances the actions of the chemical mediators of the sympathetic nervous system. Through this and other means, thyroid hormone indirectly increases cardiac output. Finally, thyroid hormone is essential for normal growth as well as for development and function of the nervous system.

Adrenal Glands

Each of the pair of **adrenal glands** consists of two separate endocrine organs-an outer steroid-secreting **adrenal cortex** and an inner catecholamine-secreting **adrenal medulla.** The adrenal cortex secretes three different categories of steroid hormones: (1) **mineralocorticoids** (primarily aldosterone); (2) **glucocorticoids** (primarily cortisol); and (3) **adrenal sex hormones** (primarily the weak androgen, dehydroepiandrosterone). Excessive production of: (1) mineralocorticoids gives rise to **Conn syndrome**, (2) glucocorticoids yields **Cushing syndrome**, and (3) sex hormones produce the **masculinization** of women. A deficiency of adrenocortical hormones is known as **Addison disease**.

Aldosterone regulates Na^+ and K^+ balance and is important for blood pressure homeostasis, which is accomplished secondarily as a result of the osmotic effect of Na^+ in maintaining the plasma volume, a life-saving effect. Control of aldosterone secretion is related to Na^+ and K^+ balance and blood pressure regulation and is not influenced by ACTH.

Cortisol helps to regulate intermediary metabolism and is important in stress adaptation. It increases the blood levels of glucose, amino acids, and fatty acids and spares glucose for use by the glucose-dependent brain. The mobilized organic molecules are available for use as needed for energy or for repair of injured tissues. Cortisol secretion is regulated by a negative-feedback loop involving hypothalamic corticotropin-releasing hormone (CRH) and pituitary ACTH. The most potent stimulus for increasing activity of the CRH/ACTH/cortisol axis is stress.

Dehydroepiandrosterone is responsible in women for the sex drive and growth of pubertal hair.

The **adrenal medulla** consists of modified sympathetic postganglionic neurons, which secrete the catecholamine **epinephrine** into the blood in response to sympathetic stimulation. For the most part, epinephrine reinforces the sympathetic system in its general systemic "fight or flight" responses and in its maintenance of arterial blood pressure. Epinephrine also exerts important metabolic effects, namely, increasing blood glucose and blood fatty acids. The primary stimulus for increased adrenomedullary secretion is activation of the sympathetic system by stress.

Endocrine Control of Fuel Metabolism

Intermediary or fuel metabolism refers collectively to the synthesis (**anabolism**), breakdown (**catabolism**), and **transformations** of the three classes of energy-rich organic nutrients-**carbohydrate, fat,** and **protein**-within the body. Glucose and fatty acids derived respectively from carbohydrates and fats are used primarily as metabolic fuels, whereas amino acids derived from proteins are used primarily for the synthesis of structural and enzymatic proteins.

During the **absorptive state** after a meal, the excess absorbed nutrients not immediately needed for energy production or protein synthesis are stored to a limited extent as glycogen in the liver and muscle but mainly as triglycerides in adipose tissue. During the **postabsorptive state** between meals when no new nutrients are entering the blood, the glycogen and triglyceride stores are catabolized to release nutrient molecules into the blood. If necessary, body proteins are degraded to release amino acids for conversion into glucose. The blood glucose concentration must be maintained above a critical level even during the postabsorptive state, because the brain depends on blood-delivered glucose as its energy source. Tissues that do not depend on glucose switch to fatty acids as their metabolic fuel and thus spare glucose for the brain.

These shifts in metabolic pathways between the absorptive and postabsorptive state are hormonally controlled. The most important hormone in this regard is insulin. **Insulin** is secreted by the beta cells of the **islets of Langerhans,** the **endocrine portion of the pancreas**. The other major pancreatic hormone, **glucagon**, is secreted by the alpha cells of the islets. Insulin, the "hormone of feasting," is an anabolic hormone; it promotes the cellular uptake of glucose, fatty acids, and amino acids and enhances their conversion into glycogen, triglycerides, and proteins, respectively. In doing so, it lowers the blood concentrations of the small organic molecules. Insulin secretion is increased during the absorptive state, primarily by a direct effect of an elevated blood glucose on the beta cells, and is mainly responsible for directing the organic traffic into cells during this state.

Glucagon, the "hormone of fasting," mobilizes the energy-rich molecules from their stores during the postabsorptive state to keep up the blood glucose level between meals. Glucagon, which is secreted in response to a direct effect of a fall in blood glucose on the pancreatic alpha cells, in general opposes the actions of insulin.

Endocrine Control of Calcium Metabolism

Changes in the concentration of free, diffusible plasma Ca^{2+}, the biologically active form of this ion, produce profound and life-threatening effects, most notably on neuromuscular excitability. **Hypercalcemia** reduces excitability, whereas **hypocalcemia** brings about overexcitability of nerves and muscles, if severe enough to the point of fatal spastic contractions of respiratory muscle.

Three hormones regulate the plasma concentration of Ca^{2+} (and concurrently regulate PO_4^{3-})-parathyroid hormone (PTH), calcitonin, and vitamin D. **PTH,** whose secretion is directly increased by a fall in plasma Ca^{2+} concentration, acts on bone, kidneys, and the intestine to raise the plasma Ca^{2+} concentration. In so doing, it is essential for life by preventing the fatal consequences of hypocalcemia. The specific effects of PTH on bone are to promote Ca^{2+} movement from the bone fluid into the plasma in the short term and to promote localized dissolution of bone by enhancing activity of the osteoclasts (bone-dissolving cells) in the long term. Dissolution of the calcium phosphate bone crystals releases PO_4^{3-} as well as Ca^{2+} into the plasma. PTH acts on the kidneys to enhance the reabsorption of filtered Ca^{2+}, thus reducing the urinary excretion of Ca^{2+} and increasing its plasma concentration. Simultaneously, PTH reduces renal PO_4^{3-} reabsorption, in this way increasing PO_4^{3-} excretion and lowering plasma PO_4^{3-} levels. This is important because a rise in plasma PO_4^{3-} would force the deposition of some of the plasma Ca^{2+} back into the bone. Furthermore, PTH facilitates the activation of **vitamin D,** which in turn stimulates Ca^{2+} and PO_4^{3-} absorption from the intestine.

Calcitonin, a hormone produced by the C cells of the thyroid gland, is the third factor that regulates Ca^{2+}. In negative-feedback fashion, calcitonin is secreted in response to an increase in plasma Ca^{2+} concentration and acts to lower plasma Ca^{2+} levels by inhibiting activity of bone osteoclasts. Calcitonin is unimportant, except during the rare condition of hypercalcemia.

REPRODUCTIVE SYSTEM

Both sexes produce **gametes** (reproductive cells)-*sperm* in males and *ova* (eggs) in females-each of which bears one member of each of the 23 pairs of chromosomes present in human cells. Union of a sperm and an ovum at fertilization results in the beginning of a new individual with 23 complete pairs of chromosomes, half from the father and half from the mother.

The **reproductive system** is anatomically and functionally distinct in males and females, befitting their different roles in the reproductive process. Males produce sperm and deliver them into the female. Females produce ova, accept sperm delivery, and provide a suitable environment for supporting development of a fertilized ovum until the new individual can survive independently in the external world. In both sexes, the reproductive system consists of: (1) a pair of **gonads,** testes in males and ovaries in females, which are the primary reproductive organs that produce the gametes and secrete sex hormones, and (2) a **reproductive tract** composed of a system of ducts and associated glands that respectively provide a passageway and supportive secretions for the gametes. The externally visible portions of the reproductive system constitute the **external genitalia.**

Sex determination is a genetic phenomenon dependent on the combination of **sex chromosomes** at the time of fertilization, an XY combination being a genetic male and an XX combination a genetic female. **Sex differentiation** refers to the embryonic development of the gonads, reproductive tract, and external genitalia along male or female lines, which gives rise to the apparent anatomic sex of the individual. In the presence of masculinizing factors, a male reproductive system develops; in their absence, a female system develops.

Male Reproductive Physiology

Spermatogenesis (sperm production) occurs in the highly coiled seminiferous tubules within the testes. **Leydig cells** located in the interstitial spaces between these tubules se-

crete the male sex hormone **testosterone** into the blood. Testosterone is secreted before birth to masculinize the developing reproductive system, then its secretion ceases until puberty, at which time it begins once again and continues throughout life. Testosterone is responsible for maturation and maintenance of the entire male reproductive tract, for development of secondary sexual characteristics, and for stimulating libido.

The **testes** are regulated by the anterior pituitary hormones, **LH** and **FSH**. These gonadotropic hormones, in turn, are under control of hypothalamic **gonadotropin-releasing hormone (GnRH)**. Testosterone secretion is regulated by LH stimulation of the Leydig cells and, in negative-feedback fashion, testosterone inhibits gonadotropin secretion. Spermatogenesis requires both testosterone and FSH. Testosterone stimulates the mitotic and meiotic divisions required to transform the undifferentiated diploid germ cells, the spermatogonia, into undifferentiated haploid spermatids. The remodeling of spermatids into highly specialized motile spermatozoa is stimulated by FSH. A spermatozoon consists only of a DNA-packed head bearing an enzyme-filled acrosome at its tip for penetrating the ovum, a midpiece containing the metabolic machinery for energy production, and a whip-like motile tail. Also present in the **seminiferous tubules** are **Sertoli cells,** which protect, nurse, and enhance the germ cells throughout their development. Sertoli cells also secrete **inhibin,** a hormone that inhibits FSH secretion, thus completing the negative-feedback loop.

The still immature sperm are flushed out of the seminiferous tubules into the **epididymis** by fluid secreted by the Sertoli cells. The epididymis and **ductus deferens** store and concentrate the sperm and increase their motility and fertility before **ejaculation**. During ejaculation, the sperm are mixed with secretions released by the accessory glands, which contribute the bulk of the **semen**. The **seminal vesicles** supply fructose for energy and **prostaglandins,** which promote smooth muscle motility in both the male and female reproductive tract to enhance sperm transport. The **prostate gland** contributes an alkaline fluid for neutralizing the acidic vaginal secretions. The **bulbourethral** glands release lubricating mucus.

Sexual Intercourse Between Men and Women

The male sex act consists of **erection** and **ejaculation,** which are part of a much broader systemic, emotional response that typifies the male sexual response cycle. Erection is a hardening of the normally flaccid penis that enables it to penetrate the female vagina. Erection is accomplished by marked vasocongestion of the penis brought about by reflexly induced vasodilation of the arterioles supplying the penile erectile tissue. When sexual excitation reaches a critical peak, ejaculation, which consists of two stages, occurs: (1) **emission,** the emptying of semen (sperm and accessory sex gland secretions) into the urethra, and (2) **expulsion** of semen from the penis. The latter is accompanied by a set of characteristic systemic responses and intense pleasure referred to as **orgasm.**

Women experience a sexual cycle similar to that of men; both have excitation, plateau, orgasmic, and resolution phases. The major differences are that women do not ejaculate and they are capable of multiple orgasms. During the female sexual response, the outer third of the vagina constricts to grip the penis while the inner two thirds expands to create space for sperm deposition.

Female Reproductive Physiology

In the nonpregnant state, female reproductive function is controlled by a complex, cyclical negative-feedback control system between the hypothalamus (GnRH), anterior pituitary (FSH and LH), and ovaries (estrogen, progesterone, and inhibin). During pregnancy, placental hormones become the main controlling factors.

The **ovaries** perform the dual and interrelated functions of **oogenesis** (producing ova) and secretion of the female sex hormones **estrogen** and **progesterone.** Two related ovarian endocrine units sequentially accomplish these functions: the **follicle** and the **corpus luteum.** Oogenesis and estrogen secretion occur within an ovarian follicle during the first half of each reproductive cycle (the **follicular phase**). At approximately midcycle, the maturing follicle releases a single ovum (**ovulation**). The empty follicle is then converted into a corpus luteum, which produces progesterone as well as estrogen during the last half of the cycle (the **luteal phase**). This endocrine unit is responsible for preparing the uterus as a suitable site for implantation if the released ovum is fertilized. If fertilization and implantation do not occur, the corpus luteum degenerates. The consequent withdrawal of hormonal support for the highly developed uterine lining causes it to disintegrate and slough, producing **menstrual flow.** Simultaneously, a new follicular phase is initiated. Menstruation ceases, and the uterine lining (**endometrium**) repairs itself under the influence of rising estrogen levels from the newly maturing follicle.

If **fertilization** does take place, it occurs in the oviduct as the released egg and sperm deposited in the vagina are both transported to this site. The fertilized ovum begins to divide mitotically. Within 1 week, it grows and differentiates into a **blastocyst** capable of implantation. Meanwhile, the endometrium has become richly vascularized and stocked with stored glycogen under the influence of luteal-phase progesterone. It is into this especially prepared lining that the blastocyst implants by means of enzymes released by the blastocyst's outer layer. These enzymes digest the nutrient-rich endometrial tissue, accomplishing the dual function of carving out a hole in the endometrium for **implantation** of the blastocyst while at the same time releasing nutrients from the endometrial cells for use by the developing **embryo.**

After implantation, an interlocking combination of fetal and maternal tissues, the **placenta,** develops. The placenta is the organ of exchange between the maternal and fetal blood and also acts as a transient, complex endocrine organ that secretes a number of hormones essential for pregnancy, the most important of which are **human chorionic gonadotropin, estrogen,** and **progesterone.** Human chorionic **gonadotropin stimulates and maintains the corpus luteum of pregnancy**, which continues to secrete estrogen and progesterone for the first trimester of pregnancy until the placenta takes over this function for the last two trimesters. Human chorionic gonadotropin is the chemical in the urine that is detected by pregnancy diagnosis kits.

At **parturition,** rhythmic contractions of increasing strength, duration, and frequency accomplish the three stages of **labor: dilation of the cervix, birth of the baby, and delivery of the placenta (afterbirth).** Once the contractions are initiated at the onset of labor, a positive-feedback cycle is established that progressively increases their force. As contractions push the fetus against the cervix, secretion of **oxytocin,** a powerful uterine muscle stimulant, is reflexly increased. The extra oxytocin causes stronger contractions, giving rise to even greater release of oxytocin. This positive-feedback cycle progressively intensifies until cervical dilation and delivery are accomplished.

During **gestation** (pregnancy), the breasts are specially prepared for **lactation** (milk production). The elevated levels of placental estrogen and progesterone, respectively, promote development of the ducts and alveoli in the **mammary glands** (breasts). **Prolactin,** from the anterior pituitary, stimulates the synthesis of enzymes essential for milk production by the alveolar epithelial cells. However, the high gestational level of estrogen and progesterone prevents prolactin from promoting milk production. Withdrawal of the placental steroids at parturition initiates lactation. Lactation is sustained by suckling, which triggers the release of oxytocin and prolactin. Oxytocin causes milk ejection by stimulating the myopithelial cells surrounding the alveoli to squeeze the secreted milk out through the ducts. Prolactin stimulates the production of more milk to replace the milk ejected as the baby nurses.

Suggested Sources

Sherwood L: Fundamentals of Human Physiology, 2nd ed. West Publishing Company, 1995.

Sherwood L: Human Physiology: From Cells to Systems, 4th ed. Brooks/Cole, 2001.

Questions and Answers

Questions

1. Which of the following systems serves as a protective barrier between the external environment and the remainder of the body?
   A. Skeletal
   B. Integumentary
   C. Immune
   D. Respiratory

2. Which of the following organelles is referred to as the energy source of the cell?
   A. Vaults
   B. Lysosomes
   C. Mitochondria
   D. Peroxisomes

3. When appropriately triggered, nerve and muscle cell membranes undergo brief, rapid reversals of membrane potential, these reversals serve as electrical signals known as
   _____.
   A. resting potential.
   B. peak potential.
   C. action potential.
   D. threshold potential.

4. Which of the following lobes houses the auditory cortex of the brain?
   A. Occipital
   B. Temporal
   C. Parietal
   D. Frontal

5. Which of the following structures regulates temperature, thirst, and urine output?
   A. Hypothalamus
   B. Thalamus
   C. Cerebellum
   D. Pituitary

6. Parasympathetic stimulation of the exocrine glands produces a large volume of thick saliva that is rich in mucus.
   A. True.
   B. False.
   C. The parasympathetic has no effect on the exocrine glands.

7. The cardiac impulse originates at the sinoatrial node. This area of the heart is referred to as the pacemaker of the heart and has the fastest rate of spontaneous depolarization to threshold.
   A.   The first statement is true; the second statement is false.
   B.   The first statement is false; the second statement is true.

   C.   Both statements are true.
   D.   Both statements are false.

8. Which of the following terms defines the peak pressure exerted by ejected blood against vessel walls?
   A. Resistance
   B. Flow rate
   C. Diastolic pressure
   D. Systolic pressure

9. The major component of blood is _____.
   A. water.
   B. erythrocytes.
   C. plasma.
   D. platelets.

10. Which of the following cells are responsible for attacking parasites and play a key role in allergic responses?
    A. Monocytes
    B. Lymphocytes
    C. Basophils
    D. Eosinophils

11. Which of the following terms refers to the stretching force of exerted across the lung wall?
    A. Pulmonary compliance
    B. Airway resistance
    C. Elastic recoil
    D. Tidal volume

12. The urine-forming functional component of the kidney is the
    _____.
    A. glomerulus.
    B. nephron.
    C. renal pelvis.
    D. Bowman capsule.

13. Which of the following enzymes is found in saliva and initiates the digestion of polysaccharides?
    A. Amylase
    B. Sucrase
    C. Lactase
    D. Maltase

14. All of the following are gastric secretions in the stomach lumen except one. The exception is _____.
    A. HCl.
    B. pepsinogen.
    C. lipase.
    D. intrinsic factor.

15. Bile is stored and concentrated in the _____.
    A. liver.
    B. gallbladder.
    C. spleen.
    D. kidney.

16. All of the following are physical means by which heat is exchanged between the body and the external environment except one. The exception is:_____.
    A. radiation.
    B. conduction.
    C. convection.
    D. ventilation.

17. A deficiency of adrenocortical hormones is known as:
    A. Conn syndrome.
    B. Cushing syndrome.
    C. Addison disease.
    D. Graves disease.

18. All of the following hormones are responsible for regulating the plasma concentration of calcium except one. The exception is _____.
    A. parathyroid hormone.
    B. vitamin D.
    C. calcitonin.
    D. aldosterone.

19. Leydig cells located in the interstitial spaces between the seminiferous tubules secrete which of the following hormones?
    A. Luteinizing
    B. Gonadotropin
    C. Estrogen
    D. Testosterone

20. The chemical in urine detected by pregnancy diagnosis kits is _____.
    A. prolactin.
    B. oxytocin.
    C. corpus luteum.
    D. human chorionic gonadotropin.

ANSWERS

1. **B**. The skin or integument is the only barrier that separates the body from the environment.

2. **C**. Mitochondria generate ATP; vaults perform RNA transport; lysosomes are responsible for digestion; and peroxisomes detoxify wastes.

3. **C**. An action potential is the entire rapid change in potential from threshold to peak reversal and back to resting.

4. **B**. The visual cortex is located in the occipital lobe. The frontal lobe houses intellect, emotions, behavior and personality and the parietal lobe houses sensation.

5. **A**. The thalamus processes sensory input.

6. **B**. The parasympathetic causes the production of a large volume of watery saliva that is rich in enzymes.

7. **C**. Impulses pass from the atria to the ventricles through the AV node.

8. **D**. Diastolic pressure refers to the minimum force exerted on a vessel wall during relaxation.

9. **C**. Plasma constitutes 55% to 58% of blood volume; erythrocytes comprise 42% to 45%.

10. **D**. Eosinophils are the only white blood cells that specialize in attacking parasitic infections.

11. **A**. Pulmonary compliance refers to the distensibility of the lungs.

12. **B**. The nephron consists of a vascular component (glomerulus and peritubular capillaries) and a tubular component (the Bowman capsule and renal pelvis).

13. **A**. Polysaccharides are broken down into disaccharides in the mouth by salivary amylase. Maltase, sucrase, and lactase break down disaccharides into monosaccharides in the small intestine.

14. **C**. Lipase is the enzyme responsible for the digestion of fats.

15. **B**. The gallbladder is hormonally stimulated to contract and empty bile into the duodenum during digestion of a meal.

16. **D**. Evaporation is the fourth mechanism for heat exchange.

17. **C**. Graves disease is a result of hyperthyroidism, Conn syndrome results from excessive production of mineralocorticoids, and Cushing syndrome occurs from an excessive production of glucocorticoids.

18. **D**. Aldosterone regulates Na^+ and K^+ balance.

19. **D**. Testosterone secretion is regulated by luteinizing hormone stimulation of the Leydig cells and, in negative-feedback fashion, testosterone inhibits gonadotropin secretion.

20. **D**. Human chorionic gonadotropin stimulates and maintains the corpus luteum of pregnancy, which continues to secrete estrogen and progesterone for the first trimester of pregnancy until the placenta takes over this function for the last two trimesters. Prolactin and oxytocin are related to milk production or lactation.

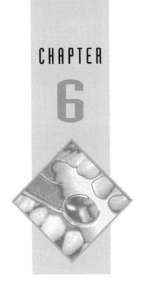

CHAPTER
6

Nutrition

CHRISTINA B. DEBIASE, BSDH, MA, EdD
DINA AGNONE VAUGHAN, BSDH, MS

 NUTRITION AND DIGESTION

Nutrition is the process whereby living things use **nutrients** obtained from food for growth, development, maintenance, repair, energy, metabolism, and homeostasis. Nutrients are divided into six categories: proteins, fats, carbohydrates, vitamins, minerals, and water.

Digestion is the process whereby foods that have been eaten break down into nutrients that can subsequently be **absorbed** into the circulation and **metabolized** into their final state for use by the body. There are two types of digestion: mechanical digestion and chemical digestion. **Mechanical digestion** includes **mastication** or chewing food and mixing it with saliva (**insalivation**), churning of food in the stomach and mixing it with gastric juices until it reaches a liquid consistency referred to as **chyme,** and **peristalsis** or the rhythmic contraction of the intestines to propel the food mass through the intestines. **Chemical digestion** involves the mixing of food with digestive juices and the breakdown of food into simpler forms by the action of **enzymes**. Enzymes cause the chemical changes of food into usable nutrients that can be absorbed and metabolized by the body. Gastric juices consist of **hydrochloric acid** and the enzymes **protease, lipase, and rennin**. Most digestive activity occurs in the **small intestine** through the action of bile and pancreatic and intestinal juices.

A calorie is the unit used to measure energy needs and use. One **calorie** is the amount of heat necessary to raise the temperature of 1 g of water 1°C. A **Calorie** or a **kilocalorie** = 1 calorie × 1000.

- 1 g of protein = 4 calories
- 1 g of carbohydrates = 4 calories
- 1 g of fat = 9 calories

Foods that provide energy but have no nutrient value are referred to as **empty calories**. Examples of empty calories are soft drinks, alcohol, and candy. One gram of alcohol yields 7 calories.

 PROTEINS

Proteins are large molecules that primarily contain hydrogen, oxygen, carbon, and nitrogen atoms arranged into amino acids. Their primary function is to build new tissue and repair damaged tissues. As the **fundamental building block of cells**, proteins are the only nutrients that perform this function. In addition, proteins manufacture hormones and enzymes, build antibodies to fight infection, regulate body fluids, transport oxygen and nutrients in the blood, and aid in blood clotting and muscle contraction. The structure of collagen, bone, keratin, and tooth matrix (primarily pulp tissue) is comprised of protein.

The structural units of proteins are referred to as **amino acids**. Billions of proteins are derived from combinations of 22 different amino acids. There are **nine essential amino acids (EAAs)**, which can only be obtained from the diet. These EAAs are tryptophan, histidine, lysine, leucine, isoleucine, valine, threonine, phenylalanine, and methionine. Foods that supply adequate amounts of the nine EAAs to maintain nitrogen balance and foster growth are referred to as **high-quality** or **high biologic value proteins. Non-essential amino acids (NEAAs)** are also required but can be synthesized by the body from EAAs. The liver is the main site for the metabolism of amino acids.

A **complete protein** is one that contains all of the EAAs. Complete proteins are found in animal foods such as eggs, milk, cheese, fish, and meat. An **incomplete protein** is one that lacks one or more of the EAAs and is derived from plant foods such as grains, legumes, and vegetables. **Complementary proteins** are incomplete proteins that are derived from various sources that work together to function as complete proteins (e.g., corn and beans). These combinations enable true vegetarians to obtain sufficient amounts of protein in their diets.

If a diet is deficient in calories from carbohydrates and fats, dietary protein may be burned to supply energy. Unfortunately, dietary protein cannot be stored by the body. When dietary protein is also deficient, the body tissues are utilized for energy, resulting in body wasting or **cachexia**. **Protein-energy malnutrition (PEM)** is common in Third World countries where high-quality protein and caloric intake are deficient. Proteins should comprise approximately 10% to 15% of the total daily caloric intake.

 # FATS

Fats or **lipids** are insoluble in water and contain the elements carbon, hydrogen, and oxygen. Because of their structure (less oxygen), fats provide more energy per gram than do proteins or carbohydrates. Lipids can be divided into two types:

1. **Simple lipids**, which are found in foods and can be manufactured by the body
2. **Structural lipids,** which are produced by the body for certain functions

Dietary lipids include cholesterol, triglycerides, fatty acids, and phospholipids. **Cholesterol** is a fatty substance produced by the body and regulated by the liver. Approximately 30% of cholesterol is obtained exogenously (from the diet) via animal-derived foods. Cholesterol is a component of brain and nervous tissue, bile salts, teeth, and cell membranes and is a precursor of vitamin D and sex and adrenal hormones.

Glycerides (mono-, di-, and tri-) consist of fatty acids and glycerol. **Triglycerides** are the most common fat found in animal or protein foods. **Monoglycerides** and **diglycerides** are found in the small intestine and result from the hydrolysis of triglycerides during digestion.

A **fatty acid** is a chain of carbon atoms attached to hydrogen atoms with an acid group on one end. Fatty acids are classified based on their degree of **saturation** (the number of hydrogen atoms attached to a carbon). A **saturated fat** has two hydrogen atoms attached to each carbon. The length of the carbon chain and the level of saturation determine the flavor and melting point of fats. Most animal or saturated fats are solid at room temperature (e.g., butter); whereas short chained fatty acids (12 carbons) are liquid at room temperature (i.e., oils). **Unsaturated fats** result when hydrogen atoms are missing. When adjacent carbon atoms are joined by a double bond instead of two hydrogen bonds, the fatty acid is **monounsaturated**. If numerous carbons are connected by double bonds, the fatty acid is **polyunsaturated**. By a process called **hydrogenation** (adding hydrogen atoms), a polyunsaturated vegetable oil can be changed into solid shortening. The only essential fatty acids that must be obtained from the diet are **linoleic acid, linolenic acid,** and **arachidonic acid.** These fatty acids are the precursors for **prostaglandins** (a hormone-like compound that has the ability to stimulate uterine contractions and other smooth muscle, lower blood pressure, regulate body temperature, regulate stomach acid secretion, promote platelet aggregation, and control inflammation and vascular permeability).

In addition to triglycerides, plant and animal fats contain phospholipids, cholesterol, sphingolipids, glycolipids, and phytosterols. **Phospholipids** are the second most prevalent fat in the body and are believed to be responsible for the mineralization and calcification of bones and teeth. Phospholipids, like cholesterol, constitute a structural component of cell membranes and teeth.

Lipoproteins are compound lipids that consist of cholesterol, triglycerides, and phospholipids combined with protein. The liver and the intestinal mucosa produce lipoproteins, which transport insoluble fats throughout the body. Four lipoproteins are found in the blood. They are **high-density lipoproteins (HDLs), low-density lipoproteins (LDLs), very low density lipoproteins (VLDLs),** and **chylomicrons. Hyperlipidemia,** a major risk factor in coronary heart disease, refers to increased plasma cholesterol and LDL levels. LDL picks up cholesterol from ingested fats and from cells that synthesize it in the body and deliver it to blood vessels and muscles where it is deposited in the cells. The concentration of cholesterol in the cells within the linings of the arteries contributes to the accumulation of atherosclerotic plaque, which eventually narrows the arteries. A dietary reduction of saturated fats usually lowers these blood levels. High HDL levels promote the removal of excess cholesterol from the cells. Exercise usually increases HDL levels. Additional risk factors for coronary heart disease are included in **Table 6-1**.

Approximately 30% to 40% of the average caloric intake consists of fat. Fats provide fatty acids for normal growth and skin care, give flavor and consistency to foods, provide satiation because they remain in the stomach longer, and serve as a carrier for fat-soluble vitamins. From a dental health standpoint, fats are not only a part of the tooth structure, but also fats such as nuts and cheese, which are consumed after fermentable carbohydrate ingestion, may serve to raise the oral pH thus reducing the dissolution of hydroxyapatite by acids. The retention of sticky carbohydrates, which are responsible for promoting caries, may be more readily cleared from the oral cavity by concurrently consuming fats. Because fats delay gastric emptying, the ab-

TABLE 6–1 High Risk Factors for Heart Disease

WITHOUT CONTROL	WITHIN OUR CONTROL
Family history	Smokers* are at the highest risk
Gender	High cholesterol
Age	Hypertension
	Low exercise
	Low high-density lipoproteins
	Type A behavior
	Diabetes
	Periodontal disease†

*Smokers who exercise lower their risk considerably.
†Smoking and periodontal disease are known to increase serum lipid levels.

sorption of **fluoride-rich foods** (e.g., tea, fish) and supplemental fluorides may be enhanced by fat intake.

Excess fat intake results in fat storage and the formation of adipose tissue. The functions of **adipose tissue** are to maintain body temperature, help protect vital organs, and provide a concentrated source of energy.

 # CARBOHYDRATES

Carbohydrates are the most important source of energy. They consist of carbon, hydrogen, and oxygen. The number of carbon atoms in the molecule dictates the type of carbohydrate: **monosaccharides** have 2 to 6 carbon atoms; **disaccharides** have 12 atoms; and **polysaccharides** have >12 carbons. The position of hydroxyl (-OH) groups determines properties such as sweetness and absorption. **Complex carbohydrates** contain naturally occurring sugars and provide other nutrients such as vitamins and minerals. **Refined carbohydrates** supply only empty calories in foods such as cookies, cakes, soft drinks, and alcoholic beverages.

Monosaccharides (i.e., **glucose, fructose,** and **galactose)** are the simplest carbohydrates and are absorbed without further digestion. Glucose, which is also referred to as *dextrose* or corn sweetener, is formed by the digestion of disaccharides and polysaccharides. Glucose supplies energy to the cells via the bloodstream, and excesses are stored in the liver and muscles as **glycogen.** Glycogen, which is stored in the heart muscle, is critical to normal cardiac functioning. Once the storage capacity of glycogen is reached, it converts to fat and is stored as adipose tissue. Fructose (levulose) or fruit sugar is the sweetest monosaccharide and results from the digestion of sucrose. Galactose results from digestion of lactose and is also produced from glucose during lactation in the synthesis of lactose.

Disaccharides (i.e., **sucrose, maltose,** and **lactose**) only contribute to metabolism after they have been digested and broken down into monosaccharides. Sucrose or table sugar is metabolized into glucose and fructose. The presence of sucrose in the oral cavity increases the amount and rate of plaque accumulation. *Streptococcus mutans* in the presence of a highly sucrose environment promotes the formation of polysaccharides known as **glucans,** which enable plaque colonies to adhere to the teeth. Sucrose lowers the pH of the plaque and dissolution of the enamel by acids occurs. The result is **dental caries.** Other monosaccharides and disaccharides such as lactose are also readily metabolized by oral microorganisms, which is the case in nursing bottle caries. The total amount of **fermentable carbohydrates** (i.e., sugars or cooked starch) in the diet is less significant in causing dental caries than the form in which it is consumed and the frequency of intake.

Maltose or malt sugar is created in bread or beer making. It is metabolized into glucose by the action of the enzyme **maltase.** Lactose is found only in milk. The enzyme **lactase** breaks down lactose in the intestine to form glucose and galactose. Individuals who are lactose-intolerant have a deficiency of lactase.

Polysaccharides are the complex carbohydrates, which include **starch, cellulose,** and **glycogen**. Starch is broken down into simple sugars during digestion, but the process takes longer than monosaccharide or disaccharide metabolism. Consequently, the energy from starches is released more slowly into the body. Starches are not considered to have caries-causing potential, except when cooked. Cooked and refined starches are more easily hydrolyzed by salivary and plaque **amylase** to form maltose, which can then reduce the oral pH and demineralize the enamel. Cellulose is a polysaccharide vegetable fiber that is not digested by humans. Glycogen is the animal equivalent source of starch.

Dietary fiber refers to indigestible carbohydrates such as cellulose, hemicellulose, lignin, pectin, pentosan, and gum. Fiber is essential for providing the bulk that enhances peristalsis and the elimination of wastes. Fiber is low in calories and has been shown to reduce the risk of certain diseases such as colon cancer and cardiovascular disease. Fibrous foods include the complex carbohydrates such as grains and cereals. **Soluble fibers** combined with a diet low in saturated fat may reduce blood cholesterol. These fibers are found in oat bran, barley, prunes, apples, and beans. **Insoluble fibers** found in whole grains and wheat bran are the forms of roughage that may fight colon cancer. Foods that are low in fiber include fats, sweets, meats, and dairy products.

Sugar alcohols (i.e., **sorbitol, mannitol,** and **xylitol)** are synthetic sweeteners composed of sugars and cellulose. Because the digestive system metabolizes these sugar alcohols very slowly, they are not converted to a simple sugar in the mouth. Consequently, these sweeteners are used in chewing gum. Xylitol is anticariogenic because oral bacteria lack the enzymes to ferment it.

Non-nutritive sweeteners (i.e., **aspartame, saccharin, cyclamates**) differ from sugar alcohols because they do not contribute nutrients or calories. Aspartame contains phenylalanine, and labels warn people who have **phenylketonuria** to avoid using it. During pregnancy, aspartame is preferred over saccharin because it is metabolized like other amino acids. Saccharin is known to cross the placental barrier.

An average of 50% to 60% of an individual's caloric intake should be derived from carbohydrates. In the absence of dietary carbohydrates, the body resorts to ketone bodies burned from fatty acids to produce energy. Because carbohydrates are needed to completely burn fats, **acidosis** or a high level of acid in the blood occurs. **Ketosis** is the resultant clinical condition characterized by sweet acetone breath odor.

 # VITAMINS

Vitamins are the catalysts for all metabolic reactions utilizing proteins, fats, and carbohydrates for energy, proper growth and development, and cell maintenance and repair.

Vitamins also assist in the formation of blood cells, hormones, genes, and neurotransmitter substances. Vitamins may be destroyed by smoking, alcohol, caffeine, some medications, stress, and surgery.

Vitamins are divided into two categories:

1. **Water-soluble** (i.e., **vitamins B-complex, C, folic acid, pantothenic acid**, and **biotin**)
2. **Fat-soluble** (i.e., **vitamins A, D, E**, and **K**)

Vitamins required for calcified structures are vitamins A, D, E, K, and C. Oral soft tissues and salivary glands require vitamins A, B-complex, and C.

Water-Soluble Vitamins

Water-soluble vitamins are not stored in the body, thus an adequate supply must be consumed daily. Water-soluble vitamins are usually absorbed in the jejunum. Although these vitamins are naturally supplied in food, they can easily be destroyed during food preparation.

Vitamin C, also known as ascorbic acid, is an antioxidant. An **antioxidant** is a substance that slows down the deterioration process caused by free radicals during oxidation. Vitamin C aids in the formation of collagen; promotes immunity, wound healing, and capillary integrity; facilitates erythrocyte development by aiding in the absorption of iron; assists the body in utilizing folate and vitamin B_{12}; and assists in the development and maintenance of teeth and bones by the formation of fibroblasts, osteoblasts, and odontoblasts. Steroids, salicylates, and antibiotics may increase the excretion of vitamin C.

B-complex vitamins include: B_1-thiamin; B_2-riboflavin; B_3-niacin; B_6-pyridoxine; and B_{12}-cyanocobalamin. These vitamins are found in similar foods and have similar functions. They differ from vitamin C and the fat-soluble vitamins, because they contain nitrogen.

Thiamin releases energy from carbohydrates and helps to synthesize various nervous system chemicals. It also aids in the synthesis of niacin and the regulation of appetite. **Riboflavin** also aids in the release of energy from carbohydrates, assists in protein metabolism for growth and repair, helps to maintain healthy mucous membranes and eyes, and is needed for the synthesis of niacin and pyridoxine. Congenital facial abnormalities may occur if maternal riboflavin deficiency exists at the time of conception. Vegetarians and persons on long-term phenothiazine or antibiotic therapy are at risk for developing vitamin B_2 deficiency. **Niacin** is also referred to as **nicotinic acid** and **nicotinamide**. It serves as a coenzyme to facilitate the metabolism of energy nutrients and tissue respiration in cells. Niacin is critical to the nervous system, muscle, and heart function. Interestingly, niacin is essential for the growth of cariogenic oral bacteria. It also functions in the enzymes that degrade sucrose to produce acids. The body can convert the amino acid tryptophan into niacin. **Pyridoxine, pyridoxal,** and **pyridoxamine** are three related compounds that form vitamin B_6. The functions of

vitamin B_6 include: serving as a coenzyme in protein metabolism; synthesizing niacin, hemoglobin, antibodies, and unsaturated fatty acid; producing energy from glycogen, and maintaining the nervous system. **Vitamin B_{12}** is the only vitamin that contains a mineral-cobalt. It is a coenzyme that functions with folate to synthesize nucleic acids and is essential for the formation of erythrocytes and myelin.

Folic acid or **folate** (a compound similar to folic acid) is a coenzyme that is critical for the synthesis of DNA and RNA. Along with vitamins B_{12} and C, folic acid maintains normal erythrocyte levels. **Pantothenic acid** is also involved in protein, fat, and carbohydrate metabolism. It also aids in the formation of hormones and nerve-regulating substances. **Biotin** also functions as a coenzyme in the metabolism of proteins, fats, and carbohydrates. Biotin is synthesized by intestinal microflora. Prolonged antibiotic therapy may destroy intestinal flora and lead to a biotin deficiency.

Fat-Soluble Vitamins

Larger amounts of fat-soluble vitamins can be stored by the body. Although these vitamins (A, D, E, and K) differ in function, source, and utilization, they are similar in several ways. They are soluble in fat and stable during cooking. Fat-soluble vitamins do not contain nitrogen; they require bile for absorption and are absorbed in the intestine along with other dietary fats.

Vitamin A is also known as retinol (dietary animal source) and β-carotene (dietary plant source). Vitamin A is necessary for normal growth and development of teeth, bones, and salivary glands. It also promotes healthy soft tissues (i.e., hair, mucous membranes, nails, and skin). Good vision and a healthy immune system can also be attributed to vitamin A.

Because **vitamin D** is essential for the regulation of calcium and phosphorus, it primarily functions in the mineralization of bones and teeth. Vitamin D is sometimes referred to as the sunshine vitamin because it can be obtained from sunlight. Fat malabsorption impairs the absorption of vitamin D.

Vitamin E is an antioxidant that includes four different **tocopherols**. Vitamin E protects the integrity of cell membranes, protects erythrocytes from hemolysis, and prevents the oxidation of vitamin A and unsaturated fatty acids. Vitamin E has been shown to improve the immune response by increasing the production of prostaglandins.

Vitamin E interferes with vitamin K activity; therefore, supplements should not be taken by individuals with a coagulation disorder or vitamin K deficiency or by those taking anticoagulants.

Vitamin K is a member of the group of chemical compounds known as **quinones**. Vitamin K_1 occurs in green plants; K_2 is found in animal tissues and is formed by *Escherichia coli* in the large intestine; and K_3 is a synthetic form of the vitamin. Because antibiotic therapy destroys bacteria in the colon, bacterial production of vitamin K may be diminished. Vitamin K binds calcium and may be involved in bone crystallization. This vitamin's major function is the synthesis of blood-clotting factors.

MINERALS

The minerals of greatest significance are the **electrolytes,** which disassociate in solution and are referred to as **cations** because they are positively charged. These minerals are sodium, potassium, calcium, and magnesium. Most phosphorus is present as phosphate, which is an **anion** (negatively charged). Other anions include chloride and bicarbonate. Iron, zinc, and iodine are also important minerals in health maintenance.

Sodium functions by regulating water distribution in the body by maintaining extracellular fluid (ECF) concentration, regulating acid-base balance, and facilitating nerve and muscle fiber impulse transmission.

Potassium regulates water distribution in the body by maintaining intracellular fluid (ICF) concentration, specifically affects cardiac muscle contractions and the electrical conductivity of the heart, assists in nerve impulse transmission, and also regulates acid-base balance.

Calcium is essential for the proper development of bones and teeth. Calcium maintains bone strength and muscle contractions; regulates heartbeat, nerve impulse transmission, and blood clotting; and maintains cell membranes and enzyme reactions. Calcium must be accompanied by vitamins C and D for proper absorption. The body absorbs calcium best no more than 600 mg at a time. Therefore, calcium supplements should be spread out over the course of a day. If taken as calcium carbonate, only 40% is absorbed as elemental calcium (600 mg of calcium carbonate yields 240 mg of usable calcium).

Magnesium assists in bone growth and the production of proteins. It also aids in the release of energy from the muscles in the form of glycogen and muscle nerve impulse conduction.

Phosphorus is also important for the development of bones and teeth and the release of energy from carbohydrates, fats, and proteins. Phosphorus also contributes to the formation of enzymes, cell membranes, and genetic material.

Chloride is the anion counterpart of sodium, which is necessary for maintaining ECF balance, osmotic equilibrium, and electrolyte balance. Chlorine is found in gastric secretions for protein digestion and the production of acid to enhance iron and calcium absorption and inhibit the growth of bacteria.

Iron is integral in the formation of hemoglobin in blood and myoglobulin in muscles, both of which are responsible for supplying oxygen to the cells.

Zinc has numerous functions. It is a cofactor in more than 100 enzymes that are responsible for cell growth and replication, immune responses, night vision, fertility, taste, and appetite. Zinc is required for DNA, RNA, and protein synthesis.

Iodine is essential for normal reproduction and is the part of thyroid hormones that regulates basal metabolic rate.

WATER

Water is the most abundant and essential component of the human body. A person's total body weight at birth consists of as much as 75% to 80% water; this amount decreases to 50% to 60% in adults. The body contains less water when greater amounts of adipose tissue are present. Body fluids are both intracellular and extracellular. The semipermeable membrane of the cell separates these body fluids but allows the passage of certain substances or **solutes** (i.e., glucose oxygen). **Osmotic pressure** serves to equalize the solute concentration inside and outside the cell by moving water in the direction of greatest solute concentration. The functions of water are the promotion of body processes, tissue building, the regulation of body temperature, and the preservation of the body's fluid balance. Coffee, tea, and alcohol have diuretic properties that result in increased urination.

It is important to consume additional water during warm weather, increased physical activity, and periods of illness and repair (e.g., burns, infections, wound healing). Cool water is absorbed more quickly than is warm water. Coffee, tea, soda pop, and alcoholic beverages can cause water to be lost from the body, thus increasing the need for water.

Table 6-2 is a comprehensive list of nutrients by food source, daily requirement to maintain health, deficiencies that may result from insufficient intake of these nutrients, the clinical manifestations of each deficiency, and the disorders and clinical manifestations that may occur from excessive intake of each of these nutrients.

NUTRITIONAL NEEDS FOR ORAL HEALTH THROUGH THE LIFESTYLE

Throughout the life span, various nutrients are in greater demand and required in higher concentration to sustain a healthy existence. A summary of the calories, protein, supplements, common nutritional problems, counseling recommendations, and dental considerations needed for each stage is outlined in **Table 6-3.**

INFANT NUTRITION (BIRTH TO 3 YEARS)

During infancy, adequate nutrition is essential for the promotion of normal growth and development. This stage of life (between birth and approximately 2 years of age) is second only to the fetal stage in developmental progress. Consequently, en-

TABLE 6–2 Comprehensive List of Nutrients

NUTRIENT	DIETARY SOURCES	DAILY REQUIREMENTS FOR THE AVERAGE ADULT	DEFICIENCY	EXCESS
Fiber	Whole grains, fruits, and vegetables	20–35 g	Colon cancer	• ↓ absorption of calcium, iron, and zinc • Cramps, constipation, and diarrhea
Water	Water	2500–3000 ml (10–12 cups)	Fluid volume deficit from: inadequate intake, loss of fluids from the GI tract, urinary tract, or skin; fever, anorexia, nausea, or fatigue	Fluid volume excess from congestive heart failure, kidney failure, chronic liver disease, or high levels of steroids
Protein	Meat, milk and milk products, eggs, poultry, peanut butter, grains, fruits, and vegetables	0.8 g/kg body weight	• PEM • Kwashiorkor • In children → delayed eruption and exfoliation, ↑ dental caries • Low IgA levels → mucosal infections • Negative nitrogen balance	• ↑ fat stores → obesity • Fluid imbalance • Stress on the kidneys
Carbohydrates	Milk products, grains, fruits, and vegetables	50–100 g digestible CHO	Concurrent deficiency of B vitamins, iron, and fiber	Diets high in sugar are less likely to be nutritious
Fats	Meat and milk products, nuts, and oils	3–6 g of essential fatty acids	• Low resistance to infection, • Poor reproductive capacity • Anorexia nervosa: dry skin, dull hair, thin, sensitive to cold, poor growth, and dermatitis	• Cardiovascular disease • Hyperlipidemia • Obesity • Breast, colon, and prostate cancers
Vitamin A	Liver, butter, cheese, cream, egg yolks, margarine, fortified and dried milk, and kidneys	800–1000 μg	• Night blindness, dry eyes, rough skin and mucous membranes, • Poor dental development (enamel hypoplasia), • Impaired growth and development • Low resistance to infection	Cracked bleeding lips, inflamed oral mucosa, double vision, headaches, insomnia, vomiting, diarrhea, skin rashes, alopecia, liver damage, joint pain, abnormal bone growth, menstrual irregularities, birth defects, and injury to the brain and nervous system
β-Carotene	Yellow and dark green vegetables, broccoli, carrots, sweet potatoes, squash, apricots, and cantaloupes	5–6 mg		
Vitamin D	Fortified milk products	5 μg	• Rickets in children • Osteomalacia in adults • Hypocalcemia • Osteoporosis • Enamel hypoplasia	• Calcium deposits in the kidneys and blood; ↑ bone density (hypercalcemia) • Cardiovascular damage
Vitamin E	Vegetable oils, margarine	8–10 mg	Prolonged impairment of fat absorption	Interferes with vitamin K activity
Vitamin K	Green leafy vegetables	65–80 μg	Impaired blood clotting	None observed
Vitamin C	Citrus fruits, tomatoes, cabbage, cauliflower, melons, strawberries, and dark green vegetables	60 mg	Scurvy: poor wound healing; capillary bleeding (petechia); degenerating muscles; brown, rough, dry skin; gingival enlargement and bleeding, irritability	• Diarrhea and kidney and bladder stones • Impaired blood clotting • Vitamin B_{12} deficiency may result
B-Complex Vitamins: B_1 (Thiamin)	Organ meats, pork, and enriched and whole grain products	1.1–1.5 mg	Beriberi: cardiovascular, muscle, and nervous systems are affected	—
B_2 (Riboflavin)	Meats, poultry, fish, dairy products, enriched and fortified cereals, pasta and bread	1.3–1.7 mg	Ariboflavinosis: cheilosis and glossitis, burning itchy eyes, blurred vision, photophobia, and dermatitis	—
B_3 (Niacin)	Liver, poultry, meat, tuna, eggs, whole-grain and enriched cereals, pasta, and bread	15–19 mg	Pellagra: 4Ds–diarrhea (GI upset), dermatitis (glossitis), dementia, and death	• Abnormal liver function • Gout
B_6 (Pyridoxine)	Chicken, fish, kidney, liver, pork, egg, unmilled rice, soybeans, oats, whole-wheat products, peanuts, and walnuts	1.6–2 mg	CNS abnormalities • Dermatitis with cheilosis and glossitis, • Impaired immune response • Anemia	• Tingling, shooting pains in the arms and legs; numbness of the hands and feet • Depression and headaches • Kidney damage
Folic Acid	Green leafy vegetables, legumes, liver, oranges, peanuts, sunflower seeds, and wheat-germ	180–200 μg	• Glossitis, cheilosis • Impaired immune response • Megaloblastic anemia • Pregnancy • Spina bifida, anencephaly	• Masks symptoms of B_{12} deficiency

Continued

TABLE 6–2 Comprehensive List of Nutrients (Completed)

NUTRIENT	DIETARY SOURCES	DAILY REQUIREMENTS FOR THE AVERAGE ADULT	DEFICIENCY	EXCESS
B_{12} (Cobalamin)	Liver, kidney, meat, fish, eggs, dairy products, oysters, and nutritional yeast	2 μg	• Pernicious anemia: tip and margins of the tongue may be red, smooth, and numb or have a burning sensation; spinal cord degeneration • Vegetarians *or* the body cannot absorb the vitamin (lack of intrinsic factor)	—
Biotin	Liver, egg yolk, soy flour, and cereals	30–100 μg	Ingestion of avidin (↑ uncooked egg white) → anorexia, pallor, nausea, vomiting, glossitis, dermatitis, and depression	—
Pantothenic Acid	Meat, whole-grain cereals, and legumes	4–7 mg	—	—
Calcium	Milk and milk products, sardines, oysters, canned salmon, dark green leafy vegetables, citrus fruits, dried beans and peas, and figs	1200 mg	In children → rickets and distorted bone growth In adults → osteoporosis	• Drowsiness, extreme lethargy, and impaired absorption of zinc, iron, and manganese • Calcium deposits in tissues
Phosporus	Meat, poultry, fish, eggs, dried beans and peas, milk and milk products, and soft drinks	700 mg	Hypophosphatemia muscle weakness, loss of appetite, malaise, and bone pain • Prolonged use of antacids	Hyperphosphatemia— calcium deficiency, tetany, and convulsions
Magnesium	Raw green leafy vegetables, nuts, soybeans, seeds, and whole grains	320–420 mg	• Muscle twitching and tremors, irregular heartbeat, insomnia, muscle weakness, and leg and foot cramps • May occur in persons with *prolonged* diarrhea, diabetes, kidney disease, epilepsy, alcoholism, or diuretic use	• Impaired nervous system function • Kidney failure
Iron	Liver, kidney, red meats, egg yolk, green leafy vegetables, dried fruits, dried beans and peas, potatoes, molasses, and enriched whole-grain cereals	10–15 mg	Iron deficiency anemia: fatigue, weakness, pallor, shortness of breath, glossitis, xerostomia, and delayed wound healing	• Heart disease • Toxic accumulation of iron in the heart, liver, and pancreas
Zinc	Meat, liver, eggs, poultry, seafood, and whole-grain cereals	12–15 mg	• Delayed wound healing, skin lesions, decreased taste, loss of appetite, and impaired immune system • In children → impaired sexual development • Prenatally → abnormal brain development	• Nausea and vomiting, anemia, and gastric bleeding • Premature births and stillbirth
Iodine	Seafood, iodized salt, saltwater fish, seaweed, and sea salt	150 μg	• Goiter • Prenatally → cretinism (stunted body growth and mental development)	• Iodine poisoning • Sensitivity reaction
Manganese	Nuts, whole grains, vegetables and fruits, tea, instant coffee,	2–5 mg	Unknown in humans	Mask-like facial expression, slurred laughing, spastic gait, and hand tremors
Potassium	Orange juice, bananas, fresh fruits, meats, bran, peanut butter, dried beans and peas, potatoes, coffee, tea, and cocoa	1600–2000 mg	• Abnormal heart rhythm, muscular weakness, lethargy, and kidney and lung failure • May result from dehydration due to prolonged use of diuretics or laxatives, or exposure to the sun while working or exercising	• Muscular paralysis • Abnormal heart rhythm
Sodium	Prepared foods, table salt	<3000 mg	• Heavy perspiration, injury, chronic diarrhea, or renal disease • Muscle cramps, weakness, nausea, and diarrhea	• Hypertension • Heart disease • Stroke
Chloride	Table salt or sea salt	750 mg	• Disturbed acid-base balance in the body	• Disturbed acid-base balance

CHO, carbohydrate; CNS, central nervous system; GI, gastrointestinal; Ig, immunoglobulin; PEM, protein-energy malnutrition.

ergy requirements are greatest at birth and then decline rapidly during the first year of life. During the first year of life, caloric needs range from 108 to 115 kcal/kg of body weight.

Protein requirements correlate with growth rate. For an infant from birth to 6 months of age, protein needs are generally 2.2 g/kg of body weight. This requirement decreases to 1.6 g/kg of body weight from 6 to 12 months. Iron supplements should begin at 4 to 6 months, when the infant's fetal store of iron is diminished. Iron-fortified formulas and cereals provide adequate supplementation.

Under normal circumstances, multivitamins and mineral supplements are not required for the growing child, with the exception of vitamin K for all newborns just after birth to prevent hemorrhagic disease. Fluoride supplements are recommended for all children younger than 8 years of age if their water supply contains less than 0.3 ppm of fluoride (see Chapter 14). Iron supplementation is suggested if it is not provided in formula.

Breast Milk

Breast-feeding is considered the best choice for feeding the normal full-term infant. Human milk is unique in nutrients and contains other substances, such as enzymes, hormones, and growth factors. Breast milk is normally thin and looks slightly blue. It is high in lactose and relatively low in protein. Specific protein fractions synthesized in the breast tissue help to protect against gastrointestinal (GI) infections.

Breast milk primarily contains unsaturated fatty acids. Its saturated fatty acid content is lower than that of cow's milk. The enzyme, **lipase**, is inherent in breast milk and improves fat digestion. Human milk contains only 20% of its protein as **casein** and the rest as whey protein. **Whey protein** is soluble in acid and consists primarily of **lactalbumin** and **lactoglobulin**.

Human milk has a relatively low mineral content, which is ideal for the infant's immature kidneys. Although the iron content is low, approximately 50% to 75% is absorbed. Because of the high bioavailability of iron, additional sources of iron are unnecessary during the infant's first 4 to 6 months. Breast milk is adequate to meet the infant's needs for at least 4 months. Supplemental foods during that time may reduce iron absorption.

Vitamin D supplementation (400 IU) is advised in breast fed infants who live in areas that receive limited exposure to sunlight. Breast milk from strict vegetarian mothers is likely to be deficient in vitamin B_{12}, therefore, these infants should receive supplements of this vitamin.

Infant Formulas

Formula composition contains fat, carbohydrate, protein, minerals, vitamins, and water in amounts sufficient to meet the needs of a healthy growing infant.

As established by the guidelines of the American Academy of Pediatrics, the electrolyte, mineral, and vitamin contents are similar to those of breast milk. Adequate amounts of these nutrients are furnished if the infant receives 150 to 180 ml/kg/day. Fluoride is no longer added to formulas because of the high variability of fluoride in the water supply.

Lactase, the disaccharide found in almost all mammalian milk, is the most common sugar found in infant formula. It is absorbed less efficiently than are other sugars, thus allowing a small amount to enter the distal bowel, where it is fermented by intestinal bacteria, resulting in a lower pH in the intestinal lumen. Lactose also seems to enhance the absorption of calcium.

Most infant formulas use vegetable oil as their source of fat. These oils are generally polyunsaturated and free of cholesterol. This is distinctly different from cow's milk, which contains saturated fat and cholesterol.

Infant formulas are so well balanced that the only supplement of real concern is iron. Iron-fortified formulas are recommended after 2 to 3 months of age. Commercial formulas are more appropriate for infants than is milk from cows or goats. Formulas can be discontinued at approximately 1 year of age, but the milk provided thereafter should be whole milk.

Oral Problems in Infancy

Baby Bottle Tooth Decay. A leading oral health problem among children younger than 3 years of age is **baby bottle tooth decay (BBTD)**, which is also known as nursing bottle caries. This nutritional disease, which is associated with inappropriate feeding practices, is characterized by early rampant decay. BBTD occurs when sweetened liquids (e.g., fruit juice, milk, sweetened water) stay on the teeth for an extended period while a child is sleeping. This leads to demineralization of the enamel. Frequent bottle feedings and excessive breast-feeding can contribute to BBTD. Other contributing factors include: (1) a decrease in the flow of saliva while sleeping, which diminishes the cleaning action; (2) a more viscous saliva in children, which enhances plaque adhesion on the teeth; and (3) a warm oral environment during sleep, which provides a cultural medium for bacterial growth. Colonization of S. mutans occurs after the teeth erupt. Infection with S. mutans occurs through transmission of the pathogen from caregiver to infant by sharing utensils that are contaminated with saliva during feeding or by kissing. Preventive measures include: (1) holding the child while feeding him or her so that if the child falls asleep, feeding can be discontinued; (2) put the child to bed without a bottle or with a bottle filled with plain water; (3) avoid dipping a pacifier in a sweetened liquid; (4) clean the child's teeth with gauze or a washcloth as soon as the first tooth erupts; (5) consult with a pediatric dentist or physician to assess the child's need for fluoride supplements; (6) become knowledgeable about the sugar content in commercial formulas and baby food; and (7) discontinue nursing as soon as the child can drink from a cup (see Chapter 14).

Cleft Palate/Lip. Each year in the United States, 1 in every 700 to 1,000 infants is born with a **cleft palate/lip**. Many scientists believe than many factors may contribute to this condition, such as malnutrition, drugs, disease, or heredity. Because an opening exists in the roof of the mouth and the floor of the nasal cavity, the negative pressure needed for sucking cannot be created and the infant may not receive adequate nutrition. An infant with cleft palate/lip adapts better to breast-feeding than to bottle-feeding. These infants should be fed at a 60- to 80-degree angle with a pulse bottle or an elongated nipple with an enlarged hole (see Chapter 12).

NUTRITION FOR TODDLERS AND PRESCHOOL CHILDREN (4 TO 6 YEARS)

Most preschoolers do not appear to be as interested in eating as they were when they were infants. The loss of appetite might be related to a decrease in the growth rate during early childhood. Nutritional needs during childhood depend on

TABLE 6–3 Nutrition Through the Life Cycle

LIFE CYCLE	CALORIC REQUIREMENTS/ BODY WEIGHT	PROTEIN REQUIREMENTS/ BODY WEIGHT	DENTAL CONSIDERATIONS	COUNSELING	SUPPLEMENTAL REQUIREMENTS	MOST COMMON NUTRITIONAL PROBLEM
Infancy	108-115kcal/kg	• 0-6 months: 2.2g/kg • 6-12 months: 1.6 g/kg	• Development and ewruption of primary teeth • Baby bottle tooth decay • Cleft lip/palate	• Diet/caries histories of both parents to reveal eating/ decay patterns • Analysis of carbo-hydrate intake	• Vitamin K just after birth to prevent hemorrhagic disease • Iron supple-mentation should begin at 4-6 months	
Toddlers/ preschoolers	• 1-3 years: 102 kcal/kg • 4-6 years: 90 kcal/kg	• 1-3 years: 1.2 g/kg • 4-6 years: 1.1 g/kg	• Dental caries • Gingivitis • Eruption of primary teeth • Development of permanent teeth	• Meals should be be encouraged at regular times • Clarify any misconceptions	• Calcium and vitamin D • Some may experience deficiencies in vitamins A and C, calcium, and zinc	Iron deficiencies and dental caries
School-aged	70 kcal/kg	1 g/kg	• Exfoliation of primary teeth • Eruption of permanent teeth	Involve them in meal preparation	• Iron	Iron deficiencies and obesity
Adolescence	• 11-14 years: 55 kcal/kg-males 47 kcal/kg-females • 15-18 years: 45 kcal/kg-males 40 kcal/kg-	• 11-14 years: 1 g/kg • 15-18 years: 0.9 g/kg-males 0.8 g/kg-females	• Dental caries • Malocclusion • Periodontal disease	• Appeal to their physical image • Praise good food choices and discourage harmful practices	• Iron, and calcium • Poor dietary habits result in inadequate folate, ribo-flavin, vitamins B6, A, and C, iron and calcium	Eating disorders
Adulthood	40 kcal/kg-males 35 kcal/kg-females	1 g/kg-males 0.8 g/kg-females	Periodontal disease	• Frequency of snacking • Retentiveness of foods • Amount of sugar to food and drinks		
Elderly	2300-kcal males 1900-cal females	0.8 g/kg	• Periodontal disease • Root caries	• Based on the individual needs of the patient • Address the need for socialization at mealtimes • Consume prepared foods high in fat and firm CHO	• Calcium, vitamin C, vitamin B12, zinc • A well-balanced diet depending on ndividual needs medical require-quirements	• Ill-fitting dentures • Dietary inade-quacies-thiamin, riboflavin, vitamins C and B6, folate, calcium, and zinc

the child's stage and rate of growth, physical activity, body size, basal metabolism, and health. The average caloric requirement for children who are 1 to 3 years of age is 102 kcal/kg of body weight. This requirement decreases to 90 kcal/kg of body weight for children who are 4 to 6 years of age and 70 kcal/kg of body weight for children who are 7 to 10 years of age. Proteins needs are 16 g/day, or 1.2 g/kg of body weight, for children aged 1 to 3; 24 g/day or 1.1 g/kg of body weight for children aged 4 to 6; and 28 g/day or 1 g/kg of body weight for children who are 7 to 10 years of age. A balanced and individualized diet is essential. Poor nutritional status is generally more prevalent in lower socioeconomic status groups. Approximately 10% of all children, regardless of socioeconomic status, may have an iron deficiency. Iron deficiencies and dental caries are the most common nutritional problems encountered in children. Some children may also experience deficiencies in vitamins A and C, calcium, and zinc. However, healthy children who consume well-balanced diets do not require routine supplementation of vitamins and minerals.

During the second year of life, development of fine motor skills results in toddlers feeding themselves. Finger feeding may be preferred to spoon-feeding; some finger foods should be provided at very meal. By 18 months of age, the toddler can manipulate a cup. Rotary chewing skills develop in the second year, therefore more solid foods can be introduced; foods that can be aspirated such as nuts and grapes should be avoided. Regularity of meal times is important for a toddler to avoid fatigue and malnutrition. Toddlers often demonstrate erratic and unpredictable appetites and may try to attract attention by refusing to eat. Parents should not force children to eat when they are not hungry. By compensating at subsequent meals, little variability in total energy intake results. At this age, new foods should be offered frequently with a variety of healthy snacks to promote successful feeding and adequate nutrients.

As children move into the preschool years, they are relatively independent at the table and can feed themselves. Preschoolers generally prefer their foods separate and foods that can be chewed easily. By allowing children to eat with adults, they will imitate others in both manners and food habits. Snacking is also an area of concern, because most snacks that are appealing to children are high in sodium, fat, and fermentable carbohydrates. Parents, teachers, and sitters must be made aware of "good" and "bad" snacks. They should read labels; avoid sucrose, fructose, glucose, corn sweeteners, honey, and molasses. Different sugars react differently in relation to decay. A table of relative cariogenicity of various sugars follows (**Table 6-4**).

Foods considered to have low caries producing potential are cheese, peanuts, yogurt, corn chips, pizza, bologna, raw carrots, celery, popcorn, and pretzels. If fermentable carbohydrates are going to be eaten, they should be consumed with a meal to buffer acid production and reduce their cariogenicity. Liquids have the most rapid clearance time and are least harmful, even though they may contain a high percentage of sucrose. The most cariogenic foods are those containing natural or refined sugars in a highly retentive form. Sticky caramel candy is highly cariogenic, along with raisins and dried fruits. Consistently restricting a child's intake of simple sugars early will teach good snacking habits.

Oral Problems of Toddlers and Preschool Children

Most children experience some form of dental disease, whereas some experience a high rate of caries. Because tooth formation begins before birth (~6 weeks in utero) and is not completed until approximately 12 years of age, the actual structure of the tooth is affected by food intake during this time. A clear relationship has been shown between nutritional deficiencies during tooth development and anomalies in tooth size, shape, and composition; time of tooth eruption; and susceptibility to caries. Calcium and vitamin D must be present for proper calcification of dentin and enamel.

 SCHOOL-AGED CHILDREN (7 TO 12 YEARS OLD)

Throughout this period, the child continues to require a diet that meets nutritional needs and establishes lifelong eating habits. During this time, food has social, emotional, and psychological implications. Favorite foods often remain favorites throughout life. Comfort foods that were given when a child was ill are still regarded as comfort foods when that child grows up. The child's diet is greatly influenced by the family. Parents need to take an active role in healthy choices

---

TABLE 6–4 Relative Cariogenicity of Sugars

CARIOGENICITY	MEDIUM TO LOW CARIOGENICITY	MEDIUM CARIOGENICITY	HIGH CARIOGENICITY
Sorbitol	Maltose	Lactose	Sucrose
	Mannitol	Glucose	
	Xylitol	Fructose	
	Starch		

for their child. The child who is given sweets as a reward will continue to think of sugar as a reward in adulthood. Otherwise, children can concede to social pressures that can challenge a child's dietary practices. Vending machines at school, convenience stores, and radio and television commercials are constant enticements for the child to eat unhealthy foods. Teaching children at this age about the fat and sugar content of foods, how to read ingredient labels, identify hidden sugars, and prepare foods that they enjoy by substituting artificial sweeteners and polyunsaturated fats is valuable in assisting the child with healthy decision-making. Although eating habits and food preferences are firmly established by late childhood, parents can counterbalance the effects of school activities and the media by purchasing and preparing healthy foods. Foods that are high in sucrose, sodium, and fat should not be kept in the house. Family meals, particularly breakfast, should not be skipped. Meals should not be eaten on the go, in shifts, in front of the television, or at fast food establishments. Schools can also modify their nutritional practices by eliminating cariogenic foodstuffs from the vending machines and lunch programs.

At approximately 12 years of age, there is an increase in activity and metabolism that requires additional high-energy foods incorporated into a well-balanced diet consisting of all food groups. Almost all foods are liked; vegetables are the least favorite. Planning menus around food groups is important in order to include all the necessary nutrients. The appetite is usually good, but food habits and intake may suffer because children do not take time for meals. Enforcement of a specific amount of time at the table may prevent the child from forming the habit of eating too fast.

The two most common nutritional disorders in the United States are **obesity** and **iron deficiency anemia**. Iron deficiency anemia affects significant numbers of children and adolescents, primarily females. This condition can be attributed to the start of menstruation and self-imposed dieting.

The number of children who are overweight has almost doubled in the last 25 years. Obesity in childhood and subsequent adulthood is associated with excessive caloric intake in infancy through bottle feeding and early weaning. It is believed that by breast-feeding, solid foods are introduced much later, thus decreasing the risk of overfeeding. Normal growth can be disturbed if weight loss for the obese child is not monitored carefully. Common practices among parents that increase their child's risk of becoming obese are giving a child large portions, recommending that the child eats more, forcing him or her to clean the plates, and giving food as a reward for desired behaviors.

Dental Considerations for the School-Aged Child

This age range marks the exfoliation of primary teeth and the eruption of permanent teeth. Therefore, administration of fluoride is vital for several reasons: (1) the crowns of numerous permanent teeth are still forming during this developmental period, (2) the permanent molars and premolars are highly susceptible to decay as they erupt, and (3) children are acquiring their independence and are becoming increasingly responsible for their own oral hygiene. At this age, topical fluoride becomes as important as systemic fluoride. To provide maximum protection, systemic fluoride is recommended through age 14 for those in nonfluoridated areas. Sealants should also be considered at this time to protect the pits and fissures of newly erupted premolars and molars, particularly if the patient experienced a high caries rate in the primary dentition.

 ## ADOLESCENCE (13 TO 20 YEARS OLD)

Adolescence is known as the period of growth and development when an individual moves from childhood to adulthood. It is a period of very rapid physical growth and development, which is second only to infancy. Adolescence is often described as beginning with the onset of puberty and ending when morphologic and physiologic growth and development are largely completed. Growth spurts may be observed during adolescence with an increase in muscle mass, body fat distribution, and skeletal growth. The average child can expect a 20% to 25% increase in height and a 100% gain in weight during this period. Due to the biologic, social, psychological, and cognitive changes during adolescence, 17% of U.S. teenagers are considered to be at nutritional risk. Many are susceptible to nutritional deficiencies, due to rapid growth spurts.

Adolescents' food habits are unique and are characterized by an increased tendency to skip meals, snacking, dieting, vegetarianism, and increased consumption of fast foods. These behaviors can be explained by their newly found independence, poor body image, search of self-identity and peer acceptance, and difficulty conforming to the existing value system that is expected of them.

Most adolescents are faced with continual changes as they try to understand their identity. This stress can decrease the utilization of several nutrients, particularly vitamin C and calcium. Approximately 25% of an adolescent's calories come from high-calorie, low-nutrient dense foods, which makes it easy to overeat.

Although the RDAs provide recommended nutrient intakes by chronologic age, nutrient needs closely parallel physical development. For example, adolescent girls need to increase their energy intake sooner and decrease it more quickly than boys because of earlier onset of puberty and lower total body weight once adulthood is reached.

Particular care needs to be taken to provide adequate intake of calcium, iron, and zinc. Forty-five percent of adult skeletal mass is formed during adolescence. Calcium needs are greater during adolescence than during any other time of life. Calcium intake during adolescence promotes calcium retention and bone mineral density. An increase in calcium intake by adolescent females from 800 to 1300 mg/day may increase hip bone density by 6%. The expansion of blood volume, increase in red blood cell mass and muscle mass (especially in boys), and the need to replace the iron losses associated with menstruation in girls require increased iron. Participation in sports activities leads to red blood cell destruction. Poor dietary habits result in inadequate folate; riboflavin; vitamins B_6, A, and C; iron; and calcium intake. Tobacco use, often experimented with or adopted at this time, has a deleterious effect on the absorption of nutrients.

Adolescent Health Concerns

Eating Disorders-Anorexia Nervosa and Bulimia

Increasing numbers of children and adolescents are overweight. Adolescents, especially girls, are often obsessed about their body image and have a desire to be thin. They are eager to try fad diets and other unsafe weight-loss methods that may lack nutrients. This is unfortunate, because nutrients during this period are necessary to build and strengthen their bodies. Obesity, anorexia nervosa, and bulimia are serious health concerns that are amenable to early treatment.

Anorexia nervosa and bulimia are two different conditions, but they have several similarities. Anorexia nervosa is primarily a disease that affects adolescent girls who have an exaggerated, intense fear of becoming fat. Stringent self-imposed dieting leads to extreme weight loss.

Criteria for a diagnosis of **anorexia nervosa** include a weight loss equal to or exceeding 15% below expected or original body weight, amenorrhea (for premenopausal women), and an intense desire for slimness with a distorted body image (Diagnostic Criteria for Anorexia Nervosa). Dental complications in advanced stages of malnutrition are generally observed in clients with anorexia nervosa.

Bulimia occurs more frequently than does anorexia nervosa. Persons with bulimia do not exhibit significant weight loss (Diagnostic Criteria for Bulimia Nervosa). A bulimic person might even be normal or slightly overweight and appear healthy. Bulimia is characterized by intentional, although not necessarily controllable, secret **binges** usually followed by **purging (Figure 6-1).**

Oral Manifestations

A patient who suffers from either eating disorder might exhibit one or more of the following: perimylolysis, an increase in pit and fissure and smooth surface caries, oral mucosal irritation, cheilosis, xerostomia, and chronic swelling of the parotid glands.

Perimylolysis is the erosion of enamel on the lingual, occlusal, or incisal surfaces of the teeth, primarily the maxillary incisors **(Figure 6-2).** This occurs as a result of the chronic regurgitation of low-pH gastric contents. Particularly in prolonged cases of bulimia, the teeth appear stained

from exposed dentin and the incisal edges of anterior teeth have a "moth-eaten" appearance **(Figure 6-3)**. The loss of enamel from the occlusal surfaces of restored teeth gives the filling material the appearance of being elevated (i.e., amalgam islands) **(Figure 6-4)**. Teeth with erosion also experience thermal sensitivity due to dentinal exposure.

Dental caries activity can increase due to an increase in carbohydrate consumption during binging, a decrease in the salivary pH, a decrease in the quantity and buffering capacity of the saliva, and poor oral hygiene. The perioral area, intraoral mucous membranes, and the periodontal tissues can be inflamed and dry from existing vitamin deficiencies and from xerostomia, which serves to dehydrate the oral mucosa. An iron deficiency will produce atrophy of the filiform papillae of the tongue and pallor of the lips, tongue, and mucous membranes. A B-complex deficiency causes glossitis, papillary hypertrophy of the tongue, and angular cheilosis. Bleeding gingivae are often observed in individuals with a vitamin C deficiency. Sore throat, burning tongue, and cheilosis can also be caused directly by the eating disorder if the oral environment remains acidic from frequent vomiting. Furthermore, the throat can be sore due to abrasions on the pharyngeal wall from using fingers or other objects to induce vomiting.

Enlargement of the salivary glands, although not fully understood, appears to be related to nutritional deficiencies and atypical eating behaviors. The cheeks look puffy, and pain can be present **(Figure 6-5)**. In particular, the parotid gland undergoes work hypertrophy because it is taxed from repeated abrupt binging episodes and irritated by gastric juices flowing through the opening and lining of the ducts. Xerostomia might be associated with parotid swelling, but it is directly related to the loss of body fluids from vomiting and diuretic abuse. Depression and anxiety can also decrease salivary output. Certain visual signs are descriptive of the malady, such as enamel erosion, tooth abrasion, or calluses across the knuckles of the dominant hand used to initiate the gag reflex **(Figure 6-6)**.

Counseling the patient not only requires knowledge of the signs and symptoms of an eating disorder, but more important, it demands communication, which reflects support, respect, and empathy for the individual's predicament. Many individuals become extremely relieved when they can share the burden of their problem with someone who will not pass judgment on them. People with eating disorders cannot resolve their condition until they admit its presence and willingly accept and remain in treatment.

Dental intervention procedures begin with a complete dental evaluation to assess a patient's orodental involvement. Patients who exhibit eating disorders also need nutritional guidance in order to make alternative noncariogenic food choices. Although meticulous oral hygiene is paramount, toothbrushing after emesis is contraindicated. The acids from the vomitus will demineralize the tooth, and immediate toothbrushing can abrade the weakened outer enamel surfaces, expediting erosion. Rinsing with a sodium

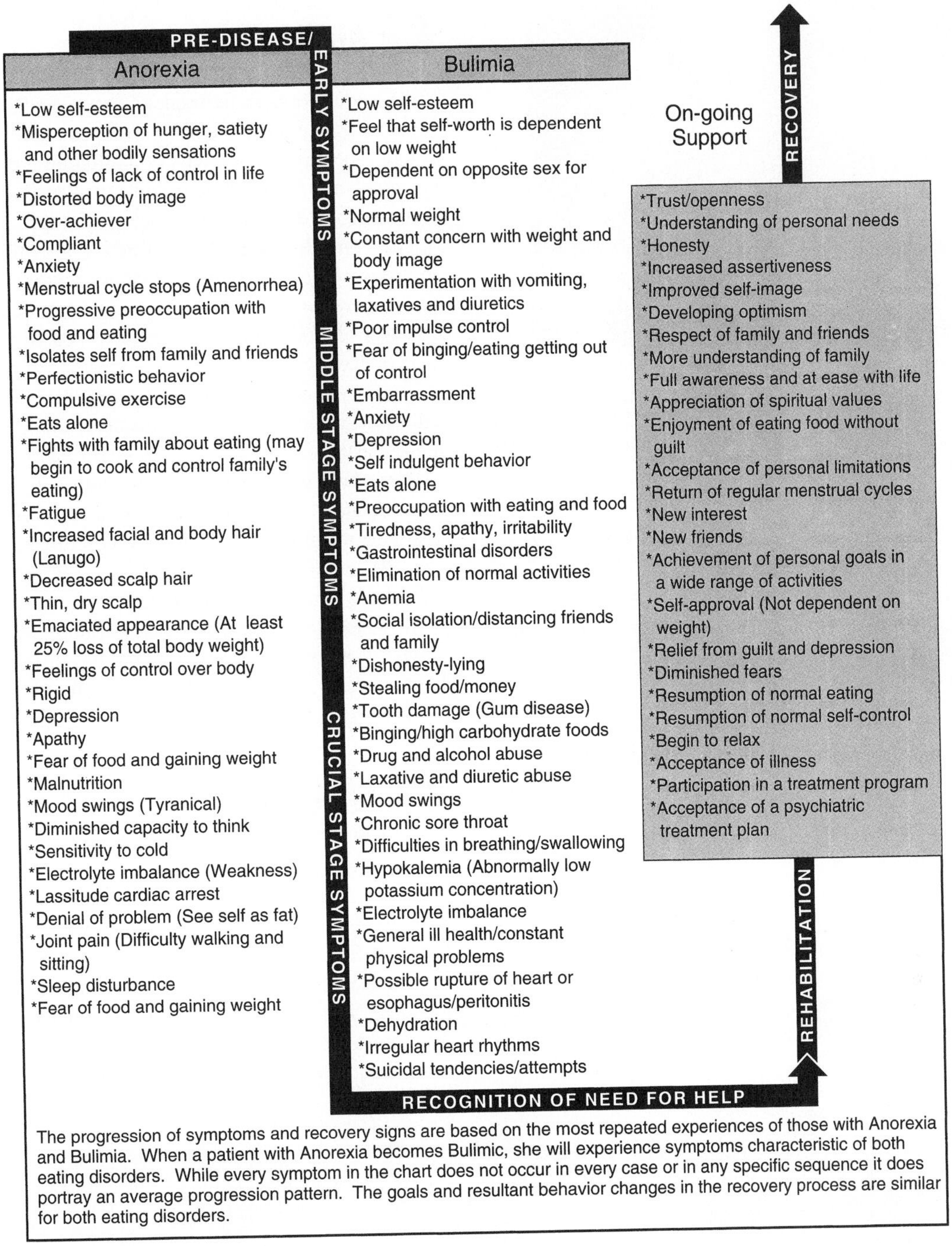

Figure 6-1. Anorexia nervosa-bulimia: A multidimensional profile. (From Stegeman CA: The Dental Hygienist's Guide to Nutritional Care. Philadelphia, WB Saunders, 1998, p 356.)

bicarbonate solution or allowing antacid tablets to dissolve the mouth immediately after vomiting will neutralize residual gastric acids in the oral cavity. A daily neutral sodium fluoride rinse in a 0.05% concentration or a fluoride gel (0.4% stannous fluoride or 2% neutral sodium fluoride) applied daily with a toothbrush or a custom tray in conjunction with a fluoride dentifrice are advised to prevent decay and minimize enamel erosion and subsequent tooth sensitivity. Therapeutic fabrication of a dental prosthesis to prevent the progression of enamel erosion from routine vomiting can also be employed (**Figure 6-7**).

Extensive restorative dental treatment to stabilize the condition of the oral cavity should not commence until the eating disorder is controlled. The preventive approach, which includes the application of sealants, is usually adequate for the patient with minimal erosion, whereas moderate enamel loss can require a bonded composite resin. Composites are esthetic and also serve to improve the patient's

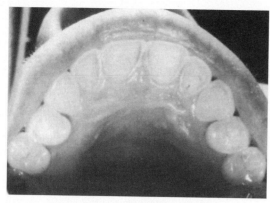

Figure 6-2. Perimylolysis. Note the flat lingual surface created by the enamel erosion. (Courtesy of JE Bouquot, DDS, MS, West Virginia University, Morgantown, WV. From DeBiase CB: Dental Health Education: Theory and Practice. Philadelphia, Lea & Febiger, 1991, pp 111-117.)

self-image. Permanent crowns become necessary when the patient has experienced severe erosion. The teeth and restorations should be examined for new caries, recurrences, and defects that harbor plaque, on an average of 1 to 3 months depending on the patient's needs. Fluoride therapy should also be monitored.

Dental Considerations for the Adolescent

Dentistry for the adolescent usually begins after the eruption of the permanent premolars and canines. Orthodontic intervention initiated during late childhood is a common form of dental therapy for this age group. Other dental concerns such as caries and periodontal disease seem to be the most severe during the teenage years. Hormonal changes, rapid growth, and the quest for independence as exemplified by poor oral hygiene and erratic eating patterns have been implicated as plausible causes (see Chapters 13 and 14).

 ADULTHOOD

Young adulthood is defined as the period from 18 to 40 years of age; middle adulthood ranges from 40 to 65 years of age. The nutritional goals of adulthood include maintaining good nutritional intake and an ideal body weight and preventing or delaying the onset of illness and disease.

The bones are in a phase of active growth from birth to approximately age 18 or 20. Active growth is characterized by an increase in bone length and width. Peak bone mass, however, is probably not attained before age 25. Bone growth and shaping of the growing skeleton generally cease at maturity, but adult bone is constantly being remodeled. This bone remodeling is what makes adult orthodontic treatment feasible.

Remodeling is the result of a continuous process of existing bone reabsorption (loss) and new bone deposition (growth) to replace that which was removed. Between the ages 30 and 40, the reabsorption of existing bone is greater than the formation of new bone, resulting in a net loss of bone. Osteoclastic activity occurs in both men and women. Once this activity is begun, it continues throughout life. **Osteoporosis** is the result of excessive bone loss and is discussed in the section on the elderly.

 PREGNANCY

During pregnancy, the diet should supply the nutrients necessary for maternal and fetal tissue formation. Calorie and protein needs are greatest during the last trimester, when the fetus experiences maximal growth. The recommended daily kilocalorie allowance is 300 kcal above the nonpregnant allowance. The recommended daily allowance for protein is 30 g more than for the nonpregnant woman. Increased protein intake is needed to support the rapid fetal growth, pla-

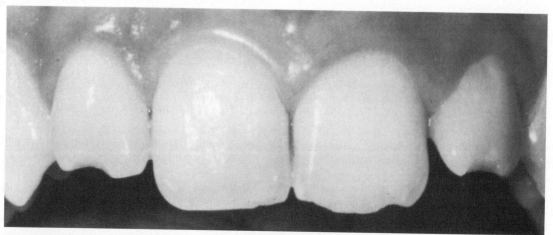

Figure 6-3. "Moth-eaten" appearance of incisal edges due to enamel erosion. (Courtesy of CA Spear, BSDH, MS, West Virginia University, Morgantown, WV. From DeBiase CB: Dental Health Education: Theory and Practice. Philadelphia, Lea & Febiger, 1991, pp 111-117.)

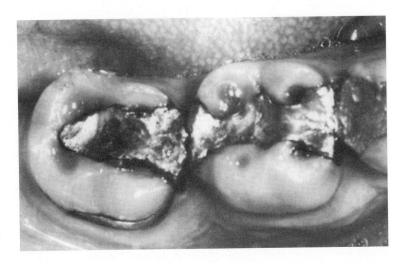

Figure 6-4. "Amalgam islands" resulting from occlusal erosion. (Courtesy of CA Spear, BSDH, MS, West Virginia University, Morgantown, WV. From DeBiase CB: Dental Health Education: Theory and Practice. Philadelphia, Lea & Febiger, 1991, pp 111-117.)

cental development, enlarging maternal tissue, increased maternal blood volume, and formation of amniotic fluid. Efficient use of protein depends on adequate energy intake. If calories are reduced, protein requirements are increased.

Recommended weight gain during pregnancy is at least 25 lb. Weight gain should be about 1 lb each month during the first trimester and 1 lb/wk during the second and third trimesters.

Minerals

Edema alone does not indicate the need for salt restriction or the use of diuretics. In fact, edema is normal in pregnancy, particularly when the fetus is large. If a sudden, excessive weight gain arises from edema, it could signal **pregnancy-induced hypertension (PIH).**

Calcium and phosphorus must be increased by the pregnant mother to promote mineralization of the fetal skeleton. The recommended calcium and phosphorus intake is approximately 400 mg higher than that for the nonpregnant woman. If dairy products are deficient in the pregnant woman's diet, calcium supplementation is recommended. A fetus will draw upon the mother's calcium stores in bone (not teeth) when a dietary calcium deficiency exists. Phosphorus requirements are easily met by consuming the typical American diet. Adequate intake of calcium and phosphorus appears to lessen the incidence of PIH.

Iron is needed for the increased manufacture of hemoglobin in the mother and fetus. Iron is another nutrient that the fetus draws from the mother at her expense if intake is inadequate. The fetus accumulates most of its iron during the last trimester; therefore, the preterm newborn may experience iron deficiency anemia. Supplementation is generally recommended to prevent depletion of maternal iron stores and to ensure that the fetal iron stores are adequate for the first year. The recommended level of supplementation is 30 to 60 mg/day throughout pregnancy and for 2 to 3 months after delivery.

Zinc deficiency may result in an increased risk of congenital malformation, an infant that is small for its gestational age, spontaneous abortion, and PIH. The recommended allowance for zinc during pregnancy is 5 mg above the level of the nonpregnant woman. This level is easily met if protein needs are satisfied. Pregnancy also requires an increased need for iodine, magnesium, and copper, but supplements are usually unnecessary.

Vitamins

Vitamin needs are increased during pregnancy. Multivitamin supplements are usually not necessary when an adequate diet is consumed, although folate supplementation is recommended. In a normal pregnancy, folate turnover is increased in the expanding maternal and fetal tissues; and folate deficiency is strongly correlated with neural tube defects in the fetus and with iron deficiency anemia.

Although still controversial, a deficiency of vitamin B_6 in pregnant women has been reported to cause nausea and depression as well as low **Apgar** scores (an assessment of the baby's color, respiration, heart rate, reflexes, and muscle

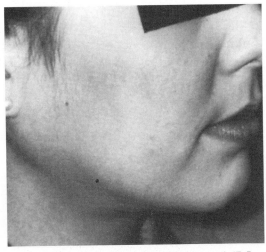

Figure 6-5. Parotid gland enlargement. (Courtesy of JE Bouquot, DDS, MS, West Virginia University, Morgantown, WV. From DeBiase CB: Dental Health Education: Theory and Practice. Philadelphia, Lea & Febiger, 1991, pp 111-117.)

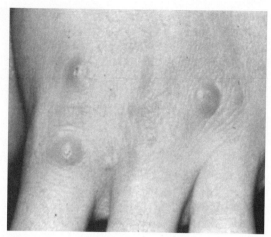

Figure 6-6. Knuckle callouses from chronically inducing vomiting. (Courtesy of JE Bouquot, DDS, MS, West Virginia University, Morgantown, WV. From DeBiase CB: Dental Health Education: Theory and Practice. Philadelphia, Lea & Febiger, 1991, pp 111-117.)

tone; a score >4 indicates severe asphyxia with a likelihood of neurologic damage).

A deficiency of thiamin, riboflavin, or niacin may result in congenital malformation, retarded growth, and fetal death. The requirements for these nutrients are directly proportional to caloric intake. As caloric intake increases during pregnancy, so does the requirement for vitamins B_1, B_2, and B_3.

Because vitamin C induces the production of enzymes in the fetus for catabolism of the vitamin, the newborn infant, upon delivery, may begin to exhibit a deficient state.

Excessive intake of vitamin A may be teratogenic and cause urogenital and central nervous system malformations, such as microcephaly. Vitamin D is required for calcium and phosphorus absorption and mineralization of bone tissue of the fetus, although an excess may promote neonatal hypercalcemia and abnormal skull development. Vitamin D deficiency can lead to poor tooth enamel development and hypocalcemia in the fetus. If the pregnant woman is exposed

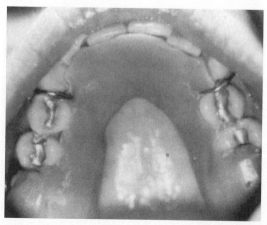

Figure 6-7. Preventive appliance to be worn during vomiting episodes to cover and protect those surfaces most affected by erosion. (From Ruff JC, Abrams RA: Preventive dental prosthesis for the patient with bulimia. Sp Care Dent 7:218-220, 1987.)

to sunlight or increases her dietary intake of fortified milk, the increased needs for vitamin D are generally met.

Special Considerations

The pregnant adolescent is at high nutritional risk. Adequate energy, protein, and micronutrients are needed to support rapid growth and maturation of the adolescent and the rapidly growing fetus. Many of the adverse outcomes of the adolescent pregnancy can be prevented through active nutrition and health care intervention. Nutritional counseling should begin as soon as possible.

Alcohol crosses the placenta to the fetus. There is evidence that even small amounts of alcohol during pregnancy may be harmful. **Fetal alcohol syndrome** is the term used to describe the adverse effects of excessive alcohol consumption on the infant. Characteristics of the infant with fetal alcohol syndrome include abnormalities of the eyes, nose, heart, and central nervous system; growth retardation; small head circumference; failure to thrive; and mental retardation. These characteristics are most pronounced in the babies of mothers with a long history of heavy drinking.

Low birth weight is a major contributing factor in approximately two thirds of all infant deaths as well as in mental retardation. Factors that influence birth weight are maternal weight, weight gain and nutritional status during pregnancy, maternal age, number of pregnancies, smoking, periodontal disease, hypertension, diabetes, and neonatal infection. The better the nutritional status of the woman entering pregnancy, the more successful will be the outcome.

Pregnant women with diabetes mellitus are advised to divide their diet into several small meals throughout the day. If the diabetes is difficult to control, every meal and snack should contain protein and carbohydrate and should be eaten at consistent intervals each day. Intake of sucrose should be minimized. Carbohydrate intolerance experienced during pregnancy is referred to as **gestational diabetes**. Pregnant women should be screened for glucose intolerance, because undetected hyperglycemia places the fetus at greater risk for intrauterine death.

PIH is often called preeclampsia or eclampsia. **Preeclampsia** is characterized by hypertension, protein in the urine, and edema. **Eclampsia,** which is more severe, includes convulsions or coma. PIH is most likely to occur among underweight women who fail to gain appropriately during pregnancy.

Additional concerns associated with pregnancy include: morning sickness, which is usually seen in early pregnancy and is best treated with small, frequent meals, easily digested foods, and liquids between meals; constipation, which is best treated by increasing intake of fluids, whole grains, fruits, and vegetables rather than the use of laxatives; hemorrhoids, which may be aided by rest and warm baths; and heartburn or a full feeling, especially likely during the last trimester, which is usually rectified by eating small, frequent meals, chewing well, and eating slowly.

Maternal Dietary Requirements

Lactation (breast-feeding) requires approximately 500 calories a day beyond that needed by nonpregnant women. Most lactating women, however, consume only 200 to 300 extra calories each day while producing ample quantities of milk. Many women experience a very gradual weight loss during lactation. In addition to extra calories, breast-feeding requires approximately 20 g of additional protein and varying amounts of other nutrients. Calcium needs are elevated during lactation. Lactating women should consume 1200 mg/day of calcium from dietary sources. Protein, caloric, and calcium needs may be met through the addition of 3 to 3.5 servings of dairy products to the diet daily. For women who are unable to consume adequate amounts of dietary calcium, supplements (~600 mg/day) are recommended to prevent bone loss. The needs for ascorbic acid, vitamin E, and folic acid are also increased during lactation and can be met with foods such as fruits, whole grains, and leafy green vegetables. Iron supplementation may be needed to replenish iron stores if the diet during pregnancy was deficient in iron.

 ## ELDERLY

As people age, their energy requirements are less. Many elderly tend to eat less or consume more of foods that have low nutritional value. Unless food is carefully selected, the intake of essential micronutrients may fall below desired levels. This is compounded by: (1) personal habits: there appear to be many reasons why elderly individuals may impose certain dietary restrictions upon themselves. Unfortunately, in time, such restrictions can compromise nutritional status and ultimately place an individual's health at risk; (2) economic limitations: limited financial resources strongly influence food choices; (3) sociologic factors: living alone, the difficulty of getting to the grocery store, and a decreased interest in preparing and eating meals alone have a negative impact on food choices; (4) medications: the elderly constitute 13% of the population (this figure will rise to about 22% by 2030), receive 31% of all prescription drugs, and are more likely to take medications for an extended period of time; (5) lack of knowledge: many of the elderly are not aware that good nutrition can still enhance their quality of life; and (6) a "too late now" attitude: some elderly people think that it is too late to change to a more nutritious diet, but this is not true. Improved nutrition can help at any age. Consequently, the elderly represent a nutritionally vulnerable population.

With aging, there is a decrease in body weight and a change in body composition, which is reflected by a decrease in lean body mass and a relative increase in fat. It is estimated that there is a 6% decrease in lean body mass, mainly skeletal muscle, with each decade after 30 years of age. There is a slight decline in the need for calories. Men older than 50 require 2300 kcal/day, and women older than 50 years of age need approximately 1900 kcal/day. Protein for adults older than 50 years of age is approximately 0.8 g/kg of ideal body weight (IBW). The RDA for vitamins and minerals remains stable from the middle adult years. However, menopausal women may require additional calcium to prevent osteoporosis. **Osteoporosis** is a condition in which excessive loss of bone mass or density occurs with the result that bones become weak and brittle. Eventually, this weakening of the bones leads to fractures of the hip, wrist, ankle, and spleen. This disorder afflicts older people, although women are more susceptible to it than are men. It has been estimated that one third of American women older than 50 years of age have osteoporosis. Apparently, menopause marks the onset of an acute change in the calcium balance and rapid bone loss in women; the most rapid bone loss occurs during the first 5 years after menopause. Some researchers have suggested that the progressive loss of alveolar bone, leading to tooth loss, may be a manifestation of osteoporosis. Research shows that women in their 60s who have osteoporosis require new dentures because of excessive ridge reabsorption, which occurs three times more frequently when compared with women who do not have osteoporosis. However, edentulism has decreased to about one third of persons 65 to 74 years of age.

The prevention of osteoporosis begins early in life with the formation and maintenance of strong bones. Later in life, a three-step prevention program is important.

- **Exercise**-the kind that makes the muscles and bones work against gravity-can strengthen the skeleton (e.g., walking, tennis, and running). Although swimming is an excellent aerobic exercise, it lacks the weight-bearing stress that builds bone mass.
- **Adequate calcium** intake is essential throughout life. Before 30 years of age, calcium helps to build bone mass. After age 30, adequate calcium intake has a role in preventing calcium loss from the bones. The National Institute of Health recommends that women consume 1000 mg/day of elemental calcium before menopause and 1500 mg/day afterward. Women who take estrogen are usually advised to take 1000 mg.
- **Estrogen replacement therapy** slows the loss of calcium from the bones. It may also help to protect postmenopausal women against heart attacks. However, the benefits of replacement hormones must be weighed against a possible increase in the patient's risk of certain cancers.

The nutritional needs of most older people are satisfied by well-balanced diets. Physiologic changes that occur during the aging process may have nutritional implications. These include decreased taste acuity, impaired sense of smell, poor dentition or periodontal disease, decreased gastric secretion of hydrochloric acid, decreased gastrointestinal motility, frequent or multiple drug prescriptions, and impaired motor abilities. Psychosocial changes such as lack of socialization, economic problems caused by fixed incomes, and poor dentition or ill-fitting dentures may also affect eating habits. Consequently, common dietary inadequacies among the elderly include thiamin, riboflavin, vitamin C, vitamin B_6, folate, calcium, and zinc.

Nutritional Recommendations

Although the elderly require the same nutrients as do other age groups, the amounts of nutrient may need to be adjusted. Fluid intake is a concern for the elderly. They are susceptible to fluid imbalances that can lead to cardiac impairments. Dehydration is also a common cause of confusion in the elderly.

Dietary mineral intake may also need to be adjusted, based on assessment of the nutritional status of the elderly patient. Elderly patients usually have a negative calcium balance and lose bone mass, leading to spontaneous fractures, and subsequent disabilities. This is a result of decreased calcium intake and genetic, hormonal, and environmental factors. Decreased physical activity contributes to calcium loss over the years. The combined use of alcohol, antacids, and drugs also compromises calcium reserves. The elderly tend to have a lower exposure to sunlight, which results in a reduced synthesis of vitamin D in their skin. Calcium levels in the elderly often fall because of a lower intake of milk, dairy products, and other calcium sources. The elderly may have a slight deficiency in zinc due to a decrease in protein consumption.

Dairy products, fruits, and vegetables are frequently lacking in the diet, especially for those who live alone. Low vitamin C levels in the blood and **scurvy** may be observed in the elderly, who often avoid eating fruits and vegetables that could serve as a source of vitamin C.

Soft foods are often chosen due to a decrease in chewing function from ill-fitting prostheses, and a preference for foods that are easy to eat and prepare and that cost less. The choice of softer food usually results in a decrease in protein and intake of more fat and refined carbohydrates. In general, people with less education and income; the housebound, especially those who live alone; those with physical disabilities, depression, and other mental disorders; those with recent drastic lifestyle changes; and those who do not have regularly cooked meals are considered to be at risk of developing malnutrition.

Nutrition and Dental Health

Xerostomia is a condition that is commonly found in the elderly. It is not a direct consequence of the aging process but may result from one or more factors that affect salivary secretion. A decrease in salivary flow can lead to poor oral health. Emotions, neuroses, organic brain disorders, and drug therapy can all cause xerostomia. Xerostomia is characterized by diminished or absent salivary flow or a change in the viscosity of saliva. Xerostomia serves many functions, and if the gland is not producing saliva, it can have a negative impact on oral tissues and dietary intake. Saliva functions to: (1) lubricate oral tissues, (2) assist in chewing, swallowing, and digestion, (3) remove debris from teeth, (4) have an antibacterial action, (5) neutralize the bacterial acids, (6) aid in the remineralization of enamel, (7) increase taste, and (8) allow for ease of talking.

Many groups of drugs including antihypertensives, anticonvulsives, antidepressants, antihistamines, tranquilizers, analgesics, anti-inflammatory agents, decongestants, bronchodilators, and diuretics can cause dry mouth as a side effect. Other causes of xerostomia include: salivary gland obstruction caused by obstruction of the salivary duct with a salivary stone; chemotherapy and radiation for head and neck cancer; infection such as mumps; autoimmune disorders; lupus erythematosus; biliary cirrhosis; systemic diseases; stress and depression; significant vitamin A, vitamin C, and protein deficiency; liquid diets; and dehydration.

Dry mouth can cause pain and discomfort in the oral cavity, difficulty swallowing, decreased taste perception, increased root caries, sticky, tacky saliva, low tolerance to spicy foods, ulcerations, angular cheilosis (cracking or burning at the corners of the mouth), dentinal hypersensitivity, dry nose, dry throat, and shiny mucosa.

Due to the consequences of xerostomia, appropriate intervention strategies must be implemented. Each patient will have different causes of dry mouth and varied symptoms. Therapy should be individualized to relieve symptoms and decrease discomfort. Recommended therapies may involve artificial salivas; lip balm to moisten the lips; use of a humidifier; frequent fluids; sugar-free items; nutrient-dense, soft, moist foods; and tart foods.

A painful, burning tongue known as **glossitis** is often encountered in nutritional anemias associated with deficiencies of vitamin B_{12}, folic acid, or iron. Vitamin B_{12} deficiencies are seen frequently in older people, particularly in women. Most cases of vitamin B_{12} deficiencies observed in the United States are the result of impaired absorption of the vitamin caused by **pernicious anemia**. This deficiency is characterized by many symptoms such as: generalized weakness; a sore, painful tongue; and numbness or tingling of the extremities. The tongue is red instead of pink and is characterized by a gradual atrophy of the papillae, which results in a smooth, or bald, tongue. In anemic patients, the oral mucosa becomes sensitive and intolerant to dentures.

 NUTRITIONAL COUNSELING

When giving dietary counseling, attaining a balanced diet should be emphasized for people in all age groups. Food choices and eating habits merit attention. From a dental viewpoint, include the frequency of between-meal snacking, the physical form and retentiveness of sugar-sweetened snacks on and between the teeth, and the amount of sugar added to food or beverages for sweetening. The length of intimate contact of fermentable carbohydrate with plaque bacteria determines the relative cariogenic potential. Sugar-sweetened foods in both solid and liquid form, combined with dental plaque, can produce tooth decay. The sequence of food intake during a meal can influence the incidence of dental caries. Eating cheese or peanuts before or after sugar-containing foods reduces the cariogenicity of the latter. Furthermore, meats, eggs, some types of nuts, and some dairy products do not produce an acidic plaque pH. Milk and certain cheeses (e.g., cheddar, Swiss, Monterey jack, mozzarella, Brie, and Gouda) produce little or no plaque acid. Whenever possible, the diet counselor should make the following recommendations: (1) provide a nutritionally balanced varied diet from the basic food groups (**Figure 6-8**); (2) eliminate high-sugar snacks whenever possible; (3) restrict sugar-containing foods to mealtime (when the organic acids formed may undergo neutralization) if they must be included for providing energy; and (4) suggest hard cheeses and nuts as between-meal snacks.

Dietary counseling should begin at pregnancy. Diet histories of both parents should be taken to reveal cariogenic eating patterns that can be transferred to the newborn infant. An analysis of the frequency of fermentable carbohydrates intake and oral hygiene habits can be instrumental in creating an awareness of a potential problem for the parent. Intercepting and modifying damaging health practices before birth can prevent BBTD and possibly the development of caries later on.

During the preschool years, parents should be encouraged to have meals at regular times, and they should offer new foods frequently. Clarifying any misconceptions that may interfere with a child's ability to consume foods that meet his or her nutritional needs for growth and development is important. As children move into the school-age years, they should be involved in meal preparation and should be encouraged to have good oral hygiene techniques.

The best tactic for nutritional counseling among adolescents is to appeal to their physical image or their muscular development for sports. The earlier information is presented, the more likely it is to be accepted and used later in life. When helping adolescents to improve their eating patterns, the best approach is to praise good food choices, ignore those that are neutral, and discourage harmful practices.

NUTRITIONAL FADS

Fad diets are both numerous and popular in the United States as Americans continue to search for a gimmick to lose weight. According to promoters of weight-loss diets, specific foods or food combinations facilitate weight loss by oxidizing body fat, increasing the metabolic rate, or controlling hunger. These diets are often deficient in essential nutrients. Results of fad diets can be fatal. Benefits, such as rapid weight loss, may not be long-lasting.

Unconventional procedures for nutritional assessment are numerous. **Hair analysis** is used to recommend vitamin and mineral supplements. Although hair analysis can indicate exposure to toxic heavy metals, vitamins are not present in hair except in the roots below the skin. Furthermore, hair mineral content can be affected by shampoos, bleach, dye, and many other factors, including environmental and geographic factors.

Herbal medicine has merit but should be approached with caution. Herbs, including herbal teas, and other plant-based

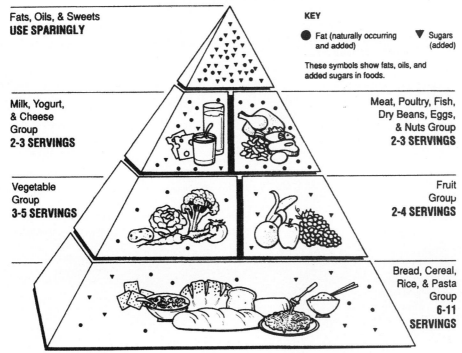

Figure 6-8. The Food Pyramid is a visual guide to healthier living. (Courtesy of the U.S. Department of Agriculture.)

formulations are marketed to prevent and cure numerous conditions. Several severe health problems, such as cardiovascular disease, cirrhosis, and renal failure have occurred from use of herbal preparations in the United States. A woman can reduce these risks by: (1) avoiding herbs if pregnant or nursing (herbs should not be given to infants), (2) not taking large amounts of any single herbal preparation on a daily basis, (3) buying only preparations that list all ingredients on the label (but this is still no guarantee of safety), and (4) avoiding any preparation that contains comfrey.

A unique point regarding herbs is that they cannot be patented. That is why they are widespread and widely used. Many herbs have side effects and can interact with current medications. Dental professionals need to research herbs and supplements. **Table 6-5** provides a list of some herbs and supplements that may be encountered in a dental office, along with their purpose, side effects, and contraindications.

Vegetarian Diets

Vegetarian diets may either totally exclude meat, fish, eggs, and dairy products (**vegan**) or rely upon fish (**pesco-vegetarian**), eggs (**ovo-vegetarian**), or dairy products (**lacto-vegetarian**) as a source of protein. Meatless diets can provide adequate nutrients and also offer certain health advantages. Vegetarian diets may lower risk factors for: (1) heart disease by lowering serum cholesterol levels and controlling body weight, and (2) cancer because of the low fat and high fiber content of the diet, and the high intake of β-carotene-containing vegetables and fruits.

Legumes (dried beans, dried peas, and lentils) can be combined with grains, nuts, or seeds to provide all EAAs. Vitamin B_{12}, which is found only in animal products, may be supplied through tablet supplementation or through fortified soybean products if no animal products are consumed.

Plant-based diets that include one or a combination of dairy products, eggs, or fish can be nutritionally similar to diets containing meats if menus are planned to provide sufficient calories, EAAs, and adequate sources of calcium, riboflavin, iron, and vitamins A, D, and B_{12}.

Health Foods

The terms organic, natural, and health foods are loosely defined and are often used interchangeably. No scientific basis exists for claiming that organic foods are more nutritious than are conventional foods; however, many consumers believe these foods are the answer to good health. Food grown by chemical processes does not necessarily differ in taste, appearance, or nutrient content from those that are grown organically.

TABLE 6-5 Herbs: Their Uses and Contraindications

HERB	PURPOSE	SIDE EFFECTS	CONTRAINDICATIONS
Echinacea	Immune booster		Avoid with autoimmune diseases, influenza, and respiratory tract infection
Ginkgo biloba	Short-term memory; antioxidant; depression	Headaches, dizziness, GI problems– if taken with Prozac	Bleeding disorders or anticoagulants
St. John's wort	Antidepressant	GI irritation, photosensitivity, reduced iron absorption	Psychoactive drugs (Prozac and Diazepam); reduces the bioavailability of digoxin, cyclosporine, warfarin, estrogen, oral contraceptives
Ginseng	Anticoagulant	Headache, insomnia, anxiety, skin rashes, diarrhea	High blood pressure, diabetes, Nardil, warfarin
Valerian	Sedative	Headache, nausea, morning grogginess, blurred vision with overdose	Sedative aids; may prolong general anesthesia
Kava kava	Tranquilizer, muscle relaxant	Scaly dermatitis with long-term use	Generally safe; may prolong general anesthesia
Ephedra-ma huang	Decongestant; pseudo epinephrine	Increased blood pressure, palpitations, nervousness	High blood pressure, thyroid disease, diabetes, and antidepressant drugs; found in weight loss products
Dong quai	Menopause, PMS	Photosensitivity	Anticoagulants
Garlic	Antibiotic, anticoagulant properties	GI irritation	Anticoagulants
Coenzyme Q 10	Antioxidant, immune enhancer, cardiac and periodontal applications		
Melatonin	Hormone		May counteract effect of steroids; may exaggerate an autoimmune response; and may suppress fertility
Glucosamine sulfate	Anti-inflammatory	None	Diabetes

Vitamin Supplementation

Although most Americans who consume a varied diet do not require vitamin supplementation, such supplements are routinely consumed by them. In some subgroups, such as the elderly, use of vitamins may be even higher.

Indications for vitamin supplementation include pregnancy, infancy, vegans, anorectics, persons of low socioeconomic status, and those who cannot metabolize nutrients properly.

THERAPEUTIC DIETS

Diet therapy is the most important approach to many disease and recovery states. In some cases, diet therapy can replace drug therapy. **Therapeutic diets** represent components of the general diet, which provide optimal health for patients who require dietary modifications to treat specific conditions. Examples follow.

- Water-modified: restricted fluid intake in severe heart failure, kidney failure
- Carbohydrate-modified: carbohydrate-controlled diet for diabetes and hypertriglyceridemia
- Protein-modified: low protein for the unstressed patient with chronic kidney failure; high protein for the stressed patient
- Fat-modified: low total and saturated fat and low cholesterol for hypercholesterolemia; low total fat for malabsorption syndromes
- Vitamin-modified: restricted vitamin A in renal failure; increased vitamin C in the infected or injured patient
- Mineral-modified: low sodium, potassium, and phosphorus in kidney failure; increased zinc in the infected or injured patient
- Other substances: restricted alcohol intake for hypertriglyceridemia

In addition, therapeutic diets may be modified in consistency or texture. Common examples include **soft** and **liquid diets** for patients with no teeth, post oral maxillofacial surgery, post anesthesia, and GI disorders and **high-fiber (high-residue) diets** for patients with constipation.

Soft and Liquid Diets

A **soft diet** is a normal diet excluding foods that are difficult to eat, such as such as steak, toast, and crackers. Soft foods in their natural state are eaten. Foods are not liquefied as in the full liquid diet.

A **clear liquid diet,** which consists of broths, gelatin, and clear liquids that the patient can consume comfortably, is most often used in a hospital setting and is not generally required by patients with dental problems outside of that setting.

A **full liquid diet** is one that includes a wider range of foods. These foods are liquid at room temperature or liquefy at body temperature. A full liquid diet also includes foods that have been liquefied by processing in a blender. A patient with dental problems who requires a liquid diet is usually given it for only a few days.

Liquid formula foods are commercially available preparations (e.g., canned supplements) that are prepared to include all necessary nutrients in a form that ranges from 300 to 3000 calories/day. Depending on the patient's nutritional status, these foods may be prescribed for a period of time before and after surgery.

Another variation in therapeutic diets involves the sequence in which they are used. The **refeeding diet** is used in patients who have been without **enteral feeding** for an extended period and who usually have some digestive dysfunction. The refeeding regimen is a graduated approach to the reintroduction of foods into the diet.

Enteral Feeding

Oral intake is the preferred method of nutritional support. If after 3 to 5 days oral intake is not possible, **enteral nutrition,** which is commonly referred to as tube feeding, can be initiated if the GI tract is functional. Its use is widespread in hospitals in the United States and fairly common in the nursing home and homebound settings, because the patient or caregiver can easily care for an external stoma, the cost is lower, fewer complications arise, and there is greater likelihood of maintaining GI mucosal integrity.

The selection of tubes and pumps designed specifically for feeding is quite broad. Small-gauge feeding tubes should always be used for enteral feeding, because of their pliability and long-term tolerance. Because gastric contents cannot be reliably aspirated through the soft, small-bore tubes, the need to monitor gastric retention may justify the use of standard large-bore **nasogastric** tubes in certain patients who are at risk for pulmonary aspiration.

Although soft nasogastric tubes have been used safely for months and even years in some patients, long-term tube feeding is usually best accomplished through a **percutaneous endoscopic gastrostomy (PEG).** This method of gastrostomy placement, in most cases, is preferred over surgical gastrostomies because of low morbidity and cost. A PEG tube is placed by passing an endoscope with a light source into the patient's stomach. The light is viewed through the skin and an incision is made under local anesthesia. The PEG tube is inserted directly through the incision, or directed down the esophagus and out the incision, and secured. Because the risk of pulmonary aspiration is not appreciably lower with gastrostomies than with nasogastric tubes, in patients at high risk for aspiration, duodenal intubation either through the nose or through a PEG tube is advised.

In patients who are not at high risk for aspiration (i.e., those who are alert and have a normal gag reflex), it is not necessary to confirm tube placement radiographically before beginning feeding. Insufflation of air and auscultation over the stomach and return of bile or gastric contents, followed by monitoring during the first hour of feeding, are usually adequate, and avoid delay of feeding.

Formula Selection

The choices of enteral feeding formulas have increased. Important criteria for selection of formulas include caloric density, protein content, route of administration, and cost.

Lactose-containing formulas should not be used in acutely ill patients because of the common problem of lactase deficiency. Most of the commonly used formulas for tube feeding are highly caloric and lactose free (which practically eliminates consideration of lactose content as a criterion for selection). Formulas that provide more than 20% of calories as protein are considered high in protein. Almost all hospitals have discontinued the preparation of formulas in a blender for inpatient use because of higher personnel cost, poorer quality control, and greater potential for clogging of fine-bore feeding tubes.

Tube-Feeding Methods

Continuous Feeding

Preference is given to the continuous drip method with a closed, aseptic system. A pump should always be used to avoid accidental infusions of dangerously large volumes. Continuous feeding ensures reliable nutrient delivery and reduces the risk of diarrhea, gastric distention, and pulmonary aspiration of the feeding formula.

The initial infusion rate should vary depending on the patient's overall condition. Patients with impaired mental status or prolonged lack of use of the GI tract (>2 weeks) should have feedings introduced and increased more slowly than alert patients whose intestines have been properly functioning recently.

Bolus Feeding

This method involves infusing a certain volume of formula into the feeding tube by gravity, over several minutes several times a day. It is most useful for long-term feeding in stable patients and is commonly used in homes and nursing homes. It allows mobility and reduces the cost, because a pump and infusion set are not needed.

Overall, the complications of tube feeding include diarrhea, gastric retention, hyperglycemia, dehydration, and pulmonary aspiration of gastric contents.

Parenteral Nutrition

Parental nutrition, or intravenous feeding, has been referred to as to **total parenteral nutrition (TPN)** and as **hyperalimentation (hyperal, or HA)**. It can also be described more specifically as **central venous alimentation (CVA)** or **peripheral venous alimentation (PVA)**.

With parenteral nutrition, calories are supplied by carbo-

hydrates (in the form of dextrose) and fat (in the form of vegetable-oil emulsions). Protein is supplied by crystalline amino acids. Vitamins, minerals, and trace elements are added in chemical form. Certain medications, such as insulin, can be added to the TPN solution when necessary.

Some of the indications for parenteral nutrition include: (1) a nonfunctioning GI tract due to conditions such as short bowel syndrome from trauma, infection, or infarction resulting in surgical resection; (2) conditions in which bowel rest is desirable such as inflammatory bowel disease or intestinal fistulas; (3) certain cases of severe malnutrition before surgery, and (4) certain cases of severe chemotherapy-induced nausea and vomiting. Parenteral nutrition is usually used when oral or enteral intake is inadequate to meet the patient's needs for more than 3 to 5 days.

The contraindications to parenteral nutrition are all relative; there are no situations in which a person should absolutely not be fed. Relative contraindications include the presence of a functional GI tract, intended use for less than 3 to 5 days, and a patient who will die imminently due to underlying disease. Specific exceptions to these can be cited, therefore each case should be evaluated on an individual basis.

These solutions must be infused into central veins, where they are rapidly diluted by high blood flow rates. Typically, the catheter tip is introduced into the superior vena cava via the subclavian or internal jugular vein. When central venous catheterization is undesirable or when parenteral nutrition is desired for short periods, more dilute solutions can be infused into peripheral veins.

 ## PICA

The persistent ingestion of non-food item such as cigarettes, dirt, and laundry starch is called *pica*. This practice is often exhibited in the mentally retarded or poor. Complications of pica may include interference with the absorption of certain minerals such as iron, lead poisoning, hemolytic anemia of the fetus if practiced by a pregnant women, and parasitic infections.

Suggested Sources

Davis JR, Stegeman CA: The Dental Hygienist's Guide to Nutritional Care. Philadelphia, WB Saunders, 1998.

DeBiase C: Dental Health Education: Theory and Practice. Malvern, PA, Lea & Febiger, 1991.

Ehrlich A: Nutritional and Dental Health. Albany, NY, Delmar, 1987.

Nizel A, Papas A: Nutrition in Clinical Dentistry. Philadelphia, WB Saunders, 1989.

Oral Health Care for Older Adults. Bethesda, MD, The National Oral Health Information Clearinghouse, 1998.

www.fns.usda.gov/fns.

www.usda.gov/cnpp.

Weinsier R, Moran S: Fundamentals of Clinical Nutrition. St. Louis, MO, CV Mosby, 1993.

Zambito R, Black H, et al: Hospital Dentistry Practice and Education. St. Louis, MO, CV Mosby, 1997.

Questions and Answers

Questions

1. Which of the following vitamins is essential for normal growth and function of the salivary glands?
   A. E
   B. C
   C. A
   D. K

2. Glossitis may result from all of the following except one. The exception is _____.
   A. iron.
   B. folic acid.
   C. niacin.
   D. zinc.

3. Intrinsic factor is necessary for the absorption of _____.
   A. B_1.
   B. B_2.
   C. B_3.
   D. B_6.
   E. B_{12}.

4. Glucose is stored in the liver as _____.
   A. iron.
   B. glycogen.
   C. cellulose.
   D. galactose.

5. Which of the following vitamins are recommended to prevent spina bifida and other neural tube defects?
   A. A
   B. K
   C. Pantothenic acid
   D. Folic acid

6. All of the following herbs and supplements are contraindicated when taking anticoagulants EXCEPT one. The exception is _____.
   A. gingko biloba.
   B. echinacea.
   C. dong quai.
   D. garlic.

7. Which of the following types of fiber may be helpful in reducing serum cholesterol?
   A. Insoluble
   B. Soluble
   C. Incomplete
   D. Complete

8. Which of the following conditions results when there are not enough carbohydrates in the diet to completely burn fats?
   A. Ketosis
   B. Acidosis
   C. Glycogenesis
   D. Lipogenesis

9. Linoleic and arachidonic essential fatty acids are considered the precursors for the development of which of the following compounds?
   A. Phospholipids
   B. Lipoproteins
   C. Triglycerides
   D. Cholesterol
   E. Prostaglandins

10. Dried apricots and prunes are good sources of _____.
    A. iron.
    B. zinc.
    C. phosphorus.
    D. magnesium.

11. A patient with bulimia should be instructed to do which of the following immediately after a vomiting episode?
    A. Brush teeth thoroughly.
    B. Rinse with a commercial mouth rinse.
    C. Rinse with a baking soda solution.
    D. Apply topical fluoride to the teeth with a cotton swab.

12. Postmenopausal women have a tendency to develop signs and symptoms of osteoporosis. Recommended preventive measures for osteoporosis include exercise, calcium supplementation, and estrogen replacement therapy.
    A. Statement one is true; statements two is false.
    B. Statement one is false; statement two is true.
    C. Both statements are true.
    D. Both statements are false.

13. Which of the following foods would be included in a full liquid diet?
    A. Chunky applesauce
    B. Plain yogurt
    C. Dried cereal softened in milk
    D. Mashed banana

14. One gram of fat contains _____ calories.
    A. three.
    B. four.
    C. seven.
    D. nine.

15. Which of the following vitamins contributes to the formation of hemoglobin on red blood cells and infection-fighting antibodies?
    A. B_6
    B. B_{12}
    C. C
    D. D

16. Which of the following minerals, found in nuts, tea, and instant coffee, is a trace element that is needed for functioning of the central nervous system?
    A. Phosphorus
    B. Manganese
    C. Magnesium
    D. Iodine

17. How many servings are recommended daily for foods listed at the tip of the Food Pyramid (fats, oils, and sweets)?
    A. None
    B. One
    C. Two
    D. Three

18. Which of the following digestive juices contains hydrochloric acid?
    A. Intestinal
    B. Pancreatic
    C. Gastric
    D. Hepatic

19. Which of the following terms refers to the chemical change that determines the final use of individual nutrients by the body?
    A. Absorption
    B. Digestion
    C. Metabolism
    D. Insalivation

20. Preeclampsia is characterized by all of the following signs except one. The exception is _____.
    A. hypertension.
    B. convulsions.
    C. edema.
    D. protein in the urine.

ANSWERS

1. **C.** Vitamin A is essential for growth and development of teeth, bones, salivary glands, and oral soft tissues.

2. **D.** Iron, folic acid, and niacin deficiencies all result in glossitis.

3. **E.** People who lack gastric intrinsic factor can only absorb B_{12} by injections that bypass the stomach.

4. **B.** If energy is not needed by the body, it is stored in the liver and muscles as glycogen.

5. **D.** Research indicates that a deficiency in folic acid during pregnancy may contribute to neural defects such as spina bifida (the spinal cord is not properly encased in bone) and anencephaly (part of the brain does not develop).

6. **B.** Echinacea is purported to boost the immune system to avert colds and flu.

7. **B.** Insoluble fiber is found primarily in whole grains and wheat bran. It provides roughage, which enhances elimination and may help to protect against colon cancer.

8. **B.** Carbohydrates are needed to burn fat completely. Acidosis results when there is insufficient dietary carbohydrate to completely burn the fat. Ketosis is a clinical condition characterized by fruity acetone breath and occurs in the absence of carbohydrates. Excessive breakdown of tissue protein, loss of sodium, and involuntary dehydration are consequences of this condition.

9. **E.** Lipoproteins consist of cholesterol, triglycerides, and phospholipids.

10. **A.** Iron is one of the few nutrients found in dried fruits.

11. **C.** By toothbrushing or exposing the teeth to acid (fluoride or mouthrinse) after a vomiting episode, further enamel breakdown will occur.

12. **C.** Menopause marks the onset of an acute change in the calcium balance, and rapid bone loss may result. Preventive measures can be very successful in averting osteoporosis if these measures are initiated early in life.

13. **B.** Plain yogurt is the only food mentioned that is liquid at room temperature.

14. **D.** One gram of protein or carbohydrate equals 4 calories. One gram of alcohol is equal to 7 calories.

15. **A.** Vitamin B_6 contributes to the formation of erythrocytes and plasma cells.

16. **B.** Manganese is the only mineral found in the food sources listed. Manganese is found uniquely in instant coffee.

17. **A.** No servings are listed for fats, oils, and sweets, which should be used sparingly.

18. **C.** Pancreatic juice contains trypsin, lipase, and amylase. Intestinal juice contains the enzymes peptidases, sucrase, maltase, and lactase.

19. **C.** Digestion is the process of breaking down food into nutrients. Absorption is the process of moving these nutrients into the bloodstream where they can be utilized by the body. The process of mixing food with saliva is called insalivation.

20. **B.** Convulsions are characteristic of eclampsia.

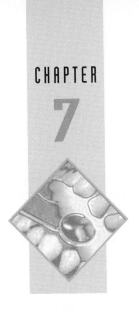

CHAPTER

7

Microbiology and Immunology

JOHN G. THOMAS, MS, PhD   CHRISTINA B. DeBIASE, BSDH, MA, EdD

More bacterial cells exist in the human body than the total number of human cells. In the mouth, this is exemplified by tremendous microbial diversity. It is estimated that there are at least 500 species, and only approximately half of these species have been identified. The relationship of organisms to the environment of the oral cavity should be discussed as an oral ecosystem, where factors and variations in location contribute to the environment and create unique niches.

Today, it is recognized that the germ theory has evolved to the community theory. The **germ theory,** amplified and organized by Koch (known as Koch's postulates), emphasized the importance of a single organism as a significant pathogen. The Centers for Disease Control and Prevention (CDC) state that >80% of infections identified in hospitalized patients are due to an imbalance in the ecosystem, which is caused by contributions from several organisms. This concept is referred to as the **community theory**.

With the evolution and clarification of the impact of ecosystems and their influence on **pathogenicity,** terminology has expanded. The language of the microbiologist has changed considerably but reflects the understanding of the ecosystems and the specific interrelationship of multiple organisms **(polymicrobes)** with the environment **(Table 7-1)**. In fact, the **ecosystem** is a multispecies consortia that has established architecture, methods of communication, and responses to environmental stress that are coordinated for the purpose of survival. **Biodiversity** provides a means of survival.

NORMAL MICROBIAL FLORA (ECOSYSTEM) AND BACTERIAL LOAD OR BIOBURDEN

Microorganisms that are usually noninvasive and harmless to the host and that normally reside in various locations in the body are referred to as the **normal flora (Table 7-2)**.

The type and numbers vary in different locations, depending on the host's age, diet, and factors such as temperature and acidity. These organisms help to prevent invasion, **colonization,** and infection by pathogenic microorganisms. Some of the normal flora help to synthesize vitamin K, aid in absorption of certain nutrients, and help to convert bile pigments and acids in the intestine. Although harmless in their usual sites, they may produce disease if introduced into other areas of the body. Such organisms are referred to as **opportunistic pathogens**.

Microbial Ecosystem of the Human Body

As defined in **Table 7-3**, there are four natural, microbial reservoirs of the human body or **biofilms** that make up the human ecosystem. This ecosystem is predominantly anaerobic and consists of >500 distinct, diverse, heterogeneous symbiotic microbes. The reservoirs are not compartmentalized or separated from each other but rather represent a continuum of each biofilm in its entirety-all with a common ancestry.

The development of the ecosystem defines its heterogeneity and complexity. Within hours of birth, oral, vaginal, gut, and skin flora are established as a complex microbial, heterogeneous ecosystem (with architectural structure) that becomes more complex with further acquisition of species and development of colonies during the first two decades of life. Because these four anatomic reservoirs are essentially sterile at birth, microbial colonization is acquired from the environment, formula, or caregiver and brings with it the existing characteristics of those organisms (e.g., resistance to antibiotics).

Table 7-4 compares the overall gram-positive and gram-negative facultative anaerobic and aerobic flora of the four reservoirs or ecosystems, emphasizing similarities and the common ancestry of the bacterial communities. The organisms listed also reflect those recently associated with periodontal disease and gingivitis.

TABLE 7-1 Key Definitions and Vocabulary

Colonization: The establishment of bacteria in a living host
Opportunistic pathogens: Microorganisms that gain access to a normally sterile area of the body and produce disease
Infectious disease: Organisms producing damage to the host with manifestation of clinical signs and symptoms
Pathogenicity: The capacity of organisms to produce disease
Virulence: The degree of pathogenicity

Biofilms

Biofilms have been known to exist in nature for some time, but their significance in human infections and the ecology have been misunderstood for the most part. Now it is recognized that biofilms represent the standard organization of microbes and that 99% of microbial communities exist as biofilms both in nature and in the ecosystem of humans. In fact, it is the exception for an organism to exist alone. In the broadest sense, **biofilms exist in nature, industry, and medicine at interphase boundaries and proliferate at these positions**. The preferred site for biofilm formation is a liquid-solid junction. In the strictest sense, as emphasized in periodontal disease, the biofilm is an intimate association of organisms on a solid substrate that is maximized through binding and inclusion within a polymer matrix.

The architecture of the biofilm contains **domains** that give rise to a mosaic of microenvironments or an ecologic homeostasis. Diseases that exist in biofilm communities are diseases of imbalance or ecologic shifts within these domains and can be defined as community behavior based on stress, antibiotics, and so forth (**Figure 7-1**).

BASIC MICROBIOLOGY

Classification

The purpose of classifying organisms is to arrange organisms with similar characteristics into groups, establish criteria for identification, determine evolutionary relationships, and minimize confusion in communication.

The **linnean system of classification** subdivides organisms into a hierarchy of nonoverlapping, successively smaller groups with increasingly more precise characteristics. The hierarchy as applied to bacteria includes:

Kingdom
  Phylum (in zoology) of division (in botany and bacteriology)
    Class
      Order
        Family
          Genus
            Species
              Strain, type, etc. (often indicated by letters, numbers, geographic names, etc.

Types of Cells

All cells can be divided into two broad types: eukaryotic cells and prokaryotic cells. The term **eukaryotic** means having a true nucleus; that is, a nucleus surrounded by a membrane. In contrast, **prokaryotic** cells have no nucleus. The terms eukaryotic and prokaryotic, which are used in this way without capital letters, are descriptive terms and are not official names of groups. In contrast, when these words are capitalized, they are currently the accepted names of a kingdom.

The **eukaryotes (i.e., fungi, protozoa, and algae)** contain a nucleus surrounded by a nuclear membrane. Their genetic material consists of multiple chromosomes with histones. **Histones** are proteins attached to the DNA of eukaryotes; these histones allow the DNA to be packaged into chromosomes. A mitotic apparatus exists to ensure equal distribution of the products of chromosomal replication to the two daughter cells. They contain numerous membrane-bound organelles in the cytoplasm (e.g., mitochondria, endoplasmic reticulum, lysosomes). **Eukaryotes include both animal and plant cells.**

Prokaryotes (bacterial cells) contain a primitive nucleus. Nuclear (genetic) material is present in a nuclear area, but the nuclear material is not enclosed in a membrane. The nuclear material consists of a single, circular chromosome that has no histones associated with it. No mitotic spindles are apparent in the nuclear area during cell division. No membrane-bound intracellular structures (e.g., mitochondria, endoplasmic reticulum, lysosomes) are found. Plant cells, fungi, algae, and most bacteria have a rigid cell wall, whereas animal cells do not. Plant cell walls contain cellulose, whereas the walls of bacterial cells contain peptidoglycan as a distinctive component. This kingdom does not include fungi, algae, protozoa, or viruses. **Viruses are considered to be acellular; they consist of protein and nucleic acid (Table 7-5).**

Structures of Bacterial Cells

The basic shapes and arrangements of bacterial cells include three types: (1) cocci, (2) rods, and (3) spirals .

Structure = function = survivability

BACTERIAL FORMS WITH CELL WALLS

The most external limiting structure of all bacteria is the **cell wall** (except the mycoplasma and L forms of bacteria that have no cell wall). The cell wall functions by:

- **Protecting the cell from a number of noxious substances.** The cell is relatively porous and does not restrict the flow of small molecules to and from the cytoplasmic

TABLE 7–2 Normal Flora by Anatomic Site

I. NORMAL FLORA OF THE MOUTH
  A. AT BIRTH
     Flora corresponds to organisms in the mother's vagina
     (usually a mixture of micrococci, streptococci, coliforms, and
     Lactobacillus acidophilus)
  B. AFTER THE NEWBORN PERIOD
     1. α-Hemolytic streptococci (*viridans* group)
     2. *Neisseria catarrhalis*
     3. *Staphylococcus epidermidis*
     4. *Haemophilus hemolyticus*
     5. *Streptococcus pneumoniae*
     6. Nonhemolytic streptococci
     7. Diphtheroids
     8. Coliforms
     9. β-Hemolytic streptococci other than group A
     10. Micrococci
     11. *Veillonella*
     12. Treponemas
     13. *Fusobacterium*
     14. *Actinomyces israelii*
     15. Yeasts (*Candida albicans, Geotrichum*)
     16. *Leptotrichia buccalis*
     17. *Eikenella corrodens*
  C. GUMS, TOOTH POCKETS, AND TONSILLAR CRYPTS
     (Anaerobic flora)
     1. Anaerobic micrococci
     2. Anaerobic streptococci
     3. *Vibrios*
     4. *Fusobacterium*
     5. Spirochetes (*Treponema microdentium*)
II. NORMAL FLORA OF RESPIRATORY TRACT
  A. NASAL PASSAGES
     1. Diphtheroids
     2. *Staphylococcus epidermidis*
     3. *Staphylococcus aureus* (20–80% of population)
     4. *Streptococcus pneumoniae* (5–15% of population)
     5. *Haemophilus influenzae* (5–210% of population)
     6. *Neisseria* sp (0–15% of population)
     7. *Neisseria meningitidis* (0–4% of population)
     8. Streptococci
  B. NASOPHARYNX (Sterile at birth)
     1. Streptococci (*viridans* group)
     2. Nonhemolytic streptococci
     3. *Neisseria* sp (90–100%)
     4. Staphylococci (few)
     5. *Haemophilus influenzae* (40–80% of the population)
     6. *Streptococcus pneumoniae* (20–40% of the population)
     7. β-Hemolytic streptococci (5–15% of the population)
     8. *Neisseria meningitidis* (5–20% of the population)
     9. *Haemophilus parainfluenzae*
     10. *Pseudomonas aeruginosa*
     11. *Escherichia coli*
     12. *Proteus* sp
     13. Paracolons
     14. Diphtheroids
     15. *Mycoplasma pneumoniae*
     16. *Bacteriodes*
  C. TRACHEA, BRONCHI, LUNGS, AND SINUSES:
     (Normally sterile)
III. NORMAL FLORA OF THE GASTROINTESTINAL TRACT
  A. ESOPHAGUS
     Microorganisms from the mouth, pharynx, and ingested food
  B. STOMACH

  1. Minimal numbers (10^3–10^5 bacteria/Gm. of contents)
  2. In obstruction with food retention, characteristic flora
     includes: *Sarcina*, yeasts, and *Lactobacillus acidophilus*
  3. With hypoacidity and carcinoma, *Sarcina* proliferates
  C. DUODENUM
     1. Minimal numbers (10^3–10^5 bacteria/Gm.)
     2. Gallbladder infection may expel organisms into the
        duodenum
  D. JEJUNUM AND UPPER ILEUM: very few organisms
     1. Lactobacilli
     2. Enterococci
  E. LOWER ILEUM: (10^8–10^{10} bacteria/Gm.)
     1. Streptococci (*viridans* group)
     2. *Streptococcus faecalis* (*enterococcus*)
     3. Staphylococci
     4. Lactobacilli
     5. *Clostridium perfringens*
     6. *Veillonella*
     7. *Escherichia coli* (occasionally)
  F. LARGE INTESTINE: (10^{11}–10^{12}) bacteria/Gm. of contents)
     1. *Bacteroides*
     2. Diphtheroids
     3. Coliforms (*Escherichia coli, Enterobacter aerogenes,
        Klebsiella*)
     4. Enterococci
     5. *Staphylococci* (coagulase-positive and coagulase-negative)
     6. *Lactobacillus* (*acidophilus* and *brevis*)
     7. Spirochetes
     8. Yeasts (*Candida, Geotrichum, Cryptococcus, Penicillium,
        Aspergillus*)
     9. *Proteus*
     10. *Pseudomonas*
     11. *Bacillus subtilis*
     12. *Actinomyces*
     13. *Borrelia*
     14. *Fusobacterium*
     15. *Clostridium* sp
  G. INTESTINAL FLORA OF BREAST-FED INFANTS
     1. *Lactobacillus bifidus* (*Bifidobacterium*)
     2. Enterococci and coliforms (few)
     3. Staphylococci (few)
  H. INTESTINAL FLORA OF BOTTLE-FED INFANTS
     1. *Lactobacillus acidophilus*
     2. Coliforms
     3. Enterococci
     4. *Bacillus* sp
     5. *Clostridium* sp
  I. MECONIUM: Usually sterile
IV. FLORA OF NORMAL VOIDED URINE
   Usually sterile of <1000 colonies/ml. The following organisms
   are most often found in normal urine and are probably
   "contaminants" from the urethra and adjacent areas.
   1. *Staphylococcus epidermidis*
   2. Diphtheroids
   3. Coliforms
   4. Enterococci
   5. *Proteus* sp
   6. Lactobacilli
   7. Streptococci (α- and β-hemolytic)
   8. Yeasts
   9. *Bacillus* sp
   (depends on age, glycogen content, pH, enzymes)

(Continued)

TABLE 7–2 Normal Flora by Anatomic Site (Continued)

A. NEWBORN: Sterile
B. 24 HOURS to 3 DAYS
    1. Staphylococci
    2. Enterococci
    3. Diphtheroids
    4. *Mycobacterium smegmatis*
C. 3 DAYS TO A FEW WEEKS
    1. *Lactobacillus acidophilus* (Doderlein bacillus)
D. PREPUBERTAL
    1. Micrococci
    2. Streptococci (α-hemolytic and nonhemolytic)
    3. Coliforms
    4. Diphtheroids
E. ADULT
    1. *Lactobacillus acidophilus*
    2. *Staphylococcus epidermidis*
    3. Streptococci (α-hemolytic and nonhemolytic)
    4. *Escherichia coli*
    5. Diphtheroids
    6. Yeasts
    7. Anaerobic streptococci
    8. *Listeria* sp
    9. *Clostridium* sp
F. PREGNANCY: Increased numbers of:
    1. *Staphylococcus epidermidis*
    2. Lactobacilli
    3. Yeasts
G. POSTMENOPAUSAL
    1. Similar to prepubertal flora
V. NORMAL FLORA OF THE SKIN
    A. *Staphylococcus epidermidis*
    B. *Staphylococcus aureus*
    C. *Sarcina*
    D. Coliforms
    E. *Proteus*
    F. Diphtheroids
    G. *Bacillus subtilis*
    H. Mycobacteria (external auditory canal, genital and axillary regions)

    I. *Candida albicans*
    J. Cryptococci
    K. Streptococci (*viridans* group)
    L. Enterococci
    M. Mima
VI. NORMAL FLORA OF THE EYE
    A. *Corynebacterium xerosis* (diphtheroids)
    B. *Staphylococcus epidermidis*
    C. *Sarcina*
    D. Saprophytic fungi
    E. *Neisseria* sp
    F. *Moraxella* sp
    G. Nonhemolytic streptococci
VII. NORMAL FLORA OF THE EAR
    A. *Staphylococcus epidermidis*
    B. Diphtheroids
    C. *Gaffkya tetragena (peptococci)*
    D. *Bacillus* sp
    E. Saprophytic fungi
VIII. NORMAL FLORA OF THE URETHRA
    A. MALES
        1. *Staphylococcus epidermidis*
        2. Diphtheroids
        3. *Mycoplasma* sp
    B. FEMALES (Usually sterile)
        1. Few nonpathogenic gram-positive cocci
        2. *Mycoplasma* sp
IX. NORMAL FLORA OF SMEGMA
    A. *Mycobacterium smegmatis*
X. NORMAL FLORA OF CERVIX
    A. Usually sterile or contains microorganisms similar to those in the upper vagina
XI. NORMAL FLORA OF SPINAL FLUID
    A. Sterile
XII. NORMAL FLORA OF BLOOD AND TISSUES
    A. Sterile or only transients

membrane beneath. Larger molecules, which include some enzymes, are not allowed to pass. Because of this restriction, some enzymes that are secreted by the bacterial cell accumulate within the matrix of the cell wall.

- **Maintaining rigidity, thus giving the bacterium its characteristic shape.**
- **Protecting the cell from osmotic lysis.**
  Cytoplasm contains a high concentration of salts and nutrients. The high concentration of dissolved solids makes the internal osmotic pressure equal to 5 to 20 atmospheres (atm). A high internal osmotic pressure would tend to make water enter the cell in amounts large enough to burst the cell. The cell wall provides mechanical containment for the cytoplasmic membrane and its contents and thus prevents lysis (i.e., bursting). **The cell wall IS NOT the osmotic barrier,** because the cell wall does not restrict diffusion of the solute (i.e., material dissolved in the solvent) into and out of the cell; **the cytoplasmic membrane is the osmotic barrier.**

- **Carrying antigens that participate in protective immunity**.
- **Serving an essential role in cell division**.
- **Acting as a primer for its own biosynthesis**. New peptidoglycan is added to the old structure; however, without some peptidoglycan present to which the new structure can be added, the new cell wall either cannot be made or is made with difficulty.
- **Protecting the cell from detrimental enzymes such as lysozymes and from various potentially toxic chemicals including disinfectants and antibiotics.** The high lipid content of the outer layer of gram-negative and acid-fast cell walls is especially effective in performing this protective mechanism. The outer layer of gram-negative cell walls contains a toxic **lipopolysaccharide (LPS)** called **endotoxin.**

The **cytoplasmic membrane** contributes 2% to 40% of the dry weight of the cell. The chemical composition of pep-

TABLE 7–3 Origin of the Microbial Human Ecosystem and the Four Biofilm Reservoirs

MICROBIAL RESERVOIRS/ ECOSYSTEMS	"BIOBURDEN" OR COLONY-FORMING UNITS	SOURCE	AEROBE TO ANAEROBE RATIO	ORIGIN
GI	$1 \times 10^{11-12}$	Stool	1:1000	Formula-fed/caregiver
GU	$1 \times 10^{8-9}$	Invagination	1:100	Environmental
Mouth	2×10^{11}	Crypt	1:10	Vaginal/caregiver
Skin	$1 \times 10^{4-6}$	Sweat gland	1:10	Vaginal

GI, gastrointestinal; GU, genitourinary.

tidoglycan in the cell wall is unique to bacteria. **Peptidoglycan** is a single, giant, bag-shaped polymer that covers the entire bacterium and is found only in bacteria. It is found in almost all bacteria, including both gram-positive and gram-negative bacteria. All pathogenic bacteria that have a cell wall have peptidoglycan in the cell wall. Peptidoglycan is made up of three linking parts: (1) a backbone, (2) a tetrapeptide side chain, and (3) a peptide bridge. This link in bacteria is hydrolyzed by **lysozyme**, which is an enzyme found in tears, white blood cells, and egg white. Lysozyme functions in white blood cells and tears as part of the normal host defense mechanism to help control bacteria.

The cell walls of **gram-positive bacteria** are dense; they are more or less uniform; and they look like a single layer under the electron microscope. The thickness in different bacteria ranges from 20 to 80 nanometers (nm). As many as 40 layers of peptidoglycan occur. Up to 80% of the cell wall is peptidoglycan; the remainder is mainly teichoic acid. **Teichoic acid**, which is one of the major surface antigens in some gram-positive bacteria, functions by acting as a receptor for the attachment of some bacteriophages (bacterial

viruses), binding magnesium ion and supplying that ion to the cell, and by promoting cell stability and reproduction. Some teichoic acids vary with changes in nutrients in the environment. Not many other structural components vary with the environment. Variation may have an important role in stability or pathogenesis.

Cell walls of **gram-negative bacteria** appear bilayered by electronic microscopy. The thickness in different bacteria ranges from 10 to 30 nm. The four identifiable layers that tend to overlap (starting from the interior) are: peptidoglycan, lipoprotein, outer membrane, and LPS. **Peptidoglycan** is comparable in structure and composition to peptidoglycan in gram-positive bacteria. With fewer cross-links than gram-positive peptidoglycan, this peptidoglycan more closely resembles a gel.

The **outer membrane** is a phospholipid bilayer that helps to contain enzymes and other solutes in the gel. It restricts diffusion of lipophilic compounds, including many antibiotics, disinfectants, and detergents. It also restricts diffusion of enzymes such as lysozyme and thus protects the peptidoglycan by making gram-negative bacteria more resistant to

TABLE 7–4 Anatomic Distribution of Common Flora for Four Reservoirs/Ecosystems

ORGANISMS	MICROBIAL RESERVOIRS OR ECOSYSTEMS			
	GI	GU	SKIN	MOUTH
Streptococcus salivarius	+	0	+	+++
S. sanguis	+	0	0	++
S. mitis	+	0	0	++
S. milleri	+	0	0	++
S. mutans	++	+	+	++
Lactobacillus sp	+++	++	+	++
Actinomyces sp	+	+	0	+++
Fusobacterium sp	++	++	0	+++
Capnocytophaga	++	++	0	++
Treponema sp	+	+	0	++
Prevotella melaninogenica	++	+	+	0
Porphyromonas gingivalis	++	+	0	0
Actinobacillus actinomycetemcomitans	+	0	0	+
Veillonella	++	+	+	+

This table compares the overall gram-positive and gram-negative facultative anaerobic and aerobic flora of the four reservoirs or ecosystems, emphasizing similarities and common ancestry of the bacterial communities. The organisms listed also reflect those recently associated with periodontal disease and gingivitis.
GI, gastrointestinal; GU, genitourinary.

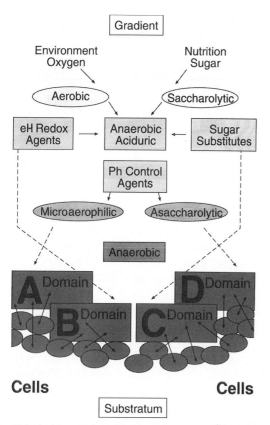

Figure 7-1. Architectural organization of plaque biofilm influenced by the gradient of four selected pressures: O_2, carbohydrate source, pH, and eH.

The lipid portion of the LPS is embedded in the outer leaflet of the outer membrane so that the polysaccharide portion extends into the extracellular space. The LPS consists of three portions: lipid A (central structure), core (branched polysaccharide made on a chain of seven units), and terminal repeat units (repeating series of sugars that are repeated up to 25 times). Every gram-negative bacterium contains a highly toxic component called endotoxin. The endotoxin is identical to LPS. When LPS is hydrolyzed into lipid A and polysaccharide, toxicity is associated with lipid A. The relative toxicity of LPS from different bacteria varies, but all are toxic and all have the same types of biologic activities. **O antigen** is the major surface antigen of gram-negative bacteria. This antigen is located in the terminal repeat units of the LPS. The variation of polysaccharides makes numerous specificities possible. For example, >1000 antigenic types of the genus *Salmonella* have been described. O antigen provides protective immunity in this species.

Cytoplasmic Membrane

The **cytoplasmic membrane** is also referred to as the **protoplasmic membrane** or **plasma membrane** and is located just beneath the cell wall. It is similar in structure and function to all biologic membranes in cells of all kingdoms. The presence of hydrophobic and hydrophilic ends on the phospholipids causes them to orient themselves into a fluid membrane in which the various proteins embedded in the membrane are free to move around. This creates an **osmotic barrier,** thus allowing the passage of water through a semipermeable membrane that restricts passage of solute. Water tends to move from a lower to a higher concentration of solute. Because the concentration of dissolved materials inside bacteria is generally higher than the concentration outside, water tends to enter bacteria from most aqueous environments. The entrance of water into the bacterial cell by osmosis is held at equilibrium because of the corset effect of the cell wall.

Capsule

Capsules are viscous accumulations of polymers outside the cell wall that form a distinct layer of seemingly unstructured material. A capsule functions by:

injurious agents than gram-positive bacteria. Some of the major proteins of the outer membrane are called porins. **Porins** form relatively nonspecific pores that permit free diffusion of small hydrophilic molecules up to a molecular weight of 600. Minor proteins of the outer membrane function in specific transport of small molecules (e.g., vitamin B_{12}) in a manner similar to that of the carrier transport systems of the cytoplasmic (inner) membrane.

Lipoprotein cross-links the peptidoglycan to the outer membrane and is inserted noncovalently into the outer membrane. The lipoprotein is held there by lipophilic attraction to both lipid and protein and by divalent metal cations such as magnesium and binds the outer membrane to the cell wall. Free lipoprotein occurs within the outer membrane in approximately twice the concentration as the bound form.

TABLE 7–5 Comparison of Eukaryotes and Prokaryotes

CHARACTERISTIC	EUKARYOTES	PROKARYOTES
Membrane-bound	Yes	No
Mitotic spindles	Yes	No
Membrane-bound	Yes	No
Contain sterols	Yes (cholesterol in animals, ergosterol in plants)	Only in mycoplasma
Rigid cell wall	Yes in plants, fungi, and algae	Most do
	Not in animals	
Peptidoglycan in the cell wall	No	Most bacteria do

1. Acting as a virulence factor that contributes to the invasiveness of the bacterium
2. Protecting bacteria from engulfment (i.e., by phagocytosis) by scavenger phagocytic cells
3. Developing the protective immunity that can be attributed to capsular antigens

Glycocalyx

Glycocalyx is a loose mesh network of polysaccharide fibrils that enclose the cell and appear to extend from the cell surface into the extracellular space. It functions by allowing bacteria to adhere to surfaces. In order for a bacterium to infect an animal or plant, it must first adhere to the cells of that animal or plant. *Streptococcus mutans* uses the glycocalyx to adhere to tooth enamel, where it converts sucrose to acidic products that cause dental caries. This binding action is specific, because these bacteria adhere poorly to cells of the gingiva or tongue.

Flagella

Flagella are hair-like appendages that extend from the cell surface. They have a helical structure, and the wavelength is a genetic characteristic of the genus. Bacteria may have none, one, some, or several hundred flagella per cell; the number and location are characteristic of the genus. They originate from a hooked organelle in a basal body in the cytoplasmic membrane. Because the diameter of 12 to 20 nm is smaller than the light microscope can detect, flagella are not visible in routinely stained smears of bacteria. Flagella function as an organ of locomotion or motility. Motile bacteria have flagella; nonmotile bacteria do not. The flagella rotate and drive the bacteria through a liquid medium in a direction determined by the direction of rotation. The direction changes from time to time and is partially dependent on the environment. Motile bacteria exhibit chemotaxis. In **chemotaxis**, bacteria move toward a chemical attractant such as a nutrient or away from a chemical repellent such as a disinfectant. Flagella consist of protein subunits called **flagellin**. Bacteria synthesize the subunits, which aggregate spontaneously to form the flagella. If flagella are removed mechanically from bacteria, new flagella are made and motility is restored in minutes. Flagella contribute modestly to virulence but are not essential for growth or virulence. Some bacteria never have flagella. Nonmotile mutants of bacteria that usually have flagella still survive and cause disease, but some are slightly less capable of inducing disease than are their flagellated counterparts. Flagella are antigenic and stimulate the immune system. Some contribute modestly to protective immunity. Antigenic specificity varies even within a species.

Pili

Also called **fimbriae** or **microfibrils, pili** are filamentous appendages that extend from the foreface of bacteria. Pili

TABLE 7–6 Classification of Bacteria by Morphotype

1. **Morphology (Shape) and Arrangement (Grouping)**
   a. As exhibited by the predominant population but not necessarily by every individual in that population
   b. Three morphologic types observed
      Cocci
      Generally spherical or approaching spherical
      Grouping of cells is determined partly by the orientation of the plane of cell division and partly whether cells adhere after division has occurred
      Types of cocci (terms are descriptive and not official names)
         Diplococci
            Typically occur in pairs
            Vertical plane of division
            Pairs of cells separate after division
         Streptococci
            Typically in chains
            Vertical plane of division
            Cells tend to adhere after division
         Tetrads
            Typically in packets of four
            Vertical and horizontal plane of division
         Sarcinae
            Typically in packets of eight
            Plane of division vertical, horizontal, and in the plane of the paper
         Staphylococci
            Typically in grape-like clusters
            Random planes of division
      Rods
      Casually referred to as bacilli (singular, bacillus)
      May be large or small, long or short
      Spirals
      May be long or short, fat or thin, flexible or rigid, tightly coiled or loosely coiled, many or few turns

are shorter, thinner, and straighter than flagella and are visible only by electron microscopy. They are common in gram-negative bacteria but also occur in a few genera of gram-positive bacteria. They originate in the cytoplasmic membrane and do not contribute to motility. Pili consist of protein subunits called **pilin**. When removed mechanically, pili are regenerated. The pili allow the organism to adhere to cells that line an anatomic structure. Binding of pili to host cells can be prevented by antibodies produced by an immune response to the pili antigens. From 100 to 200 pili are evenly distributed over the cell surface.

Nuclear Material

Nuclear material consists of **DNA** that contains the genome (i.e., genetic information) of the organism. Attachment of the DNA to the cytoplasmic membrane ensures that one DNA molecule is included in each new cell during division. The DNA is not distributed throughout the cytoplasm of the cell but is concentrated in a nuclear area. Only a thin fibrillar network of DNA is demonstrable by electron microscopy.

Ribosomes

Ribosomes are the site of protein synthesis similar to that found in eukaryotic cells. Bacterial ribosomes contain 30% protein and 70% **ribonucleic acid (RNA)**. That accounts for 40% of the protein and 90% of the RNA in the cell and means that many ribosomes are present in a bacterial cell. This fact is confirmed by electron microscopy. Whole bacterial cells stain intensely with basic dyes such as crystal violet and safranin O due to the number of ribosomes present and their acidic nature. DNA is also acidic but is present in smaller quantities than RNA.

Inclusions

Some bacteria store materials such as sulfur, lipid, glycogen, and starch in their cytoplasm. Poly-β-hydroxybutyric acid, a lipid-like compound, is a common storage material. Polymers of metaphosphate also occur in the cytoplasm of some bacteria. These molecules are used as a source of phosphate for formation of the high-energy molecule adenosine triphosphate (**ATP**). These molecules are also called **volutin granules**. Stored materials may represent either nutrient or waste materials. Chemical content of stored material is typical of a genus or species.

Endospores

Endospores (or simply **spores**) are a differentiated form of bacteria that resist heat, drying, toxic chemicals, and irradiation. Endospores are a resting form of bacteria. No metabolic activity occurs while the bacteria exist as spores. Endospores are designed for long-term survival in injurious or sparse conditions. All members of that family are gram-positive.

BACTERIAL FORMS WITHOUT CELL WALLS

Protoplasts and **spheroplasts** are variants of wall-defective bacteria that are produced artificially in the laboratory. Protoplasts result from treatment of gram-positive bacteria, and no recognizable cell wall remains. Spheroplasts result from treatment of gram-negative bacteria. At least the outer membrane and LPS remain. **L forms** or **L phase variants** are wall-defective variants of typical bacteria and are identified and differentiated from protoplasts and spheroplasts by their ability to replicate in a laboratory medium. **Mycoplasma** is a type of bacterium that never has a cell wall or any cell wall components and never originates from or reverts to a conventional bacterial form. These bacteria are always resistant to penicillin but are often susceptible to antibiotics that function by methods other than inhibition of cell wall synthesis. In humans, *Mycoplasma pneumoniae* is one cause of pneumonia and is similar to gonorrhea; other species of *Mycoplasma* are often found in the mouth and urogenital tract of healthy humans but are rarely associated with disease.

BACTERIAL GROWTH

It is important to recognize that the same nutrient and physical requirements are similar for all living species, including humans. However, the molecular form of these requirements may vary greatly among different bacteria or between bacteria and humans. For example, whereas some bacteria synthesize all of their own amino acids and vitamins from carbon dioxide and ammonia, humans require many of their nutrients to be preformed. On the other hand, both bacteria and humans need the same vitamins and amino acids to survive.

Bacteria are more diverse in their metabolic preferences and capabilities than are humans. Because of that diversity, they play an important role in maintaining the ecology of the various reservoirs in humans. Generally, requirements for survival are defined by nutritional and physical conditions. These requirements are outlined in **Tables 7-7 and 7-8**.

Uptake of Nutrients

Nutrients are supplied from extracellular sources to be used by the cell. The nutrients must pass through the cytoplasmic membrane into the cell. Large molecules such as proteins or polysaccharides must be at least partially hydrolyzed before they can be used by the cell. Hydrolytic enzymes must be available to cleave the molecules outside the membrane. Nutrients do not cross the cell membrane freely. They are often present in higher concentrations inside rather than outside the cell and may enter the cell against such a concentration. Transport across the cell membrane is an active process; it does not result from simple diffusion.

Growth Rate

Binary fission results in successive doubling of the population. **Generation time** is the statistic often used to express rate of growth; that is, time for an average cell to divide and also time for the population to double. It is influenced by cultural conditions and varies among species. Generally, the term **reproduction** is used to indicate an increase in cell numbers, whereas the term **growth** is used to indicate an increase in cell mass, which might include an increase in cell number or cell size.

Growth Curve

Growth curve is a signature of population dynamics. It consists of the following: (1) **lag phase**, (2) **logarithmic (exponential) phase**, (3) **stationary phase**, and (4) **death phase**. The **lag phase** consists of active synthesis of enzymes and cellular components, and cells divide at the end of this phase. **In the logarithmic (exponential) phase** (almost a

TABLE 7–7 Nutritional Requirements of Bacteria

Energy	Phototrophs: use radiant energy (light)
	Chemotrophs: oxidize chemical compounds
Carbon	Autotrophs: require only CO_2 as a carbon source
	Simple requirements; complex synthetic mechanisms
	Photoautotrophs acquire energy from light
	Chemoautrophs acquire energy from oxidation of chemical compounds
	Heterotrophs
	Require organic compounds as a carbon source
	Include the disease-producing bacteria
Nitrogen sources	Atmospheric-nitrogen fixation in soil
	Inorganic (e.g., NH_4^+, NO_3^-)
	Organic (amino acids, nucleic acids)
Nonmetallic elements	Sulfur
	Phosphorus
Metallic elements	K, Ca, Mg, Mn, Fe, Zn, Co, Mo
Vitamins	Nutritional requirements for growth of all bacteria
	Some or all may be synthesized endogenously
	Others must be supplied from an external (exogenous) source
	Commercial production of vitamins (or amino acids) is usually achieved with microorganisms
	that make an excessive amount
Water	The universal solvent

straight line when log numbers are plotted), cell division is at a constant rate, and cells are smallest at this time with less time for maximum synthesis. In the **stationary phase,** nutrients become exhausted, toxic products accumulate, and cell division is equal to cell death. The maximum synthesis of byproducts usually occurs during this phase. In the **death phase,** cell death exceeds cell division. A classic growth is shown in **Figure 7-2.**

BACTERIAL METABOLISM

The ability of an organism to survive and to utilize its energy sources may, quite by accident, have significant impact on the community as well as on the host tissues. This is true in the case of *S. mutans* and *S. sanguis* (the new trend is to reverse bacteria names; both are acceptable) in the normal flora of the mouth.

Organisms that are tolerant of acid (i.e., **aciduric**) survive in a low pH. In contrast, organisms that produce acid (i.e., **acidogenic**) cause an environmental change and a pH reduction. Both *S. sanguis* and *S. mutans* can ferment sugars at a low pH. However, in an alkaline environment, *S. sanguis* preferentially ferments sugar more rapidly than does *S. mutans*. The reverse is true at a lower pH; *S. mutans* ferments sugar more rapidly than does *S. sanguis*. The short-term impact is that sugar consumption by either results in a lower pH. However, the long-term effect of sugar consumption is much more deleterious. There is a selection of *S. mutans* in plaque that is acid tolerant and continues to produce acid at the lower pH. There is, therefore, a deselection of the alkaline-generating organism such as *S. sanguis*. Because the natural competition for nutrients is removed and the sen-

tinel capacity of *S. sanguis* is reduced, an overproduction of *S. mutans* results. Hence, the multispecies consortia due to the selective environmental pressures and change in pH favors the overgrowth of an organism, which has the capacity to reduce pH, live in that environment, and result in greater production of caries. **Figure 7-3** describes this cycle.

BACTERIAL GENETICS

It is the expected truth that in replication, offspring will resemble their parents in color, size, shape, and so forth. Exceptions are known to occur.

In understanding microbial genetics, two specific terms must be defined: genotype and phenotype. **Genotype** is based on the entire layer of genes possessed by a cell. In contrast, **phenotype** is the array of properties expressed by a cell.

Phenotypic Changes (Modifications, Adaptations)

The following types of changes may be observed-morphology of the cell, formation of spores, formation of a capsule, formation of flagella, pigment production, physiology of the cell, inducible enzymes synthesized only when another substance is present in the environment, contrasted with constitutive enzymes, and enzymes present continuously.

Genotypic Changes

A mutation is a permanent, heritable change in genotype; some of these changes are said to be "spontaneous" changes,

TABLE 7–8 Physical Conditions that Affect Growth of Bacteria

Temperature Requirements

   Psychrophiles
      Optimum temperature for growth = 15–20°C
      Will grow at 0°C
   Mesophiles
      Optimum 25–40°C
      Disease-producing organisms
   Thermophiles
      Optimum 45–60°C
      Also tend to be heat resistant and to survive in canned food

Oxygen Requirements (eH)

   Groups
      Aerobic: grow in the presence of oxygen (generally required)
      Anaerobic: grow only in the absence of oxygen
      Facultative anaerobes: either
      Microaerophilic: grow in a small amount of oxygen

pH Requirements

   Optimum and tolerated levels vary widely
   Preservation of food by pickling with lactic and acetic acids
      (e.g., pickles or sauerkraut)

Osmotic Pressure

   NaCl
      Used for preservation of food (e.g., salt fish, salt port)
      Halophilic organisms
      Thrive in the high NaCl concentrations of oceans and salt lakes
      Often require medium or high osmotic pressure for growth
   Sucrose
      High concentrations preserve food (e.g., jelly, syrup)

Water

   Required for metabolism and growth

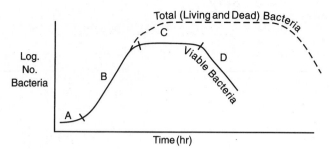

Figure 7-2. *A,* Specialized structures may become significant as the organism finds its "niche." (C, capsule; F, flagella; P, pili; CM, cell membrane; CW, cell wall; N, nucleus, R, release.) *B, Neisseria gonorrhoeae* with proteins I, II, and III; pili (T1-T5); lipopolysaccharide (endotoxin); O-antigen (also called somatic antigen). (From Mahon CR, Manuselis G: Textbook of Diagnostic Microbiology, 2nd ed. Philadelphia, WB Saunders, 2000, p 15.)

cell wall membrane and undergo recombination with a recipient chromosome by a double crossover. **Transduction** is the movement from one cell to another via a viral agent (bacteriophage).

ORAL MICROBIOLOGY

Oral Flora Organisms

Indigenous Oral Flora and Development of Dental Plaque. Bacteria colonize most of the surface of the human body. Their populations are particularly dense in the oral cavity and the intestinal tract. For many years, the bacteria of the mouth were largely ignored and were considered to be harmless and uninteresting. It is now known that organisms of this "normal" flora can cause disease such as subacute bacterial endocarditis, mixed anaerobic infections of various body tissues, and actinomycosis. Of greater interest to the dental profession is the recognition that oral bacteria are the etiologic agents of caries and periodontal disease.

Large numbers of bacteria of diverse genera and species inhabit the mouth. These organisms may be divided into in-

whereas others may be induced by known mutagens. Changes in the bacterium's own genes (DNA) occur by any of three mechanisms: **substitution, insertion (addition),** and **deletion. Mutagens**, chemicals, and irradiation are also generally carcinogenic, although notable exceptions are known. Brief descriptions are as follows: insertion/addition-a section of genetic material that is inserted into an existing gene sequence *or* the mutational process producing a genetic insertion; deletion-the absence of a section of material from a chromosome *or* the mutational process that results in a deletion; mutagen-an agent that tends to increase the frequency or extent of mutation.

Briefly, **conjugation** is the transfer of genetic material (i.e., DNA) between bacteria through specialized (sex) pili. In a more elaborate definition, conjugation is the fusion of similar gametes with the ultimate union of their nuclei, which among lower thallophytes (fungi) replaces the typical fertilization of higher forms. **Transformation** is the transfer of *free* bacterial DNA. DNA must penetrate the

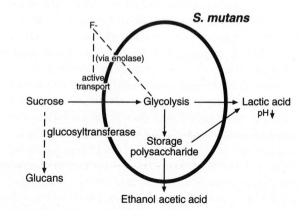

Figure 7-3. Pathophysiology of *Streptococcus mutans.* (Modified from 3-day Review Course, University of Virginia.)

TABLE 7–9 Intraoral Site Distribution of Various Indigenous and Transient Members of the Oral Biofilm Community

ORAL FLORA COMMUNITY SPECIES	AEROTOLLERANCE	SALIVA	TONGUE	PLAQUE SUPRAGINGIVAL	SUBGINGIVAL
Streptococcus salivarius	+++	+++	+++		
Streptococcus sanguis	+++	++	++	+++	+
Streptococcus mitis	++	++	++	++	++
Streptococcus milleri	++	+/−	+/−	+ to +++	0
Streptococcus mutans	++	+/− to +	+/−	+ to +++	0
Lactobacillus sp	+	+	+	+	+/−
Actinomyces sp	+/−	0	+	++	+/− to ++
Actinomyces actinomycetemcomitans	+/−	+	0	+/−	0 to +
Veillonella	+/−	0	+	++	++
Fusobacterium sp	0	0	0	+/−	+/− to ++
Capnocytophaga	−	0	0	+/−	+/− to +
Bacteroides melaninogenicus	−	0	0	+/−	+/− to +
Porphyromonas gingivalis	−	0	0	0	0 to +
Treponema sp	−	0	0	0	0 to +

Semiquantitative Bioburden: 0 = not usually detected; +/− = rarely present; + = usually present in low proportions; ++ = usually present in moderate proportions; +++ = usually present in high proportions. **Corresponding Culturable Colony-Forming Units (Viable):** $<10^3$, $\geq10^3$–$<10^5$, $\geq10^5$–$<10^6$, and $\geq10^6$

digenous, supplemental, and transient flora. As the name implies, **transient flora** microbes are merely "passing through." This flora is usually present in small numbers, and any given organism is present in only a few individuals. On the other hand, the **indigenous flora** consists of bacteria that are found in large numbers in almost all individuals. The **supplemental flora** consists of bacteria that are almost always present in all individuals but in low numbers.

Members of the indigenous flora occupy different ecologic areas in the mouth (**Table 7-9**). Bacteria in saliva represent the wash-off from oral surfaces and most closely resemble the flora of the tongue. The tongue, buccal mucosa, and teeth have flora characteristic for their site in terms of the types of bacteria present. The specific composition of the flora at these sites varies from one person to another, and in the case of dental plaque from tooth to tooth in the same mouth. In addition, some bacteria tend to colonize only certain areas of a tooth. For example *S. mutans* preferentially colonizes occlusal fissures and interproximal sites.

The major factors that control the colonization of oral surfaces are: (1) **the ability of an organism to attach to the surface,** and (2) **its ability to grow once attached (Table 7-10).** Bacterial attachment to surfaces is highly specific, and this specificity is largely responsible for the varying composition of the flora in different sites. **Subsequent growth of an attached organism is dependent on the availability of nutrients, the pH, and the oxidation-reduction potential (eH) of a given site.**

The types and numbers of organisms found in the mouth are limited by mechanical cleansing of the salivary flow and desquamation of mucosal cells. In addition, saliva also contains antibodies that inhibit attachment of some bacteria and enzymes (e.g., lysozymes that may inhibit growth).

Occlusal fissures, interproximal areas, and the area at the gingival margin are protected to some extent from the normal cleansing mechanisms of the mouth. Bacteria accumulate in these areas very quickly. The ability to colonize these retentive sites is less dependent on the adherence mechanism than is the colonization of smooth surfaces. In addition, bacterial colonization changes throughout life.

Development

At birth, the oral cavity is sterile. Flora begin to develop within hours. Within a few days, the following microorganisms are present-*Streptococcus* sp, *Neisseria sp*, *Staphylococcus* sp, *Veillonella* sp, *Lactobacillus* sp, and coliform bacteria (which are transient and disappear). As teeth erupt, the following microorganisms appear: *Actinomyces* sp, *Bacteroides* sp, *Fusobacterium* sp, *Leptothrix*, spirochetes, *S. mutans*, *S. salivarius*, *S. sanguis*, and *Nocardia* sp (**Table 7-11**)

Bacterial Plaque Biofilm/ Bacterial Reservoir

Acquired pellicle is structurally a homogenous, organic, tenacious film that forms on exposed oral surfaces from 0.1 to 0.8 μm thick. It forms within minutes after plaque is removed and is free from microorganisms until plaque attaches to it. The composition of pellicle is primarily glycoproteins from saliva that aid in the adherence of microbes.

Bacterial plaque is an organized mass of microorganisms that are held together by a gel-like intermicrobial matrix. Plaque is nonmineralized and found on teeth and other oral surfaces. Plaque may contain inflammatory and epithelial cells but consists mainly of water (80%) and solids

TABLE 7–10 Microorganisms* of the Oral Biofilm Community, Gram Stain Morphotype and Relationship to O$_2$ Redox Potential (eH)

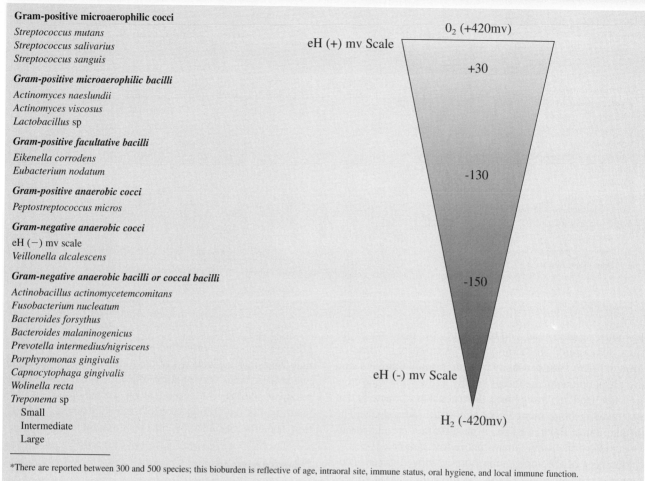

Gram-positive microaerophilic cocci

Streptococcus mutans
Streptococcus salivarius
Streptococcus sanguis

Gram-positive microaerophilic bacilli

Actinomyces naeslundii
Actinomyces viscosus
Lactobacillus sp

Gram-positive facultative bacilli

Eikenella corrodens
Eubacterium nodatum

Gram-positive anaerobic cocci

Peptostreptococcus micros

Gram-negative anaerobic cocci

eH (−) mv scale
Veillonella alcalescens

Gram-negative anaerobic bacilli or coccal bacilli

Actinobacillus actinomycetemcomitans
Fusobacterium nucleatum
Bacteroides forsythus
Bacteroides malaninogenicus
Prevotella intermedius/nigriscens
Porphyromonas gingivalis
Capnocytophaga gingivalis
Wolinella recta
Treponema sp
   Small
   Intermediate
   Large

eH (+) mv Scale

O$_2$ (+420mv)

+30

-130

-150

eH (-) mv Scale

H$_2$ (-420mv)

*There are reported between 300 and 500 species; this bioburden is reflective of age, intraoral site, immune status, oral hygiene, and local immune function.

(20%) (e.g., bacteria and extracellular polysaccharides-sticky substances like dextrans and levans that contribute to colonization). The formation of **plaque biofilm** is very organized **(Table 7-12)**

Materia alba is a white material that consists of an informal collection of microorganisms and cellular debris. It forms a soft deposit over acquired pellicle and microbial plaque. Materia alba may contain desquamated epithelial cells, living and dead bacteria, disintegrating white blood cells, salivary proteins, and food debris. As plaque ages, the inner layers become more and more anaerobic (i.e., lower eH) (see Chapter 13).

The predominant bacteria in **supragingival plaque** are *S. sanguis, A. viscosus,* and *A. naeslundii*. Other bacteria include *A. israelii, S. mutans, Veillonella* sp, and *Fusobacterium* sp. The predominant bacteria in **crevicular fluid** are *S. mitis, S. sanguis, S. epidermidis, Rothia dentocariosa, A. viscosus, A. naeslundii,* and small spirochetes. **Subgingival plaque attached to teeth** is similar to supragingival plaque. Inner layers consist mainly of gram-positive cocci and rods and gram-negative cocci and rods. Apical portions consist mainly of gram-negative rods and filamentous forms. Subgingival plaque is associated with calculus formation, root caries, and periodontal disease. These bacteria may invade the soft and hard tissues, making them more difficult to destroy. **Loosely adherent or epithelial associated plaque** extends from the gingival margin apical to the junctional epithelium, adjacent to the gingival epithelium or pocket lumen. Predominantly gram-negative cocci and rods, motile forms, and spirochetes reside in loose plaque.

Plaque types are different, because they relate to disease. For example, **cariogenic plaque** is associated with the initiation of caries. A high-sucrose diet favors cariogenic plaque. Periodontal disease-producing plaque promotes inflammatory responses demonstrated by gingivitis, periodontitis, and other periodontal infections. **Calculogenic plaque** leads to the mineralization of plaque and results in calculus. Factors that influence the composition and maturation of bacterial plaque are listed in **Table 7-13.**

TABLE 7–11 Changes in Oral Flora Associated with Eruption of Teeth

ORGANISM	PREDENTATE INFANTS	DENTATE INFANTS
Streptococcus sanguis	Not detectable	Always detectable
Streptococcus mutans	Not detectable	Often detected
Bacteroides sp	Infrequently detected	Often detected
Fusobacterium sp	Infrequently detected	Often detected
Actinomyces sp	Infrequently detected	Often detected

Calculus: An Alternative Reservoir

Calculus is mineralized plaque that covers the exterior surface of nonmineralized plaque. It consists of shed bacteria, desquamated epithelial cells, blood cells, and salts from saliva.

Subgingival plaque forms by extension of supragingival plaque; however, each mineralizes separately. Calculus results from the deposition of minerals into a plaque organic mixture. Three steps are necessary:

1. Pellicle formation
2. Plaque formation
3. Mineralization: within 24 to 48 hours, foci develop close to the underlying tooth surface and eventually unite. Mineralization of plaque first occurs with the deposition of minerals. The supragingival mineral sources are gingival sulcus fluid and inflammatory exudate. Mineralization of hydroxyapatite crystals form in the intercellular matrix or on the bacterial surface.

The time elapsing between primary soft deposit to the mature mineralized stage of calculus is 10 to 20 days. The average time is approximately 12 days. Subgingival calculus is the result of pocket formation; it is not the cause. In a pocket, calculus can help retain toxins and contribute to inflammation. The role of calculus in disease is unclear; however, mineralization does the following:

1. Brings bacterial matter closer to supporting tissues
2. Interferes with local self-cleaning mechanisms
3. Makes removal of plaque more difficult

ORAL INFECTIONS/DENTAL INFECTIONS

The adult oral cavity (one of the four primary reservoirs) has a dense diverse indigenous microbiota/ecosystem that consists of protozoa, yeast, viruses, and bacteria (see Table 7-4). Of the more than 500 bacterial species found in the oral cavity, about 22 identified genera predominate.

Table 7-14 lists oral microbial pathogens. These pathogens constitute organisms traditionally recognized as meeting Koch's postulates (i.e., the germ theory) and those more recently associated with the community theory or an imbalance in the oral microbiota or ecosystem. Streptococcal pharyngitis, non-streptococcal pharyngitis, infectious dermatitis, rhinoscleroderma, and mechanical ventilation associated with medical devices are classic germ theory or single organism diseases. This means that when the single pathogen is eradicated, the disease process is reversed. However, thrush, epiglottitis, periodontitis, sinusitis, and deep space infections are associated with the emerging community theory in which an imbalance of a group of organisms within the multispecies microconsortia predominates and is associated with disease. In this case, it is almost never possible to eradicate all the organisms, but rather bring them back into the more normal biodistribution relative to the age and normal health of the tissue associated with these organisms.

Of significance, the following infections are associated with the dental community and defined generally by specific anatomic locations or tooth locations. These infections are

TABLE 7–12 Maturation of Plaque

Days 2–4	Early or immune plaque-mainly cocci—*Streptococcus mutans, S. sanguis* Cocci (*Streptococcus* sp, *Veillonella* sp) predominate; increasing numbers of filamentous (*Actinomyces* sp) forms and slender rods. Neutrophils increase.
Days 4–7	Increasing numbers of filamentous forms, rods, and *Fusobacterium* sp near the gingival margin. In this area, plaque is thicker and develops a more mature flora sooner than in other areas. Some spirochetes and vibrios are present. As plaque spreads coronally, new plaque has coccal forms. Increasing numbers of white blood cells (T lymphocytes). Increasing numbers of gram-negative-anaerobic organisms (*Bacteroides* sp). Inflammation is observed in the gingiva.
Days 14–21	Older or mature plaque; predominantly vibrious and spirochetes; some cocci and filamentous forms; increased B lymphocytes and plasma cells; gingivitis clearly evident

TABLE 7–13 Factors Influencing the Composition and Maturation of Bacterial Plaque

Factors of Bacterial Growth

Extracellular products
 Glucans (skeleton of plaque)
 Fructans (energy resources)
Bacterial interactions: coaggregation reactions
Plaque ecology
 Dietary changes: sucrose intake—aciduric bacteria
 Oxygen environment: anaerobic bacteria
 Nutritional interactions: bacterial succession
 Bacteriocin production

Host-Derived Factors

Mechanical oral cleaning mechanisms
Saliva
 pH, lactoperoxidase, lactoferrin, lysozyme
 Salivary glycoproteins: adhesion mechanisms
Host immune responses
 Oral secretions-IgA
 Crevicular fluid: leukocytes, IgG, IgM, complement, etc.

addressed separately as caries microbiology, gingival/periodontal microbiology, endodontic microbiology emphasizing infected root canals and periapical infections, and lastly infections associated with implants. These implants act as indwelling medical devices and demonstrate the same consequences of an uncontrolled microbiota that is associated with chronic infections.

Dental Infections/An Imbalance

Enamel/Caries

Bacterial diseases of dental **calcified structures (i.e., enamel, dentin, cementum)** involve the demineralization of mineral components and dissolution of organic matrix. Demineralization requires cariogenic bacteria, a substrate, and a host. **Caries** is a multifactorial disease requiring the interaction of: (1) the causative agent-bacteria, (2) a susceptible host, and (3) the environment-substrate. A susceptible host eating a cariogenic diet will not get caries unless the appropriate bacteria are present. Similarly, these bacteria will not cause caries in a susceptible host if carogenic dietary factors are absent.

Cariogenic Bacteria

1. Able to adhere to tooth surfaces, form a protective matrix
2. Aciduric-can tolerate an acid environment
3. Acidogenic-produce acid from the metabolism of sugars
   - *S. mutans* produces lactic acid from fructose; is associated with smooth surface caries
   - *A. viscosus* and *A. naeslundii* produce lactic acid from glucose; involved in root surface caries
4. Normal pH of oral cavity is 6.2 to 7.0. The pH will be lower in caries-susceptible people and higher in caries-resistant people. Cariogenic bacteria tolerance of a pH of

5.2 to 5.6-the pH at which decalcification occurs or the critical pH.

5. Predominant cariogenic bacteria by location:
   - Smooth surface-*S. mutans*
   - Root surface-*A. viscosus, A. naeslundii,* other filamentous rods
   - Pit and fissures-*S. mutans, Lactobacillus* sp.
   - Deep dentin-*Lactobacillus* sp, *A. naeslundii,* other filamentous rods

Host: Oral Cavity

1. Tooth morphology: deep occlusal pits and fissures
2. Saliva: washes away food particles; buffers acid; higher flow rate contributes to an increased pH
3. Antibacterial functions: IgA, lysozyme, and salivary peroxidase

Host Factors

Genetics. Epidemiologic surveys of caries incidence demonstrate differences in caries experience among groups of people. These differences were thought to be genetic, and people with a low caries experience were referred to as "caries-resistant" or "caries-immune." Some of the differences in these epidemiologic studies were due to differences in: (1) the degree of infection with *S. mutans*, (2) diet, and (3) exposure to fluoride. The best evidence for a genetic factor in caries susceptibility is that identical twins show fewer differences in caries experience than do fraternal twins.

Salivary Flow. Reduced salivary flow increases caries susceptibility.

Age of the Tooth. In experimental animals, weanlings are much more susceptible to caries than are older animals. In humans, occlusal caries is primarily a disease found in children.

Tooth Composition. Teeth with enamel containing fluoride are more resistant to caries. The availability of fluoride is more accurately described as an environmental factor.

Substrate

Diet. Diet is the most important of the environmental factors. Carbohydrate is necessary for acid production by oral bacteria. An increase in the consumption of refined sugar (sucrose) results in an increased incidence of caries. The **frequency of eating** and the **consistency of the food** are more important than are the presence or absence of sugar in the diet. Sucrose in solid form is more cariogenic.

Substrate-sucrose (source is dietary sugar) is the single most important factor contributing to caries in caries-susceptible people.

Sucrose (glucose) plus *S. mutans* in the presence of glucosyltransferase leads to the production of dextran and lactic acid.

TABLE 7–14 Oral Pharyngeal Microbial Pathogens and Associated Syndromes

ORAL INFECTION OR SYNDROME	PUTATIVE PATHOGENS	SPECIAL INSTRUCTIONS
1. Streptococcal pharyngitis	*Streptococcus pyogenes* (GABHS)	Routine microbiology culture
2. Nonstreptococcal pharyngitis	*Mycoplasma pneumoniae, Chlamydia pneumoniae, Bordetella pertussis, B. parapertussis, Corynebacterium diphtheriae, Neisseria gonorrhoeae* Respiratory viruses *Acranobacterium hemolyticum*	Tests for viral pharyngitis (other than EBV or CMV serology) are not usually performed. *C. diphtheriae* is enhanced by culturing both the throat and the nasopharynx. PCR is recommended for *B. pertussis*.
With immune compromise	Enterobacteriaceae, *S. aureus,* or *Candida* sp	
3. Mechanical ventilation and medical associated devices	Enterobacteriaceae, *S. aureus, Candida*	Biofilm analysis (MBEC)
4. Epiglottitis	*Haemophilus influenzae*	Routine microbiology culture
5. Vincent angina and gingivitis	*Fusobacterium necrophorum* plus other mixed anaerobes (including *Bacteroides* sp)	Culture not usually helpful; GS is best.
With peritonsillar abscess		For abscess, culture purulent scraping aerobically and anaerobically
6. Thrush	*Candida albicans* and other yeast	Scraping of exudate for fungal culture and smear + CW
7. Infectious stomatitis	HSV	Culture or DFA of scraping from the lesion for virus
8. Purulent nasopharyngitis	Mixed oral flora	Culture not usually helpful
9. Rhinoscleroma	*Klebsiella rhinoscleromatis*	Routine microbiology culture and GS
10. Ozaena	*Klebsiella ozaenae*	Routine microbiology culture and GS
11. Periodontitis	*Porphyromonas gingivalis, Bacteroides forsythus, Treponema denticola, Prevotella intermedia, Peptostreptococcus micros, Actinobacillus actinomycetemcomitans, Wolinella recta, Eikenella corrodens,* other spirochetes	Scraping of plaque shows numerous spirochetes using darkfield microscopy; culture and susceptibility testing of subgingival plaque
12. Dental infections, including periapical abscess and osteomyelitis	*Peptostreptococcus* sp, *Veillonella* sp, *B. fragilis* group, *Prevotella* and *Porphyromonas* sp, and *Fusobacterium* sp	Routine anaerobic microbiology culture on abscess material
13. Actinomycosis, or "lumpy jaw"	*Actinomyces israelii*	Notify laboratory that condition is suspected for optimal testing
14. Sialadenitis	*S. aureus*	Routine microbiology culture
15. Parotitis	Mumps virus, influenza virus, enteroviruses, *M. tuberculosis*	Vial culture and serology, or a culture for *M. tuberculosis*
16. Acute sinusitis	*H. influenzae, S pneumoniae, S. pyogenes, M. catarrhalis, P. acnes,* rhinovirus, influenza virus, and parainfluenza virus and fungi	Routine microbiology culture on purulent sinus material
17. Chronic sinusitis	Mixed oral flora anaerobes, *M. catarrhalis* and fungi	Routine microbiology culture on purulent sinus material emphasizing fungi and CW*
18. Deep space infections	*S. pyogenes, S. aureus, Peptostreptococcus* sp, *Bacteroides, Prevotella, Porphyromonas* sp, *Fusobacterium* sp, *Actinomyces israelii,* and viridans group streptococci	Routine microbiology culture on aspirated purulent material emphasizing anaerobes and CW*
19. Bacterial tracheitis	*S. aureus* and streptococci	Routine microbiology culture on aspirated purulent material

*CW, calcofluor white: stain for chitin found in fungi; HSV, herpes simplex virus; direct fluorescent antibody (DFA); gram stain (GS); minimal biofilm eradication concentration (MBEC).
From Rutkauskas JS: Infect Dis Clin North Am Dec 1999.

Gingivitis and Periodontitis Diseases

Gingivitis and periodontitis (Table 7-15) are infectious diseases based on community theory (i.e., imbalance). Factors contributing to the disease process are:

- Nature of bacterial flora
- Ability of bacteria to be virulent-produce toxins, enzymes, and chemotactic factor
- Capability of bacteria to be protected by capsules from the host response mechanism
- Intensity of the host response to the bacteria

The anaerobic infections found most frequently in the oral cavity are gingivoperiodontal diseases and pulpal and periapical infections. The different clinical forms of gingivitis are generally infections that affect the soft tissues. **Periodontitis** comprises a group of diseases characterized

TABLE 7–15 Putative Oral Pathogens Associated with Carious Lesions, Gingivitis, and Periodontal Diseases

DISEASE	MORPHOTYPES AND IMMUNE FEATURES	PREDOMINANT CULTIVABLE SPECIES
Healthy	Gram-positive cocci and rods, few motile rods, few spirochetes	*Streptococcus* sp
		Actinomyces sp
Smooth surface caries		*Streptococcus mutans*
Root surface caries		*Actinomyces viscosus*
		Actinomyces naeslundii
Gingivitis	Gram-positive cocci and rods, gram-negative cocci and rods, few motile rods, few spirochetes	*Streptococcus* sp
		Actinomyces sp
		Fusobacterium
		Veillonella
Necrotizing ulcerative gingivitis and necrotizing ulcerative periodontitis	Intermediate-sized spirochetes invade tissue; gram-negative primarily	*Prevotella intermedia*
		Fusobacterium nucleatum
Pregnancy gingivitis		*Prevotella intermedia*
Generalized/localized juvenile periodontitis (aggressive periodontitis)	Significant treponema; subgingival gram-negative anaerobes, soft tissue invasion by gram-negative organism in the pocket wall; depressed neutrophil function	*Actinobacillus actinomycetemcomitans*
Adult periodontitis (chronic periodontitis)	Subgingival plaque; gram-negative anaerobic, motile, complex, flora—cocci, rods, spirals; intermediate and small spirochetes	*Prevotella intermedia*
		Porphyromonas gingivalis
		Capnocytophaga sp
Refractory or recurrent periodontitis	Significant treponema	*Actinobacillus actinomycetemcomitans*
		Bacteroides forsythus
		Fusobacterium sp
		Capnocytophaga sp
		Eikenella corrodens
		Porphyromonas gingivalis
		Prevotella intermedia
		Wolinella recta
Rapid progressive periodontitis	Gram-negative anaerobes; depressed neutrophil function; small spirochetes	*Actinobacillus actinomycetemcomitans*

by connective tissue attachment loss and bone loss. **Subgingival microbiota is a complex multispecies consortia (biofilm), but there is a prevalence of** *Porphyromonas gingivalis, Prevotella intermedia/nigrescens, Actinobacillus actinomycetemcomitans, Bacteroides forsythus, Peptostreptococcus micros, Campylobacter rectus,* species of *Fusobacterium, Eikenella,* and *Treponema.* The treponemes can be subclassified into three groups based on size by darkfield microscopy: small (Sm), intermediate (In), and large (Lg). Small treponemes are considered to be the most pathogenic and correlate with disease progression.

Figure 7-4 defines the organization and multispecies architecture of oral flora associated with gingivitis (supragingival plaque) and periodontitis (subgingival plaque). In the former, the germ theory (postulated by Robert Koch) is addressed because of a limited number of free-floating (planktonic) bacteria, primarily gram-positive microaerophilic organisms. Planktonic organisms are associated with less virulence and are obviously more easily disrupted. In the latter, the community theory is in operation, defining a multispecies consortia organized into domains of the biofilm composed of attached (sessile) gram-negative anaerobic rods. Subgingival sessile organisms are more resistant to removal and biomass degradation.

In 1988, Shah and Collins proposed the reclassification of *Bacteroides asaccharolyticus, B. gingivalis,* and *B. endodontalis* into a new genus called *Porphyromonas.* Reclassification was based on the fact that members of these asaccharolytic black-pigmented *Bacteroides/Porphyromonas* form a homogenous group that differs remarkably in biochemical and chemical properties from the type species of *Bacteroides (B. fragilis).* In addition, the saccharolytic black-pigmented *Bacteroides* have been reclassified for similar reasons into a new genus called *Prevotella* following a proposal by Shah and Collins in 1990. In 1991, *P. nigrescens* was separated from the species *P. intermedia.* Nine species of black-pigmented bacteria (BPB) have now been isolated from humans, and several other species have been isolated from animals. Microbial species can change over time so that an acute exacerbation can occur. The present nomenclature for human species of BPB is as follows:

Black-pigmented *Porphyromonas* (asaccharolytic *Bacteroides* sp)

• *P. asaccharolytica* (usually nonoral)

Clinical Comparison: Planktonic vs Sessile Life Forms

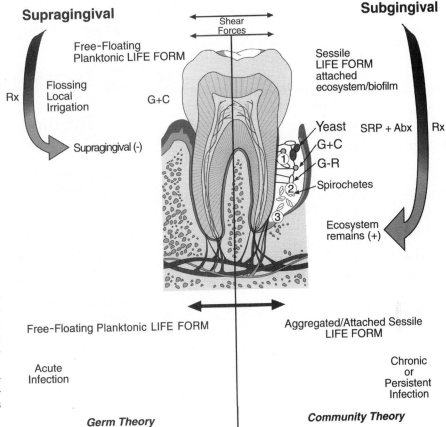

Figure 7-4. Clinical comparison of planktonic and sessile life forms in supragingival and subgingival biofilms.

Planktonic organisms are more often associated with low virulence and less pathogenicity as in supragingival plaque. Subgingival plaque is composed, generally, of a multi-species consortia whose architecture via adherence and coaggregation is manifested as a sessile community. In fact, in periodontal disease we now know there are three biofilms: (1) that attached to the cementum, (2) that which is called flux and a free-floating community and (3) that which is attached to the tissue.

Planktonic, or free-floating organisms are obviously more easily disrupted potentially eradicated whereas sessile are not.

- *P. gingivalis*
- *P. endodontalis*

Black-pigmented *Prevotella* (saccharolytic *Bacteroides* sp)

- *P. melaninogenica*
- *P. denticola*
- *P. loescheii*
- *P. intermedia*
- *P. nigrescens*
- *P. corporis*
- *P. tannerae* (most recently detected in 1997)

Nonpigmented *Prevotella* isolated from infections of endodontic origin include:

- *P. buccae*-associated with acute symptoms
- *P. bivia*
- *P. oralis*
- *P. oris*
- *P. oulorum*
- *P. ruminicola*

Other bacteria implicated with clinical signs and symptoms but without an absolute correlation include *P. buccae* and species of *Peptococcus, Peptostreptococcus, Eubacterium, Actinomyces*, and *Fusobacterium*.

Strict anaerobes often isolated from infections of endodontic origin:

1. Black-pigmented bacteria: gram-negative, coccal/bacillary, nonmotile
2. *Fusobacterium*: gram-negative fusiform, nonmotile
3. *Veillonella parvula*: gram-negative cocci, nonmotile
4. *Peptostreptococcus*: gram-positive cocci, nonmotile
5. *Eubacterium*: gram-positive rod, nonmotile
6. *Actinomyces israelii*: gram-positive branching rods, nonmotile
7. *Lactobacillus*: gram-positive rod, nonmotile

Yeasts and viruses have been isolated.

Infection of the Pulp and Periapical Tissues: Endodontics

Dental pulp may respond to various irritants-mechanical, thermal, chemical, electrical, and microbial. By far the most important of these is microbial infection. Therefore, a **principal function of treating and filling root canals is to eliminate bacteria from the canal and periapical region.** Inflammation is the basic response of the pulp to any injurious agent. Viable bacteria and their products (i.e., enzymes, toxins) induce an inflammatory response. Components of the bacterial cell released after the death of the cell can also irritate tissues and perpetuate chronic periapical lesions. Immunologic responses (both humoral and cellular) to viable bacteria, their products, or necrotic pulp tissue antigens may play a role in the pathogenesis of periapical lesions.

There is a similarity between the genera identified in periodontal pockets and infected root canals and periapical infections. However, some species are more prevalent than others in both infections. The following were observed predominantly inside the root canals: *P. intermedia/nigrescens, Peptostreptococcus anaerobius, P. micros, Eubacterium lentum, E. alactolyticum,* and *Porphyromonas endodontalis,* with strong associations among some species.

Bacteria may infect dental pulp (by):

1. Extension of a carious lesions through the enamel and dentin
2. After trauma with fracture of the crown
3. After trauma in which the crown remains intact. Bacteria in the bloodstream localize in the injured pulp tissue. This process is called anachoresis.
4. Extension of bacteria in the periodontal pocket along the periodontal ligament
5. Extension of bacteria from periapical lesion on an adjacent tooth

The most important of these routes of infection is the extension of carious lesions into the pulp. The bacteria found in infected pulp chambers are a reflection of the normal flora of the oral cavity. The technique, which is used most often for culturing root canals, involves placing a sterile paper point in the canal for 1 minute and then placing it in either brain heart infusion broth with 0.1% agar or trypticase soy broth with 0.1% agar. This technique allows the growth of most of the common facultative bacteria found in root canals but does not permit the growth of strictly anaerobic species.

The facultative bacteria most commonly found in infected root canals are species of α-hemolytic streptococci. If *S. salivarius* is found, it is probably due to contamination of the specimen with saliva.

When adequate anaerobic techniques are used, anaerobes are found in most necrotic pulps. In some cases, only anaerobic organisms are found, but mixed infections with anaerobic and facultative bacteria are more common.

Implants

Since the development of implants as a means to replace lost dentition, two types of infection have been described: **mucositis** and **periimplantitis.** These are named according to whether the infection involves inflammation of soft tissues or inflammation and bone loss. The microflora associated with periimplant infections is similar to the microflora found in periodontal diseases, particularly in partially edentulous patients. **Implant placement is, therefore, not recommended for patients who present with uncontrolled periodontal disease.**

Pericoronitis is another infection associated with anaerobic gram-negative bacilli and treponemes. Treponemes have been observed in almost all the cases of chronic pericoronitis of the third lower molar. There are numerous methods for microbiologic diagnosis, and treatment of some oral infections depends on a close interaction between the microbiologist and the dentist.

SYSTEMIC INFECTIOUS DISEASES ASSOCIATED WITH THE ORAL ECOSYSTEM

The number of organisms and potential infectious diseases associated with the oral passage are significant. Listed in **Table 7-16** are some of the more common infectious diseases and their usual route of transmission, which are of concern to the dental community. **Table 7-17** lists organisms/disease via target organ systems or potential proximity to the ecosystems of humans. Of major concern is the fact that it may not be the primary infection that is significant, but the developing **sequelae** that presents itself as the first characteristic of a disease recognized by a member of the dental team. This is particularly true for cardiovascular diseases (e.g., infective endocarditis) and selected staphylococcal infections (e.g., toxic shock syndrome). For ease of discussion, however, the specific oral diseases are emphasized by their general microbial category (i.e., bacterial, fungal, or viral).

Lastly, it is also important to remember that not only the presenting clinical signs and symptoms may be those of a sequelae from a primary infection sometime earlier, but the patient may also acquire multiple organisms and present with signs and symptoms that are difficult to evaluate. Hence, thrush may be an indicator of human immunodeficiency virus (HIV).

Types of Infection

Generally, the types of infections developing can be classified by their length of presentation reflecting the **incubation phase.** An **acute infection** is an infection with a rapid onset, short course, and pronounced symptoms. In contrast, a **chronic infection** is an infection that progresses slowly and continues for a long time. **Localized infections** are those that are restricted or limited to one tissue or organ system. **Generalized infections,** on the other hand, are multisystemic or infections where the organism is distributed widely, although not necessarily uniformly, throughout the host. It is often referred to as a **systemic infection** and may have multiple presentations. A **latent infection** is an infection wherein symptoms are not apparent. The infecting agent does not actively reproduce in a detectable manner. Lastly, the **carrier state** is a condition wherein an infected person harbors a specific agent in the absence of discernible clinical symptoms and serves as a potential source of infection for those who are in close contact.

TABLE 7–16 Infectious Agents Transmissible to Patients and Personnel in the Dental Operatory

AGENT	ROUTE	ESTIMATED SURVIVAL
Viruses		
Respiratory	Secretions/saliva	Hours
Herpes zoster/varicella	Saliva/vesicles	Hours
Mumps	Saliva/secretions	Hours
Herpes simplex 1 and 2	Saliva/secretions	Minutes
Hepatitis A	Feces/blood	Hours/days
Hepatitis B	Saliva/blood	Hours/days
Epstein-Barr	Saliva	Seconds/minutes
Cytomegalovirus	Saliva	Seconds/minutes
Bacteria		
Mycobacterium tuberculosis	Saliva/sputum	Days/week
Staphyloccus aureus	Exudates/saliva/skin	Days
Streptococcus pyogenes	Saliva/secretions	Hours/days
Mycoplasma pneumoniae	Saliva/secretions	Seconds/minutes
Treponema (pallidum)	Exudates/mucosa	Minutes

Sources of Infection/Routes of Transmission

Infectious diseases can be further classified by their route of acquisition, their method of transmission, and the type of pathogen involved. The routes of acquisition are shown theoretically in **Figure 7-5**, which describes the various portals of entry. There are seven and these include:

1. Direct penetration by trauma (tetanus)
2. Direct penetration by an arthropod bite (Lyme disease)
3. Direct penetration by a needle stick (drug abuser)
4. Direct penetration by a pathogen (hookworm)
5. Transplacental passage (rubella)
6. Transplacental inoculation of sexually transmitted organisms (gonorrhea)
7. Dissemination by aerosols (tuberculosis)

In the broader sense, this acquisition is defined as being **endogenous** (i.e., acquired from the host as a normal flora) or as **exogenous** (i.e., acquired from the community). Generally, those agents acquired via the exogenous reservoir are associated with the germ theory and more attributable to Koch's postulates.

Transmission is generally described as horizontal or vertical. Whereas **horizontal transmission** describes person-to-person and **vertical** mother-to-offspring. In infections transmitted by airborne particles, via the horizontal route, there are three types of carriers: droplet, droplet nuclei, and dust. **Droplets** are usually greater than 10 mc in diameter and emanate from the nose or mouth during coughing and sneezing. Most droplets do not travel more than 1 M from the source. In contrast, **droplet nuclei** are small residues arising from dry deposits of approximately 20 mc in diameter. These can readily spread through a room by air currents, and infectivity depends on the resistance of the organisms to

drying and the bioburden of the challenge. In contrast to the two mechanisms mentioned, **dust** is a large particle on the floor or bedding that can be resuspended in air by agitation. Dust may have inherent microorganisms associated with particles (e.g., dried sputum, fungal spores).

Types of pathogens can be described as **extracellular, facultative intracellular,** or **obligate intracellular.** Examples of each include extracellular group A β-streptococcus, facultative intracellular mycoplasma, *Legionella pneumophila* in legionnaires' disease, and obligate intracellular influenza virus. Generally, these types of pathogens can also be described as 20% viral, 7% streptococcal, 1% bacteria, and the greater proportion (~72%) unknown.

There are, however, general characteristics of respiratory tract infections that can help delineate the possible causative agent. Respiratory infections are most often seasonal; they occur commonly in the winter and early spring when there is close contact with humans. Respiratory infections are more common in children than in adults given that repeated exposure may help to induce some degree of protective immunity. Given the rapid dissemination of infected organisms with any community, these organisms are not associated with a single infection, but rather with numerous infections. Lastly, the most common route is via airborne particles or mechanically via hand to hand or hand to eye.

Ultimately, whether an infectious disease process or infection develops depends on a number of competing factors. For each organism, it is important to recognize that the pathogenicity and the potential consequence can be defined by the following events:

- Portal of entry?
- Attachment?
- Virulence of the pathogen?
- Penetration/replication/spread?

TABLE 7–17 Diseases and Microorganisms Grouped by Organ System

Respiratory disease:	Streptococcal pharyngitis
	Tuberculosis
	Pneumonia
	Pneumococcal (multidrug resistant)
	Mycoplasmal
	Chlamydial
	Legionnaires' disease
	Viral including influenza, RSV, parainfluenza
Cardiovascular:	Bacteremia/septicemia
	Infective endocarditis
	Infections of prostheses
	Infectious mononucleosis (EBV and CMV)
Neurologic:	Meningitis (bacterial)
	Encephalitis (HSV)
	Tetanus
Skin and eye:	Herpes simplex 1 and 2 (vesicular eruptions)
	Varicella-zoster
	Staphylococcal and streptococcal infections
	Toxic shock and toxic shock-like
	Herpes keratitis
	Adenovirus keratoconjunctivitis
Hepatitis:	A (infective)
	B (serum)
	C (non-A non-B)
	D
	E
	F
	G
	H
Multiorgan System:	HIV
	CMV
Urogenital:	HSV 1 or 2
	Chlamydia trachomatis
	Human papillomavirus
	Gonorrhea

CMV, cytomegalovirus; EBV, Epstein-Barr virus; HIV, human immunodeficiency virus; HSV, herpes simplex virus; RSV, respiratory syncytial virus.

- Toxigenicity?
- Host response?
- Antibiotic resistance?

Another method of measuring the possible consequences of the exposure of an organism is to put it into an equation. The potential of developing an infection depends on three factors, which can be expressed as an equation:

$$\text{Infection} = \frac{\text{Number of organisms} \times \text{virulence of organism(s)}}{\text{Resistance of host (local and systemic)}}$$
$$\text{(bioburden or biomass)}$$

This quantifies the significance of the bioburden or biomass and virulence plus the impact of local or systemic immunity. Another method of highlighting the potential outcome is to recognize the events as a "cascade" and whether exposure will result in infection depends on a number of events associated with the route of exposure, the size of the inoculum (i.e., bioburden), repeated exposures, and the cofactor.

Specific Oral Diseases of Interest

Bacterial Infections

Bacterial infections include:

- Group A β-hemolytic streptococcus-pharyngitis, rheumatic fever
- *Streptococcus pneumoniae*-multidrug-resistant community acquired pneumonia (CAP)
- Streptococcal infections non-group A-bacterial endocarditis-α-hemolytic streptococcus
- *Mycobacteria* tuberculosis and *Mycobacterium* other than tuberculosis (MOTTS), often called *M. avium intracellulare* (MAI) complex

Streptococci are spherical cocci that are gram-positive and divide in a plane that generally results in pairs or chains

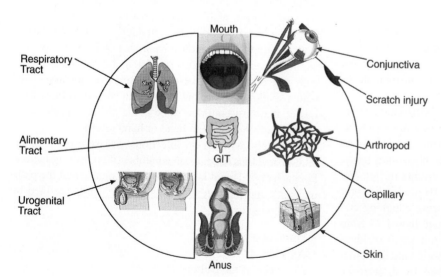

Figure 7-5. Routes of acquisition. Microorganisms have taken advantage of or devised methods that penetrate or bypass protective barriers.

of organisms. The most important pathogens of the genus streptococci include *S. pyogenes.* Group A is associated with serious infections in humans, such as pharyngitis. *S. agalactiae* (group B) is associated with the newborn via vertical transmission. *S. faecalis* (group D) is a common urinary pathogen in which vancomycin resistance (VRE) is becoming problematic. The viridans group, including *S. pneumoniae*, is the most common cause of community acquired pneumonia.

Mycobacterial infections are still the most frequent infectious diseases resulting in the most serious sequelae in the world, followed by malaria. Of course, HIV is beginning to erode this position, but in the 1990s *M. tuberculosis* was the single most causative destructive agent with >30 million deaths worldwide. The structure is unique, because it contains a lipid-enriched cell wall that is defined by its laboratory characteristic of acid-fast bacillus. The single most important point, however, is recognition that the only **aerosol communicable** mycobacterium is *M. tuberculosis*. This represents a real exposure potential in the office or community. However, initial culture methods may not define which mycobacterium is present but only that an acid-fast bacillus-positive specimen has been received in the laboratory. Hence, it is routine policy to address all acid-fast bacillus-positive specimens as being potentially *M. tuberculosis* and represent a foci for aerosol transmission.

Fungal Infections

Yeast-*Candida albicans*-Thrush

Yeast infections are **endogenous** in source and reflect an imbalance of the microbiota and structured architecture of the biofilm. *Candida albicans* (i.e., thrush) is the result of overgrowth from an organism that routinely inhabits the mouth. The most common genus is *Candida,* and several species may reflect the immune status of the host. Again, note the concept of community and recognize that organisms are markers for disease process or failure of local immunity. The most common of the *Candida* species is *C. albicans,* which represents approximately 85% of those isolates in immunosuppressed or immunomodulated patients.

Molds-Aspergillus and Penicillium

Fungal infections associated with molds (where there is an aerial mycelium and no yeast form) are evident in selected communities where employment and aerosol, environmental, and industrial exposure may indicate an unusual risk factor. Black lung is an example. Here, *Penicillium* and *Aspergillus* may be associated with continued immunosuppression as a chronic infection.

Aspergillus sp. Members of this genus are reported to cause ear infections. Many species produce mycotoxins, which may be associated with disease in humans and animals. Toxin production is dependent on the species or a strain within a species and on the food source for the fungus. Some of these toxins have been found to be carcinogenic in animal species. Several toxins are considered to be potential human carcinogens and a common cause of extrinsic asthma (immediate-type hypersensitivity: type I). Acute symptoms include edema and bronchospasms; patients with chronic cases may develop pulmonary emphysema.

Penicillium sp. A wide number of organisms have been placed in this genus. They are often found in aerosol samples and are commonly found in soil, food, cellulose, and grains. It is also found in paint and compost piles. *Penicillium* may cause hypersensitivity pneumonitis or allergic alveolitis in susceptible individuals. It is reported to be allergenic (skin). It is commonly found in carpet, wallpaper, and in interior fiberglass duct insulation. Some species can produce mycotoxins. It is a common cause of extrinsic asthma (immediate-type hypersensitivity: type I). Acute symptoms include edema and bronchospasms. Patients with chronic cases may develop pulmonary emphysema.

Viral Infections

Viral infections focus on respiratory agents, including **influenzae, respiratory syncytial virus (RSV), parainfluenzae, herpangina (enterovirus),** and **herpes simplex virus (HSV).**

Additionally, multisystem viral diseases presenting potential exposure risks to the dental community are addressed, including: **hepatitis A, hepatitis B, non-A non-B hepatitis viruses (hepatitis C), hepatitis D-H, HIV-1, and mumps virus.** Key characteristics and corresponding tables follow.

Viruses are obligate intracellular pathogens smaller than bacteria that basically include a nucleic acid covered by a protein (i.e., a nuclear capsid). Large viruses are usually **enveloped**; viruses less than 70 nm are **non-enveloped** and defined as small viruses. The structure and size of viruses are very important. An interrelationship to pathogenicity and route of exposure may best be defined as "structure equal function." Generally, smaller viruses are stable in the environment; they are transmitted by **fomites** and can pass through the gastrointestinal (GI) system without destruction. In contrast, viruses that are **enveloped** are environmentally unstable; they cannot pass through the gut but rather they focus on respiratory organ systems. These two defining characteristics of "structure equals function" are shown in **Tables 7-18** and **7-19.**

Historically, viruses have also been divided into DNA **(Table 7-20)** viruses or RNA **(Table 7-21)** viruses, representing the fact that viruses have only generally one nucleic acid compared with bacteria. This is a rather artificial system based on demographics of the viral genetic material, but it is an organizational scheme that has been used for years in

TABLE 7–18 Structure: Naked Capsid (Non-enveloped)

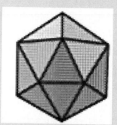

COMPONENTS	PROPERTIES
Protein	Environmentally stable
	Temperature
	Acid
	Proteases
	Detergents
	Drying
	Released from the cell by lysis

Clinical Consequences

1. Can be spread easily—on formites, hand to hand, dusts, small droplets
2. Can dry out and retain infectivity
3. Can survive the adverse conditions of the gut
4. Can be resistant to detergents and poor sewage treatment
5. Resistant to commonly used solvents (e.g., acetone, alcohol)
6. Elicit a protective antibody response

Examples

Poliovirus
Rotavirus
Adenovirus (fecal-oral, Table 7–22)

TABLE 7–19 Virus Structure Enveloped

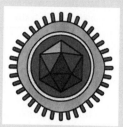

COMPONENTS	PROPERTIES
Membrane	Environmentally labile
Lipids	Disrupted by acid
Proteins	Disrupted by detergent
Glycoproteins	Disrupted by drying
	Disrupted by heat
	Modify cell membrane during replication
	Released by budding and cell lysis

Clinical Consequences

1. Must stay wet
2. Cannot survive the gut
3. Spreads in large droplets, secretions, and organ or blood transplants
4. Does not need to kill the cell to spread
5. Initiates a cell-mediated immune response
6. Antibody- and cell-mediated immune response may be necessary for protection and control
7. Pathogenesis often due to hypersensitivity and inflammation initiated by CMI

Examples

Measles
Mumps
Herpes
Influenza (respiratory, see Table 7–22)

teaching microbiology/virology. The reality is that viruses are transmitted clinically, not by their DNA or RNA material but rather by their seasonality and the routes by which they are transmitted-both of which are often interrelated.

In keeping with the tradition of a clinical focus, the route of transmission is also a means by which viruses may be grouped (**Table 7-22**). Viruses may be bloodborne; they may also be spread by close contact, fecal/oral contamination, the respiratory route, or **zoonoses**, where animal vectors play an important role.

Figure 7-6 describes the **seasonality** of certain viral diseases; that is, the predictability that these viruses will surface based on temperatures. These viruses spread via two target organ systems: respiratory and GI. This, in turn, is related to the definition of "structure equals function." Those that are respiratory viruses are transmitted predominantly via aerosol, based on their large envelope and attachment to droplets. In contrast, viruses that are transmitted via the GI system and fecal/oral route are usually small non-envelope viruses that may exist and maintain viability in passing through the relatively stringent environment of the GI system. As outlined in Figure 7-6, respiratory

viruses have a periodicity and are generally heralded by parainfluenza in early December followed by RSV and subsequently influenza in early to mid-January. Rhinovirus is the last of the respiratory viruses and is associated with a long-term presentation. In counterdistinction, viruses associated with the fecal/oral route are seen with periodicity that may not be recognized. Rotavirus, the most common

TABLE 7–20 DNA Viruses

FAMILY	IMPORTANT HUMAN VIRAL PATHOGENS
Pox	Smallpox, vaccinia
Herpes	Herpes simplex types 1 and 2, varicella-zoster, Epstein-Barr, cytomegalovirus, human herpes virus VI, VII
Adeno	Adenovirus
Ahepadna	Hepatitis B
Hepadna	JC virus, BK virus, simian virus 40 (SV40), Papova, papillomavirus
Parvo MRVO	Lu111, B19 virus, adeno-associated virus

TABLE 7–21 RNA Viruses

FAMILY	IMPORTANT HUMAN VIRAL PATHOGENS
Paramyxo	Parainfluenza Measles, mumps
Pneumovirus	Respiratory syncytial
Orthomyxo	Influenza types A and B
Arena	Lassa fever virus, Tacaribe virus complex (Junin virus and Machupo virus), lymphocytic choriomeningitis
Rhabdo	Rabies, vehicular stomatitis virus
Bunya	La Crosse (California encephalitis), sandfly fever, Crimean-Congo hemorrhagic fever
Retro	Human T cell leukemia types I and II, human immunodeficiency, Visna, etc.
Reo	Reto, Reo, California tick fever
Pico	Rhino, polio, ECHO, Coxsackie, encephalomyocarditis
Toga	Rubella, western, eastern, Venezuelan, equine encephalitis, Ross River, Sindbis, Semliki Forest
Flavi	Yellow fever, dengue, St. Louis encephalitis
Norwalk/calici	Norwalk agent
Delta	Delta agent

ECHO, enteric cytopathogenic human orphan.

cause of viral diarrhea in infants, starts predictably in the United States in Southwest Texas in October and migrates across the United States; its final presentation is in Maine in late March or early April.

Key Characteristics of Selected Viruses

Hepatitis B virus (HBV)

- Old terminology-Dane particle, serum hepatitis
- Dental health care workers at high risk for infection
- Vaccine available (adults can receive the first dose of the vaccine at any time; second dose at 1 to 2 months after the first dose; and the third dose 4 to 6 months after the first dose)
- Carrier state-5% to 10%
- Use of universal precautions and proper sterilization minimizes the risk of infection.
- Resistant virus that is difficult to destroy
- Present in many body fluids; transmissible through saliva as well as blood
- Comparative features of hepatitis viruses (Table 7-23)

AIDS-HIV = HIV-1 and HIV-2

- Depletion of T_4 helper cells/inducer lymphocytes
- Transmission through: blood transfusions, sharing needles for intravenous drug use; sexual contact-both homosexual and heterosexual; perinatal-from a mother to her baby across the placenta in utero, during birth, or via breast milk. There is no known transmission via saliva. Antibody

develops 3 to 10 weeks after exposure but may take as long as 6 months.

- Latent period-after exposure, before symptoms develop-3 months to 10 years
- Dental health care workers at low risk for infection
- Universal precautions and proper sterilization minimize risk.
- Symptomatic and asymptomatic patients with AIDS and AIDS-related complex (ARC) may present for dental treatment with oral symptoms, including oral candidiasis, various viral infections, bacterial periodontal infections, and neoplasms.

Herpes viruses

- These viruses are characterized by a latent stage that follows the initial infection.
- Reactivation from the latent phase may be triggered by stress, sunlight, or trauma.
- HSV type 1 (HSV-1) (oral) and HSV-2 (genital). Types 1 and 2 present the same clinically. The virus is latent in the trigeminal nerve. The viral reservoir is sulcular epithelium. Treat the virus with acyclovir during the prodromal phase. Lesions are infectious. Herpetic whitlow is a herpes infection of the fingers.
- Chickenpox/shingles-varicella-zoster virus (VZV). Chickenpox is the initial infection. Shingles is the recurrent form.
- Mononucleosis-Epstein-Barr virus (EBV). There is a latent period, and reactivation is possible.
- Cytomegalovirus infections-cytomegalovirus (CMV). CMV causes a mononucleosis-like illness in adults and severe illness in infants. It can also cause significant opportunistic infection in patients with AIDS. The virus is found in the tumor cells of Kaposi sarcoma. Routes of transmission include blood, sexual contact, saliva, droplet, and perinatal contact.

Mumps-mumps virus

- This virus is spread by droplets (saliva).

Immunology-The Immune System/Components

The consequences of microbial challenge to a multiorgan system is best described as a cascade of events. Over time, this cascade has been quantified and specialized so that selected cells respond to challenges by potential pathogenic organisms. This is a choreographed event that has evolved as the microorganisms have become more specialized and adapted to survival. When discussing this multisequence of events, it is convenient to organize them into the subsets that are coordinated but often sometimes act independently.

Disease barriers can first be divided into nonspecific resistance. These include mechanical and chemical barriers, the most important of which is intact skin. This involves intact mucous membranes, the nasal hairs, coughing and sneezing reflexes, tears and eyelashes, and secretions in microorganisms, particularly of the normal flora.

TABLE 7–22 Routes of Viral Transmission

A. BLOOD-BORNE VIRUSES

Family	Viruses	Disease
Hepadna virus	Hepatitis B	Hepatitis
Flavivirus	Hepatitis C	Non-A, non-B hepatitis
Retrovirus	Human immunodeficiency virus	AIDS
Retrovirus	Human T lymphotropic virus type 1	Leukemia, tropical spastic paraparesis
Herpes	Cytomegalovirus	Mononucleosis syndrome, pneumonia, hepatitis, febrile illness
Parvoviridae	Parvo B19	Fifth disease (erythema infectiosum), hydrops fetalis, transient aplastic crisis, acute parvo B19 infection

B. CLOSE CONTACT

Family	Virus	Disease
Herpes	Herpes simplex virus types 1 and 2	Oral/genital herpes, gingivostomatitis, pharyngitis, whitlow (finger), keratoconjunctivitis (eye), encephalitis/meningitis (CNS)
Herpes	Varicella-zoster*	Varicella (chickenpox) zoster (shingles)
Herpes	Epstein-Barr virus	Infectious mononucleosis
Herpes	Cytomegalovirus†	Mononucleosis syndrome
Herpes	Human herpes virus 6	Exanthem subitum (roseola)
Papova	Papilloma	Warts

C. FECAL-ORAL VIRUSES

Family	Virus	Disease
Picorna	Polio	Paralytic polia
Picorna	Hepatitis A	Hepatitis
Picorna	Coxsackie A virus‡	Herpangina, common cold, hand, foot and mouth disease, meningitis, paralysis
Picorna	Coxsackie B virus‡	Myocarditis, pleurodynia, common cold
Picorna	ECHO‡	Common cold, myocarditis
Reovirus	Rotavirus	Infantile diarrhea, gastroenteritis
Calici-?	Hepatitis E	Non-A, non-B hepatitis

D. RESPIRATORY VIRUSES

Family	Virus	Disease
Picorna	Rhinovirus	Common cold
Orthomyxo	Influenza	Influenza, common cold, croup, tracheobronchitis, pneumonia
Paramyxo	Parainfluenza	Croup, tracheobronchitis, bronchiolitis, pneumonia
Pneumovirus	Respiratory syncytial virus	Bronchiolitis, pneumonia (infants)
Paramyxo	Mumps	Mumps, encephalitis
Paramyxo	Measles	Measles, encephalitis, pneumonia
Adenovirus	Adenovirus!!	Pharyngitis, tracheobronchitis, keratoconjunctivitis, common cold, acute respiratory distress
Gastroenteritis		(type 40/41) Pneumonia

E. ZOONOSES

Family	Virus	Vector	Disease
Arboviruses	Venezuelan equine encephalitis	Aedes, Culex	Mild systemic or severe encephalitis
Alphaviruses	Eastern equine encephalitis	Aedes, Culiseta	Mild systemic; encephalitis
	Western equine encephalitis	Culex, Culiseta	Mild systemic; encephalitis
Flaviviruses	Dengue	Aedes	Mild systemic; dengue hemorrhagic fever/shock syndrome
	Yellow fever	Aedes	Hepatitis, hemorrhagic fever
	St. Louis encephalitis	Culex	Encephalitis; usually in adults
	Powassan	Ixodes ticks	Encephalitis
Bunyaviruses	California encephalitis virus/La Crosse virus	*Aedes triseriatus*	Mild systemic or encephalitis; usually in children
Rhabdoviruses	Rabies	Infected mammal	Fatal encephalitis
Arenaviruses	Lassa fever virus	Mastssomysnatalensis (large African rodent)	Hemorrhagic fever

*Spread mainly by respiratory means.
†Also spread in blood and organ transplants.
‡Certain types spread by respiratory route.
!!Also spread by the fecal-oral route.
AIDS, acquired immunodeficiency syndrome;

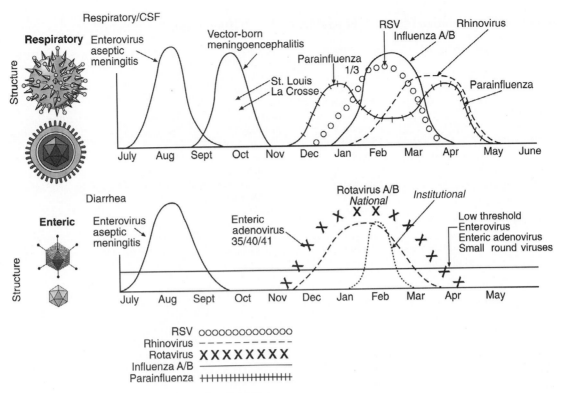

Figure 7-6. Seasonality of diseases involving viruses (predictability).

The normal or indigenous microflora/biofilm is a very significant barrier to invasion by potential putative pathogens. Pathogens need energy sources, and there is significant competition for selected nutrients and environmental and receptor sites on the targeted host cells. The normal or indigenous microflora consists of highly specialized bacteria that have become highly adapted to commensalism. These organism communities under the biofilm arrangement cause minimal damage under normal conditions. When the ecologic balance of the biofilm is disturbed, infections can occur, but the competition and biodiversity of the biofilm present a significant barrier to invasion by potential pathogens.

Inflammation is a nonspecific but predictable response of challenged cells. It includes a series of events that represent a dynamic process. Inflammation of sudden onset and short duration is characterized as acute; in contrast, chronic inflammation involves a significant length of time. It is important to remember that inflammation occurs only in living cells. Necrotic or dead tissues cannot mount an inflammatory response.

An important part of the inflammatory process is immigration of the white blood cells (leukocytes) from the blood vessels into the site of injury. There are six different kinds of white blood cells: neutrophils, monocytes, lymphocytes, plasma cells, eosinophils, and mast cells. The neutrophil [polymorphonuclear neutrophil (PMN) or leukocyte] is the first cell to immigrate to the site of injury and is a primary cell involved in acute inflammation. The monocyte or macrophage is the second cell to participate in the inflammatory response. The lymphocyte and plasma cells are involved in both chronic inflammation and immune response; the eosinophil and mast cell participate in both inflammatory and immune responses.

Mediators of inflammation are a group of chemicals that cause vasodilation, neutrophil migration, **chemotaxis**, and vascular permeability. Three integrated systems in the blood may be activated during the process. These include the kinin system, the clotting mechanism, and the complement system. The **kinin system** mediates inflammation by causing increased dilation. The **clotting mechanism** functions primarily in the clotting of blood. The **complement system** is a complicated interaction of at least 22 serum proteins that act in a sequential cascade and function in both inflammation and immunity. As shown in **Figure 7-7**, complement may be activated at C1 by an antigen-antibody complex or at C3 by endotoxins. Components of the complement system cause selected **mast cells** to release granules in the cytoplasm that contain the chemical histamine. **Histamine** causes an increase in vascular permeability and vasodilation.

An important and emerging group is a ubiquitous family of "prostaglandins" and "leukotrienes" derived from arachidonic acid known as the **eicosanoids.** This family consists of long chain components composed of polyunsaturated fatty acids synthesized in or on cells from arachidonic acid. The term *prostaglandin* was coined by early investigators who mistakenly believed that the prostate gland was the major source.

TABLE 7–23 Comparative Features of Hepatitis A, B, C, D (Delta), and E

FEATURE	HEPATITIS A	HEPATITIS B	HEPATITIS C	HEPATITIS D	HEPATITIS E
Taxonomy	Enterovirus 72 (Picornavirus)	Hepadeviridae (reverse transcriptase)	Flavivirus (enveloped)		Calicivirus (Picornavirus)
Incubation period	2–6 wk	4–26 wk	2–20 wk	4–8 wk	2–9 wk
Virus	27 nm/RNA	42 nm/DNA (incomplete/DNA)	30–60 nm/RNA	Incomplete/RNA	27–34 nm/RNA
Onset	Acute (variable)	Insidious	Insidious (variable)	Variable	Acute (variable)
Transmission	Fecal-oral	Parenteral (or equivalent)	Parenteral (or equivalent) STD/perinatal	Parenteral (or equivalent)	Fecal-oral
Severity	Mild	Moderate to severe	Variable	Severe	Variable
Fulminant hepatitis	Rare (<0.1%)	1–2%	0.5–1% (est.)	Common	0.1–0.5% (est.)
Symptoms	Fever, malaise, headache, anorexia, vomiting, dark urine, jaundice	Same as A, but 10–20% with serum sickness-like reaction	As with A	As with A	As with A
Carrier state	None	Yes	Yes	Yes	None
Chronicity (%)	0	5–10	50–70	Coinfection: 2–5; superinfection: >90	0
Association with blood transfusion (%)	Very rare	5–10	50–90	Unknown	0
Serology	Anti-HAV IgM fraction IgG fraction	HbsAg HbeAg Anti-HBs Anti-HBc IgM fraction IgG fraction Anti-HBe HBV	Anti-HCV 1°C 100-3 polypeptide (bloodbank) 2°C 1000 C22/33 polypeptide RIBA or confirmation	Anti-Delta IgM fraction IgG fraction Delta antigen Delta DNA	None
Postexposure prophylaxis	IG	HBIG + hepatitis B vaccine	Probably IG	Prevent type B	Unknown
Mortality rate (%)	<0.5	1–2	Unknown ?	Very high	1–2 (hospitalized patients) 10–20 (pregnancy)
Mechanism of hepatic injury	Cytotoxic antibody response	T lymphocyte cytotoxicity	Unknown	Probably direct viral hepatotoxicity	Unknown
Special notations	—	—	Cirrhosis 25%	—	Cholestasis more common

STD, sexually transmitted disease; HAV, hepatitis A virus; HBV, hepatitis B virus; HCV, hepatitis C virus; RIBA, recombinant immunoblot assay; IG, immunoglobulin; HBIG, hepatitis B immunoglobulin.

Prostaglandins are not stored but are produced when stimulated by cell damage or during cell activation. In general, the prostaglandins most commonly found in the body are:

- PGE_2
- PGF_2
- PGI_2

Recently, there has been growing awareness that these may be significantly involved in the association of periodontal disease as a risk factor for low birth weight babies.

Inflammation may be classified in clinical practice according to four parameters: (1) duration, (2) etiology, (3) location, and (4) morphology or pathologic characteristics. Inflammation is most often classified by duration. Acute inflammation lasts for a few hours to a few days and is usually considered to be severe and recurrent. Chronic inflammation, in contrast, may represent: (1) one extension of an acute inflammation,

(2) prolonged healing after acute inflammation, or (3) persistence of causative agents. Chronic inflammation also develops in response to foreign substances. For instance, a foreign body granuloma will develop around thorns in subcutaneous tissue. Likewise, people exposed to dust containing silica particles develop chronic lung silicosis.

Immune Response

The immune response has two different forms: a relatively nonspecific set of natural protective mechanisms and a complex system of cellular and **humoral** reactions (immunity in a body fluid) that evolve in response to repeated exposures to foreign substances-acquired immunity.

Natural immunity is made up of mechanical and chemical barriers, the most important of which includes intact skin and the four reservoirs of normal microbial flora.

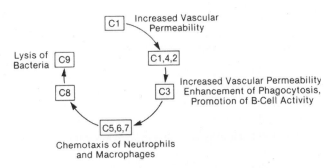

Figure 7-7. Complement system. Simplified scheme of sequential activation of the complement system and the functional activities related to periodontal disease. (From Allen DL, McFall WT, Jenzano J: Periodontics for the Dental Hygienist, 4th ed. Philadelphia, Lea & Febiger, 1987, p 48.)

Acquired immunity is based on specific responses elicited by foreign substances that act as **antigens.** The initial antigen-antibody reaction is amplified by a series of events that involve the cells of the immune system and closely related helper cells such as macrophages, basophils, and eosinophils. Importantly, acquired immunity is based on the ability of the body's immune system to distinguish self from non-self, to generate an immunologic memory, and to mount an integrated reaction of various cells. The ability of the body to mount an appropriate immune response is called **immunocompetence.**

The bone marrow stem cells give rise to two major cell lineages: lymphoid cells and all other hematopoietic cells. Descendants of the lymphoidal stem cells migrate to the thymus and mature into **T lymphocytes** and **B lymphocytes.** The bone marrow and thymus are called primary lymphoid organs, and the differentiation of T and B cells in them is developmentally programmed and unrelated to antigen stimulation. From the primary lymphoid organs, the T and B lymphocytes enter the blood circulation and colonize various secondary lymphoid organs. T and B lymphocytes have distinct functions even though morphologically they cannot be distinguished by light or electron microscopy.

There are two types of B lymphocytes. One type becomes the **plasma cell,** when stimulated by the antigen. The plasma cell produces the specific antibody needed to fight that targeted antigen. The other type of B lymphocyte is the **B memory cell.**

Plasma cells produce proteins called **antibodies.** Antibodies are called **immunoglobulins** and are carried in the blood. There are five different types of antibodies produced as shown in **Table 7-24.** Although they all have the same basic structure, they are arranged differently to accomplish this targeted task. This variation allows each type of antibody to function differently. The structure, the molecular weight, the percentage of the antibody in serum, the average half-life in serum, and the biologic functions are outlined in Table 7-24.

The T lymphocytes take their name from their association with the thymus. Different types of T lymphocytes have different functions. Some are memory cells; others are effectors or regular types, such as T helper cells that increase the function of the B lymphocytes. T suppressor cells suppress the functioning of the B lymphocytes.

TABLE 7–24 Humoral Components and Characteristics of the Immunoglobulin (Ig) Classes

CLASS COMPONENT	IGG MONOMER	IGG DIMER, MONOMER	IGM PENTAMER	IGD MONOMER	IGE MONOMER
Number of Antigen Binding Sites	2	4 2	10	2	2
Molecular Weight	150,000	170,000–385,000	900,000	180,000	200,000
Percent of Total Antibody in Serum	80%	13%	6%	1%	0.002%
Average Life in Serum (Days)	23	6	5	3	2.5
Crosses Placenta?	Yes	No	No	No	No
Binds Complement ?	Yes	No	Yes	No	No
Complement Binds To	Phagocytes	Phagocytes	B lymphocytes	B lymphocytes	Mast cells and basophils
Biological Functions	Long-term immunity; memory Abs	Secretory Ab; on mucous membrane	Produced at first response to Ag; can serve as B-cell receptor	Receptor on B cells	Antibody of some type of allergy; worm infections

IgG   IgA (dimer only)   IgM   IgD   IgE

Cytokines are messenger molecules of the immune system. The induction and regulation of the immune system involve multiple interactions among lymphocytes, monocytes, inflammatory cells, and endothelial cells. Many such interactions are mediated by short-acting cell mediators. Cytokines that are a soluble product of lymphocytes are called **lymphokines. Table 7-25** lists a number of the important cytokines and their main functions. Interleukin-1 (IL-1) is considered to be one of the most important **interleukins,** and its multiple functions are listed in **Table 7-26.**

When challenged, B lymphocytes and the production of antibodies respond either as a first exposure or a second exposure to the recognized and processed antigen. The primary response involves a latent period while the antigen is processed and the immune system is stimulated. The IgM is the first antibody to rise followed by an IgG, of which the total response is less than the second response, when the antigen is recognized by plasma cells. In the anamnestic response, the total antibody production is considerably higher, and the time frame for which the antigen exposure to mount a challenge of the antibody is significantly shorter. This is a reflection of the memory cells that had been produced in the first exposure.

Immune responses (humoral or cellular) to antigen stimulation of either endogenous or exogenous source can cause tissue-damaging reactions. Clinically, these are called **hypersensitivity reactions,** and the resultant tissue lesions are referred to as **hypersensitivity disease.** Hypersensitivity diseases are best classified on the basis of the immunologic mechanism mediating the disease. This is important, because it clarifies the manner in which the immune response ultimately causes tissue injury and damage. The four types of immune mediated disorders are outlined in **Table 7-27.**

There are also diseases of self-recognition or failure of the immune system that are called **autoimmune diseases,** and there are diseases where the immune system does not function at all or at a lower rate called **immunodeficiency diseases.**

Oral Immunology

General Host Defense Mechanism

Mechanical processes are a major factor in **defense mechanisms** of the oral cavity. They include the flow of saliva; desquamation of the oral mucosa; and motion of the lips, cheeks, and tongue.

Saliva contributes to defense in ways other than mechanical ones, because saliva contains a number of antibacterial substances, such as lysozyme, lactoferrin, and lactoperoxidase. Some salivary glycoproteins bind to bacteria and may prevent their adherence to the tooth. Saliva also contains immunoglobulins. The main immunoglobulin in saliva is secretory IgA (see Table 7-24). **Salivary IgA** may contribute to immunity in the mouth by preventing adherence of bacteria. Other immunoglobulins found in the gingival fluid include **IgG, IgA,** and **IgM.** Crevicular fluid also contains complement and phagocytic cells (mainly PMNs).

Prostaglandins are found in gingival tissue. The concentration of prostaglandin E_2 is higher in inflamed gingival tissue than in normal tissue. Both prostaglandins E_1 and E_2 stimulate bone reabsorption in experimental animals.

Interactions between the complex microflora of the oral cavity may also contribute to host defenses. α-Hemolytic streptococci are antagonistic to colonization of the oropharynx by *S. pyogenes, S. pneumoniae,* and *C. albicans.*

Disease-Specific Immunology

Immediate Hypersensitivity. PMNs, lymphocytes, plasma cells, and immunoglobulins in gingival tissue may reflect normal host defenses and may be protective. Some investigators think that they are related to destructive hypersensitivity reactions. Antigen-antibody reactions could result in complement activation, IgE mediated hypersensitivity, or Arthus reaction. Mast cells decrease in

TABLE 7–25 Main Functions of the Interleukins and Major Cytokines

CYTOKINE	BIOLOGIC EFFECTS
IL-1	Acute phase response, fever, T cell and macrophage activation, stimulation of bone marrow
IL-2	Growth factor for B and T cells; activates cytotoxic lymphocytes; enhances NK cell function
IL-3	Proliferation of pluripotent stem cells in marrow
IL-4	Induces IgE synthesis, T cell growth factor
IL-5	Eosinophil growth factor
IL-6	Differentiation of activated B cells
IL-7	Growth factor for immature B and T cells
IL-8	Neutrophil activator
IL-11	Megakaryocyte growth factor
Interferon (α, β, γ)	Interferes with viral replication
TNF-α	Acute-phase response, antitumor and leukocyte adherence
TNF-β	Increases release of IL-1, TNF, and other cytokines

IL, interleukin; NK, natural killer; TNF, tumor necrosis factor.

TABLE 7–26 Major Action of Interleukin-1

Inflammatory

Chemotactic for neutrophils, lymphocytes, and monocytes
Increased collagen synthesis
Increased collagen and proteoglycanase synthesis
PGE_2 production by synovial fibroblasts
Increased bone reabsorption via osteoclast-activating factor
Stimulates degranulation and release of nitric oxide

Immunologic

T cell activation: production of IL-2
B cell activation: acts as B cell growth factor
Lymphokine production increased: IL-2, IL-3, interferons

Systemic

CNS:	Fever
	Increased corticosteroid production
	Decreased appetite
	Increased slow-wave sleep
Metabolic:	Increased acute-phase proteins
	Amino acid release
	Decreased albumin synthesis
	Reduced serum iron and zinc levels
Hematologic:	Neutrophilia
	Lymphopenia
Vascular:	Increased adherence of leukocytes
	Increased PGI and PGE synthesis
	Increased platelet activating factor

CNS, central nervous system; IL, interleukin; PGE, prostaglandin E; PGI, prostaglandin I.

number in inflamed gingiva, perhaps due to degranulation. Histamine levels are elevated in inflamed gingiva.

Cell-Mediated Immune Response. Ivanyi and Lehner first demonstrated that lymphocytes from patients with periodontal disease were stimulated by antigen from dental plaque and from plaque bacteria and measured by blastogenic response. The degree of the blastogenic response was correlated with the degree of disease in cases of gingivitis and mild periodontitis. The response was reduced in patients who had severe periodontitis. Later, a blocking factor was found in patients with severe disease.

Some subsequent studies have confirmed the observations of Ivanyi and Lehner, whereas others have failed to show a correlation between lymphocyte blastogenesis and disease. Both B and T lymphocytes from patients with periodontal disease can be stimulated by antigen(s) from plaque bacteria to synthesize and release lymphokines.

Immune Mechanisms

The response of the host to plaque bacteria is thought by many workers to be the major mechanism of tissue destruction in periodontal disease.

Periodontal disease is initiated by several putative periodontal pathogens. The response mounted by the host to these pathogens includes recruitment of the host's inflammatory cells, such as neutrophils in the acute phase and monocytes or macrophages in the more chronic phase of the disease process. The periodontal pathogens incite these infiltrating inflammatory cells and also resident cells of the periodontium, such as fibroblasts, epithelial cells, and osteoblasts, to produce a number of host-derived mediators including cytokines and chemokines, which drive the inflammatory response. This host response is designed primarily to eliminate the pathogens associated with the periodontal infection. However, the broad spectrum of proteolytic enzymes that are released by the host cells can lead to breakdown of host tissues and the classic clinical manifestations of periodontal disease.

Matrix metalloproteinases (MMPs) are a family of at least 12 different zinc-dependent, neutral endopeptidases that can act together or with other biologic factors to degrade various components of the extracellular connective tissue matrix. In health, a balance of MMP activity along with naturally occurring inhibitors facilitates turnover of normal tissue. In response to the infection and inflammation characteristic of periodontal disease, the levels of these enzymes can greatly exceed the capacity of the constitutive

TABLE 7–27 Mechanisms of Immunologically Mediated Disorders

TYPE	PROTOTYPE DISORDER	IMMUNE MECHANISM
I Anaphylactic type	Anaphylaxis, some forms of bronchial asthma	Formation of IgE (cytotropic) antibody—release of vasoactive amines and other mediators from basophils and mast cells followed by recruitment of other inflammatory cells
II Cytotoxic type	Autoimmune hemolytic anemia, erythroblastosis fetalis, Goodpasture disease, pemphigus vulgaris	Formation of IgG, IgM—binds to antigen on the target cell surfaces—phagocytosis of the target cell or lysis of the target cell by C8, C9 fraction of the activated complement or antibody dependent cell-mediated cytotoxicity
III Immune complex disease	Arthus reaction, serum sickness, systemic lupus erythematosus, certain forms of acute glomerulonephritis	Antigen-antibody complexes—activated complement—attracted neutrophils—release of lysosomal enzymes and other toxic moieties
IV Cell-mediated (delayed) hypersensitivity	Tuberculosis, contact dermatitis, transplant rejection	Sensitized T lymphocytes—release of lymphokines and T cell–mediated cytotoxicity

regulatory mechanisms, resulting in degradation of periodontal tissues. Members of the MMP family include the collagenases, gelatinases, and stromelysins.

Bacteria in the Gingival Sulcus

The oral microbiota is unusually diverse; it consists of several hundred taxa, many of which reside on the tooth surface both above and below the gingival margin in a complex biofilm known as plaque. A subset of these species has been implicated in the pathogenesis of periodontal disease, and certain subspecies of these putative pathogens may be more virulent than other pathogens. Three of these microorganisms are commonly referred to as periodontal pathogens in the periodontal literature; these are *Actinobacillus actinomycetemcomitans* (Aa), *Porphyromonas gingivalis* (Pg), and *Prevotella intermedia* (Pi). Aa is most often associated with early-onset periodontitis, whereas Pg and Pi are more often associated with adult-onset periodontitis. Many other oral organisms have also been implicated in the pathogenic process. Some of these bacteria can invade directly into the periodontal tissues, rendering them extremely difficult to eliminate using traditional periodontal approaches such as scaling.

PMN collagenase and gelatinase (MMPs 8 and 9), which are thought to be responsible for most of the connective tissue breakdown, are evident in periodontitis.

Cell-to-Cell Mediators

Upon interaction with bacterial LPS, the monocytes, lymphocytes, and plasma cells release a number of substances that serve to regulate the function of other cells as well as the releasing cell types. These substances include cytokines (e.g., TNF and IL-1), chemokines, and prostanoids [e.g., prostaglandin E_2 (PGE$_2$)]. Cytokines specific to monocytes are called monokines; those specific to lymphocytes are called lymphokines. These chemical signaling substances induce the formation, secretion, and activation of MMPs from certain infiltrating and resident cells of the periodontium.

TNF, IL-1, and PGE$_2$ have all been implicated in the cascade of degradative activity that follows LPS stimulation of macrophages, and are thought to act synergistically with LPS to induce bone reabsorption. For example, IL-1 has been shown to promote PMN adherence to endothelium, induce procollagenase mRNA transcription in fibroblasts, autoinduce its own production by macrophages, stimulate PGE production by fibroblasts, and stimulate bone reabsorption by osteoclasts.

A wide variety of other cytokines, growth factors, and other immune cell products may be involved in periodontal breakdown. This complicated network of host cells and their mediators is the subject of numerous research programs worldwide. However, the cytokines may prove to be useful markers of the active phase of periodontal disease and facilitate the selection of appropriate treatment regimens. Overexpression of some of these substances as a result of genetic polymorphism may prove to be a significant risk factor in the development of the disease.

Procollagenase from Resident Cells

MMPs are expressed by resident cells as pro-enzymes, which are devoid of collagenolytic activity. Extracellular activation is required in order to produce functional enzyme. Pro-collagenases have a basic 5-domain structure, with the regions of the enzyme typically referred to as a signal peptide, a propeptide, a catalytic site, a hinge region, and a pepsin-like domain. Fibroblasts are the primary source for fibroblast type collagenase (MMP-1), which is the enzyme typically expressed constitutively in normal tissue turnover. Other MMPs expressed by resident cells of the periodontium include gelatinase (MMP-2), stromelysin (MMP-3), and the recently described osteoblast.

Breakdown of Collagen Matrix

Although the precise course remains to be fully elucidated, the cascade of events appears to culminate in the methodical destruction of the connective tissue of the periodontium, mediated by the MMPs. First, stomelysins remove the proteoglycan and fibronectin portions of the matrix, making the collagen fibril accessible to proteolytic degradation by the collagenases. Once cleaved, the collagen fiber begins to unfold and becomes susceptible to further degradation by gelatinases. As the disease progresses, bone reabsorption, mediated by osteoclast activation, results in the characteristic bone loss associated with periodontitis. Sub-antimicrobial doses of doxycycline (Periostat) inhibits the cascade of enzymes involved in this destructive process. Periostat has been approved by the FDA as an adjunctive antiinflammatory therapy in the treatment of periodontal disease.

 # MANAGEMENT/THERAPY AND USE OF ANTI-INFECTIVE AGENTS

There has been a growing awareness by the public as a whole and the medical community specifically that antibiotics have been overused, misused, and used in perhaps deleterious adjunctive means (e.g., their use as a food additive in agriculture). All this has contributed to a growing awareness that **resistance** is emerging and that there is a significant consequence and cost to the misuse and overuse of antibiotics, whether it is by the medical or dental community.

Limiting Microbial Growth

Antiseptics/Antimicrobials/ Anti-infective Agents

Antiseptics and antibiotics have been used to treat oral infections for some time. Although antiseptics and antibiotics have antibacterial properties, they represent two distinct and separate categories for agents. **Antiseptics** or chemical antimicrobial agents were administered locally, usually as a wash, whereas **antimicrobial agents** could be administered either topically or systemically for more serious infections. A third category has now arisen for the local delivery of antimicrobial agents. This **sustained-release delivery** makes it possible to use antimicrobial agents to augment the benefits of mechanical periodontal therapy. Each of these is discussed later with emphasis on dental management.

In dentistry, **antiseptics** are chemical antimicrobial agents that are applied topically or subgingivally to mucous membranes, wounds, or intact dermal surfaces to inhibit microorganisms, their reproduction, or their metabolism. Most are bactericidal, although some are bacteriostatic. In general, they are used in various topically applied products in conjunction with a mechanical cleansing or débridement. Effectiveness depends on formulation, concentration, and quantity and varies widely among agents utilized. Antiseptics are usually available without prescription, because they have an excellent safety profile and result in no significant bacterial resistance. **Table 7-28** is a summary of differences between antiseptics and antibiotics.

The most commonly used disinfectants in dentistry are discussed in Chapter 12.

Antibiotics

Antibiotics are organic substances that can destroy and inhibit the growth of bacteria and other organisms by targeting specific sites of action. Most antibiotics have been isolated and purified from their natural source and are prepared synthetically or semisynthetically. In contrast to antiseptics, they are administered orally (PO), parenterally (IM or IV), and most recently via sustained-release local delivery systems.

Antimicrobial activity varies according to the agent selected, dosage, route of administration, whether the organism responds to the antibiotic, and whether the antibiotic can reach the site of infection. Some antibiotics are effective against selected gram-positive organisms, and some attack gram-negative bacteria. Some are most effective against aerobic bacteria, and others are most effective against anaerobic bacteria. **Table 7-29** lists the most frequently used oral antibiotics in dentistry and the organisms that are responsive to them. The number of classes of antimicrobial agents continues to grow as emerging bacterial resistance reduces the effectiveness of earlier generations. **Resistance** refers to the ability of an organism to resist the effects of an antagonistic agent (e.g., a bacterial pathogen immune to an antibiotic). The most commonly prescribed antimicrobial agents in dentistry include the penicillins, tetracy-

clines, metronidazole, clindamycin, and the quinolones. Remarkably, in this era of antibiotic resistance, most oral infections that require antibiotics in addition to surgical therapy still respond well to a simple penicillin or an early generation cephalosporin. However, the evidence shows that this is changing. Resistance has an impact on decisions made relative to the dosing frequency, the amount of antibiotic, and the length of time. Obviously, there is no optimum for one antibiotic, and each must be evaluated in the clinical picture of the patient, the age, the site of the infection, and the potential organisms present at that site (i.e., the composition of the biofilm). However, principles and strategies that minimize the development of resistance while maximizing the benefit of anti-infective therapy including: (1) antisepsis, (2) antibiotics (local or systemic), or (3) adjunctive therapy (local delivery, sustained release) are being evaluated.

Spectrum of Activity

Classification of antibiotics may be based on a number of characteristics, which may include antibiotic class, mode of action, and whether or not the ultimate outcome of the action is a bacteriostatic or bactericidal impact on the microbial target. **Table 7-30** lists the antibiotic class segregated by mode of action and ultimate bacterial activity.

Bacteriostatic Versus Bactericidal Antibiotics

Antibiotics are classified primarily as bacteriostatic or bactericidal agents based on their mode of action and cellular target site. **Bacteriostatic drugs** inhibit the growth and replication of microorganisms. The final eradication of the pathogen is accomplished by the immune system of the host. **Bactericidal drugs** kill and thus eradicate the organisms. In critical infections, where host defenses are impaired and drug levels may be moderate, the complete killing and lysis of bacteria by bactericidal agents is preferred to rapidly control the infection and prevent a relapse or recurrent infection. With in vivo testing, the bactericidal effect often results in sharp end points of growth or no growth. Depending on the organism involved and the drug pharmacodynamics/pharmacokinetics, an antibiotic may have bacteriostatic, bactericidal, or a combination of both types of activity. The distinction between bacteriostatic and bactericidal activity can be relative; at high enough con-

TABLE 7–28 Summary of Differences Between Antiseptics and Antibiotics

	PRESCRIPTION REQUIRED	INCIDENCE OF ADVERSE EFFECTS	DEVELOPMENT OF RESISTANCE	SPECTRUM OF ACTION	SAFE FOR FREQUENT USE	MOST COMMON ROUTE OF ADMINISTRATION
Antiseptics	No	Low	Rare	Broad	Yes	Local
Antibiotics	Yes	Moderate	Low-moderate	Limited	No	Oral or systemic

TABLE 7–29 Antibiotics Used in Oral Infections

	ACTIVITY		
ANTIBIOTIC CLASS	G + A	G + ANA	G − ANA
1. Oral penicillins	+	+	+/−
2. Oral cephalosporins	+	−	−
3. Oral macrolides			
Old (erythromycin)	+	−	−
New (Biax/azithromycin)	+	+/−	+
4. Oral (other)			
Clindamycin	+	−	+
Metronidazole	−	−	+
Tetracyclines	−	−	+/−
5. Oral fluoroquinolones			
Old (ciprofloxacin)	+	−	+/−
New (ofloxacin)	+	+	+

G + A, gram-positive aerobe; G + ANA, gram-positive anaerobe; G − ANA, gram-negative anaerobe. + = active; − = inactive; +/− = variable.

centrations, some bacteriostatic agents can achieve bactericidal action.

ANTIBIOTICS AND SUSTAINED RELEASE LOCAL DELIVERY

Given the growing concerns with resistance and the need for targeted concentrated antimicrobial agents, local delivery systems have been formulated and approved by the Food and Drug Administration (FDA). Presently, four products have been approved in the United States: Actisite, Atridox, Arestin, and Periochip. Three of these products use a tetracycline or a tetracycline analog, whereas the fourth uses chlorhexidine gluconate. It is important to remember that these products are recommended as adjunctive therapy to traditional periodontal débridement. Although Periostat is doxycycline, it is administered systemically in a subantimicrobial dose and is considered an immune modulating therapy rather than an anti-infective. (See Chapter 13.)

PHARMACOKINETICS OF ANTIBIOTIC USE

Principles of Antibiotic Dosing for Orofacial Infections

- Employ **high doses** for a short time. Successful use of antibiotics depends on maintaining the blood and tissue concentrations above the minimal inhibitory concentration for the organism. High concentrations are more critical with aminoglycosides, metronidazole, and quinolones (i.e., concentration-dependent antibiotics), whereas prolonged exposure of the organism to the antimicrobial agent is more critical with the β-lactams (i.e., time-dependent an-

tibiotics). Prolonged dosing beyond what is necessary only increases antibiotic toxicity, allergy, and selection of resistant microorganisms.
- Use an oral antibiotic loading dose. Without a loading dose, it takes 6 to 12 hours to achieve maximum therapeutic blood and tissue levels via oral administration.
- Achieve **blood levels** of the antibiotic at two to eight times the minimal inhibitory concentration. Such blood levels are necessary to compensate for the tissue barriers that impede antibiotic penetration into the site of the infection.
- Use **frequent dosing intervals.** This is important with the older β-lactam antibiotics, such as penicillin V and the first-generation cephalosporins (e.g., cephalexin, cephradine) in order to maintain relatively constant blood levels.
- Determine the duration of therapy by the remission of disease. The antimicrobial agent is terminated when the patient's host defenses have gained control of the infection and the infection is reasonably certain to resolve or has resolved.

As continually emphasized, there is a growing recognition of antibiotic resistance and the need to use antibiotics appropriately. Re-evaluation and design of antibiotic utilization are outlined in the following points.

Duration of Antibiotic Therapy

A significant misconception in antibiotic therapy is that use of an antibiotic requires a "complete course" of therapy. Conceptual errors about a preordained "course" of antimicrobial therapy emanate from several faulty assumptions:

- Prolonged antimicrobial therapy destroys resistant microorganisms. This is a contradiction in terms, because antimicrobial agents cannot affect microorganisms that are resistant to them (i.e., the definition of microbial resistance), and the prolonged use of antimicrobial agents only serves to select for these resistant species.
- Prolonged antibiotic therapy is necessary for "rebound" infections that recur, because the organisms are suppressed but are not eliminated. Acute orofacial infections do not rebound, particularly if the source of the infection is properly eradicated.
- Antibiotic dosages and duration of therapy can be extrapolated from one infection to another. This is not possible given the variability in infectious processes.

The ideal duration of antibiotic therapy is the shortest that will prevent both clinical and microbiologic relapse. The only practical guide for determining the effectiveness of antimicrobial treatment, and hence the duration of therapy, is clinical improvement of the patient as judged by remission of the infection.

Acute orofacial infections have a rapid onset and relatively short duration of 2 to 7 days or less, particularly if the offending cause is treated or eliminated. If clinical experience and the nature of the infection dictate that its anticipated course will be 3 days, then 3 days of antibiotic therapy

TABLE 7–30 Spectrum of Activity by Antibiotic Class and Mode of Action

MODE OF ANTIBIOTIC ACTION	BACTERIAL ACTIVITY: BACTERICIDAL VS BACTERIOSTATIC	ANTIBIOTIC CLASS
Interference with cell wall synthesis	Bactericidal	Penicillins Cephalosporins β-Lactamase inhibitor combinations Monobactams Carbapenems Glycopeptides Fosfomycin
Interference with DNA replication	Bactericidal	Quinolones Metronidazole Rifampicin
Interference with protein synthesis	Bactericidal Bacteriostatic	Aminoglycosides Tetracyclines Streptogramins Oxazolidinones Chloramphenicol
	Bacteriostatic or bactericidal*	Macrolides Lincomycin Clindamycin
Interference with folic acid synthesis	Bacteriostatic	Sulfonamides Trimethoprim Sulfonamide and trimethoprim combination may sometimes have bactericidal activity

*Depends on the pathogen and drug concentration.

is enough; if 5 days, then 5 days of therapy, and so forth. When clinical evidence indicates that the infection is reasonably certain to resolve or is resolved, the antibiotic therapy should be terminated.

Unfortunately, there is limited information on the current dosage, dosing interval, or duration of dosing for the antimicrobial management of periodontopathic microorganisms. These infections may not differ substantially from other infections; therefore, until sound clinical data exist to the contrary, the antimicrobial pharmacokinetic principles of vigorous dosage and short duration should be applied. Also, due consideration should be given to risks of antimicrobial allergy and toxicity and alterations in the patient's microbial ecology.

Failures in Antibiotic Therapy

Clinical Reasons for Antibiotic Failure

- Inappropriate choice of antibiotic (the microorganism is not susceptible)
- Emergence of antibiotic-resistant microorganisms (rebound infections, superinfections, and selection of resistant microbes)
- A blood concentration of the antibiotic that is too low (faulty dosing)
- Slow growth rate of microorganisms (β-lactams require dividing organisms for activity; older abscesses have a slow microbial growth rate)

- Impaired host defenses (suboptimal activity of the patient's immune and inflammatory systems)
- Patient noncompliance (failure to take antibiotics properly)
- Antibiotic antagonism (if multiple antibiotics are used)
- Inability of the antibiotic to penetrate to the site of the infection (purulence, tissue barriers, inoculum effect, and glycocalyx production)
- Limited vascularity or decreased blood flow (foreign bodies or implants: heart implants, orthopedic devices, dental implants, diabetic limbs, and osteomyelitis)
- Unfavorable local factors (decreased tissue pH or oxygen tension)
- Failure to eradicate the source of the infection (lack of incision and drainage)

Premedication for Dental Procedures: Prophylaxis Revisited

For the past 40 years, anecdotal information has suggested a link between dental procedures and the onset of endocarditis, which is a potentially deadly inflammation of the heart's lining or valves caused by bacterial infection. As a result, professional guidelines issued jointly by the American Heart Association (AHA) and the American Dental Association (ADA) have recommended the administration of prophylactic antibiotics to dental patients who are considered to be at risk for the development of endocarditis (e.g., patients with known heart valvular cardiac problems, including mitral valve prolapse with regurgitation and organic heart murmurs).

Endocarditis prophylaxis is recommended for the following cardiac conditions:

High-risk category
- Posthetic cardiac valves
- History of previous bacterial endocarditis
- Complex cyanotic congenital heart disease (e.g., tetralogy of Fallot)
- Surgically constructed systemic pulmonary shunts

Moderate risk category
- Most other congenital cardiac malformations
- Acquired valvular dysfunction (e.g., rheumatic heart disease)
- Hypertrophic cardiomyopathy
- Mitral valve prolapse with valvular regurgitation or thickened leaflets

Antibiotic prophylaxis is recommended for following dental procedures in susceptible patients:

Dental extractions
Periodontal procedures including surgery, scaling, and root planing, probing, and recall maintenance
Placement of dental implants
Endodontic surgery, instrumentation beyond the apex
Initial placement of orthodontic bands
Intraligamentary local anesthetic injections

Antibiotic prophylaxis is not routinely indicated for most dental patients with total joint replacements and is also not routinely indicated pins, plates, and screws. Antibiotic prophylaxis is suggested for patients who are at increased risk of hematogenous joint infection. They include patients with the following criteria: immunocompromised/immunosuppressed, insulin-dependent (type 1) diabetes, the first 2 years after joint replacement, previous prosthetic joint infection, malnourishment, and hemophilia (see Chapter 12).

Prophylactic Antibiotic Regimens for Dental Procedures

Situation	Agent	Regimen
• Standard prophylaxis	Amoxicillin	2 g PO 1 hr before the procedure
• Unable to take oral medications	Ampicillin	2 g IM/IV 30 minutes before the procedure
• Allergic to penicillin	Clindamycin	600 mg PO 1 hr before the procedure
• Allergic to penicillin and unable to take oral medications	Clindamycin *or* Cefazolin	600 mg IV 30 minutes before the procedure / 1 g IM or IV 30 minutes before the procedure

From Dajani AS, et al: Prevention of bacterial endocarditis: Recommendations of the American Heart Association. JAMA 277(22):1794-1801, 1997.

Laboratory Assessment/Techniques

Infections of the oral cavity are common and cause approximately 1% of all persons to visit a physician each year. The best diagnostic approach begins with a careful history and physical examination followed by specific laboratory tests to detect suspected pathogens.

Given the current economic environment and the recognition that laboratory tests may be expensive, a cascade approach can be utilized. This approach is based on the species of the potential pathogen(s) suspected and whether or not this is a potential pathogen based on Koch's postulates versus the Germ Theory. The following laboratory tests are categorized by type; the least expensive methodologies are listed first, and those that require greater expertise, cost, and time are listed last. With the numerous molecular methodologies emerging and rapid antigen detection feasible using monoclonal antibodies, cost-effective strategies with rapid turnaround are emerging. These strategies enhance the ability of a diagnostic laboratory to rapidly detect the causative organism or mixed species consortia.

Bacterial Screening

Tests for Caries Activity

Lactobacillus Count. Saliva is diluted and plated on a subjective medium for lactobacilli (e.g., Rogosa agar), then the number of colony-forming units are counted after a suitable incubation period.

The advantage is that salivary lactobacilli generally reflect the disease status of people with high caries and very low caries activity.

The disadvantage is that **salivary lactobacillus counts** do not correlate well in people with moderate caries activity; these counts cannot be used successfully to predict caries. This test counts total lactobacilli, but all species may not be equally cariogenic.

Snyder Test. **In the Snyder test,** 1 ml of saliva is placed in melted **Snyder agar** and mixed; the medium is allowed to solidify. The medium, which consists of nutrient agar at a pH of 5.0, contains a pH indicator that turns yellow below a pH of 4.0. If the medium turns yellow after being incubated for 24 to 48 hours, acid has been produced and the test result is positive.

The Snyder test is essentially a simplified relative lactobacillus count. The advantages and disadvantages are already listed. There is a statistically significant correlation between caries activity and a positive result on a Snyder test in large groups of people. The correlation is not good when individuals are evaluated.

Saliva Acidity. Several tests (e.g., Karshan, Swerdlove, Turner, and Crane) directly measure the acidity of saliva. Other tests (e.g., Rickles' test) measure the acidity of saliva after several hours of incubation with a carbohydrate.

The advantage is that the test should measure acidity produced by all acidogenic bacteria in saliva and not just the aciduric types.

In terms of the disadvantages, only a few clinical trials have been done and the available results are inconsistent. Because the most numerous acidogenic organism in saliva (i.e., *S. salivarius*) is seldom found in plaque and the carcinogenic *S. mutans* is found mainly in plaque, the ability of saliva to produce acid may not reflect the carcinogenic potential of plaque. Such tests will probably prove useless as predictors of susceptibility to caries.

Detection of Streptococcus mutans in Interproximal Areas or on Tooth Surfaces

Orion Diagnostica Site Strip. The Dentocult SM Site Strip is used to estimate the presence of *S. mutans* in interproximal areas or on tooth surfaces. The locations that best represent the extent of *mutans* colonization are usually the buccal and proximal sites of maxillary posterior teeth. Furthermore, restored surfaces are normally more colonized by *S. mutans* than are sound surfaces.

Tests for Bacteria Associated with Periodontal Disease

Screening **PERIOSCAN** reagent cards and strips are in vitro tests indicated for use on patients with clinical evidence of periodontal disease:

- To detect a BANA-hydrolase from *Porphyromonas (Bacteroides) gingivalis, Bacteroides forsythus,* and *Treponema denticola,* anaerobic bacteria associated with adult periodontal disease in discrete oral sites
- As an adjunct to clinical observations in the diagnosis and management of adult periodontal disease
- As an adjunct to clinical observations in the monitoring of sites during periodontal therapy or on maintenance recall

Cultivable Oral Microbiology

The purpose of periodontal microbiology testing is to identify microorganisms associated with periodontitis and test their susceptibility and resistance to various antibiotics to aid in periodontal treatment planning, particularly with regard to the use of antibiotics.

Cases to Culture

- Early onset: prepubertal periodontitis, juvenile periodontitis, rapidly progressive periodontitis
- Rapidly progressive: periodontitis associated with some systemic diseases
- Refractory

- Patients with poor plaque control should not be considered good candidates for microbial testing. Local factors should be controlled before sampling is done.

Time to Culture

All samples are to be taken before débridement:
- At baseline to aid in treatment planning
- 1 month after débridement for those who have not responded to mechanical therapy
- At least 1 month (preferably 3 months) after antibiotic treatment to determine antibiotic efficacy

Preparation

Identify one to three sites to be cultured. For cases with multiple sites, collect a representative sample. Use sites that are at least 5 mm in depth and that bleed upon probing.

Normally, cultural techniques attempt to recover the following organisms: *Actinobacillus actinomycetemcomitans, Capnocytophaga* sp, *Prevotella intermedia, Eikenella corrodens, Enterococcus* sp, *Peptostreptococcus micros, B. forsythus, Porphyromonas gingivalis, Staphylococcus* sp, gram-negative enterics, and yeast. The total anaerobic count from the subgingival plaque sample as well as the facultative anaerobic count is calculated, and the proportion of isolates is assessed.

Susceptibility Testing

With the growing concern of antibiotic resistance and the potential consequence of misuse or overuse of antibiotics, directed therapy based on susceptibility testing is now becoming more significant. Several procedures are available to determine whether an organism is susceptible, intermediate, or resistant. It is important, however, to remember that standards have been established by the **National Committee for Clinical Laboratory Standards** (NCCLS) that specifically quantify the amount of antibiotic necessary to categorize whether an antibiotic and the organism interaction would have a clinical response equivalent to qualify as susceptible, intermediate, or resistant. Guidelines, which are published annually, update the "breakpoints" that establish the three categories described as S, I, and R. Given that most periopathogens are anaerobic, susceptibility testing involves additional technical difficulties and requires some expertise. Various methods have evolved, including agar dilution. The newest method is the **Etest** (AB Biodisk, Sweden). This test allows for evaluation of 30 concentrations on an impregnated strip where antibiotic concentrations are layered and not dependent on two-fold concentrations (as in the traditional two-fold dilution assay used in traditional susceptibility testing).

Darkfield Microscopy

Before a subgingival plaque specimen is inoculated onto selective and differential blood agar plates, the specimen is examined under the darkfield microscope. **Darkfield microscopy** is used instead of the traditional Gram stain so that the spirochetes (small, intermediate, and large) may be visualized. It is important to remember that although *Treponema denticola* is potentially cultable, there is a ratio of small, intermediate, and large that has the greatest prediction as to the impact of treponemes on the periodontal process and the staging of the event.

Non-cultable Techniques

Non-cultable techniques include direct detection by molecular probes or immunofluorescence (antigen-antibody).

Given that most organisms associated with periodontal disease may be difficult to recover and may require extensive expertise in anaerobic bacteriology, alternative methods have arisen. Some researchers utilize **DNA probe**-based tests that detect conserved gene sequences within a target nucleic acid of periodontal pathogens. A commercial system utilizes this approach. Other researchers in academic environments such as the Forsyth Dental School, Boston, MA) use a checkboard assay for identifying and quantifying the amount of DNA for selected pathogens. Others have found **immunofluorescence** to be particularly appropriate for *B. forsythus* and *P. gingivalis,* suggesting that these two species are not reliably recovered by traditional cultures.

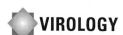

VIROLOGY

Several oral infections are not bacterial but have a viral etiology. These infections may include herpangina associated with enteroviruses, vesicular eruptions associated with HSVs, and recovery from sputum or pharyngeal cultures for RSV in pediatrics and influenza virus in pediatrics or adults. Most viral infections are of an acute nature (as described earlier) and have as a unique feature the fact that in the pro-

drome or incubation period, the highest viral bioburden is evident. Once infection has resulted in clinical symptoms, the number of viral particles is reduced given the essential response of the immune system. Within **5 to 7 days** after symptomatology, the amount of viral particles present is generally beyond the level of detection for most clinical laboratories. Therefore, timing of viral specimens is paramount, and those generally collected after the 10th day of clinical presentation are very low in yielding positive clinical correlatable results. Specimens for highest yield for culturable viruses should be collected within 5 days of acute onset. At the same time, an acute phase serum may be drawn that would allow for, in certain cases, the detection of **IgM** specimen marker by fluorescent antibody technique. In traditional assays, measuring the change between the acute serum and that collected approximately **10 to 21** days in the convalescent stage allows for a measurable change in the antibody titer.

Table 7-31 shows the significance of positive viral cultures. For example, herpes virus infections may lower the resistance of the periodontal tissue, thus increasing the risk for periodontopathic bacterial overgrowth. In general, viruses increase an individual's vulnerability to superinfection. Recovery of a virus is not always directly related to pathogenicity. There are three categories of diagnostic virology and the recovery of virus. These are **diagnostic** where the virus is not considered normal flora, **probable** where it correlates best with viral surveillance or seasonality, and **possible** where the viral recovery is only predictive of disease when augmented with additional laboratory detection methods, usually serologic.

Suggested Readings

Arrona G, De Rosa A, Rossa F, et al: A biocompatibility study and the effects of slow-release antibiotic materials in the treatment of periodontal disease. The biocompatibility of cellulose acetate charged with 25% tetracycline hydrochloride. A clinical and scanning microscopic study of a case. Minerva Stomatol 47(10):553-557, 1998.

TABLE 7–31 Significance of Positive Viral Culture Results

SOURCE OF POSITIVE CULTURE STUDIES/COMMENTS	INTERPRETATION	ADDITION
1. Skin lesion, vesicular fluid; cervix; eye; cerebrospinal fluid; blood (buffy coat); other body fluids; tissue or biopsy material	DIAGNOSTIC of infection in site culture	Viruses are not considered normal flora at any of these sites
2. Throat, bronchial washings; urine	PROBABLE cause of clinical disease	Correlates best with viral surveillance in area. Viruses can be cultured during subclinical infection and during incubation after exposure. Latent viruses may be reactivated and detectable even in the absence of clinical disease. Serology studies are of limited value.
3. Stool; fecal swabs	POSSIBLE association with clinical illness and may NOT be associated with disease; same viral isolate from other sites; serologic conversion to homologous viruses	Adenoviruses and enteroviruses must be interpreted cautiously in children

Barone A, Sbordone L, Ramaglia L, Ciaglia RN: Microbiotica associated with refractory peridontitis: Prevalence and antibiotic susceptibility. Minerva Stomatol 48(5):191-201, 1996.

Blandizzi C, Malizia T, Lupetti A, et al: Periodontal tissue disposition of Axithromycin in patients affected by chronic inflammatory periodontal diseases. J Periodontol 70(9):960-966, 1999.

Caton JG: Evaluation of Periostat for patient management. Comp Cont Educ Dentistry 20(5):451-456, 1999.

Ciancio SG: Antiseptics and antibiotics as chemotherapeutic agents for periodontitis management. Comp Cont Educ Dentistry 21(1):59-76, 2000.

Colombo AP, Haffajee AD, Smith CM, et al: Discrimination of refractory periodontitis subjects using clinical and laboratory parameters alone and in combination. J Clin Periodontol 26(9):569-576, 1999.

Colombo AP, Sakellari D, Haffajee AD, et al: Serum antibodies reacting with subgingival species in refractory periodontitis subjects. J Clin Periodontol 25(7):596-604, 1998.

Contreras A, Umeda M, Chen C, et al: J Periodontol 70(5):478-484, 1999.

Darby ML: Microbiology in Mosby's Comprehensive Review of Dental Hygiene, 4th ed. St. Louis, CV Mosby, 1998, pp 246-323.

Guggenheim Z, Shapiro S (eds): Oral Biology at the Turn of the Century: Misconceptions, Truths, Challenges, and Prospects. Basel, Switzerland, S. Karger, 1998.

Jorgensen MG, Slots J: Practical antimicrobial periodontal therapy. Comp Cont Educ Dentistry 21(2):111-112, 2000.

Killoy WJ, Polson AM: Controlled local delivery of antimicrobials in the treatment of periodontitis. Dent Clin North Am 42(2):263-283, 1998.

Kinane DF, Radvar M: A six-month comparison of three periodontal local antimicrobial therapies in persistent periodontal pockets. J Periodontol 70(1):1-7, 1999.

Lang NP, Nyman SR (eds): Implant and crown and bridge therapy in the periodontally compromised patient. Periodontology 2000. Copenhagen, Munksgaard International Publishers, 1994, Vol 4, pp 1-159.

Lo Bue AM, Nicoletti G, Toscano MA, et al: *Porphyromonas gingivalis*: Prevalence related to other microorganisms in adult refractory periodontitis. New Microbiol 22(3):209-218, 1999.

Lo Bue AM, Rosseti B, Cali G, et al: Antimicrobial Interference of a subinhibitory concentration of azithromycin on fimbrial production of *Porphyromonas gingivalis*. J Antimicrob Chemother 40(5):653-657, 1997.

Schuster GS: Oral flora and pathogenic organisms. Infect Dis Clin North Am 13(4):757-774, 1999.

Murdoch DA: Gram-positive anaerobic cocci. Clin Microbiol Rev 11(1):81-120, 1998.

Newman HN, Wilson M (eds): Dental Plaque Revisited: Oral Biofilms in Health and Disease. London, University College, Eastman Dental Institute, 1999.

Nisengard RJ, Newman MG: Oral Microbiology and Immunology, 2nd ed. Philadelphia, WB Saunders, 1994, pp 319-513.

Oral and Dental Diseases. In Clinical Infectious Diseases, Vol. 25 (Suppl 2) September, 1997. Proceedings of the 1996 Meeting of the Anaerobic Society of the Americas, July 19-21, Chicago, IL.

Seymour RA, Heasman PA: Pharmacological control of periodontal disease. II: Antimicrobial agents. J Dent 23(1):5-14, 1995.

Slots J, Rams TE (eds): Systemic and topical antimicrobial therapy in periodontics. Periodontology 2000. Copenhagen, Munksgaard International Publishers, Vol 10, 1996, pp 5-159.

Socransky SS, Haffajee AD (eds): Microbiology and immunology of periodontal diseases. Periodontology 2000. Copenhagen, Munksgaard International Publishers, Vol 5, 1994, pp 7-168.

Soder B, Nedlich U, Jin LJ: Longitudinal effect of non-surgical treatment and systemic metronidazole for 1 week in smokers and non-smokers with refractory periodontitis: A 5-year study. J Periodontol 70:761-771, 1999.

Soskolne WA, Chajek T, Flashner M, et al: An in vivo study of the chlorhexidine release profile of the Periochip in the gingival crevicular fluid, plasma, and urine. J Clin Periodontol 25(12):1017-1021, 1998.

Van Dyke TE (ed): Special patient categories. Periodontology 2000. Copenhagen, Munksgaard International Publishers, Vol 6, 1994, pp 7-124.

Vandekerckhove BN, Quirynen M, van Steen berghe D: The use of tetracycline-containing controlled-release fibers in the treatment of refractory periodontitis. J Periodontol 68(4):353-361, 1997.

Varvara G, D'Arcangelo C: The evaluation of the clinical efficacy and tolerance of azithromycin in odontostomatological infections. Minerva Stomatol 47(1-2):57-62, 1998.

Questions and Answers

Questions

Microbiology/Epidemiology

1. Which of the following genera are gram-negative bacteria that grow well at -150 mV (eH) and are strongly associated with periodontal disease?
   A. *Treponema* sp
   B. *Actinomyces* sp
   C. *Streptococcus* sp
   D. *Porphyromonas* sp

2. In periodontal disease, which morphotype size of the treponema spirochete is most commonly associated with advancing periodontal disease?
   A. Small, S, treponema
   B. Intermediate, I, treponema
   C. Large, L, treponema
   D. *Treponema denticola*

3. Which of the following reasons explains why *Streptococcus mutans* is a cariogenic pathogen?
   A. It grows most efficiently in a positive eH (+30 mV) oxygen-enriched environment.
   B. It is a strict anaerobe.
   C. It is a gram-negative bacterium associated with endotoxin production.
   D. It survives in a very low pH similar to that of *Lactobacillus* sp.

4. The established number of oral flora totals _____ microbes?
   A. <100
   B. 300-550
   C. >700
   D. Unknown

Oral Plaque/Biofilm

5. Which morphotype of the organism is most often associated with progressive periodontal disease, defining a deep pocket and highly anaerobic environment measured as -150 to 170 mV (eH)?
   A. Cocci
   B. Budding yeast
   C. Short gram-negative rods
   D. Filamentous gram-positive rods

6. A biofilm is a "community" of microbes from many species that live in a coordinated environment that is responsive to stress. Which of the following statements is most indicative of this biofilm?
   A. Its biomass becomes greater in the presence of antibiotics.
   B. Bacteria within the biofilm represent a "sessile" community of microbes in contrast to free-floating "planktonic" microbes.
   C. It is much more resistant to topical as well as systemic antibiotics.
   D. All of the above are true.

7. Which of the following describes the origin of microbes that comprise approximately 20% of plaque?
   A. Vaginal vault, if vaginally delivered
   B. Caregiver, if delivered by a cesarean section
   C. Are well established within 3 days after birth
   D. All of the above

8. Multispecies organisms comprising the flora of the tongue are most likely characterized in which manner?
   A. Predominantly aerobic and gram-positive cocci in morphotype
   B. Primarily anaerobic and gram-negative in morphotype
   C. Primarily gram-positive cocci that are anaerobic in eH potential
   D. None of the above

Antibiotics

9. In empirical selection of an antibiotic that focuses on oral infections, which of the following features should be considered significant?
   A. Its spectrum of activity, including aerobic/anaerobic organisms
   B. Its efficacy in various pH-determined environments
   C. Its association with low development of resistance
   D. All of the above

10. Which of the following classes of antibiotics has had limited application in oral infectious disease management?
    A. Penicillins
    B. Tetracyclines
    C. Metronidazole
    D. Cephalosporins

11. Antibiotic therapy in the management of an oral facial infectious disease is considered:
    A. Critical and should be used as a sole form of management.
    B. As "adjunctive therapy," complementary to other forms of management.
    C. Best when at least two broad-spectrum antibiotics are prescribed.
    D. All of the above.

12. Of the three recently approved local and systemic antibiotic treatments for periodontal disease, which broad-spectrum anaerobic-focused antibiotic do all three treatments use?

A. Penicillin

B. Ciprofloxacin

C. Erythromycin

D. Tetracycline

Viruses

13. Which of the following statements can be associated with large, enveloped viruses (>70 nm)?

    A. They are often associated with respiratory secretions or transmission via close contact.

    B. They are released from infected cells slowly, thus they do not cause the cells to rupture.

    C. They are environmentally unstable.

    D. All of the above are true.

14. Viruses that are "small" (<70 nm) have essentially no envelope and are best associated with which of the following characteristics?

    A. Gastrointestinal (GI) diseases

    B. Potential long-term viability on inanimate surfaces

    C. Are released in a "large burst" from the infected cell and, thus, produce enough antigen to be potentially good sources of vaccine

    D. All of the above

15. When evaluating a newly discovered virus, which of the following characteristics would suggest its degree of "communicability"?

    A. Size and lipid envelope development

    B. Nucleic acid content (i.e., DNA vs RNA)

    C. Its shape

    D. None of the above

16. Which of the following viruses does not belong to the group of herpes viruses?

    A. Herpes simplex virus (HSV)

    B. Cytomegalovirus (CMV)

    C. Varicella-zoster virus (VZV)

    D. Retrovirus

Immunology

17. Which of the following antibody "classes" is most often associated with "acute response" and defines an early phase in the infectious disease process?

    A. IgM

    B. IgG

    C. IgE

    D. IgA

18. In respiratory viral infections, which class of immunoglobulins is most often associated with prevention of epithelial associated attachment?

    A. IgA

    B. IgM

    C. IgG

    D. IgE

ANSWERS

1. **D.** *P. gingivalis* is one of the four most strongly associated periopathogens. It appears late in the process and defines a lowered eH.

2. **A.** Of the three morphotypes, S (Small) is the most periopathogenic *Treponema* sp and is a marker of disease progression.

3. **A.** It utilizes selected carbohydrates and survives best in a (+) mV environment (eH).

4. **B.** Although the numbers vary to some degree for "transient flora," the established microbiota is 300 to 550 "rich," which ensures the "survival" of the species.

5. **D.** The *Bacteroides* sp containing *B. forsythus*, *Porphyromonas*, and *Prevotella* are most viable at a low eH (-150 to 170 mV).

6. **D.** A biofilm is an enriched ecosystem that is much more resistant to removal than planktonic microbes and grows in the presence of antibiotics

7. **D.** We live in a "microbial world" that is transferred early in life and established in four reservoirs by 72 hours: gastrointestinal, genitourinary, mouth, and skin.

8. **A.** The organisms of a particular site reflect: (a) the environment (eH), (b) the acidity (pH), and (c) the energy source (C).

9. **D.** Empirical selection recognizes the multispecies probability of the target organism.

10. **D.** Cephalosporins have limited efficacy against the multispecies targeted organisms, particularly anaerobes.

11. **B.** In infectious disease, antibiotics are generally considered to be complimentary to mechanical reduction of the bioburden and improved immunologic functions.

12. **D.** Tetracyclines (e.g., doxy minocycline) are used as broad-spectrum antibiotics, with low side effects, broad anaerobic coverage, and modulation of the immune system in low doses.

13. **D.** Structure = function in virology; large enveloped viruses are produced slowly by budding from the cell surface.

14. **D.** Small viruses are environmentally stable, including acid environments (i.e., GI); they produce a large bioburden on the immune system and thus are rapidly recognized by plasma cells and are good for diagnostic serology.

15. **A.** "Communicability" is a function of "survivability," which is associated with smallness (size) and a less complicated capsid/envelope covering the nucleic acid.

16. **D.** There are now eight members of the herpes group; none contains a reverse transcriptase or is an RNA virus.

17. **A.** IgM is the first of the immune cascades associated with plasma cells and the humoral response; it is generally detected in 5 to 10 days and disappears within 2 to 3 weeks.

18. **A.** IgA is a predominantly respiratory-associated immunoglobulin that is very important in preventing a "triphasic" upper respiratory cascade: (1) virus, then (2) routine bacterial pathogen, and then (3) a complicating sequelae.

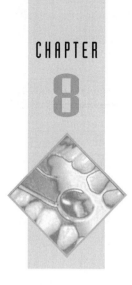

CHAPTER

8

Pathology

ROBERT M. HOWELL, DDS, MSD

The recognition of disease is generally based on detecting a deviation from normal. This deviation may be expressed as a **sign** (a measure of physiologic functions such as temperature or heart rate or clinical appearance) or a **symptom** (the patient's subjective expression of wellness such as "not feeling well" or "tired all the time.") Therefore, to determine if a disease exists, it is important to have some understanding of the normal physiologic functions and response mechanisms.

The body does not have an infinite number of responses to call upon in the face of disease. In fact, a relatively small number of functions play a role in most disease states. Therefore, fundamental knowledge of these more common functions is necessary in order to interpret many disease states.

 INFLAMMATION

The **inflammatory response** is probably the most important defense mechanism of the body (**Figure 8-1**). This response is used to fight infections, damage resulting from trauma, responses to immune-challenging stimuli, and, to some extent, tumor growth. Even in ancient cultures in which there was no understanding of microbial organisms, the signs and symptoms associated with infection were recognized. The main signs of inflammation have been referred to as the **cardinal signs of inflammation**: redness, swelling, pain, and **increased temperature** (to the local site). Some people also include **loss of function** among the cardinal signs. Each of these signs represents one or more response mechanisms to an injurious stimulus.

Redness

Immediately after an injury, a vascular reflex causes **vasoconstriction**. Clinically, this action is seen as a transient blanching of the tissue in the area of injury. The injured cells release vasoactive substances, which then result in and sustain **vasodilation**. Vasodilation increases the quantity of blood flowing into the area, which we perceive clinically as redness.

Swelling

When small-caliber vessels and capillaries dilate, the wall of these vessels becomes stretched and gaps open between the endothelial cells that line the vessels. Initially, the gaps are small but are large enough to permit an increase in the permeability of the vessel wall and allow fluid to escape (**Figure 8-2**). As fluid accumulates in the surrounding tissue, swelling becomes clinically obvious. Various chemical mediators known as **cytokines** and **chemokines** intensify and sustain the dilation, widening the gap and further increasing the permeability of the vessel wall. This leakage of fluid into the tissue spaces is called **transudate**. As these gaps get larger, proteins and high molecular weight electrolytes leak out into the tissues. The accumulation of these higher molecular weight proteins and electrolytes changes the local tissue osmotic pressure, which attracts even more intravascular fluids into the tissue compartment, thus creating more swelling, which is clinically referred to as **edema**.

Vasodilation increases the internal diameter of the blood vessel, thus causing a drop in the intravascular blood pressure. This results in a slowing of the rate of blood flow through the area or **sludging**. With this decrease in the flow rate of blood in the vessel, the white blood cells (WBCs) begin to migrate toward the vessel wall (**margination**). WBCs have surface adhesion molecules that allow them to attach to the cells lining the blood vessels, resulting in **pavementing** of the WBCs on the internal surface wall of the vessel (**Figure 8-3**). Eventually, the WBCs begin to migrate through the vessel wall (a process known as **transmigration**) into the adjacent tissue along with everything else that has leaked out of the vessel, thus creating an **exudate**. Injured cells and other inflammatory cells also release sub-

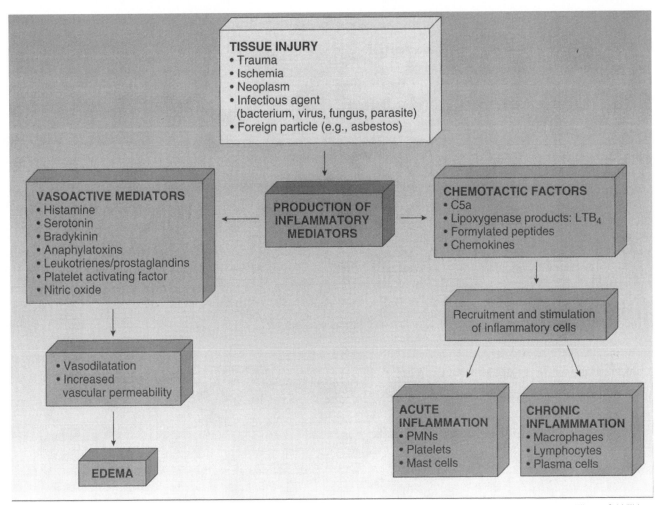

Figure 8-1. Mediators of the inflammatory response. (From Rubin E, Farber JL: Pathology, 3rd ed. Philadelphia, Lippincott Williams & Wilkins, 1999, p 40.)

stances called chemotaxins, which attract more WBCs to the site of injury. This response of WBCs to chemical mediators is called **chemotaxis**.

Increased Temperature

As the quantity of blood flowing into the area increases, the blood brings with it additional warmth from the body's core. Cytokines that were released by the injured cells also react on the hypothalamus (i.e., the part of the brain that regulates body temperature) and cause a fever. **Fever**, which is an abnormal rise in body temperature, is thought to occur to increase the body's metabolic activity and further stimulate the inflammatory reaction. Cold-blooded animals are known to position themselves to gather more sunlight in an attempt to raise their internal body temperatures when they are ill.

Pain

When injury to tissue occurs, various inflammatory substances known as **kinins**, such as bradykinin, are released.

In addition to prolonging the inflammatory response, kinins may also cause local pain. Furthermore, while injured cells die, they release various substances that can create significant destruction to local tissue. This, along with local edema, can also act on nerve fibers in the area to cause pain.

Loss of Function

Loss of function is more difficult to explain. In some organ systems, inflammation may compromise normal function. In other organ systems, loss of function may be related to pain and interference with neurotransmission. Because of the wide range of possible explanations for loss of function, not all authors include this in the list of cardinal signs.

Nature of the Inflammatory Reaction

The inflammatory reaction can be classified in two ways: (1) by its clinical course, or (2) by the microscopic pattern of the inflammatory infiltrate.

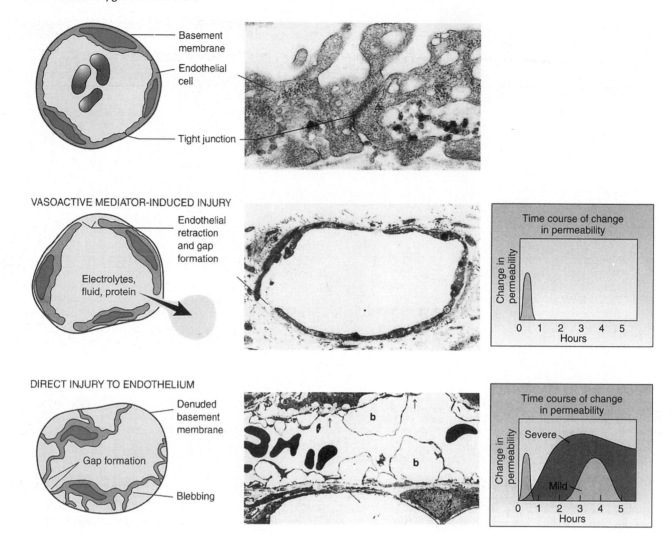

Figure 8-2. Small vessel response to inflammation that results in edema. (Modified from Rubin E, Farber JL: Pathology, 3rd ed. Philadelphia, Lippincott Williams & Wilkins, 1999, p 42.)

When the onset of a disease is sudden and intense, it is referred to as **acute** inflammation. If the onset is slow, insidious, and protracted, it is classified as **chronic** inflammation. **Subacute** inflammation is used to describe those reactions that lie in between acute and chronic. Also, during an inflammatory reaction, local factors change constantly, thus causing an acute response to become chronic or a chronic response to become acute. It is not unusual for the pattern to shift several times during a disease process, especially if the underlying disease process is untreated or inappropriately treated.

Inflammatory reactions are also classified by the type of inflammatory cells that populate the site of disease. In general, the clinical presentation and the types of cells present histologically are consistent. Microscopically, in an acute response, one finds a predominance of **polymorphonucleated leukocytes** (referred to as neutrophils or **PMNs**). PMNs, which are the first line of defense in the inflammatory response, are the predominant WBCs in the bloodstream and account for 50% to 70% of circulating WBCs. PMNs are also the most mobile WBCs and can release **chemotaxins** to attract more PMNs to the area.

PMNs, in addition to being phagocytic, also contain enzymes known as **lysozymes,** which can break up proteins and destroy bacteria. All of these strong defense forces come with a price, however, which may ultimately result in the death of the PMN. As the PMN breaks down, all the enzymes and other substances that are contained within it are released into the area. This action causes more tissue injury, and more PMNs are recruited to the area. As the injury or infection is controlled, either by treatment or the host's own immune response, the local environment changes to favor other types of WBCs.

In a chronic inflammatory reaction, PMNs are uncommon and the population of WBCs changes to predominantly **lymphocytes** and **monocytes**. These WBCs are normally present in smaller numbers within the bloodstream. Because these WBCs are less mobile than neutrophils, they are not present in the initial acute phase of the inflammatory reaction.

Lymphocytes are part of the immune system of defense. Generally, each lymphocyte is highly specific to a specific foreign substance, referred to as an **antigen.** Lymphocytes rely on monocytes (also known as **macrophages** or **histio-**

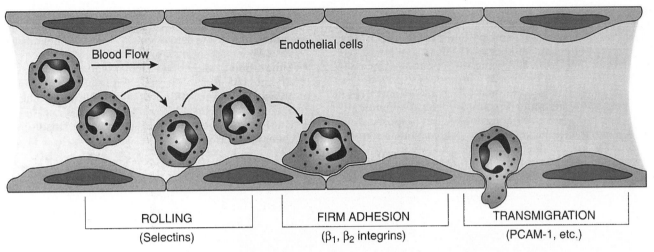

Figure 8-3. Process of leukocyte migration from the vessel into adjacent tissues. (From Rubin E, Farber JL: Pathology, 3rd ed. Philadelphia, Lippincott Williams & Wilkins, 1999, p 56.)

cytes outside of the bloodstream) to present antigens on their cell surfaces so that lymphocytes can recognize and attack the antigens. To be useful in the inflammatory process, lymphocytes must be activated and reproduced in large numbers. For this reason, the chronic inflammatory process takes longer to become a force, and lymphocytes are usually the predominant cell type later in the inflammatory process.

In subacute inflammatory reactions, there is a mixture of acute cells (i.e., PMNs) and chronic cells (i.e., lymphocytes, plasma cells, and macrophages). The ratio of acute to chronic WBCs in a subacute reaction is not exact.

There are two other WBCs in the bloodstream; however, they are generally not present in large numbers in most inflammatory reactions. These WBCs are **basophils** and **eosinophils**, which are named in terms of how they are stained in a blood smear. Their exact roles are not completely understood, but a few general features are known about them. Basophils, when found in tissue, are called **mast cells** and their primary role appears to be the release of **histamines** and other substances that are used to sustain the inflammatory response. Basophils make up less than 2% of WBCs. Eosinophils are usually found in significant numbers in allergic reactions, parasitic infections, muscle injury, and Hodgkin lymphoma. The role that they play in these diverse diseases is not well understood. Eosinophils constitute less than 1% of the WBCs in the bloodstream.

Clinical Application

Redness, swelling, increased temperature in the involved area, and pain are clear signs of the body's attempt to modify the course of an injury. As resolution of the inflammation occurs, these signs diminish over time until the changes at the cellular level have returned to normal. To facilitate **healing**, it is necessary to clinically alter the processes. Consider what is going on at the cellular level and what could be done to alter the process. For example, to limit the inflammatory response,

it would be necessary to identify and remove the causative agents or insult that initiated the process. A basic goal of **therapy**, therefore, is to modify local conditions that either initiated or might be prolonging the inflammatory process. By intervening in this process, the balance is tipped in favor of the host's natural responses, thus allowing the body to heal itself.

HEALING AND REPAIR

When an injury occurs that results in tissue destruction, one of two main healing processes takes place. If damaged tissue heals itself by replacing the destroyed cells with the same kind of cells, this process is referred to as **regeneration**. If, on the other hand, the destroyed cells cannot be regenerated by their own kind, the body attempts to close the void with scar tissue. This process is called **repair**. In addition to the type of tissue involved, the physical nature of the injury also plays a role in which process dominates healing. For example, cardiac muscle has little potential to regenerate; therefore, in a heart attack, damaged cardiac muscle will mainly be replaced by scar tissue. The liver, on the other hand, has excellent potential to regenerate. However, if the size of the injury is very large, scar tissue will form, which is seen in cirrhosis of the liver.

Skin is another tissue with an excellent potential to regenerate. A good example is a surgical wound **(Figure 8-4).** If the wound margins are clean and meticulously sutured closed, generally little scar formation occurs. This is referred to as healing by **primary intent**. If, however, the wound is large and not sutured closed or if the wound becomes infected causing more tissue damage, the wound will fill in with granulation tissue and be replaced by dense fibrous tissue to form a very visible scar. This process is called healing by **secondary intent**. Very large scars on the skin are referred to as **keloids** **(Figure 8-5).**

Sites of tooth removal offer another perspective of the healing process. When a tooth is removed, the empty socket

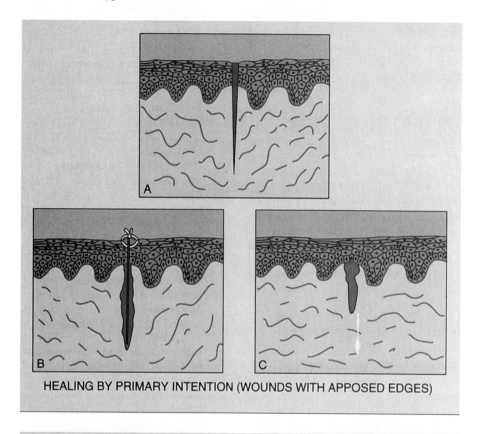

HEALING BY PRIMARY INTENTION (WOUNDS WITH APPOSED EDGES)

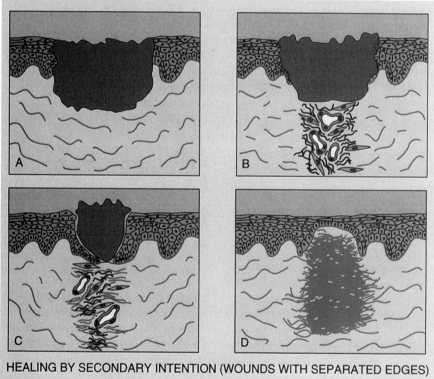

HEALING BY SECONDARY INTENTION (WOUNDS WITH SEPARATED EDGES)

Figure 8-4. Wound healing sequence of primary and secondary intent. (From Rubin E, Farber JL: Pathology, 3rd ed. Philadelphia, Lippincott Williams & Wilkins, 1999, p 97.)

fills in with blood and forms a **clot**. The clot is gradually replaced by granulation tissue that grows in from the edges of the socket. Bone eventually grows in to replace the granulation tissue, thus filling the defect. In this example, regener-

ation takes place over a long period due to the slow nature of bone growth. Occasionally, the socket does not heal with bone but retains its connective tissue scar, which results in a **fibrous defect**. At other times, the reaction may produce

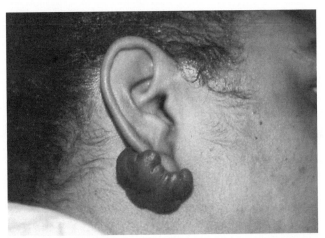

Figure 8-5. Keloid. Exaggerated scar formation. (From Rubin E, Farber JL: Pathology, 3rd ed. Philadelphia, Lippincott Williams & Wilkins, 1999, p 99.)

very dense bone, thus creating a bone scar or **osteosclerosis**. In rare cases, an extraction site may fill with bone marrow and create an **osteoporotic marrow defect**.

 NEOPLASIA

Neoplasia literally means "new growth." This new growth, however, differs from replacement new growth such as hair or nails. Neoplasia is used to define growth that is abnormal. Another term that is often used for a **neoplasm** is **tumor**. Whichever term is used, the key features are that **growth is both unregulated and relentless**. Before going into detail about neoplasia, however, there are two other types of changes in growth that must also be covered-**hypertrophy** and **hyperplasia**. Clinically, they may appear somewhat like neoplasia, but they represent reactive growth; that is, some external force is stimulating the growth. When this stimulus is removed, the growth stops. Neoplasia either does not have an external force or if neoplasia was initiated by one, it no longer needs that external force for continued growth.

Hypertrophy

The first of the two terms used to describe non-neoplastic growth is hypertrophy. Hypertrophy is growth that occurs when the cells of a tissue have increased in **size** but not nec-

essarily in number. A good example of this type of growth is skeletal muscle. When one exercises, muscles enlarge; however, this enlargement is caused by an increase in the size of the individual muscle fibers. Even though hypertrophy has been used to describe tissue enlargement in the oral cavity, such growth is uncommon.

Hyperplasia

The other type of non-neoplastic tissue enlargement is hyperplasia. Hyperplasia is from growth resulting from an increase in the **number** of cells present. This differs from neoplasia in that it is a reactive growth. Once the stimulus that initiated it is removed, the growth stops and usually regresses. An example of hyperplasia in the oral cavity would be gingival hyperplasia associated with neglect of oral hygiene. Once proper oral hygiene is established, the gingiva generally returns to a more normal size and contour.

Characteristics of Neoplasia

Neoplasms are divided into two categories-**benign** and **malignant**. The term *benign* come from the root word for "kind"; however, not all benign neoplasms are always kind. Benign denotes a pattern of growth that is usually slow and nonaggressive. However, a benign tumor in the wrong place, such as in the brain, can be fatal. The term *malignant* is derived from the root word for "malicious." Although there is a commonly held belief that all malignant neoplasms grow rapidly and spread throughout the body, some grow very slowly and do not readily spread. These inconsistencies can create confusion when one is trying to designate a neoplasm as benign or malignant. **Table 8-1** outlines some of the differences between benign and malignant neoplasms. With the exception of metastatic potential, none of the others is absolute. Benign tumors, by definition, do not have the potential to metastasize.

The causes of neoplasia are varied. Some are induced by physical damage to cells (e.g., by radiation), chemicals, or viruses. Whatever the cause, some alteration of the genetic code results in uncontrolled cellular reproduction. Furthermore, tumor cells, even malignant ones, do not always multiply faster than do normal (non-neoplastic) cells. Some malignant neoplasias are notorious for being fatal within months after a diagnosis has been made (e.g., a small cell carcinoma of the lung), whereas others may not be fatal for years (e.g.,

 TABLE 8–1 Characteristics of Growth for Benign and Malignant Neoplasms

CHARACTERISTICS OF GROWTH	BENIGN	MALIGNANT
Rate of growth	Slow growth, few mitoses	Rapid growth; mitoses common
Differentiation	Resembles parent tissue; structured growth	Disorganized; may not resemble parent tissue
Pattern of growth	Grows by expansion; pushes adjacent tissue aside	Grows by invasion; grows into the adjacent tissue
Metastatic potential	None	Has potential but may not always do so

prostate carcinomas). After childhood, cells are stimulated to replace those that are worn out and damaged. Due to the genetic mutation, tumor cells are programmed to replicate continuously, resulting in more cells being produced than are being lost. The end result is uncontrolled growth-a neoplasm.

Nomenclature

Neoplasms are classified or named predominantly in terms of the tissue from which they arise. The suffix **-oma** is appended to the name of the tissue of origin to designate a benign tumor. Malignant tumors have either the word **carcinoma** or **sarcoma** added to the name of the tissue of origin. Carcinoma is added to the name when the tissue of origin is epithelium. Sarcoma is added if the malignancy is of nonepithelial origin. **Table 8-2** lists a few examples of benign and malignant neoplasms.

There are notable exceptions to this naming convention, however. In Table 8-2, the term **papilloma** is used to designate a benign neoplasm of squamous epithelial origin. Other significant exceptions are neoplasms of lymph nodes and melanin-producing cells. There are no benign melanomas (nevus is used to designate a variety of benign pigmented lesions). Likewise, there are no benign lymphomas (benign tumors of lymph node origin). Some neoplasms also have historically had a person's name attached to them. Often, this was done because the tissue of origin was uncertain when neoplasms were first described. For better or worse, these eponyms have persisted. Examples of neoplasms designated by a person's name are Hodgkin lymphoma, Burkitt lymphoma, Kaposi sarcoma, and Pindborg tumor. Other neoplasms are named after the site or region in which they have occurred or the configuration in which they grow. Examples of these neoplasms are thymoma, carotid body tumor, clear cell carcinoma, and verrucous carcinoma.

Spread of Neoplasia

Benign and malignant neoplasms may share many growth characteristics but differ in one significant feature-**metas-**

tasis. As mentioned earlier, benign tumors, by definition, cannot metastasize. Malignant tumors can spread to another structure by direct invasion, by way of the lymphatic system, or by way of the bloodstream (hematogenous spread). It is not uncommon for a malignant neoplasm to spread by more than one route. Basal cell carcinoma (BCC) is an example of a malignant neoplasm that tends to spread primarily by local invasion. Epithelial malignancies tend to spread first by way of the lymphatic system, whereas malignant neoplasms of nonepithelial origin favor a hematogenous route first.

Carcinomas account for approximately 90% of all oral cancers. When carcinomas of oral origin metastasize, they commonly do so by way of regional lymph nodes. If a carcinoma develops on the lateral border of the tongue, it generally metastasizes to the submental or submandibular region on the same side (**ipsilateral** side) (**Figure 8-6**). When a carcinoma arises near the midline, however, it may metastasize to either or both sides. Toward the more posterior portion of the oral cavity, carcinomas commonly metastasize to the cervical chain of lymph nodes. Once a carcinoma metastasizes, it may further metastasize to contiguous lymph nodes further down the chain. If not treated early, carcinomas become blood-borne and spread to involve extranodal organs. Carcinoma of the gingiva or palate often becomes blood-borne early on due to early invasion into the bone marrow and spread to the lungs and other distant organs.

Sarcomas, which are nonepithelial malignancies, account for only approximately 10% of all oral malignancies. Whereas sarcomas may metastasize by way of the lymphatics, the more common route is by way of the bloodstream. For this reason, they are found more often in distant organs such as the lungs and bone marrow early in their occurrence.

TABLE 8–2 Benign and Malignant Neoplasms by Tissue of Origin

TISSUE OF ORIGIN	BENIGN	MALIGNANT
Epithelium (glandular)	Aden*oma*	Adeno*carcinoma*
Squamous epithelium	Papill*oma**	squamous cell *carcinoma*
Fibrous connective tissue	Fibr*oma*	Fibro*sarcoma*
Bone	Oste*oma*	Osteo*sarcoma*
Pigmented nevus	Nevus	Melanoma* (or malignant melanoma)
Lymph node	*	Lymphoma* (or malignant lymphoma)

*Exceptions to the rule.

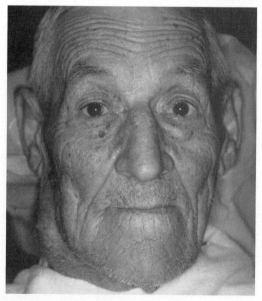

Figure 8-6. Ipsilateral metastasis. The swollen lymph node on the right side of the patient's neck is from a squamous cell carcinoma on the right side of the tongue.

Another, less common malignancy, which is found in the oral cavity, is a neoplasm that has metastasized to the jawbone. Carcinomas of the breast, lung, and kidney have commonly been reported to metastasize to the jaws. The most common site for cancer metastasizing to the jaws is the body of the mandible. Whereas cancers may metastasize to the maxilla, this location generally accounts for less than 20% of all metastases to the jaws.

 ## INTRAORAL LESIONS

Lesions of the Mucosal Surfaces of the Lips

The most common diseases that affect the mucosal surface of the lower lip are the **mucocele** and **actinic** or **solar keratosis**. Owing to the abundance of minor salivary gland tissue and the frequency of trauma to the lower lip, mucoceles are found most commonly in the lower lip (**Figure 8-7**). Neoplasms of minor salivary gland origin in the lower lip are uncommon and account for only approximately 10% of the swellings found there. This is in direct contrast to swellings of the upper lip. Benign tumors of minor salivary gland origin account for about 90% of swellings there, the most common being **monomorphic adenoma (Figure 8-8)**, whereas mucoceles of the upper lip account for less than 10% of upper lip swellings.

Actinic or solar keratosis is a common mucosal epithelial change of the vermillion surface of the lips, which is caused by chronic exposure to ultraviolet radiation present in sunlight (**Figure 8-9**). This form of radiation injury is uncommon on the mucosal surface of the upper lip, because it is somewhat protected from direct sunlight. These changes are often found on the lower lip, especially in older persons who have spent a lot of time outside. The lower lip is one of the

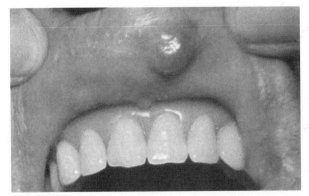

Figure 8-8. Monomorphic adenoma. A swelling of the upper lip, which is of salivary gland origin, is more likely to be a monomorphic adenoma than a mucocele. (From Langlais RP, Miller CS: Color Atlas of Common Oral Diseases, 2nd ed. Philadelphia, Lippincott Williams & Wilkins, 1998, p 65.)

most common sites for oral cancer, and people who have actinic cheilitis are considered to be at risk of having malignant transformation to **squamous cell carcinoma (Figure 8-10)**. However, due to the ease of early detection, it also has one of the best long-term prognoses.

Lesions of the Perioral Skin

On the skin surfaces of the face, **nevi** (pigmented "moles"), **seborrheic keratosis** (pigmented, senile changes of the skin induced by chronic exposure to ultraviolet radiation) (**Figure 8-11**) and **BCCs** (the most common form of skin cancer) are frequently encountered lesions. BCCs may occur on any sun-exposed skin surfaces, especially the face. BCCs appear as shallow ulcerative lesions with a rolled margin, and they commonly exhibit dilated blood vessels known as **telangiectasia (Figure 8-12)**. BCCs metastasize infrequently but will grow large if they are not treated. A BCC

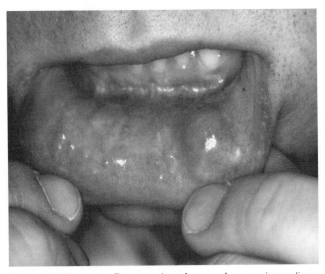

Figure 8-7. Mucocele. Extravasation of mucus from a minor salivary gland on the lip caused by trauma.

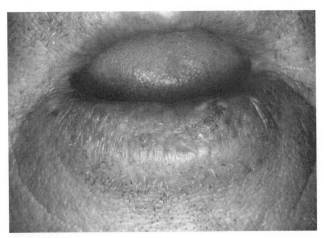

Figure 8-9. Actinic or solar cheilosis. Epithelial atrophy on the vermillion surface of the lower lip from chronic exposure to ultraviolet radiation.

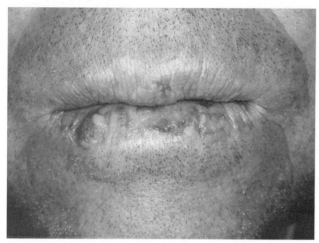

Figure 8-10. Squamous cell carcinoma. Early malignant transformation on the lower lip with pre-existing actinic cheilitis.

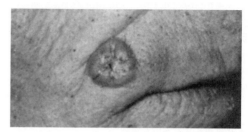

Figure 8-12. Basal cell carcinoma. Note the rolled margin and telangiectasia (thin spider web-like blood vessels) on the surface. (From Eversole LR: Clinical Outline of Oral Pathology, 3rd ed. Philadelphia, Lea & Febiger, 1992, p 218.)

generally has an excellent prognosis as long as it does not extend into a vital structure such as the brain. BCCs also respond equally well to surgery or radiation therapy.

Nevi and seborrheic keratoses are both pigmented lesions but differ in their clinical presentation. Seborrheic keratoses are usually darkly pigmented lesions that have an almost waxy surface; they look as if they were pasted on the surface of the skin. There is probably some slight risk of seborrheic keratoses transforming into a carcinoma, mainly because they are induced by chronic exposure to sunlight.

Nevi usually appear to be within the skin. Nevi on sun-exposed skin appear to have a higher risk of transformation into a **malignant melanoma.** Melanoma has become a common form of skin cancer, and incidences have been increasing at a higher rate than other forms of skin cancer.

Pigmented Mucosal Lesions

Most flat, pigmented lesions or **macules** represent areas of the accumulation of melanin pigment, such as a freckle or **ephelis.** On the lips, these lesions are referred to as **labial melanotic macules (Figure 8-13).** When they occur intrao-

rally, they are referred to as **oral melanotic macules.** Unless these macules exhibit growth or suddenly change appearance, they do not generally require treatment.

Other sources of pigmentation on mucosal surfaces include **smoker's melanosis, drug-induced melanosis** (as seen with the use of minocycline), **amalgam tattoo,** and less common diseases such as **Addison disease, Peutz-Jeghers syndrome,** and the **café au lait** spots associated with **neurofibromatosis** (von Recklinghausen disease of the skin) and **polyostotic fibrous dysplasia** (McCune-Albright disease).

Nevi may also occur within the oral cavity, although less commonly than in the skin. Most nevi have little potential for malignant transformation; however, the ratio of malignant to benign nevi is higher in the oral cavity than on the skin. For this reason, intraoral pigmented lesions should be evaluated and should not be ignored.

White Lesions of Oral Mucous Membranes

The wide range of oral diseases may clinically present as white lesions of mucous membranes. **Leukoplakia** is the

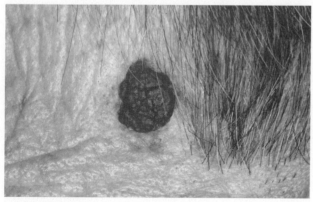

Figure 8-11. Seborrheic keratosis. This lesion may be induced by chronic ultraviolet radiation.

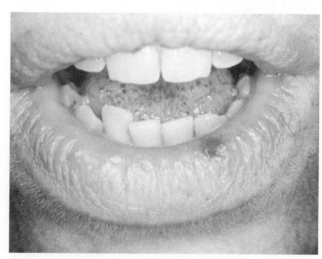

Figure 8-13. Labial melanotic macule. A flat, freckle-like lesion on the lower lip.

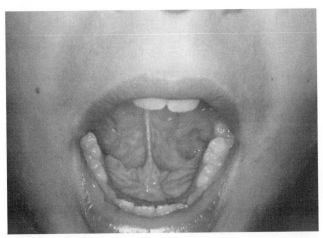

Figure 8-14. White sponge nevus. People who have this autosomal dominant disorder have the thick, white lesions on the mucosal surfaces.

term used to describe a white, flat lesion. Leukoplakia is a descriptive name and is not a diagnosis. The most common causes of leukoplakia in the oral cavity are related to trauma such as alcohol or tobacco use and chemical or thermal burns. For the most part, white lesions have a moderately low risk of malignant transformation, unless certain risk factors are present, most notably tobacco and alcohol abuse.

White sponge nevus (Cannon disease, white folded nevus), a hereditary disorder, is characterized by thickened, white surfaces. The degree of thickening can be quite striking and worrisome when first viewed. The key features to recognizing this condition are its wide distribution (involving any mucosal surface and often bilateral) and a history of early onset or other members of the family who have similar lesions (**Figure 8-14**).

Treatment for white lesions varies. Those lesions that are of obvious traumatic origin are best treated by removing the irritant and monitoring the patient until the lesion resolves. Most white lesions are simply thickening of the epithelium

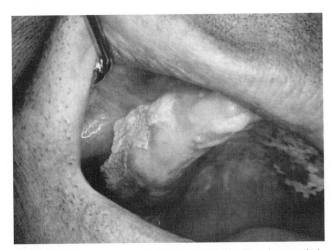

Figure 8-15. Proliferative verrucous leukoplakia. The characteristic feature of this lesion is its rough, corrugated, white surface.

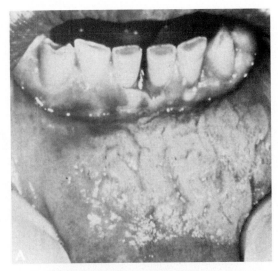

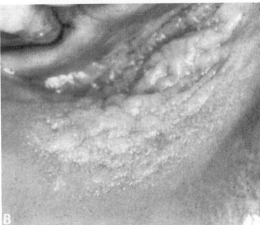

Figure 8-16. "Snuff pouch." This white, folded mucosal surface is where this patient holds his smokeless tobacco. (From DeBiase C: Dental Health Education: Theory and Practice. Malvern, PA, Lea & Febiger, 1991, p 122.)

(e.g., **hyperkeratosis, hyperparakeratosis, acanthosis,** or **leukoedema**). Lesions that fail to show signs of resolving in a reasonable period of time (2-6 weeks) may be signs of **epithelial dysplasia. Proliferative verrucous leukoplakia** is a flat lesion with a rough or warty-looking surface (**Figure 8-15**). This lesion is considered by many to have greater risk of malignant transformation than most other forms of leukoplakia. Lesions that appear to be the result of tobacco use (e.g., **nicotine stomatitis** or a "**snuff pouch**") should regress if the use of tobacco is stopped (**Figure 8-16**). If regression is not observed, a biopsy should be considered.

Patients with mucosal burns will, most often, remember the event (e.g., pizza; a hot beverage; or exposure to some chemical, such as aspirin or one of many chemicals commonly used in dentistry) (**Figure 8-17**).

Lichen planus, which is a common skin disease, also occurs in the oral cavity. This disease most often presents orally as bilateral, lacy white lesions known as the **striae of Wickham (Figure 8-18**). Lichen planus on the gingiva and

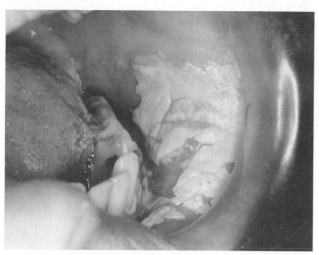

Figure 8-17. Burn caused by an aspirin. This patient held an aspirin in the area in an attempt to relieve a toothache. This white plaque is burned, necrotic epithelium.

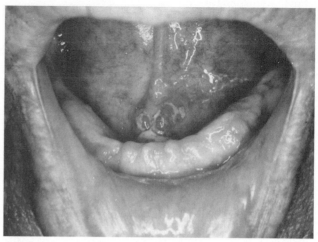

Figure 8-19. Speckled leukoplakia. The speckling of a white lesion, as seen here on the sublinual caruncle, should be considered a serious change until proved otherwise by biopsy.

dorsal surface of the tongue may be more difficult to recognize owing to the heavy keratinization on these surfaces. In general, lichen planus does not require a biopsy unless the clinical features appear atypical. Some controversy exists with regard to whether lichen planus undergoes a malignant transformation. Some believe that lichen planus may become malignant, whereas others believe that the cancer arose in **lichenoid dysplasia**, a dysplasia that mimics lichen planus clinically. This latter group believes that patients who have lichenoid dysplasia may have an increased risk of malignant transformation; however, this risk does not apply to patients with lichen planus.

Candida infections can also cause white lesions intraorally. Whereas the typical candida infection presents as a white membrane that can be wiped away leaving a reddened surface, candida can also present as true leukoplakia (hyperkeratosis), which cannot be removed by wiping. In this case, a biopsy may be necessary to diagnose candidiasis.

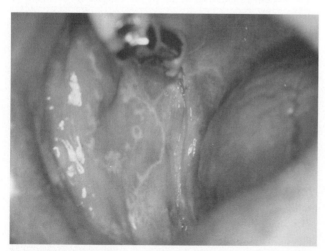

Figure 8-18. Lichen planus. The reticulated pattern of the lacy white lines is characteristic of lichen planus.

A variation of leukoplakia is **speckled leukoplakia (Figure 8-19)**. Speckled leukoplakia is used to describe a lesion that exhibits features of both red (see **erythroplakia**) and white (**leukoplakia**) changes in the mucosa and should be viewed with suspicion.

Red Lesions of the Oral Mucous Membranes

Small, discrete, bright red lesions on mucosal surfaces most often represent vascular anomalies or developmental vascular lesions, such as **hemangiomas** of arterial origin that may blanch under pressure. Venous hemangiomas, on the other hand, appear dark blue and may not blanch. Many hemangiomas are congenital and do not need to be removed.

A more serious red lesion is **erythroplakia**. Erythroplakia is a term used to describe a mainly red, velvety lesion that has no apparent cause. These lesions must be correctly identified, because most are premalignant or malignant at the time of diagnosis.

Erythema migrans (benign migratory glossitis, geographic tongue) is a common red lesion of the tongue. The exact cause of this lesion is unknown. The characteristic feature of erythema migrans is the presence of a whitish ring or halo surrounding a patch denuded of its filiform papillae **(Figure 8-20)**. This lesion can be seen occasionally on mucosal surfaces other than the tongue; similar to the tongue lesions, erythema migrans presents as a white halo surrounding an erythematous patch.

Median rhomboid glossitis (Figure 8-21) is an uncommon condition that is another form of candidiasis. In this case, the lesion is located in the midline of the tongue, back toward the circumvallate papillae. These lesions usually present clinically as a reddened plaque-like lesion or an elevated lesion. Generally, a biopsy is unnecessary unless the lesion fails to respond to antifungal medications.

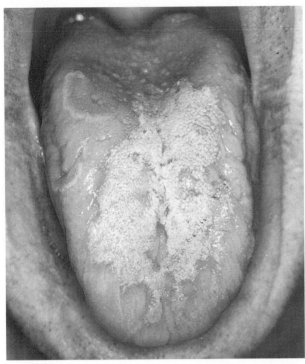

Figure 8-20. Erythema migrans. The characteristic features of this lesion are the prominent white border, loss of the filiform papillae in the central part of the lesions, and a changing surface pattern. They are commonly multiple.

Ulcerative Lesions of the Mucous Membranes

The most common ulcerative conditions in the oral cavity are aphthous and traumatic ulcers. Other lesions that present as oral ulcers include **herpes simplex** and erosive lichen planus and early lesions of squamous cell carcinoma.

The most common form of **aphthous stomatitis** is the **minor aphthous** (also known as the **canker sore**) (**Figure 8-22**). Minor aphthous ulcers are generally small (<1 cm in

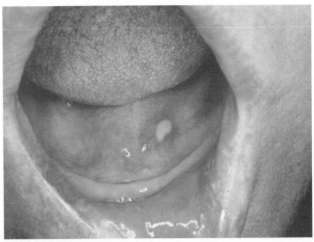

Figure 8-22. Minor aphthous ulcer. Ulcers of unknown origin occur mainly on unattached mucosal surfaces. Many may be traumatically induced.

diameter), isolated, and superficial and heal without scarring. They occur predominantly on unattached mucosal surfaces such as the lip, tongue, and vestibular mucosa. As a general rule, most minor aphthous ulcers heal within 2 weeks without intervention, but topical anesthetics can provide palliative relief. **Major aphthous ulcers** present as deep ulcers that often last for weeks at a time and frequently heal with scarring (**Figure 8-23**). Major aphthous ulcers often require the use of topical steroids. A third, uncommon form of aphthous stomatitis, is **herpetiform aphthous**. This lesion is so named because it occurs as a cluster of small ulcers that resemble herpes simplex clinically. As the etiology of aphthous stomatitis is highly variable, effective treatment can be challenging.

Traumatic ulcers are for the most part indistinguishable from minor aphthous ulcers. Many patients who have aphthous ulcers have a history of trauma to the area (e.g., during

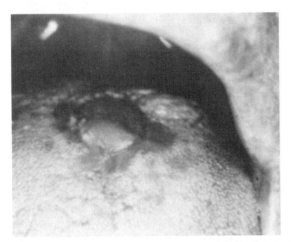

Figure 8-21. Median rhomboid glossitis. This localized lesion on the midline of the tongue was caused by *Candida albicans*. (From Eversole LR: Clinical Outline of Oral Pathology, 3rd ed. Philadelphia, Lea & Febiger, 1992, p 145.)

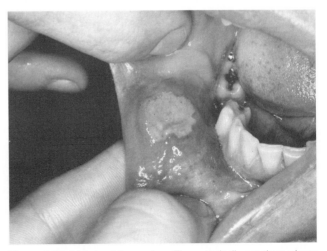

Figure 8-23. Major aphthous ulcer. These typically are deep ulcers that heal with scarring. Many may require treatment in order to heal.

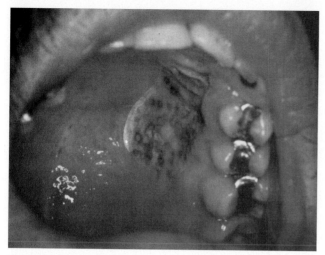

Figure 8-24. Recurrent *Herpes simplex*. Herpes typically occurs as a cluster of small ulcers on attached mucosal surfaces.

radiographic film placement, scaling procedures, or the site of an injection) before an ulcer appears. Traumatic ulcers may occur on any mucosal surface; they generally heal without scarring and are treated like minor aphthous ulcers.

Herpes simplex in adults occurs as small clusters of punctate ulcers that may run together (i.e., **coalesce**) to form larger irregular areas of ulceration (**Figure 8-24**). Individual ulcers are usually 2 to 3 mm in diameter with a shallow, whitish center surrounded by a red halo. Herpetic ulcers occur predominantly, but not exclusively, on attached mucosa such as the gingiva and palate. As with minor aphthous ulcers, most resolve within 2 weeks without intervention. Antiviral agents may be helpful; however, they are most efficacious when taken in the early stages of the disease. **Herpetic whitlow**, a herpetic infection of the distal portion of a finger or nail bed and **herpes keratitis**, a herpetic infection of the cornea of the eye, have been reported as practitioner-acquired infections. Fortunately, since the adoption of universal precautions, these conditions are rarely seen today.

Other, but less common diseases that may exhibit oral ulcers include **lupus erythematosus**, **erythema multiforme** (including **Stevens-Johnson syndrome**, which may occur as a reaction to a drug), **Crohn disease, cyclic neutropenia, Behçet syndrome,** and **Reiter syndrome.**

Bullovesicular Diseases

The ulcerative diseases covered in the previous section may also present as **vesicles** (blisters) or lesions that the patient recalls as epithelium sloughing off of the mucosal surface. This is especially true of the viral diseases such as herpes, zoster, and herpangina. There is another group of immune-related diseases that present as vesicles. The two more commonly encountered in the oral cavity are **pemphigus vulgaris** and **mucous membrane pemphigoid**. Both of these autoimmune diseases affect how the epithelial cells attach to each other or to the basement membrane. A feature that often leads to the

final diagnosis is the ability to create a blister by gentle finger pressure across, what appears to be, normal mucosa. This phenomenon is known as the **Nikolsky sign**.

Pemphigus vulgaris, which means "common" or "ordinary" pemphigus, is the most form of pemphigus and is an autoimmune disease that involves the desmisomes (which permit epithelial cells to attach to each other). This allows the epithelial cells to pull apart, thus creating an **intraepithelial** cleft that presents clinically as a blister. These blisters are very thin; they rupture immediately and only last for minutes to a few hours. The distinctive feature of pemphigus vulgaris is the presence of free-floating epithelial cells within the blister, which are referred to as **Tzanck cells**. This type of intraepithelial pulling apart is called **acantholysis**. This disease can affect both the skin and mucous membranes.

Mucous membrane pemphigoid, which is also an autoimmune disease, is similar to pemphigus vulgaris except that the reaction is against the attachment of the epithelium to the basement membrane. This creates a blister that is made up of the full thickness of the epithelium. For this reason, patients may have blisters that last for several hours or even a few days. Pemphigoid is a disease that involves mucous membranes more often than skin. The eyes are also involved and can lead to scarring and loss of vision if left untreated.

Both pemphigus and pemphigoid often present with gingival lesions, and they, along with lichen planus, account for the majority of the lesions that are known as desquamative gingivitis. Both of these conditions require medical intervention in the form of steroids. Occasionally, other immunosuppressive drugs such as methotrexate and azathioprine are given.

In addition to pemphigus vulgaris and mucous membrane pemphigoid, a hereditary disease that also exhibits vesicle formation or sloughing is **epidermolysis bullosa** (EB). This uncommon disease can have an autosomal dominant or recessive inheritance pattern. Blistering and shearing of the skin can occur from even gentle friction or daily activities. More than 20 different subtypes of EB exist with varying degrees of severity, ranging from a mild to an incapacitating (and sometimes fatal) condition.

 # INFECTIONS OF THE ORAL CAVITY

Bacterial Infections

Excluding some of the bacteria associated with periodontal disease, gingivitis, and dental caries, the most bacterial infections of the oral cavity are caused by **gram-positive cocci** (i.e., *Streptococcus* and *Staphylococcus*). Whereas much is made of oral infections from *Mycobacterium tuberculosis*, *Actinomyces*, *Treponema pallidum*, and *Neisseria gonorrhoeae*, these organisms are not a frequent primary cause of oral infections.

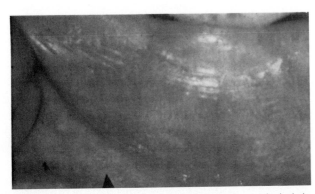

Figure 8-25. Parulis. The sinus tract from a gingival or periapical abscess is seen.

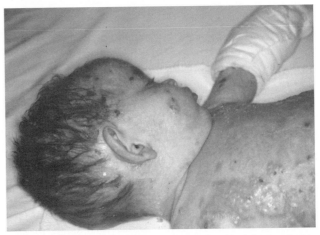

Figure 8-26. Impetigo. Impetigo is a pustular skin infection that is often caused by *Staphylococcus aureus*.

Streptococcus

Streptococcus pyogenes is a β-hemolytic bacterium that is often associated with **acute pharyngitis** (i.e., sore throat) and tonsillitis. *Streptococcus viridans*, an α-hemolytic organism that is associated with **subacute bacterial endocarditis**, is a common inhabitant of the oral cavity.

Staphlococcus

Staphlococcus aureus is often present in acute dental infections, especially **abscesses**. Terms that are frequently used to designate the sinus tract from a draining abscess are **parulis** or **gumboil**, which is so-named because dental abscesses commonly drain intraorally on or near the gingiva (**Figure 8-25**). *S. aureus* is also commonly found in suppurative **osteomyelitis** and some skin infections such as **impetigo (Figure 8-26).**

Actinomyces

Cervicofacial actinomycosis (i.e., abscesses of the face and upper neck) is most commonly caused by *Actinomyces israelii*. *Actinomyces israelii* is a facultative anaerobe that is commonly found in the oral cavity. "**Sulfur granules,**" which are colonies of the organism found in abscesses and sinus tracts, are a distinctive clinical feature of this less common oral infection.

Fungal Infections

Of all the fungi known to infect the oral cavity, by far the most common are from the genus *Candida*. Other organisms that are known to cause intraoral infections include *Histoplasmosis capsulatum*, *Cryptococcus neoformans*, **North American** *Blastomycosis dermatitidis*, and *Coccidioides immitus*. These organisms are generally much less common than *Candida* and tend to occur in rather specific regions of the United States. One characteristic feature that most of these organisms share is that they are **granulomatous infections** and they present with a rough, pebbly surface.

Saprophytic fungal infections of the maxillary sinuses can have significant clinical implications. These types of infections occur primarily in medically compromised patients and may cause necrosis of the palate. They have also been known to cause death due to a fungal embolism. Organisms most often found in this type of infection are members of the phylum *Zygomycetes*. Two frequently encountered members of this phylum are *Mucor* and *Rhizopus*. Another fungal organism that is known to occur in this location is **aspergillosis**. These organisms preferentially select nonliving material to grow on; the organisms do not normally infect healthy people unless these people are exposed to extremely large quantities. However, patients with poorly controlled **diabetes mellitus** or immunosuppression are susceptible **(Figure 8-27).**

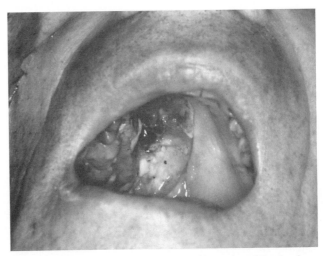

Figure 8-27. Mucor. This fistula is caused by a sinus infection from a member of the phylum *Zygomycetes*. This type of infection is associated with chronic, uncontrolled diabetes mellitus or immunosuppression.

Candida

Candida albicans is the most commonly encounter species of the genus *Candida* in the oral cavity. Candidiasis may present in one of several forms. The "classic" form is **pseudomembranous candidiasis** in which a pseudomembrane of desquamated epithelial cells and tangled *Candida* pseudohyphae forms (**Figure 8-28**). When this pseudomembrane is wiped away, an erythematous and often hemorrhagic, denuded surface is exposed.

Atrophic candidiasis is another variant of candidiasis. In this form, which is commonly seen under a denture, the mucosa appears erythematous and atrophic. Other examples of atrophic candidiasis are **median rhomboid glossitis,** which appears as a plaque-like, erythematous lesion on the midline dorsal surface of the tongue (see Figure 8-21) and **angular cheilitis,** which is also known as **perlèche** (**Figure 8-29**). Angular cheilitis is found most often in people who wear dentures or in those who have overclosure as a result of loss of the posterior teeth.

Hyperplastic candidiasis is less often recognized. It presents as a plaque-like area of epithelial thickening, often with hyperkeratosis or parakeratosis that cannot be wiped away. It may also clinically look like "speckled leukoplakia."

An uncommon presentation of candidiasis is the **granulomatous** form, which is usually found in people who are taking long-term antibiotics or who are immunosuppressed.

Viral Infections

The four most common groups of viruses involving the oral cavity are: (1) the **herpes virus type 1** [(HSV-1) or herpes simplex], (2) **coxsackievirus** (enterovirus pharyngitis), (3) **infectious parotitis** (mumps), and (4) **human papillomavirus** (HPV). Other viral infections that occasionally present with oral lesions are **Koplik spots,** which are seen in

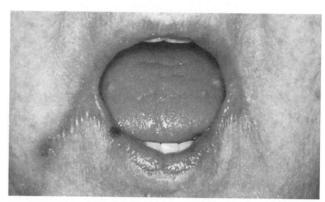

Figure 8-29. Angular cheilitis. This is usually found in denture wearers. Overclosure causes deep creases at the corners of the mouth, which stay moist and enhance the growth of candida. (From Langlais RP, Miller CS: Color Atlas of Common Oral Diseases, 2nd ed. Philadelphia, Lippincott Williams & Wilkins, 1998, p 63.)

measles, and the **human immunodeficiency virus** (HIV), which is associated with periodontal disease.

Herpes Virus

The human herpesvirus family of viruses includes several strains that often produce oral lesions. Of these, herpes simplex is the most common. Other members of this family include **varicella-zoster virus** (human herpesvirus type 3), **Epstein-Barr virus** (human herpesvirus type 4), and **cytomegalovirus** (human herpesvirus type 5). Most recently, human herpesvirus type 8 has been implicated as the cause of Kaposi sarcoma, which is a malignancy that is associated with the **aquired immunodeficiency syndrome** (AIDS).

Primary herpetic infections usually occur in young children; however, they can affect teenagers and adults. The infection is manifested by generalized vesicles over the gingiva, lips, or oral cavity in general and lasts for 7 to 10 days. The mouth is sore, and the condition is contagious. Treatment is palliative and requires adequate fluid intake and rest (**Figure 8-30**). Of the adult population, 90% are estimated to have circulating antibodies to HSV-1. Oral lesions vary from a few labial lesions to an acute pharyngotonsilliar eruption. HSV-2, genital herpes, is primarily a sexually transmitted disease but may occur in the oral cavity. In some areas of the United States of America, HSV-1 infections in the genital area occur as frequently as they do in the oral cavity. There are no significant clinical features that would allow one to differentiate between these two viruses.

Recurrent herpes is the most common form of oral HSV-1, even though only about 10% of persons who have antibodies to HSV-1 remember having the primary form. Recurrent herpes, also known as a **cold sore,** occurs most commonly on the lips (**herpes labialis**) (**Figure 8-31**). Intraorally, lesions are found most often on attached mucosa and occur characteristically as clusters of small ulcers.

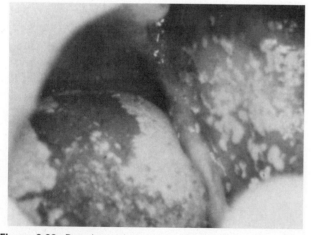

Figure 8-28. Pseudomembranous candidiasis. This pseudomembrane is actually a tangled mass of candida organisms and necrotic epithelium. When wiped away, a raw, bleeding surface is exposed. (From Eversole LR: Clinical Outline of Oral Pathology, 3rd ed. Philadelphia, Lea & Febiger, 1992, p 27.)

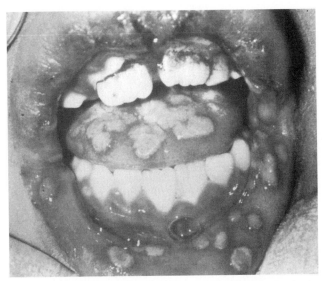

Figure 8-30. Primary herpetic infection. Primary herpes simplex infections occur mainly in children; however, most initial infections are much less severe. Primary lesions are seen occasionally in people who have an immune-compromising disease.

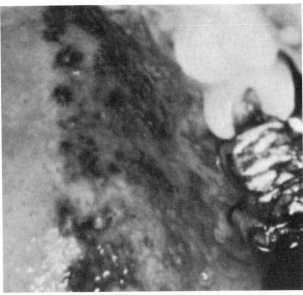

Figure 8-32. Herpes zoster. Herpes zoster, which is the recurrent form of chickenpox, occurs when the herpes zoster virus is reactivated. Herpes zoster virus commonly follows the distribution of the trigeminal nerve. Its unilateral distribution is considered to be a hallmark of the disease. (From Eversole LR: Clinical Outline of Oral Pathology, 3rd ed. Philadelphia, Lea & Febiger, 1992, p 96.)

Herpes Zoster-Varicella Virus

The herpesvirus, HSV-3, is responsible for **varicella** or **chickenpox** and **zoster**. Oral lesions are not especially common in varicella. When they do appear, they resemble lesions seen in HSV-1 but are usually more widely distributed. Recurrent lesions (**zoster** or "**shingles**"), although uncommon, appear mainly in older adults or immunocompromised persons. This virus, like other members of the herpesvirus family, resides quiescent within neural ganglion cells until triggered to reproduce. The characteristic feature of zoster is the striking **unilateral distribution of the vesicles** (**Figure 8-32**). Patients may also have persistent pain in affected areas following resolution of the outbreak of oral or skin lesions.

Epstein-Barr Virus

The most notable oral infections caused by Epstein-Barr virus (HSV-4) are **infectious mononucleosis** and **hairy leukoplakia**. Oral lesions of infectious mononucleosis usually present as **petechiae** on the soft palate. "Hairy" leukoplakia presents as a white plaque-like lesion on the lateral borders of the tongue, which may have a characteristic vertical strip-like pattern (**Figure 8-33**). The occurrence of hairy leukoplakia is considered to be a sign of significantly diminished immunity in persons who are HIV positive.

Coxsackievirus

The most frequently encountered oral coxsackie infections are **hand, foot, and mouth disease** and **herpangina**. Hand, foot, and mouth disease is suitably named. It presents with small vesicles on the hands and feet and is also found intraorally. Herpangina gets its name from the fact that the lesions resemble herpes, occurring in clusters in the posterior oropharynx, a pattern that is also seen in an unrelated disease-**herpetiform aphthous ulcers**.

Human Papillomavirus

Various strains of HPV are thought to be responsible for many epithelial growths ranging from warts to carcinoma of the cervix. Although HPV can readily be identified in lesions such as **verruca vulgaris** (i.e., warts) and **condyloma acuminatum** (i.e., venereal warts), they are not detected in all occurrences of the common oral wart-like growth, **squa-**

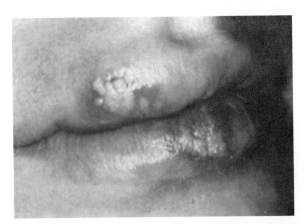

Figure 8-31. Recurrent herpes. Recurrent herpes commonly occurs on the lips. The reasons for this reactivation of the herpes virus vary. (From Eversole LR: Clinical Outline of Oral Pathology, 3rd ed. Philadelphia, Lea & Febiger, 1992, p 98.)

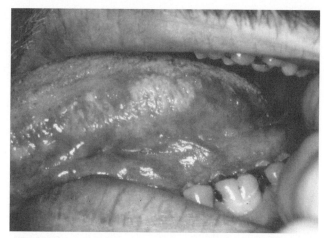

Figure 8-33. Hairy leukoplakia. Hairy leukoplakia is induced by the Epstein-Barr virus. It has been considered to be a marker for the transition of a person's HIV-positive status to that of AIDS.

mous papilloma. This virus is, however, thought to be the most likely causative agent.

Human Immunodeficiency Virus

HIV, owing to its specificity to the CD4 receptor sites on T lymphocytes, usually results in severe immunosuppression over time and the emergence of numerous diseases that are not normally found in persons with competent immune systems, including the occurrence of certain neoplasms. Kaposi sarcoma **(Figure 8-34),** carcinoma of the human female cervix, B cell lymphoma of the gastrointestinal tract, and hairy leukoplakia are all likely to have been initiated by viruses that express themselves because of immunosuppression. These diseases are now used as indicators for the conversion from HIV-positive status to AIDS. Other diseases found in people who have HIV/AIDS (and other immunosuppressed people) include candidiasis, gingivitis, periodontitis, and recurrent aphthous ulcers.

RADIOPAQUE LESIONS OF THE JAWS

Radiographic opacities are caused by either an increase in bone density or the presence of a substance of greater density than bone, such as a **foreign substance (Figure 8-35).** Foreign substances are generally easier to recognize than is some bony disease process, such as a bone-producing neoplasm or a reactive lesion stimulating additional bone deposition.

Bone-Producing Lesions

True bone-producing neoplasms are not common in the jaws; however, two common lesions (neither of which are neoplasms) are **exostosis (Figure 8-36),** which is generally found on the facial aspect of the jaw bone, and **torus,** which is midpalatal **(Figure 8-37)** and lingual of the mandible in the canine-premolar area **(Figure 8-38).** These lesions are often seen on radiographs and, when projected over the alveolus, may be confused for a neoplasm. Their location and long-standing history separate these from true neoplasms.

Two bone diseases that exhibit some degree of radiopacity are **ossifying fibroma** and **fibrous dysplasia.** Most often, these two lesions have a **ground-glass** radiographic pattern. This pattern is created by the displacement of normal trabecular bone by the deposition of new, less organized bone. The distinguishing feature of an ossifying fibroma is the presence of a distinct margin. Lesions of fibrous dysplasia seem to fade into the normal bony trabecular pattern.

Another, less common neoplasm that may appear radiopaque is **osteosarcoma.** The classic **sunburst** or **sun ray** pattern is usually a late radiographic finding. An early feature of osteosarcoma that involves the teeth is widening of the periodontal ligament. This feature is also shared with

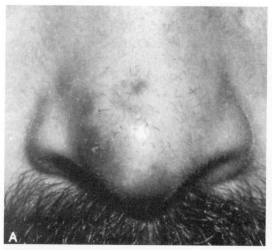
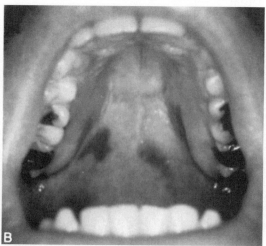

Figure 8-34. Kaposi sarcoma. A. Extra oral lesion of the nose. B. The dark area on the palate is Kaposi sarcoma in a person with AIDS. Kaposi sarcoma is now thought to be caused by herpes virus type 8. (From DeBiase C: Dental Health Education: Theory and Practice. Malvern, PA, Lea & Febiger, 1991, p 128.)

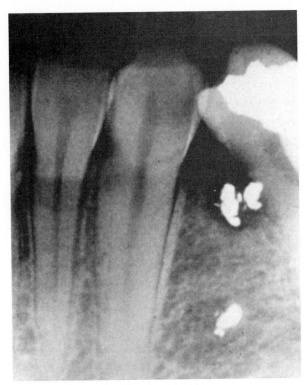

Figure 8-35. Foreign body. These radiopaque masses are fragments of amalgam. (From Eversole LR: Clinical Outline of Oral Pathology, 3rd ed. Philadelphia, Lea & Febiger, 1992, p 324.)

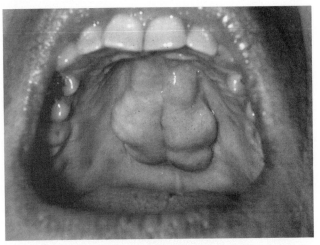

Figure 8-37. Maxillary torus. Midpalatal non-neoplastic bony protuberances are known as maxillary tori.

chondrosarcoma, which is a rare lesion of the jaw. Histologically, this widening represents invasion of the ligament by the malignant neoplasm.

Another disease that often presents as a radiopacity is **osteitis deformans (Paget disease of bone)**. Whereas Paget disease is not rare, less than 20% have jaw involvement. The maxilla is involved about seven times more often than is the mandible. A characteristic radiographic finding is thickening of the cementum on the roots of teeth in the affected jaw.

This does not seem to occur if the jaws are not affected. Lesions in bone are described as being **punched-out** radiolucencies with a **cotton wool** filling, a term used to describe loose cotton or cotton pulled from a bat or roll.

Reactive lesions that present as radiopaque lesions are **focal cemento-osseous dysplasia [(COD) or focal sclerosing ostemyelitis]**, **florid COD** or **diffuse sclerosing osteomyelitis**, and **periapical cemental dysplasia [(PCD) or cementoma]**.

PCD differs from the other two in that it occurs predominantly in the anterior mandible of middle-aged women of African-American origin (**Figure 8-39**). These lesions are described as having three rather distinct stages of development: (1) the osteolytic stage, (2) the cementoblastic stage, and the mature stage. In the osteolytic stage, the lesion appears as a radiolucent lesion at the apical portion of a mandibular anterior tooth (which is usually vital). In the cementoblastic stage, deposition of calcified material is present, usually beginning in the center of the radiolucency and

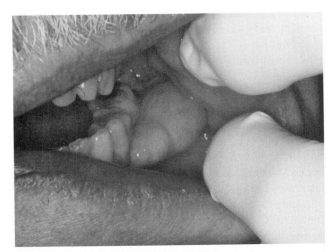

Figure 8-36. Exostosis. Bony, non-neoplastic protuberances on the alveolar processes are known as exostoses.

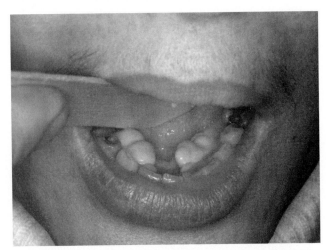

Figure 8-38. Mandibular tori. Exostoses on the lingual surface of the mandibular ridge are known as mandibular tori. Occurrences in fam-

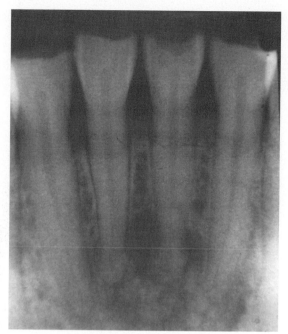

Figure 8-39. Periapical cemental dysplasia. Periapical cemental dysplasia is more commonly (but not exclusively) found in the mandibular anterior region in black women older than 40 years of age.

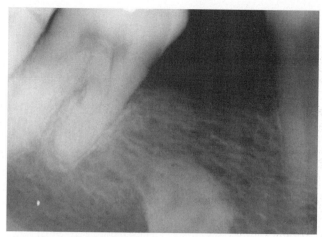

Figure 8-40. Condensing osteitis. Condensing osteitis is a sclerotic process of bone or a bone scar.

spreading outward toward the periphery. In the mature stage, the radiolucency is largely replaced by a radiopaque mass. Blunting of the apices of teeth associated with these lesions is also a common finding.

Focal COD is most often seen in the posterior portion of the jaws, especially the mandible. This lesion is predominantly found in women between the ages of 20 and 50 years. Unlike PCD, focal COD is seen more often in whites than blacks. Focal COD is generally thought to be a reactive lesion that arises from the periodontal ligament and is not neoplastic in origin.

Florid COD appears to be a process similar to the focal COD, except that larger segments of the jaw are involved and there is a significant predilection for blacks. The term *florid* is used to denote a generalize distribution of radiolucent and radiopaque masses in more than one focal area, involving dentulous and edentulous areas.

The **cementoblastoma** (a true cementoma) is a radiopaque lesion that is found predominantly in the posterior portion of the mandible, usually in the mandibular premolar-molar area. Unlike the periapical cemental dysplasia and focal COD, the cementoblastoma is attached to the root of the tooth and is probably a true cementum neoplasm. Radiographically, a well-delineated radiopaque mass is seen engulfing and reabsorbing the root of the affected tooth. About half of the patients with cementoblastoma have pain. These lesions are found most often in patients in their late teens or early 20s.

Condensing osteitis (sclerosing osteomyelitis) is an inflammatory lesion of bone. Inflammation of bone is usually a destructive process, but if the inflammatory process is very mild, bone may be stimulated to be laid down (**Figure 8-40**).

This lesion is found mainly at the apex of a nonvital tooth or at the site of a previous extraction. This lesion is predominantly a focal process; however, in the case of chronic periodontal disease, it may appear radiographically as a florid process. These focal and florid lesions can easily be mistaken for focal COD and florid COD, which were presented earlier. The most important radiographic feature that distinguishes COD lesions from condensing osteitis is that condensing osteitis does not exhibit a well-defined margin.

Lesions That Produce Tooth Substance

The quantity of calcified material produced by odontogenic lesions varies. Lesions that typically produce only fine calcified particles are: the **adenomatoid odontogenic tumor (AOT)**, the **calcifying epithelial odontogenic tumor (CEOT)**, and the **calcifying odontogenic cyst (COC)**. The AOT is found mainly in the anterior maxilla of women in their teens, usually in the canine area. The CEOT and the COC are found predominantly in people between 20 and 40 years of age with no gender predilection. All three lesions are commonly associated with an unerupted tooth.

Odontoma is, for the most part, not a true neoplasm but rather should be thought of as an unerupted, grossly abnormal supernumerary tooth. An odontoma may or may not resemble a tooth radiographically; however, a mixture of densities similar to dentin and enamel are usually distinguishable (**Figure 8-41**). Odontomas are found more commonly in the early years of life when tooth development is occurring. Although uncommon, odontogenic lesion such as ameloblastomas and keratocysts have been known to develop in odontomas, because they are like any other unerupted tooth.

Ameloblastic fibroma (AF) and **ameloblastic fibro-odontoma** (AF-O) are generally considered by most authorities to be true neoplasms. Some consider them to be "soft" odontomas or odontomas with little or no calcified tooth substance. AFs do not produce large, calcified particles; they may pro-

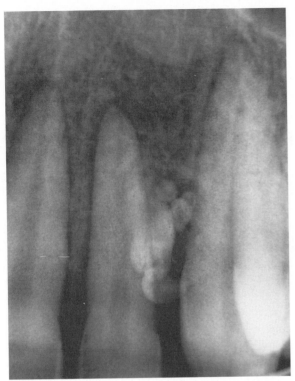

Figure 8-41. Odontoma. Odontomas are commonly found in children or young adults. They are distinguished radiographically by the varying densities created by the dentin and enamel of which they are made.

duce small quantities of tooth substance. Radiographically, an AF-O commonly presents as a predominantly radiolucent lesion with scattered small calcified structures (**Figure 8-42**). AFs and AF-Os occur more commonly in the young.

One of the most common radiopaque abnormalities to be encountered in the jaws is a **retained root tip** (**Figure 8-43**). Residual root tips may result from fracture of a root during surgery or from incomplete root reabsorption of a deciduous

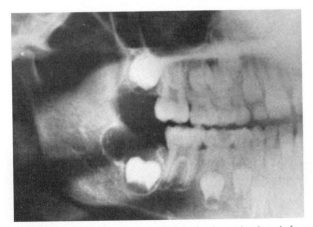

Figure 8-42. Ameloblastic fibroma. This lesion is predominantly found in children and young adults. Although they consist of toothbud-like tissue, these lesions produce little or no calcified products. (From Eversole LR: Clinical Outline of Oral Pathology, 3rd ed. Philadelphia, Lea & Febiger, 1992, p 259.)

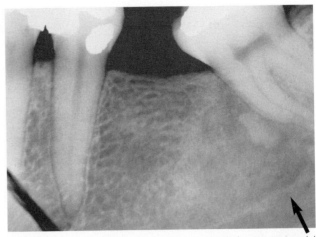

Figure 8-43. Retained root tip. A retained root tip is present mesial to the mandibular molar root. Retained root tips are often mistaken for sclerotic bone.

tooth. Retained deciduous root fragments may be perplexing if there are no missing permanent teeth clinically. The same holds true for amalgam fragments left from restored deciduous teeth when the permanent teeth have no restoration. It is easy to forget about the primary dentition when examining an adult.

A soft tissue radiodensity that is found occasionally on panoramic radiographs is the **mucus retention cyst** or **pseudocyst of the maxillary sinus**. This inflammatory lesion is not unlike a mucocele on the lower lip. This lesion appears as a dome-shaped mass on the floor of the maxillary sinus. It does not contain any calcified material; it appears somewhat opaque on panoramic radiographs because it is a soft tissue mass within an otherwise empty cavity (the maxillary sinus).

RADIOLUCENT LESIONS OF THE JAWS

Unilocular Radiolucent Lesions

Radiolucencies in bone indicate something displacing normal cortical or trabecular bone. The **submandibular salivary gland depression (Staphne cyst)** is an example of a depression in the lingual cortical plate that is caused by the submanibular gland. This focal thinning of the mandible causes it to appear as a radiolucent lesion within the bone. The characteristic feature of the submandibular salivary gland depression is its location. This lesion appears as a sharply demarcated radiolucency in the posterior mandible, below the mandibular canal (**Figure 8-44**).

Occasionally, when teeth are removed, the empty tooth socket fills in with hematopoietic marrow instead of normal trabecular bone. Because bone marrow is less dense than trabecular bone, the area appears as a radiolucency. This lesion is referred to as an **osteoporotic bone marrow defect**. These are more commonly seen in the posterior mandible and in women.

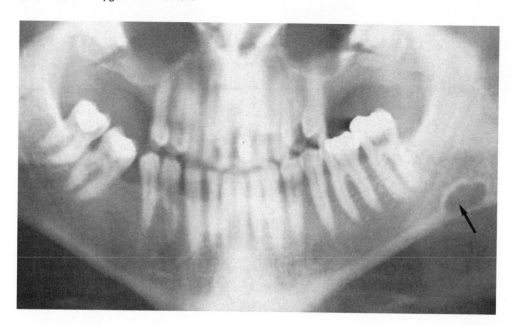

Figure 8-44. Submandibular salivary gland depression. Also known as a Staphne cyst, this is actually a depression in the lingual surface of the mandible. Its distinguishing feature is the sharply demarcated radiolucent lesion that is located below the mandibular canal. (From Eversole LR: Clinical Outline of Oral Pathology, 3rd ed. Philadelphia, Lea & Febiger, 1992, p 235.)

The **radicular** or **periapical cyst** is the most common radiolucency of the jaws (**Figure 8-45**). If the nonvital tooth that initiated this lesion is removed but the cyst is left behind, it is referred to as a **residual cyst** (**Figure 8-46**). Occasionally, this cyst may be located more laterally on the root of the nonvital tooth mimicking a lateral periodontal cyst.

A **lateral periodontal cyst** most often presents as a **unilocular or multilocular** lesion (**Figure 8-47**) and are referred to occasionally as **botryoid odontogenic cysts** (resembling a cluster of grapes). Lateral periodontal cysts are most commonly encountered in the mandibular premolar area.

After the periapical cyst and residual cyst, the most frequently encountered unilocular radiolucency is probably the **dentigerous cyst.** They are most often associated with unerupted mandibular third molars (**Figure 8-48**) followed in frequency by unerupted maxillary canines. Confusion often exists regarding radiolucency surrounding the crown of an

unerupted tooth. Should it be called a dentigerous cyst or a tooth follicle? The following, slightly less than scientific criteria seem adequate in most cases. If the radiolucency is small, it is a dental follicle. If it is large, it is a dentigerous cyst.

The **traumatic bone cyst** (**idiopathic bone cavity, hemorrhagic bone cavity,** and **simple bone cyst** are some of the other names for this lesion) is a lesion that is found mainly in the mandible of people between the ages of 10 and 20 years. The origin of this lesion and its name often causes confusion, because it is not a cyst (the cavity is not lined by epithelium), and many (if not most) patients have no recollection of trauma to the area. The characteristic radiographic feature of this lesion is the scalloped margins that are seen as it interdigitates between the roots of the teeth in the involved area without causing root reabsorption (**Figure 8-49**).

Clinically, the most significant lesions that occur as radiolucencies of the jaws are primary neoplasms of bone or neo-

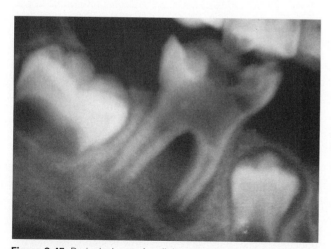

Figure 8-45. Periapical cyst. A radiolucency associated with the root of a nonvital tooth is most likely to be either a periapical cyst or a periapical granuloma. When these cysts are 1 cm or less in diameter, it is impossible to distinguish between them radiographically.

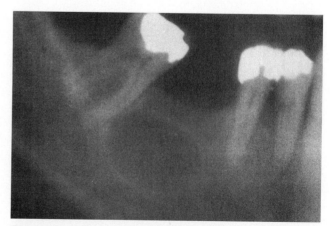

Figure 8-46. Residual cyst. A cyst (or fragments of a cyst) was left behind when the involved tooth was removed. In this case, it resembles a lateral periodontal cyst radiographically. (From Neville BW, Damm DD, White DK: Color Atlas of Clinical Oral Pathology, 2nd ed. Baltimore, Lippincott Williams & Wilkins, 1999, p 97.)

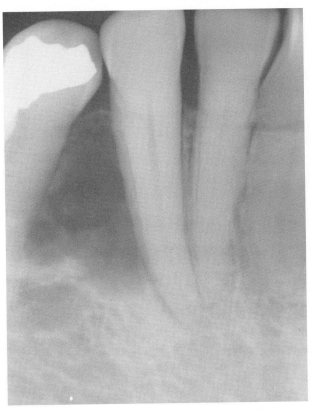

Figure 8-47. Lateral periodontal cyst. Lateral periodontal cysts may be unilocular or multilocular radiographically. Note the "soap bubble" multilocular appearance of this lesion.

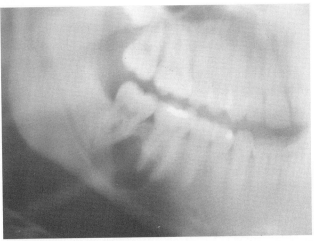

Figure 8-49. Traumatic bone "cyst." The characteristic feature of this lesion is the scalloping or ballooning of the radiolucency up between the roots of the teeth.

plasms that have metastasized to the jaws. Of the many neoplasms of bone that present as radiolucent lesions, **multiple myeloma**, **Langerhans cell granuloma** and **metastatic neoplasm to the jaws** should be considered. These lesions most commonly present as ill-defined radiolucencies; however, occasionally, they may be unilocular lesions.

Multiple myeloma and malignant neoplasms that have metastasized to the jaws are predominantly diseases found in older adults. The radiographic pattern of multiple myeloma is often described as **punched-out** radiolucencies or **floating teeth** (**Figure 8-50**). The pattern that is often ascribed to neoplasms metastatic to the jaws is one of an ill-defined destructive lesion that creates a **moth-eaten** appearance of the bone. Reabsorption of the roots of the teeth in the area is also a common finding. Another significant clinical finding is **paresthesia** or **anesthesia** caused by destruction of sensory nerve fibers in the area.

Langerhans cell granuloma (**histiocytosis X, eosinophilic granuloma,** and **Langerhans cell disease** are other names used for this entity) usually occurs in people younger

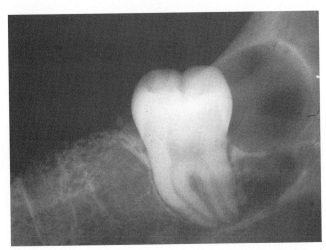

Figure 8-48. Dentigerous cyst. This lesion is present about and distal to the crown of an unerupted third molar, which is a common site.

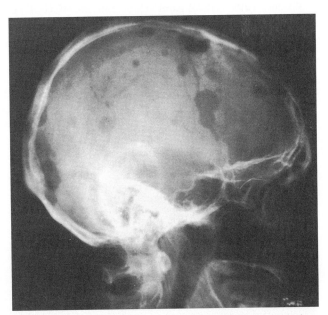

Figure 8-50. Multiple myeloma. Punched-out radiolucent lesions such as those seen in this skull film and floating teeth on dental radiographs are common in multiple myeloma. (From Rubin E, Farber JL: Pathology, 3rd ed. Philadelphia, Lippincott Williams & Wilkins, 1999, p 1149.)

than 20 years of age. Variants of this disease occur in different age groups. The chronic unifocal form mainly affects adults. The multifocal form occurs mainly in older children; and the acute disseminated form occurs in very young children. Floating teeth is a common radiographic finding in children with this disease (**Figure 8-51**).

Multilocular Radiolucencies of the Jaws

In a discussion of multilocular lesions, one should remember that these lesions may appear unilocular in the early stages of their development. They, however, usually progress to become multilocular in time.

Odontogenic keratocyst often present as multilocular radiolucencies, especially when they are large. They may or may not be associated with an unerupted tooth. Most of these lesions occur in the mandible between the ages of early teens and late 30s (**Figure 8-52**).

Ameloblastoma is not a very common neoplasm. The average age of occurrence is early to mid-30s, although these neoplasms may occur over a wide age range. There is no gender predilection for this neoplasm. Most of these lesions occur in the mandible associated with an unerupted tooth and are common among the molars. Radiographically, these lesions are described has having a **soap bubble** appearance (**Figure 8-53**). A variant of the ameloblastoma is the **unicystic ameloblastoma**. As its name implies, it does not have the usual soap bubble radiographic pattern. It also differs from ameloblastoma in that it occurs at a younger age and has a much lower recurrence rate.

A third lesion that commonly presents as a multilocular radiolucency is the **central giant cell granuloma [(CGCG)** or **giant cell tumor** or **giant cell lesion**]. Most CGCGs occur in the mandible, mainly anterior to the molar teeth, and in women who are an average age of 21 years (**Figure 8-54**). They may become quite large and may cause reabsorption of the roots of

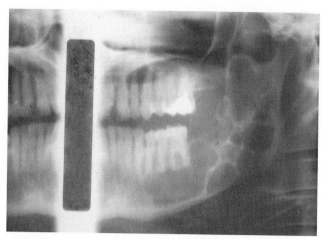

Figure 8-52. Odontogenic keratocyst. Large lesions commonly present as multilocular lesions. This radiograph depicts a recurrent cyst. Recurrence is more common in keratocysts than in dentigerous cysts.

teeth in the involved area. A CGCG-like lesion (**brown tumor of hyperparathyroidism** or **von Recklinghausen disease of bone**) also occurs. Therefore, any patient with a CGCG should be tested for hyperparathyroidism.

Cherubism, an hereditary condition with an autosomal dominant pattern, is usually recognized in the first decade of life. The characteristic cherub face is due to the presence of bilateral multilocular lesions radiographically, which result

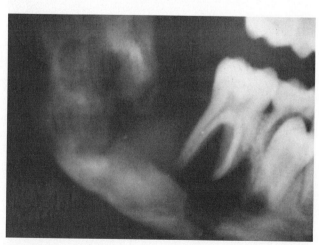

Figure 8-51. Langerhans cell granuloma. This is primarily a disease of children and young adults. Jaw involvement is commonly present as floating teeth.

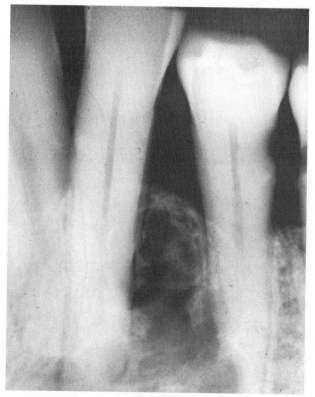

Figure 8-53. Ameloblastoma. Typically, ameloblastomas present as multilocular lesions, especially when they grow large.

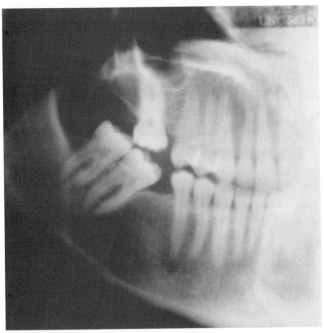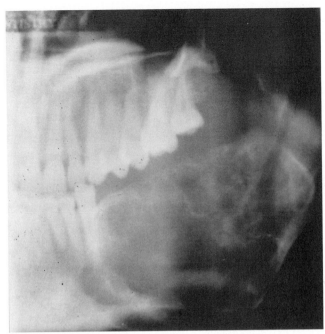

Figure 8-54. Central giant cell granuloma. Like the keratocyst and the ameloblastoma, these lesions are multilocular radiographically.

in a progressive bilateral facial swelling with displacement of the eyes when the maxilla is involved. **Hypertelorism** (increased distance between the eyes) is also characteristic of cherubism. Although mandibular lesions are most common, any or all quadrants may be involved.

A rare lesion that may occur in the mandible and that typically appears as a multilocular radiolucent lesion is **central hemangioma**. It is not uncommon for these lesions to have a significant arterial component with blood flow sounds (**bruit**) that can be heard with a stethoscope. Radiographically, this lesion is usually associated with the mandibular canal; however, the lesion can also be large and can involve a large portion of the mandible on that side.

 DENTAL DEFECTS

Defects or anomalies in tooth formation result from some incident or disease, which occurs during one or more stages of tooth development. These stages in order are **initiation, proliferation, histodifferentiation, morphodifferentiation, apposition,** and **calcification.** Once calcification is complete, the morphology of the tooth is set, leaving only environmental influences such as caries, erosion, abrasion, or attrition (or combinations of these) to alter the tooth structure.

Defects of Enamel

Many conditions can result in defects of enamel. During the initiation phase when the teeth begin to form (see the bud stage in Chapter 4), interferences such as radiation exposure or a hereditary disturbance like ectodermal dysplasia can result in the complete absence of teeth (**anodontia**) or partial

absence of teeth (**oligodontia**). A developmental disturbance creating increased cellular activity during this stage can result in the development of extra teeth or **supernumerary teeth**. The most common site is between the maxillary central incisors and is referred to as a **mesiodens. Natal teeth** are supernumerary teeth that are present at birth. They are defective and their removal is generally recommended, particularly if mobility poses the threat of aspiration. In contrast, primary teeth that erupt prematurely (during the first few weeks of life) are known as **neonatal teeth**. These teeth are usually normal primary teeth and should be retained. A radiograph should be exposed to confirm the differential diagnosis.

The proliferation stage is characterized by a rapid multiplication of cells (see the cap stage in Chapter 4). Interference during this stage of development may cause the formation of teeth with fewer or more cusps or roots than normal. Anomalies such as fusion and gemination may occur. **Fusion** involves the union of two normally separate tooth germs leading to a single large tooth. **Gemination** is a single tooth that incompletely divides into what appears to be two teeth with two separate pulp chambers and one pulp canal (**Figure 8-55**).

Differentiation of cells of developing teeth into specialized components refers to the histodifferentiation stage (see the bell stage in Chapter 4). Amelogenesis imperfecta may result if interference occurs during this stage of tooth development. **Amelogenesis imperfecta (Figure 8-56)** is a hereditary condition that has several modes of inheritance, both dominant and recessive, autosomal and X-linked, creating more than a dozen variants. In the most simplistic classification, these can be divided into four types: **hypocalcified, hypoplastic, hypomaturation,** and associated with **taurodontism**. In the hypocalcified form, cal-

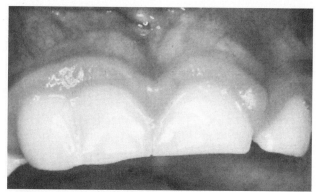

Figure 8-55. Gemination. Gemination of the primary maxillary right central incisor is present. (Courtesy of JE Bouquot, DDS, MS, West Virginia University, Morgantown, WV. From DeBiase C: Dental Health Education: Theory and Practice. Malvern, PA, Lea & Febiger, 1991, p 54.)

cium uptake by the forming enamel crystal is altered and causes "soft" enamel that is easily damaged. In the hypoplastic form, the ability of the developing tooth to form adequate enamel matrix during morphodifferentiation is compromised, and thin or pitted enamel results. The hypomaturation form is the result of a lack in maturation of the enamel or its ability to calcify appropriately. This results in an altered crystal density of the enamel, which causes light to be reflected differently and is seen as discoloration of the enamel similar to that found in fluorosis. There can be significant variation in the severity of this condition from a very mild hypoplastic type showing only pitting of the surface to a severe hypocalcified type where the enamel can be removed with a scaler or curet.

During the morphodifferentiation stage, the specialized cells arrange themselves in a manner that dictates the final size and shape of the tooth. Anomalies associated with interference during this stage of development are **taurodontism**, **dens-in-dente** (tooth within a tooth), **microdontia** [unusually small teeth (maxillary laterals and third molars most commonly)], **macrodontia** [unusually large teeth (fu-

sion, gemination)], and **dilaceration** (a sharp bend or curve in the crown or root). Taurodontism is occasionally associated with a subgroup of amelogenesis imperfecta with a combination of hypoplasia and hypomaturation defects. The malformed roots of taurodontism associated with this form of amelogenesis imperfecta probably results from an alteration in the **Hertwig epithelial root sheath,** which is derived from the reduced enamel epithelium of the developing crown. Taurodontism is also characterized by elongated pulp chambers and defined pulp horns. Two other enamel defects, which are associated with congenital syphilis, are **mulberry molars** and **Hutchinson incisors.**

The appositional stage involves the deposition of enamel matrix by ameloblasts and dentin matrix by odontoblasts. **Hypoplasia** may occur during this stage of development from local insults (e.g., periapical infection or trauma) or systemic diseases (e.g., rickets, fevers, cerebral palsy, Down or Hurler syndromes, epidermolysis bullosa, and hypoparathyroidism) (**Figure 8-57**). Pits or linear depressions void of enamel mark when the interference occurred. **Turner tooth** is a form of localized **odontodysplasia** that affects a developing tooth, most often a permanent tooth injured by an odontogenic infection of the overlying primary tooth during the development stage of the crown (**Figure 8-58**). When the injury is mild, only the enamel is involved; if, however, the injury is severe, the entire crown may become malformed. Hereditary defects such as amelogenesis and dentinogenesis imperfecta can also develop during this stage. **Fluorosis** is probably the most common systemically induced enamel defect. In severe forms, it may damage the enamel formation and result in pitting or other deformities of the enamel surface.

During the calcification stage, hydroxyapatite crystals are precipitated into the enamel matrix to mineralize or harden it. Hypomineralized (hypocalcified) enamel results from interference during this stage of tooth development. Clinically, these hypomineralized areas manifest as white opaque spots. In mild forms, fluoride alters the crystal structure of the enamel and affects the way that light is transmitted and reflected by enamel.

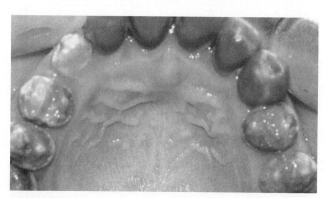

Figure 8-56. Amelogenesis imperfecta. There are many forms of amelogenesis imperfecta, which range from moderate enamel hypoplasia to this severe form in which the enamel poorly calcifies and easily worn away. (From Langlais RP, Miller CS: Color Atlas of Common Oral Diseases, 2nd ed. Philadelphia, Lippincott Williams & Wilkins, 1998, p 33.)

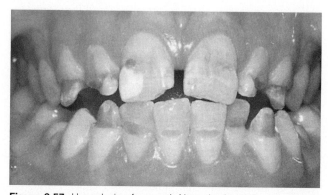

Figure 8-57. Hypoplasia of enamel. Note the band-like hypoplastic defect in the enamel of the teeth. This pattern is characteristic of a systemic disorder that disturbed the development of these teeth. (From Langlais RP, Miller CS: Color Atlas of Common Oral Diseases, 2nd ed. Philadelphia, Lippincott Williams & Wilkins, 1998, p 33.)

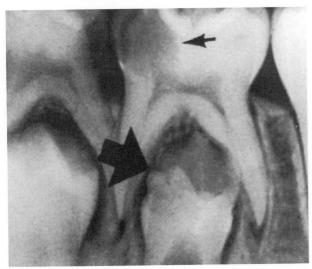

Figure 8-58. Turner tooth. This localized example of hypoplasia results from a dental infection of the primary tooth, which involves the developing permanent tooth bud below. (From DeBiase C: Dental Health Education: Theory and Practice. Malvern, PA, Lea & Febiger, 1991, p 57.)

This may cause teeth to appear to be darker or have white spots.

Defects in Dentin

Dentinogenesis imperfecta (hereditary opalescent dentin) is an autosomal dominant trait that sometimes occurs with **osteogenesis imperfecta**; however, it is not thought of as a part of osteogenesis imperfecta. In this condition, teeth have abnormal dentin that probably developed during the apposition stage of formation. Enamel is not generally abnormal.

Because the dentin has abnormal tubule formation, the reflective index of the dentin is abnormal and reflects light differently. Teeth appear to have a darker, often brown color with an opal-like quality created by the translucency of normal enamel over abnormal dentin.

Clinically, the enamel may fracture away because it is not well supported by or well attached to the abnormal dentin. The exposed soft dentin wears away and creates scooped-out occlusal surfaces. Radiographically, the teeth in dentinogenesis imperfecta appear to have normal-sized crowns; however, a narrowing of the root causes a **tightly cinched belt** look at the cervical margin of the tooth with thin, spiked roots (**Figure 8-59**). The pulp chambers and root canals are obliterated; however, in one variant, the pulp chambers and canals are larger than normal and create a shell-like tooth radiographically.

Dentin dysplasia type I (rootless teeth, radicular dentin dysplasia) clinically appears normal. Histologically, crowns initially appear normal; however, something happens during the later stages of root development, and the apposition and formation of dentin become greatly disorganized. This results in short and weakened roots that may fracture. Radiographic findings in dentin dysplasia type I are

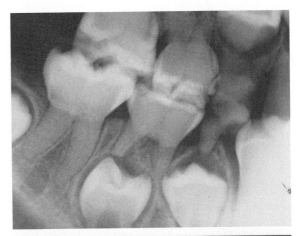

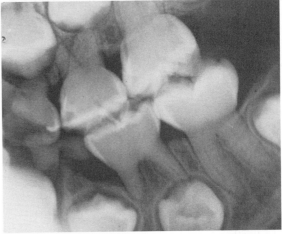

Figure 8-59. Dentinogenesis imperfecta. The distinguishing radiographic features of dentinogenesis imperfecta are obliteration of the pulp chambers and spiked roots.

striking. In addition to shortened roots, pulp chambers and root canals of the teeth are compressed, thus creating a thin horizontal line that has been likened to a **chevron** (a V-shaped strip) (**Figure 8-60**).

In **dentin dysplasia type II (coronal dentin dysplasia)**, the pulp chambers of the teeth are much larger than normal, which has been described radiographically as resembling the stem of a **thistle** (a large hollow tube). Most often, large pulp stones are seen in these enlarged pulp chambers (**Figure 8-61**).

Defects That Involve Both Dentin and Enamel

Regional odontodysplasia may involve one tooth or several teeth that are localized in a single quadrant. The exact cause is unknown; however, its localized nature would tend to rule out heredity or systemic disorders. Clinically, the teeth usually have distorted crowns and are very fragile. Radiographically, the affected teeth appear as **shell teeth** or "**ghost**" **teeth** with only a rim or shell of tooth substance (**Figure 8-62**). This more likely is the result of localized alteration during the apposition stage of tooth development.

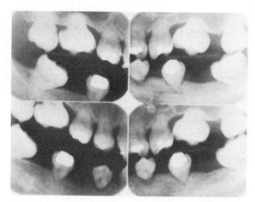

Figure 8-60. Dentin dysplasia, type I. Note the lack of root formation and abnormal pulp shapes. (From Eversole LR: Clinical Outline of Oral Pathology, 3rd ed. Philadelphia, Lea & Febiger, 1992, p 363.)

Defects of Cementum

Hypophosphatasia is a familial skeletal disease characterized by low levels of serum alkaline phosphatase. Early loss of primary teeth due to a lack of cementum is commonly seen.

ORAL SWELLINGS

Focal Swellings of the Gingiva and Alveolar Ridge

Several rather common lesions present as discrete, focal swellings of the gingiva. Probably the most common are **parulis** (mentioned earlier), **fibroma, pyogenic granuloma, peripheral giant cell granuloma, mandibular torus, facial exostoses, focal fibrous hyperplasia (epulis),** and **peripheral ossifying fibroma.** Other diseases and neoplasms may occur in this location, however, they are less common.

True **fibromas** of the oral cavity are very uncommon (**Figure 8-63**). Most lesions called fibromas are actually reactive

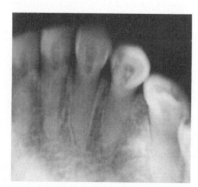

Figure 8-61. Dentin dysplasia, type II. The key features of this abnormality are the enlarged pulp chambers and pulpal calcifications (denticles). (From Langlais RP, Miller CS: Color Atlas of Common Oral Diseases, 2nd ed. Philadelphia, Lippincott Williams & Wilkins, 1998, p 33.)

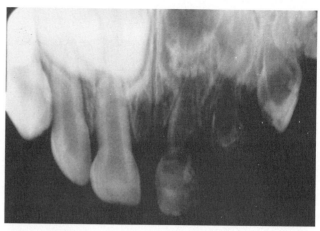

Figure 8-62. Regional odontodysplasia. The characteristic features are the "ghost" or shell-like appearance of the teeth radiographically and the regional presentation (one quadrant).

responses to local irritation. They may be found on any mucosal surface. Oral "fibromas" consist of dense fibrous connective tissue that is firm to the touch; they have a smooth surface and are usually slightly pale to normal in color.

Pyogenic granuloma, contrary to its name, is not a **suppurative** (pus-forming) lesion. Like the fibroma, this lesion is a reactive lesion. Unlike the fibroma, however, this lesion consists of granulation tissue instead of dense fibrous connective tissue. The surface is usually ulcerated, which causes it to appear erythematous (**Figure 8-64**). Pyogenic granuloma may also be hemorrhagic. When removing these lesions, it is important also to eliminate the local factors that initiated its growth. Some of these may eventually **sclerose** (i.e., form scar tissue). When this happens, they clinically become fibroma-like lesions.

The **peripheral giant cell granuloma** is also a reactive lesion; however, unlike pyogenic granuloma, it contains numerous multinucleated giant cells. These lesions are thought to arise from the periodontal membrane, because they are found only on tooth-bearing surfaces. Histologically, they exhibit a

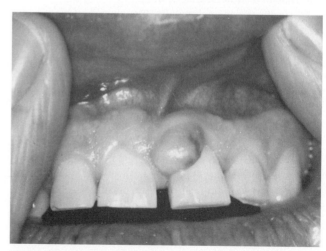

Figure 8-63. Fibroma. These lesions have a smooth surface; they appear slightly pale and are rubbery to firm on palpation.

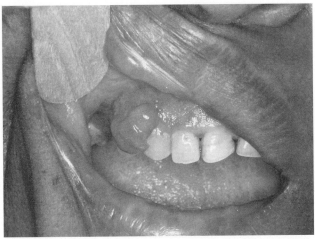

Figure 8-64. Pyogenic granuloma. The distinguishing features of pyogenic granuloma are its reddish color and its history of bleeding easily. Local irritants are the common etiology, and these may occur anywhere.

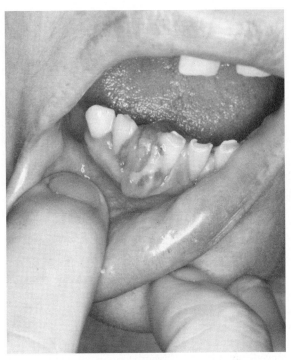

Figure 8-65. Peripheral giant cell granuloma. This lesion may resemble a pyogenic granuloma; however, it tends to be more purplish and often displaces teeth as it grows. Also, the lesion occurs only occur on tooth-bearing surfaces.

rich vascular stroma and abundant hemosiderin pigment and often have an intact surface layer of squamous epithelium. Clinically, this lesion usually appears as a smooth-surfaced gingival swelling that is not unlike a fibroma; however, it appears blue to purple (**Figure 8-65**). Peripheral giant cell granulomas may recur if they are inadequately removed.

Mandibular tori and **exostoses** are very common swellings of the alveolar ridges (see Figures 8-36 and 8-38). They are generally not removed unless they interfere with function or for prosthetic reasons. The exact cause of these bony projections is unknown; however, in some cases, they appear to be hereditary.

Focal fibrous hyperplasia (**epulis**) is generally found in patients who wear dental prostheses. These lesions are also reactive and may vary in appearance from pale (fibroma-like) to erythematous (pyogenic granuloma-like). They may also be referred to as **epulis fissuratum,** because they are often lobulated or have a creased surface that surrounds a portion of the denture flange (**Figure 8-66**).

The **peripheral ossifying fibroma** is a lesion that clinically resembles a pyogenic granuloma. Histologically, varying amounts of bone and occasionally multinucleated giant cells are seen. Whereas the amount of bone produced is usually small, particles of bone on dental radiographs may sometimes be detected. This lesion most likely arises from the periosteum, which accounts for its histologic appearance and its occurrence on alveolar surfaces. It is more frequently seen in young adult women.

Diffuse or Generalized Swellings of the Gingiva and Alveolar Ridge Mucosa

A diffuse fibrous swelling on the gingiva or alveolar ridge may be related to various causes. Examples include **drug-in-**

duced gingival hyperplasia, hyperplasia from local irritation, hereditary gingival fibromatosis, and the oral manifestations of an underlying systemic disease (**Figure 8-67**).

Phenytoin (dilantin) was one of the first drugs associated with gingival hyperplasia. More recently, **cyclosporine** (a drug taken by organ transplant patients to reduce the likelihood of rejection) and calcium channel blocking agents such as **nifedipine** (an antihypertensive medication) have been documented to cause gingival hyperplasia. No clinical features can be used to distinguish among these other than a history of taking one of these drugs.

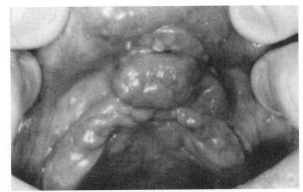

Figure 8-66. Focal fibrous hyperplasia (epulis). Focal fibrous hyperplasia may appear like a fibroma or a pyogenic granuloma and is seen most often in people who wear dentures. (From Eversole LR: Clinical Outline of Oral Pathology, 3rd ed. Philadelphia, Lea & Febiger, 1992, p 119.)

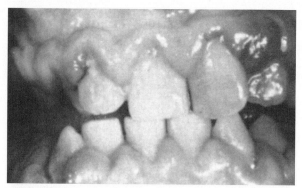

Figure 8-67. Generalized gingival hyperplasia is most commonly induced by drugs, especially by phenytoin, nifedipine, and cyclosporin. (From Eversole LR: Clinical Outline of Oral Pathology, 3rd ed. Philadelphia, Lea & Febiger, 1992, p 124.)

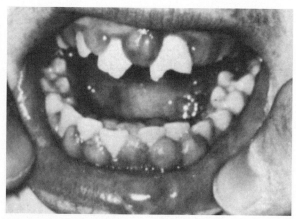

Figure 8-69. Leukemic infiltrate is present in the gingiva. (From Eversole LR: Clinical Outline of Oral Pathology, 3rd ed. Philadelphia, Lea & Febiger, 1992, p 126.)

Occasionally, one encounters a patient with generalized gingival inflammation that has produced widespread gingival swelling and is usually associated with heavy plaque accumulation. Its presentation is consistent with its inflammatory origin, such as chronic gingivitis.

Hereditary gingival fibromatosis is an uncommon disease. It has no particular characteristic clinical features to distinguish it from drug-induced hyperplasia other than a family history and the fact that the patient is not taking a gingival hyperplasia-inducing drug.

Some systemic conditions may result in gingival swelling. Patients who have **poorly controlled diabetes mellitus** may have a generalized gingival inflammation or multiple abscesses of gingival or periodontal origin (**Figure 8-68**). This is probably due to a compromised inflammatory response, which is often found in patients who have unstable diabetes.

Gingival enlargement may also be a finding in a patient who has **leukemia**. Enlargement results from a massive infiltrate of leukemic cells or from the lack of normal inflammatory cells (displaced by the atypical leukemic cells repopulating the bone marrow) resulting in a generalized gingival infection (**Figure 8-69**).

Gingival hyperplasia is also seen in **pregnancy** and is thought to result from the altered hormonal state and its influences on tissue responses.

Wegener granulomatosis is an uncommon disease that has a fairly characteristic gingival presentation. This disease is suspected to be an immune disorder that commonly involves multiple organs; however, when gingival lesions occur, the disease has a somewhat unique appearance that is referred to as "**strawberry**" **gingivitis**. It is so named because of its erythematous, knobby surface that resembles a strawberry.

Verrucous carcinoma is commonly found in the vestibules and involves the gingiva or alveolar ridge (**Figure 8-70**). These cancers are commonly associated with use of smokeless tobacco. As a general rule, they tend to be slightly less aggressive than are squamous cell carcinomas.

Swellings of the Lip

Swellings of the lower lip are more common than those of the upper lip. Most **lower lip** swellings are the result of traumatically induced extravasation of mucus (**mucocele**) (see Figure 8-7). Minor salivary gland neoplasms account for less than 10% of lower lip swellings. This is in direct contrast to the upper lip, where benign neoplasms of minor salivary glands outnumber mucoceles by 9:1. The most common neoplasms of salivary gland origin in the upper lip are the **pleomorphic adenoma** (**mixed tumor**) and the **monomorphic adenoma** (see Figure 8-8).

Hemangioma and **lymphangioma**, swellings of vascular origin, for the most part are congenital vascular anomalies of the lip, tongue, and face, which are first recognized early in life. The lower lip is also a common site for **squamous cell carcinoma**, which is found mainly in people older than 50 years of age (see Figure 8-10). Squamous

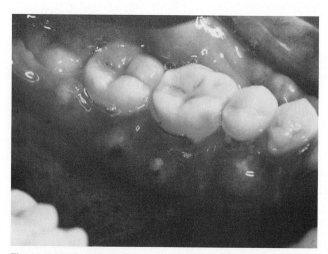

Figure 8-68. Gingival/periodontal abscesses. These abscesses are generally associated with some underlying systemic disease process. In this case, the cause is poorly controlled diabetes mellitus.

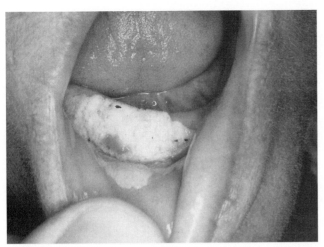

Figure 8-70. Verrucous carcinoma. This lesion commonly grows as a slightly flat lesion in the early stages. Its rough, warty-like surface is characteristic. Oral verrucous carcinoma is commonly associated with tobacco use, especially smokeless tobacco.

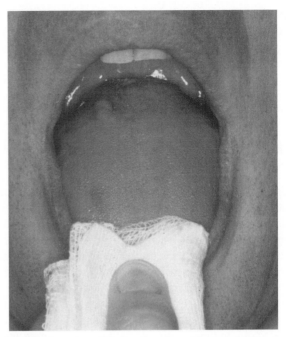

Figure 8-71. Granular cell lesion. Granular cell lesions, benign nerve neoplasms, and vascular lesions are the most common tumors that occur on the tongue. Color is often helpful in distinguishing among them.

cell carcinoma accounts for approximately 90% of all oral malignancies.

An uncommon lesion of the mucosal surface of the lower lip is **keratoacanthoma**, which is a growth that occurs more commonly on sun-exposed skin. Characteristically, it is a discrete nodular lesion that is shaped slightly like a crater and is filled with a central plug of keratin. Clinically, this lesion may resemble squamous cell carcinoma; however, the lesion is known to regress spontaneously if untreated.

Swellings of the Tongue

The most frequently encountered swellings of the tongue are of vascular or neural origin. The tongue is a common oral site for the occurrence of congenital **hemangiomas** and **lymphangiomas**. Clinically, these swellings may have a deep bluish to red color, and patients have been aware of them for many years with little or no growth. On palpation, they are generally compressible.

The most common neoplasms of neural origin in the tongue are **neurofibroma, neurilemoma,** and **granular cell tumor (Figure 8-71).** Neurofibroma is usually a solitary neoplasm; however, it may also represent the "tip of the iceberg" of a hereditary condition known as **neurofibromatosis, type 1** (or **von Recklinghausen disease of the skin**). Patients with this condition may have literally hundreds of neurofibromas scattered throughout the body. There is some increased risk of malignant transformation in one of these neurofibromas in this syndrome.

Neurofibromas are clinically firm to the touch and painless and have a normal mucosal color. This is also true for a neurilemoma. There are no clinical features to distinguish between a neurofibroma and a neurilemoma. The diagnosis is ultimately made microscopically.

The granular cell tumor is thought to be of **neuroectodermal** origin with the tongue being the most common oral site. Clinically, they are firm swellings and look yellow.

Another lesion, which is histologically similar to the granular cell tumor but occurs on the alveolar ridge of newborn children, is the **congenital epulis of the newborn (Figure 8-72).**

Infrequently, trauma to the tip of the tongue may damage the ducts of the minor salivary glands of **Blandin and Nuhn** and result in a mucocele.

The tongue is one of the more common sites for intraoral cancer; the vast majority being squamous cell carcinoma. They usually present as firm, indurated, and ulcerative le-

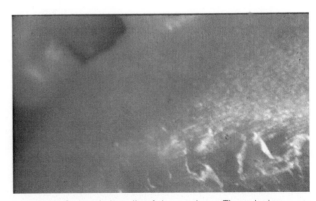

Figure 8-72. Congenital epulis of the newborn. These lesions may occur occasionally on both jaws. (Courtesy of Dr. Sheryl Hunter. From Langlais RP, Miller CS: Color Atlas of Common Oral Diseases, 2nd ed. Philadelphia, Lippincott Williams & Wilkins, 1998, p 23.)

sions that may not be especially painful in the early stages. The lesions rather rapidly become large fungating ulcers. Approximately one half of people with squamous cell carcinoma of the tongue will have already have metastasis to lymph nodes of the cervical neck at the time of diagnosis. Cervical lymph nodes that are involved are usually firm and nonmovable (i.e., **fixed**).

Swellings in the Floor of the Mouth

Swellings in the floor of the mouth may be the result of **developmental cysts** (i.e., **dermoid, epidermoid, lymphoepithelial**, or **thyroglossal duct cysts**) **(Figure 8-73)**, **neoplasia**, **mucus spillage (extravasation)**, or **infection. Ludwig angina** is a potentially fatal **space infection** that involves the floor of the mouth. Edema, which results from an infection in this anatomic space, causes the floor of the mouth to become elevated and forces the tongue to occlude the airway, which often requires a tracheotomy. This condition may be fatal if the infection descends into the chest.

Dermoid and epidermoid cysts occur most often above the mylohyoid muscle in the floor of the mouth. If large, these cysts can also cause displacement of the tongue, thus making speech and eating difficult to accomplish. These swellings are generally somewhat compressible but may be "tense" on palpation. The distinction between the dermoid and epidermoid cysts can only be made microscopically.

Lymphoepithelial cysts occur more commonly in areas where lymphoid tissue is abundant, such as the tonsillar region. A common site is near the lingual frenum in the floor of the mouth. Clinically, these cysts appear as compressible, slightly yellow swellings, which may drain a keratin-rich fluid that resembles pus.

The **thyroglossal duct cyst** (or **thyroglossal tract cyst**) is an uncommon cyst that developed from remnants of the thyroglossal tract. Although this lesion may appear as a swelling in the floor of the mouth, it presents more commonly as midline swellings in the neck near or below the hyoid bone.

Swellings of the Palate

The most common swelling of the palate is the **maxillary torus** (see Figure 8-37). This lesion usually becomes obvious in early adulthood and may grow slowly for several years. The lesion is characterized by its presence in the midline and bony hard feel to the touch.

Another frequent swelling on the palate is a draining **sinus tract** from an **abscess**. (This lesion has also been referred to as a **fistulous tract**; however, unless the maxillary sinus is involved, it should not be called a fistula.) This is more common in the posterior segment, where the palatal roots of the molar teeth are adjacent to the lingual cortical plate of the palate. In the anterior segment, drainage tracts are found more often in the labial vestibular area where the facial cortical plate covering the roots of the anterior teeth is very thin.

In the midline, anterior portion of the maxilla, **cysts of the incisive papilla** present as palatal swellings. **Cysts of the incisive canal** (i.e., **nasopalatine duct cysts**), unless very large, do not usually create much palatal swelling but can readily be detected on radiographs **(Figure 8-74)**. **Minor salivary gland neoplasms** are also a frequent cause of palatal swellings. Statistically, a **minor salivary gland neoplasm on the palate has about an equal chance of being benign or malignant**. A few clinical clues may help to differentiate benign from malignant lesions. Most benign palatal salivary gland neoplasms exhibit slow growth and, unless traumatized, they do not exhibit surface ulceration. Malignant neoplasms, because they grow more rapidly, often exhibit central necrosis and surface ulceration. Another characteristic feature that is seen in early malignant minor salivary gland neoplasms on the palate is surface **telangiectasia** (i.e., dilated, superficial blood vessels over the swelling).

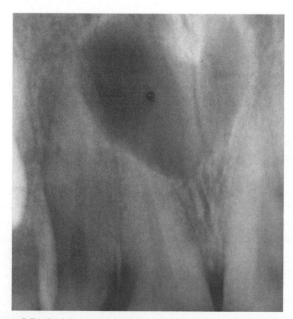

Figure 8-74. Incisive canal cyst (nasopalatine duct cyst). The heart-shaped radiolucency, which is situated between the roots of central incisors, is typical.

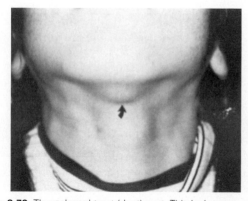

Figure 8-73. Thyroglossal tract (duct) cyst. This lesion presents as a midline swelling, usually below the hyoid bone. (From Eversole LR: Clinical Outline of Oral Pathology, 3rd ed. Philadelphia, Lea & Febiger, 1992, p 213.)

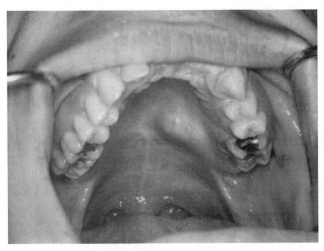

Figure 8-75. Pleomorphic adenoma. A smooth, dome-shaped mass is present with no telangiectasia.

The most common benign minor salivary gland tumor of the palate is the **mixed tumor** (or **pleomorphic adenoma**) (**Figure 8-75**). The **mucoepidermoid carcinoma** is the most frequent malignant salivary gland neoplasm of the palate. A second, but less common malignant salivary gland tumor of the palate is the **adenoid cystic carcinoma**. Squamous cell carcinoma of the palate is also seen. As a general rule, malignant neoplasms of the palate do not have a good prognosis.

A rare lesion that has a predilection for the hard palate is **necrotizing sialometaplasia**. Although the exact cause of this lesion is unknown, focal **ischemia** resulting in **infarction** of the gland is the favored theory. A characteristic clinical feature is the sudden appearance of a swelling, which sloughs and leaves a deep crater-like lesion. Healing is usually uneventful but may take several weeks if the lesion is large.

Swellings of the Buccal Mucosa

A common swelling of the buccal mucosa is the **fibroma** (see Figure 8-63). As noted earlier, this lesion is usually reactive and is not neoplastic (which its name implies). Because these lesions consist of dense, almost scar-like fibrous connective tissue, they do not often completely resolve following removal of the initiating irritant and must be removed surgically.

Another, but less common, swelling of the buccal mucosa results from **herniation of adipose tissue from the buccal fat pad** through the buccinator muscle. These lesions appear yellowish and are soft when palpated.

Neoplasms of minor salivary gland origin also occur on the buccal mucosa, the most common being the **mixed tumor (pleomorphic adenoma)**. **Mucoepidermoid carcinoma** is the most common malignant salivary gland neoplasm.

Neural lesions also occur on the buccal mucosa. The more common ones are **traumatic neuroma, neurilemoma,** and **neurofibroma** (either solitary or as part of **neurofibro-**matosis, type 1). Other than a history of trauma or pain (for the traumatic neuroma) or of multiple lesions (for neurofibromatosis), there is little clinically to help distinguish these lesions from one another.

Hematomas are the result of injury with spillage of blood into tissue spaces. Hemangiomas and **lymphangiomas** are mainly congenital lesions and appear bluish-purple.

Squamous cell carcinoma and a variant, **verrucous carcinoma,** are almost always found in patients who have a history of long-term tobacco use. Squamous cell carcinomas may appear **red**, **white,** or **speckled** and present as a firm, **indurated,** and ulcerated mass. Verrucous carcinoma is generally white, has a rough, wart-like surface texture, and is named for its wart-like (**verruca**) appearance. Verrucous carcinoma is generally superficial in the early stages; however, if untreated, it will eventually invade deeply. Verrucous carcinomas are almost always associated with tobacco use and are found more often in the **lower vestibular area** and the buccal mucosa.

Swellings of the Neck and Face

Swellings of the neck include a wide range of lesions, many of which are developmental. Examples of developmental swellings include **benign lymphoepithelial cysts** (arising from epithelium trapped within lymph nodes), **dermoid** or **epidermoid cysts** (arising from accessory skin structures such as hair follicles), and **thyroglossal duct** or **tract cysts** (which occur in the midline of the neck between the hyoid bone and the thyroid gland). These swellings tend to be compressible, although they may be tense and feel slightly firm on palpation. For the most part, they exhibit a normal skin color.

Swellings of the face, especially the upper, sun-exposed skin, may represent skin cancer. **BCC,** the most common form of skin cancer, appears as a slow-growing ulcerative lesion with "rolled" margins and a central depressed crater that repeatedly scabs over and then sloughs (see Figure 8-12). BCCs are slow-growing lesions and infrequently metastasize.

Malignant melanoma, which is another form of skin cancer, is increasing in incidence more rapidly than any other form of skin cancer and is the predominant cause of death from skin cancers. Most are thought to be caused by chronic exposure to sunlight or, more specifically, by the ultraviolet portion of the spectrum. Pre-existing nevi on sun-exposed skin are the most common site for melanomas of the skin. A melanoma is more likely to be fatal than a BCC, because a melanoma commonly metastasizes. A malignant melanoma often has irregular margins and variations in color (**Figure 8-76**).

In the preauricular area, a swelling is most likely to represent some disease of the parotid gland. In addition to neoplasms, chronic inflammatory diseases are not uncommon. **Chronic sialadenitis** often occurs when the parotid duct becomes occluded with a salivary stone (**sialolith**). Swelling is also seen in cases of acute sialadenitis, such as **infective parotitis (mumps)**. If persistent bilateral parotid swelling oc-

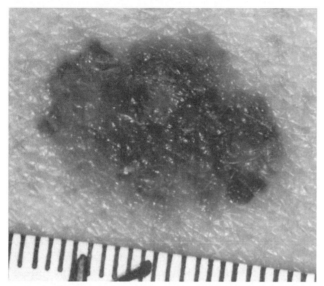

Figure 8-76. Malignant melanoma. The clinical features that are common to melanoma are recent color change, irregular margins, recent enlargement, and ulceration or nodularity. (From Rubin E, Farber JL: Pathology, 3rd ed. Philadelphia, Lippincott Williams & Wilkins, 1999, p 128.)

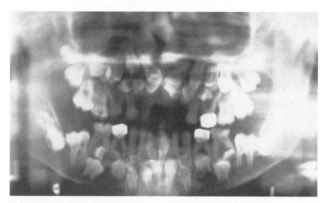

Figure 8-78. Cleidocranial dysplasia. Multiple unerupted teeth (both normal dentition as well as supernumerary teeth) and the primary dentition fail to shed. (From Langlais RP, Miller CS: Color Atlas of Common Oral Diseases, 2nd ed. Philadelphia, Lippincott Williams & Wilkins, 1998, p 31.)

curs, the autoimmune inflammatory disease **Sjögren syndrome** should be considered, especially if the patient has a history of another immune disorder such as **rheumatoid arthritis**. **Xerostomia** and **xerophthalmia** (dry eyes) are common complaints of patients who have Sjögren syndrome.

Salivary gland neoplasms are common in the parotid gland. (**Figure 8-77**). Approximately two thirds of all benign and one half of all malignant salivary gland tumors involve the parotid gland. If all salivary tumors of the parotid gland are considered, about two thirds are benign. The most common benign salivary gland tumor in the parotid gland is the **mixed tumor (pleomorphic adenoma)**. The most common malignant salivary gland neoplasms of the parotid are the **mucoepidermoid carcinoma** and the **acinic cell carcinoma**; however, the acinic cell carcinoma is relatively uncommon in other salivary glands.

 SYNDROMES

Syndromes That Affect the Teeth or Bones of the Face

Cleidocranial dysplasia is an autosomal dominant trait that includes alteration in the shape of the skull (**brachycephaly**) and frontal bossing, flattening of the bridge of the nose, clinical **oligodontia** (there is a delay or failure of teeth to erupt, including **supernumary teeth**) (**Figure 8-78**), and partial or complete lack of development of the clavicles (**Figure 8-79**). The clavicular abnormality allows these people to approximate the shoulders forward, often to the point of the shoulders touching.

Craniofacial dysostosis (**Crouzon syndrome**) is an autosomal dominant trait that is characterized by midfacial depression with relative prognathism, exophthalmos (bulging eyes), and hypertelorism (wide-spaced eyes) (**Figure 8-80**).

Mandibulofacial dysostosis (**Treacher Collins syndrome**) is an autosomal dominant trait that results in abnormal growth in the first and second branchial arches. People

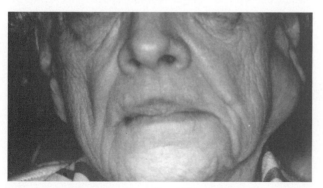

Figure 8-77. Salivary gland neoplasm. This salivary gland tumor occurs in the parotid gland.

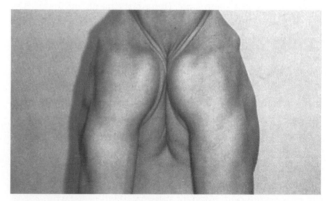

Figure 8-79. Cleidocranial dysplasia. Lack of adequate development of the clavicles brings the shoulders together. (From Langlais RP, Miller CS: Color Atlas of Common Oral Diseases, 2nd ed. Philadelphia, Lippincott Williams & Wilkins, 1998, p 31.)

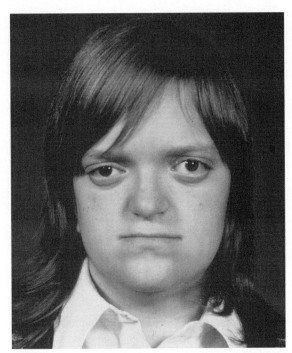

Figure 8-80. Craniofacial dysostosis (Crouzon syndrome). Hypertelorism, exophthalmos, and midface depression are distinguishing features of this autosomal dominant trait.

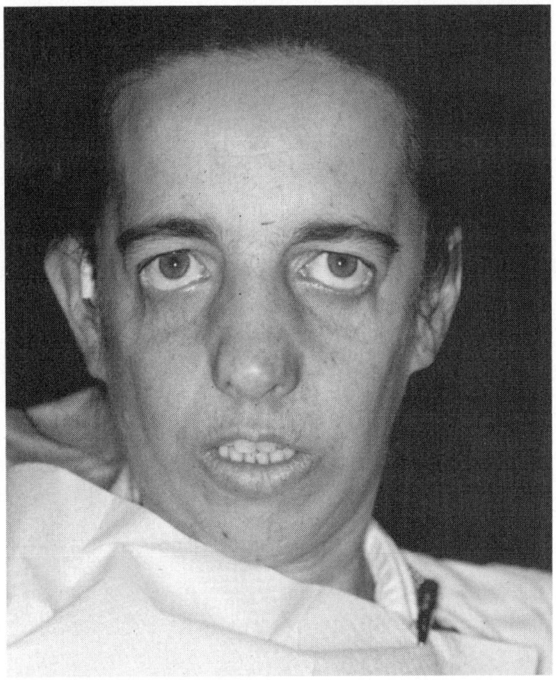

Figure 8-81. Mandibulofacial dysostosis (Treacher Collins syndrome). Lack of adequate growth of the first and second arches results in retrognathia, malformed ears, and zygomatic process of the maxilla. Loss of hearing may also occur.

with this syndrome have malformed ears (often with some hearing loss), an underdeveloped mandible (**retrognathia**), underdevelopment of the maxilla and zygomas, and notching or drooping of the lower eyelids (**colobomas**) (**Figure 8-81**). **Cleft palate** is also seen in some people with this syndrome.

Robin sequence (also published under the name of **Pierre Robin syndrome**) is an uncommon developmental defect of unknown etiology. The sequence of events that creates this condition appear to begin with inability of the tongue to drop out of the way of the palatal halves, thus preventing closure of the palate during embryogenesis. Failure of the tongue to move into its proper location also affects mandibular growth. Failure of this normal sequence of developmental events to take place results in the three defects that make up the Robin sequence-**micrognathia** (small mandible), **glossoptosis** (displacement of the tongue into the posterior oropharynx), and **cleft palate**. Because these children often have eating and breathing problems, surgical management is often required.

Cleft palate and **cleft lip** are not uncommon and occur in about 1 in 700 to 1000 births. The incidence in different countries varies as does the incidence in some racial and ethnic groups. The combination of cleft lip and palate occurs more commonly than either an isolated cleft of the lip or of the palate. A significant percentage of cases of cleft lip and palate appear to exhibit a hereditary pattern. In its mildest form, cleft palate appears as a **bifid uvula** (**Figure 8-82**).

Gardner syndrome is another autosomal dominant trait that affects the face. People with this syndrome have **osteomas,** which may occur in the jaws and epithelial inclusion cysts of the skin. The most significant aspect of this syndrome is the occurrence of intestinal polyps of the large bowel, which become malignant. Currently, it is recommended that persons with this syndrome have the large bowel removed as a precaution, because the incidence of malignant transformation is approximately **100%**.

Osteogenesis imperfecta is an autosomal hereditary condition that results in defective bone development. There are subsets of this syndrome, some of which are **dominant** and

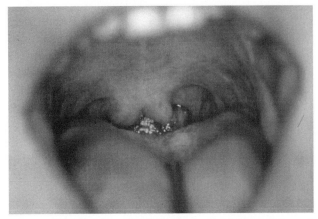

Figure 8-82. Bifid uvula. This may represent clefting of the soft palate.

some of which are **recessive** traits. The severity of the syndrome varies from a **lethal** condition resulting in stillbirth or death shortly after birth to a mild form exhibiting some skeletal deformity, with and without **blue sclera** of the eyes. The significance of this syndrome, dentally, is that some people with this disease also have an analogous condition called **dentinogenesis imperfecta (hereditary opalescent dentin).**

Ectodermal dysplasia is another disease with more than one hereditary pattern, both autosomal and X-linked. People with this disease have **oligodontia,** and the teeth that develop are often conical (**Figure 8-83**). Other characteristics include sparse hair that is coarser than normal and fewer than normal sweat glands. **Papillon-Lefèvre syndrome** is an inherited autosomal recessive disease characterized by hyperkeratotic skin lesions, severe destruction of the periodontium, and calcification of the dura. By age 15, the child is usually edentulous.

Hurler's Syndrome is transmitted as an autosomal recessive trait and is the trypical form of mucopolysaccharidosis. The condition is referred to as gargoyleson, because the face has a gargoyle-like appearance. Other manifestations of the condition include dwarfism, severe somatic and skeletal changes, mental retardation, deafness, cardionvascular defects, hepatosplenomegaly and joint contractures.

Syndromes That Affect Soft Tissues of the Face

Neurofibromatosis, type 1 (von Recklinghausen disease of skin, NF-1) is an autosomal dominant trait (although mutations without a family history have been reported) that is characterized by the formation on **multiple neurofibromas** (**Figure 8-84**). These neurofibromas may be small or extremely large and pendulous and number into the hundreds. Oral lesions are not uncommon. In addition to the neurofibromas, a prominent feature is the presence of **café au lait** spots (the color of coffee with milk). These spots differ from those seen in fibrous dysplasia in that they tend to be **more**

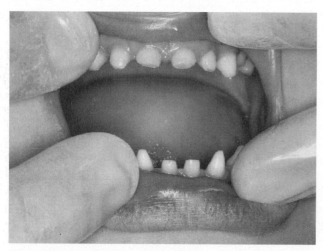

Figure 8-83. Ectodermal dysplasia. Malformed or missing teeth are characteristic of this hereditary disorder.

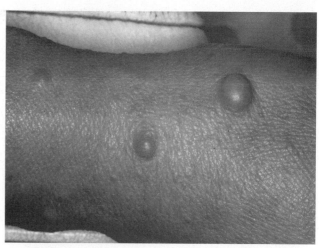

Figure 8-84. Neurofibromatosis (von Recklinghausen disease of skin). Multiple neuromas and café au lait spots are seen in this condition.

frequent and also they have a **smooth border.** A few people with this disease experience malignant transformation of one or more of the numerous neurofibromas.

Multiple endocrine neoplasia (MEN) syndrome is an uncommon condition. People with this condition develop neoplasms or functional hyperplasia in one or more endocrine glands. There are three variations of this condition; however, the one with significant oral lesions is known as **type 2B** in some textbooks or **type III** in others. The characteristic oral lesions are **multiple neuromas on the tongue.** People with this condition also have a predisposition to develop a certain type of **malignant thyroid tumor.** Many people also develop functional adrenal gland tumors, which secrete catecholamines that may result in life-threatening hypertension.

Two congenital vascular defects that have oral involvement are **encephalotrigeminal angiomatosis (Sturge-Weber angiomatosis)** and **hereditary hemorrhagic telangiectasia (Rendu-Osler-Weber or Osler-Weber-Rendu syndrome).**

Encephalotrigeminal angiomatosis (**EtA**) is a nonhereditary condition in which vascular anomalies are dispersed along the distribution of the **trigeminal nerve (Figure 8-85).** People with EtA have hemangiomas that involve both the brain at the origin of the trigeminal nerve and of the face and oral cavity. Large congenital vascular lesions of the face that do not follow the distribution of cranial nerve V are commonly referred to as a **port wine stain.** People with this condition often have seizures as a result of the intracranial lesions.

Hereditary hemorrhagic telangiectasia (**HHT**) is an autosomal dominant trait. People with the condition have numerous small dilated capillary-like lesions that involve multiple organ systems, including the skin and oral mucosa (**Figure 8-86**). A frequent complaint of people with HHT is recurrent episodes of nosebleed (**epistaxis**); although, oral bleeds are not generally significant.

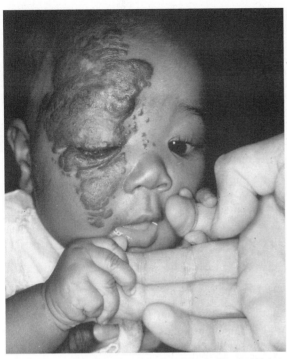

Figure 8-85. Encephalotrigeminal angiomatosis (Sturge-Weber angiomatosis). Unilateral facial and oral angiomas following the distribution of cranial nerve V are the features of this condition.

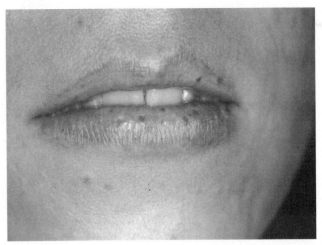

Figure 8-86. Hereditary hemorrhagic telangiectasia. Multiple petechial-like lesions are the hallmark of this autosomal dominant trait.

 HEMATOLOGIC DISORDERS

Conditions That Affect Hemostasis

In order to prevent a complete loss of all our blood following an injury, the body has two separate mechanisms that work in unison to achieve **hemostasis** (control of hemorrhage)-a **platelet** and a **coagulation** system. A defect in either mechanism will make hemostasis difficult and may even be life threatening if the condition is not treated.

When an injury occurs to the endothelial lining of a blood vessel, platelets adhere to the exposed collagen in the connective tissue and release a substance that attracts more platelets. This is referred to as platelet **aggregation**. Platelets also act as a frame or scaffold on which **fibrin** from the coagulation system sticks. **This mixture of platelets and fibrin creates the blood clot**. If something decreases the number of platelets available in the blood (**thrombocytopenia**) or the ability of the platelets to stick together (**thrombocytopathy**), increased bleeding occurs at the site of injury. Platelet disorders may be hereditary or acquired. **Nonsteroidal anti-inflammatory drugs (NSAIDs)** inhibit platelet function by interfering the enzyme cyclooxygenase, one of the key enzymes in the inflammatory reaction. This is one reason why people who take high-dose NSAIDs (e.g., people with significant arthritis) have a **tendency to bruise easily** or to have **prolonged bleeding after a cut**. This is also the reason why a low dose of aspirin is used to decrease the risk of heart attack. It helps to reduce the formation of

clots within the arteries of the heart. It is, therefore, important that the initial health history and every periodic update should include questions about bleeding tendencies or ease of bruising.

Signs and symptoms associated with platelet dysfunctions include small, pinpoint-sized bleeds under the skin, which are referred to as **petechial hemorrhages**, frequent nosebleeds (**epistaxis**), large areas of bleeding under the skin (**purpura**), or **prolonged bleeding** (often seen in dental health care as continued oozing of blood following subgingival instrumentation or extraction of a tooth).

Several steps in the process of blood coagulation are referred to as the **coagulation cascade**. The end product of the process leading up to the formation of a blood clot is the formation of **fibrin**. Most of the common defects in the coagulation mechanism, however, involve a missing coagulation factor or the inability of a coagulation factor to be activated in the **extrinsic** pathway of the process. The most frequently encountered defect in the coagulation system is the lack of **factor VIII** (the **antihemophilic factor**). A severe lack of this protein causes **hemophilia** (**hemophilia A** or **classic hemophilia**). Missing **factor IX** also causes hemophilia, which is known as **hemophilia B (Christmas disease)** and is the second most common disease involving a coagulation factor. Another less common disorder is **von Willebrand disease,** which is caused by a deficiency in **von Willebrand factor**, a cofactor with factor VIII. These conditions are X-linked hereditary disorders. If one of these factors is missing, or if any of the other coagulation factors in the **intrinsic pathway (factor VII)** or the **common pathway** (where the intrinsic and extrinsic arms merge) are missing or cannot be activated, blood will not coagulate. People with these conditions are usually recognized early in life; therefore, a family history is very important in order to identify these individuals.

Testing for suspected bleeding problems may involve a variety of tests; however, three commonly used tests to screen for hemorrhagic disorders are the bleeding time (**BT**), prothrombin time (**PT**), and the activated partial thromboplastin time (**APTT**). **Table 8-3** indicates the condition that is most likely associated with an abnormal test.

If utilizing the PT, patients should be treated with a result that is twice the normal reading. The **international normalized ratio (INR)** is the patient's PT tested with a standardized reagent and compared with the national average. An INR of 3 is acceptable for most dental procedures.

Neoplastic Diseases of Lymph Nodes

Although there are some nonaggressive lymphoproliferative disorders, neoplasms of the lymph nodes are mainly malignant. Several classifications for lymph node neoplasms exist; however, in the most simplistic scheme, lymph node tumors can be divided into **Hodgkin** and **non-Hodgkin** lymphomas. The reason for this division is based on the fact that Hodgkin lymphomas seemed to be different from other lymphomas in their behavior and response to treatment. Cervical lymphadenopathy is a very common sign in lymphoma (**Figure 8-87**).

Of the four types of Hodgkin lymphoma, **nodular sclerosing** (NS) is the most common and generally has the better prognosis. One of the most common early clinical signs in NS is **lymph node swelling in the neck**. The characteristic and essential histologic finding in all forms of Hodgkin lymphoma is the presence of **Reed-Sternberg cells**.

Non-Hodgkin lymphomas (NHLs), as a group, tend to be more aggressive and respond less well to therapy than do Hodgkin lymphomas; NHLs contain a larger variety of tumors. Although uncommon in the United States, the NHL that is most likely to involve the head and neck region routinely is **Burkitt** lymphoma. Mandibular involvement is almost a universal finding in people who have Burkitt lymphoma. Two unusual features of Burkitt lymphoma are its occurrence in young children and the geographic region of Africa where it was originally identified. This distinctive geographic distribution has led researchers to speculate that Burkitt lymphoma may be spread by mosquitoes.

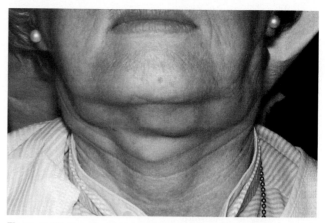

Figure 8-87. Non-Hodgkin lymphoma. Cervical lymphadenopathy is common in both non-Hodgkin and Hodgkin lymphomas. (From Neville BW, Damm DD, White DK: Color Atlas of Clinical Oral Pathology, 2nd ed. Philadelphia, Lippincott Williams & Wilkins, 1999, p 323.)

Another disease that may have frequent jaw involvement is **multiple myeloma**, which is a neoplasm of plasma cells (transformed B cells). Radiographically, this disease exhibits **multiple punched-out** radiolucencies or **floating teeth** (see Figure 8-50). Multiple myeloma is primarily a disease found among older adults. Arising from plasma cells, these neoplasms produce large quantities of immunoglobulins that result in **elevated serum immunoglobulin levels**. **Bence Jones protein** in the urine is seen in neoplasms, which produce large quantities of **light chain** fragments of immunoglobulins.

Neoplasms of bone marrow differ from lymphomas in that they are considered **non-solid** tumors. **Leukemias**, for example, arise in the bone marrow and involve the bloodstream, a fluid compartment, and not a single "solid" organ or structure. The most simplistic classification of leukemias divides them into **acute** and **chronic**, depending on their clinical behavior. Leukemias are labelled as **lymphocytic** if they are derived from cells that give rise to bloodstream lymphocytes and **myelogenous** if they arise from the stem cells in the bone marrow, which produce red blood cells. The eventual outcome of leukemia is the production of abnormal cells, which eventually displace the normal cellular components of the bone marrow and bloodstream. Death usually results from an infection or from **thrombocytopenia** (i.e., widespread bleeding caused by the displacement of **megokaryocytes**, the cells that produce platelets). Generally, acute leukemias occur more frequently in children, and chronic leukemias occur more often in adults.

Suggested Sources

Eversole LR: Clinical Outline of Oral Pathology. Philadelphia, Lea & Febiger, 1992.
http://dir.yahoo.com/Health/
  General links are given to other health sites.
http://www.dental.washington.edu/ob510/ch9menu.html
  This site includes information on developmental anomalies of the teeth.

TABLE 8–3 Screening Test for Hemorrhagic Disorders

POSITIVE TEST RESULT	CONDITION
Prolonged BT, normal PT and APTT	Platelet disorder or deficiency
Prolonged PT, normal aPTT and BT	Deficiency of factor VII
Prolonged APTT, normal PT and BT	Hemophilia; patient on anticoagulant therapy; patients with liver disease
Prolonged APTT and PT, normal BT	Fibrinogen, prothrombin, or factor X deficiency
Prolonged BT, PT, and APTT	Disseminated intravascular coagulopathy (DIC)

http://www.dermis.net/bildb/index_e.html
   This is an English translation of diseases of the skin.
http://www.freemedicaljournals.com
   The article abstracts for numerous journals.
http://www.healthlinks.net
   General links are provided to health sites.
http://rarediseases.org
   Uncommon diseases are presented.
http://www.telemedice.org
   Topics on dermatology are included.

http://www.uiowa.edu/~oprm/AtlasHome.html
   This university site focuses on oral pathology.
http://www.usc.edu/hsc/dental/opath
   This university site focuses on oral pathology.
Langlais RP, Miller CS: Color Atlas of Common Oral Conditions. Philadelphia, Lippincott Williams & Wilkins, 1998.
Neville BW, Damm DD, White DK: Color Atlas of Clinical Oral Pathology, 2nd ed. Baltimore, Lippincott Williams & Wilkins, 1999.

Questions and Answers

Questions

1. All of the following are signs of inflammation EXCEPT one. Which is the exception?
   A. Redness
   B. Paresthesia
   C. Swelling
   D. Increased temperature

2. Which term best describes a swelling resulting from the presence of fluids within soft tissues that contain high molecular weight proteins and some inflammatory cells?
   A. Transudate
   B. Sludging
   C. Exudate
   D. Suppuration

3. Which of the following is the predominant cell in an acute inflammatory response?
   A. Lymphocyte
   B. Monocyte
   C. Eosinophil
   D. Neutrophil

4. A wound that heals by replacing the damaged tissue with cells of the same kind is referred to as which type of healing?
   A. Primary intent
   B. Secondary intent
   C. Regeneration
   D. Repair

5. An increase in the size of a tissue or structure resulting from an increase in the size, but not number, of cells refers to which of the following terms?
   A. Hypertrophy
   B. Hyperplasia
   C. Neoplasia
   D. Dysplasia

6. Adenocarcinoma is the term used to describe which of the following tumors?
   A. A benign tumor of nerve tissue origin
   B. A malignant tumor of salivary gland origin
   C. A malignant tumor of ovarian origin
   D. A benign tumor of the brain

7. Which of the following is the more common lesion on the lower lip?
   A. Monomorphic adenoma
   B. Pleomorphic adenoma
   C. Mucoepidermoid carcinoma
   D. Mucocele

8. Café au lait spots are associated with which of the following?
   A. Fibrous dysplasia
   B. Addison disease
   C. Peutz-Jeghers syndrome
   D. Minocycline use

9. Striae of Wickham are seen with which of the following diseases?
   A. Pemphigus vulgaris
   B. Mucous membrane pemphigoid
   C. Lichen planus
   D. Erythema multiforme

10. A patient has a cluster of small ulcers on the hard palate, none of which are larger than 2 mm in diameter. Which virus is most likely to be the causative agent?
    A. Cytomegalovirus
    B. Measles virus
    C. Coxsackievirus
    D. Herpesvirus

11. A patient has a draining sinus tract on the skin over the body of the mandible. In the suppuration, you note small yellow granules. Which organism is most likely to cause this abscess?
    A. Candida
    B. Actinomyces
    C. Mucor
    D. Histoplasmosis

12. Median rhomboid glossitis is caused by which organism?
    A. *Cryptococcus*
    B. *Blastomyces*
    C. *Aspergillus*
    D. *Candida*

13. A "cotton wool" radiographic bony pattern most often suggests which disease?
    A. Paget disease of bone
    B. Osteosarcoma
    C. Multiple myeloma
    D. Fibrous dysplasia

14. Which of the following is most like to occur at the anterior mandible of middle-aged women?
    A. Cementoblastoma
    B. Periapical cemental dysplasia
    C. Fibrous dysplasia
    D. Chondrosarcoma

15. A 12-year-old girl has a radiolucent lesion in the anterior maxilla that is associated with an unerupted canine. Within the radiolucency are small specks of calcified material. Which is the most likely diagnosis?
    A. Odontoma
    B. Dentigerous cyst
    C. Adenomatoid odontogenic tumor
    D. Ameloblastoma

16. Which of the following is more likely to appear as a multilocular radiolucency?
    A. Dentigerous cyst
    B. Traumatic bone "cyst"
    C. Odontogenic keratocyst
    D. Radicular cyst

17. Bence Jones protein is found in which disease?
    A. Osteosarcoma
    B. Langerhans cell granuloma
    C. Multiple myeloma
    D. Lipoid proteinosis

18. In which of the following is it important to rule out hyperparathyroidism?
    A. Central giant cell granuloma
    B. Paget disease of bone
    C. Cherubism
    D. Fibrous dysplasia

19. Which of the following is associated with taurodontism?
    A. Dentin dysplasia
    B. Amelogenesis imperfecta
    C. Dentinogenesis imperfecta
    D. Odontodysplasia

20. In which of the following would you find teeth that exhibit constricted cervical areas, thin pointed roots, and obliterated pulp chambers?
    A. Dentin dysplasia
    B. Amelogenesis imperfecta
    C. Dentinogenesis imperfecta
    D. Odontodysplasia

21. A patient has several teeth in the maxillary left quadrant that are malformed and appear as "shell" teeth. The rest of the dentition appears to be normal. Which is the most likely diagnosis?
    A. Dentin dysplasia
    B. Amelogenesis imperfecta
    C. Dentinogenesis imperfecta
    D. Odontodysplasia

22. A patient presents with a gingival swelling between teeth numbers 9 and 10. The lesion is blue, and the surface does not appear ulcerated. The mass has moved these two teeth apart. Which is the most likely diagnosis?
    A. Fibroma
    B. Pyogenic granuloma
    C. Peripheral giant cell granuloma
    D. Peripheral ossifying fibroma

23. All of the following drugs have been known to cause gingival hyperplasia EXCEPT one. Which is the exception?
    A. Minocycline
    B. Phenytoin
    C. Cyclosporin
    D. Nifedipine

24. A patient has a 5-mm mass on the lateral border of the tongue. It is neither ulcerated nor painful. It is yellow and has grown very slowly during the past 10 months. Which is the most likely diagnosis?
    A. Traumatic neuroma
    B. Hemangioma
    C. Mucocele
    D. Granular cell tumor

25. A patient has a painless, nonulcerated swelling on the hard palate. You suspect that the swelling is a salivary gland lesion. Which of the following statements best matches these clinical signs and symptoms?
    A. The lesion is probably necrotizing sialometaplasia.
    B. The tumor has about an equal chance of being malignant or benign.
    C. The most common tumor in this location would be acinic cell carcinoma.
    D. It would be important to rule out Sjögren disease.

ANSWERS

1. **B**. Redness, swelling, and increased temperature are three of the four cardinal signs of inflammation. Paresthesia may be a residual effect of inflammation but is not a sign. Pain is a sign.

2. **C**. An exudate consists of fluids, proteins, and cells that have escaped due to increased vascular permeability.

3. **D**. Neutrophils (PMNs or polys) are the most mobile of the inflammatory cells and are found in larger numbers in the circulating blood.

4. **C**. Repair involves the formation of scar tissue. Regeneration is replacement of damaged cells by cells of the same type. Primary and secondary intent healing represents the difference between an open wound and a sutured wound, the latter resulting in less scar formation.

5. **A**. Hypertrophy is only cell enlargement. Hyperplasia involves increasing the number of cells (and possibly some small increase in cell size). Neoplasia is unorganized growth. Dysplasia is atypical growth but is not neoplastic.

6. **B**. Adeno- refers to glandular tissue, and -carcinoma refers to an epithelial malignancy.

7. **D**. Mucoceles are much more common on the lower lip than either benign or malignant salivary gland neoplasms.

8. **A.** All these conditions may have increased pigmentation; however, only fibrous dysplasia has café au lait spots. Addison disease and minocycline generally have more diffuse pigmentation. Peutz-Jeghers syndrome has small, periorifice melanotic spots.

9. **C.** The lacy, reticulated pattern of white lines known as the striae of Wickham is classic for lichen planus.

10. **D.** Whereas small ulcers may be seen in coxsackievirus, clusters are most commonly seen with herpes virus. Cytomegalovirus, which is a member of the herpes family of viruses, does not present as clusters of small ulcers.

11. **B.** Sulfa granules, which are small aggregates of actinomyces in a "sea" of pus, are distinctive for this organism.

12. **D.** Median rhomboid glossitis, which was once thought to be a developmental defect, has been shown to be a localized candidal infection.

13. **A.** The cotton wool pattern in bone is characteristic for Paget disease. Osteosarcomas produce tumor masses of bone. Multiple myeloma produces punched-out radiolucencies. Fibrous dysplasia produces a ground-glass pattern radiographically.

14. **B.** Of the four lesions, periapical cemental dysplasia typically occurs more often in people older than 40 years of age and in the anterior segment of the mandible.

15. **C.** Approximately 70% of adenomatoid odontogenic tumors (AOT) occur in females younger than 20 years of age. Most tumors involve the anterior portion of the jaws (usually the maxilla). Because they are frequently associated with an unerupted tooth, an AOT often resembles a dentigerous cyst. However, the AOT extends beyond the CEJ and can involve more than half of the root. As calcifications form within the tumor, they can be seen as radiopaque areas radiographically.

16. **C.** A characteristic feature of the odontogenic keratocyst (OKC) is the tendency to exhibit a multiocular radiolucent radiographic pattern. OKCs microscopically produce satellite cysts that create the honeycomb or multiocular appearance.

17. **C.** Bence Jones protein is found in people with multiple myeloma. In multiple myeloma (caused by abnormal plasma cells), large quantities of immunoglobulins are produced and spill out in the urine; they are known as Bence Jones protein.

18. **A.** In hyperparathyroidism, excess parathyroid hormone is produced. This results in the breakdown of bone to release calcium and phosphates by osteoclasts. The lesions (also known as the brown tumors of hyperparathyroidism) are indistinguishable from central giant cell granulomas of bone.

19. **B.** Taurodontism is found in certain types of amelogenesis imperfecta. Dentin dysplasia type 2 may also exhibit enlarged pulp chambers; however, it is not the same as taurodontism.

20. **C.** Obliteration of pulp chambers and root canals is the characteristic radiographic pattern in dentinogenesis imperfecta. A constricted cervical portion with a relatively normal occlusal surface is also a characteristic radiographic pattern.

21. **D.** Shell or ghost teeth are the diagnostic features of odontodysplasia. It is the result of some unknown disruption of the odontogenic process just after the initiation of the calcification process so that only a thin shell of tooth substance is formed.

22. **C.** All of these lesions are commonly found on the gingiva. The fibroma is usually normal mucosal colored. The pyogenic granuloma is most often erythematous and hemorrhagic. The peripheral ossifying fibroma generally appears either like a fibroma or a pyogenic granuloma. Owing to the hemosiderin found in the peripheral giant cell granuloma, these lesions tend to appear purple, and their association with the periodontal structures tends to move teeth as they enlarge.

23. **A.** Of the four drugs listed, only minocycline has not been associated with gingival enlargement. Minocycline, has however, been reported to cause hyperpigmentation of the gingiva.

24. **D.** Hemangiomas, being vascular in origin, are red to bluish in color. Mucoceles have a bluish-tinged, translucent look, because they contain mucus. Traumatic neuromas usually have a normal color. The granular cell tumor, comprised of foamy-looking macrophages, has a yellowish clinical appearance.

25. **B.** This lesion is nonulcerated, which would rule out necrotizing sialometaplasia. Acinic cell carcinoma is not the most common malignant salivary gland neoplasm of the palate. None of the common clinical signs and symptoms such as xerostomia and xerophthalmia is present, which reduces the likelihood that this single, isolated swelling is caused by Sjögren disease. Minor salivary gland neoplasms have about an equal chance of being benign or malignant.

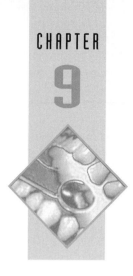

Pharmacology

PEGGY W. COLEMAN, PhD

The dental hygienist interacts with many patients who are receiving medication. This chapter reviews the properties and effects of drugs or, in a more general sense, the interactions of drugs with living systems to produce biologic effects.

Orientation

A **drug** is defined as any chemical that can affect living processes. By this broad definition, most chemicals can be considered drugs. **Pharmacology** is defined as the study of drugs and their interactions with living systems. **Therapeutics** is defined as the use of drugs to diagnose, prevent, or treat disease or to prevent pregnancy. The focus of this chapter is to understand the use of drugs as therapeutic agents.

An **ideal drug** should have certain characteristics. The three most important characteristics are **effectiveness, safety**, and **selectivity**. An effective drug is one that produces the responses for which it has been administered. A safe drug would not produce a harmful effect, even when given in very high doses. However, there is no such thing as a safe drug, because all drugs have the ability to cause injury. A selective drug elicits only those responses for which it is given and produces no side effects, but all medications produce side effects. There appears to be no such thing as an ideal drug. The hygienist must take care to maximize therapeutic effects and minimize harmful effects.

Additional properties of an ideal drug include reversible action, predictability, ease of administration, freedom from drug interactions, low cost, chemical stability, and possession of a simple generic name.

Drug Names

Drugs have three types of names. The **chemical name** is a description of a drug using chemical nomenclature. Chemical names are long, complex, and inappropriate for daily use. *N*-acetyl-para-aminophenol is the chemical name for acetaminophen. **Generic names** are assigned by the United States Adopted Names Council, and each drug has only one generic name (e.g., acetaminophen). The generic name is known as the nonproprietary name. **Trade names** or brand names are the names under which a drug is marketed. These names are created by the drug companies and are usually easy to remember. A drug can have many trade names. Tylenol, Panadol, and Neopap are examples of trade names for acetaminophen.

BASIC PRINCIPLES OF PHARMACOLOGY

Pharmacokinetics

Pharmacokinetics is the study of how drugs move through the body. The four basic pharmacokinetic processes are **absorption**, **distribution**, **metabolism**, and **excretion**. Drugs must cross membranes to enter into the blood from their site of administration and to reach their site of action. Drugs must also cross membranes to undergo metabolism and excretion. The three most important ways by which drugs cross cell membranes are: (1) passage through channels and pores in the cell membrane, (2) active transport across the cell membrane, and (3) direct penetration of the membrane. Very few drugs are small enough to enter cells via channels or pores. Small ions such as sodium and potassium have the ability to cross membranes via channels. Active transport systems are important for movement of some drugs across cell membranes. All transport systems are selective and usually carry just one drug. Most drugs are too large to pass through channels or pores and lack a transport system. For these drugs, movement throughout the body is dependent on their ability to directly penetrate cell membranes. A drug must be lipid soluble in order to directly penetrate membranes.

Many drugs are either weak organic acids or weak organic bases and can exist in charged (ionized) and uncharged (non-ionized) forms. **The more that a drug is ionized, the less the drug is absorbed; the less a drug is ionized, the more the drug is absorbed.** The extent to which a weak base or weak acid becomes ionized is determined by the pH of the medium in which it is dissolved. Acids tend to ionize in basic media, and bases tend to ionize in acidic media. Aspirin is a weak acid, and in the stomach (an acidic medium) most of the aspirin molecules are nonionized and can be absorbed across the membranes of the stomach.

Absorption is the movement of a drug from its site of administration into the blood. Factors that affect drug absorption are the rate of dissolution, surface area, blood flow, and lipid solubility. Absorption depends on the rate of dissolution. Drugs that dissolve rapidly have a faster onset of action. The amount of surface area available for absorption influences absorption. The larger the surface area, the faster is the rate of absorption. Absorption of drugs occurs most rapidly from sites where blood flow is high. Highly lipid-soluble drugs are absorbed more rapidly than are drugs with low lipid solubility.

Distribution is defined as the movement of drugs throughout the body. Distribution is determined by three factors: (1) blood flow to tissues, (2) the ability of a drug to exit the vascular system, and (3) the ability of a drug to enter cells.

Metabolism of drugs, which is also known as biotransformation, is the enzymatic alteration of the structure of the drug. Most drugs are metabolized by the hepatic microsomal enzyme system, which is also known as the P-450 system.

Excretion is the removal of drugs from the body. Most drugs and their metabolites are excreted by the kidneys. A few drugs exit the body in bile, saliva, sweat, breast milk, and expired air.

Pharmacodynamics

Pharmacodynamics (drug action) is defined as the study of the effects that drugs have on the body and how they produce their effects. Dose-response relationships determine the minimum amount of drug needed to produce an effect and the maximum response that a drug can elicit. If the dose of the drug is plotted on a logarithmic scale and the response is traced on a linear scale (log dose-effect curve), a curve is produced from which the potency and efficacy of a drug's action may be determined. **Potency** refers to the amount of the drug that must be given to produce an effect. The concept of potency is shown by the curves A and B in **Figure 9-1**. The potency of drug A is greater, because the dose required to produce its effect is smaller. Drug B is less potent than drug A, because a larger dose of drug B is required to produce the same effect as that of drug A.

Efficacy is defined as the largest effect that can be produced by a drug. The efficacy increases as the height of the curve increases (see Figure 9-1). The efficacy of drugs A and B are greater than that of drug C.

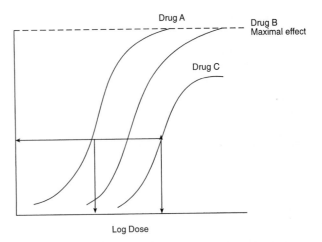

Figure 9-1. Comparison of potencies and effectiveness of three drugs. Drug A is more potent than drug B or drug C. Drugs A and B are more effective than drug C.

The **therapeutic index (TI)** is a measure of a drug's safety. The TI is based on experiments that are performed in lower animals and clinical trials conducted in humans. The TI is the ratio of a drug's LD50 to its ED50. The LD50 is the dose that is lethal to 50% of the animals treated. The ED50 is defined as the dose that is required to produce a defined therapeutic response in 50% of the population. A large TI indicates that the drug is safe. If the TI is small, the drug is more likely to be toxic.

The **half-life (t½)** of a drug is the amount of time required for the concentration of a drug to decrease one half of its blood level at any given time. A drug with a short half-life has a short duration of action, because it is removed from the body quickly.

Adverse Drug Reactions

Adverse drug reactions are defined as any undesirable response to a drug. A **toxic reaction** is an adverse drug reaction caused by excessive dosing. A **side effect** is a reaction that is not part of the desired therapeutic outcome. An **allergic reaction** is an immune response. For an allergic reaction to occur, the person must have been previously exposed to the drug. An **idiosyncratic reaction** is an uncommon reaction resulting from a genetic predisposition. A **teratogenic effect** is a drug-induced birth defect.

 AUTONOMIC NERVOUS SYSTEM DRUGS

Physiology of the Autonomic Nervous System

The **autonomic nervous system** (ANS) has three major functions: (1) regulation of blood pressure and heart rate; (2) regulation of salivary, gastric, sweat, and bronchial glands; and (3) regulation of smooth muscles of the bronchi, blood vessels, urogenital system, and gastrointestinal (GI) tract. These regulatory functions are shared between the two divisions of the ANS-the **sympathetic nervous system** and the **parasympathetic nervous system**.

The ANS relies on three neurotransmitters and several different types of receptors in the target tissues to regulate physiologic responses. The neurotransmitters are **acetylcholine** (ACh), **norepinephrine** (NE), and **epinephrine** (Epi). This information is summarized in **Figure 9-2**.

As Figure 9-2 indicates, acetylcholine is the transmitter released at most junctions of the peripheral nervous system. Acetylcholine is the transmitter released at all: (1) preganglionic neurons of the sympathetic and parasympathetic nervous system, (2) all postganglionic neurons of the parasympathetic nervous system, and (3) all motor neurons to skeletal muscle.

Norepinephrine is the transmitter released by most postganglionic neurons of the sympathetic nervous system. The adrenal medulla releases epinephrine (80%) and norepinephrine (20%) into the bloodstream, which produces effects similar to those occurring in response to stimulating the sympathetic nervous system.

Two major categories of receptors are associated with the peripheral nervous system. **Cholinergic receptors** mediate responses at all junctions where acetylcholine is the transmitter. **Adrenergic receptors** mediate responses to norepinephrine and epinephrine (i.e., adrenaline).

For each of these major receptor categories, there are receptor subtypes. The three major subtypes of cholinergic receptors are **muscarinic, nicotinic N** (N_N), and **nicotinic M** (N_M). The four major subtypes of adrenergic receptors are α_1, α_2, β_1, and β_2 (see Figure 9-2).

Drugs are selective for specific receptor subtypes. We can group responses to cholinergic receptor action based on the receptor subtype involved. Activation of **muscarinic** receptors causes: (1) increased secretions from gastric, intestinal,

pulmonary, and sweat glands; (2) contraction of bronchial smooth muscle; (3) decreased heart rate; (4) focusing of the lens of the eye for near vision; and (5) miosis (reduction of the pupillary diameter).

Activation of **nicotinic M** receptors causes contraction of skeletal muscle. Activation of **nicotinic N** receptors produces ganglionic transmission at the ganglia of both sympathetic and parasympathetic nerves.

β_1-Adrenergic receptors are located in the eyes, arterioles, veins, and male sex organs. Stimulation of β_1-adrenergic receptors in the eye causes the pupil to enlarge or mydriasis. Activation of b_1-adrenergic receptors in arterioles and veins produces vasoconstriction. Activation of β_1-adrenergic receptors in the male sexual apparatus causes ejaculation.

α_2-Adrenergic receptors are located presynaptically and regulate transmitter release. When these receptors are stimulated further, release of norepinephrine is suppressed. β_1-Adrenergic receptors are located in the heart and kidney. Activation of β_1-adrenergic receptors in the heart increases heart rate, increases the force of contraction, and increases conduction velocity through the atrioventricular (AV) node. In the kidney, activation of β_1-adrenergic receptors causes the release of renin.

Activation of β_2-adrenergic receptors in bronchioles results in bronchial dilation. β_2-Adrenergic receptors are located in the arterioles of the heart, lungs, and skeletal muscle. Activation of these receptors causes vasodilation. Activation of β_1-adrenergic receptors in the liver and skeletal muscle results in the breakdown of glycogen to glucose, thus increasing blood levels of glucose.

The ANS drugs basically fall into four groups. Drugs can stimulate or mimic the parasympathetic nervous system and are called muscarinic agonists or parasympathomimetic agents. Drugs that inhibit or block the effect of the parasympathetic nervous system are called parasympatholytic drugs or anticholinergic agents. Drugs that stimulate or mimic the sympathetic nervous system are referred to as sympathomimetics and drugs that inhibit or block the sympathetic nervous system are called sympatholytics or adrenergic blockers.

⬡ CHOLINERGIC DRUGS

Muscarinic Agonist and Antagonists

Muscarinic agonists directly activate muscarinic cholinergic receptors. These drugs cause increased secretion from sweat, salivary, gastric, and bronchial glands. Muscarinic agonists decrease heart rate and increase contraction of intestinal, urinary tract, and bronchial smooth muscle. Activation of muscarinic receptors in the eye produces miosis and accommodation for near vision. **Bethanechol** (Urecholine) is a direct-acting muscarinic agonist that is used to relieve urinary retention.

The adverse reactions associated with administration of acting muscarinic agonists are extensions of their pharma-

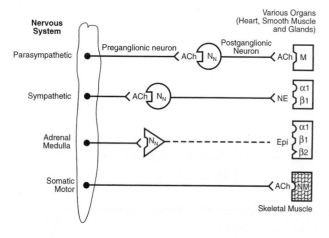

Figure 9-2. Anatomy and locations of receptor subtypes activated by acetylcholine (ACh), norepinephrine (NE), and epinephrine (Epi) in the autonomic nervous system (ANS). Cholinergic receptor subtypes are muscarinic (M), nicotinic$_N$ (N_N) and nicotinic$_M$ (N_M). Adrenergic receptors of the peripheral ANS are α_1, β_1, or β_2.

cologic effect. Excessive salivation, increased secretion of gastric acid, abdominal cramps, diarrhea, and urination are side effects observed with muscarinic agonists.

Muscarinic antagonists block the action of acetylcholine at muscarinic receptors. **Atropine** is a muscarinic antagonist that prevents the action of acetylcholine at the postganglionic parasympathetic endings.

Atropine blocks muscarinic receptors, and its effects are opposite to those produced by muscarinic activation. Atropine increases heart rate, decreases salivation, relaxes bronchial smooth muscle, decreases urinary bladder tone, and decreases motility of the GI tract. Atropine acts in the eye to cause mydriasis and cycloplegia.

Important uses of atropine and other muscarinic antagonists include preoperative medication to reduce secretions of saliva and bronchial mucus, ophthalmic examinations, reversal of bradycardia, and treatment of muscarinic agonist poisoning. In dentistry, muscarinic antagonists can be used to produce a dry field before some dental procedures.

Adverse effects of atropine and other muscarinic antagonists are dry mouth (xerostomia), constipation, blurred vision, urinary retention, tachycardia, elevation of intraocular pressure, and reduced sweating.

Cholinesterase Inhibitors

Acetylcholinesterase is an enzyme that is present on the surface of postjunctional cells and degrades acetylcholine into inactive products. **Cholinesterase inhibitors** are drugs that bind to acetylcholinesterase and prevent the degradation of acetylcholine. Some cholinesterase inhibitors are reversible, whereas some are irreversible. Acetylcholine accumulates in all junctions where acetylcholine is the transmitter when these drugs are administered. Muscarinic receptors, nicotinic receptors in ganglia, and the neuromuscular junction (NMJ) are stimulated. Cholinesterase inhibitors have limited therapeutic applications because of this lack of specificity.

The major use of reversible cholinesterase inhibitors such as **neostigmine** (Prostigmine) and **physostigmine** (Eserine) is treatment for myasthenia gravis. Other uses for reversible cholinesterase inhibitors are reversal of nondepolarizing neuromuscular blockade and treatment of glaucoma.

The irreversible cholinesterase inhibitors produce the same pharmacologic responses as do the reversible inhibitors. The responses to the irreversible inhibitors last longer. **Echothiophate** (Phospholine Iodide) is an irreversible cholinesterase inhibitor that is used for glaucoma.

Adverse effects of cholinesterase inhibitors result in excessive salivation, increased tone and motility of the GI tract, increased gastric secretions, urinary urgency, miosis, and sweating.

Neuromuscular-Blocking Agents

Neuromuscular-blocking agents block nicotinic N receptors at the neuromuscular junction. These receptors are blocked and cannot be activated by acetylcholine, thus producing muscle relaxation. The neuromuscular-blocking agents can be classified according to their mechanism of action as nondepolarizing and depolarizing.

The only depolarizing neuromuscular blocker in use is **succinylcholine** (Aectine). Succinylcholine binds to nicotinic M receptors and causes the motor end-plate to depolarize and remain in a state of depolarization. Depolarization produces a brief period of muscle contraction followed by flaccid paralysis.

Succinylcholine is used primarily when muscle relaxation is only needed for short periods of time, such as endotracheal intubation, endoscopy, and electroconvulsive therapy. Neuromuscular-blocking agents do not reduce pain or consciousness.

People with low pseudocholinesterase activity are unable to degrade succinylcholine, and paralysis can persist for hours instead of a few minutes. Malignant hyperthermia can also be triggered by succinylcholine.

Tubocurare is the oldest nondepolarizing neuromuscular blocker. It competes with acetylcholine at nicotinic M receptors on the motor end-plate. Tubocurarine binds to the nicotinic M receptors and blocks the action of acetylcholine. Tubocurare does not activate the receptors, thus there is no muscle contraction and a state of flaccid paralyis is produced. Tubocurare's duration of action lasts between 20 minutes and 2 hours.

Most adverse effects of tubocurare involve the cardiovascular and respiratory systems. Tubocurare paralyzes the muscles of respiration and can produce respiratory arrest. Tubocurare can cause hypotension.

 ## ADRENERGIC DRUGS

Adrenergic Agonists

Adrenergic agonists activate adrenergic receptors and produce effects that mimic the sympathetic nervous system. These drugs are also known as sympathomimetics. Most adrenergic agonists produce their effects by binding to adrenergic receptors and mimicking the actions of natural transmitters. Adrenergic agonists vary in their ability to stimulate the receptor subtypes. A few drugs act on sympathetic nerve terminals to promote release of norepinephrine. Some adrenergic agonists block reuptake of norepinephrine into the nerve terminal, and some inhibit epinephrine degradation by monoamine oxidase (MAO) and catechol-o-methyltransferase (COMT).

Adrenergic agonists are classified as catecholamines or noncatecholamines. Catecholamines cannot be taken orally; they have a short duration of action and cannot cross the blood-brain barrier. Noncatecholamines can be taken orally; these drugs are metabolized slowly and penetrate the blood-brain barrier.

Epinephrine is an adrenergic agonist that activates all four receptor subtypes (α_1, α_2, β_1, and β_2 receptors). Epinephrine is added to local anesthetics solutions to delay absorption and reduce systemic toxicity. It is also used to control superficial bleeding, reduce nasal congestion, and elevate blood pressure. Epinephrine is the drug of choice for anaphylaxis and acute bronchial attacks. It is also used to treat patients with cardiac arrest.

Epinephrine may be administered by injection, topical application, and inhalation. This drug cannot be given orally, because it is destroyed by MAO and COMT, which are located in the intestinal wall and the liver. It also has a very short plasma half-life owing to enzymatic degradation.

Epinephrine produces many adverse effects, because it activates all four receptor subtypes, and can produce a dangerous increase in blood pressure, dysrhythmias, angina pectoris, and hyperglycemia.

Levonordefrin (Neo-Cobefrin) is a synthetic vasoconstrictor that is often added to local anesthetic solutions. Levonordefrin is similar to epinephrine in many respects; however, this agent produces less cardiac stimulation and bronchial dilation.

Isoproterenol (Isuprel) is a synthetic catecholamine that stimulates only β-adrenergic receptors. Isoproterenol can help to overcome AV heart block and restart the heart by activating β_1-receptors in the heart. Following its introduction, isoproterenol was used to treat asthma because it activates β_2-receptors. Its use in the treatment of asthma has declined owing to the development of agonists that are more selective β_2-adrenergic receptors.

Phenylephrine (Neo-Synephrine) is a noncatecholamine whose action is limited to α_1-receptors. Phenylephrine can be administered locally to reduce nasal congestion. Phenylephrine is used as a vasoconstrictor in local anesthetics.

Terbutaline (Brethaire) is a noncatecholamine specific for β_2-adrenergic receptors. This drug can be used to treat asthma and to delay preterm labor.

Adrenergic Antagonists

Adrenergic antagonists or adrenergic-blocking agents directly block adrenergic receptors. Adrenergic blocking agents can be divided into two groups: (1) drugs that selectively block α-adrenergic receptors, and (2) drugs that selectively block β-adrenergic receptors.

Phenoxybenzamine (Dibenzyline) and **phentolamine** (Regitine) are nonselective α-adrenergic blockers. These drugs competitively inhibit vasoconstriction by norepinephrine and epinephrine at α_1-adrenergic receptors on blood vessels causing vasodilation. They are used in the treatment of pheochromocytoma and peripheral vascular disease, such as Raynaud disease.

Phenoxybenzamine and phentolamine can produce orthostatic hypotension, reflex tachycardia, nasal congestion, and inhibition of ejaculation.

Prazosin (Minipress) and **terazosin** (Hytrin) are competitive blockers of α_1-adrenergic receptors and are used to treat hypertension. These agents are also used in the treatment of benign prostatic hyperplasia to increase ease of urination.

Adverse effects of α_1-blockade include orthostatic hypotension, reflex tachycardia, nasal congestion, and inhibition of ejaculation.

The β-adrenergic blocking drugs competitively block β-receptors. The β-adrenergic antagonists may be classified as nonselective or cardioselective. Nonselective agents such as propranolol block β_1 and β_2 receptors. Cardioselective β-blockers represented by metoprolol selectively block β_1-receptors. Most of the therapeutic effects of the β-adrenergic antagonists result from blockade of β_1-receptors in the heart. Therapeutic applications of β_1-adrenergic blockade include hypertension, angina pectoris, and cardiac dysrhythmias.

Adverse effects of β_1-adrenergic blockade include bradycardia, reduced cardiac output, precipitation of heart failure, and AV heart block. Adverse effects of β_2-adrenergic blockade are bronchoconstriction and inhibition of glycogenolysis.

Indirect-Acting Antiadrenergic Agents

Indirect-acting antiadrenergic drugs work by mechanisms that do not involve direct receptor activation. There are two categories of indirect-acting antiadrenergic drugs. Drugs that decrease the release of norepinephrine from nerve terminals are called adrenergic neuron-blocking agents. Drugs that act in the central nervous system (CNS) to decrease the sympathetic outflow are called centrally acting α_2-agonists.

Adrenergic neuron-blocking agents are drugs that prevent the release of norepinephrine from sympathetic neurons. **Reserpine** (Novoreserpine) acts by depleting norepinephrine from adrenergic postganglionic nerve terminals, resulting in decreased stimulation of adrenergic receptors. Reserpine also causes depletion of transmitters from neurons in the CNS.

The main therapeutic indication for reserpine is hypertension. Adverse effects include depression, bradycardia, orthostatic hypotension, nasal congestion, and diarrhea.

Guanethidine (Ismelin) is an adrenergic neuron-blocking agent that blocks the release of norepinephrine from sympathetic neurons. This drug has hypotensive actions that are similar to those of reserpine. The only indication for guanethidine is in the treatment of hypertension. It is usually reserved for patients whose blood pressure cannot be controlled with other medications.

Guanethidine cannot cross the blood-brain barrier and does not have adverse CNS effects. Adverse effects of guanethidine are diarrhea and orthostatic hypotension.

The **centrally acting agonists** stimulate α_2-receptors in the CNS and reduce sympathetic outflow to blood vessels and the heart. **Clonidine** (Catapres) and **methyldopa** (Aldomet) are both centrally acting agonists that are used to treat hypertension.

The most commonly observed adverse effects of clonidine are drowsiness and xerostomia. Rebound hypertension has occurred when clonidine is abruptly withdrawn. Methyldopa produces a positive result on a Coombs' test in 10% to 20% of patients taking the drug chronically. Other adverse effects of methyldopa are hepatotoxicity and xerostomia.

 # CENTRAL NERVOUS SYSTEM DRUGS

Drugs for Epilepsy

The goal in treating epilepsy is to reduce seizures to a level that allows the patient to live a normal or near-normal life. Identification of the particular type of seizure is important, because most antiseizure drugs are selective for particular seizures.

Phenytoin (Dilantin) is used to treat both partial and tonic-clonic seizures; however, it is not useful in the treatment of absence seizures. Phenytoin is the drug of choice to treat tonic-clonic seizures in adults and older children. Phenytoin is also used to treat digitalis-induced cardiac dysrhythmias.

At therapeutic drug levels, phenytoin produces very little sedation and other CNS effects. CNS effects that can occur when blood levels of phenytoin are elevated are nystagmus, sedation ataxia, diplopia, and cognitive impairment. Reducing the dose can usually control these effects.

Gingival hyperplasia occurs in more than 20% of all chronic users. Good oral hygiene can minimize the hyperplasia.

Other adverse effects of phenytoin include skin rashes, hirsutism, and interference with vitamin D metabolism.

Phenobarbital (Luminal) is one of the most commonly used antiseizure medications. Phenobarbital, an anticonvulsant barbiturate, suppresses seizures without causing sedation. This drug is effective against generalized tonic-clonic seizures and partial seizures but is ineffective against absence seizures. Phenobarbital is used alone or in combination with other antiseizure medications.

The most common CNS side effect associated with phenobarbital is drowsiness. With continued drug use, tolerance to sedation develops. Instead of becoming sedated, some children become hyperactive and irritable.

The drug metabolizing enzymes of the liver are stimulated by phenobarbital. The rate at which other drugs are metabolized can be increased and their effects decreased. Oral contraceptives and warfarin are metabolized by the liver, and their effects would be reduced if they were taken concurrently with phenobarbital.

Carbamazepine (Tegretol) is used to treat tonic-clonic, simple partial, and complex partial seizures. This drug is not used to treat absence seizures. The drug has fewer adverse effects than do phenobarbital and phenytoin and is often preferred to these drugs. Carbamazepine is used in dentistry to treat trigeminal and glossopharyngeal neuralgias. The drug is also used to treat bipolar disorder and is often effective in patients refractory to lithium.

Even though carbamazepine has minimal effects on cognitive function, it can cause various neurologic effects including dizziness, vertigo, confusion, and headache. Tolerance to these effects usually develops with continued drug use. Fatal blood dyscrasias including agranulocytosis and aplastic anemia have been reported but are rare. Other adverse effects include dry mouth, glossitis, stomatitis, rashes, and photosensitivity.

Like phenobarbital, carbamazepine induces the hepatic drug-metabolizing enzymes and can increase the metabolism of other drugs.

Valproic acid (Depakote) is active against various seizures including tonic-clonic, atonic, and myoclonic seizures. Valproic acid is effective in the treatment of absence seizures. The drug has fewer side effects than phenytoin or phenobarbital.

Valproic acid has few serious side effects, but death from liver failure has occurred. Most common adverse effects associated with valproic acid include nausea, vomiting, and indigestion.

The drug of choice for the treatment of absence seizures is **ethosuximide** (Zarontin). It is ineffective against partial seizures and tonic-clonic seizures.

Ethosuximide has few serious side effects. During the initial phase of treatment, the drug may cause drowsiness and lethargy. These effects usually diminish with continued use. Other adverse effects include nausea, vomiting, and diarrhea. Oral effects reported with ethosuximide include gingival enlargement and swelling of the tongue.

Antipsychotic Agents and Their Use in Schizophrenia

Antipsychotic agents are used to treat a broad spectrum of psychotic disorders including schizophrenia, acute mania, depressive psychoses, drug-induced psychoses, and delusional disorders. In addition, the antipsychotic agents are used to treat Tourette syndrome and Huntington chorea and also to suppress emesis.

The antipsychotics are divided into two major groups: traditional antipsychotics and atypical antipsychotics. The traditional antipsychotic agents block dopamine receptors in the CNS and can cause serious movement disorders called extrapyramidal side effects. The atypical antipsychotics also block dopamine receptors but in a manner different from the traditional antipsychotic. The atypical drugs have a low incidence of extrapyramidal reactions. Therapeutic responses to antipsychotic drugs develop slowly and may require several months to achieve maximal effects.

The traditional antipsychotic agents can be classified as low potency, medium potency, or high potency. Although the traditional antipsychotics vary according to potency, they are essentially equal in their ability to relieve symptoms of psychoses; however, they differ significantly in their side effects. In general, the lower potency agents such as **chlorpromazine** (Thorazine) produce more sedation and anticholinergic effects, whereas the high-potency agents like **haloperidol** (Haldol) have a higher incidence of extrapyramidal effects and less anticholinergic effects.

The primary indication for antipsychotic drugs is treatment of schizophrenia. These agents suppress symptoms during acute psychotic episodes. Positive symptoms such as hallucinations and delusions respond better to these agents than negative symptoms (e.g., emotional and social withdrawal).

Antipsychotic agents may also be used to manage patients going through a severe manic phase of bipolar disorder to suppress the severe symptoms of Tourette syndrome and to suppress vomiting associated with cancer chemotherapy and other conditions.

The antipsychotic agents produce various adverse effects. The most troublesome ones are extrapyramidal side effects, especially tardive dyskinesia. Other adverse effects include neuroleptic malignant syndrome, anticholinergic effects, orthostatic hypotension, sedation, gynecomastia, galactorrhea, seizures, sexual dysfunction, dermatologic effects, and agranulocytosis.

Atypical antipsychotic agents cause few or no extrapyramidal symptoms and can relieve positive and negative symptoms of schizophrenia. The first atypical antipsychotic introduced in the United States was **clozapine** (Clozaril).

Atypical antipsychotics are indicated for patients with schizophrenia who cannot tolerate the extrapyramidal effects or have not responded to traditional agents.

Clozapine produces potentially life-threatening agranulocytosis. Frequent white blood cell counts are required during therapy. **Olanzapine** (Zyprexa) is a new atypical antipsychotic approved for schizophrenia and other psychotic disorders but does not cause agranulocytosis.

Antidepressants

Antidepressants are drugs used to treat major depression and can benefit patients with chronic insomnia, attention-deficit/hyperactivity disorder, and panic disorder. Antidepressants currently available include **tricyclic antidepressants** [tricyclic antidepressants (TCAs)], **selective serotonin reuptake inhibitors** (SSRIs), and several new atypical antidepressants. Therapeutic responses to antidepressant agents develop slowly with initial responses occurring in 1 to 3 weeks. One or 2 months may be needed for maximal responses to develop.

TCAs such as **amitriptyline** (Elavil) were the first agents available for treating major depression. These agents are inexpensive, effective, easy to administer, and relatively safe. TCAs block reuptake of norepinephrine and serotonin into nerve terminals and intensify their effects.

Some of the diverse adverse reactions associated with TCAs are sedation, orthostatic hypotension, and anticholinergic effects (e.g., dry mouth, constipation). The most serious adverse effect associated with the TCAs is cardiac toxicity, which can be lethal when an overdose is taken.

The SSRIs selectively block the reuptake of serotonin. **Fluoxetine** (Prozac), an SSRI, is the most widely prescribed antidepressant in the United States. Other SSRIs are sertraline (Zoloft), fluvoxamine (Luvox), and paroxetine (Paxil). These agents are as effective as the TCAs but do not cause sedation, hypotension, or anticholinergic effects. They do not cause cardiotoxicity when taken in overdose. Compared with the TCAs, the SSRIs tend to produce CNS stimulation rather than CNS depression.

Fluoxetine is used primarily to treat major depression. Antidepressant effects are observed in 1 to 3 weeks. Fluoxetine has been approved by the Food and Drug Administration (FDA) for obsessive-compulsive disorder.

Adverse effects include nausea, diarrhea, anxiety, and insomnia. Sexual dysfunction is more common with SSRIs than with other antidepressants. Oral adverse effects include xerostomia, taste changes, glossitis, and aphthous stomatitis.

Drugs for Bipolar Disorder

The main agent used to treat **bipolar disorder** or manic-depressive illness is **lithium.** Both the manic phase and the depressed phase are controlled by lithium. When taken prophylactically, lithium reduces the severity and frequency of recurrent depressive and manic episodes.

Adverse effects that occur at therapeutic levels include fine hand tremor, thirst, muscle weakness, and polyuria. Serious toxicities occur when plasma levels exceed 1.5 mEq/L, and death has resulted. Lithium is teratogenic and is contraindicated during the first trimester of pregnancy.

Lithium excretion is reduced when sodium levels are reduced. Diuretics cause loss of sodium and can increase the risk of toxicity.

Drugs for Anxiety and Insomnia

Drugs used to relieve anxiety are called antianxiety agents, anxiolytics, or tranquilizers. Hypnotics are drugs that promote sleep. A single drug may be used to treat insomnia and anxiety, because some drugs alleviate anxiety in low doses and induce sleep in higher doses. A wide variety of agents have the ability to depress the functions of the CNS, thus sedating and calming the patient. The benzodiazepines were introduced in the early 1960s and soon became the drugs of first choice for treating anxiety and insomnia. Benzodiazepines include familiar agents such as **diazepam** (Valium), **lorazepam** (Ativan), and **alprazolam** (Xanax). The benzodiazepines are much safer than the barbiturates or other general CNS depressants; they have a lower abuse potential, cause less tolerance and dependence, and do not induce hepatic drug-metabolizing enzymes.

Gamma-aminobutyric acid (GABA), an inhibitory neurotransmitter found in the CNS, is potentiated by the benzodiazepines. These agents only enhance the actions of endogenous GABA and do not directly mimic GABA; therefore, there is a limit to how much CNS depression these drugs can produce.

The benzodiazepines are used primarily to treat insomnia, anxiety, and seizure disorders. In addition, these drugs are used: (1) to relieve muscle spasms, (2) to facilitate withdrawal from alcohol, (3) to treat panic disorder, and (4) to induce anesthesia.

The benzodiazepines are safe drugs, and adverse reactions are rare. The main adverse effects are daytime sedation and anterograde amnesia. The benzodiazepines are very weak respiratory depressants, and the abuse potential is much lower than that of the barbiturates.

The barbiturates were widely used before the benzodiazepines became available. Although the barbiturates have undesirable properties, they are valuable in seizure control and anesthesia.

The barbiturates are classified on the basis of duration of action: (1) long-acting, (2) short-intermediate-acting, and (3) ultra-short-acting. **Phenobarbital** (Luminal) and **mephobarbital** (Mebaral) are members of the long-acting group. These agents are used primarily in the treatment of epilepsy (see the section on epilepsy). Short-intermediate-acting barbiturates such as **amobarbital** (Amytal), **aprobarbital** (Alurate), and **secobarbital** (Seconal) are useful as sedatives. Ultrashort-acting barbiturates-**methohexital** (Brevital) and **thiopental** (Pentothal)-are used for induction of anesthesia. The barbiturates mimic the actions of GABA as well as enhance the inhibitory effects of GABA in the CNS.

These drugs have many undesirable qualities. Barbiturates: (1) are powerful respiratory depressants, (2) have a high potential for abuse, (3) induce tolerance and physical dependence, and (4) induce synthesis of hepatic drug-metabolizing enzymes.

Analgesics and Anesthetics

Drugs that alleviate pain without causing loss of consciousness are called analgesics. Opioid (narcotic) analgesics are the most effective analgesics available. The term opioid is used to include drugs derived from the opioid poppy and other chemicals that produce opiate effects. Commonly used opioid analgesics include **morphine, codeine, meperidine** (Demerol), **oxycodone** (Percodan, Percocet), and **propoxyphene** (Darvon).

The opioids are classified on the basis of how they affect receptor function. At the receptor, a drug can act as a pure opioid agonist (e.g., morphine, codeine), agonist-antagonist opioid (e.g., pentazocine), or pure opioid antagonist (e.g., naloxone).

Morphine is the prototype of the opioid agonists and is the standard by which newer opioids are measured. By mimicking actions of endogenous peptides in the CNS, morphine relieves pain.

Morphine and other opioid agonists are used therapeutically to relieve pain. Morphine is the drug of choice for the relief of moderate-to-severe pain. Morphine can relieve the chronic pain of cancer, the pain of myocardial infarction, and postoperative pain. Morphine also produces sedation, reduces anxiety, and produces a sense of well-being (euphoria). The opioid agonists suppress cough and are used clinically for their antitussive action. Doses that produce antitussive effects are much lower than those needed for analgesia, thus less potent agents such as codeine are used. The opioids decrease propulsive intestinal contractions and motility of the intestinal tract and are used for the symptomatic relief of diarrhea.

The most serious adverse effect of morphine and other pure opioid agonists is respiratory depression. Death from overdose is usually caused by respiratory arrest.

Other adverse effects include constipation, urinary retention, orthostatic hypotension, cough suppression, biliary colic, emesis, miosis, and elevation of intracranial pressure.

Tolerance and physical dependence can occur with morphine and all opioid agonists. With prolonged use, tolerance develops to sedation, analgesia, euphoria, and respiratory depression. Tolerance does not develop to miosis and constipation.

Pentazocine (Talwin) is an agonist-antagonist opioid and will serve as the prototype for this group. The agonist-antagonist opioids produce less analgesia, have a lower potential for abuse, and produce less respiratory depression compared with the pure opioid agonist.

Pentazocine is used to treat mild-to-moderate pain but is less effective than morphine against severe pain. Respiratory depression is limited with the agonist-antagonist opioids, and they have a low potential for abuse.

Adverse reactions of pentazocine include sedation, dizziness, nausea, vomiting, and headache. Unlike morphine, pentazocine can increase both blood pressure and heart rate.

Opioid antagonists competitively block the effects of opioid agonists. **Naloxone** (Narcan) is a pure opioid antagonist and prevents the agonist from producing effects. Naloxone can reverse respiratory depression, coma, and analgesia produced by opioids.

Naloxone is used in the treatment of opioid overdose, management of opioid addiction, and reversal of postoperative opioid effects. Naloxone has no significant effects when administered alone. If naloxone is given to an opioid addict, an immediate withdrawal reaction will precipitate.

CNS drugs are usually high on the controlled substance chart based on their abuse potential **(Table 9-1).**

Local Anesthetics

Local anesthetics are substances that produce a loss of sensation in a circumscribed area of the body. Local anesthetics block conduction of the nerve impulse by decreasing the

TABLE 9-1 Schedule of Controlled Substances

SCHEDULE	DRUGS
I	Heroin, LSD, marijuana
II	Opium, morphine, meperidine, oxycodone, cocaine, codeine (single drug), short-acting barbiturates, amphetamines
III	Codeine combinations, androgens
IV	Benzodiazepines, phenobarbital, chloral hydrate, meprobamate
V	Antitussives and antidiarrheals with opioid derivatives (OTC)

$$\langle \rangle - \overset{O}{\underset{\|}{N}}HC - R_1 - \overset{R_2}{\underset{R_3}{N}} + H^+ \rightleftharpoons \langle \rangle - \overset{O}{\underset{\|}{N}}HC - R_1 - \overset{R_2}{\underset{R_3}{N}} + H^+$$

pH > 7
Free base
Lipid soluble
Penetrates nerve cell
Form present in normal tissue

pH < 7
Salt
Water soluble
Active form at site of action
Form present in inflammation

Figure 9-3. Effect of pH on the properties of a local anesthetic.

permeability to sodium ions. Local anesthetics bind to specific sodium receptors on the sodium channels in the nerve membrane and prevent the influx of sodium. By blocking sodium channels in the axonal membrane, the propagation of action potentials is prevented and nerve conduction fails. Small, unmyelinated nerves are blocked more readily than are large, myelinated nerves.

Most local anesthetics fall into one of two chemical groups-esters or amides. A patient who is allergic to one chemical group is very likely to be allergic to other agents in that group. All local anesthetic agents have a **hydrophilic amino group** and **hydrophobic component** that are separated by an intermediate hydrocarbon chain containing either an **ester** or **amide** linkage. The hydrophobic group consists of an aromatic nucleus and allows the anesthetic agent to penetrate the lipid membrane where the receptor sites for these drugs are located. The hydrophobic component makes the local anesthetic water soluble. This allows the anesthetic to diffuse through the extracellular fluid and come in contact with the nerve.

All of the local anesthetics are synthetic with the exception of cocaine. These drugs are weak bases, fat-soluble viscous liquids, and solids are unstable on exposure to air. These fat-soluble bases are combined with acids to form salts to form clinically useful compounds. In this form, the local anesthetics are water-soluble and relatively stable when exposed to air. Solutions for injection can be prepared by dissolving the local anesthetic salt in either saline or sterile water.

Local anesthetics must be in the free base form to have a nerve-blocking effect. The pH of a local anesthetic solution and of the tissue into which it is injected determines how much of the drug is in the ionized form or the free base form (nonionized). The lower the pH or the more acidic the solution, the greater is the proportion of the drug in the ionized form. Local anesthetic solutions available for injection have a pH of 5 to 6, and most of the drug is in the ionized form. The pH of normal tissue is 7.4, and once injected the amount of anesthetic in the free base form increases. Infection or inflammation produces acidic

products, and the acidity of the inflamed area reduces the amount of the drug in the effective form **(Figure 9-3).**

Onset of anesthesia is determined primarily by the molecular properties of the anesthetic. Agents with a low molecular weight, high lipid solubility, and in the nonionized form cross the nerve axon with ease.

Local anesthesia is terminated when the molecules of anesthetic diffuse out of the axon and are carried away in the blood. Local anesthetic agents possessing vasodilating properties will increase the systemic absorption of the local anesthetic agent and terminate anesthesia. A vasoconstrictor like epinephrine will delay systemic absorption and prolong anesthesia.

The ester local anesthetics are primarily hydrolyzed and **inactivated by plasma pseudocholinesterases.** Para-aminobenzoic acid (PABA) is the major metabolic product of ester hydrolysis and is excreted in the urine. Most allergic reactions that occur following administration of an ester local anesthetic are in response to PABA.

The amide local anesthetics are metabolized in the liver by microsomal enzymes. Patients with severe liver disease and alcoholics may accumulate amide local anesthetics.

Local anesthetics can be absorbed in quantities sufficient to cause systemic toxicity. Toxicity from local anesthetics can produce myocardial depression and cardiac arrest. Toxic amounts of local anesthetic agents cause CNS excitation followed by depression.

Local anesthetic solutions within the dental cartridge usually contain several components, including the local anesthetic agent, a vasoconstrictor, an antioxidant for vasopressor, sodium chloride, and distilled water. Local anesthetic agents in dental cartridges are given in **Table 9-2.**

General Anesthetics

General anesthetics produce a reversible loss of consciousness and insensitivity to painful stimuli. In the dental office, general anesthesia is an indispensable tool for oral and maxillofacial surgery as well as for patients with special needs. Drug combinations are used to produce general anesthesia in order to minimize adverse reactions.

The degree of CNS depression produced by general anesthetics has been described in four stages. These stages were

TABLE 9–2 Local Anesthetics Available in Dental Cartridges

LOCAL AGENT	CONCENTRATION	DURATION OF ACTION	VASOCONSTRICTOR
Articaine hydrochloride	4%	Intermediate	Epinephrine 1:100,000
Articaine hydrochloride	4%	Intermediate	Epinephrine 1:200,000
Bupivacaine hydrochloride	0.5%	Long	Epinephrine 1:200,000
Etidocaine hydrochloride	1.5%	Long	Epinephrine 1:200,000
Lidocaine hydrochloride	2%	Short	None
Lidocaine hydrochloride	2%	Intermediate	Epinephrine 1:50,000
Lidocaine hydrochloride	2%	Intermediate	Epinephrine 1: 100,000
Mepivacaine hydrochloride	3%	Short/Intermediate	None
Mepivacaine hydrochloride	2%	Intermediate	Levonordefrin 1:200,000
Mepivacaine hydrochloride	2%	Intermediate	Epinephrine 1:200,000
Prilocaine hydrochloride	4%	Short	None
Prilocaine hydrochloride	4%	Long	Epinephrine 1:200,000

described for patients undergoing anesthesia with ether by Guedel (1920) and are given in **Table 9-3**.

Classification of Anesthetic Agents

General anesthetics can be classified into two groups: (1) inhalation anesthetics, and (2) intravenous anesthetics. Inhalation anesthetics can be divided into volatile liquids and gases.

The gases exist in gaseous state at atmospheric pressure. The anesthetic gases are **nitrous oxide, cyclopropane,** and **ethylene**. Nitrous oxide is the only anesthetic gas used extensively.

The volatile liquids exist in a liquid state at atmospheric pressure but can easily be converted to the volatile state. The volatile liquids include **halothane, enflurane, isoflurane, methoxyflurane, desflurane,** and **sevoflurane.**

Intravenous anesthetics may be used alone or with inhalation agents. When combined with inhalation anesthetics, they permit dosage of the inhalation agent to be reduced and they produce anesthesia that cannot be achieved with an inhalation agent alone. Intravenous agents include short-acting barbiturates, **benzodiazepines, ketamine,** and **opioids**.

Nitrous oxide (N_2O) is a colorless gas with little or no odor. The anesthetic potency of nitrous oxide is very low, and surgical anesthesia cannot be produced using nitrous oxide alone. Despite its low potency, nitrous oxide is a widely used anesthetic agent. Most patients receiving general anesthesia receive nitrous oxide as a supplement to the primary anesthetic. The analgesic potency of nitrous oxide is very high.

Use of a nitrous oxide-oxygen (N_2O-O_2) combination is routinely used by dentists to provide anxiety relief with analgesia. This combination makes the patient slightly sedated and relaxed, and the patient is conscious with protective reflexes intact. This combination of nitrous oxide and oxygen has many advantages, including rapid onset of action, and it is easy to administer.

DIURETICS

Diuretics are used to treat hypertension and mobilization of edematous fluid. The three major classes of diuretics are: (1) high ceiling or loop diuretics, (2) thiazide diuretics, and (3) potassium-sparing diuretics.

The most frequently prescribed loop diuretic is **furosemide** (Lasix). Furosemide blocks the reabsorption of sodium and chloride in the ascending limb of the loop of Henle, thus preventing the passive reabsorption of water. Furosemide is a very potent diuretic that is used for rapid or massive mobilization of fluid.

Most adverse effects are due to excessive loss of electrolytes and fluid. Hyponatremia, hypochloremia, and severe dehydration can result. Furosemide can cause hypotension, which is a result of fluid volume depletion and relaxation of the venous smooth muscle.

Furosemide and other loop diuretics can cause hypokalemia. Eating potassium rich foods, taking potassium supplements, or adding a potassium-sparing diuretic can minimize potassium loss. Hypokalemia is a problem for patients taking cardiac gylcosides. Hyperglycemia, hypocalcemia, and hyperuricemia are other adverse effects. Hyperuricemia is a special problem if the patient is predisposed to gout. Furosemide can also cause hearing loss. Deafness is usually transient.

The effects produced by the thiazide diuretics are similar to those of the loop diuretics. The most widely used thiazide diuretic is **hydrochlorothiazide** (e.g., HydroDIURIL). The thiazide diuretics increase the renal excretion of sodium, chloride, and potassium. Loss of potassium can increase the risk of dysrhythmias for patients receiving cardiac glycosides. The thiazide diuretics cause a loss of water but produce less diuresis compared with the loop diuretics.

Thiazide diuretics are often the drugs of choice for treatment of mild hypertension. For patients requiring multiple drug therapy, a thiazide diuretic may be included. Thiazide diuretics are utilized for mobilizing edema associated with

TABLE 9–3 Stages of Ether Anesthesia

	MAIN FEATURE	REFLEXES	RESPIRATION	BLOOD PRESSURE
Stage I	Analgesia	Present	Slow and deep	Elevated
Stage II	Delirium	Present	Irregular; abdominal and thoracic	Elevated
Stage III	Surgical stage	Absent	Slow and regular;shallow; abdominal	Normal-falling
Stage IV	Medullary paralysis	Absent	Paralysis	Low

mild-to-moderate heart failure. Thiazide diuretics also cause hyperglycemia and hyperuricemia; however, they do not cause hearing loss.

Thiazides lower blood pressure and can enhance the effects of other antihypertensive drugs. Nonsteroidal anti-inflammatory drugs (NSAIDs) can reduce the hypotensive effect of thiazides when taken concurrently for several days since thiazide diuretics do not cause loss of hearing, can be combined with ototoxic drugs, such as aminoglycosides

Potassium-sparing diuretics are weak diuretics and are seldom used alone to promote diuresis. Potassium excretion is decreased by these drugs, which are used to counteract the potassium loss produced by loop and thiazide diuretics. Spironolactone and triamterene are potassium-sparing diuretics.

Spironolactone (Aldactone) is a competitive antagonist of aldosterone. By inhibiting aldosterone, spironolactone causes potassium retention and sodium depletion with scanty diuresis. Spironolactone is used to treat hypertension and edema. The drug is usually combined with a thiazide or loop diuretic.

Triamterene (Dyrenium) is also a potassium-sparing diuretic. Triamterene directly inhibits the sodium-potassium exchange mechanism in the distal and cortical collecting tubules. The net effect is a loss of sodium and retention of potassium.

Triamterene is used to treat hypertension and edema. Triamterene is combined with thiazide and loop diuretics to counteract the potassium-wasting effects. The combination of hydrochlorothiazide and triamterene (Dyazide, Maxzide) is often used. Hyperkalemia is the most dangerous adverse effect. Common side effects include nausea, vomiting, leg cramps, and dizziness.

CARDIOVASCULAR DRUGS

Drugs Acting on the Renin-Angiotensin System

The angiotensin-converting enzyme (ACE) inhibitors and angiotensin II receptor antagonists produce their effects by interfering with the renin-angiotensin system (RAS). ACE inhibitors are used to treat hypertension and heart failure. The angiotensin II receptor antagonists are only approved for the treatment of hypertension.

The RAS is a complex system that plays an important role in the regulation of blood pressure, blood volume, and fluid and electrolyte balance. The liver produces angiotensinogen, an inactive molecule, which is present in the blood at all times. When a decrease occurs in blood pressure or blood flow to the kidneys, they release renin, which catalyzes angiotensinogen to angiotensin I (inactive). Angiotensin I is converted to angiotensin II (active) by ACE. ACE is found on the luminal surface of blood vessels, especially those of the lungs.

Angiotensin II is a potent vasoconstrictor of arterioles and causes blood pressure to rise. Angiotensin II stimulates the release of aldosterone from the adrenal cortex. Aldosterone stimulates the kidneys to retain sodium and excrete potassium, which facilitates water retention and thus increases blood pressure.

The ACE inhibitors are used to treat hypertension, congestive heart failure, myocardial infarction, and diabetic and nondiabetic nephropathy. The ACE inhibitors include **captopril** (Capoten), **enalapril** (Vasotec), **lisinopril** (Prinivil), and **ramipril** (Altace). The ACE inhibitors block the formation of angiotensin II. This results in vasodilation and a decrease in blood volume.

Captopril (Captoten) was the first ACE inhibitor to be marketed. Captopril is used in the treatment of hypertension, congestive heart failure, myocardial infarction, and diabetic nephropathy. Captopril is absorbed following oral administration.

Captopril may produce first-dose hypotension. An abrupt lowering of angiotensin II levels causes widespread vasodilation. Captopril and other ACE inhibitors produce a dry, nonproductive cough in 5% of patients. ACE inhibitors can cause hyperkalemia, renal failure, and angioedema. Dysgeusia (i.e., a bad taste in the mouth) and rash are common. Dysgeusia occurs in approximately 4% of patients, and a rash occurs in up to 10% of patients.

Enalapril (Vasotec) was the second ACE inhibitor to be approved in the United States. Enalapril is a prodrut that is not highly active and must be converted by the liver to enalaprilate, its active form. Enalaprilate is a highly potent inhibitor of ACE.

Enalapril has the same mechanism of action and therapeutic uses as captopril. The pharmacokinetics and adverse effects are similar.

Newer ACE inhibitors are **benazepril, fosinopril, lisinopril, moexipril, quinapril, ramipril,** and **trandolapril.** These Ace inhibitors have the same mechanism of action as captopril, and produce similar pharmacologic and adverse effects.

Losartan (Cozaar) and **valsartan** (Diovan) are angiotensin II receptor blockers. The therapeutic effects of the angiotensin II receptor blockers are very similar to those of ACE inhibitors. The angiotensin II receptor blockers do not cause an increase in potassium levels, angioedema, or cough.

Calcium Channel Blockers

Calcium channel blockers are drugs that inhibit the movement of extracellular calcium ions into vascular smooth muscle cells and cardiac cells. Movement of extracellular calcium into vascular smooth muscle cells is necessary for contraction resulting in vasoconstriction. Calcium channel blockers cause blood vessels to dilate. They act selectively on arteries and arterioles with no significant effect on veins. In cardiac muscle cells, influx of calcium increases heart rate, AV conduction, and myocardial contractility. Calcium channel blockers produce an opposite effect.

The calcium channel blockers are used to treat hypertension, cardiac dysrhythmias, and angina pectoris. **Nifedipine** (Procardia), **diltiazem** (Cardizem), and **verapamil** (Calan) are commonly used calcium channel blocking agents.

Nifedipine blocks calcium channels primarily on arterioles, resulting in vasodilation and lowering arterial pressure. This drug has very little effect on calcium channels in the heart. Fast-acting preparations activate the baroreceptor reflex and result in tachycardia. With sustained-release formulations, blood pressure is slowly lowered and the baroreceptor reflex is not activated.

Nifedipine is used to treat essential hypertension and hypertensive emergencies. Only the sustained-release formulation is used in hypertension. Nifedipine is also used to treat angina pectoris. A β_1-adrenergic blocking agent can be used to prevent reflex tachycardia.

Adverse effects of nifedipine include dizziness, headache, peripheral edema, and flushing. Adverse oral effects include xerostomia, dysgeusia, and gingival hyperplasia. Nifedipine causes reflex tachycardia and can increase pain for patients with angina pectoris.

Diltiazem and verapamil block calcium channels in the heart and blood vessels. Blocking calcium channels in peripheral arterioles causes vasodilation and lowers blood pressure. Dilation of coronary arterioles increases blood flow to the heart. Blockade of calcium channels in the AV node reduces AV conduction, and blockade in the myocardium reduces force of contraction. Diltiazem and verapamil are useful for treating cardiac dysrhythmias, hypertension, migraines, and angina pectoris.

Adverse effects include dizziness, headache, flushing, and edema of the feet and ankles. Gingival hyperplasia, xerostomia, and dysgeusia are oral manifestations of the calcium channel blockers. Constipation is a frequent complaint with verapamil.

Drugs for Hypertension

Arterial pressure = cardiac output (CO) $\times$ total peripheral resistance (TPR). Cardiac output is determined by heart rate, myocardial contractility, blood volume, and venous return. TPR is determined by arteriolar constriction. Drugs used to treat hypertension alter some factor that controls blood pressure.

The 10 principal sites at which antihypertensive drugs act are: (1) brainstem, (2) sympathetic ganglia, (3) adrenergic nerve terminals, (4) cardiac β_1-adrenergic receptors, (5) vascular α_1-adrenergic receptors, (6) renal tubules, (7) vascular smooth muscle, (8) β_1-adrenergic receptors on juxtaglomerular cells, (9) ACE, and (10) angiotensin II receptors. **Table 9-4** lists antihypertensive agents at these specific sites.

The treatment of hypertension is usually initiated with a diuretic or a β_1-adrenergic blocker. Calcium channel blockers, ACE inhibitors, α_1-adrenergic blockers, or β_1-adrenergic blockers are alternate drugs for initial therapy. If the therapeutic response to these agents is inadequate, a centrally acting sympatholytic, adrenergic neuron blocker or direct-acting vasodilator can be used.

Drugs for Angina Pectoris

Angina pectoris is the severe chest pain that occurs when coronary blood flow is inadequate to supply the oxygen required by the heart. The most frequent cause of angina is occlusion of coronary arteries by atherosclerotic plaques. The main way to relieve the pain of angina is to decrease cardiac oxygen demand.

Three classes of drugs are used to treat angina. The organic nitrates (e.g., **nitroglycerine**) are the most frequently used antianginal drugs. **Calcium channel blockers** and β_1-adrenergic blocking agents are also useful for treating angina.

Nitroglycerine and other organic nitrates relax vascular smooth muscle and produce vasodilation. At therapeutic blood levels, nitroglycerine acts primarily on the veins. Arterioles are dilated much less than veins. By dilating veins, venous capacitance is increased venous return to the heart is decreased, which decreases preload and decreases oxygen demand.

Nitroglycerine is very lipid soluble and easily crosses cell membranes. Nitroglycerine can be administered by various routes (e.g., sublingual, transdermal, buccal, intravenous, and oral). This drug is rapidly metabolized by hepatic enzymes, and bioavailability by the oral route is usually less than 10% to 20%. The sublingual route avoids the first-pass effect and temporarily avoids metabolism. Effects of sublin-

TABLE 9–4 Drugs for Treatment of Hypertension

RENIN-ANGIOTENSIN SYSTEM	ADRENERGIC ANTAGONISTS	DIURETICS	OTHERS
ACE Inhibitors	**β-Blockers**	**Thiazides and Related Diuretics**	**Calcium Channel Blockers**
Benazepril	Acebutolol	Bendroflumethiazide	Amlodipine
Captopril	Atenolol	Benzthiazide	Diltiazem
Enalapril	Betaxolol	Chlorothiazide	Felodipine
Fosinopril	Bisoprolol	Cyclothiazide	Isradipine
Lisinopril	Metoprolol	Hydrochlorothiazide	Nifedipine
Moexipril	Nadolol	Hydroflumethiazide	Nicardipine
Quinapril	Penbutolol	Indapamide	Nimodipine
Ramipril	Pindolol	Methyclothiazide	Nislodipine
Trandolapril	Propranolol	Metolazone	Verapamil
	Timolol	Polythiazide	
		Quinethazone	
		Trichlormethiazide	
Angiotensin II Receptor Antagonists	**α₂-Blockers**	**Loop Diuretics**	**Direct-Acting Vasodilators**
Candesartan	Doxazosin	Furosemide	Hydralazine
Irbesartan	Prazosin	Ethacrynic acid	Minoxidil
Losartan	Terazosin	Bumetanide	
Valsartan		Torsemide	
	α/β-Blockers	**Potassium-Sparing Diuretics**	**Centrally Acting α₂-Agonists**
	Labetalol	Spironolactone	Clonidine
	Carvedilol	Triamterene	Methyldopa
		Amiloride	Guanabenz
			Guanfacine
	Adrenergic Neuron Blockers		
	Guanethidine		
	Guanadrel		
	Reserpine		

ACE, angiotensin-converting enzyme.

gual nitroglycerine begin in 1 to 3 minutes and last for up to 1 hour.

The adverse effects of nitroglycerine are an extension of therapeutic vasodilation. Initial therapy can produce a throbbing headache. Other adverse effects are orthostatic hypotension and reflex tachycardia.

β_1-Adrenergic blockers (e.g., **metoprolol, propranolol**) are very useful in the management of angina pectoris. The β_1-adrenergic blockers decrease heart rate, blood pressure, and contractility, which decrease myocardial oxygen demand.

All calcium channel blocking agents relax smooth muscle in arterioles, thus decreasing the work of the heart. Verapamil and diltiazem reduce heart rate and contractility, thus decreasing myocardial oxygen demand.

Drugs for Heart Failure

In congestive heart failure, there is a reduction in ventricular contractility that results in inadequate cardiac output and unsatisfactory circulation. Over time, the compensatory responses lead to the following: (1) cardiac dilation, (2) in-creased sympathetic tone, (3) activation of the renin-angiotensin-aldosterone system, (4) retention of water, and (5) increased blood volume.

Congestive heart failure is treated with three classes of drugs: (1) vasodilators, (2) inotropic agents, and (3) diuretics.

Vasodilators are the only class of drugs used for long-term therapy of congestive heart failure that have been shown to reduce mortality. ACE inhibitors (e.g., enalapril and captopril) are preferred for long-term therapy (see ACE inhibitors). Patients who cannot tolerate ACE inhibitors are treated with a combination of **hydralazine-isosorbide dinitrate** (see inorganic nitrates).

Inotropic drugs increase the force of myocardial contraction. The cardiac glycosides are the only inotropic agents suitable for long-term use. **Digoxin** (Lanoxin) and **digitoxin** (Crystodigin) are the only two cardiac glycosides available in the United States.

Digoxin increases the force of ventricular contraction (positive inotropic effect). The heart becomes a more efficient pump, and cardiac output is increased. Digoxin inhibits the enzyme sodium, potassium-ATPase and by an indirect process promotes accumulation of calcium in cardiac muscle cells. The extra calcium increases cardiac muscle contraction. By improving cardiac output, digoxin can reverse the symptoms of congestive heart failure.

Digoxin is absorbed orally, but absorption is variable. This drug undergoes distribution throughout the body and is eliminated primarily by renal excretion. The half-life of digoxin is 1.5 days.

Digoxin has a very narrow TI. and toxic effects are common. Early noncardiac signs of digoxin toxicity include anorexia, nausea, and vomiting. Neurologic signs of toxicity include headache, fatigue, and visual disturbances (e.g., blurred vision and yellow and green tinge to vision).

Digoxin can cause almost all types of dysrhythmias. The most common cause of dysrhythmias in patients receiving digoxin is hypokalemia. Thiazide and loop diuretics produce hypokalemia, and they are often used in the treatment of congestive heart failure.

Digitoxin (Crystodigin) has the same mechanism of action, the same applications, and produces the same adverse effects. Digitoxin is more lipid soluble; this drug is excreted by the liver and has a half-life of 7 days.

Patients with volume overload are treated with diuretics. These drugs decrease pulmonary edema, peripheral edema, cardiac dilation, and venous pressure by reducing blood volume. Thiazide and loop diuretics cause hypokalemia, which can predispose a patient to serious arrhythmias (see diuretics).

Antidysrhythmic Drugs

There are many types of dysrhythmias that produce abnormalities in the rhythm of the heartbeat. Alterations in the normal electrical impulses regulating cardiac rhythm cause dysrhythmias. Antidysrhythmic drugs correct or compensate for the alteration. Most dysrhythmias can be divided into two major groups: supraventricular dysrhythmias and ventricular dysrhythmias, depending on the origin of the dysrhythmia. Ventricular dysrhythmias can be very dangerous.

There are four classes of antidysrhythmic agents, designated by Roman numerals, I to IV. The classes are determined by ion movements during the phases of cardiac action potentials.

Class I antidysrhythmic drugs decrease the rate of entry of sodium ions into cardiac muscle cells. This slows impulse conduction through the atria, ventricles, and His-Purkinje system. Class I agents include **quinidine** (Quinidex), **procainamide** (Pronestyl), and **lidocaine** (Xylocaine).

Quinidine is useful in treating supraventricular and ventricular dysrhythmias. Quinidine is indicated for the long-term suppression of dysrhythmias. Quinidine widens the QRS complex and prolongs the QT interval of the electrocardiogram (ECG). Quinidine has an anticholinergic effect on the sinoatrial node resulting in an increased heart rate. Quinidine causes diarrhea other GI effects in about 33% of patients. Quinidine can also produce all types of dysrhythmias.

Procainamide (Pronestyl) is similar to quinidine in applications and actions. It is useful against a broad spectrum of dysrhythmias. Procainamide has minimal anticholinergic effects. Serious adverse effects (systemic lupus erythematosus-like syndrome and blood dyscrasias) frequently limit the use of procainamide.

Lidocaine (Xylocaine) is a dysrhythmic agent that is used only by the intravenous route. It has a low incidence of toxicity and high degree of effectiveness against ventricular dysrhythmias, including those associated with myocardial infarction. It is not effective against supraventricular dysrhythmias. Lidocaine's most common adverse effects are on the CNS: tremor, nausea, confusion, and drowsiness.

Class II dysrhythmic agents consist of β-adrenergic blocking agents (see adrenergic antagonists). Propranolol (Inderal), **acebutolol** (Sectral), **esmolol** (Brevibloc), and **sotalol** (Betapace) are the only four β-blocking agents approved for treating dysrhythmias. These drugs block cardiac β_1-receptors and reduce sympathetic stimulation of the heart. These drugs are useful in treating dysrhythmias caused by excessive sympathetic stimulation of the heart.

Class III drugs prolong action potentials by blocking potassium channels. As a result, they prolong the action potential. **Bretylium** (Bretylol) is usually used in an emergency setting for severe ventricular dysrhythmias.

Class IV dysrhythmics block calcium channels in cardiac muscle cells. The calcium channels blocking agents used to treat dysrhythmias are verapamil (Calan) and diltiazem (Cardizem) (see calcium channel blocking agents). Diltiazem and verapamil suppress AV nodal conduction and are used for patients with atrial fibrillation or atrial flutter to terminated supraventricular tachycardia.

ANTICOAGULANTS

Oral anticoagulants are used to prevent formation of blood clots. **Warfarin (Coumadin)** is the most important member of the oral anticoagulant family. Warfarin is used therapeutically for long-term prophylaxis of thrombosis.

Warfarin prevents clotting by antagonizing vitamin K. Blocking vitamin K interferes with the synthesis of four clotting factors (factors VII, IX, X, and prothrombin).

Warfarin is absorbed following oral administration. After absorption, 99% of warfarin is bound to plasma albumin leaving only 1% free. Warfarin is metabolized by the hepatic microsomal enzyme system and excreted by the kidneys.

Anticoagulant responses to warfarin are delayed when therapy is initiated and discontinued. Warfarin has no effect on existing clotting factors. Coagulation is not affected until these factors are depleted and takes several days. After warfarin therapy is discontinued, coagulation is inhibited for several days.

The major adverse effect of warfarin therapy is bleeding. Warfarin overdose is treated with vitamin K.

Drug interactions involving oral anticoagulants are numerous. The combination of warfarin and aspirin should be avoided because bleeding and hemorrhagic disasters can occur.

Barbiturates induce the hepatic drug metabolizing enzymes and can increase the hepatic metabolism of warfarin. The anticoagulant effect of warfarin is decreased.

DRUGS THAT LOWER LDL-CHOLESTEROL LEVELS

Drugs used to lower low-density lipoproteins (LDLs) are hydroxymethylglutaryl coenzyme A (HMG CoA) reductase inhibitors, nicotinic acid and bile acid-binding resins. LDLs is referred to a "bad cholesterol."

The HMG CoA reductase inhibitors are the most effective with the least adverse effects. Examples of HMG CoA reductase inhibitors are **lovastatin** (Mevacor), **fluvastatin** (Lescol), **atorvastatin** (Lipitor), **cerivastatin** (Baycol), **pravastatin** (Pravachol), and **simvastatin** (Zocor). These agents are often referred to as "statins," because their generic names end in statin.

The statins decrease cholesterol levels by inhibiting HMG-CoA reductase. This lowers very low density lipoproteins (VLDL) levels as well as LDL levels. High-density lipoproteins (HDL) levels are raised by 8% by the statins.

Adverse effects of HMG CoA reductase inhibitors are uncommon. Headache, rash, or GI disturbances have been reported. These effects are usually mild and transient. Hepatoxicity has been reported in 1% to 2% of patients treated for 1 year or longer. Myopathy develops in less than 0.5% of patients.

Cholestyramine (Questran) and **colestipol** (Colestid) are bile acid-binding resins. These agents cause a reduction in LDL-cholesterol. These drugs are similar in most respects and extremely safe.

The bile acid-binding resins bind with bile acids in the intestines to form an insoluble product that is lost from the intestinal tract through the feces. This loss of bile acids refults in a reduction of cholestrerol levels.

Adverse effects are minimal, because the resins are not absorbed from the GI tract. Constipation is the most common side effect.

Niacin (nicotinic acid) is a B vitamin. In large doses, it reduces LDL and VLDL levels and raises HDL levels. These large doses cause frequent adverse effects. Intense flushing of the face and neck occurs in most patients. Hepatoxicity, allergic reactions, and cholestasis have been reported.

Gemfibrozil (Lopid) lowers VLDL levels and increases HDL levels. This drug is used to treat hypertriglyceridemia. Adverse effects are minimal. Rashes and GI disturbances are most common.

ENDOCRINE AGENTS

Drugs for Thyroid Disorders

The thyroid gland produces two hormones that have profound effects on metabolism, cardiac function, growth, and development. These hormones are triiodothyronine (T_3) and thyroxine (T_4).

Thyroid function is regulated by the hypothalamus and pituitary. The hypothalamus produces and releases thyroid-releasing hormone (TRH), which stimulates the release of thyroid-stimulating hormone (TSH) from the anterior pituitary. TSH causes the thyroid to make and release T_3 and T_4, which act on the pituitary and hypothalamus to suppress release of TSH and TRH.

Hypothyroidism can occur at any age. Mild deficiency of thyroid hormone in the adult is referred to as hypothyroidism and severe deficiency is called myxedema. If hypothyroidism occurs in infancy, the condition is called myxedema.

Hypothyroidism requires replacement therapy with thyroid hormones. Preparations containing T_3, T_4, or both hormones are administered to mimic normal thyroid function. In most cases, treatment must be continued throughout life. Synthetic thyroxine-**levothyroxine** (Levothyroid, Synthroid)-is the drug of choice for most patients requiring thyroid hormone replacement. Liothyronine (Cytomel) is a synthetic triiodothyronine. Liothyronine has a shorter half-life and a more rapid onset of action and is more expensive than levothyroxine. **Liotrix** (Euthyroid, Thyrolar) is a mixture of synthetic T_3 and T_4.

Hyperthyroidism can be treated with antithyroid drugs, by partial thyroidectomy, or destruction of thyroid tissue with radioactive iodine.

Propylthiouracil (PTU) is an antithyroid drug that inhibits thyroid synthesis. PTU can be used alone in the treatment of hyperthyroidism, as an adjunct to radiation therapy, and can be used to suppress thyroid function in patients awaiting surgery.

^{131}I is a radioactive isotope used to destroy thyroid tissue in patients with hyperthyroidism. Full effects of ^{131}I require 2 to 3 months to develop. Patients older than 30 years of age are candidates for ^{131}I therapy.

Drugs for Diabetes Mellitus

Diabetes mellitus is basically a disorder of carbohydrate metabolism. The principal sign of diabetes is inappropriate hyperglycemia, which causes polydipsia, polyuria, polyphagia, weight loss, and ketonuria. Long-term complications of diabetes include hypertension, heart disease, blindness, renal failure, neuropathy, amputations, impotence, and gastroparesis. Patients with uncontrolled diabetes are more prone to periodontal disease, are more susceptible to dental caries, and have xerostomia.

Diabetes mellitus is currently classified as **insulin-dependent diabetes mellitus (IDDM)** or **type I** and **noninsulin-dependent diabetes mellitus (NIDDM)** or **type II**. IDDM results from an autoimmune destruction of the pancreatic beta cells and is associated with a complete lack of insulin secretion. Patients with NIDDM are capable of insulin secretion, but there is cellular resistance to insulin's actions. Patients with IDDM and NIDDM share the same long-term complications.

IDDM is treated with **insulin replacement**. Five forms of insulin are available in the United States, and the major difference among the currently used insulins is their duration of action. Regular insulin has a rapid onset and short duration; lispro insulin has a very rapid onset and short duration; NPH insulin and lente insulin have intermediate duration; and ultralente insulin has a prolonged duration.

Insulin is administered by injection. Insulin is a peptide and would be inactivated by the digestive system if taken orally. All insulins may be injected subcutaneously. Only regular insulin may be administered intramuscularly and intravenously.

The most common adverse effect of insulin therapy is hypoglycemia. Symptoms include palpitations, sweating, headache, mental confusion, drowsiness, and fatigue. Severe hypoglycemia can eventually produce coma, convulsions, and death. Insulin-induced hypoglycemia must be treated rapidly with a fast-acting oral sugar or intravenous glucose.

NIDDM is treated with **oral hypoglycemic agents** and/or insulin. There are four families or oral hypoglycemic drugs: sulfonylureas, biguanides, α-glucosidase inhibitors, and thiazolidinediones. Oral hypoglycemic agents are only used in the treatment of NIDDM.

The **sulfonylurea agents** fall into two groups: first-generation agents **tolbutamide** (Orinase) and second-generation agents **glipizide** (Glucotrol). Both generations are equally effective in reducing blood glucose levels; however, the second-generation agents produce their effects at much lower doses than first-generation agents. The sulfonylureas stimulate release of insulin from the beta cells of the pancreas and increase cellular sensitivity of the target tissues to insulin. Adverse effects of the sulfonylureas include hypoglycemia, blood dyscrasias, and GI disturbances.

Metformin (Glucophage) is a biguanide that is used to lower blood glucose levels in NIDDM. Metformin lowers blood glucose levels by decreasing production of glucose by the liver and enhances glucose utilization by muscle. The most common adverse effects are nausea, diarrhea, and decreased appetite.

Acarbose (Precose) is an α-glucosidase inhibitor that delays absorption of dietary carbohydrates. Ingested polysaccharides and complex carbohydrates must be broken down into monosaccharides by α-glucosidase, an enzyme located on the brush border of intestinal cells in order to be absorbed. Acarbose inhibits this enzyme and slows digestion of carbohydrates and postprandial increase in blood glucose.

Acarbose can be used alone or with other agents including insulin, biguanides and sulfonylureas. Adverse effects of acarbose include flatulence, cramps, abdominal distention, and diarrhea. Hypoglycemia does not occur when acarbose is used alone but may develop if combined with a sulfonylurea or insulin.

Troglitazone (Rezulin) was the first member of the new class of antihypoglycemic agents known as thiazolidinediones. Troglitazone decreases insulin resistance at the target cells, resulting in an increase in glucose uptake by muscle and a decrease production of glucose by the liver. Troglitazone is only approved for patients with NIDDM who are currently taking insulin but remain hyperglycemic. Adverse effects are usually mild or absent. Troglitazone can cause hypoglycemia, but only in the presence of excessive insulin.

Drugs for Disorders of the Adrenal Cortex

The adrenal cortex produces two major classes of steroid hormones: the **glucocorticoids** and **mineralocorticoids**. The term adrenocorticoids may be used when referring to either the glucocorticoids or mineralocorticoids.

Glucocorticoids influence the metabolism of carbohydrates, proteins, and fats. During times of stress, glucocorticoids are essential for survival. The major glucocorticoid in the body is cortisol (hydrocortisone).

The mineralocorticoids affect water and electrolyte composition of the body. The major mineralocorticoid, aldosterone, stimulates the kidney to retain sodium and water and excrete potassium.

Excess levels of circulating glucocorticoids cause signs and symptoms of Cushing syndrome. Major causes of excess glucocorticoids are: (1) hypersecretion of ACTH by pituitary adenomas, (2) hypersecretion of glucocorticoids by adrenal carcinomas and adenomas, and (3) administration of large doses of glucocorticoids to treat arthritis and other nonendocrine diseases.

Treatment of Cushing syndrome is directed at the cause. Surgical removal of the adrenal gland is the treatment of choice for adrenal carcinoma and adenoma. Mitotane (Lysodren) is indicated for patients with inoperable adrenal carcinoma. Mitotane is an anticancer agent that produces selective destruction of adrenocortical cells. Partial removal of the pituitary is the preferred treatment of Cushing syndrome caused by pituitary adenoma.

Two drugs-**ketoconazole** (Nizoral) and **aminoglutethimide** (Cytadren)-can relieve symptoms of Cushing syndrome by inhibiting corticosteroid synthesis. These drugs are usually employed as an adjunct to surgery or radiation.

Hyperaldosteronism is usually caused by an aldosterone-secreting adrenal adenoma, and treatment is surgical removal of the adrenal. When adrenal hyperplasia causes hyperaldosteronism, an aldosterone antagonist is the preferred treatment. The most frequently used drug is spironolactone, which is a potassium-sparing diuretic.

Insufficiency of adrenal hormone can result from many causes and requires lifelong replacement therapy. All patients with adrenal insufficiency require treatment with a glucocorticoid, and some patients may also require treatment with a mineralocorticoid. Cortisone and hydrocortisone are the glucocorticoids of first choice. Fludrocortisone is the mineralocorticoid of choice.

When glucocorticoids are given in low doses for replacement therapy, no adverse effects occur. When used chronically in high doses for nonendocrine diseases, such as rheumatoid arthritis and systemic lupus erythematosus, glucocorticoids can cause severe side effects.

 # NONSTEROIDAL ANTI-INFLAMMATORY DRUGS

The nonsteroidal anti-inflammatory drugs (NSAIDs) are used clinically for: (1) relief of mild-to-moderate pain, (2) suppression of inflammation, and (3) relief of fever. This family of drugs consists of aspirin and a large number of related compounds.

Aspirin or acetylsalicylic acid is a member of the chemical family known as salicylates. Other salicylates are **choline salicylate** (Arthropan)**, magnesium salicylate** (Magan), **sodium salicylate**, **salsalate** (Disalcid), and **diflunisal** (Dolobid). Aspirin will serve as the prototype salicylate.

Aspirin inhibits cyclooxygenase, an enzyme necessary for the synthesis of prostaglandins, prostacyclin, and thromboxane A_2. Cyclooxygenase has two forms: cyclooxygenase-1 (COX-1) and cyclooxygenase-2 (COX-2). The therapeutic benefits of inhibiting COX-1 are analgesia and reduction of fever. Inhibition of COX-2 is responsible for decreasing inflammation.

Aspirin has many therapeutic uses. It is the initial drug of choice for rheumatoid arthritis, osteoarthritis, and juvenile arthritis. Aspirin is also indicated for other inflammatory disorders.

Aspirin is widely used to relieve mild-to-moderate pain. It is most active against joint pain, muscle pain, and headache. Aspirin can be as effective as an opioid for the relief of some types of postoperative pain. Aspirin is also the drug of choice for reducing fever. Aspirin does not lower normal body temperature nor body temperature elevated in response to exercise. Aspirin is valuable for the relief of pain associated with dysmenorrhea. By inhibiting prostaglandin synthesis in uterine smooth muscle, aspirin relieves dysmenorrhea.

Thromboxane A_2 is necessary for platelet aggregation. Aspirin irreversibly inhibits the enzyme necessary for production of thromboxane A_2. Aspirin is used in the treatment or prophylaxis of diseases associated with excessive platelet aggregation, such as coronary artery disease and postopera-

tive deep vein thrombosis. Low doses of aspirin following myocardial infarction decrease the risk of reinfarction and death.

The most common adverse effects are GI in nature and are from direct gastric irritation or from inhibition of COX-2. Heartburn, nausea, vomiting, and gastric bleeding have been observed. Gastric ulceration occurs in 25% of patients on long-term, high-dose therapy.

At therapeutic doses (2 aspirin tablets), aspirin inhibits platelet aggregation. Platelets are affected until new ones are formed (~1 week). Aspirin therapy should be discontinued at least 1 week before surgery.

The use of aspirin in children who have chickenpox or influenza has been epidemiologically associated with Reye syndrome. Aspirin and other NSAIDs should be avoided in pediatric patients suspected of having influenza or chickenpox.

The incidence of hypersensitivity reactions to aspirin is less than 1%. Most allergic reactions occur in adults with asthma, hay fever, chronic urticaria, or nasal polyps.

When aspirin levels exceed therapeutic levels, a toxic reaction referred to as salicylism occurs. Signs of salicylism include tinnitus, sweating, headache, vomiting, and dizziness.

Aspirin overdose can produce serious effects and may even be fatal. Aspirin overdose causes respiratory depression, acidosis, hyperthermia, and dehydration. Death usually results from respiratory failure.

A large number of NSAIDs with actions similar to aspirin have been produced. These agents, which are often referred to as traditional NSAIDs, inhibit both COX-1 and COX-2 and their pharmacologic effects and adverse reactions are similar to those of aspirin. In comparison with aspirin, the NSAIDs cause reversible inhibition of platelet aggregation. Examples of traditional NSAIDs are **ibuprofen** (Advil), **flurbiprofen** (Ansaid), **naproxen** (Naprosyn), **diclofenac** (Voltaren), and **diflunisal** (Dolobid).

The NSAIDs are used therapeutically for: (1) suppression of inflammation, (2) relief of pain, and (3) reduction of fever. These actions result from inhibition of prostaglandin synthesis by inhibiting cyclooxygenase.

The NSAIDs are used in the treatment of rheumatoid arthritis and other inflammatory disorders. These drugs are also used to treat fever, mild-to-moderate pain, primary dysmenorrhea, tendinitis, and bursitis.

Adverse effects of NSAIDs are similar to those of aspirin. GI pain, irritation, and bleeding can occur with all NSAIDs. NSAIDs have caused renal failure, cystitis, and an increased incidence of urinary tract infections (UTIs). Patients who are hypersensitive to aspirin are likely to be cross-hypersensitive to NSAIDs.

NSAIDs that selectively inhibit COX-2 are now available. COX-2 inhibitors reduce inflammation without causing adverse effects associated with inhibition of COX-1. **Celecoxib** (Celebrex) and **rofecoxib** (Vioxx) are selective COX-2 inhibitors.

Both agents are used therapeutically to relieve signs and symptoms of osteoarthritis and rheumatoid arthritis. Celecoxib had been approved for reducing intestinal polyps in patients with familial adenomatous polyposis. Rofecoxib has analgesic effects and can be used to relieve acute pain in adults, including dental pain.

Adverse effects include dizziness, fatigue, and headache. Oral manifestations reported include xerostomia and stomatitis.

These agents are contraindicated for patients who have experienced allergic reactions to aspirin or other NSAIDs.

Acetaminophen (Tylenol) is an effective analgesic and antipyretic agent but is devoid of anti-inflammatory and antirheumatic actions. The analgesic and antipyretic effects of acetaminophen are equal to those of aspirin. In comparison with aspirin, acetaminophen does not suppress platelet aggregation and does not produce gastric bleeding.

Acetaminophen inhibits prostaglandin synthesis in the CNS and reduces pain and fever. The agent has very little effect on prostaglandin synthesis outside the CNS.

Acetaminophen is absorbed from the GI tract and widely distributed throughout the body. Most of the drug is metabolized by the liver, and metabolites are eliminated by the kidneys.

Acetaminophen is metabolized in the liver by two pathways. Metabolism by the major pathway produces nontoxic metabolites, whereas the minor pathway produces a highly reactive and toxic compound. At therapeutic doses, most of the drug is converted to nontoxic metabolites. When large doses are taken, a larger amount of the drug is processed by the minor pathway and produces large quantities of the toxic compound. Accumulation of the toxic compound causes liver damage.

Adverse effects of acetaminophen at therapeutic doses are rare. Toxic levels of acetaminophen cause hepatic necrosis. Liver damage can be minimized by administering **acetylcysteine** (Mucomyst). Nephrotoxicity has been associated with long-term use of acetaminophen. The risk of liver damage is increased by consumption of alcohol. Alcohol stimulates the enzymes that metabolize acetaminophen to its toxic metabolite.

ANTIHISTAMINES: H₁ ANTAGONISTS

Histamine is stored in mast cells and basophils. Mast cells are located in the skin and other soft tissues, and basophils are present in the bloodstream. Histamine is released from the tissues in the body in response to allergic reactions or the administration of certain drugs. Histamine activates two types of receptors-H_1 receptors and H_2 receptors. Stimulation of H_1 receptors causes vasodilation of arterioles and venules, increased capillary permeability, bronchoconstriction, pain, and itching. Stimulation of H_2 receptors increases gastric acid secretion.

The **antihistamines** are classified as H_1 receptor antagonists and H_2 receptor antagonists. The term antihistamine refers to drugs that are H_1 antagonists.

The H_1 antagonists are classified as first-generation H_1 antagonists and second-generation antagonists. The first-generation antihistamines have a highly sedating effect, whereas the second-generation antihistamines have little or no sedative effect.

H_1 antihistamines bind to H_1 histamine receptors and antagonize the effects of histamine. In arterioles and venules, H_1 antihistamines prevent vasodilation. In capillary beds, H_1 antihistamines decrease permeability and reduce pain and itching at sensory nerve endings. Antihistamines usually produce CNS depression. These effects are more pronounced with the first-generation antihistamines. Some antihistamines suppress nausea and vomiting.

The H_1 antihistamines are used for a wide variety of purposes. Antihistamines alleviate the symptoms of type I hypersensitivity reactions. They provide dramatic relief of the symptoms of seasonal allergic rhinitis or allergic conjunctivitis. The antihistamines are employed as adjuncts in the treatment of anaphylaxis. Epinephrine is the drug of choice for management of anaphylaxis.

Several of the antihistamines, such as **dimenhydrinate** (Dramamine) and **promethazine** (Phenergan), are effective for nausea associated with motion sickness. The antihistamine must be given 30 minutes before departure for travel.

The antihistamines are used as sleep aids in over-the-counter preparations. **Diphenhydramine** (Benadryl) or promethazine (Phenergan) are very sedating and are usually selected for this application.

The H_1 antihistamines produce a wide array of adverse effects. Sedation is the most common side effect of the H_1 antihistamines. Patients should be warned against operating motor vehicles and engaging in hazardous activities.

GI disturbances include nausea, vomiting, and constipation. Administration of antihistamines with meals reduces GI disturbances.

The H_1 antihistamines have weak anticholinergic properties. These anticholinergic effects produce xerostomia and drying of the mucous membranes of the nasal passages and throat.

Loratidine (Claritin) and **fexofenadine** (Allegra) are examples of second-generation antihistamines. These drugs do not produce sedation, because they are unable to cross the blood-brain barrier. The nonsedative antihistamines are usually well tolerated.

DRUGS FOR PEPTIC ULCER DISEASE

The drugs for treating ulcers are: (1) antibiotics, (2) mucosal protectants, (3) antisecretory agents, and (4) antisecretory agents that enhance mucosal defenses. Antibiotics are used to eradicate *Helicobacter pylori*. Antisecretory agents and antacids are used to reduce gastric acidity, and mucosal protectants are used to enhance mucosal defense mechanisms.

All patients with duodenal or gastric ulcers and confirmed infection with *H. pylori* should be treated with antibiotics. Antibiotics most frequently used are **tetracycline, bismuth, metronidazole, amoxicillin,** and **clarithromycin** (see the section on antibiotics). Single-agent therapy of *H. pylori* has proved ineffective and has led to drug resistance. Regimens for eradicating *H. pylori* employ at least two or three antibiotics.

The H$_2$-receptor antagonists (H$_2$RAs) compete with histamine at the H$_2$ receptors, which are located on the parietal cells of the stomach. Four H$_2$RAs are available: **cimetidine** (Tagamet), **ranitidine** (Zantac), **famotidine** (Pepcid), and **nizatidine** (Axid). All four H$_2$RAs are equally effective in decreasing gastric acid secretion and the incidence of serious adverse effects is low.

Cimetidine binds to and blocks androgen receptors, which may result in impotence, reduced libido, and gynecomastia. These effects are reversible.

Cimetidine inhibits hepatic drug-metabolizing enzymes and can cause plasma levels of many drugs to rise. In contrast to cimetidine, ranitidine, famotidine, and nizatidine have little effect on drug-metabolizing enzymes and do not have antiandrogenic effects.

The most effective inhibitors of gastric acid secretion are the proton pump inhibitors. These drugs inhibit gastric H$^+$, K$^+$-ATPase, which is the enzyme that generates gastric acid. **Omeprazole** (Prilosec) and **lansoprazole** (Prevacid) are proton pump inhibitors approved for treatment of duodenal ulcers, gastric ulcers, gastroesophageal reflux disease, and Zollinger-Ellison syndrome.

The proton pump inhibitors produce minimal adverse effects. Headache, nausea, vomiting, and diarrhea have been reported in less than 1% of patients. Oral adverse effects include xerostomia, mucosal atrophy of tongue, and taste perversion.

Sucralfate (Carafate) forms a sticky gel that adheres to the ulcer and creates a protective barrier against gastric acid. Sucralfate is approved for treatment of duodenal ulcers. Sucralfate has no serious adverse effects. The major side effect is constipation, which occurs in 2% of patients.

CHEMOTHERAPY OF INFECTIOUS DISEASES

Basic Principles of Antimicrobial Therapy

An **antibiotic** is a chemical produced by one microorganism that has the ability to harm other microbes. An antimicrobial drug is defined as any chemical, natural or synthetic that has the ability to kill or suppress growth of microorganisms. Common usage often extends the term antibiotics to include synthetic dentibacterial agents.

Antibiotics are **selectively toxic**. The term selective toxicity refers to the ability of a drug to injure invading microbes without injuring cells of the host. Antibiotics can be highly toxic to microbes without affecting host cells, because the cellular chemistry of mammals and microbes are different.

Antibiotics can be classified by their antimicrobial activity. Antibiotics that are active against only a few microorganisms are called narrow-spectrum antibiotics, whereas broad-spectrum antibiotics are active against a wide array of microbes. Antibiotics that kill microbes are called **bactericidal**, whereas drugs that only suppress growth are **bacteriostatic.**

Over time, a microbe can develop resistance to an antibiotic and lose sensitivity to the drug entirely. Acquired resistance is a major concern in that it can make effective drugs useless in treating certain diseases. Resistance to antibiotics can be acquired by spontaneous mutation or by conjugation. Spontaneous mutation produces random changes in the microbe's DNA. Usually resistance to only one drug is produced by spontaneous mutations. Most bacteria acquire resistance by conjugation, a process by which extrachromosomal DNA is transferred one microbe to another. Conjugation often results in multiple drug resistance and gram-negative bacteria are most frequently involved. Antibiotics promote the emergence of resistance by favoring overgrowth of microbes that are resistant.

When treating an infection, the most appropriate antibiotic should be selected. The identity of the infecting organism and drug sensitivity should be determined as soon as possible.

Combinations of antibiotics should usually be avoided, but in some situations a combination may be life saving. When two antibiotics are used together, the effects can be **additive, potentiative, or antagonistic**. When the effect of a combination of drugs is equal to the sum of the effects of the two drugs alone, the effect is additive (1 + 1 = 2). If the effects of a combination of antibiotics is greater than the sum of the effects of the individual agents, the interaction is potentiative (1 + 1 > 2). If a combination of two antibiotics is less effective than either agent alone, the reduced response is antagonistic (1 + 1 < 2).

Situations exist where antimicrobial prophylaxis is both appropriate and effective. Patients with a history of rheumatic or congenital heart disease or the presence of heart valve prosthesis should receive prophylactic antibiotics before dental procedures.

All antibiotics can produce suprainfections. A suprainfection is a new infection that appears during the course of treatment of the original infection.

Antimicrobial agents can produce a wide variety of GI complaints, including diarrhea, nausea, and stomach pain. The incidence depends on the antibiotic, the dose of the drug, and the presence of food in the stomach.

Antimicrobial agents can interact with other drugs. Many antimicrobial agents may reduce the effectiveness of oral contraceptives and can also potentiate the effect of oral anticoagulants such as warfarin.

Antibiotics can interact with other antibiotics. Two antibiotics that act on the same receptor would compete for the receptor and be less effective. A bacteriostatic drug would slow the growth of microbes and inhibit the effects of a bactericidal agent.

Penicillins

The **penicillins** are known as **β-lactam** antibiotics because they have a β-lactam ring in their structure. The penicillins and all β-lactam antibiotics share the same mechanism of action.

Penicillins weaken the bacterial cell wall by inhibiting transpeptidases and activating autolysins. Transpeptidases are necessary for cell wall synthesis, and autolysins promote destruction of the cell wall. These combined actions weaken the cell wall causing lysis and death. The penicillins are usually bactericidal and more effective against rapidly growing bacteria.

Resistance to penicillin is determined primarily by two mechanisms. Some bacteria produce β-lactamases, enzymes that inactivate penicillins and other β-lactam antibiotics. β-Lactamases that act on penicillins are called penicillinases. Some penicillins cannot penetrate the gram-negative envelope and reach target enzymes. Most penicillins are inactive against gram-negative bacteria.

The penicillins can be divided into four major groups based on the antimicrobial spectrum. The first group contains **penicillin G** and **V**, narrow-spectrum penicillins that are sensitive to penicillinase. The second group consists of narrow-spectrum penicillins that are resistant to penicillinase. This group includes **oxacillin** and **cloxacillin**. The third group includes **amoxicillin** and **ampicillin,** and these agents are classified as broad-spectrum penicillins. The fourth group consists of extended-spectrum penicillins and includes **carbenicillin indanyl** and **ticarcillin**.

Penicillins are very safe antibiotics. The major adverse effect of penicillins is the production of allergic reactions. These allergic reactions range from mild rashes to life-threatening anaphylaxis. Patients allergic to one penicillin are usually cross-allergic to other penicillins. Some patients (5%-10%) who are allergic to penicillin are also allergic to cephalosporins.

Penicillin G is considered a narrow antibacterial spectrum. It is most effective against gram-positive bacteria, gram-negative cocci, anaerobic bacteria, and spirochetes. Penicillin G is unstable in stomach acid and destroyed by penicillinase. Penicillin G is distributed to most tissues and body fluids, except the meninges. If the meninges are inflamed, penicillin G will enter the cerebrospinal fluid (CSF). Penicillin G is rapidly eliminated from the body by the kidneys, mainly as the unchanged drug. Impaired renal function can increase plasma levels of penicillin. Probenecid competes with penicillin for active tubular transport and delays renal excretion of penicillin.

The spectrum of action of penicillin V is similar to that of penicillin G. Penicillin V is stable in stomach acid; when given orally, it produces higher blood levels than an equivalent amount of penicillin G. Because of the higher blood levels, penicillin V is used to treat many dental infections.

Oxacillin and cloxacillin are penicillinase resistance and are acid stable. The penicillinase-resistant penicillins produce more adverse effects such as GI distress, renal failure, and bone marrow depression. They are usually reserved for treatment of infections caused by penicillinase-producing staphylococci.

Ampicillin, amoxicillin, and bacampicillin are broad-spectrum penicillins. All the broad-spectrum penicillins are inactivated by penicillinase. Ampicillin and amoxicillin can produce various allergic reactions. Ampicillin is more likely to produce rashes compared with other penicillins.

Ticarcillin and carbenicillin indanyl sodium are extended-spectrum penicillins or antipseudomonal penicillins. The extended penicillins are used primarily for infections with *Psuedomonas aeruginosa.*

Penicillins are sometimes combined with a β-lactamase inhibitor such as clavulanic acid to increase their activity against β-lactamase-producing bacteria. Amoxicillin plus clavulanic acid is sold as **Augmentin.**

Cephalosporins and Other Inhibitors of Cell Wall Synthesis

The **cephalosporins** are β-lactam antibiotics that inhibit cell wall synthesis. They bind to cell membrane enzymes involved in cell wall synthesis, causing lysis and death. Like the penicillins, the cephalosporins are bactericidal and active against a broad-spectrum of microbes.

There are four generations of cephalosporins based on general features of antimicrobial activity. Progressing from first-generation cephalosporins to fourth-generation cephalosporins: (1) there is increased activity against gram-negative microbes and anaerobes, (2) more resistance to destruction by β-lactamases, and (3) increased distribution to CSF.

The cephalosporins can be administered orally, intravenously, or intramuscularly. After absorption, the cephalosporins are distributed to most tissue and body fluids. Third- and fourth-generation cephalosporins penetrate the meninges and CSF levels are sufficient for bactericidal effects. Almost all the cephalosporins are eliminated by the kidney by glomerular filtration and tubular secretion.

The cephalosporins are well tolerated, and serious adverse effects are rare. Hypersensitivity reactions are the most frequent adverse effects. These reactions include fever, rashes, and anaphylaxis. Penicillins and cephalosporins have structural similarities, and patients who are allergic to this type of drug may be cross-allergic with the other. The incidence of cross allergenicity is low with approximately 5% to 10% of penicillin-allergic patients being allergic to cephalosporins. Adverse GI effects are common and include diarrhea, nausea, vomiting, and abdominal pain. Other adverse effects include nephrotoxicity, superinfection, and bleeding.

First-generation cephalosporins, represented by **cephalothin** (Keflin) and **cephalexin** (Keflex), are indicated for infections caused by gram-positive microbes. The first-generation agents are employed for prophylaxis for patients with "at risk" joints undergoing dental procedures.

Second-generation cephalosporins have increased activity against gram-negative microorganisms but are much less active than the third-generation agents. **Cefaclor** (Ceclor) and **cefamandole** (Mandol) are second-generation cephalosporins.

Third-generation cephalosporins have high activity against gram-negative organisms and can penetrate the CSF. They are the drugs of choice for meningitis caused by enteric, gram-negative bacilli. **Cefotaxime** (Claforan) has been utilized for meningitis caused by *H. influenzae*.

Cefepime (Maxipime) is effective against both gram-positive and gram-negative pathogens. It is used in the treatment of uncomplicated and complicated UTIs.

Imipenem (Primaxin) has the broadest antimicrobial spectrum of any agent available. It is marketed in combination with cilastatin, a compound that inhibits degradation of imipenem by the kidneys. Imipenem inhibits cell wall synthesis. Because of its broad spectrum and low toxicity, it is effective in a wide variety of infections including mixed infections caused by nosocomial organisms.

Vancomycin (Lyphocin) has a narrow spectrum of activity against many gram-positive cocci. It acts by inhibiting cell wall synthesis and is bactericidal. It is a potentially toxic drug and is reserved for treatment of: (1) antibiotic associated pseudomembranous colitis, and (2) treatment of serious infections in patients allergic to penicillins.

Bacteriostatic Inhibitors of Protein Synthesis

The **tetracyclines** are **broad-spectrum** antibiotics active against a wide variety of gram-positive and gram-negative bacteria. The tetracyclines interfere with bacterial growth by inhibiting protein synthesis by binding to the 30S ribosomal subunit. Tetracyclines inhibit bacterial growth and replication and are bacteriostatic. The six tetracyclines available for systemic used in the United States are **tetracycline, oxytetracycline, demeclocycline, methacycline, doxycycline,** and **minocycline.**

All six tetracyclines are similar in structure, antimicrobial spectrum, and adverse effects.

All of the tetracyclines are absorbed following oral administration. They are distributed to most body fluids and tissues. The tetracyclines accumulate in bone and the enamel and dentin of unerupted teeth.

The tetracyclines form insoluble compounds with calcium, magnesium, iron, zinc, and aluminum. These insoluble compounds are not absorbed. Tetracyclines should not be administered with milk products, calcium supplements, iron supplements, laxatives containing magnesium, or antacids containing aluminum or magnesium.

The most common adverse effect of tetracycline therapy is GI distress. The adverse effects include nausea, vomiting, diarrhea, glossitis, stomatitis, and xerostomia.

Tetracyclines bind to calcium in the dentin and enamel of developing teeth. They can produce permanent yellow or brown discoloration and enamel hypoplasia. Tetracyclines should not be used during the last half of pregnancy or in children younger than 8 or 9 years of age.

Minocycline can cause black pigmentation of the hard palate and of maxillary and mandibular alveolar bone. This pigmentation appears bluish through the mucosa.

Tetracyclines increase the sensitivity of the skin to ultraviolet light, and patients taking tetracyclines sometimes react with an exaggerated sunburn. The tetracyclines may lead to the development of suprainfections. Overgrowth of *Candida albicans* in the mouth, vagina, bowel, and pharynx has been observed during tetracycline therapy. Pseudomembranous colitis, a suprainfection of the bowel that can be life threatening, can be caused by tetracyclines.

Other adverse effects include hepatotoxicity, renal toxicity, and vestibular toxicity. The renal toxic effects of tetracyclines are additive with that of other drugs.

The macrolides act by inhibiting bacterial protein synthesis by binding to the 50S ribosomal subunit and blocking the addition of new amino acids to the growing peptide chain. The macrolides are broad-spectrum antibiotics and include **erythromycin, azithromycin, clarithromycin,** and **dirithromycin.**

Erythromycin has a spectrum of action similar to that of penicillin V. It is active against most gram-positive bacteria as well as some gram-negative microbes. Erythromycin is the drug of choice for several infections, including *Bordetella pertussis, Legionella pneumophila,* and *Mycoplasma pneumoniae.* Patients who are allergic to penicillin G can be treated with erythromycin. This drug is ineffective against the anaerobes that are typically found in dental infections.

Erythromycin is distributed to most tissues and body fluids and is excreted in the bile. It is then partially reabsorbed via the enterohepatic circulation, before final excretion in the feces and urine.

GI disturbances are the most common adverse effects of erythromycin. Cholestatic hepatitis is the most serious adverse effect and is caused by erythromycin estolate.

In addition to activity against the same microorganisms as erythromycin, azithromycin and clarithromycin have some activity against anaerobes. They can be used as alternative antibiotics in the treatment of orofacial infections caused by susceptible aerobic and anaerobes. Most adverse effects are GI, including abdominal pain, nausea, and diarrhea.

Clindamycin (Cleocin) is a bacteriostatic antibiotic that inhibits bacterial protein synthesis. Clindamycin is active against most gram-positive aerobes and most gram-positive and gram-negative anaerobes. Clindamycin is the preferred drug for pelvic infections caused by *Bacteroides fragilis*. This drug can be used as a substitute for penicillin in prophylaxis for bacterial endocarditis.

The most common adverse effects associated with clindamycin are diarrhea and hypersensitivity reactions, especially rashes. Clindamycin causes a high incidence of antibiotic-associated pseudomembranous colitis.

Aminoglycosides: Bacterial Inhibitors of Protein Synthesis

The aminoglycosides are narrow-spectrum antibiotics that are used primarily to treat serious infections caused by aerobic gram-negative bacilli. Microorganisms sensitive to the aminoglycosides include *Proteus mirabilis, Pseudomonas aeruginosa, Escherichia coli, and Klebsiella pneumoniae*. They bind to the 30S ribosomal subunit; inhibit protein synthesis; and cause the formation of abnormal proteins. They are bactericidal. The aminoglycosides are similar in their pharmacokinetics, adverse effects, and uses. **Gentamicin** (Garamycin), **tobramycin** (Nebcin), **amikacin** (Amikin), **neomycin** (Netromycin), **kanamycin** (Kantrex), **streptomycin**, and **paromomycin** (Humatin) are aminoglycosides.

The aminoglycosides are polycations; they do not cross over cell membranes. They are not absorbed from the GI tract and must be administered intravenously or intramuscularly for systemic effects. Aminoglycosides do not enter into the CSF, and they are eliminated primarily by the kidneys.

The aminoglycosides can produce serious adverse effects that limit their clinical use. All aminoglycosides are toxic to the eighth cranial nerve and can lead to impaired hearing and balance. Damage to the cells of the inner ear may be irreversible, and hearing impairment and deafness may be permanent. They cause kidney damage by damaging cells of the proximal renal tubules, but injury to the kidney is usually reversible.

Sulfonamides and Trimethoprim

The **sulfonamides** and **trimethoprim** have a wide range of antimicrobial activity against both gram-positive and gram-negative bacteria. Both agents prevent bacteria from utilizing para-aminobenzoic acid (PABA) for the synthesis of folic acid, a compound required by all cells for the formation of DNA and RNA.

The sulfonamides are bacteriostatic. Even though resistant strains have become common in recent years, sulfonamides are indicated for the treatment of many UTIs. These agents are often used to treat acute otitis media, which is caused by *H. influenzae* in children and chronic bronchitis caused by *S pneumoniae* in adults.

The most common adverse reactions of the sulfonamides are hypersensitivity reactions. Rash, photosensitivity, and drug fever are mild reactions. Stevens-Johnson syndrome is a severe hypersensitivity reaction that has a mortality rate of 25% (See Ch. 8). Other adverse effects include acute hemolytic anemia, kernicterus, and renal damage from crystalluria.

Sulfisoxazole (Gantrisin) is rapidly absorbed and rapidly excreted. This drug is very water-soluble and reduces the risk of crystalluria. It is the preferred sulfonamide for treatment of UTIs.

The clinical uses of **sulfamethoxazole** (Gantanol) are the same as those for sulfisoxazole. This drug is indicated for both systemic infections and UTIs.

Trimethoprim (Proloprim) is effective against most gram-positive and gram-negative microorganisms. Trimethoprim may be bacteriostatic or bactericidal. Trimethoprim inhibits bacterial dihydrofolate reductase, the enzyme that converts dihydrofolic acid into folic acid. Trimethoprim is only approved for treatment of uncomplicated UTIs.

The most frequently reported adverse effects of trimethoprim are rash and itching. Serious, but rare, adverse effects (neutropenia, megaloblastic anemia, and thrombocytopenia) have occurred in patients with pre-existing folic acid deficiency.

A fixed-dose combination of trimethoprim (TMP) and sulfamethoxazole (SMZ) (Bactrim) are marketed together. These two drugs act on sequential steps in bacterial folic acid synthesis and the result of their combination is synergistic. TMP-SMZ is effective against both gram-negative and gram-positive bacteria.

TMP-SMZ is effective in the treatment of chronic and recurrent UTIs as well as uncomplicated UTIs. TMP-SMZ is effective for acute exacerbations of chronic bronchitis and is the treatment of choice for pneumonia and other infections caused by *Pneumocystis carinii* in immunocompromised patients.

The adverse effects of TMP-SMZ are similar to those caused by sulfonamides. The most common adverse effects are nausea, vomiting, and rash.

Miscellaneous Antibacterial Drugs

Metronidazole (Flagyl) is used in the treatment of infections caused by obligate anaerobic bacteria and protozoal infections. Metronidazole is the drug of choice for infection with *Trichomonas vaginalis*. Because it is effective against *Bacteroides* species, it is useful in the treatment of many periodontal infections. The combination of amoxicillin with metronidazole is useful in the treatment of juvenile or refractory periodontitis.

Metronidazole is converted to a more chemically reactive form by microbes. This reactive form causes microbial DNA to break and the helical structure is lost, thus impairing the function of DNA.

The most common adverse effects of metronidazole are GI tract effects. Nausea, vomiting, dry mouth, and an unpleasant sharp metallic taste have been reported.

Dizziness, vertigo, convulsions, and ataxia have been reported and warrant discontinuation of metronidazole. Metronidazole can produce a disulfiram-like effect in some patients. These patients experience abdominal distress, vomiting, flushing, and headache if they drink alcoholic beverages during therapy with metronidazole.

Antituberculosis Agents

Tuberculosis (TB) is a chronic disease caused by *Mycobacterium tuberculosis,* which is also known as *tubercle bacillus.* Treatment of tuberculosis is always done with two or more drugs to reduce emergence of resistant strains. Treatment of tuberculosis is long term and lasts from 6 months to 2 years or longer. Treatment is difficult, because the incidence of resistance to one or more drugs is increasing and many patients with TB often have inadequate defense mechanisms [e.g., acquired immunodeficiency syndrome (AIDS)].

Drugs used in the treatment of tuberculosis are divided into two main categories: first-line drugs and second-line drugs. First-line agents have the greatest efficacy with the least toxicity. First-line drugs include **isoniazid** (Laniazid), **rifampin** (Rifadin), **pyrazinamide,** and **ethambutol** (Myambutol). Of these, isoniazid and rifampin are the most important. Most patients with tuberculosis can be successfully treated with these drugs. For the first 2 months, treatment is usually with isoniazid, rifampin, and pyrazinamide followed by isoniazid and rifampin. Isoniazid and rifampin are continued daily for 9 to 12 months.

Isoniazid is the primary drug for treatment of tuberculosis, and all patients with isoniazid-sensitive strains of TB should receive the drug if they can tolerate it. Isoniazid is also the only antituberculosis drug effective for preventive therapy. Isoniazid is very selective for mycobacteria. It is bacteriostatic for "resting" bacilli and bactericidal for rapidly dividing microorganisms.

The mechanism of action of isoniazid is unknown. It has been suggested that isoniazid inhibits the biosynthesis of mycolic acids, important components of the mycobacterial cell wall.

Tubercle bacilli can develop resistance to isoniazid during treatment. Multiple drug therapy decreases the emergence of resistant strains.

Isoniazid can be administered orally or by intramuscular injection. The drug is absorbed by either route and is distributed to all body fluids and cells. Isoniazid is inactivated by the liver, and the metabolites are excreted in the urine.

The most common adverse effects involve the nervous system. Numbness, tingling, burning, and pain of the hands and feet are most common. Muscle twitching, restlessness, sedation, incoordination, and convulsions have been re-

ported. These neurotoxic symptoms can be reversed by administering pyridoxine.

Approximately 1% of patients taking isoniazid exhibit clinical hepatitis, and 10% develop abnormal laboratory values. Severe hepatic damage, leading to death, has occurred in patients receiving isoniazid. Age is the most important factor in determining the risk of hepatic toxicity. The incidence of isoniazid-induced hepatic toxicity increases with increasing age.

Rifampin (Rifadin) is bactericidal to *Mycobacterium tuberculosis* and inhibits the growth of most gram-positive bacteria as well as many gram-negative organisms. Rifampin inhibits RNA polymerase, preventing the synthesis of RNA and consequently protein synthesis.

Mycobacteria may develop resistance to rifampin rapidly when used alone in the treatment of tuberculosis. The drug is always employed in combination with at least one other agent to treat tuberculosis.

Rifampin is absorbed from the GI tract and distributed to all body fluids and tissues. Rifampin is eliminated by hepatic metabolism.

Common adverse reactions include anorexia, stomach distress, nausea, vomiting, and diarrhea. Rifampin is toxic to the liver and may cause jaundice and hepatitis. The incidence of hepatitis is less than 1%. Rifampin gives a red-orange color to sweat, saliva, tears, and urine.

Pyrazinamide is bactericidal to *Mycobacterium tuberculosis.* The mechanism of action of the drug is unknown. The combination of rifampin, isoniazid, and pyrazinamide is considered to be the regimen of choice for initial therapy of tuberculosis caused by nonresistant bacteria. After 2 months, treatment with pyrazinamide is discontinued whereas rifampin and isoniazid are continued for another 4 months.

Pyrazinamide is well absorbed from the GI tract and widely distributed throughout the body. The drug is excreted by the kidneys.

Liver injury is the most common and serious adverse effect of pyrazinamide. Symptoms of hepatic disease occur in approximately 15% of patients; jaundice occurs in 2% to 3%. Death due to hepatic necrosis has occurred in rare cases.

Second-line drugs are used only for treatment of tuberculosis caused by resistant microorganisms or by nontuberculous mycobacteraia. These drugs are generally less effective and more toxic than the first-line drugs. They must all be given parenterally. Second-line drugs include **para-aminosalicylic acid** (PAS)**, kanamycin, amikacin, capreomycin, ethionamide, cycloserine, ciprofloxacin,** and **ofloxacin.** These agents are potentially ototoxic and nephrotoxic, and no two drugs from this group should be used simultaneously. A second-line drug is used in combination with other antituberculous drugs.

Antifungal Agents

Antifungal agents can be divided into two major groups: (1) drugs for superficial mycoses, and (2) drugs for systemic mycoses. Some agents may be used systemically or topically. The dental health care provider is usually treating mucosal lesions of the oral cavity.

The superficial fungal infections are caused by two groups of organisms: (1) *Candida* species, and (2) dermatophytes or tinea. *Candida* infections usually occur on moist skin and mucous membranes. Dental health care providers primarily manage oral infections caused by *C. albicans*. Infections with tinea affect the skin and cause athlete's foot or ringworm.

Oral infections caused by *C. albicans* are managed with **nystatin, clotrimazole**, **ketoconazole**, or **fluconazole**. Infections with tinea are managed with a variety of over-the-counter preparations and prescription products.

Nystatin (Mycostatin, Nilstat) is a polyene macrolide antibiotic that is useful only to treat candidiasis. Nystatin is fungicidal and fungistatic agent. Nystatin binds to components of the fungal cell membrane, thus increasing permeability and reducing viability. Nystatin can be administered topically and orally. The drug is not absorbed from the GI tract, skin, or mucous membranes.

Nystatin produces few adverse effects. Topical application may produce local irritation. Higher doses of nystatin taken orally have caused nausea, vomiting, and diarrhea.

Clotrimazole (Mycelex) is a synthetic antifungal agent available for oral and vaginal use. Clotrimazole is primarily effective against the *Candida* species. Clotrimazole alters cell membrane permeability. The cell membrane loses its function, and cellular components are lost.

Clotrimazole is available for oral use as a slowly dissolving lozenge for the treatment of oropharyngeal candidiasis. The amount of clotrimazole absorbed by this route is unknown.

When clotrimazole is applied to the skin, it may cause stinging, erythema, edema, and desquamation. When applied to the vagina, lower abdominal cramps and slight increase in urinary frequency have been reported.

Ketoconazole (Nizoral) is an imidazole approved for both oral and topical therapy of superficial mycoses as well as systemic mycoses. The drug inhibits the synthesis of ergosterol, a component of the fungal cytoplasmic membrane. Membrane permeability is increased, and cellular components leak out.

Ketoconazole requires an acidic enviornment for the absorption. Drugs that reduce gastric acidity (e.g., proton pump inhibitors, antacids, H_2 antihistamines) decrease absorption. Ketoconazole is eliminated by hepatic metabolism. Ketoconazole is used in the treatment and management of mucocutaneous and oropharyngeal candidiasis. Ketoconazole has many adverse reactions and should only be used after other topical antifungal agents have been ineffective.

Hepatotoxicity is the most serious adverse reaction associated with ketoconazole. Fatal hepatic necrosis has occurred rarely. In males, ketoconazole has caused gyneco-mastia, decreased libido, and reduced potency. In females, menstrual irregularities have occurred. Other adverse effects include nausea, vomiting, itching, fever, and chills.

Fluconazole (Diflucan) is used to treat oropharyngeal and esophageal *Candida* infections. The drug is used prophylactically against candidiasis in immunocompromised patients. Fluconazole has become the drug of choice for treatment of meningitis caused by *Coccidioides immitis* and is used to prevent relapse of cryptococcal meningitis in patients with AIDS.

Fluconazole inhibits ergosterol synthesis in fungal cell membranes resulting in damage to the cell membrane. The drug is primarily fungistatic. Fluconazole is almost completely absorbed from the GI tract and distributed to all body tissues and fluids. The drug is eliminated unchanged in the urine.

Fluconazole is less toxic than ketoconazole. The most common adverse effects are nausea, headache, vomiting, skin rash, abdominal pain, and diarrhea. Rare cases of death due to hepatic failure have been reported.

 ANTIVIRAL AGENTS: DRUGS FOR NON-HIV VIRAL INFECTIONS

The antiviral agents can be divided into two groups: drugs for non-human immunodeficiency virus (HIV) type I infections and drugs for HIV infection and related opportunistic infections. Agents for treating non-HIV viral infections are active against a narrow spectrum of viruses and are useful for treating a limited number of infections.

Acyclovir (Zovirax) is the drug of choice for infections caused by herpes simplex viruses (HSV) and varicella-zoster virus. Acyclovir is selectively activated by herpes enzymes to an acyclovir triphosphate. Acyclovir triphosphate inhibits viral DNA replication, thus suppressing viral reproduction. Acyclovir does not affect human DNA, thus host cells are minimally affected.

Acyclovir can be administered orally, topically, and intravenously. Acyclovir is not absorbed when applied topically. Acyclovir is distributed to all body fluids following absorption. The drug is not metabolized and is eliminated by the kidneys.

Acyclovir is used to treat *herpes simplex genitalis*. Initial infections of genital herpes are treated with topical acyclovir. Oral acyclovir is superior for treating recurrent infections. Oral acyclovir can be used to treat primary *herpes simplex* infections of the gingiva and mouth. Taken prophylactically, oral acyclovir can prevent recurrent herpes labialis. In older adults, acyclovir is effective in the treatment of herpes zoster.

Acyclovir has few serious adverse reactions. The type of adverse reaction experienced depends on the route of administration. When applied topically, acyclovir causes transient burning or stinging. The most common adverse effects to oral acyclovir are headache, vertigo, nausea, vomiting, and diarrhea. Phlebitis and inflammation at the site of injection are the most common adverse reactions following intravenous therapy. Intravenous acyclovir can cause renal damage.

Ganciclovir (Cytovene, Vitasert) is a synthetic antiviral effective against herpesviruses including cytomegalovirus (CMV). Ganciclovir inhibits viral DNA synthesis and is currently approved for: (1) treatment and chronic suppression of cytomegalovirus (CMV) retinitis in immunocompromised patients, and (2) prevention of CMV disease in transplant patients.

The major serious adverse effects of ganciclovir are neutropenia and thrombocytopenia. CNS side effects ranging from headache to convulsions and coma occur in 5% to 20% of patients. Because of these serious side effects, use of ganciclovir should be restricted to prevention and treatment of CMV infection in the immunocompromised host.

Amantadine (Symmetrel, Symadine) is a synthetic antiviral agent. Amantadine prevents influenza A virus from entering host cells and inhibits uncoating of viruses following penetration into host cells.

Amantadine is used in the prevention of influenza A virus infection during epidemics, especially in high-risk patients. Amantadine can be used for treatment of active influenza A infection. It is most effective when therapy is instituted within 48 hours after the onset of influenza symptoms.

Amantadine is absorbed from the GI tract and distributed widely to body tissues and fluids. The drug is excreted unmetabolized via the kidneys. Amantadine produces little toxicity. The most frequent serious reactions include depression, psychosis, orthostatic hypotension and congestive heart failure.

Drugs for HIV Infection

HIV is a retrovirus that has RNA as its genetic material. The disease produced by infection with HIV is AIDS.

There are three classes of antiretroviral drugs: (1) nucleoside reverse transcriptase inhibitors (NRTIs), (2) non-nucleoside reverse transcriptase inhibitors (NNRTIs), and (3) protease inhibitors. Management of HIV infection is with multidrug therapy. Patients usually take three drugs for HIV itself-usually a protease inhibitor and two NRTIs. These drugs do not cure HIV but reduce levels of HIV.

Zidovudine (Retrovir) was the first NRTI used in the treatment of HIV infection. The drug is an analog of the naturally occurring nucleoside, thymidine. Abbreviations for this drug are AZT for azidothymidine, its original name and ZDV for zidovudine.

Zidovudine inhibits HIV replication in infected individuals. It becomes incorporated into the viral DNA strand and prevents synthesis of DNA.

Zidovudine is absorbed following oral administration and distributed to all body tissues including the CNS. Zidovudine is inactivated by the liver, and the metabolites are excreted by the kidneys.

Zidovudine's principal toxic effects are related to bone marrow depression, which can lead to severe anemia, granulocytopenia, and thrombocytopenia. GI adverse effects that have been reported are nausea, vomiting, diarrhea, and abdominal pain.

Other NRTIs are **didanosine** (Videx), **lamivudine** (Epivir), **stavudine** (Zerit), and **zalcitabine** (Hivid).

The non-nucleoside reverse transcriptase inhibitors (NNRTIs) bind to the active center of reverse transcriptase and directly inhibit HIV-1 replication. These drugs are usually active against AZT-resistant HIV-1 variants but lack activity against HIV-2.

Nevirapine (Viramune) is an NNRTI that inhibits reverse transcriptase HIV-1 and is approved for treating infection with HIV-1. Nevirapine should never be used alone, because the likelihood of resistance increases. The drug does not affect human DNA polymerase and is harmless to humans.

Nevirapine is absorbed following oral administration and is distributed to all body fluids and tissues. The drug is metabolized by the liver, and metabolites are excreted in the urine.

A rash is the most common adverse effect and can benign or severe and life threatening. A mild rash can be managed with antihistamines or glucocorticoids. If a severe rash develops, nevirapine should be withdrawn.

The most effective antiretroviral drugs available are the protease inhibitors. These drugs bind to the active site of HIV protease and prevent the release of structural proteins and enzymes. The virus remains immature and noninfectious.

TABLE 9–5 Abbreviations Relevant to Pharmacology

- bid = twice a day
- tid = three times a day
- qid = four times a day
- ac = before meals
- ad lib = as desired
- hs = at bedtime
- po = by mouth
- prn = as needed
- qh = every hour
- q6h = every 6 hours
- rx = therapy, treatment, prescription
- ss = one half
- stat = immediately
- qd = every day

Saquinavir (Invirase) was the first protease inhibitor to be approved for treatment of HIV infection. The drug is usually combined with at least one NRTI to reduce the emergence of resistance.

Saquinavir is administered orally but is poorly absorbed and has an extensive first pass metabolism. This drug is metabolized by the hepatic microsomal enzyme system, and metabolites are excreted in the feces.

Adverse effects include headache, nausea, diarrhea, and abdominal pain. Oral adverse reactions include buccal mucosal ulceration, dry mouth, taste alteration, and stomatitis.

DRUG/PRESCRIPTION ABBREVIATIONS

Abbreviations commonly used in prescription writing are outlined in **Table 9-5**.

Suggested Sources

Gage TW, Pickett FA : Dental Drug Reference, 5th ed. St. Louis, CV Mosby, 2001.

Hardman JG, et al: Goodman and Gilman's The Pharmacological Basis of Therapeutics, 9th ed. New York, McGraw-Hill, 1996.

Haveles EB: Pharmacology for Dental Hygiene Practice. Albany, Delmar, 1997.

Katzung BG: Basic and Clinical Pharmacology, 7th ed. Stamford, Appleton & Lange, 1998.

Lehne RA: Pharmacology for Nursing Care, 4th ed. Philadelphia, WB Saunders, 2001.

Requa-Clark B: Applied Pharmacology for the Dental Hygienist, 4th ed. St. Louis, CV Mosby, 2000.

Vander A, Sherman J, Luciano D: Human Physiology the Mechanisms of Body Function, 7th ed. New York, McGraw-Hill, 1998.

Websites

www.rxlist.com
www.druginfonet.com
www.rxmed.com

Questions and Answers

Questions

1. All of the following medications cause gingival hyperplasia EXCEPT one. Which one is the EXCEPTION?
   A. Nifedipine
   B. Diltiazem
   C. Verapamil
   D. Phenytoin
   E. Captopril

2. Which of the following characteristics will increase the absorption of a drug from the lumen of the small intestines?
   A. Weak acid and high lipid solubility
   B. Weak base and high lipid solubility
   C. Weak acid and low lipid solubility
   D. Weak base and low lipid solubility

3. What is the neurotransmitter released from the postganglionic neurons of the parasympathetic nervous system?
   A. Acetylcholine
   B. Norepinephrine
   C. Epinephrine
   D. Serotonin
   E. Dopamine

4. Which of the following medications will reduce secretions of saliva and bronchial mucus and can be used to produce a dry field before some dental procedures?
   A. Isoproterenol
   B. Terbutaline
   C. Norepinephrine
   D. Bethanechol
   E. Atropine

5. The dental hygienist should be aware that guanethidine (Ismelin) is especially likely to produce which of the following adverse effects?
   A. Dehydration
   B. Bronchospasm
   C. Tachycardia
   D. Orthostatic hypotension
   E. Sedation and depression

6. Your patient is currently being treated with haloperidol. Which of the following conditions is the primary indication for this medication?
   A. Schizophrenia
   B. Angina pectoris
   C. Hypertension
   D. Depression
   E. Anxiety

7. Which of the following drugs can be used to reverse respiratory depression produced by opioids?
   A. Epinephrine
   B. Naloxone
   C. Probenecid
   D. Trimethoprim
   E. Loratidine

8. Which of the following statements explains why the effectiveness of a local anesthetic may be reduced in the presence of infection?
   A. The low pH of the area may inhibit the liberation of the salt.

B. The low pH of the area may inhibit the liberation of the free base.

C. The high pH of the area may inhibit the liberation of the salt.

D. The high pH of the area may inhibit the liberation of the free base.

9. The ester local anesthetics are primarily inactivated in the plasma. The amide local anesthetics are metabolized primarily by the liver.
   A. Both statements are true.
   B. Both statements are false.
   C. The first statement is true; the second one is false.
   D. The first statement is false; the second one is true.

10. Which of the following is the most serious electrolyte imbalance associated with thiazide diuretic therapy?
   A. Sodium depletion
   B. Sodium retention
   C. Potassium depletion
   D. Potassium retention
   E. Calcium depletion

11. A person allergic to the penicillins might also be allergic to which of the following antibiotics?
   A. Tetracyclines
   B. Cephalosporins
   C. Aminoglycosides
   D. Sulfonamides
   F. Erythromycin

12. The patient's history indicates that he is taking isoniazid, rifampin, and ethambutol. The hygienist would know that this person is being treated for _____.
   A. severe acne vulgaris
   B. herpes simplex viruses
   C. legionnaires' disease
   D. juvenile periodontitis
   E. tuberculosis

13. Which of the following is the drug of choice for treating acute anginal attacks?
   A. Epinephrine
   B. Norepinephrine
   C. Quinidine
   D. Nitroglycerine
   F. Digoxin

14. All of the following medications are effective antirheumatic and anti-inflammatory agents EXCEPT one. Which one is the EXCEPTION?
   A. Aspirin
   B. Ibuprofen
   C. Acetaminophen
   D. Celecoxib

15. Which of the following drugs would be useful in treating allergic rhinitis?
   A. Loratidine
   B. Cimetidine
   C. Ibuprofen
   D. Omeprazole
   E. Imipenem

16. _____ is the drug of choice for treatment of anaphylactic shock?
   A. Diphenhydramine
   B. Epinephrine
   C. Norepinephrine
   D. Terbutaline
   F. Prazosin

17. Which of the following antibiotics can be used for prophylaxis for infective endocarditis in a patient with a history of penicillin allergy?
   A. Amoxicillin
   B. Acyclovir
   C. Cefaclor
   D. Rifampin
   E. Clindamycin

18. The most important drug interaction of aspirin is that which occurs with_____.
   A. oral anticoagulants
   B. oral hypoglycemic agents
   C. antineoplastic agents
   D. thyroid drugs
   E. penicillin

19. The most common adverse effect of the H_1 antihistamines is

   _____.
   A. gastric bleeding
   B. blurred vision
   C. sedation
   D. apnea
   E. nausea

20. Patients should not rely on oral contraceptives when taken concurrently with barbiturates such as phenobarbital because_____.
   A. the combination affects coagulation and may lead to blood clots.
   B. Interaction of oral contraceptives with barbiturates can cause paradoxic excitation
   C. Barbiturates increase the blood flow to the ovaries and counteracts the contraceptive effects.
   D. Barbiturates induce the liver metabolizing enzymes and increase the metabolism of oral contraceptives

ANSWERS

1. **E.** Gingival hyperplasia has not been associated with captopril. Gingival hyperplasia is an adverse effect of nifedipine, diltiazem, verapamil, and phenytoin.

2. **B.** Nonionized and high lipid-soluble drugs are more readily absorbed across cell membranes. The pH of the small intestine is basic. A basic drug will be nonionized in the basic pH of the small intestine. Acids and low lipid soluble drugs are less likely to be absorbed across cell membranes. Acids are in the ionized form in the small intestine. A base would be in the nonionized form, but low lipid solubility would inhibit absorption.

3. **A.** Acetylcholine is the neurotransmitter at the postganglionic parasympathetic nerve endings. Norepinephrine is the

neurotransmitter at the postganglionic sympathetic nerve endings. Epinephrine is released from the adrenal medulla. Serotonin and dopamine are neurotransmitters in the CNS.

4. **E.** Acetylcholine increases secretion of saliva, and atropine is an antagonist of acetylcholine producing opposite effects such as a dry mouth. Isoproterenol, terbutaline, and norepinephrine are drugs that affect the sympathetic nervous system and do not decrease the outflow of saliva. Bethanechol mimics the action of acetylcholine and would increase the outflow of saliva.

5. **D.** Guanethidine induced orthostatic hypotension can be very severe. Blood pressure may fall so low that the brain and heart receive inadequate oxygen. Dehydration, bronchial spasm, tachycardia, sedation, and depression are not adverse effects of guanethidine.

6. **A.** Schizophrenia is the primary indication for antipsychotic agents such as haloperidol. Angina pectoris, hypertension, depression, and anxiety cannot be treated with haloperidol.

7. **B.** Naloxone is a pure opioid antagonist and can reverse respiratory depression, coma, and analgesia produced by opioids. Epinephrine is the drug of choice for treatment of anaphylactic shock. Probenecid competes with penicillin for active tubular transport and delays renal excretion of penicillin. The combination of trimethoprim and sulfamethoxazole is synergistic, and the combination is used to treat UTIs. Loratidine is a nonsedating antihistamine that is used to alleviate symptoms of type I hypersensitivity reactions.

8. **B.** The local anesthetics must be in the free base form (nonionized form) to have nerve-blocking effect. Local anesthetic solutions have a pH of 5 to 6, and most of the drug is in the ionized form. The pH of normal tissue is 7.4, and once injected the amount of the anesthetic in the free base form increases. Infection produces acidic products, yielding a low pH; the amount of the drug in the effective form (nonionized) is reduced.

9. **A.** Both statements are true. The ester local anesthetics are primarily hydrolyzed and inactivated by plasma pseudocholinesterases. The amide local anesthetics are metabolized in the liver by microsomal enzymes.

10. **C.** The thiazide diuretics increase the renal excretion of sodium, chloride, and potassium. Loss of potassium can increase the risk of dysrhythmias. If serum potassium falls below 3.5 mEq/L, fatal dysrhythmias may result. Thiazide diuretics cause loss of sodium, but impact on sodium is small and usually insignificant. Thiazide diuretics do not cause retention of sodium or potassium. Thiazide diuretics reduce urinary excretion of calcium.

11. **B.** Penicillins and cephalosporins have structural similarities, and patients who are allergic to one type of drug may be cross-allergic with the other type. Tetracyclines, aminoglycosides, sulfonamides, and erythromycin are not structurally related to the penicillins, and cross-allergic reactions have not been reported.

12. **E.** Treatment of tuberculosis is always with two or more drugs, and isoniazid, rifampin, and ethambutol have the greatest efficacy and least toxicity. Severe acne vulgaris is usually treated with a tetracycline. Acyclovir is the drug of choice to treat infections caused by herpes simplex viruses. Erythromycin is the drug of choice to treat legionnaires' disease. Metronidazole in combination with amoxicillin is useful in the treatment of juvenile or refractory periodontitis.

13. **D.** Nitroglycerine is effective, fast-acting, and inexpensive and remains the drug of choice for relieving acute anginal attacks. Epinephrine and norepinephrine would make an angina attack worse. Quinidine is the used to treat arrhythmias. Digoxin is used in the treatment of congestive heart failure.

14. **C.** Acetaminophen is an effective analgesic and antipyretic agent but is devoid of anti-inflammatory and antirheumatic actions. Aspirin, ibuprofen, and celecoxib are effective anti-inflammatory and antirheumatic agents.

15. **A.** Loratidine is a nonsedative antihistamine that is used in the treatment of allergic rhinitis. Cimetidine and omeprazole are used to treat peptic ulcer disease. Ibuprofen is an NSAID. Imipenem is a broad-spectrum antibiotic.

16. **B.** Epinephrine activates all four adrenergic receptor subtypes and causes a rise in blood pressure, bronchial dilation, and constriction of arterioles. Diphenhydramine is an antihistamine and alleviates the symptoms of type I hypersensitivity reactions, but it has no effect on bronchial constriction. This drug can be used as an adjunct in the treatment of anaphylaxis. Norepinephrine has no effect on bronchial constriction but would elevate blood pressure. Terbutaline is specific for β_2-receptors and would have no effect on blood pressure. Prazosin is a competitive blocker of α_1-receptors.

17. **E.** Clindamycin is effective against both gram-positive and gram-negative anaerobes and can be used as a substitute for penicillin in prophylaxis for bacterial endocarditis. A patient who is allergic to one penicillin is usually cross-allergic to other penicillins such as amoxicillin. Acyclovir is an antiviral agent. Some patients who are allergic to penicillin are also allergic to cephalosporins. Rifampin is used to treat tuberculosis.

18. **A.** The combination of warfarin, an oral anticoagulant, and aspirin should be avoided, because bleeding and hemorrhagic disasters have occurred. There are no important reactions between aspirin and oral hypoglycemic agents, antineoplastic agents, thyroid drugs, or penicillin.

19. **C.** The major adverse effect of the H_1 antihistamines is sedation. Gastric bleeding, blurred vision, nausea, and apnea are not common adverse effects of H_1 antihistamines.

20. **D.** The drug metabolizing enzymes of the liver are stimulated by barbiturates, and the effects of oral contraceptives would be reduced if taken concurrently with phenobarbital. The combination of oral contraceptives and barbiturates does not lead to blood clots. Paradoxic excitation is not caused by the interaction of barbiturates and oral contraceptives. Barbiturates do not increase the blood flow to the ovaries.

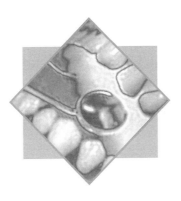

PART III

Provision of Clinical Dental Hygiene Services

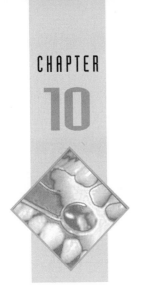

Assessing Patient Characteristics

LOUISE T. VESELICKY, DDS, MDS, MED
CAROL SPEAR, BSDH, MSDH
CHRISTINA B. DeBIASE, BSDH, MA, EDD

 ## ASSESSMENT

Patient assessment is one of the key roles of a dental hygienist. The concept of **assessment** includes gathering, organizing, and analyzing data from several sources. These sources include the medical history, dental history, personal dialogue with the patient, vital signs, radiographs, intraoral and extraoral examination, study casts, periodontal chartings (e.g., assessments of inflammation, probing depths, recession, mobility, furcations), and dental chartings (e.g., assessments of caries, existing restorations, tooth loss, occlusion).

Medical History

The medical history is essential, because it serves as a document for:

- **Planning and implementing a patient's individualized care** (by assisting with determining the etiology and diagnosis of oral conditions and by revealing medical and psychosocial conditions that warrant additions, alterations, or deletions to a care plan to avoid harm or potential emergency situations).
- **Establishing baseline information** about a patient's history for reference when changes are found at subsequent follow-up appointments,
- **Establishing a referral base** in the event that a patient requires the services of a physician, social worker, etc.
- **Providing answers to legal questions** if they arise. Because medical histories are legal documents, all responses and changes should be entered in indelible ink. If an error is made in documentation, a single line should be drawn through the written error; the error should be initialed by the interviewer; and the correct information should follow. Errors in documentation should not be obscured by correction fluid or ink. Patients should sign

the document to verify the information contained in it. Information obtained from the patient during a health history assessment is confidential and can be shared with appropriate health personnel with the patient's permission. Health histories should be updated at each visit.

Various medical history forms are utilized by health care providers. They usually involve a combination of the questionnaire and the interview for clarification of questions that receive an affirmative response from the patient. Ample space should be provided to take notes pertaining to a patient's current medications, allergies, and so forth. A **disease-oriented history that is subdivided into body systems** is a thorough approach to designing a medical history.

When reviewing the patient's medical history, it is important to remember that certain diseases are associated with: (1) oral manifestations (i.e., periodontal disease, xerostomia, gingival hyperplasia), and (2) a risk for potential medical emergencies (e.g., seizures, angina, hypoglycemia) (see Chapters 7, 8, 9, 11, 12, and 13).

For example, it has been shown that patients who have uncontrolled **diabetes** (i.e., persons who have a difficult time controlling their blood glucose levels) are at an increased risk for periodontal disease. In addition, diabetic patients with periodontal disease have a more difficult time controlling their blood glucose levels. The incidence of periodontal disease in the diabetic population increases as the patient goes through puberty and older adulthood. Periodontal disease has also been shown to be more frequent and severe in diabetic patients who have advanced systemic complications. However, the increased incidence of periodontal disease in the diabetic population does not coincide with increased plaque and calculus levels. Conversely, epidemiologic studies have also shown that patients with periodontal disease are at an increased risk of developing diabetes. Patients who are not diabetic and who only have a family history of diabetes may have a polymorphonuclear neutrophil (PMN) chemotactic defect.

Additionally, the patient who is about to have an organ **transplant** should be free of overt periodontal disease before the surgery. Patients who have had a transplant are at an increased risk of developing infection and must be monitored closely to prevent or control periodontal disease.

Recent evidence has also suggested a positive association between the presence of periodontal infection and **cardiovascular disease (CVD)/cerebrovascular accident (CVA; i.e., stroke)**. Patients with periodontal disease have a 1.5- to 2-fold greater risk of incurring fatal CVD than do patients with no periodontal disease. Dental infections appear to increase the risk for developing coronary artery disease similar to other risk factors such as hypertension, diabetes, age, smoking, and elevated serum triglycerides. The exact mechanism for this association is unclear at this time. However, a few proposed mechanisms should be mentioned. Bacterial products, such as the lipopolysaccharide endotoxins from gram-negative bacteria, stimulate the release of inflammatory cells. The inflammatory response that is characteristic of periodontal disease, marked by high levels of inflammatory mediators, appears to exacerbate the process of atherogenesis. Another proposed mechanism is that certain oral bacterial strains of *Streptococcus sanguis* as well as *Porphyromonas gingivalis* induce the aggregation of platelets, which may increase the risk for thromboembolic events.

Increased evidence suggests that pregnant women who have periodontal disease may be seven times more likely to have a **pre-term, low-birthweight baby**. It is thought that prostaglandins and tumor necrosis factor-α, which are present during a normal pregnancy, are raised to an abnormally high level that may induce early labor. Women who are contemplating pregnancy should have a complete oral examination to rule out periodontal disease or treat it, if present. This should be an integral part of prenatal care.

In addition, **smoking** is a major risk factor for periodontal disease. Smoking may not only alter the pathogenesis of the disease but may also cause the disease to become refractory to treatment.

Patients who take certain **medications** may have gingival hyperplasia. Other medications lead to dry mouth, which can increase the incidence of 1) caries by reducing the ability of the oral cavity to buffer acids and 2) gingival disease by decreasing the secretory IgA, which is part of normal saliva. Numerous patients will have conditions such as valvular replacement, mitral valve prolapse with regurgitation, or immunosuppressive conditions or medications that warrant antibiotic premedication before periodontal débridement therapy. In addition, some medications that are normally prescribed in dentistry may be contraindicated (e.g., with liver or renal disease).

Patients with certain **blood** and **autoimmune** diseases are also at an increased risk for developing periodontal disease. Patients with a defective host response may overreact to the bacterial challenge imposed by the presence of plaque. This results in local changes such as excessive gingival inflammation and a potential alteration in the microbial flora; subsequent systemic complications of bacteremia may become life threatening to these individuals. These individuals may also be at risk for abnormal bleeding during dental procedures.

Patients with **impairments (mental or physical)** may have difficulty performing preventive measures against oral bacteria and dietary substrate, resulting in an increased risk for developing oral/dental complications. People with Down syndrome have defective neutrophil chemotaxis, which predisposes them to periodontal disease.

Dental History

Information obtained from the dental history, combined with the medical history, contributes significantly to planning the dental treatment and procedures required for the patient. Depending on the treatment to be rendered, a dental history may be brief or quite extensive. Any **dental history** should provide information on the immediate or chief complaint, previous and present dental hygiene and dental care, and routine personal oral health practices. See **Table 10-1** for items that may be included in a dental history.

Questioning the patient about the items noted earlier in the dental history is essential to the overall assessment of the patient. Missing teeth, root reabsorption, and even some bone and attachment loss may be associated with previous orthodontic treatment.

A tooth with deep pocketing and attachment loss should be evaluated for vitality. An endodontic or periodontal lesion may be present. The treatment of the endodontic lesion should be done first, before any periodontal therapy is attempted.

TABLE 10–1 Suggested Items for the Dental History

1. Reason for the appointment (i.e., chief complaint)
2. Regularity of dental hygiene and dental appointments
3. Previous dental treatment
4. Oral radiation history
5. Family dental history
6. Unusual dental experiences
7. Adverse reactions to anesthetics, latex
8. Injuries to the face or teeth
9. Tooth, gum, or mouth pain or sensitivity
10. Temporomandibular joint pain or treatment
11. Dry mouth
12. Oral habits (e.g., bruxism, cheekbiting, biting objects)
13. Frequency of eating sweets
14. Tobacco use
15. Availability of water fluoridation/fluoride history
16. Oral hygiene practices, including dental products used
17. Any other concerns not covered by the above

*Adapted from Wilkins EM: Clinical Practice of the Dental Hygienist. Philadelphia, Lippincott Williams & Wilkins, 1999, pp 94–95.

Previous periodontal therapy should be determined, such as which specific procedures were done and when and also whether the patient has continued with maintenance treatment. An overcontoured restoration serves as a plaque trap that can accentuate periodontal disease in these areas.

The presence of fluoride in the patient's drinking water, caries history, existing caries and restorations, and diet must be assessed to determine a prevention plan for the patient.

Personal History

The patient's personal history includes **biographical information** such as:

- Name, address, telephone numbers (work and home)
- Birth date, place of birth
- Gender
- Marital status
- If a child, the name of the parent or guardian; if a parent, the age and gender of the children
- Occupation
- Physician
- Referring dentist, if applicable
- Insurance carrier; if applicable

Vital Signs

Vital signs should always be included in the medical history and updated with each visit. The technique for measuring vital signs; the normal values for **respiration, blood pressure, body temperature**, and **pulse**; and management of emergency situations are outlined in Chapter 12.

Extraoral and Intraoral Assessment

Assessment Instruments

Mouth mirrors, explorers, and periodontal probes (described under periodontal assessment) are essential in the process of assessing the patient's oral/dental status and determining the appropriate treatment plan.

Mouth Mirror

The mouth mirror is an examination instrument. It is essential in the process of assessing the soft tissue, hard tissue, and periodontal status of the patient in order to determine the appropriate treatment plan. The **mouth mirror** consists of a handle, shank, and working end. Handles are available in various diameters. Larger diameter handles are more ergonomically sound and contribute to a more controlled and less strained grasp. The mirror or working end is attached to the shank, which is screwed into the cone socket handle. Mirror diameters range in size from 1 to 2 inches and are denoted in numbers such as 4, 5, 7, and 8. The diameters increase as the number increases.

Three types of mouth mirror working ends are available: **front surface, concave**, and **plane surface**. A front surface mirror produces a true image of objects reflected and is most often the preferred mirror for intraoral dental procedures. See **Table 10-2** for a description of each type of mirror.

The mouth mirror may be used for the following: **indirect vision; retraction** of the cheeks, lips, and tongue; **illumination**, or reflecting light onto an area; and **transillumination**, which is the reflecting of light through the teeth. It is held with a **modified pen grasp** and usually in the **nondominant hand**. This entails grasping the handle between the pads of the thumb and index finger and the side of the middle finger.

Explorers

Explorers are used for examining the supra- and subgingival surfaces of the teeth in order to detect calculus, demineralized or carious surfaces, and irregularities of tooth surfaces or restorations. The basic parts of an explorer include a handle; a shank, which may be straight, curved, or angled; and a wire-like working end, which is a circular tip that tapers to a fine point. They may be designed as single-ended, double-ended mirror image paired, or double-ended dissimilar instruments. Several types of explorers are available and vary in terms of the angle and length of the shank and the shape and length of the tip. **More angled shanks** allow for easy access to posterior teeth, whereas straighter shanks allow access primarily to the anterior teeth. **Long shanks** allow for better access to pockets than do short shanks, and curved working ends enhance proximal calculus detection.

Positioning of the **terminal shank**, which is the section of the entire shank that is closest to the tip, is an important factor in correct adaptation of the working end to the tooth. A visual cue for correct adaptation for detection of calculus with an explorer is that the **terminal shank should be positioned parallel to, but not touching, the surface to be explored. In addition, only the side of the point should touch the tooth.** If the entire tip is placed against the tooth surface, the actual point will be against sulcular tissue, which results in pain and laceration, and the clinician will be unable to feel the surface of the tooth (**Figure 10-1**).

TABLE 10-2 Mouth Mirrors

TYPE	CHARACTERISTICS
Front surface	• Reflecting surface on the front surface of the lens • Produces a clear, true image
Plane (flat) surface	• Reflecting surface on the back surface of the lens • Produces a "ghost" image
Concave	• Produces a magnified image that may be distorted

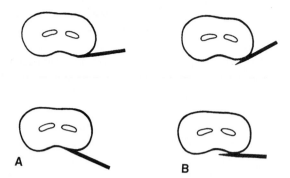

Figure 10–1. Instrument adaptation. Cross-section of a maxillary first permanent premolar to show adaptation of the tip of an explorer. *A,* Appropriate adaptation in which the tip of the explorer is maintained on the tooth surface in a series of strokes to explore around a line angle. *B,* Incorrect adaptation with the tip of the explorer extended away from the surface of the tooth. (From Wilkins EM: Clinical Practice of the Dental Hygienist, 8th ed. Philadelphia, Lippincott Williams & Wilkins, 1999, p 524.)

The **exploring stroke** for detection of calculus involves vertical insertion of the tip subgingivally to the coronal edge of the junctional epithelium. With the side of the point against the tooth at all times, the tip is moved vertically or diagonally along the entire facial or lingual tooth surface. A light secure grasp allows for tactile sensitivity and is essential during the entire process of exploring.

Components and Technique of Assessment

Assessment procedures require a comprehensive evaluation of the patient. This includes a visual assessment of the body that includes:

- Gait for ability to ambulate, use of a cane, walker, or wheelchair
- Dexterity for paralysis or arthritis
- Speech for oral clefts, slurring, stuttering, cough, or hoarseness
- Skin for symmetry, contour, texture, discoloration, swelling, or induration
- Eyes for corrective lenses, pupil size, discoloration, or protrusion
- Face for skin changes, expression, movement, paralysis, injury, or breath odor

The face is the most descriptive area of the body. It may provide clues to underlying diseases. In addition to observation of the face, a thorough assessment of the face involves palpation. **Palpation** involves an examination with the hands using the sense of touch. The types of palpation include:

- **Bimanual:** Tissue is pressed gently between the fingers of two hands, as is done for the floor of the mouth.
- **Bidigital:** Tissue is pressed and gently rolled between the fingers of the same hand, which is done with the gingiva,

lips, tongue, buccal mucosa, thyroid, and cervical lymph nodes. The patient should turn the head to each side, making the sternocleidomastoid muscle on the opposite side of the neck more prominent for examination.
- **Digital:** Tissue is palpated using the finger of one hand, which is done for the facial gingiva of the posterior teeth when palpating an exostosis.
- **Bilateral:** Two hands are used simultaneously to examine the same structures on each side of the head and neck, which is done for the temporomandibular joint (TMJ) and, for example, the preauricular and postauricular nodes.

Establishing a sequence for performing an examination of the head, neck, and oral cavity is recommended to alleviate skipping an area inadvertently, to save time, and to promote patient confidence. After examination of the patient's gait, dexterity, speech, skin, eyes, and face, the following structures should be assessed:

- Lymph nodes for enlargement or induration **(Figure 10-2)**
- TMJ for crepitus (noise), deviation, or limitations of movement, and tenderness
- Lips for skin changes
- Labial and buccal mucosa (Stensen duct, vestibule, and frena) for skin changes, moistness, and tobacco use
- Tongue (lateral borders, dorsum and ventral surfaces) for skin changes, papillae, movement, and piercing
- Floor of the mouth (submandibular and sublingual salivary ducts, and frenum) for skin changes and flow of saliva
- Saliva for quantity and consistency
- Hard palate for skin changes
- Soft palate and uvula for skin changes
- Tonsillar region and throat for skin changes

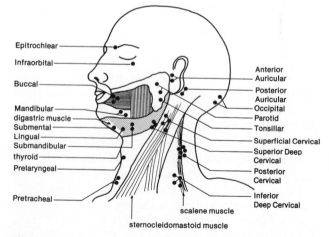

Figure 10–2. Lymph nodes of the head and neck. (From DeBiase C: Dental Health Education: Theory and Practice. Philadelphia, Lea & Febiger, 1991, p 156.)

Description of Soft Tissue Lesions

During an oral examination, the clinician must recognize any soft tissue abnormalities. Often, the specific diagnosis of an abnormality may not be known. However, an accurate description of the lesion, which includes its size, color, morphology (i.e., shape, texture), location, and history, should be documented. The periodontal probe is an excellent measuring tool for documentation of the size of noted lesions.

Most lesions can be classified as **elevated, flat,** or **depressed**. Elevated lesions are above the plane of mucosa, whereas flat lesions are level with the surface of mucosa and depressed lesions are below the level of mucosa. Elevated lesions may be categorized as either **blisterform** (containing fluid and of a soft consistency) or **nonblisterform** (solid containing no fluid and of a firm consistency). All three categories may have regular or irregular margins and may appear as either single or multiple lesions. See **Table 10-3** for a list of terms that describe lesions.

Periodontal Evaluation

The assessment of the condition of the gingival tissues as well as performing nonsurgical therapy to prevent and control gingival diseases are essential roles of the dental hygienist.

Gingival Assessment

When assessing a patient's periodontal condition, it is necessary to evaluate the appearance of the gingival tissues (i.e., their color, contour, consistency, and texture).

The **color** of the healthy gingiva is usually coral pink. There can also be physiologic pigmentation, which gives the tissues a brownish color (see Chapter 8). In the presence of gingival disease, such as gingivitis or periodontitis, the gingival tissues usually lose their coral pink color and appear either red, blue, or gray. The color changes may be localized such as along the gingival margin, in the papilla, or diffusely spread throughout the gingival tissues.

The **contour** of the gingival tissues is usually dependent upon the shape of the teeth, their position in the arch, and the underlying anatomy. Healthy gingival tissues usually have knife-edged margins. In the presence of gingivitis or periodontitis, the gingival contour may be bulbous, blunted, or cratered. The margins are usually rolled.

The **consistency** of the gingival tissues in health is usually firm and resilient. In the presence of gingival disease (e.g., gingivitis or periodontitis), the gingival tissues are usually soft and spongy with a loss of resiliency. Sometimes in the presence of long-standing, chronic disease, the tissues may appear firm due to the maturation of the granulation tissue. This type of tissue is called fibrotic.

A stippling appearance is usually associated with the surface **texture** of healthy gingiva. The **stippling** looks like an orange peel (see the Histology section in Chapter 4). In the

TABLE 10–3 Glossary of Oral Lesions and Descriptive Terms

1. Macule: flat circumscribed alteration of tissue that may vary in size, shape, or color (e.g., amalgam tattoo, petechia, freckles)
2. Plaque: a 5-mm or more slightly raised lesion with a broad, flat top
3. Papule: circumscribed superficial pinhead to 5-mm elevation of tissue (e.g., tiny mole)
4. Nodule: 5 mm–1 cm solid elevation of tissue that is usually deep seated and involves the submucosa
5. Tumor: a 2-cm or greater enlargement or swelling of tissue (malignant or benign)
6. Vesicle: elevated 1 cm or less alteration of tissue containing fluid, such as serum, mucin, or blood (e.g., blister, secondary herpes)
7. Bulla: similar to a vesicle but larger (>1 cm), deep seated, and more resistant to rupture
8. Pustule: pus-containing elevation of tissue
9. Keratosis: an abnormal thickening of the outer layers of epithelium (e.g., linea alba, cheekbite, leukoplakia)
10. Erosion/abrasion: a shallow depressed lesion characterized by a loss of the outer layer of the mucosa (e.g., lichen planus, toothbrush trauma)
11. Ulcer: a deep defect that extends below the epithelium (e.g., aphthous ulcer)
12. Pseudomembrane: a false membrane formed as a response to a necrotizing agent (e.g., covering over an ulcer)
13. Desquamation: shedding of epithelial cells in sheets
14. Petechiae: pinpoint submucosal hemorrhage (e.g., nicotine stomatitis)
15. Ecchymosis: large submucosal hemorrhage (e.g., bruise)
16. Induration: hardness or firmness of the soft tissue
17. Sessile: having a broad base of attachment
18. Pedunculated: having a narrow or stalk-like base of attachment
19. Erythematous: redness, inflammation
20. Granular: composed of or resembling granules (e.g., Fordyce granules/spots)
21. Exophytic: outward growing or projecting (e.g., exostosis, tori)
22. Fungating: growing exuberantly, like a fungus
23. Verrucous: wart-like appearance
24. Papillomatous: a cauliflower-like appearance
25. Fissured: cracked appearance
26. Corrugated: wrinkled texture
27. Crusted: dry or scab-like texture
28. Circumscribed: well defined or demarcated
29. Patent: open, unobstructed

presence of gingival disease, such as gingivitis or periodontitis, the gingival tissues usually lose their stippling and appear smooth and shiny. Gingival characteristics are part of the overall periodontal assessment process; however, a definitive periodontal diagnosis cannot be made based on the appearance of the gingival tissues alone.

The **width of the attached tissue** should be determined as well as the **amount of keratinized** tissue present. If a patient has minimal keratinized tissue, studies have shown that the tissue can remain healthy and stable for a long time. However, if subgingival restoration margins are to be placed in an area of minimal (<2 mm) keratinized gingiva, a tissue graft procedure should be done to ensure adequate healthy keratinized gingiva. The presence of a **low or high frenum**

attachment should be noted as well as any gingival changes associated with the frenum pull. If the marginal gingiva is moved by the frenum pull, a frenectomy with a soft tissue graft is indicated. The presence of **recession** as well as the amount of recession should be recorded.

Periodontal Assessment

A complete periodontal evaluation must include periodontal probing. Patients who require periodontal therapy and also patients on maintenance therapy who have had periodontal therapy should have complete probing evaluations performed. **The anatomic (histologically determined) gingival sulcus** extends from the gingival margin to the coronal end of the junctional epithelium. The periodontal probe, when used in its traditional manner in relation to the gingival sulcus or pocket, will penetrate to varying depths beyond the gingival margin. Thus, measurements of histologic pocket depth do not always coincide with clinical pocket depth. Several variables may affect the penetration of the periodontal probe: the amount of inflammation present in the sulcus/pocket, the pressure applied to the probe (probing force), the amount of deposits present on the tooth, and the diameter of the probe. Other difficulties associated with probing may include angulation of the probe, shape of the teeth, errors in visual assessment, access to the area, the segment of the dentition involved, subgingival deposits, and the cooperation of the patient. Studies that have evaluated the forces used during periodontal probing have shown that a 20- to 30-g force range is the ideal range for probing forces resulting in reproducible probing depth readings. Probing depths on six areas of each tooth should be recorded: mesiofacial, midfacial, distofacial, mesiolingual, midlingual, and distolingual. A conventional periodontal probe should be used.

Periodontal Probing

The **conventional periodontal probe** is an examination instrument that has a working end that is calibrated in millimeters and is similar to a ruler. There are a variety of probe designs and calibration patterns **(Figure 10-3)**.

The working end may be round and tapered with a blunt, rounded, or ball tip, or it may be flat with a blunt tip. The millimeter markings on the working end are either indentations or color bands at millimeter intervals. Although there is an advantage to using a probe with each millimeter demarcated, the clinician may be more comfortable with another design. The most important factor is that the measurements are consistent and accurate.

The conventional periodontal probe is utilized in measuring the **sulcus** or **probing depth**, which is the distance between the coronal aspects of the junctional epithelium (the apical depth of the periodontal probe tip penetration) and the crest of the gingival margin. **Clinical attachment level** is measured as the distance from the cementoenamel junction to the apical depth of the periodontal probe tip penetration. To obtain the **total attachment loss**, the clinician should also measure the amount of recession and add this to the probing depth **(Figure 10-4)**. It is important to distinguish between the probing depth and the clinical attachment level. Because probing depth is affected in part by the location of the gingival margin, and the level of this margin may fluctuate with the state of the tissue (i.e., inflammation, hypertrophy, recession), the term **"attachment level"** may better describe and relate in more precise terms the state of the sulcus.

The **technique for probing** involves lightly inserting the tip of the probe subgingivally to the coronal edge of the junctional epithelium and keeping it as parallel as possible to the tooth surface. After inserting the probe into the sulcus, it is "walked" up and down in the sulcus around the entire facial and lingual surfaces of each tooth. Six sulcus/pocket depths are recorded for each tooth: facial distal, facial, facial mesial, lingual distal, lingual, and lingual mesial. The lingual and facial readings recorded are the deepest readings detected along the entire facial and lingual surfaces of a tooth. To ensure accurate proximal readings, the probe tip must be parallel to the tooth surface and tilted slightly so that the tip is directed beneath the contact point of the tooth.

Shallow, healthy probing depths usually range from 1 to 3 mm. These depths are usually associated with lack of

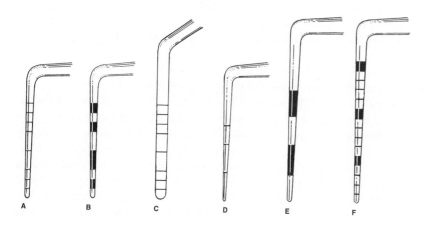

Figure 10–3. Examples of probes. Names and calibrated markings shown are: *A*, Williams (1-1-1-2-2-1-1-1); *B*, Williams, color-coded; *C*, Goldman-Fox (1-1-1-2-2-1-1-1); *D*, Michigan O (3-3-2); *E*, Hu-Friedy or Marquis Color-coded (3-3-3-3 or 3-3-2-3); and *F*, Hu-Friedy PCPUNC 15 (each millimeter to 15), color coded at 5-10-15. (From Wilkins EM: Clinical Practice of the Dental Hygienist, 8th ed. Philadelphia, Lippincott Williams & Wilkins, 1999, p 205.)

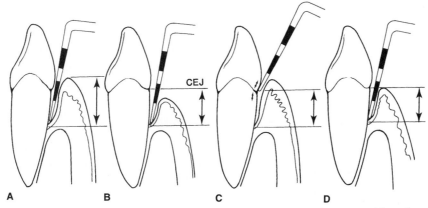

Figure 10–4. Clinical attachment level. *A*, Probing depth: the pocket is measured from the gingival margin to the attached periodontal tissue. *B*, Clinical attachment level in the presence of gingival recession is measured directly from the cementoenamel junction (CEJ) to the attached tissue. *C*, Clinical attachment level when the gingival margin covers the CEJ: first, the CEJ is located as shown, and then the distance to the CEJ is measured and subtracted from the probing depth. *D*, The clinical attachment level is equal to the probing depth when the gingival margin is at the level of the CEJ. (From Wilkins EM: Clinical Practice of the Dental Hygienist, 8th ed. Philadelphia, Lippincott Williams & Wilkins, 1999, p 210.)

future disease progression. It is important to note that deeper probing depths (≥ 4 mm) at a single examination will not necessarily be a predictor for future attachment loss or a marker of the presence of active disease.

There may be difficulty in locating the CEJ with conventional clinical methods, especially if the landmark is subgingival. **Acrylic stents** have been constructed and used as landmarks for assessing attachment loss over time. Studies have shown that the use of stents provided better reproducibility of probing attachment level than with the use of probing and visual assessment of the CEJ alone. These stents are cumbersome and time consuming. They can distort with time as teeth are lost or restored. They would be impractical for mass in-office use to aid in attachment level assessment. An automated probe may be more helpful to serve this purpose.

Several **automated probing systems** have been developed. Some of the main systems are described in reference to their major features and method of operation. The **Foster Miller Alabama Probe** has been used in research clinical trials. It has been shown to exhibit good repeatability compared with the conventional probe. The CEJ is detected using the probe tip when measuring attachment levels. It is currently used as a research tool. The **Florida Probe** has been compared with the conventional probe. The standard deviation of repeated pocket depth measurements was less than that of the conventional probe. When measuring attachment levels, a stent is placed over the occlusal surfaces of the teeth. The height of the tooth is incorporated into the measurement. Thus, by not using the CEJ as a fixed reference, the severity of the attachment loss is not seen by looking at the readings alone. The **Interprobe** is an automated probing system that has shown repeatability similar to the conventional probe. The ability to duplicate probe position when using these automated systems is a concern. Some of the systems may use stents to help to accomplish this. There is a voice-activated computer probe called the **Simplesoft Voice Chart**. This probe utilizes voice-activated computer software for charting. The operator uses conventional methods for performing the periodontal examination and speaks into the system for recording data. There is also a **thermocouple probe** that combines the use of the conventional probe with a sulcus/pocket temperature measurement. This probe measures a core sublingual temperature and then compares sulcular temperatures to the sublingual reading.

Periodontal Screening and Recording

A simple, efficient, and cost-effective method of screening for the presence of periodontal disease is by using the **periodontal screening and recording (PSR) system**. A special color-coded **periodontal screening probe** is used with a ball end of 0.5 mm in diameter. It is calibrated in 0.5, 3.5, 5.5, 8.5, and 11.5 demarcations. A color-coded area on this probe extends from 3.5 to 5.5 mm. This type of probe is utilized for quickly assessing the periodontal status and treatment plan of patients. The dentition is divided into sextants. All areas on each tooth are probed, and the deepest area in each sextant is given a code and recorded in the box delineating each sextant (**Figure 10-5**). The code ranges from 0 to 4, and specific patient treatment guidelines are indicated by each code. The coding system for the PSR is as follows:

0 = All probing depths in the sextant are within the first clear band.

1 = All probing depths in the sextant are within the first clear band with bleeding upon probing.

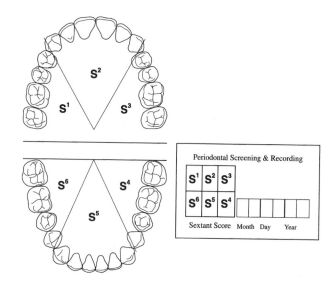

Figure 10–5. The procedure for performing a periodontal screening and recording involves dividing the mouth into sextants, probing all teeth in each sextant, assigning a code to the deepest probing depth in the sextant, and recording the code in the box provided.

2 = All probing depths in the sextant are within the first clear band, and there is either calculus present or an overhanging margin.

3 = The probing depths within the sextant fall within the black markings on the probe.

4 = The probing depths within the sextant are deeper than the end of the black marking on the probe.

* = Any notable feature such as furcation involvement, mobility, or recession

If one sextant has a 3, that sextant needs a comprehensive periodontal examination. If one sextant has a 4, or 2 or more sextants have a 3, a comprehensive periodontal examination is indicated. The PSR serves as a periodontal screening tool only. The PSR does not provide a tooth by tooth measurement of attachment levels. It does not take the place of a comprehensive periodontal examination.

Tooth Mobility

Tooth mobility has been referred to as a degree of looseness of a tooth beyond physiologic movement. The term **fremitus** is a palpable or visible movement in the tooth determined when occlusal forces are placed on the tooth. The etiology of mobility may include gingival or periodontal inflammation, parafunctional habits, occlusal prematurities, and traumatic forces applied to teeth by removable appliances. Mobility of the teeth tends to decrease after nonsurgical periodontal therapy. This is due mainly to the decrease in inflammation. Mobility recordings are graded by classifying the amount of movement when the tooth is checked; this is done by attempting to move a tooth between two metal instruments in all directions. The most commonly used index of tooth mobility is the Miller index. The majority of pathologic mobility occurs in the faciolingual direction. **Grade I** mobil-

ity is said to be slight or the first noticeable sign of movement in any direction greater than normal. **Grade II** mobility is considered up to 1 mm of total movement in any direction. **Grade III** mobility is the most advanced mobility, because there is >1 mm mobility in any direction as well as the tooth being depressible in a vertical dimension.

Fremitus

Fremitus or increasing mobility may be a sign of occlusal trauma. **Occlusal trauma** is defined as an injury to the tooth or its attachment as a result of excessive occlusal forces. **Primary occlusal trauma** refers to occlusal trauma resulting from excessive occlusal forces to a tooth or teeth with normal periodontal support. **Secondary occlusal trauma** is trauma or injury to a tooth or teeth with inadequate periodontal support. Most studies have shown that excessive occlusal forces do NOT initiate periodontal diseases, including connective tissue attachment loss. There is some evidence that in the presence of periodontal disease, occlusal traumatism may lead to greater attachment loss than in cases where no occlusal trauma exists.

Furcation Involvement

Furcation involvement should be determined. Classification of furcation involvement can be divided into four grades. If the furcation can be entered with a furcation probe by up to 2 mm, it is classified as a **grade I**. When tissue destruction in a furcation area is such that the furcation probe can be placed deep into the furcation but cannot be passed all the way through, it is called a **grade II**. When the destruction is such that the furcation probe can be placed through and through the furcation, it is classified as a **grade III**. A **grade IV** furcation is referred to as similar to a class III in that there is through-and-through destruction, but gingival recession is present exposing the furcation **(Figure 10-6)**.

Mucogingival Line

The **mucogingival junction** demarcates the connection between the alveolar mucosa and the attached gingiva. Healthy attached gingiva is pink and keratinized, whereas the alveolar mucosa is smooth and vascular. The **mucogingival line** is located on all facial surfaces and lingual surfaces of the mandibular arch only.

Bleeding

During periodontal probing, the presence of bleeding upon probing should also be noted. A dot above the probing reading in which the bleeding occurred is simple and easy to compare with past and future periodontal assessments. The presence of bleeding upon gentle probing is a marker for the presence of inflammation in the sulcus. However, the presence of bleeding upon probing is not an entity that can pre-

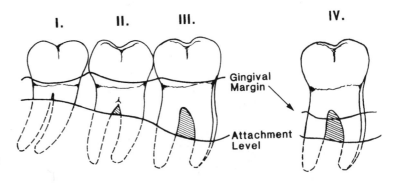

Figure 10–6. Classification of furcations. I, Early, beginning involvement. II, Moderate involvement, in which the furcation can be probed but not through and through. III, Severe involvement, when the bone between the roots is destroyed and a probe can be passed through. IV, Same as III, with clinical exposure resulting from gingival recession. (From Wilkins EM: Clinical Practice of the Dental Hygienist, 8th ed. Philadelphia, Lippincott Williams & Wilkins, 1999, p 230.)

dict the presence of current disease activity or future attachment loss in that site.

Dental Deposits

Materia alba is a loosely adherent unstructured white mass of oral debris (e.g., food, sloughed tissue) and bacteria. It adheres loosely to the teeth and can be removed by vigorous rinsing or irrigation. This is usually a sign of poor oral hygiene.

Dental plaque is the colonization and attachment of oral bacteria to the tooth surface. Oral bacteria colonize in the acquired pellicle that is attached to the tooth surface. The **acquired pellicle** is a film of denatured protein that is derived from the saliva. Depending on the type of bacteria dominating the plaque and the presence or absence of sucrose in the oral cavity, dental plaque bacteria may initiate periodontal disease or dental caries. The removal of plaque is accomplished by the use of mechanical devices (e.g., brush, floss) and antimicrobial agents.

Freshly deposited plaque is transparent and difficult to see. Older mature unstained plaque may be seen if the tooth is dried with compressed air. Food, tobacco, or other pigments can stain plaque and, thus, allow for easy visual detection. However, plaque is usually colorless and is most readily detected by the application of a disclosing agent to the teeth.

Calculus is a term used to describe hardened or calcified dental plaque. This plaque can occur supragingivally or subgingivally and adheres to the tooth surface. The source of minerals for calculus formation is the saliva for supragingival calculus and sulcular fluid for subgingival calculus. It may occur localized or generalized on one or more teeth and can form as spicules, bands, thin layers, or sheets on a crown or root surface. **Supragingival** calculus occurs on the clinical crown and is usually white to yellow or gray but may be stained darker from food, tobacco, or other pigments. **Subgingival** calculus occurs subgingivally on the root surface and usually ranges in color from light brown to black because of staining from blood pigments in the inflamed pocket.

Stained supragingival calculus may be seen directly; however, unstained supragingival calculus is difficult to see when it is wet with saliva. Drying the tooth with compressed air allows for distinguishing the dry calculus from the translucent tooth surface. An explorer may be used for detection when visual examination is not adequate.

Most generally, subgingival calculus is best detected with an explorer or periodontal probe. Often, dark edges of calculus may be seen through the free gingiva, or the diseased marginal gingiva can be reflected with air and reveal subgingival calculus.

The physical presence of calculus on a tooth is not a mechanical irritant to the soft tissue. Calculus has clinical significance, because its rough and porous surface allows for plaque accumulation and retention. Therefore, detection and removal of calculus is an important function that permits gingival tissue to resume a healthy state.

Discoloration or **staining** of the teeth occurs by adhering directly to the tooth surface, adhering to calculus or plaque, or incorporating within the tooth structure. Stain is significant primarily because of its cosmetic effect. It can be classified according to its location or its origin (**Table 10-4**).

There are numerous types of extrinsic stain, which are primarily associated with food and tobacco, although some have no known etiology. Some types are more common than are others, and some occur on specific areas of the teeth. Intrinsic stains may occur as a result of interrupted tooth development, disease, or systemic use of antibiotics (**Table 10-5**).

Endogenous intrinsic stains may result from medications, imperfect tooth development, or nonvital teeth.

Nonvital teeth, which are untreated or in which endodontic root canal therapy has failed, may become discolored due

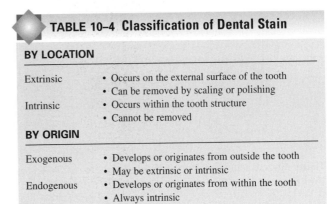

TABLE 10-4 Classification of Dental Stain

BY LOCATION	
Extrinsic	• Occurs on the external surface of the tooth
	• Can be removed by scaling or polishing
Intrinsic	• Occurs within the tooth structure
	• Cannot be removed
BY ORIGIN	
Exogenous	• Develops or originates from outside the tooth
	• May be extrinsic or intrinsic
Endogenous	• Develops or originates from within the tooth
	• Always intrinsic

⬢ **TABLE 10–5 Extrinsic Stains—Location and Etiology**

STAIN	PRIMARY LOCATION	ETIOLOGY
Yellow	Any tooth	Food pigments
Green	Facial cervical third	Chromogenic bacteria
	Mx anteriors	Blood pigments
		Marijuana
Black line	Follows the line of the gingival crest on the facial and lingual surfaces; occurs most often in females	Unknown, usually in clean mouths
Tobacco	Cervical third, lingual surfaces	Tar products and brown pigments from tobacco
Other brown stain	Any tooth surface	Coffee, tea, cola, soy sauce, chlorhexidine rinses, betel nut
Orange and red	Anterior facial and lingual	Chromogenic bacteria
Metal stains	Anterior cervical third	Inhaling of metal dust; ingestion of drugs (e.g., iron)

to blood hemorrhages in the pulp chamber. The stain may range from yellow-brown, slate gray, bluish-black, to black.

Systemic **tetracycline**, if administered during tooth development, has an affinity for mineralized tissues and is absorbed by the teeth and bones. Discoloration, ranging from light green to dark yellow or gray, can occur generalized or on individual teeth.

Imperfect tooth development as a result of genetic or environmental factors can result in endogenous intrinsic stain. **Amelogenesis imperfecta** results in partial or completely missing enamel and gives the teeth a yellow-brown or gray-brown appearance. **Dentinogenesis imperfecta** results in abnormal development of the dentin and gives the teeth a translucent or opalescent gray to bluish-brown color.

Enamel hypoplasia occurs because of a disturbance in the ameloblastic activity during enamel formation and results in pitting of the teeth. This may be caused by illness or excessive ingestion of fluoride during formation of the enamel. If caused by excessive fluoride, it is called **dental fluorosis**. If illness or ingestion of excessive fluoride occurs during the calcification of enamel, **hypocalcification** occurs and results in white spots or areas on mature teeth. These pits or white spots later become discolored from food or other pigments or stain (see Chapter 8).

Exogenous intrinsic stain may originate from various extrinsic stains. Restorative materials such as amalgam can impart a gray to black discoloration to the tooth adjacent to a restoration. Likewise, topically applied stannous fluoride can result in a brown stain along the margins of restorations or in areas of decalcification.

Once a complete periodontal examination or assessment is performed, it is important to develop a diagnosis, prognosis, and definitive periodontal treatment plan before therapy is started. A complete series of radiographs along with vertical bitewings is needed before any definitive periodontal care plan can be developed.

Dental Chartings

Facial injuries/ jaw fractures (see Chapter 12) may include injury to the teeth. Tooth fractures are classified by the location and extent of the fracture (**Figure 10-7**). Three additional forms of injury include:

- **Luxation** or the loosening of a tooth with displacement, or loosening without displacement called **subluxation**
- **Intrusion** of the tooth into the alveolar bone with subsequent fracture of the socket or **extrusion** (partial displacement)

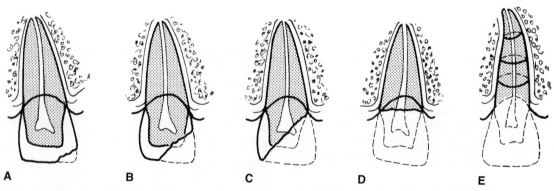

Figure 10–7. Fractures of teeth. A, Enamel fracture. B, Crown fracture without pulpal involvement. C, Crown fracture with pulpal involvement. D, Fracture of the crown and root near the neck of the tooth. E, Root fractures involving the cementum, dentin, and pulp may occur in the apical, middle, or coronal third of the root.(From Wilkins EM: Clinical Practice of the Dental Hygienist, 8th ed. Philadelphia, Lippincott Williams & Wilkins, 1999, p 245.)

- **Avulsion** of the tooth, which is the complete loss of a tooth out of its socket

Caries

Assessment for caries can be found in **Chapter 14**.

Occlusion

Adult Occlusion

In the early 1900s, Edward H. angle developed a system for classifying the occlusion of permanent teeth and based it on the relationship of the mandibular and maxillary first permanent molars. This system describes the first molar and canine relationship and the facial profile of an individual with a normal (ideal) occlusion and designates deviations from the normal occlusion as a class of malocclusion. All three classes of malocclusion in which the relationship of the mandible to the maxilla is described can be found in (**Table 10-6, Table 10-7,** and **Figure 10-8**).

A specific facial profile is characteristic of individuals with either normal occlusion or a malocclusion (**Figure 10-9**). A **mesognathic** facial profile is relatively flat because of a slightly protruded mandible. In a **retrognathic** profile, the mandible is retruded or shifted distally, which makes the maxilla more prominent. A **prognathic** profile features a prominently protruding mandible.

Malrelations of groups of teeth and malpositions of individual teeth may occur in the dentition (**Tables 10-8** and **10-9**). These must be noted when describing the occlusion of a patient. The extent of overjet, underjet, overbite, and openbite is recorded using a periodontal probe to measure the distance in millimeters.

Pediatric Occlusion

The occlusion of the primary teeth is classified the same as the adult dentition for canine relationship, but the molar relationship is viewed somewhat differently. Very simply, an imaginary line is drawn from the distal of the maxillary primary second molar to the distal of the mandibular primary second molar when observing the teeth in occlusion from the facial aspect. If the distal surface of the mandibular pri-

TABLE 10–6 Characteristics of Normal (Ideal) Occlusion on the Permanent Dentition

Facial profile:	Mesognathic
Molar relation:	Mesiobuccal cusp of the maxillary first molar occludes with the buccal groove of the mandibular first molar
Canine relation:	Maxillary canine occludes with the distal half of the mandibular canine and the mesial half of the mandibular first premolar

TABLE 10–7 Characteristics of Three Classes of Malocclusion of the Permanent Dentition*

CLASS I (NEUTROCCLUSION)

- Facial profile: same as normal occlusion
- Molar relation: same as normal occlusion
- Canine relation: same as normal occlusion
- Difference from normal occlusion is the malposition of the teeth

CLASS II (DISTOCCLUSION)

- Facial profile: retrognathic
- Molar relation: buccal groove of the mandibular first molar is distal to the mesiobuccal cusp of the maxillary first molar by at least the width of a premolar
- Canine: distal surface of the mandibular canine[†] is distal to the mesial surface of the maxillary canine by at least the width of a premolar
- Division of class II:
  Division 1: All maxillary teeth are protruded
  Division 2: One or more maxillary teeth are retruded
- Subdivisions of class II: the right side of the dentition may be a class II and the other side a class I

CLASS III (MESIOCCLUSION)

- Facial profile: prognathic
- Molar relation: buccal groove of the mandibular first molar is mesial to the mesiobuccal cusp of the maxillary first molar by at least the width of a premolar
- Canine relation: distal surface of the mandibular canine is mesial to the mesial surface of the maxillary canine by at least the width of a premolar[‡]

*For illustrations of classes of malocclusion, see Figure 10-8.
[†]If the distance of the mandibular molar or canine relationship to the maxillary teeth is less than the width of a premolar, classify as a "tendency" toward a class II.
[‡]If the distance of the molar or canine relationship to the maxillary teeth is less than the width of a premolar, classify as a "tendency" toward a class III.

mary molar is mesial to that of the maxillary primary molar, a mesial step is created. The term **mesial step** can be viewed as synonymous to class III malocclusion (**Figure 10-10A**). Conversely, if the distal surface of the mandibular primary molar is distal to that of the maxillary, a distal step results. A distal step and can be viewed as synonymous to class II malocclusion. If the distal surfaces of both the maxillary and the mandibular molars are on the same vertical plane, it is called **flush terminal plane** (see **Figure 10-10B**).

Primate space is a diastema or gap that is often observed in the primary dentition. This spacing is normally found between the mandibular canine and first molar and the maxillary lateral incisor and canine (**Figure 10-11**). The primate space enables the primary molars to shift mesially, thus allowing adequate spacing for the eruption of the permanent first molars into proper occlusion. Without primate space, ectopic eruption of the permanent tooth may occur. **Ectopic eruption**, in this case, refers to eruption of a permanent tooth into the distal surface of the primary tooth, resulting in reabsorption of the primary tooth (**Figure 10-12**).

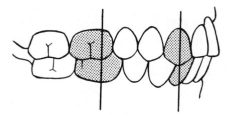

Normal (Ideal) Occlusion

Malocclusion

Class I: Neutroclusion.

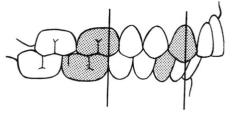

Class II: Distoclusion.

Division 1:

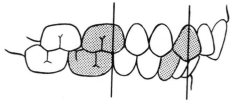

Class II: Distoclusion.

Division 2:

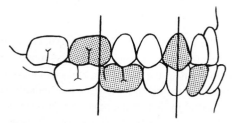

Class III: Mesioclusion.

Figure 10–8. Normal occlusion and classification of malocclusion. (From Wilkins EM: Clinical Practice of the Dental Hygienist, 8th ed. Philadelphia, Lippincott Williams & Wilkins, 1999, p 259.)

TABLE 10–8 Malrelations of Groups of Teeth

MALRELATION	DESCRIPTION
Posterior crossbite	Maxillary or mandibular teeth either facial or lingual to the normal position, may be bilateral or unilateral
Anterior crossbite	Maxillary incisors lingual to the mandibular incisors
Edge-to-edge bite	Incisal surfaces of the maxillary anterior teeth occlude with the incisal surfaces of the mandibular anterior teeth
End-to-end bite	Molars and premolars occlude cusp-to-cusp
Open bite	Lack of occlusal or incisal contact between the maxillary and mandibular teeth
Overjet	Horizontal distance between the labioincisal surfaces of the mandibular incisors and the linguoincisal surfaces of the maxillary incisors
Underjet	Maxillary incisors are lingual to the mandibular incisors; often seen in a class III malocclusion (reported as a [–])
Overbite	Vertical distance by which maxillary incisors overlap mandibular incisors; considered deep when the incisal edge of the maxillary tooth is at the level of the cervical third of the facial surface of the mandibular anterior tooth

Orthodontic intervention does not normally take place until after the mixed dentition phase at approximately 7 to 12 years of age.

Clinical Testing

Clinical Testing for Pulp Vitality

Clinical testing for pulp vitality includes **thermal tests** (cold and heat), **percussion, palpation, electrical pulp testing**, and **fiberoptic illumination**. Because of limitations inherent in most of them, it is risky to rely on a single test for confirmation of pulp vitality. Patience and the process of elimination are important factors for determining the vitality of the pulp of a specific tooth. Before any type of testing is performed, the clinician should explain the procedure to the patient and choose similar teeth for controls. Reliable responses to pulp vitality testing depend on the teeth being dry. This should be accomplished by isolating the teeth and drying them with sterile gauze.

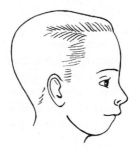

RETROGNATHIC

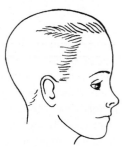

MESOGNATHIC

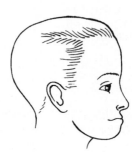

PROGNATHIC

Figure 10–9. Types of facial profiles. (From Wilkins EM: Clinical Practice of the Dental Hygienist, 8th ed. Philadelphia, Lippincott Williams & Wilkins, 1999, p 256.)

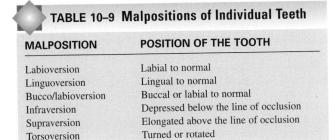

TABLE 10–9 Malpositions of Individual Teeth

MALPOSITION	POSITION OF THE TOOTH
Labioversion	Labial to normal
Linguoversion	Lingual to normal
Bucco/labioversion	Buccal or labial to normal
Infraversion	Depressed below the line of occlusion
Supraversion	Elongated above the line of occlusion
Torsoversion	Turned or rotated

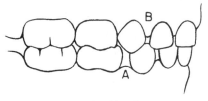

Figure 10–11. Primary teeth with primate spaces. A, Mandibular primate space between the canine and the first molar. B, Maxillary primate space between the lateral incisor and the canine. (From Wilkins EM: Clinical Practice of the Dental Hygienist, 8th ed. Philadelphia, Lippincott Williams & Wilkins, 1999, p 260.)

Methods for **cold testing** include a **cold water bath, ethyl chloride, sticks of ice**, and **carbon dioxide sticks**. Ethyl chloride and a cold bath are the most frequently used. Ethyl chloride is sprayed onto a cotton pellet, which is then applied to the middle third of the facial surface of the crown of the suspected tooth for 5 seconds or until the patient feels pain. The cold water bath requires rubber dam isolation of the tooth and spraying ice water from a syringe onto the tooth for at least 5 seconds.

Methods for **heat testing** include utilization of **warm temporary stopping** and a **hot water bath**. A stick of temporary stopping is heated over a flame and then applied for 5 seconds to the middle third of the facial surface of the tooth crown, which has been coated with petroleum jelly. The hot water bath requires rubber dam isolation of the tooth, then very warm water should be sprayed onto the tooth for 5 seconds.

Thermal testing with cold or hot water baths can be performed on unrestored teeth and also on full metal or porcelain crowns. Both methods prevent excessive damage to the tooth due to temperature change.

Four types of patient response to thermal stimulation may occur. No response may indicate a nonvital pulp or a false-negative result because of factors such as pulpal calcification or patient medication. A 1- to 2-second mild-to-moderate response is considered normal. A strong painful response that subsides within 1 to 2 seconds is characteristic of **reversible pulpitis**. A strong painful response that lingers for several seconds after the stimulus is removed is indicative of **irreversible pulpitis**.

Percussion testing is performed by tapping on the incisal or occlusal edge of a tooth with the handle of a mouth mirror. Another method is to ask the patient to bite on a hard object such as the stick of a cotton swab or a specially designed autoclavable plastic stick.

Palpation or application of pressure with a fingertip on the mucosa overlying the apex of the tooth can be utilized to determine the periapical extent of the inflammation. As in all testing, a control tooth must also be tested.

Electrical pulp testers (vitalometers) are devices (usually battery powered) that deliver a current of electricity to the facial surface of a tooth. These testers are used to determine the presence or absence of sensory nerves in the tooth. False-positive and false-negative results may occur, and these testers do not measure the degree of health or disease of the pulp. The tooth must be dried with a cotton roll and isolated. A conductor, usually toothpaste, is placed on the tip of the pulp tester and placed on the tooth while the patient touches the handle so that the circuit can be completed. The level of current is gradually increased until the patient indicates a sensation. The presence of a response usually indicates the presence of vital pulp tissue, whereas no response usually indicates pulpal necrosis. False-positive results may

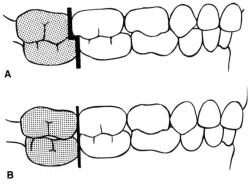

Figure 10–10. Eruption patterns of the first permanent molars. A, Terminal mesial step. The distal surface of the mandibular second primary molar is mesial to the distal surface of the maxillary second primary molar. B, Terminal plane. The distal surfaces of the mandibular and maxillary second primary molars are on the same vertical plane; permanent molars erupt in end-to-end occlusion. (From Wilkins EM: Clinical Practice of the Dental Hygienist, 8th ed. Philadelphia, Lippincott Williams & Wilkins, 1999, p 260.)

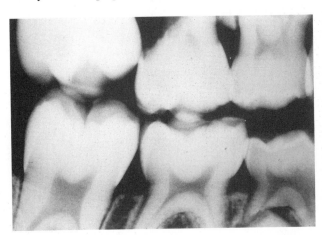

Figure 10–12. Ectopic eruption may be an indication of inadequate arch length. As the first permanent molar erupts, it resorbs the distal margin of the primary second molar. This occurs most often in the maxillary arch.

occur and are often the result of the toothpaste from the electrode touching the gingiva; therefore, complete isolation to ensure a dry tooth is essential. Another concern when utilizing electric pulp testers is that careful sterilization or disinfection of the handpiece and electrode must be followed to ensure prevention of cross-contamination among patients.

The use of **transillumination** is another valuable method for determining vertical tooth fractures, which can illicit pulpal pain. This is done by directing fiberoptic illumination from a fiberoptic handpiece at the gingival sulcus.

Sources

Annals of Periodontology: 1996 World Workshop in Periodontics, vol 1(1). Chicago, American Academy of Periodontology, 1996, p 53.

Cohen S, Burns RC: Pathways of the Pulp, 7th ed. St. Louis, CV Mosby, 1998, pp 10-14.

Darby ML, Walsh MM: Dental Hygiene Theory and Practice. Philadelphia, WB Saunders, 1995, pp 190, 282, 314-318, 354-357, 476-479.

McCann AL, Wesley RK: A method for describing soft tissue lesions. Dent Hygiene 61:219, 1987.

Periodontal Screening and Recording. Training Program. From the American Academy of Periodontology and the American Dental Association, sponsored by Procter & Gamble, 1992.

Tupta-Veselicky L, et al: A clinical study of an electronic constant force periodontal probe. J Periodontol 65:616-622, 1994.

Walton RE, Torabinejad M: Principles and Practice of Endodontics, 2nd ed. Philadelphia, WB Saunders, 1996, pp 58-61.

Wilkins EM: Clinical Practice of the Dental Hygienist, 8th ed. Philadelphia, Lippincott Williams & Wilkins, 1999, pp 87-95, 121-125, 205-219, 230, 245-246, 254-260, 264-275, 277-283, and 285-290, 296-298, 524.

Woodall IR: Comprehensive Dental Hygiene Care, 4th ed. St. Louis, CV Mosby, 1993, pp 249-255, 298-300.

Questions and Answers

Questions

1. A vesicle is a 1 cm or larger alteration of tissue that contains fluid. This is classified as a blisterform lesion.
   A. Both statements are TRUE.
   B. Both statements are FALSE.
   C. The first statement is TRUE, and the second one is FALSE.
   D. The first statement is FALSE, and the second one is TRUE.

2. A 3-mm wart-like elevation of tissue with a stalk-like attachment to the mucosa may be described as a/an:
   A. indurated sessile nodule.
   B. sessile verrucous papule.
   C. pedunculated fungating nodule.
   D. pedunculated verrucous papule.

3. Erosion of oral mucosa is a superficial lesion characterized by loss of outer epithelium. This condition is synonymous with abrasion of soft tissue.
   A. Both statements are TRUE.
   B. Both statements are FALSE.
   C. The first statement is TRUE, and the second one is FALSE.
   D. The first statement is FALSE, and the second is TRUE.

4. Pinpoint submucosal hemorrhage best describes which of the following?
   A. Vesicle
   B. Petechia
   C. Ecchymosis
   D. Hemangioma
   E. Hematoma

5. Which classification of malocclusion best describes a permanent dentition in which the mandibular teeth are crowded and overlapping and the mesial buccal groove of the mandibular first molar occludes with the mesial buccal cusp of the maxillary first molar?
   A. Class I
   B. Class II, division 1
   C. Class II, division 2
   D. Class III

6. The classification of malocclusion in which the buccal groove of the mandibular first permanent molar is distal to the mesial buccal cusp of the maxillary first permanent molar and one or more maxillary incisors are retruded.
   A. Class I
   B. Class II, division 1
   C. Class II, division 2
   D. Class III

7. When viewing the facial profile of a patient, you observe that his lower lip is resting between his maxillary and mandibular incisors and his mandible is retruded. This facial profile is:
   A. Prognathic
   B. Mesognathic
   C. Retrognathic

8. The horizontal distance between the facial surfaces of the mandibular incisors and the lingual surfaces of the maxillary incisors is called:

A. Openbite
B. Overbite
C. Underjet
D. Overjet

9. A tooth that is erupted beyond the line of occlusion is:
   A. linguoverted.
   B. buccoverted.
   C. supraverted.
   D. infraverted.

10. Calculus should be removed from the teeth because its rough surface is a mechanical irritation to the gingival tissue.
    A. Both statement and reason are correct and related.
    B. Both statement and reason are correct but NOT related.
    C. The statement is correct, but the reason is untrue.
    D. The statement is NOT correct, but the reason is an accurate statement.
    E. Neither the statement nor the reason is correct.

11. Calculus should be removed from the teeth because its rough and porous surface contributes to plaque accumulation.
    A. Neither the statement nor the reason is correct.
    B. Both the statement and the reason are correct.
    C. The statement is correct, but the reason is incorrect.
    D. The statement is incorrect, but the reason is accurate.

12. What type of extrinsic stain of unknown etiology is found characteristically on the lingual gingival third of the maxillary posterior teeth of women who have good oral hygiene?
    A. Green
    B. Betel nut
    C. Black line
    D. Tetracycline

13. Which of the following stains is considered to be an endogenous intrinsic stain?
    A. Tobacco
    B. Betel nut
    C. Tetracycline

14. Which of the following patient responses to thermal stimulation are indicative of an irreversible pulpitis?
    A. No response
    B. A 1- to 2-second mild-to-moderate response
    C. A 1- to 2-second strong painful response
    D. A strong painful response that lingers for several seconds

15. For what type of clinical pulp vitality testing is ethyl chloride used?
    A. Heat testing
    B. Cold testing
    C. Electrical pulp testing
    D. Fiberoptic testing

16. The primate space on the maxillary arch is normally found between which of the following primary teeth?
    A. Canine and first molar
    B. Canine and lateral incisor
    C. Lateral incisor and central incisor
    D. First molar and second molar

17. Which of the following types of palpation presses the tissues between the fingers of two hands to evaluate the floor of the mouth, for example?
    A. Digital
    B. Bidigital
    C. Bimanual
    D. Bilateral

18. Subluxation of a tooth differs from luxation in which of the following ways?
    A. Luxation does not involve loosening of the tooth.
    B. Subluxation does not involve loosening of the tooth.
    C. Luxation does not involve tooth displacement.
    D. Subluxation does not involve tooth displacement.

19. Each of the following procedures must be followed for accurate periodontal probing except one. Which one is the exception?
    A. Keep the probe tip parallel to the tooth surface as it is "walked" around the tooth.
    B. Tilt the probe slightly at the proximals to reach directly apical to the contact point.
    C. Determine the buccal or lingual reading after probing the entire buccal or lingual.
    D. Record the buccal or lingual reading at the center of those surfaces for each tooth.
    E. Record six probing depths for each tooth.

20. While exploring, the entire length of the explorer tip must be kept against the tooth surface. This will prevent laceration of the sulcular tissue.
    A. Both statements are TRUE.
    B. Both statements are FALSE.
    C. The first statement is TRUE; the second one is FALSE.
    D. The first statement is FALSE; the second one is TRUE.

21. When evaluating gingival characteristics, which of the following terms describes a healthy consistency or gingival tone?
    A. Coral pink
    B. Knife-edge
    C. Stippled
    D. Firm

22. When performing débridement on a patient, you notice that the furcation on tooth #30 can be seen, thus you take a furcation probe and probe through and through the defect. There is no gingival tissue occluding the furcation. What type of furcation defect does your patient have?
    A. Grade I
    B. Grade II
    C. Grade III
    D. Grade IV

23. When performing periodontal screening and recording, you determine a code of two from a code of one if:
    A. bleeding upon probing.
    B. probing depths are >3.5 mm but <5.5 mm.
    C. probing depths are <3.5 mm.
    D. probing depths are >5.5 mm.
    E. calculus is present.

24. Notation errors made while documenting a patient's medical history should be rectified by:
    A. erasing the error.
    B. using correction fluid over the error.
    C. putting a red "X" in ink through the error.
    D. drawing a single line through the error in ink.

25. Which of the following categories of information is normally included in the medical history rather than the dental history assessment?
    A. Chief complaint
    B. Water fluoridation exposure
    C. History of hospitalizations
    D. History of dental visits
    E. Adverse reactions to local anesthetics

ANSWERS

1. **D.** A vesicle is a blisterform lesion that contains fluid; however, it is 1 cm or less. The first statement actually describes a bulla.

2. **D.** A papule is a 5 mm or less elevation of tissue, whereas a nodule is larger. This leaves choices B or D; D is the answer because a stalk-like attachment is pedunculated.

3. **A.** Abrasion and erosion are synonymous terms that are used to describe loss of epithelium of soft tissue.

4. **B.** Ecchymosis and hematoma are synonymous and describe large submucosal hemorrhage. A vesicle is an elevation of tissue that contains any type of fluid; a hemangioma is an elevation of tissue that contains blood vessels.

5. **A.** The molar relationship described is that of a class I malocclusion.

6. **C.** The molar relationship described is that of a class II malocclusion. If one or more maxillary anteriors are retruded, it belongs in division 2. In division 1, all maxillary anteriors are protruded.

7. **C.** In a mesognathic profile, the lips would be together, and the lower lip would be protruded in a prognathic profile.

8. **D.** Underjet is the horizontal distance between the facial surfaces of the maxillary incisors and lingual surfaces of the mandibular incisors. Overbite is a vertical overlap of the maxillary incisors; open bite is lack of occlusal or incisal contact.

9. **C.** Infraverted describes a tooth that is depressed or not fully erupted to the line of occlusion. Linguoverted and buccoverted refer to a tooth being lingual or buccal to normal.

10. **C.** Calculus should be removed, but its roughness does not cause mechanical irritation. Its roughness creates a harbor for accumulation of plaque. The endotoxins from the plaque actually irritate the gingival tissue.

11. **B.** See the rationale for question 10.

12. **C.** Green stain and betel nut stain are extrinsic and of a known etiology. Tetracycline stain is intrinsic.

13. **C.** Tobacco and betel nut stain are exogenous stains.

14. **D.** No response may indicate either a nonvital pulp or a false-negative result. A mild to strong response that lasts for 2 seconds or less is indicative of reversible pulpitis.

15. **B.** Electrical and fiberoptic testing involve electrical current and a fiberoptic light, respectively. Heat testing is done with warm temporary slopping or a hot water bath.

16. **B.** The primate space on the maxillary arch is located between the lateral incisor and the canine. This space is located between the canine and the first molar on the mandibular arch.

17. **C.** Bilateral palpation utilizes two hands, but they are used to examine the same structures on each side of the head and neck.

18. **D.** Both luxation and subluxation result in tooth loosening, but displacement of the tooth does not occur with subluxation.

19. **D.** The center of the buccal or lingual surface may not be the deepest probing depth along each of those surfaces. To determine the deepest reading, the entire buccal or lingual surface must first be probed.

20. **B.** If the entire explorer tip is kept against the tooth, the actual point of the explorer tip will be against the sulcular tissue and will lacerate it. Only the side of the point of the explorer tip should touch the tooth surface.

21. **D.** Coral pink signifies healthy gingival color. Knife edge refers to healthy contours of the gingival tissues. Stippled refers to the surface texture of the gingival tissues.

22. **D.** This is a grade IV furcation. A through-and-through furcation is classed as a grade III or IV. When the gingival tissues are recessed and the furcation can be visualized, the furcation defect is considered to be a grade IV. A grade I barely penetrates the furcation. A grade II penetrates deeply into the furcation but does not go through and through.

23. **E.** A code of 1 in the periodontal screening and recording bleeds upon probing and has probing depths of <3.5 mm. A code of 2 has these in addition to displaying calculus or a defective restoration.

24. **D.** Deleting an error on any chart document can be made only by drawing a single line in ink through the error and writing the accurate information after it. The error should remain legible.

25. **C.** Dental histories should include information pertinent to the patient s immediate or chief complaint, previous and present dental and dental hygiene care, and routine personal oral health practices.

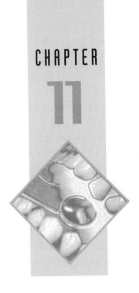

CHAPTER 11

Obtaining and Interpreting Radiographs

JOAN GIBSON-HOWELL, RDH, MSEd

Radiology is energy that defies the five senses. Because of the mysteries associated with x-radiation, it was labeled with the symbol of "x," indicating unknown. Through time, the many uses of radiation have proved its value in therapeutic and diagnostic health care.

The discovery of x-radiation is attributed to Wilhelm Konrad Roentgen on November 8, 1895 in Bavaria, Germany. Due to his outstanding contribution to the field of science and physics, Roentgen was awarded the Nobel Prize for Physics in 1901. Not long after Roentgen's discovery, Dr. Otto Walkhoff, a dentist in Brunswick, Germany, exposed and processed the first dental radiograph. Although the techniques were different, the concepts and results were similar.

The purpose of this chapter is to review the science of radiology but, more important, the integration and application of radiology knowledge into the clinical setting.

PRINCIPLES OF RADIOPHYSICS AND RADIOBIOLOGY

Radiophysics

X-radiation is an electromagnetic energy that is characterized by the following unique properties. X-rays:

1. Are invisible
2. Are weightless
3. Cannot be heard, smelled, felt, seen, or tasted
4. Travel at the speed of light
5. Travel in a straight line
6. Can be deflected
7. Have a wide range of wavelengths
8. Stray outward over a distance
9. Possess short wavelengths compared with radio waves
10. Are absorbed by matter differently, depending on the composition of the matter (This produces a negative image on the film.)
11. Cause specific objects to fluoresce (i.e., intensifying screen of extraoral films)
12. Can cause biologic changes beneficial in treatment but must be used judiciously in diagnostic radiation[1]

Significance of Ionizing Radiation

When discussing radiation, it is important to understand the concept of ionizing radiation as part of radiation biology and patient safety. Atoms lose and gain electrons in the process of converting electricity to x-ray photons. When the neutral atom loses or gains an electron (a positive or negative charge), the process is called **ionization** and the result is an **ionized atom** called an **ion**. Two types of ionizing radiation are **particulate** and **electromagnetic** radiation. Particulate radiation is used to provide irradiation therapy. Examples include alpha particles, electrons, beta particles, cathode rays, protons, and neutrons. X-rays and gamma rays are types of electromagnetic radiation that are most often used in diagnostic radiation.

Electromagnetic Radiation

Electromagnetic radiation is categorized according to its wavelength and is arranged accordingly in the **electromagnetic spectrum.** The electromagnetic spectrum, from longest to shortest wavelengths, includes **alternating current (AC)** power, radio, television, radar (these four wavelengths are visible) infrared, ultraviolet, gamma x-rays, and x-rays (these four wavelengths are not visible). These various types of electromagnetic radiation differ in **wavelength, frequency, and energy.** X-radiation, which is the shortest wavelength, has high frequency and high energy. On the opposite end of the spectrum, radio waves have the longest wavelength, the lowest frequency, and the least energy.

The electromagnetic spectrum exhibits two wavelengths:

1. Short wavelength = high frequency = high energy = high penetrating ability = the ability to penetrate thick or dense objects (i.e., x-rays).
2. Long wavelength = low frequency = low energy = low penetrating ability = does not have the ability to penetrate dense objects (i.e., radio waves).

Relationship of kVp with Wavelength and Penetrating Power

A high **kilovoltage (kVp)** (i.e., 75-90 kVp) setting produces a high-energy, high-frequency, and short wavelength x-ray. The more energy, the more conversions will occur, the more actual x-rays will be produced, and the greater will be the ability of the x-ray to penetrate thick or dense objects. The resultant radiographic film image has a **long-scale contrast** that exhibits more shades of gray, less blacks and less whites. This long-scale contrast image enables the practitioner to view details in the periodontium and the tooth layers. A **short-scale contrast** film image is the result of a low kVp setting (i.e., 65-70 kVp); this image has less energy and less ability to penetrate thick or dense objects. A short-scale contrast image has more blacks and whites and less shades of gray. The practitioner would be less able to view subtle, distinct layers of the tooth and supporting structures.

Energy conversions, which are produced by an **AC radiology machine**, alternate back and forth-AC to **direct current (DC)** and back-resulting in **heterogeneous (different) wavelengths**. This type of current has been the standard of dental radiology machines for many years. **Homogenous radiation**, on the other hand, is produced by more recent dental radiology machines. These machines produce DC with the same kinetic energies as do AC machines, but with 20% less radiation exposure to the patient.

Types of X-Ray Production

Dental radiographic machines produce two types of radiation: **general radiation (bremsstrahlung radiation)** and **characteristic radiation**. Approximately 90% of the radiation produced by dental radiology machines is called **general radiation, bremsstrahlung radiation,** or "braking radiation."

Braking radiation describes the radiation produced by the deceleration (slowing down) of high-speed electrons, which causes them to lose kinetic energy. The emitted energy is in the form of x-rays.

Characteristic radiation consists of an electron from the cathode (E1) hitting an electron on the inner shell (K) of the tungsten target atom (anode), which causes an electron (E2) to be ejected. The loss of an electron causes the tungsten atom to become unstable, excited, and ionized. Characteristic radiation makes up approximately 10% of the x-radiation emitted from the anode (tungsten atom).

How Are X-Rays Produced Inside the X-Ray Machine Tubehead?

The x-ray machine **tubehead** contains the components, cathode and anode, which generate **electrons** that eventually become x-radiation. These components magnetically attract the bundles of energy from the negative side of the tubehead-the **cathode-**to the positive side of the tubehead-the **anode-**and then direct the bundles of kinetic energy called **photons** out the tubehead opening. X-rays leave the tubehead through the **window, port,** and the **beam indicating device (BID),** or **collimator** (these phrases are interchangeable) to the patient or object.

Within the tubehead of the x-ray machine (**Figure 11-1**), the **tungsten filament** and the **molybdenum focusing cup** are located on the cathode (negative) side. When the machine is plugged into an electrical socket and the switch is turned on, the tungsten filament generates an **electron cloud** around the tungsten filament. This process is called **thermionic emission.** When the exposure button is set for the appropriate time and is activated, the anode (positive) side of the tubehead attracts the electrons from the cathode (negative) side. Once the electrons are attracted to the anode, they hit the precise spot on the **tungsten target** called the **focal point or focal spot.** The manufacturer's specifications of the focal point or spot determine the shape of the resultant x-ray beam and influence the sharpness of the resultant film image. The smaller the focal point, the sharper is the image. The focal point is the site at which electrons are transformed into x-rays.

An extensive amount of heat is generated by this electron activity. Therefore, the anode tungsten target is embedded in a **copper stem** to dissipate the heat and to prevent the tubehead from overheating. According to radiology physicists, when electrons are transformed into x-rays, 1% of this energy becomes x-radiation and 99% becomes heat. The excessive heat produced must be absorbed and dissipated through the copper stem to the **oil casing** in the **leaded, glass housing** of the x-ray tube. The heat is dissipated by the oil inside the tubehead, which is located between the leaded glass and the metal exterior of the tubehead.

The x-ray generator consists of two separate components-the **x-ray control panel** and the **tubehead assembly**. The control panel includes the on-off switch, the exposure button, the mA and kVp selector dial, the time selector, the x-ray emission light, and the pilot light. The tubehead assembly includes the low-voltage transformer, high-voltage transformer, and the x-ray tube. These components are immersed in oil owing to the excessive amount of heat generated in the tubehead.

Aluminum Filter

The remaining 1% of x-radiation leaves the x-ray tubehead by passing through an **aluminum filter** and a **lead collima-**

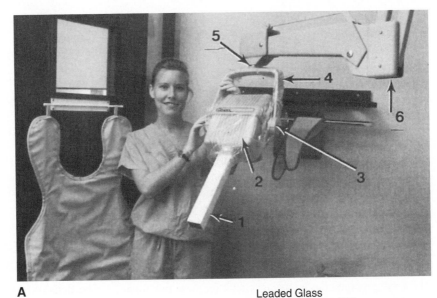

Figure 11-1. *A,* **Tubehead and extension arm of Gendex dental x-ray machine**. (1) Long, rectangular beam indicating device (BID), (2) tubehead (includes transformers and x-ray tube), (3) vertical rotation, (4) x-ray tube yoke, (5) horizontal rotation, and (6) extension arm. *B,* **Dental x-ray head, tube, and cone (BID).** The components of the x-ray generator. The x-ray tube is immersed in oil to prevent sparking from one electrical component to another and to disperse the heat from the copper sleeve of the anode. (*A* and *B,* From Langland OE, Langlais RP: Principles of Dental Imaging. Philadelphia, Williams & Wilkins, 1997, p 29.)

tor before exiting through the BID. The purpose of the aluminum filter is to absorb (filter out) the nonuseful, less penetrating, less energetic, long wavelength x-rays that are absorbed by the patient. These nonuseful x-rays increase the radiation dose to the patient in the form of **scatter radiation** and contribute to **film fog,** which decreases the sharpness of the film image.

Inherent filtration provided by the glass in the tubehead plus the **additional filtration** placed between the focal spot and the patient (the object being radiographed) can enhance the absorption of low-energy photons. The inherent and additional filtration, called **total filtration**, is expressed in **millimeters of aluminum** (mm Al). The minimum amount of total filtration is dependent upon the kVp of the x-ray machine. If the machine is 69 kVp or less, the aluminum filter must be

at least 1.5 mm of aluminum equivalent. If the machine is 70 kVp or more, the aluminum filter must be at least 2.5 mm of aluminum equivalent. These standards are established by the National Council on Radiation Protection and Measurements (NCRP report 35. Washington, D.C., NCRP, 1970).[1]

Lead Collimator

The **lead collimator** is the second layer of metal that x-radiation passes through before exiting through the BID to the patient. To **collimate** means to restrict or limit. To collimate an x-ray beam is to restrict the cross-section of the beam with a lead diaphragm to the diameter of not greater than 2.75 inches or 7 cm. Using a rectangular lead collimator (BID) reduces the overall patient exposure to radiation by

55%.[1] A rectangular collimator also reduces scatter radiation, decreases film fog, and produces a clearer film image.

Use of Electricity by the Radiology Machine

The electricity used by the x-ray machine usually operates from an AC in which the electricity runs in one direction and then reverses in the opposite direction. This is called an **AC**. However, dental x-ray machines run most efficiently on **DC** in which the electric current runs in one direction only. Therefore, the dental x-ray machine can self-rectify and change AC to DC during the production of x-rays.

The electricity used by a dental x-ray machine has two functions: (1) to boil electrons from the tungsten filament on the cathode side, and (2) to generate, accelerate, and direct the electrons from the cathode to the anode side of the tubehead. The x-ray generator has a separate circuit for these two functions. The filament circuit depends on the **step-down transformer** and the voltage circuit depends on the **step-up transformer**. A **transformer** (step-up and step-down) is a device that changes the AC from a low voltage to a high voltage or vice versa. The step-down transformer decreases the voltage from 110 to 220 volts, which provides a high current of 3 to 5 Ångstroms (Å) to heat the filament. Therefore, the step-down transformer operates primarily as the electricity comes into the tubehead. It serves to heat the tungsten filament in the x-ray tube, thus producing a high current of electrons that are attracted to the anode. The step-up transformer takes the 110 or 220 volts and increases the voltage to 65,000 to 90,000 kilovolts peak (kVp)(i.e., 65-90 kVp), which determines the speed at which the electrons in the electron cloud accelerate to the tungsten target on the opposite side. An **autotransformer** varies the voltage output on a variable kilovoltage x-ray machine.

Settings on the X-Ray Machine That Control the Energy and Number of X-Ray Electrons Produced

The common settings on an x-ray machine are the **kVp, milliamperage (mA),** and **exposure time (seconds or impulses)**. Some x-ray machines are manufactured with these three settings as variable (the operator must use available information; i.e., the type of x-ray, the x-ray exposure area, the size of the patient, the film speed, and the length of the BID to establish the setting). Other x-ray machines have preset kVp and mA settings with the exposure time being the only variable setting. The type of x-ray machine determines the protocol.

Effects of X-Ray Machine Settings on Radiographic Density and Contrast

The **density** of a radiographic film refers to the **degree of "blackness"** on the film. Density of the film depends on the amount of radiation **attenuated** or **absorbed** by the object **(Figure 11-2A).** If the object is dense (i.e., bone), very few x-rays pass through the object to bombard the **silver halide crystals** in the film emulsion, and the resultant image is **light** or **radiopaque**. If the object is not dense (i.e., soft tissue), the x-rays pass through the object and bombard the silver halide crystals in the film emulsion. The resultant radiographic image is **dark** or **radiolucent**. Density is influenced by the setting of the machine and the type of tissues irradiated. Density is controlled by mA, kVp, the source-to-film distance, film speed, processing conditions, intensifying screens, and grids.

Effect of kVp on the Film Image

The **contrast** of a radiographic film refers to the **differences in the densities** seen on the film. Contrast can also be de-

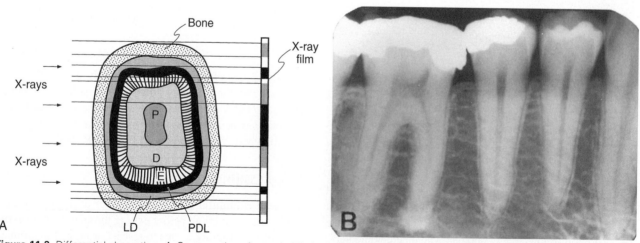

Figure 11-2. Differential absorption. *A,* Cross-section of a tooth: LD, lamina dura; PDL, periodontal ligament space; E, enamel; D, dentin; P, pulp. The enamel and lamina dura completely absorb radiation, and dentin partially absorbs radiation. Pulp and periodontal ligament transmit most of the radiation, because those tissues absorb very little radiation. *B,* Radiograph of mandibular premolar region. Pulp and periodontal ligament spaces are black (radiolucent); lamina dura and enamel are white (radiopaque). Dentin is gray. (From Langland OE, Langlais RP: Principles of Dental Imaging. Philadelphia, Williams & Wilkins, 1997, p 38.)

fined as the number of grays between the extremes of black and white. Contrast is determined primarily by the kilovolt setting and secondarily by the type of film, the processing solutions, and the type of tissue irradiated. A high kVp setting produces a long-scale contrast film image. A low kVp setting produces a short-scale contrast film image. A high kVp setting produces short wavelength primary radiation, in which the penetration of the radiation is greater and the density differences are small. This film image is better to detect subtle bone or tooth tissue changes and allows the practitioner to see more details. A low kVp setting produces long wavelength primary radiation, in which the penetration of the radiation is less and the density differences are great (**Table 11-1**). For instance, a checkered black-and-white flag to indicate the "start" of a race is an example of short-scale contrast or high contrast. High contrast is not well suited to visualize subtle or detailed changes in the bone or tooth (**Figure 11-3**)

Effect of mA on the Film Image

The **mA** primarily controls the **quantity** or the number of x-rays available to be attracted from the cathode to the anode side in the tubehead. Although the kVp setting primarily controls the film image contrast, the **density** of the film image varies directly in proportion to the mA and exposure time. An increase in the mA results in an increase in the density of the film image.

Effect of Exposure Time (S or I) on the Film Image

The **exposure time** controls the **length of time** that x-rays are **produced** and **emitted** from the tubehead toward the patient. The electronic timer is measured in **seconds** or **impulses**. The length of time x-rays are produced is directly proportional to the quantity of x-rays delivered (**beam in-**

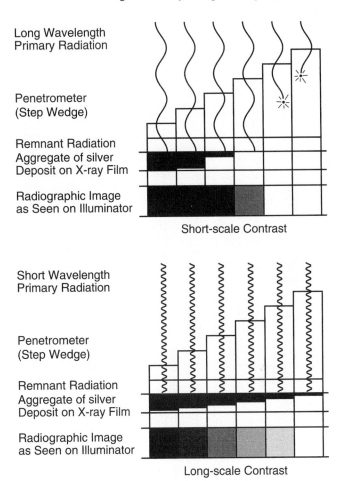

Figure 11-3. **Contrast by a penetrometer.** Comparison of long-scale and short-scale contrast using a penetrometer. *Short-Scale Contrast:* If the kVp is low (e.g., 65 kVp), a greater percentage of longer wavelengths will be produced and penetration will be less. The density differences between adjacent areas will be great, and the film will have short-scale contrast. There will be fewer shades of gray between the lighter and the darker areas of the radiographic image. *Long-Scale Contrast:* If the kVp is high (e.g., 90 kVp), a greater percentage of shorter wavelengths will be produced and the penetration of the x-rays will be greater. The density difference of adjacent areas are small, and the film will have what is called a long-scale contrast. (From Langland OE, Langlais RP: Principles of Dental Imaging. Philadelphia, Williams & Wilkins, 1997, p 52.)

tensity). Exposure time and film speed vary inversely; increasing the film speed decreases the exposure time.

Exposure Time Conversions

An x-ray machine exposure time setting is designated as either **impulses** or **seconds**. To convert seconds to impulses or impulses to seconds, a simple mathematics equation is used with the following equivalency of 60 impulses being equal to 1 second.

1. To **convert impulses to seconds**: divide the number of impulses by 60.

TABLE 11–1 Effect of Kilovoltage (kVp) on the Film Image

HIGH KVP SETTING CHARACTERISTICS	LOW KVP SETTING CHARACTERISTICS
≥75–90 kVp	<70 kVp
Short wavelength energy	Long wavelength energy
High-frequency wavelength	Low-frequency wavelength
High-energy x-rays	Low-energy x-rays
More penetrating x-rays	Less penetrating x-rays
"Hard" x-rays	"Soft" x-rays
"Useful" x-rays	"Non-useful" x-rays
Long-scale contrast	Short-scale contrast
More shades of gray	Less shades of gray
Less blacks and whites	More blacks and whites
More detail on the film	Less detail on the film
Low contrast	High contrast

TABLE 11-2 Kodak Exposure Guidelines for Kodak Ekta-Speed and Ultra-Speed Dental Film

APPROXIMATE EXPOSURE IN IMPULSES

Exposure Factors	70 kV 7 mA		65 kV 10 mA		70 kV 10 mA		80 kV 10 mA		90 kV 10 mA		65 kV 15 mA		70 kV 15 mA		80 kV 15 mA		90 kV 15 mA		Factors for This Office		
PATIENT	ADULT*	ADULT*	ADULT*	ADULT*	ADULT*	ADULT*	ADULT*	ADULT*	ADULT*	ADULT*	ADULT*	ADULT*	ADULT*	ADULT*	ADULT*	ADULT*	ADULT*	ADULT*	kV ADULT	mA ADULT	CHILD
SOURCE-IMAGE DISTANCE	8"	12"	8"	16"	8"	16"	8"	16"	8"	16"	8"	16"	8"	12"	8"	16"	12"	16"			
REGION / VERTICAL ANGLE																					
Maxillary																					
Incisor +40°	13	30	15	37	9	37	7	27	6	24	10	24	6	14	4	18	9	16			
Cuspid +45°	13	30	15	37	9	37	7	27	6	24	10	24	6	14	4	18	9	16			
Bicuspid +30°	17	38	19	47	12	47	8	34	7	30	13	30	8	18	6	23	11	20			
Molar +20°	19	43	22	54	14	54	10	39	9	35	15	35	9	20	7	26	13	23			
Mandibular																					
Incisor −15°	11	24	12	29	7	29	5	21	5	19	8	19	5	11	4	14	7	13			
Cuspid −20°	11	24	12	29	7	29	5	21	5	19	8	19	5	11	4	14	7	13			
Bicuspid −10°	11	26	13	32	8	32	6	23	5	20	8	20	5	12	4	15	8	14			
Molar −5°	13	30	15	37	9	37	7	27	6	24	10	24	6	14	4	18	9	16			
Anterior Bite-Wing																					
Size 1 Adult +8°	11	24	12	29	7	29	5	21	5	19	8	19	5	11	4	14	7	13			
Size 1 Child +8°	7	16	8	20	5	20	4	14	3	13	5	13	3	7	2	10	5	8			
Posterior Bite-Wing																					
Size 2 or 3 Adult +8°	13	30	15	37	9	37	7	27	6	24	10	24	6	14	4	18	9	16			
Size 0 Child +8°	9	20	10	25	6	25	4	18	4	16	7	16	4	9	3	12	6	10			

CONVERSION CHART

Fractions	1/60	1/30	1/20	1/15	1/12	1/10	1/8	1/6	1/5	1/4	3/10	1/3
Decimals			0.05			0.10	0.15		0.20	0.25	0.30	
Impulses	1	2	3	4	5	6	8	10	12	15	16	18	20
Fractions	7/20	3/8	2/5	5/12	9/20	7/15	1/2	7/12	3/5	5/8	13/20	2/3	7/10
Decimals	0.35	0.40	0.45	0.50	0.55	0.60	0.65	0.70
Impulses	21	24	25	27	28	30	32	33	35	36	39	40	42
Fractions	11/15	3/4	4/5	17/20	13/15	7/8	9/10	14/15	11/12	19/20	1	1-1/4	1-1/2
Decimals	0.75	0.80	0.85	0.90	0.95	1.00	1.25	1.50
Impulses	44	45	48	51	52	54	55	56	57	60	75	90

(Continued)

TABLE 11–2 Kodak Exposure Guidelines for Kodak Ekta-Speed and Ultra-Speed Dental Film (Continued)

kodak eKTASPEED

REGION / VERTICAL ANGLE		70 kV 7 mA		65 kV 10 mA	70 kV 10 mA		80 kV 10 mA		90 kV 10 mA		65 kV 15 mA		70 kV 15 mA		80 kV 15 mA		90 kV 15 mA		Factors for This Office	
EXPOSURE FACTORS																			kV	mA
PATIENT		ADULT*	ADULT	ADULT*	ADULT*	ADULT	ADULT*	ADULT	ADULT*	ADULT	ADULT*	ADULT	ADULT*	ADULT	ADULT*	ADULT	ADULT*	ADULT	ADULT	CHILD
SOURCE-IMAGE DISTANCE		8"	12"	8"	8"	16"	8"	16"	8"	16"	8"	12"	8"	12"	8"	16"	12"	16"		
		APPROXIMATE EXPOSURE IN IMPULSES																		
Maxillary																				
Incisor	+40°	7	16	8	5	20	4	14	3	13	5	12	3	7	2	10	5	8		
Cuspid	+45°	7	16	8	5	20	4	14	3	13	5	12	3	7	2	10	5	8		
Bicuspid	+30°	9	20	10	6	25	4	18	4	16	7	16	4	9	3	12	6	10		
Molar	+20°	10	22	11	7	27	5	20	4	17	7	16	5	10	3	13	6	12		
Mandibular																				
Incisor	−15°	5	12	6	4	15	3	11	2	9	4	9	2	6	2	7	4	6		
Cuspid	−20°	5	12	6	4	15	3	11	2	9	4	9	2	6	2	7	4	6		
Bicuspid	−10°	6	14	7	4	17	3	12	3	11	5	11	3	6	2	8	4	7		
Molar	−5°	7	16	8	5	20	4	14	3	13	5	11	3	7	2	10	5	8		
Anterior Bite-Wing																				
Size 1 Adult	+8°	5	12	6	4	15	3	11	2	9	4	9	2	6	2	7	4	6		
Size 1 Child	+8°	4	8	4	2	10	2	7	2	6	3	6	2	4	2	5	2	4		
Posterior Bite-Wing																				
Size 2 or 3 Adult	+8°	7	16	8	5	20	4	14	3	13	5	12	3	7	3	10	5	8		
Size 0 Child	+8°	4	10	5	3	12	2	9	2	8	3	7	2	5	2	6	3	5		

*Children: Reduce adult exposure time about one quarter. DC x-ray generators: Reduce exposure time about one third. Edentulous areas: Reduce exposure time about one third.

To avoid fractional impulses, some 8" exposure times have been rounded off to whole numbers. Mathematically, these 8" times will not comply with the inverse square law in relation to the 16" exposure times.

The above guidelines were developed following recommended time-temperature processing with Kodak chemicals. Method to compute mAs or mAi: mAs is the product of milliamperage times seconds of exposure; mAi is the product of milliamperage times the impulses of energy. If the product is the same in either case, the quantity of radiation produced is essentially the same.

Examples

mA × sec = mAs; mA × imp = mAi

10 × 1/2 = 5; 10 × 30 = 300

15 × 1/3 = 5; 15 × 20 = 300

2. To **convert seconds to impulses**: multiply the number of seconds by 60.

For example, a radiograph is exposed at 7 mA and 12 impulses. To convert the 12 impulses to seconds, divide 12 by 60, which is equal to 0.2 second. On the other hand, to convert 0.2 second to impulses, multiply by 60, which is equal to 12 impulses.

Given a conversion problem with mA and impulse settings, it is first essential to convert impulses to seconds in order to respond to a question regarding mAs. If the question requests mAi and the information is given in impulses, it is not necessary to make a conversion.

Increasing the exposure time to comply with the inverse square law is acceptable when the BID is increased from 8 to 16 inches (which occurs with new machines). It is important to use an exposure chart to guide the exposure time decisions, because the increased exposure time is inversely proportional to the longer BID. See the Kodak Exposure Chart in **Table 11-2**.

Relationship of Exposure Time to mA

Because the mA and exposure time together have a direct effect on the quantity of x-ray photons in the beam, they are combined to form one factor called **milliampere-second (mAs) or milliampere-impulse (mAi)**. This factor has the greatest effect on the quantity of radiation produced and the density of the radiographic image. The change of one factor necessitates the change of another factor to maintain appropriate film density. For example, 15 mA with a 1-second exposure time results in 15 mAs (15 × 1). Likewise, 10 mA with a 1.5-second exposure time results in 15 mAs (10 × 1.5). The higher the mA setting, the greater is the number of x-rays generated. Likewise, if the exposure time is longer, the greater is the time that x-rays will strike the film. The result is that more silver halide crystals are exposed to radiation.

An increase in mA or exposure time results in:

1. Increased quantity of x-rays produced (darker)
2. Increased intensity of the x-ray beam (darker)
3. Increased density of the film image (darker)

For example, a radiograph is exposed to 15 mA and 90 kVp with an exposure time of 0.25 second. A second radiograph is exposed with a new exposure time of 0.75 second. In order to maintain the same density, what is the new mA setting? The first film exposure, 15 mA is multiplied by 0.25 second, which equals 3.75 mAs. Now, divide the 3.75 mAs by 0.75 second, which is equal to 5 mA. The new mA setting is 5. Because the exposure time increased, the mA setting must be decreased for the two films to have the same density. Because the kVp is a constant, it is not necessary to include this variable in the calculations.

Relationship of Exposure Time to X-Ray Source to Film Distance (Length of BID)

Although increasing the exposure time is not ethically appropriate, increasing the exposure time with an increased x-ray source to film distance or the length of the BID does not expose the patient to more radiation. The increased length of the BID and the increased exposure time refer to the **inverse square law,** which maintains compliance with the **as low as reasonably achievable (ALARA) principle** (see Table 11-2). Therefore, use of the inverse square law actually exposes the patient to the lowest dose of radiation that is reasonably achievable.

The **inverse square law** is a concept that adds to the list of variables that must be considered when exposing radiographic films. The inverse square law refers to the combined effect of the **intensity of the x-ray beam** and the **exposure time**. This effect varies based on the "x-ray source to the film distance" (the length of the BID). To maintain a constant density of the film image without changing the mA or kVp, the distance of the x-ray source to the film may be changed. In other words, if you double the distance between the source of the radiation (tubehead) to the film (i.e., change the 8-inch BID to a 16-inch BID), you must increase the exposure time by 4 (i.e., multiply by 4), because the x-rays have longer "travel time." If you halve the distance between the source of the radiation (tubehead) to the film (i.e., change the 16-inch BID to an 8-inch BID), you must decrease the exposure time by one quarter (i.e., divide by 4). The "travel time" is less because the distance that the radiation travels is less.

Example 1: Office A uses an 8-inch BID, E speed film, and a chart to identify the correct exposure time based on the film exposure site. Office B uses a 16-inch BID and E speed film but does not use a chart to identify the correct exposure time per film. To calculate this exposure time change in order to comply with ALARA, use the exposure times from Office A and multiply each by 4 to appropriately expose the films on the patients in Office B. If this example were reversed, use the settings from Office B and divide by 4 to get the correct settings for Office A.

The conversions for the example cited above is as follows. A radiograph is exposed using an 8-inch BID with an exposure time of 0.5 second. A second radiograph is exposed using a 16-inch BID. What is the new exposure time? Multiply the initial $8/16$ (0.5 second) by 4, which is equal to $4/2$ or 2 seconds. The new exposure time for the 16-inch BID is 2 seconds.

Upon changing the x-ray source to film distance from 8 to 16 inches, the intensity of the x-ray beam is decreased and the exposure time should be increased. On the other hand, if the x-ray source-to-film distance is decreased from 16 to 8 inches, the intensity of the x-ray beam is increased and the exposure time should be decreased.

TABLE 11–3 Geometric Characteristics of Radiographic Films

CHARACTERISTIC	DEFINITION	DETERMINING FACTOR	RESULT OF ERROR
Sharpness	Detail resolution; definition	Focal spot size; movement of the film or the patient	Penumbra; unsharpness; blurring
Magnification	Enlargement of image	Diverging x-ray beam; target to film distance should be long; object to film distance should be short	Enlargement of image
Distortion	Image is not the true size or shape	Film alignment with object should be parallel; angle of the x-ray beam should be perpendicular to the tooth and the film	Elongation; foreshortening; enlarge or smaller image

Example 2: The first radiograph is exposed using an 8-inch BID at 4 seconds. A second radiograph is exposed using a 4-inch BID. While maintaining the same density, what is the new exposure time? According to the inverse square law, when decreasing the BID length by half, you must divide the exposure time by 4. Four seconds divided by 4 is equal to 1 second. The new exposure time is 1 second.

Relationship of Exposure Time to kVp

The exposure time and the kVp are related. If the kVp is increased by 15, the exposure time must decrease by one half to maintain an appropriate film density. Likewise, if the kVp is decreased by 15, the exposure time must be doubled to maintain an appropriate film density. This is often referred to as the **rule of 15**.

The Rule of 15

To increase contrast and maintain the original density:

1. Decrease the original kVp by 15.
2. Use twice the original exposure time.

   To decrease contrast and maintain the original density:

1. Increase the original kVp by 15.
2. Use one half of the original exposure time.

For example, a periapical film image is exposed using 75 kVp at 0.5 second. To maintain the same density for a second periapical film image exposed at 90 kVp, the exposure time would be decreased to 0.25 second.

Geometric Characteristics of Radiographic Images

The three geometric characteristics of radiographic images include sharpness, magnification, and distortion (**Table 11-3**).

1. Sharpness refers to the detail, resolution, or definition of the radiographic image that is determined by the focal size spot and by the movement of the film or movement of the patient. The error creates a **penumbra**, which is an unsharpness or blurring of the image.

2. Magnification refers to the enlargement of the image that is determined by the target-to-film distance or the object-to-film distance. The error creates an enlarged image on the x-ray film.

3. Distortion is exhibited when the image is not the true shape or size of the image. Distortion is determined by the film alignment with the object and the angle of the x-ray beam. The error creates an elongated, foreshortened, or enlarged image on the x-ray film.

Visual Characteristics of Radiographic Images

The four visual characteristics of radiographic images are radiolucency, radiopacity, contrast, and density.

The term **radiolucent** refers to a portion of the processed x-ray film that is dark or black. This becomes evident when the object in the path of the x-ray beam lacks density, thus permitting x-radiation to pass through the object to the film with little or no resistance (i.e., the maxillary sinus, mental foramen). Upon processing the film, the developing solution acts on the exposed silver halide crystals; it converts them into black metallic silver, resulting in dark areas on the film.

The term **radiopaque** refers to the area of processed x-ray film that is light or white. Due to the density of some structures, such as metal (amalgam) restoration, enamel, and bone, radiation is absorbed and does not pass through the object to the film. During film processing, the developing solution chemicals do not affect the unexposed silver halide crystal. The fixer solution washes away or clears the unexposed crystals and leaves the area on the radiographic film clear.

Radiolucent and Radiopaque Visual Characteristics with Regard to Soft and Hard Tissues, Teeth, and Materials

Soft tissues are less dense than bone or enamel and only slightly attenuate the x-ray beam as it passes through the object. Radiographically, soft tissues appear black or dark on the processed film and are called **radiolucent**. Soft tissue is not generally visible on a processed film (i.e., gingival

TABLE 11–4 Radiographic Appearance of Dental Materials: Tissues and Materials Correlated with Radiographic Appearance

TISSUES AND MATERIALS	ENAMEL	DENTIN	CEMENTUM	PULP	AMALGAM	CAST GOLD	IMPLANTS	COMPOSITE	GLASS IONOMER	CEMENTS	BANDS	GUTTA PERCHA	SEALANTS	PORCELAIN	OTHER CERAMICS
Radiographic Appearance															
Radiopaque	X	X			X	X	X	X	X	X	X	X	X		X
Radiolucent		X		X				X		X			X	X	X

Note: Certain categories have some products that are radiolucent and other products that are radiopaque.
Modified from Krouse M, Gladwin SC: Identification and management of restorative dental materials during patient prophylaxis. Dent Hyg 58:456, 1984.

papilla). The less dense the tissue or material, the less radiation is absorbed by the tissue or material. When the primary beam of radiation strikes the film, it is translated into a dark or radiolucent area on the film (see Figure 11-2B).

Hard tissues are dense and compact. Dense tissues **attenuate** (absorb) the x-ray beam. The less dense the tissue or material, the less radiation is allowed to penetrate and expose the film. The denser the tissue, the more radiation is absorbed by the tissue. This translates into a light or radiopaque area on the x-ray film (i.e., metal restoration, enamel) (**Table 11-4**).

When properly viewing the processed x-ray film, the radiologic appearance of tooth enamel is light (radiopaque). The dentin is less dense and less radiopaque than the enamel; the dental pulp is least dense and appears dark or radiolucent. The alveolar bone is a combination of trabecular bone and compact bone. The trabecular bone consists of shades of gray and a combination of opacities and lucencies. Compact bone may be considered more radiopaque than trabecular bone.

Some dental materials (metals) are opaque. Other materials have opacities similar to those of dentin and enamel. Differentiating a radiopaque dental material from enamel or dentin is accomplished by comparing the shape of the radiopacity to the expected anatomic features of the tooth. The same can be said for radiolucencies, but the possibility of caries complicates the identification. Information from the clinical examination must also be considered when differentiating opacities and lucencies from normal anatomy.

Dental caries destroys the tooth's calcified tissues. Destruction of the calcified tissues of the tooth (i.e., the enamel, dentin, and cementum) results in dental caries. Radiographically, the carious area is radiolucent when compared with enamel or dentin. The diagnostician must view the radiographs in an appropriate viewing situation with a critical eye to differentiate among normal tooth anatomy, various densities of restorations, and disease.

Dental materials that are used in restorative procedures may include amalgam, cast gold, cohesive gold (gold foil), nonprecious alloys, dental resins, porcelain crowns, porcelain fused to metal crowns, stainless steel crowns, luting cements, and cements used as bases and liners and sealants. The denser the material, the more the x-ray beam is attenuated by the material and the more opaque the object is revealed on the x-ray film.

Restorative materials that are clearly radiopaque include amalgam, cast gold, cohesive gold, nonprecious alloys, and porcelain fused to metal crowns. Stainless steel crowns and aluminum temporary crowns may be radiopaque, depending on the thickness of the material. Radiopaque restorative materials that appear as lighter shades of gray include composite resins, dental sealants, cements, and bases depending on the product.

Radiolucent restorative materials appear radiolucent due to the lack of density. These materials include temporary crowns or bridges that are made of acrylic or plastic and tooth-colored materials (e.g., resins and porcelain crowns). Due to varying compositions, cements used for luting and bases may appear darker (radiolucent) or lighter (radiopaque) than the overlying restoration. Radiolucent bases under a metal restoration, particularly amalgam, and excessive adhesive materials under composites may imitate a carious lesion on the radiograph.

Endodontic therapy is performed with various instruments. The metal materials that appear radiographically radiopaque include endodontic files, retrofill amalgams, EBM cement, rubber dam clamps and frame, metal post materials, gutta percha, silver points, endodontic sealers, a dowel pin or retentive post, and some film-holding devices.

Metal orthodontic materials used in dentistry are primarily stainless steel orthodontic bands, brackets, and wires. Other radiopaque materials used in orthodontic treatment include springs, fixed and removable retainers, space maintainers, appliances used to discourage oral habits, and bite planes.

Radiopaque surgical items include dental implants, implant fixtures, healing caps, wires, plates or screws for stabilization, and some tissue replacement materials[2] (see Table 11-4).

Density and Contrast as Visual Characteristics on Radiographs

Variables that affect both radiographic density and contrast in varying degrees include: mA, kVp, exposure time, dental anatomy, head and neck anatomy, film speed, film processing, source-to-film distance, source-to-object distance, and the inverse square law.

TECHNIQUE AND EVALUATION OF RADIOGRAPHS

Radiographic Techniques

Two common radiographic techniques include **paralleling** and **bisecting** the angle. The paralleling technique produces a radiographic image that has a better diagnostic value and is least distorted. Bisection of the angle technique produces a radiographic image that is more likely to be distorted, especially in the maxillary arch due to the anatomy of the palate. For patients who have a maxillary torus, a high narrow palate, or a small mouth, bisection of the angle technique is preferred. The mandibular arch is more conducive to the paralleling technique than is the maxilla, except when mandibular tori or a narrow anterior arch form is present.

Rules for an Accurate Radiographic Imaging Using the Paralleling Technique[1]

1. The film should be placed directly behind the teeth that are needed in the film so that it covers the particular teeth being radiographed.
2. The vertical plane of the film should be placed as parallel as possible to the long axes of the teeth that are being radiographed **(Figure 11-4)**.
3. The horizontal plane of the film must be placed parallel to the horizontal plane of the teeth. This may change slightly if the teeth differ in various parts of the mouth, because the teeth form a curved arch.
4. The vertical angulation of the BID is an open-ended, flat surface and is positioned parallel to the film packet. This angulation directs the central beam of the x-ray perpendicular to the plane of the film and the long axes of the teeth. Proper vertical angulation of the BID reduces the shape distortion of the radiographic image (i.e., elongation or foreshortening) (see Figure 11-4).
5. The horizontal positioning of the BID directs the x-rays through the embrasures or contacts between the teeth. Upon correct horizontal placement of the film, position the open-ended flat surface of the BID parallel to the horizontal placement of the film. This directs the x-rays perpendicular to the film **(Figure 11-5)**. Incorrect horizontal placement or angu-

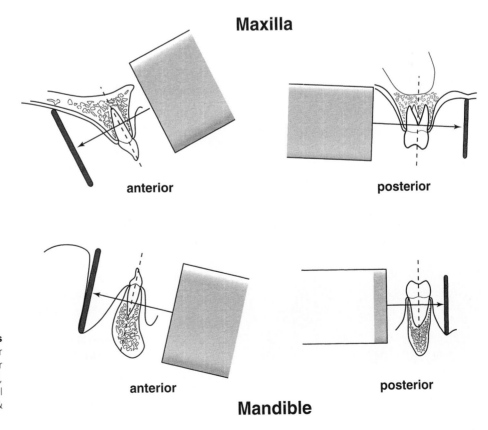

Figure 11-4. Vertical angulations of the BID. Summary of the proper vertical angulation of the BID for each region. (From Langland OE, Langlais RP: Principles of Dental Imaging. Philadelphia, Williams & Wilkins, 1997, p 100.)

Maxilla

anterior   posterior

anterior   posterior

Mandible

Maxilla

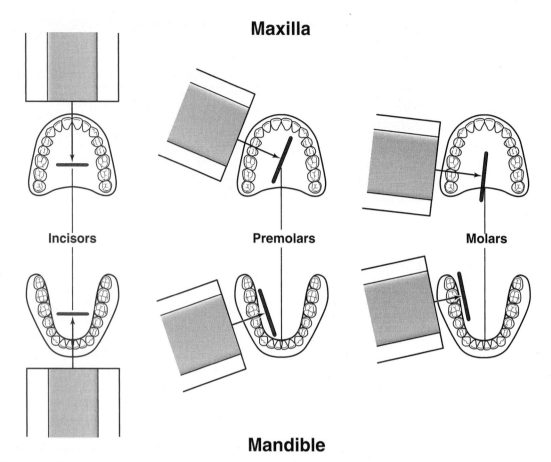

Incisors　　　Premolars　　　Molars

Mandible

Figure 11-5. Horizontal angulation (path of the central ray perpendicular to the horizontal plane of the film). Summary of proper horizontal angulations of the BID and film coverage with an x-ray beam for each region of the jaw. Note the size of the smaller rectangular BID and the size of the larger circular BID. (From Langland OE, Langlais RP: Principles of Dental Imaging. Philadelphia, Williams & Wilkins, 1997, p 93.)

lation of the BID results in horizontal overlapping of the tooth interproximal surfaces **(Figure 11-6).**

6. The central ray of the x-ray beam must be directed to the center of the film to completely cover the film. Incorrect

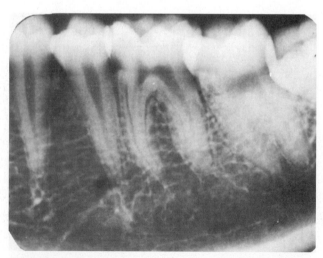

Figure 11-6. Overlapping. Overlapping of mandibular premolars and molars from improper film placement or BID placement. (From Langland OE, Langlais RP: Principles of Dental Imaging. Philadelphia, Williams & Wilkins, 1997, p 93.)

placement of the central ray results in cone-cutting or a partial image of the radiographed area **(Figure 11-7)**

Anatomic Accuracy and Proper Film Coverage in Radiographic Technique[1]

The paralleling technique reveals the following:

1. The labial and lingual cementoenamel junction (CEJ) should be superimposed.
2. The buccal and lingual cusps of posterior teeth should be superimposed.
3. The interproximal contacts between teeth should be open in at least one of the films of the series.
4. The buccal portion of the alveolar crest should be superimposed over the lingual portion of the alveolar crest on the posterior teeth.
5. The zygomatic arch should not be superimposed over the roots of the maxillary molar teeth.

Anatomic Accuracy of the Long-cone Paralleling Technique[1]

The paralleling technique reveals the following:

1. Better superimposition of buccal and lingual cusps (for better caries detection).

2. Better superimposition of the buccal position of the alveolar bone crest over the lingual portion of the alveolar bone crest (better interpretation of the crestal alveolar bone height).
3. Minimal superimposition of zygomatic bone over the roots of the maxillary molar (better for interpreting periapical pathology).
4. Better definition and less magnification (better film for overall interpretation).
5. Minimal foreshortening of the buccal roots of the molars (better for endodontic preoperative and postoperative radiographs).

Quality Radiographic Technique

A full mouth radiographic survey illustrates that specific teeth and periodontal structures need to be present in each film based on the individual needs of the patient.[1]

Radiographic Errors-Cause and Correction: Technique and Processing

Technique, processing, and handling errors constitute the major reasons for retaking radiographs. As Miles and associates state, "do it right the first time."[7]

Technique and processing errors occur for many reasons. Although it is necessary to minimize these errors, it is prudent to be familiar with what the errors looks like, what caused them, and how to correct them.

A summary of intraoral projection and technique errors is given in **Table 11-5.** A guide to the problems encountered with film processing is shown in **Table 11-6,** and a summary of the causes of film handling errors and how to correct these errors is given in **Table 11-7.**

Panoramic Radiography

It is essential to be knowledgeable and to recognize normal radiographic anatomy using the illustration (**Figure 11-8**) and a panoramic radiograph (**Figure 11-9A and B**).

The extraoral radiograph is produced by placing a screen film in a cassette with intensifying screens, placing the cassette in the machine toward the side of the patient's head or face, and projecting the x-rays from the opposite side. The screen film has emulsion on both sides and is sandwiched between the intensifying screens on both sides of the cassette. The intensifying screens contain phosphors that increase the photosensitivity of the film and convert the x-ray beam into visible light. This light then exposes the film to capture the latent image. Therefore, intensifying screens support the ALARA philosophy due to the decreased amount of radiation exposure to the patient (**Figure 11-10A and B**).

Exposing a quality panoramic radiograph necessitates skill and knowledge. From placing the panoramic film into the cassette, through patient set-up, it is essential that the practitioner is attentive to details involving the machine and

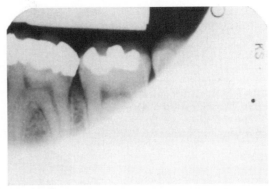

Figure 11-7. Cone-cutting or partial image error. (From Langland OE, Langlais RP: Principles of Dental Imaging. Philadelphia, Williams & Wilkins, 1997, p 174.)

patient positioning. Errors in patient positioning account for most panoramic errors, thus producing a diagnostic radiograph of minimal quality. It is important to read the manufacturer's instructions and guidelines before operating the radiology machine.

Due to the design of the rotational panoramic machine, the projection and principles of operation differ from those of the traditional radiographic machine. **Rotational panoramic radiography** is accomplished by rotating a narrow beam of radiation in the horizontal plane around an invisible rotational axis that is positioned intraorally. A narrow vertical beam is projected at a slight vertical negative angle for the beam to pass beneath the occipital portion of the base of the skull. The primary beam rotates horizontally around the patient's head onto a stationary radiographic film. The film moves in a direction opposite to the horizontal rotation of the beam. The vertical beam and the horizontal rotational center match only when the object lies within a particular plane called the **central plane** or the **image layer**. This **image layer** or **focal trough** is the **zone** or that object point at which the object is in focus (**Figure 11-11**).

When analyzing the image layer, objects that are **buccal or toward the film will be narrowed**, and objects that are **lingual or toward the source will be widened**. Because of the **negative angulation of the beam, buccal objects will be projected lower** and **lingual objects** will be **projected higher than objects in the central plane of the layer.**

These concepts are fundamental to panoramic radiography.

Concept 1: Structures are flattened and spread out.
Concept 2: Midline structures may project as single images or double images.
Concept 3: Ghost images are formed.
Concept 4: Soft tissue shadows are seen.
Concept 5: Air spaces are seen.
Concept 6: Relative radiolucencies and radiopacities are seen.[1]

The five steps of panoramic technique include: (1) request that the patient bite in the bite-block groove, (2) close the side guides bilaterally on the patient's head, (3) position the chin on the chinrest, (4) stand or seat the patient upright, and (5)

TABLE 11–5 Summary of Intraoral Projection and Technique Errors

ERROR	CAUSE	CORRECTION	L + L FIGURE/PAGE
Radiopaque artifacts on the radiograph	Leaving the dental appliance in the mouth or eyeglasses or jewelry on the patient	Ask the patient to remove removable prostheses before placing the films.	Figures 7-2 and 7-3, pp 165 and 166
Blurred image on the radiograph	Movement of the film, patient, or tubehead during exposure	Ask the patient to remain motionless during the exposure.	Figure 7-4, pp 165 and 166
Apical ends of the teeth cut off	• Film placed too close to the teeth in the maxillary arch in the paralleling technique • Too flat (insufficient) vertical angulation, which causes elongation	• Move the film farther away from the teeth in the maxillary arch. • Position the film more apically in the floor of the mouth in the mandibular arch. • Increase vertical angulation.	Figure 7-5, p 166
All of the specific region not showing	Faulty film placement (center the film over the area of interest)	Ensure that the film covers the entire area of interest.	Figure 7-6, p 166
Herringbone effect or ping-pong ball and light density	Printed back side of the film placed toward the beam of radiation (film reversed)	Ensure that the white side of the film packet is toward the BID.	Figure 7-7 A–C, p 168
Black dot in apical area	Manufacturer's identifying depression on the film placed toward the apical area of the teeth (place the "dot in slot" —XCP instrument)	The film ID dot should be placed toward the incisal/occlusal aspect of the teeth.	Figure 7-8 A and B, pp 168 and 169
Double images on radiographs	Film exposed twice to radiation; "use the film cup"	Organize the films to separate exposed and unexposed films.	Figure 7-9, pp 168 and 169
"Phalangioma" (patient's finger in the image)	When holding the film (bisecting angle technique), the finger is placed between the film and the teeth	Avoid the patient holding the film with the finger; position the film between the tongue and the teeth.	Figures 7-10 and 7-11, pp 168–170
Tongue image	Placing the film on top of the tongue		
Overlapping of teeth	• Plane of the film is not parallel to the lingual surface of the teeth • Incorrect horizontal angulation of the cone (BID)	Position the film parallel to the mean tangent of the teeth. Position the BID parallel to the film positioned in the mouth.	Figures 7-12, 7-13, and 7-14, pp 169 and 170
Foreshortening of the image	Bisecting technique: vertical angulation of the cone (BID) too steep (excessive) Paralleling technique: film not parallel with the long axes of the teeth Paralleling technique: the long cone (BID) is not positioned correctly	Decrease the vertical angulation of the BID.	Figure 7-15, pp 170–172
Dimensional distortion of the image	Inherent error in the bisecting angle technique produces elongation of the palatal roots and foreshortening of the buccal roots of the molars in the same view	Use the paralleling technique.	Figure 7-18, p 172
Image distorted severely	The film is bent as the patient bites on the film holder or bite-block.	Avoid too much biting pressure on the film; ensure that the film backing is not buckled.	Figure 7-17, pp 172 and 173
Partial image "cone-cut"	The cone (BID) of radiation is not covering the area of interest.	Ensure that the BID covers the entire film. Ensure that the entire film is immersed in the processing solutions.	Figure 7-19 A–C, pp 172, 173, and 175
Crowns of the teeth not showing	• Not enough file (¹/₈") showing below or above the crowns of the teeth • Vertical angulation too steep	• Ensure that the film covers the entire tooth. • The incisal/occlusal portion of the film should extend ¹/₈" beyond the incisal/occlusal surface of the teeth. Adjust (flatten out) the vertical angulation of the BID.	Figure 7-18 A and B, p 173

BID, beam indicating device; L + L, Langland and Langlais.
Adapted from Langland OE, Langlais RP: Principles of Dental Imaging. Baltimore, Williams & Wilkins, 1997, p 172.

TABLE 11–6 Film Processing Trouble Chart

CONDITION	CAUSE
Low-density (light) films	A. Solution temperature too low
	B. Exhausted developer (underreplenishment)
	C. Underexposed (Technique)
	D. Too much time in fixer solution
High-density (dark) films	A. Solutions overheated or too strong
	B. Light leaks in the processor cover
	C. Overexposed (Technique)
	D. Too much time in developer solution
Wet or tacky films	A. Dryer and developer temperatures too low
	B. Dryer air circulation inadequate (high humidity in dryer section)
	C. Wrong solution chemistry or film
	D. Processing too fast (higher temperature and/or faster roller speed)
Film discoloration (brown)	A. Contamination of fixer by developer solution; insufficient washing after fixing
Film discoloration (greenish yellow)	A. Fixer solution exhausted (underreplenishment)
	B. Processing too fast (higher temperature and/or faster roller speed)
	C. Wrong solution chemistry or film
Fogged films (unwanted density)	A. Incorrect or defective safe-light filter or bulb
	B. Light leaks in the darkroom
	C. Developer temperature too high
	D. Improper storage of films
Streaking (uneven density)	A. Underreplenishment
	B. Rollers encrusted with chemical deposits
	C. Dirty wash water
	D. Film not hardened properly by chemicals
Surface marks	A. Foreign materials or irregularities on the surface of the rollers
	B. Rough handling of the film before processing
Films chalky or dirty	A. No wash water or dirty wash water
	B. Fixer contaminated
Jams or failure of the film to transport	A. Chemicals contaminated or diluted
	B. Chemical temperature too high
	C. Film excessively soft and not adequately hardened; when enough gelatin lubricates the rollers, films will jam up with one another
	D. Dirty rollers
	E. Racks not seated properly
	F. Dirty wash water
	G. Incorrect dryer temperature
	H. Hesitation in the drive assembly, causing the film to pause in transit
	I. Film not tracking through the processor in a straight course (improper feeding of films)
	J. Bent film corners as the leading edge

Adapted from Langland OE, Langlais RP: Principles of Dental Imaging. Baltimore, Williams & Wilkins, 1997, p 181.

ask the patient to place the tongue on the roof of the mouth, swallow, and hold still. The exposure can then be made. Cotton rolls are helpful when there are edentulous areas.

Panoramic Technique Errors

Charts are provided to assist the practitioner in identifying panoramic patient positioning errors (**Table 11-8**) and procedural errors (**Table 11-9**).

Localization Techniques-Special Radiographic Techniques

Localization is necessary to specifically locate an object in the jaw (i.e., impacted supernumerary or unerupted teeth, salivary duct calculi, jaw fractures, foreign bodies, pathoses, retained root tip, broken instrument, broken needle, en-

dodontic tip, or filling materials. Two techniques are available for the practitioner to choose from when attempting to locate the object in the jaw. The two techniques are: (1) the tube-shift method, also called buccal object rule or Clarke rule, and the (2) right angle technique rule.

The **tube-shift method** uses two radiographs exposed at different angles. The first film is exposed using normal procedure, and the second is exposed changing the x-ray beam either horizontally or vertically.

When located horizontally aligned objects (i.e., mandibular canal) the x-ray beam must be changed vertically. The tubehead (BID) angle or x-ray beam is directed from either a positive vertical angle or a negative vertical angulation. If the x-ray beam is directed from a positive vertical angle, the object moves inferiorly (down) if it is located on the buccal; if the object is on the lingual, it will move superi-

TABLE 11–7 Summary of Film Handling Errors

ERROR	CAUSE	CORRECTION	L + L FIGURE/PAGE
Black pressure marks on the film	Teeth marks on the film (especially the pediatric occlusal film)	Request the patient to stabilize the film. Avoid biting into the film.	Figure 7-29, pp 178 and 179
Black bend lines on the film	From bending the film to reduce the patient's discomfort	Avoid excessive bending of the film corners.	Figure 7-29, pp 178 and 179
Black marks on the film	Saliva contamination of the black protective paper covering the film; caused by failure to blot the film packet with a paper towel	• Suction excessive saliva from the patient's mouth. • Wipe saliva off of the film.	Figure 7-31, pp 178 and 179
Black "lightning" or "tree-like" marks on the film	Static electricity; removing the film too rapidly from the packet or box in air with dry humidity	Avoid rapid sliding of the film; use the humidifier; wear rubber-soled shoes.	Figure 7-32, pp 178 and 179
Torn emulsion and scratches on the film	Careless handling of the film during processing when the emulsion is soft and swollen	Handle the film carefully.	Figure 7-33, p 180
Dust and powder artifacts	Film contact with dust, grit, or glove powder before processing	Handle the film with clean hands.	
Fogged film (unwanted density)			Figure 7-34, p 180
A. Light fog	1. Light leaks in the darkroom 2. Improper safe-light; check the bulb wattage, distance, and filter-film compatibility 3. Turning the overhead (white) light on too soon; (be certain that the films have cleared in the fixer first)	• Monitor and comply with the radiographic QA Program. • Comply with the manufacturer's instructions.	
B. Radiation fog	Improper storage; insufficient protection of the film next to the x-ray machine	Monitor and comply with the radiographic QA Program. Comply with the manufacturer's instructions.	
C. Processing (chemical fog)	1. Developer temperatures too high 2. Overstrength developer 3. Prolonged development for temperature 4. Contaminated developer (clean the tank routinely)	• Monitor and comply with the radiographic QA Program. • Comply with the manufacturer's instructions.	
D. Deterioration of the film	1. Temperature of the storage area too high 2. Humidity of the storage area too high 3. Strong fumes (ammonia, paint)	Store films in the refrigerator.	
White ballpoint pen marks	Writing on the front of the film packet with a ballpoint pen	Avoid writing on the film packets.	Figure 7-28, p 178

Adapted from Langland OE, Langlais RP: Principles of Dental Imaging. Baltimore, Williams & Wilkins, 1997, p 181.

orly (up). If the x-ray beam is directed from a negative vertical angle, the object moves superiorly (up) if it is on the buccal and inferiorly (down) if it is on the lingual **(Figure 11-12A)**.

In order to locate vertically aligned images (i.e., root canals), the BID must be changed horizontally. Using the **buccal-object rule** to locate vertically aligned objects, the tube-head (BID) angle or x-ray beam is directed either from a mesial or distal horizontal angulation. Thus, if the object appears to have moved in the same direction as the BID, the object is positioned lingually. If the object appears to have moved in the op-

posite direction of the BID, the object is positioned buccally (see Figure 11-12B).

The pneumonic for this rule is the SLOB rule meaning same-lingual, opposite-buccal. When the two films are compared, the BID angle change confirms the position of the object.

The second rule is the **right angle technique rule**, which compares two films exposed at right angles to each other. The two films are a periapical and an occlusal film. The occlusal film will demonstrate the object as in a buccal-lingual or anterior-posterior relationship. This technique is most commonly used to locate objects in the mandibular arch.

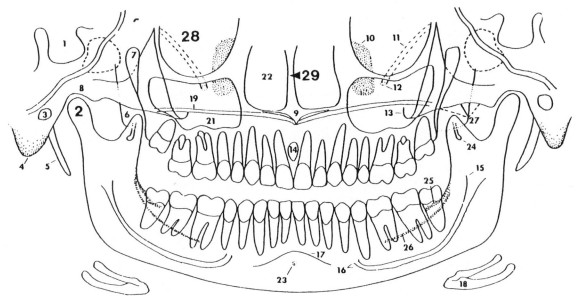

Figure 11-8. Continuous image of anatomic landmarks. Common anatomic structures. Sella turcica (1), mandibular condyle (2), external auditory meatus (3), mastoid process (4), styloid process (5), lateral pterygoid plate (6), pterygomaxillary fissure (7), articular eminence (8), anterior nasal spine (9), ethmoid sinuses (10), infraorbital canal (11), infraorbital foramen (12), zygomatic process of the maxillary (13), incisive or nasopalatine foramen (14), mandibular foramen (15), mandibular canal and mental foramen (16), mental ridge (17), hyoid bone (18), hard palate (19), maxillary sinus (21), nasal fossa (22), genial tubercles (23), hamular process (24), external oblique ridge (25), internal oblique or mylohyoid ridge (26), zygomatic arch (27), orbit (28), and nasal septum (29). (From Langland OE, Langlais RP: Principles of Dental Imaging. Philadelphia, Williams & Wilkins, 1997, p 219.)

PRINCIPLES OF RADIOLOGIC HEALTH (INCLUDING RADIATION PROTECTION AND MEASUREMENT)

Radiation Biology and Patient Safety

Radiation poses risks and harmful effects to the occupational worker, the nonoccupational worker, and the patient. Recommendations of maximum radiation exposure limits are established by the National Council on Radiation Protection and Measurements and are known as **maximum permissible dose (MPD)**. The MPD is the amount of radiation that an individual is allowed to receive from artificial sources of radiation over time, such as x-ray machines, except when the individual is a medical or dental patient. The MPD is established for two groups-the occupational worker (e.g., dental hygienist, dentist, and dental assistant) and the nonoccupational worker (e.g., office staff, family in the waiting room, and the general public). The MPD represents an acceptable low risk of harmful effects to either group. In the case of a pregnant occupational worker, the MPD is lowered to the MPD of a nonoccupational exposed person. Different organs or other body parts have specific MPDs due to their sensitivities to radiation. Refer to the graphs of MPD for various classes of exposed individuals **(Tables 11-10 and 11-11)**.

The MPD is best monitored by the employer, who may choose to subscribe to a radiation dosimetry monitoring service. The service provides an excellent way for the employer to monitor radiation exposure to the dental office staff. The badge worn by the occupational worker contains a lithium fluoride crystal insert that captures radiation exposures. The badge is clipped onto the worker's clothing over the front of the hip or chest. If the occupational worker safety rules regarding radiation exposures were not adhered to or the radiology machine was not properly functioning, the radiation reports from the monitoring service would alert the staff to identify the source of radiation and make corrective actions. The reports also provide the written documentation of staff exposures in the event that it is needed or requested for proof.

Radiation absorbed dose (rad) or **Gray (Gy)** is described as the unit of absorbed dose. It applies to any type of radiation and any absorbing material. It measures the biologic consequences of radiation or the amount of radiation deposited in a specific tissue mass. It does not refer to the radiation with regard to a specific biologic effect. Refer to the graph of conversion units for examples **(Table 11-12)**.

Radiation-equivalent man (rem) or **sievert (Sv)** is the unit of **absorbed dose** that measures the radiation with regard to a specific biologic effect based on three factors: absorbed dose, quality factors, and modifying factors. **Absorbed dose** refers to the ionizing radiation energy deposited in the object according to its size and density. This factor is multiplied by the **quality factor,** which refers to x-

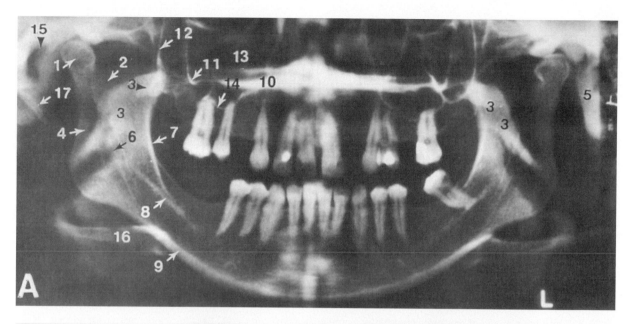

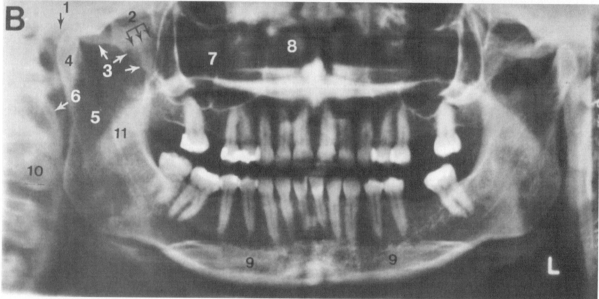

Figure 11-9. Common anatomic structures (panoramic landmarks). *A,* Condyle (1), nasopharyngeal air space (2), soft palate (3), oropharyngeal air space (4) soft tissue of ear (5), glossopalatal air space (6), external oblique ridge (7), mylohyoid (internal oblique) ridge (8), lower border of mandible (9), hard palate (10), lower border of zygomatic (malar) bone (11), posterior wall of maxillary sinus (12), maxillary sinus (antrum) (13), lower border (floor) of maxillary sinus (14), external auditory meatus (15), hyoid bone (16), and stylohyoid bone (17). *B,* Glenoid fossa (1), nasopharyngeal air space (2), zygomatic arch (3), condyle (4), oropharyngeal air space (5), stylohyoid process (6), maxillary sinus (7), inferior turbinate (8), ghost of hyoid bone (9), and spinal column. (10) (From Langland OE, Langlais RP: Principles of Dental Imaging. Philadelphia, Williams & Wilkins, 1997, p 220.)

ray, gamma rays, and alpha particles. This factor is then multiplied by the **modifying factor,** which refers to chemical, physical, and biologic agents. Another way to describe the **Sv** or **rem** is the unit dose of radiation exposure to body tissue when referring to its estimated biologic effects to an exposure of 1 roentgen (R) of x-radiation. For conversation and conversion, 1 Sv is equal to 1 Gy. Refer to graphs for conversion units **(Table 11-13).**

A prudent philosophy to adopt concerning patient safety when using ionizing radiation is the concept of **as low as reasonably achievable (ALARA).** This philosophy pertains to actions taken by the dental practitioner to comply with safety practices when exposing patients to x-radiation. In order to comply with the ALARA principle, it is essential to consider the following factors: x-ray machine settings (i.e., exposure time, mA, and kVp); use of the lead apron and thyroid shield; x-ray film size; x-ray film speed; and length, shape, size, and composition of the BID. In addition, the owner or employer of the dental practice must maintain proper functioning and inspections of the radiology ma-

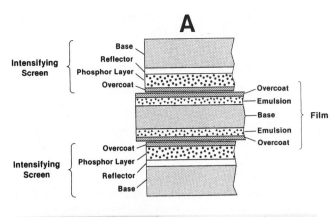

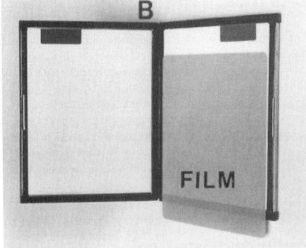

Figure 11-10. Intensifying screens and cassette. *A,* The illustration shows the double-coated film sandwiched between two intensifying screens. All components of film-0xcreen combination are shown but are not drawn to scale. For example, the thickness of the phosphor layer of the top screen may differ from that of the lower screen. *B,* Photograph of an 8 × 10 inch cassette with two white intensifying screens. The film is placed between them in the darkroom, and the cassette is closed tightly to hold the film between the two intensifying screens during exposure. (From Langland OE, Langlais RP: Principles of Dental Imaging. Philadelphia, Williams & Wilkins, 1997, p 277.)

chines in order to produce only the amount of radiation designated by the exposure time, mA, and kVp setting.

Two Types of Radiation Effects on the Biologic Tissue: Direct and Indirect

Direct effects are described as a direct exposure of radiation (a single step) that alters the biologic molecule and results in chemical changes. **Indirect effects** are referred to as an indirect exposure of radiation (two steps) in which the body's water forms free radicals, which result in chemical changes (cell damage). Indirect effects may occur at sites other than those where the radiation exposure occurred.

How Radiation Interacts with Matter at the Atomic Level in Body Tissues

Diagnostic x-ray energy is concerned with how orbital electrons interact with x-ray photons or how orbital electrons interact with the nucleus of the atom. Due to the different interactions of the orbital electrons, the resultant x-rays can either be **absorbed (attenuated)** or **scattered.** There are three types of scatter radiation: **coherent scatter, photoelectric effect,** and **Compton scatter.**

Coherent scatter or **Thomson effect** or **unmodified scatter** refers to a low-energy photon that passes close to an atom of matter, thus causing the atom to vibrate; the x-ray photon neither transfers energy to the matter nor does it harm the matter; the x-ray merely undergoes a change in direction with no energy lost or gained and no damage to the tissue itself.

Photoelectric effect results in the production of **characteristic radiation,** resulting from the movement of atoms within the tissue. This effect consists of electrically unbalanced and unstable ions. The x-ray photon bombards the tissue ejecting an electron from the atom. The x-ray photon is then completely absorbed by the tissue and gives up all of its energy. The vacated electron position is filled by an electron that has a similar or characteristic radiation energy level. This ion produces a free radical, which is the basis for radiation biologic damage to cells and tissues of living organisms.

Compton scatter or **modified scatter** refers to a type of interaction that is responsible for most of the scatter radiation encountered in diagnostic radiology. The x-ray photon collides with an outer shell electron, ejects it from its orbit (Compton electron), and continues in different directions; the x-ray photon interacts with more atoms and causes scattered photons of reduced energy. The Compton effect results in the atom absorbing the radiation energy, becoming an ion, and releasing scatter radiation.

The Compton scatter and the photoelectric effect occur in almost equal proportions in dental radiology. The ionized atoms and recoil electrons of the photoelectric and Compton effect may cause further molecular interactions in the patient's tissues. These **direct effects** may result in breaking molecules into smaller pieces, disrupting molecular bonds, forming new bonds **within** molecules, and forming new bonds **between** molecules.

Time- and Dose-Related Effects of Radiation on the Biologic Tissue

Cell sensitivity refers to the degree that a tissue or organ cell is affected by radiation. Frequently dividing, primitive cells that are most sensitive to radiation and may die after relatively low doses of radiation are referred to as **radiosensitive.** Cells that are harmed less by high doses of radiation are called **radioresistant** cells. Tissue and organ sensitivity are categorized in **Table 11-14.** Critical organs and the resultant disorders from radiation exposure are categorized in Table 11-14.

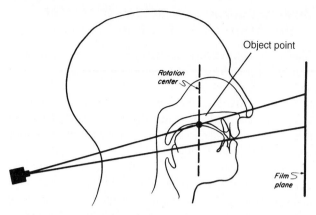

Figure 11-11. Principle of projection in the vertical dimension. The conventional projection of an intraoral radiograph is a central projection. In a central projection, the divergent rays have a common origin the object point. The film is perpendicular to the central ray. (Modified from Langland OE, Langlais RP: Principles of Dental Imaging. Philadelphia, Williams & Wilkins, 1997, p 208.)

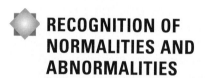

RECOGNITION OF NORMALITIES AND ABNORMALITIES

Normal Radiographic Anatomy

In order to recognize a disease, it is necessary to know what is normal, both clinically and radiographically. Therefore, to recognize periodontal disease on a radiograph, it is imperative to know normal radiographic anatomy.

Enamel is **radiopaque,** and **carious lesions** in enamel are **radiolucent. Dentin** is not as hard as enamel and radiographically appears **radiopaque,** but not as opaque as enamel. The **pulp cavity** and its component parts are **radiolucent,** and the **cementum** is usually **not radiographically apparent (Figure 11-13).**

The **periodontium** consists of: (1) the **gingiva** and **cementum,** which are **not radiographically evident;** (2) the **periodontal ligament space,** which is mainly collagen and refers to the **radiolucent** space between the root of the tooth and the lamina dura; and (3) **alveolar bone** (compact and cancellous bone), which is primarily **radiopaque** with **marrow spaces** in the **cancellous bone** that are radiographically **radiolucent.** The **lamina dura** is the thin **radiopaque** alveolar bone that begins at the alveolar crest and continues around the tooth root to make up the alveolar bone socket of a healthy tooth. The **alveolar crest** is also thin **radiopaque** alveolar bone that extends between the teeth horizontally and signifies healthy bone status. **Nutrient canals,** although normal anatomy, are more prevalent and more radiographically visible in patients who have advanced periodontal disease and hypertension. These canals are **radiolucent** anatomic spaces bordered by the **radiopaque** cortical bone. They run vertically from the interdental canals to the apices

of the tooth roots and are more readily observed in the mandibular arch **(Figure 11-14).**

Role of Radiographs in Detecting Carious Lesions

Dental caries is a pathologic condition in which the calcified portion of the tooth is destroyed. Radiographically, dental caries are less calcified and have decreased density. According to Langland and Langlais, the classification of the radiographic appearance of caries is discussed in relation to the location of the tooth caries (i.e., interproximal, occlusal, facial/lingual, pulpal, root or cemental caries; incipient, recurrent, or secondary caries; and rampant or arrested caries).[1] Because the tooth is a calcified structure, approximately **50% of the calcium and phosphorus must be destroyed** before a decrease in density can be seen radiographically.

The detection of interproximal dental caries is improved with a radiographic survey, particularly using bite-wing films. The initiation of **interproximal enamel caries** is inferior to the contact point. As it progresses, it may form a classic V-shaped radiolucent appearance with the base of the triangle at the surface of the tooth and the rounded apex pointed toward the dentinoenamel junction (DEJ). **Incipient interproximal caries** are detected radiographically as a small, cone-shaped radiolucent area in the outer enamel **(Figure 11-15). Recurrent** or **secondary caries** are seen as radiographic lesions that develop at the margins or in the vicinity of a restoration and may indicate unusual susceptibility to caries, poor oral hygiene, a deficient cavity preparation, a defective restoration, or a combination of these **(Figure 11-16). Dentinal caries** are seen as radiolucent lesions that progress to the DEJ and spread laterally, thus undermining normal enamel. In the dentin, the decay spreads rapidly in a mushroom form with the mushroom stem on the DEJ **(Figure 11-17). Occlusal caries,** which are the most prevalent caries in the oral cavity, radiographically exhibit the apex of the triangle of decay toward the outer surface (pits and fissures) of the tooth and the base of the triangle at the DEJ **(Figure 11-18). Facial and lingual caries** radiographically appear as round, radiolucent dots on the tooth surface. If a decayed pit is located on the lingual surface, it is well delineated **(Figure 11-19). Cervical caries** on the facial or lingual surface extend laterally toward the interproximal surfaces, forming a typical **crescent-shaped, semilunar cavity (Figure 11-20).** When assessing **pulpal caries,** it is prudent to remember that the caries may have progressed more than a radiographic film may reveal. Likewise, because a radiograph does not have depth, a carious lesion may be superimposed on the pulp when the carious lesion has not penetrated the pulp **(Figure 11-21).**

Overexposure of the film may result in **"burnout"** of the dentin between the pulp and carious lesion by enlarging the carious lesion **(Figures 11-22 and 11-23).** The radiographic appearance of **root caries** is described as **saucer-shaped** or having a **cupped-out appearance.** It is usually located in the

TABLE 11–8 Analysis of Panoramic Patient Positioning Errors

ERROR AND CAUSE	IDENTIFYING FEATURES	CORRECTION	L + L FIGURE/PAGE
Patient too far forward	Narrow blurred anterior teeth with a pseudospace	• Use the incisal bite guide. • Line up the incisal edge of the teeth with the notch. • Edentulous patients should bite about 5 mm behind the notch.	Figure 10-8 A, p 231. Step 1 Figure 10-13 A–F, pp 234 and 235
Patient too far back	Wide, blurred anterior teeth Ghosting of the rami, spread-out turbinates, ears, and nose in the image, condyles off the lateral edges of the film	• Use the incisal bite guide. • Line up the incisal edge of the teeth with the notch.	Figure 10-8, p 231. Step 1 Figure 10-14 A–F, pp 236 and 237
Chin tipped too low	• Excessive curving of the occlusal plane • Loss of image of the roots of the lower anterior teeth • Narrowing of the intercondylar distance and loss of the head of the condyles at the top of the film	• Tip the chin down, but the ala-tragus line should not exceed −5° to −7° downward • Use the chinrest.	Figure 10-8 B, p 231. Step 1 Figure 10-10, p 232. Step 3 Figure 10-17 A–F, pp 242 and 243
Chin raised too high	• Flattening or reverse curvature of the occlusal plane • Loss of image of the roots of the upper anterior teeth • Lengthening of the intercondylar distance and loss of the head of the condyles at the edges of the film • Hard palate shadow wider and superimposed on the apices of the maxillary teeth	• Tip the chin down −5° to −7°. • Use the chinrest.	Figure 10-8 B, p 231. Step 1 Figure 10-10, p 232. Step 3 Figure 10-18 A–F, pp 244 and 245 Figure 10-9, p 232. Step 2
Head twisted	• Unequal right-left magnification • Particularly the teeth and the ramus • Severe overlap of the contact points and blurring	• Line up the patient's midline with the middle of the incisal bite guide. • Close the side guide.	Figure 10-15 A–F, p 238
Head tilted	• The mandible appears tilted on the film. • Unequal distance exists between the mandible and the chinrest at a given point on the right and left sides. • One condyle is higher and larger than the other.	Position the chin firmly on both sides of the chinrest. Close the side guide.	Figure 10-9, p 232. Step 2 Figure 10-16 A–F, pp 240 and 241
Slumped position	Ghost image of the cervical spine superimposed on the anterior region	• Stand-up machines: have the patient step forward or place his/her feet on the markers. • All machines: be certain that the patient is sitting or standing erect.	Figure 10-11, p 233. Step 4 Figure 10-20 A–F, pp 248 and 249
Chin not on the chinrest	• Sinus not visible on the film • Top of the condyles cut off • Excessive distance between the inferior border of the mandible and the lower edge of the film	Position the chin on the chinrest.	Figure 10-8 A and B, p 231 Figure 10-19 A–E, pp 246 and 247
Bite guide not used	Incisal and occlusal surfaces of the upper and lower teeth overlapped	Use the bite guide. Compensate for missing anterior teeth with cotton rolls.	Figure 10-8 A and B, p 231 Figure 10-13 A–F, pp 234 and 235 Figure 10-14 A–F, pp 236 and 237
Tongue not on the palate	Relative radiolucency obscuring apices of the maxillary teeth (palatoglossal air space)	Place the tongue firmly against the palate. Ask the patient to swallow or suck on his/her cheeks.	
Lips open	Relative radiolucency on the coronal portion of the upper and lower teeth	Close the lips.	Figure 10-21 A–F, pp 250 and 251
Patient movement	• Wavy outline of cortex of the interior border of the mandible • Blurring of the image above the wavy cortical outline	• Ask the patient to hold still. • Explain the function of the machine to avoid startling the patient. • Be certain that the patient's clothing will not interfere.	Figure 10-12, p 233 Figure 10-22 A–F, p 252
Prostheses	• Evidence of prostheses in the image • Acrylic denture teeth and bases do not show	Remove all complete and partial dentures, eyeglasses, and jewelry	Figure 10-25 A–D, p 257

Adapted from Langland OE, Langlais RP: Principles in Dental Imaging. Baltimore, Williams & Wilkins, 1997, p 255.

TABLE 11–9 Analysis of Panoramic Procedural Errors

ERROR AND CAUSE	IDENTIFYING FEATURES	CORRECTION	L + L FIGURE/PAGE
Not starting at "home base"	A portion of the film is blank. A portion of the anatomy is lost at the edge of the film.	Align the machine and/or cassette with the starting point.	Figure 10-28, p 258
Cassette resistance	One or several dark vertical bands on the film; these represent areas of over-exposure as the cassette is stopped, but radiation continues to be emitted until the end of the cycle	• Be certain to remove thickly padded items of clothing. • In stocky patients with a short neck, the cassette may need to be raised slightly above the ideal position.	Figure 10-29, p 259
Paper or lint in screen	• Radiopacity of unusual shape, and location • Foreign object prevents complete exposure of the film by fluorescent screen	Periodically inspect and clean the screens.	Figure 10-31, pp 259 and 260
"Fingernail" artifact	Crescent-shaped radiolucency	Avoid rough handling of the film when removing from the box or cassette.	Figure 10-31, pp 259 and 260
Static electricity	• Lightning-like radiolucency; dot-like radiolucencies • Starburst and other patterns	• Dry air in the darkroom can be humid-ified with a humidifier or large bowl of water. • Avoid rapidly pulling the film from envelope-type cassettes or full box of film. • Avoid smoking near the film.	Figure 10-33, p 260
White light exposure	A portion of the film appears overex-posed	• Check other sources of light leaks in the darkroom (e.g., unsafe safe-light or radio). • Check the integrity of the cassette.	Figure 10-34, p 260
Double exposure	Two images on the same film	Always place exposed films in the same location where they may not be mis-taken for unexposed films.	Figure 7-9, p 168
Underexposed	Film too light	• Increase the kV and/or mA depending on the machine. • Place the film between screens and not to one side only. • Check the developer solution.	Figure 10-23 B, p 254 Figure 7-20, p 174 Figure 11-20 A and B, pp 277 and 278 Figure 8-9, p 195
Overexposed	Film too dark	Decrease the kV and/or mA depending on the machine.	Figure 7-21, p 174
No name	Patient's name or identification number not on the film	Use the film imprinter, special labeling tape, or special pen.	Figure 10-23, p 254

Adapted from Langland OE, Langlais RP: Principles in Dental Imaging. Baltimore, Williams & Wilkins, 1997, p 261.

area of the interproximal CEJ. **Root caries** may be **misinter-preted** as **cervical burnout,** which is also seen in the proxi-mal areas of the tooth cervix (**Figure 11-24**).

Role of Radiographs in the Diagnosis of Periodontal Disease

The value of radiographs in the diagnosis of periodontal disease is considered **adjunctive** or **complementary** to the clinical examination of the patient's oral status. It is im-perative that clinicians perceive the value of including sev-eral diagnostic aids in making an accurate diagnosis, real-izing that no single diagnostic aid is perfect. The interpretative or diagnostic limitations of radiographs in-clude: the view of a three-dimensional versus two-dimen-sional object, the angle of the position indicating device (PID), the type of film-holding device, the exposure tech-nique, and the operator's proficient use of the technique. Because of these variables, anatomic structures may not be

visible or may be superimposed or distorted rendering an image difficult to assess.

Realizing that the dental radiographic survey of a patient is a critical component of assessment and diagnosis, it is essential to remember that radiographs demonstrate the past history of a disease process, because radiographs usu-ally show less bone loss than is actually present. Radi-ographs cannot and do not accurately demonstrate the ex-tent of present disease activity or act as an indicator for future disease activity.

Sequential radiographs, when exposed over time, help the diagnostician to compare radiographic findings and monitor the progress of periodontal disease or dental caries. The comparative interpretation of the disease process assists the practitioner in determining appropriate treatment protocol. **Subtraction radiography** and **digital subtraction radiog-raphy** are more useful techniques than are conventional ra-diographic techniques in identifying the subtle differences when comparing radiographs exposed at differing times.

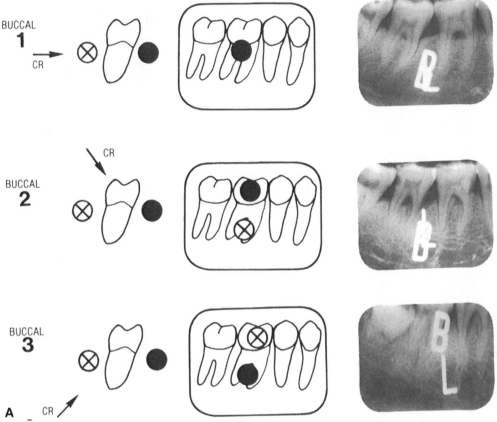

Figure 11-12. Buccal-object rule (vertical and horizontal shift). *A,* Vertical shift. Buccal and lingual foreign bodies change position with vertical shift of the x-ray beam. (1) The original radiograph. Buccal and lingual objects are superimposed. (2) The beam is directed inferiorly (positive vertical angulation). The buccal object (B) moves inferiorly while the lingual object (L) moves superiorly. (3) The beam is directed superiorly (negative vertical angulation). The buccal object (B) moves superiorly while the lingual object (L) moves inferiorly.

More information about this technique follows in the section on digital radiography.

Role of the Bite-Wing Radiograph in the Diagnosis and Monitoring of Periodontal Disease

The position of the alveolar crest on a radiograph, especially the interproximal alveolar crest in relation to the CEJ, is significant in the diagnosis of periodontal disease. The angulation of the primary beam can influence the relative position of the alveolar crest on the radiographic film. The beam angulation must be perpendicular to both the object and the film to produce an accurate image of the alveolar crest on the radiograph. The level of the radiographic alveolar crest and its position relative to the CEJ will correspond with the anatomic crest when the x-ray beam intersects the long axis of the tooth and the film at a 90-degree angle. In order for this to occur, the film must be positioned parallel to the long axis of the tooth. Therefore, bite-wing radiographs-specifically vertical bite-wing radiographs-are recommended to obtain an anatomically correct image of the position of the alveolar crest (**Figures 11-25A and B and 11-26A and B).**

Limitations of Radiographs in Diagnosing Periodontal Disease

As previously stated, radiographs have limitations when diagnosing disease. Some limitations are described in this section.

The use of the periodontal probe remains the most reliable method when determining the presence of or evaluating the current status of a periodontal pocket or a gingival sulcus. Usually "early" bone loss starts in the cancellous bone. By the time that the cortical plate is affected and identified as loss of alveolar bone height on a bite-wing radiograph by the practitioner, a great amount of disease activity has already occurred. Therefore, the usefulness of radiographs to quantify early bone loss is limited. Use of vertical bite-wing radiographs in early periodontal disease improves the diagnostic value of these films.

The use of the Nabors probe during the clinical examination remains the most reliable assessment tool to identify early furcation involvement. However, radiographs are essential to the clinical evaluation because: (1) the buccal and lingual plates of the alveolar bone are superimposed over furcation areas, and (2) the angle of the PID may produce a radiographic image that covers the disease in the furcation area.

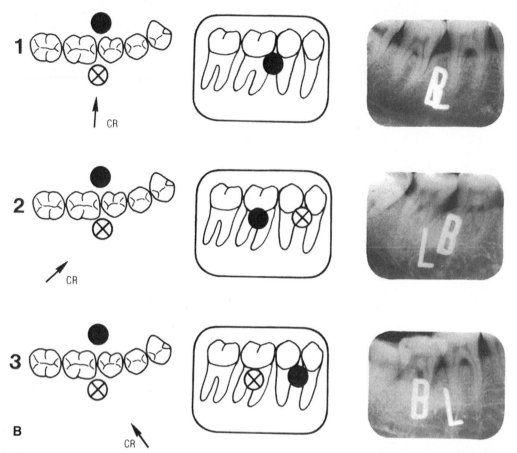

Figure 11-12. *(Continued) B*, Horizontal shift. (1) Original radiograph. Buccal and lingual objects are superimposed. (2) The beam is directed mesially. The buccal object (B) moves mesially while the lingual object (L) moves distally. (3) The beam is directed distally. The buccal object (B) moves distally while the lingual object (L) moves mesially. (From Langland OE, Langlais RP: Principles of Dental Imaging. Philadelphia, Williams & Wilkins, 1997, pp 273 and 274.)

Although bone deformities and defects can be demonstrated on a radiograph, the use of the periodontal probe and periodontal surgery are necessary to determine the shape and extent of the osseous defect. Because the radiograph does not demonstrate the tooth as a three-dimensional object, the number of walls involved in an infrabony pocket cannot be determined. A bone defect in a trifurcated or bifurcated tooth is referred to as **triangulation** or **funneling** (**Figures 11-27 and 11-28A, B,** and **C**).

Furcation involvement refers to the advancement of periodontal disease into the bone between the roots of multirooted teeth. In addition to its clinical detection, the radiographic appearance of a **furcation "arrow"** may indicate that the furcation area is diseased. The furcation arrow is a small, triangular radiographic shadow across the mesial and distal roots of some maxillary molars. Of the multirooted teeth, the maxillary first premolars are the least commonly affected and the mandibular first molars are the most commonly affected. In order for furcation involvement to be radiographically visible, the disease process must extend apically between the root division (see Figure 11-28).

An article published by Hardekopf and associates in the *Journal of Periodontology* (April 1987) states that the radi-

ographic presence of the furcation "arrow," a triangular radiographic shadow, appears to be a reliable diagnostic tool for the clinician when evaluating bony furcation involvement. The most classic presentation of the "arrow" may occur when the vertical component of bone loss is minimal. As the vertical component increases, the image broadens and become more diffuse. When this occurs, other radiographic suggestions of furcation involvement become more prominent, such as triangulation or funneling, a wedge-shaped radiolucency along the root or "through and through" involvement.[1, 5]

The absence of the furcation arrow image does not necessarily indicate the absence of a bony furcation involvement. The root morphology and the horizontal angulation of the tubehead may be factors that determine whether a given interproximal furcation defect will exhibit an "arrow."[6] Radiographic furcation involvement or the lack of it should always be combined with a clinical examination. The clinical examination should include the use of a periodontal probe, a Nabors probe, a contra-angled dental explorer, and warm air to facilitate the visual examination.

The presence of **dental calculus** may appear radiographically as a radiopaque line, spur, or spicule on the interproximal, buccal or lingual surface but must be quite heavy in

TABLE 11–10 Maximum Permissible Dose (MPD) Per Class of Exposed Individuals (rem to mSv)*

- Occupational worker (i.e., dental hygienist): annual whole body dose = 50 mSv = 0.05 SV = 5 rem (Move the decimal to the left 3 places then to the right 2 places.) (milli = 1/1000; 3 zeros = move the decimal 3 places.)
- Occupational worker who is pregnant: total dose equivalent limit during gestation period = 5 mSv = 0.005 Sv = 0.5 rem (Move the decimal to the left 3 places then to the right 2 places.) (milli = 1/1000; 3 zeros = move the decimal 3 places.)
- Occupational worker who is pregnant: dose equivalent in 1 month = 0.5 mSv = 0.0005 Sv = 0.05 rems (Move the decimal to the left 3 places then to the right 2 places.)

- Occupational worker lifetime cumulative exposure = 10 times the age in years
- Public exposure annually with continuous or frequent exposure = 1 mSv = 0.001 Sv = 0.1 rem
- Public exposure annually with infrequent exposure = 5 mSv = 0.005 Sv = 0.5 rem
- Trainees younger than 18 years of age: effective dose equivalent limit annually = 1 mSv = 0.001 Sv = 0.5 rem

*Established by the National Council on Radiation Protection and Measurements (NCRP).

order to be seen. In addition, a clinical evaluation for detection of the true extent of the calculus deposit is still necessary **(Figure 11-29)**.

A **widened periodontal ligament space** on a radiograph may indicate tooth mobility. However, tooth mobility cannot be recorded or quantified using a radiograph **(Figure 11-30)**.

Beneficial Role of Radiographs in Diagnosing Periodontal Disease

The radiographic survey, whether a complete mouth series or vertical bite-wing radiograph series, assists the clinician in identifying radiographic changes in the periodontium, which may be indicative of periodontal disease.

Radiographs provide an estimate of the amount of bone loss by demonstrating the existence of localized or generalized bone loss and the direction of bone loss, whether horizontal or vertical, by looking at the interseptal bone. It is important to identify and assess the crown-root ratio and the proximity of the root tips to each other and other anatomic structures such as the maxillary sinus. A tooth with a good crown-root ratio has a better prognosis than does one with a poor crown-root ratio. When a tooth with a thin cortical plate of bone between itself and the tooth next to it exhibits bone loss, both teeth have a more guarded prognosis **(Figure 11-31)**.

The alveolar bone height of the buccal and lingual plates of cortical or cancellous bone is often radiographically difficult to assess owing to bone density. Therefore, the radiographic evaluation has more value when assessing the interseptal bone height.

Radiographs can assist in the evaluation of a bone defect. A radiograph will demonstrate the presence of a bone defect,

TABLE 11–11 Maximum Permissible Doses per Class of Exposed Individuals (rem to mSv)

CLASS OF EXPOSED INDIVIDUAL	MAXIMUM PERMISSIBLE DOSE (MSV)
Radiation workers (e.g., dentists, assistants, hygienists) (annual) Effective dose equivalent limit (whole body)	50
Partial body dose equivalent limits	
Skin	150
Forearms	300
Hands	750
Other organs and organ systems (e.g., red bone marrow, breast, lung, and gonads)	500
Lifetime cumulative exposure	10 (multiplied by age in years)
Public exposures (annual)	
Effective dose equivalent limit, continuous or frequent exposure	1
Effective dose equivalent limit, infrequent exposure	5
Dose equivalent limits for lens of the eye, skin, and extremities	50
Trainees younger than 18 years of age (annual)	
Effective dose equivalent limit	1
Dose equivalent limit for lens of the eye, skin, and extremities	50
Pregnant women (with respect to the fetus)	
Total dose equivalent limit	5 (during gestational period)
Dose equivalent limit in 1 month	0.5

Summary of the National Council on Radiation Protection and Measurements: Exposure of the U.S. Population from Diagnostic and Medical Radiation. NCRP report 116. Washington, DC, NCRP, 1993.
Recommendations for radiation dose limits, excluding background and medical exposures but including both internal and external exposures.

TABLE 11–12 Conversion Units

MRAD (REM)	RAD (REM)	GY (SV)	MGY (MSV)
1	0.001	0.00001	0.01
1000	1	0.01	10
100	0.1	0.001	1

*Adapted from Wilkins EM: Clinical Practice of the Dental Hygienist. Philadelphia, Lippincott Williams & Wilkins, 1999, pp 94–95.

but it will not reveal its exact shape or form. The form and shape can be determined only by using the periodontal probe or by direct vision during periodontal surgery.

Bone defects characterized as osseous craters have areas of radiolucency and radiopacity. Only four wall defects are purely radiolucent, such as horizontal bone loss. These defects are thought to be the most common defect in periodontal disease and occur most often in the posterior teeth (see Figure 11-28).

Nonreabsorbable materials (e.g., ridge augmentation materials), which are used in regenerative periodontal surgery, are visible on a radiograph. Reabsorbable materials are not generally visible on radiographs; however, the healing response to these materials may be visible.

Periodontal Disease and Radiographic Interpretation Issues

The normal relationship of the interseptal bone to CEJ refers to the height of the interseptal crestal cortical bone between the teeth. The normal height of this juncture is approximately 1 to 1.5 mm below the CEJ level of the adjacent teeth (see Figure 11-25A). Most often, the crestal bone is well delineated and well mineralized in health. The crestal bone is continuous with the lamina dura. The alveolar crest is usually peaked. Blunting of this crest when teeth are rotated may give the radiographic impression that it is a vertical defect. How-

ever, the best way to assess for good bone level is to draw a line from the CEJ of one tooth to the CEJ of the adjacent tooth or teeth. Other variants of normal may not be associated with disease; that is, a widened periodontal ligament may be present around the erupting tooth of an adolescent or from a tooth being moved by orthodontic appliances (**Figure 11-32**). Categories of periodontitis, as defined by the American Academy of Periodontology and the American Dental Association, further explain the relationship of disease to the clinical and radiographic examination and its findings.

Type I: By definition, **gingivitis** exhibits no bone loss.

Type II: **Mild adult periodontitis** refers to mild areas of disease that are demonstrated radiographically as bone erosion areas. Characteristics include: blunting of the alveolar crests or the alveolar crestal bone becomes rounded; loss of normal crestal height in the anterior teeth with loss of the acute angle of the lamina dura and the alveolar crestal bone, which becomes more rounded. Significant loss of attachment must occur for 6 to 8 months before the disease is seen on a radiograph. Slight fuzziness indicates early disease process.

Type III: In **moderate adult periodontitis**, continuation of the disease process is viewed by increased areas of radiolucency that may be seen as semicircular shadows in the interseptal bone, with the apex of the shadow toward the root of the tooth or defects between the buccal and lingual plates. These defects may have a horizontal or vertical (angular) pattern. In addition to the clinical examination, the radiograph is helpful to assess the residual bone.

Horizontal bone loss describes the radiographic appearance of the height of bone remaining. The alveolar crest is still horizontal (parallel to the CEJ) but is greater than 1 to 1.5 mm from the CEJ. The buccal and lingual cortical plates are destroyed in this process. Moderate bone loss is greater than 1 mm and may extend to the midpoint of the length of the root or to the furcation level of the molars. Severe bone loss is anything greater than moderate loss.

TABLE 11–13 Conversions from Traditional Units to Systems International Units (SI)

TRADITIONAL UNITS	SYSTEMS INTERNATIONAL UNITS (SI)
Roentgen	Coulombs/kg of air
rad	Gray (Gy)
rem	Sievert (Sv)
1 GY = 100 rad (To change Gy to rads, move the decimal point to the right 2 places.) 　0.01 Gy = 1 rad 1 rad = 0.01 Gy (To change rads to Gy, move the decimal point to the left 2 places.) 　100 rad = 1 Gy 1 Sv = 100 rem (To change Sv to rems, move the decimal point to the right 2 places.) 　0.01 Sv = 1 rem	100 rems = 1 Sv (To change rems to Sv, move the decimal point to the left 2 places.) 　1 rem = 0.01 Sv Dental Radiography 　1 rad = 1 rem 　1 Gy = 1 Sv

TABLE 11–14 Critical Organs and Resultant Disorders from Radiation Tissue and Organ Sensitivity

CRITICAL ORGANS IN DENTAL RADIOGRAPHY		TISSUE AND ORGAN SENSITIVITY	
Critical Organ	Resultant Disorder	Relative Sensitivity	Tissue/Organ
Lens of the eye	Cataracts	High	Small lymphocyte
Gonads	Genetic abnormalities		Bone marrow
Fetus	Congenital defects		Reproductive cells
Bone marrow	Leukemia		Intestinal mucosa
Thyroid gland	Cancer	Fairly high	Skin
Salivary gland	Cancer		Lens of the eye
Skin	Cancer		Oral mucosa
Bone	Cancer	Medium	Connective tissue
			Small blood vessels
			Growing bone and cartilage
		Fairly low	Mature bone and cartilage
			Salivary gland
			Thyroid gland
			Kidney
			Liver
		Low	Muscle
			Nerve

Vertical bone loss or **vertical osseous defects** or **angular bone loss** refers to the type of bone loss localized between one or two teeth. The defects radiographically appear as remaining bone having an angular or oblique angulation or slope in relation to the CEJ line of the adjacent teeth.[3] Due to the radiographic superimposition of the buccal and the lingual cortical plates of alveolar bone in the mandible, it is often difficult to impossible to adequately distinguish between the involvement of infrabony defects that are one-, two- and three-walled bone defects **(see Chapter 13** and **Figures 11-33 to 11-36).**

Type IV: **Severe periodontal disease** refers to periodontal disease status in which more than one third of crestal bone loss is destroyed as measured from the CEJ. It also includes tooth mobility and drifting. Extensive vertical or horizontal bone loss may be present. The radiograph does not usually indicate the severity of the actual periodontal lesion or defect.

A **periodontal abscess** occurs when the coronal portion of a deep soft tissue pocket closes over or occludes or a foreign body is lodged in the periodontal pocket between the tooth and the gingiva. If the abscess remains without treat-

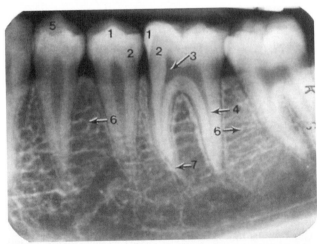

Figure 11-13. Normal anatomy of tooth and supporting structures. The enamel and dentin line of demarcation is very sharp. The enamel is whiter than dentin, because enamel is much denser. Enamel (1), dentin (2), pulp chamber (3), pulp canal (4), buccal cusp (5), alveolar bone (6), and root apex (7). (From Langland OE, Langlais RP: Principles of Dental Imaging. Philadelphia, Williams & Wilkins, 1997, p 332.)

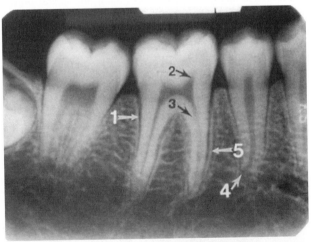

Figure 11-14. Periodontal ligament space and lamina dura. The periodontal ligament space is a distinct line just outside the root portion of the tooth and inside the lamina dura. Periodontal ligament space (1), pulp horn (2), two root canals in mesial root (3), apex of root (4), and lamina dura (5). (From Langland OE, Langlais RP: Principles of Dental Imaging. Philadelphia, Williams & Wilkins, 1997, p 332.)

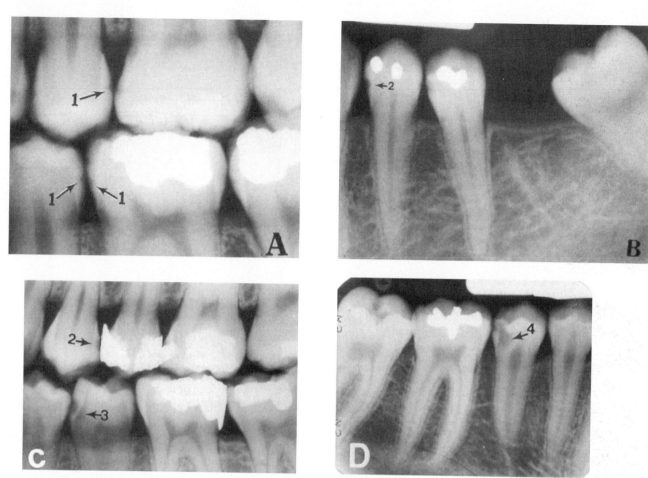

Figure 11-15. Four classes of interproximal caries penetration. *A,* Distinct Class 1 (incipient) carious lesions identified by arrows. *B,* Class 2 carious lesions on mesial of mandibular first premolar *(arrow). C,* Class 3 carious lesion on mesial surfaces of rotated mandibular second premolar. Class 2 carious lesion on distal surface of maxillary first premolar. *D,* Class 4 carious lesion on mesial surface of mandibular second premolar *(arrow).* (From Langland OE, Langlais RP: Principles of Dental Imaging. Philadelphia, Williams & Wilkins, 1997, p 399.)

ment, a radiolucent area may form along the lateral border of the root or over the tooth root apex, signifying infection and bone involvement. The tooth is usually vital. After treatment, the bone may heal.

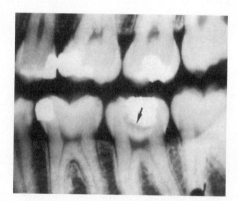

Figure 11-16. Recurrent or secondary caries. Note the radiolucent caries lesion under the radiopaque restoration. This is most likely from incomplete removal of dentinal caries before placement of the restoration. (From Langland OE, Langlais RP: Principles of Dental Imaging. Philadelphia, Williams & Wilkins, 1997, p 402.)

Early-onset periodontitis refers to the incidental, localized, or generalized forms of periodontal disease that occur in children, adolescents, and young adults. When localized, this disease is often referred to as **localized juvenile periodontitis (LPJ).** The incidental form usually affects one to three teeth and results in 3 mm or more of attachment loss. The localized form is usually seen as vertical bone loss and occurs around the incisors and first molars .The generalized form is usually seen as angular bone loss and results in rapid bone destruction with eventual tooth loss **(Figure 11-37A and B).**

Dental Conditions That May Affect the Periodontal Status of the Patient

Although the radiograph is used only as a supplemental aid in determining periodontal or occlusal trauma, **occlusal trauma** may be radiographically indicated by a **widened periodontal ligament.** It may also indicate the eruption of a tooth. The widened periodontal ligament may be a feature of an osteosarcoma, chondrosarcoma, or a systemic sclerosis. Refer to Chapter 8 for more details. It is worth noting that

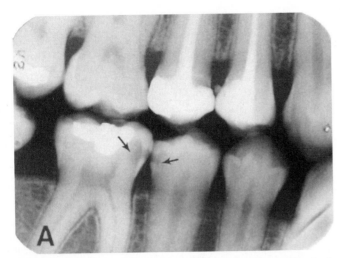

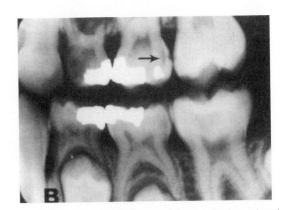

Figure 11-17. Dentinal caries. *A,* Note the dentinal carious lesions in the distal surface of the mandibular second premolar (*arrow*) and mesial of the mandibular first molar (*arrow*). *B,* Note the dentinal spreading of the carious lesion of the dentinoenamel junction of the distal surface of the maxillary second primary molar (*arrow*). (From Langland OE, Langlais RP: Principles of Dental Imaging. Philadelphia, Williams & Wilkins, 1997, p 398.)

the widened periodontal ligament may not be solely related to disease but rather to some temporary abnormality.

Subgingival dental calculus radiographically appears radiopaque. Its presence makes it difficult for the patient to adequately clean the interproximal area, which may lead to continued progression of the disease **(Figure 11-38).**

A **poor crown-root ratio refers** to the radiographic evidence of bone loss where more than one third of the tooth is no longer in the bone. As a result, there is a poor prognosis for maintaining the tooth periodontally (see Figure 11-31).

A **poor root morphology** refers to a tooth root that converges or is conical. The periodontal prognosis of this tooth is poor compared with a tooth that has widespread roots **(Figure 11-39).**

Internal root reabsorption refers to the removal of tooth structure on the inner surface of the pulp chamber and pulp canal and may extend outward through the dentin or cementum. Radiographically, it may appear radiolucent, round, oval, elongated, or as an irregular expansion of the pulp

chamber or canal within the root. The osteoclastic or odontoclastic activity of the inflamed or traumatized pulp may expand into the periodontal ligament space and open into the periodontal pocket or gingival sulcus, resulting in a pulpal infection. It may also expand through the dentin and enamel and result in perforation and pulpitis.

External root reabsorption refers to the removal of tooth, which commonly occurs in the root portion of the tooth. It often results in blunting of the root apex. Radiographically, it is less easily recognized compared with internal root reabsorption. Other dental conditions previously discussed that may affect the periodontal status of the patient include the following:

Root proximity
Furcation involvement
Pulpal or periodontal infection
Root caries, cemental caries, radicular caries, or senile
  caries
Cervical burnout

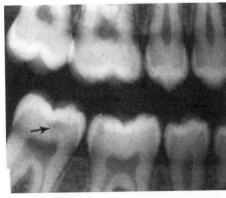

Figure 11-18. Occlusal caries. Note the occlusal caries in the mandibular second molar (*arrow*). (From Langland OE, Langlais RP: Principles of Dental Imaging. Philadelphia, Williams & Wilkins, 1997, p 401.)

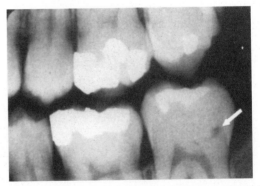

Figure 11-19. Facial/lingual caries. Note the round, black hole appearance of lingual caries on the mandibular second molar. (From Langland OE, Langlais RP: Principles of Dental Imaging. Philadelphia, Williams & Wilkins, 1997, p 401.)

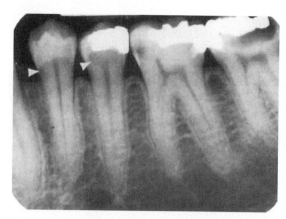

Figure 11-20. Cervical caries. Note the cervical facial caries on the first and second premolars. (From Langland OE, Langlais RP: Principles of Dental Imaging. Philadelphia, Williams & Wilkins, 1997, p 401.)

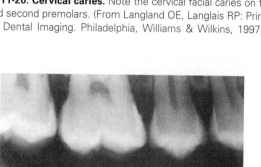

Figure 11-21. Pulpal caries. Large carious lesion of the mandibular first molar that has probably reached the pulp; however, the carious lesion could be superimposed over the pulp chamber and given an impression of a pulpal penetration. (From Langland OE, Langlais RP: Principles of Dental Imaging. Philadelphia, Williams & Wilkins, 1997, p 401.)

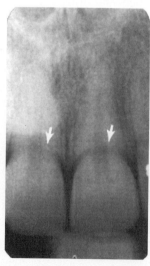

Figure 11-22. Anterior cervical burnout. Cervical burnout in the maxillary centrals. Note the dark radiolucent collar at the cervical neck of the incisors (*arrows*). (From Langland OE, Langlais RP: Principles of Dental Imaging. Philadelphia, Williams & Wilkins, 1997, p 405.)

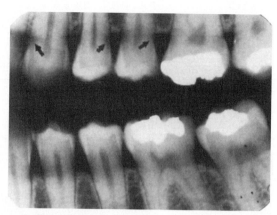

Figure 11-23. Posterior cervical burnout. Note the radiolucent areas (*arrows*) that are cervical burnout areas and not caries. (From Langland OE, Langlais RP: Principles of Dental Imaging. Philadelphia, Williams & Wilkins, 1997, p 405.)

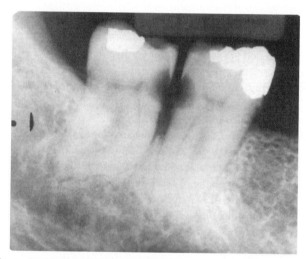

Figure 11-24. Root or cemental caries. Root or cemental caries with the characteristic cupped-out appearance, as seen between two molars. Note the loose contact and food packing between the teeth. (From Langland OE, Langlais RP: Principles of Dental Imaging. Philadelphia, Williams & Wilkins, 1997, p 402.)

Overhanging or iatrogenic restorations refer to inadequate restorative margins on a restored tooth. These restorations are often cited as a secondary etiology of gingival inflammation and periodontal disease due to bacterial plaque accumulation around them. Smooth, well-contoured margins promote complete removal of bacterial plaque, which allows for a healthier periodontium (**Figure 11-40**). When performing a periodontal examination, it is important that the clinician identifies overhanging restorations (opaque), poorly contoured margins (opaque), and open contact areas (lucent) that contribute to gingivitis and periodontitis.

Value of Radiographs When Diagnosing Periapical Lesions

In conjunction with the information gained from the patient interview and the clinical examination, radiographs are useful

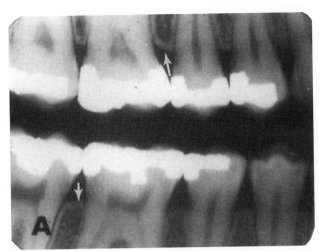
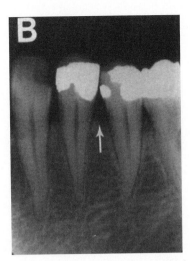

Figure 11-25. Crestal irregularities. *A*, Normal interdental alveolar crestal bone (*arrows*). The coronal border of the alveolar bone (alveolar crest) extends normally to approximately 1.5 mm from the cementoenamel junction of the teeth. *B*, Note the fuzziness and the break of continuity of the lamina dura at the crest of the alveolar bone between the first and second premolars (*arrows*). (From Langland OE, Langlais RP: Principles of Dental Imaging. Philadelphia, Williams & Wilkins, 1997, p 360.)

in diagnosis to further determine the location and extent of disease. In Chapter 8, pathologies are divided into radiopaque and radiolucent lesions. This assists in the learning and understanding of the information included in this chapter.

Radiographically, periapical lesions are demonstrated in the bone by varying degrees of **radiolucencies** and **radiopacities** depending on the abnormality, pathology, longevity of existence, and osteoblastic or osteoclastic activity.

The presence of the **lamina dura** is an indicator of health. When the lamina dura is **not present** or appears to have **lost its continuity**, **thickness**, or **degree of radiopacity**, periapical or periodontal disease may be evident. **Widening of the periodontal ligament** is also a common indicator of periodontal and periapical pathologic lesions.

According to Langland and Langlais, periapical diseases may be divided into six classifications: **acute apical peri-**

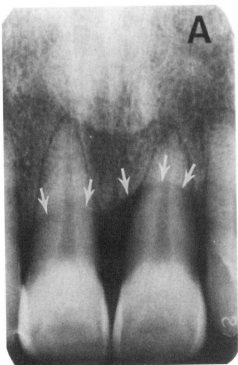
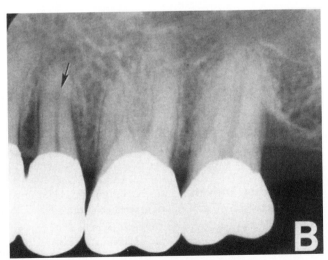

Figure 11-26. Evaluation of bone height. *A*, Note the trabecular pattern of the central incisors can be observed as the eye scans apically from the *arrows*. Below the *arrows*, the root appears denuded of bone. This is the true line of the bone height. *B*, Note the severe bone loss on lingual surface of the maxillary second premolar. This is most likely bone level on the lingual surfaces because of its clarity (*black arrow*). (From Langland OE, Langlais RP: Principles of Dental Imaging. Philadelphia, Williams & Wilkins, 1997, p 364.)

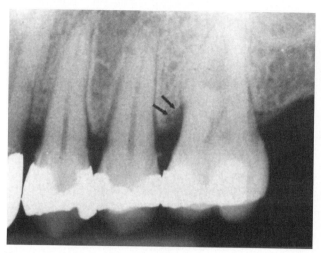

Figure 11-27. Triangulation (funneling). Note the wedge-shaped radiolucencies on the mesial aspects of the first molar (*arrows*). Spur calculus can be seen distal of the second premolar. (From Langland OE, Langlais RP: Principles of Dental Imaging. Philadelphia, Williams & Wilkins, 1997, p 360.)

odontitis (AAP), **acute apical abscess (AAA)**, **apical granuloma**, **apical cyst**, **chronic apical abscess**, and **apical condensing osteitis.**[1] As indicated by the name, *acute* implies lesions that produce pain and swelling. *Chronic* refers to lesions that have mild or no symptoms. Often an acute disease does not exhibit a significant radiographic appearance. If the radiographic technique exposure and processing is appropriate, a long-scale contrast using a higher kVp may

demonstrate subtle bone changes. A chronic disease state may exhibit a specific radiographic appearance.

The most common chronic periapical lesion is a dental granuloma, which radiographically appears radiolucent, circular to ovoid, encloses the root end, and extends periapically. The granuloma and the cyst may radiographically appear very similar. The differentiating factor may be the size. The **granuloma is usually smaller** than 1 cm in diameter, and the **cyst may be as large as 10 cm** in diameter or may fill an entire jaw. Another differentiating factor may be that the cyst is more circumscribed and is usually bound by a thin, unbroken line of sclerotic bone that contains the fluid. When infection results in an increased stimulus of trabecular bone rather than destruction, it is called **condensing osteitis** or **sclerosing osteomyelitis**. The bone appears as a **well-circumscribed radiopaque** mass of sclerotic bone surrounding and extending below the apex of one or both roots of the affected tooth. **Periapical dysplasia** or **cementoma** varies from lucent to opaque depending on its stage of maturity. **Hypercementosis** is an excessive formation of cementum that appears radiographically opaque.

Further details of oral pathologic lesions are included in Chapter 8. Recall that destruction to hard or soft tissue appears radiolucent, and a proliferation of tissue usually appears radiopaque.

Digital Radiography

Digital radiography is also called **direct radiographic imaging, computed dental radiography,** and **direct dig-**

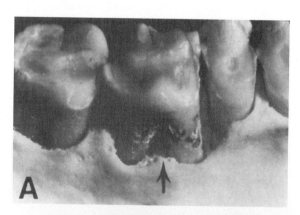

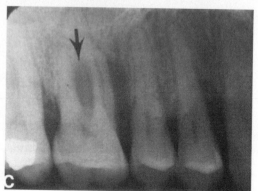

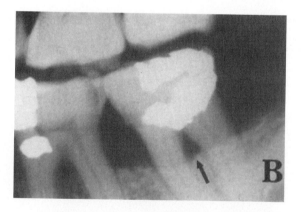

Figure 11-28. Furcation involvement. *A,* Furcation involvement of the lower first molar of a dry specimen. *B,* Radiograph of "through-and-through" bifurcation involvement of the second molar (*arrow*). C, Through-and-through trifurcation involvement of the maxillary first molar. The radiolucency is not as dark as the radiolucency of a bifurcation involvement of a lower molar because of superimposition of the palatal root of maxillary molars over the furca. (From Langland OE, Langlais RP: Principles of Dental Imaging. Philadelphia, Williams & Wilkins, 1997, p 367.)

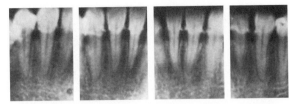

Figure 11-29. Dental calculus. Interproximal spur-like calculus in the lower anteriors. (From Langland OE, Langlais RP: Principles of Dental Imaging. Philadelphia, Williams & Wilkins, 1997, p 359.)

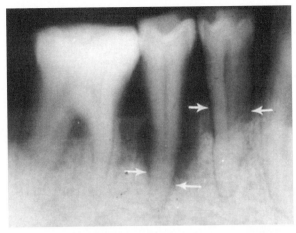

Figure 11-31. Clinical crown-root ratio. Note the poor clinical crown-root ratio of the mandibular first and second premolars (*arrows*). (From Langland OE, Langlais RP: Principles of Dental Imaging. Philadelphia, Williams & Wilkins, 1997, p 371.)

ital radiography. Digital radiography refers to a "film-less" imaging system. Instead of using film, processing solutions, and equipment, the image is captured on an intraoral sensor, stored, and digitally converted to an image. It is then processed and displayed on a computer monitor. Equipment that is necessary for direct digital imaging systems includes an x-radiation source, an intraoral sensor, a computer, and the conventional x-radiation source. Current types of direct sensor technologies are: (1) **charged-couple devices (CCDs)**, which constitute a direct digital system; (2) **complementary metal oxide semiconductor/active pixel sensor (CMOS/APS)** systems, which constitute a direct digital system; and (3) **charged injection devices (CIDs)**, which constitute an indirect digital system.

Methods of Digital Imaging

Three methods of obtaining a digital image are the **direct digital imaging**, **indirect digital imaging**, and **storage phosphor imaging**. **Direct digital imaging** consists of a sensor that is placed in the patient's mouth and exposed to radiation. The image is captured on the sensor and made visible on the computer screen within seconds. Computer software can enhance and store the image. **Indirect digital imaging** consists of a camera and a computer. The existing

x-ray film is digitized by scanning the image with the CCD camera, which converts the image to the computer monitor. The resultant image is usually of less quality and similar to a copy of an original.

The third method of digital imaging is **storage phosphor imaging**. This wireless digital system uses a reusable imaging plate coated with phosphors, which replaces the fiber-optic cable connected to a sensor. The plate is flexible and fits into the patient's mouth similar to an intraoral film. The phosphor system records the exposed image on the plate. The plate is then scanned with a laser and converted to information stored in electronic files or transferred to the computer screen to view. Owing to the laser scanning process, a

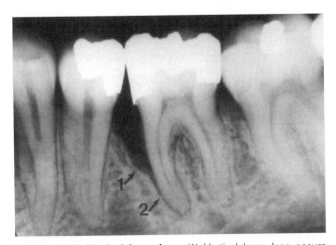

Figure 11-30. Vertical bone loss. (1) Vertical bone loss occurs when there is greater bone loss on the proximal of one tooth than the adjacent tooth. (2) Thickened periodontal ligament space. (From Langland OE, Langlais RP: Principles of Dental Imaging. Philadelphia, Williams & Wilkins, 1997, p 363.)

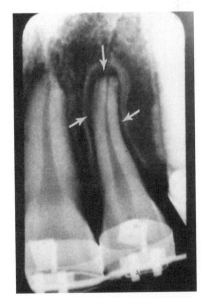

Figure 11-32. Tooth mobility from periodontal ligament (PDL) thickening. Note the thickening of the PDL and lamina dura (*arrows*) of the maxillary incisor being moved posteriorly by orthodontic appliances. (From Langland OE, Langlais RP: Principles of Dental Imaging. Philadelphia, Williams & Wilkins, 1997, p 333.)

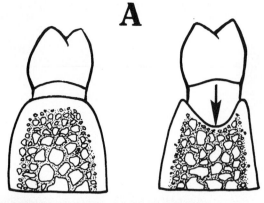

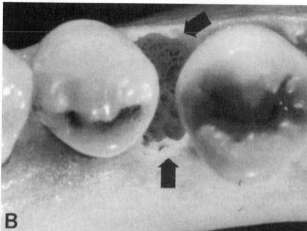

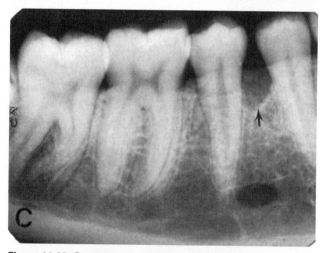

Figure 11-33. Osseous crater (two-wall bone defect). *A,* Diagram of an osseous crater between two mandibular premolars.(Left) Normal bone contour (Right) Osseous crater within interdental septal bone (*arrow*). *B,* Osseous crater between two premolars in the dry specimen. *C,* Radiographic appearance of an osseous crater between the first and second premolars. (From Langland OE, Langlais RP: Principles of Dental Imaging. Philadelphia, Williams & Wilkins, 1997, p 365.)

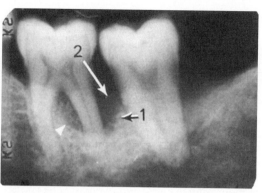

Figure 11-34. Less common two-wall bone defect. Radiograph of less frequently seen two-wall infrabony defect found here on the distal of the first molar. Distal wall (1) and lingual wall (2) were intact, with furcation involvement (*white arrowhead*) confirmed by probing. (From Langland OE, Langlais RP: Principles of Dental Imaging. Philadelphia, Williams & Wilkins, 1997, p 366.)

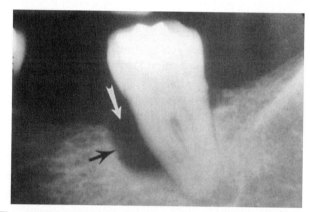

Figure 11-35. Radiograph of a two-wall bone defect with burnt-out lingual wall. Radiograph of a two-wall infrabony defect on the mesial side of the molar with the mesial wall (*black arrow*) and lingual wall (*white arrow*). The lingual remaining wall in this case is irregular and thins as well as "burnt out" and erased from the radiograph. This lingual wall was confirmed by probing. (From Langland OE, Langlais RP: Principles of Dental Imaging. Philadelphia, Williams & Wilkins, 1997, p 366.)

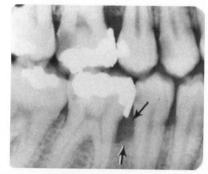

Figure 11-36. One-wall bone defect (ramp-like appearance). The defect has formed a ramp-like appearance (*arrows*), because the interdental septal bone slopes down from the facial/lingual wall crest of bone toward the crest of the destroyed facial/lingual bone. In this case, probing confirmed that the lingual wall was destroyed, and the ramping sloped down from intact facial wall toward the lingual crest of bone. (From Langland OE, Langlais RP: Principles of Dental Imaging. Philadelphia, Williams & Wilkins, 1997, p 367.)

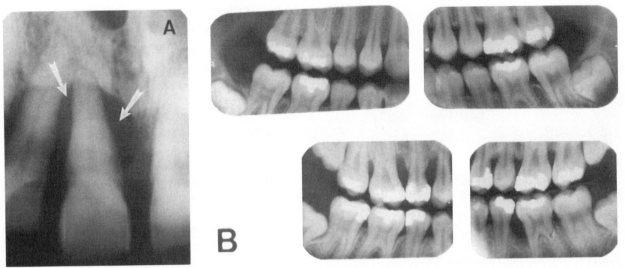

Figure 11-37. Localized juvenile periodontitis (LPJ). *A,* Classic arch-shaped anterior alveolar bone destruction found in LPJ. *B,* A 17-year-old girl with LPJ. Clinically, there were few signs and symptoms of inflammation. Upper radiographs of the patient at age 13. Lower radiographs of the patient at age 17. (Note the severe bone loss between the premolars and the molars). (From Langland OE, Langlais RP: Principles of Dental Imaging. Philadelphia, Williams & Wilkins, 1997, p 364.)

little more time is needed when compared with the direct digital imaging system.[6]

Types of Digital Imaging

The most common type of direct image sensor is the **CCD**. The CCD sensor is a detector that contains a silicon chip that is sensitive to x-radiation. When x-radiation strikes the silicon chip, excited electrons produce an electron charge. Subsequently, the electrons arrange and deposit themselves into an "electron well" known as **pixels.** (The pixel can be equated to the silver halide crystals of film emulsion that are transformed by the radiation into a latent image.) Of the 256 possible shades of gray, each pixel is assigned one shade of that gray. It is interesting to note that the human eye is only capable of distinguishing 32 shades of gray.[8] Approximately 307,000 organized pixels function to transmit, store, and

translate radiation energy to an electronic latent image.[6] This transmitted latent image is converted to a visible image on the computer screen by creating an analog output signal, which is then converted and stored in the computer.[4] This image can be visible on a computer screen, stored on a hard drive or disk, or printed on paper.

Another sensor technology is the **CMOS/APS.** The manufacturer claims 25% greater resolution. The semiconductor chip is less expensive to produce and is more durable compared with the CCD.[4]

Finally, the **CID**, is a silicon-based solid-state imaging receptor. No computer is necessary with this system. Equipment includes a CID sensor with a cord and plug inserted into the light source.[4]

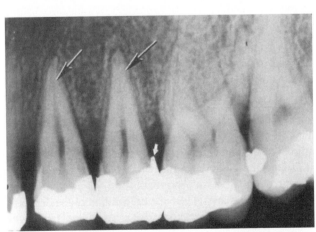

Figure 11-38. Dental calculus. Spur-like calculus of the interproximal surfaces of the lower molars and the second premolars *(arrows).* (From Langland OE, Langlais RP: Principles of Dental Imaging. Philadelphia, Williams & Wilkins, 1997, p 368.)

Figure 11-39. Spiked roots. Note the short, spiked roots of the maxillary premolars with thickened PDLS and overhanging restoration on distal of the second premolar. (From Langland OE, Langlais RP: Principles of Dental Imaging. Philadelphia, Williams & Wilkins, 1997, p 371.)

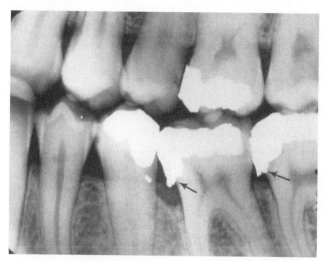

Figure 11-40. Overhanging restoration: Overhanging restorations on the mesial surfaces of the first and second molars (*arrows*). (From Langland OE, Langlais RP: Principles of Dental Imaging. Philadelphia, Williams & Wilkins, 1997, p 369.)

Digital Radiographic Procedures

Each dental staff person should read the manufacturer's information manual and instructions before using the system. Each system varies; therefore, the instructions must be carefully studied and adhered to concerning the operation, preparation of the equipment, and patient preparation and exposure.

To comply with infection control procedures, the sensor must be covered with a disposable barrier. The sensor cannot be sterilized in heat or chemicals. The sensor is placed into a sensor-holding device similar to a film-holding device and then placed appropriately into the patient's mouth. The paralleling technique and a paralleling technique film-holder device are recommended. A conventional radiographic machine exposes the sensor. The image appears on the computer monitor within seconds. The image can be stored or printed.

Advantages and Disadvantages of Digital Radiography

Advantages of the digital radiography system include: reduced radiation exposure to the patient, reduced time in producing a visible image, increased efficiency, the ability to enhance images, a superior gray-scale resolution, and overall reduced equipment and supply cost.

Disadvantages of the digital radiography system include: increased initial set-up cost, bulky sensor size, infection control, legal issues, related to manipulation of the digitized images, and overall image quality.[6]

Value of Digital Subtraction Radiography in Diagnosing Periodontal Disease

Research indicates that 30% to 50% change in mineral content of bone is necessary for bone loss to be detected on the radiograph.[9] When applying research to patient care, Webber and colleagues (1982), Jeffcoat (1984), Jeffcoat and associates (1987), and McHenry and associates (1987) confirmed that periodontal lesions with less than 5% change can be detected by digital subtraction radiography. This technique allows the practitioner to view change over time.[10-13] Simply put, this technique is accomplished by laying the images on top of one another and subtracting the information that has not changed. The information remaining on the film is called the third image or the subtracted image, which reveals the differences between the first two images. The subtle differences of the subtracted image allow the practitioner to view the diagnostically relevant information in the long-scale contrast of radiographic imaging.

Sources

1. Langland OE, Langlais RP: Principles of Dental Imaging. Philadelphia, Williams & Wilkins, 1997.
2. Gladwin MA, Bagby MA: Clinical Aspects of Dental Materials. Philadelphia, Lippincott Williams & Wilkins, 1999.
3. White SC, Pharoah MJ: Oral Radiology Principles and Interpretation, 4th ed. St. Louis, CV Mosby, 2000.
4. Razmus TF, Williamson GF: Current Oral and Maxillofacial Imaging. Philadelphia, WB Saunders, 1996.
5. Hardekopf JD, Dunlap RM, Ahl DR, Pelleu GB Jr: The "furcation arrow." A reliable radiographic image? J Periodontol 58 (4):258-261, 1987.
6. Haring JI, Jansen L: Dental Radiography Principles and Techniques, 2nd ed. Philadelphia, WB Saunders, 2000.
7. Miles DA, Van Dis ML, Jensen CW, Ferretti AB: Radiographic Imaging for Dental Auxiliaries, 3rd ed. Philadelphia, WB Saunders, 1999.
8. Platin E, Carolina Institute for Radiology Educators Workshop, University of North Carolina, Chapel Hill, NC, July 1999.
9. Early PJ, et al: Textbook of Nuclear Medicine Technology, 3rd ed. St. Louis, CV Mosby, 1979, p 379.
10. Webber RL, et al: X-ray image subtraction as the basis for assessment of periodontal changes. J Periodontal Res 17:509-517, 1982.
11. Jeffcoat MK: A new method for comparison of bone loss measurement on nonstandardized radiographs. J Periodontal Res 19:434-441, 1984.
12. Jeffcoat MK, et al: Extraoral control of geometry for digital subtraction radiology. J Periodontal Res 22:398-406, 1987.
13. McHenry K, et al: Methodical aspects and quantitative adjuncts to computerized subtraction radiology. J Periodontal Res 22:125-133, 1987.

Web sites

14. http://www.usc.edu./hsc/dental
15. http://www.dentalcare.com
16. http://www.geocities.com

Questions and Answers

Questions

1. Which of the following terms best describes x-ray energy?
   A. Photons
   B. Electrons
   C. Primary beam
   D. Thermionic emission

2. Which of the following terms best describes the most common type of radiation that is emitted from the anode of the dental radiology machine tubehead?
   A. Bremsstrahlung radiation
   B. Characteristic radiation
   C. Compton scatter radiation
   D. Coherent scatter radiation

3. The lead collimator restricts the primary beam exiting the tubehead to the maximum diameter of
   A. 2.50 cm.
   B. 7 cm.
   C. 1.75 cm.
   D. 5 cm.

4. During the assessment phase of dental hygiene periodontal treatment planning, a complete mouth series of radiographs is often recommended. All of the following film image qualities/characteristics would be appropriate EXCEPT one. Which is the EXCEPTION?
   A. High contrast
   B. Low contrast
   C. Superimposition of the buccal and lingual cusps of posterior teeth.
   D. Sharpness

5. To reduce patient exposure to radiation, it is appropriate to
   A. set a high kVp (70–90 kVp).
   B. use a short BID (8 inches round or rectangular or conical BID).
   C. use an Ultraspeed film.
   D. wear a radiation-monitoring badge.

6. The whole body maximum permissible dose (MPD) to a 34-year-old dental hygienist on an annual basis is
   A. 5.0 mSv/yr.
   B. 0.5 mSv/yr.
   C. 50 mSv/yr.
   D. 1 mSv/yr.

7. Referring to question 6, what is the MPD during gestation of this 34-year-old dental hygienist who is pregnant?
   A. 5.0 mSv during the gestation period
   B. 0.5 mSv during the gestation period
   C. 50 mSv during the gestation period
   D. 1 mSv during the gestation period

8. From the following list of body tissues, which is most radiosensitive?
   A. Thyroid gland
   B. Blood-forming tissues
   C. Cornea of the eye
   D. Mature bone and cartilage

9. All of the following reduce radiation exposure to the patient with the exception of one. Which is the exception?
   A. Rectangular collimator
   B. Ektaspeed film
   C. Radiation monitoring badge
   D. Protective lead aprons

10. All of the following determine the latent period's degree of biologic effects except one. Which is the EXCEPTION?
    A. The exposure time
    B. The type of radiation
    C. The type(s) of tissues radiated
    D. The ability to cause substances to fluoresce

11. Which of the following tissues is most radioresistant?
    A. Nerve tissue
    B. Gland tissue
    C. Skin tissue
    D. Bone marrow tissue
    E. Reproductive organ tissue

12. The main factor that controls the penetration of x-rays is
    A. film speed.
    B. exposure time.
    C. source to film distance.
    D. wavelength.

13. Radiographic intensifying screens are used for
    A. magnifying images.
    B. increasing detail of the images.
    C. reducing the exposure time to the patient.
    D. decreasing the x-ray film processing time.

14. Which of the following results in the greatest reduction of radiation to the patient?
    A. A long, round BID
    B. A conical BID
    C. A short, rectangular BID
    D. A long, rectangular BID

15. Which of the following kVp settings would produce the lowest contrast or longest scale contrast on a radiographic image?
    A. 65 kVp
    B. 75 kVp
    C. 80 kVp
    D. 90 kVp

16. The paralleling technique produces an image with
    A. more contrast.
    B. decreased density.
    C. increased density.
    D. decreased distortion.

17. The most reliable method to determine the presence of or evaluate the current status of a periodontal pocket or gingival sulcus is the
    A. radiographic film.
    B. Nabors probe.
    C. periodontal probe.
    D. dental explorer.

18. The normal relationship of the interseptal bone to the cementoenamel junction refers to the height of the interseptal crestal cortical bone between the teeth. The normal height of this juncture is approximately
    A. 2-2.5 mm.
    B. 1-1.5 mm.
    C. 1.75 mm.
    D. 7 cm.

19. Which type of bone loss describes a reduction in the height of the interseptal crestal bone.
    A. Vertical
    B. Angular
    C. Horizontal
    D. Refractory

20. A poor crown-root ratio refers to bone disease that exhibits
    A. class I furcation.
    B. class II mobility.
    C. greater than one third of the tooth existing out of the bone.
    D. sclerosing alveolar bone.

21. If a satisfactory radiograph were produced using a target-to-film distance of 8 inches and an exposure time of 0.5 second, what is the correct exposure time for a target-to-film distance of 16 inches?
    A. 1 second
    B. 2 seconds
    C. 0.5 second
    D. 0.25 second

22. What happens to the *intensity* of the x-ray beam when the BID is changed from 8 to 16 inches?
    A. Increases by 2
    B. Decreases by 2
    C. Increases by 4
    D. Decreases by 4

23. The BID is changed from a 3-inch BID to a 1-inch BID. The exposure time for the 3-inch BID is 1 second. What is the new exposure time?
    A. 6 seconds
    B. 1/6 second
    C. 1/9 second
    D. 9 seconds

24. A radiograph is exposed using an 8-inch BID. The exposure time is 4 seconds. Then, a 2-inch BID is used. What is the new exposure time?
    A. 0.36 second
    B. 0.25 second

C. 0.44 second
D. 64 seconds

25. Referring to question and answer 24, how is the intensity of the x-ray beam affected?
    A. Increased by 9
    B. Decreased by 9
    C. Increased by 16
    D. Decreased by 16

26. If a satisfactory radiograph were produced using a target-to-film distance of 8 inches and an exposure time of 0.5 second, what is the correct exposure time for a target-to-film distance of 16 inches?
    A. 0.5 second
    B. 2 seconds
    C. 0.25 second
    D. 4 seconds

ANSWERS

1. **A.** A **photon** is a unit of electromagnetic radiation that occurs as a bundle of kinetic energy or x-ray energy that travels as a wave at the speed of light and in a straight line. An electron becomes a photon when the operator pushes the radiology machine exposure button. At this time, the electromagnetic energy attracts electrons from the cathode to the anode, hits the tungsten target focal spot, and produces photons that exit the tubehead as primary and secondary beams of x-radiation.

2. **A.** Of the radiation produced by a dental radiographic machine, 70% to 90% is Bremsstrahlung radiation or general radiation. This type of radiation is also called "braking radiation," which describes the deceleration of high-speed electrons while they give up their energy in the form of x-rays. General radiation produces x-ray photons of lower energy that have many different energies and wavelengths. Characteristic radiation, which is the other radiation produced by the dental radiographic machine (10%-30% of the radiation), occurs when an electron from the cathode hits an inner shell electron of the anode and causes that electron to be ejected. The rearrangement of the electrons to fill the vacancy produces a loss of energy that results in the production of a photon.

3. **B.** 7 cm equals 2.75 inches. The federal government regulations require that the x-ray beam be collimated to a diameter of no greater that 2.75 inches as the primary beam exits the position indicating device and reaches the patient's skin.

4. **A.** This is the exception to the desirable qualities or characteristics of the radiographic films. A high-contrast film means that the film exhibits blacks and whites with few shades of gray. This film image reveals minimal alveolar bone details and subtle periodontal pathologies. A low-contrast film with many shades of gray and less blacks and whites is more desirable. This means that a higher than 70 kVp setting is needed. Superimposition of posterior teeth buccal and lingual cusps is also desirable, meaning that a more paralleling technique has been accomplished. A desirable film image sharpness is influenced by a small focal spot size, the film's crystal size, and no movement.

5. **A.** A high kVpp setting (70-90 kVp) limits the amount of radiation exposure to the patient. The use of a long position indicating device (16 inches, not 8 inches) is preferred, because there is less beam divergence. A fast-speed film (currently E+ speed film) requires half of the radiation exposure time. The use of a radiation monitoring badge assesses the radiation exposure to the operator (not to the patient).

6. **C.** The MPD to a person who has occupational exposure to radiation is 50 mSv/yr as established by the National Council on Radiation Protection and Measurements.

7. **A.** The MPD to a pregnant woman who has occupational exposure to radiation is 5 mSv during the gestation period.

8. **B.** Different tissues of the body have different sensitivities to develop radiation effects. Blood-forming tissues are very sensitive or highly sensitive to radiation. The cornea of the eye has fairly high resistance; the thyroid gland and mature bone and cartilage have fairly low resistance regarding radiation sensitivity.

9. **C.** The radiation monitoring badge registers radiation exposure to the occupationally exposed worker, because the worker wears the badge (the patient does not wear the badge). The rectangular collimator, the E+ speed film, and the lead apron protect the patient.

10. **D.** The ability to cause a substance to fluoresce is not related to the latent period's degree of biologic effects. The exposure time, the type of radiation, and the type(s) of tissues radiated are related to the latent period's degree of biologic effects.

11. **A.** Nerve tissue is considered low sensitivity to radiation. Bone marrow and reproductive organ tissue have high sensitivity. Skin tissue has fairly high sensitivity to radiation, and gland tissue exhibits fairly low sensitivity to radiation.

12. **D.** Wavelength or penetrating power of the x-ray beam determines the quality of the x-ray photons. This is a function of the kVp setting and the focal spot size. The penetration power of the x-ray beam is a measure by its half-value layer (HVL) principle, which states that 50% of the x-ray photons should penetrate through a standardized thickness of a given material (usually aluminum) depending on the kVp. The film speed and the source-to-film distance influence the sharpness of the film image, and the exposure time influences the film density.

13. **C.** The intensifying screen is used most often in the panoramic film cassette, resulting in the reduction of radiation to the patient. Magnification is most influenced by the target-to-film distance and the object-to-film distance. Detail is most influenced by the local spot size, crystal size, and movement. Processing time and intensifying screens do not have a relationship.

14. **D.** A rectangular beam indicating device (BID) complies with the collimation of not being more than 2.75 inches, but it also constricts the beam to the size of a No. 2 film. The long, rectangular BID also constricts the divergence of the beam.

15. **D.** A kVp setting of more than 70 to 90 produces a radiographic film image that has many shades of gray or low-scale contrast.

16. **D.** Decreased distortion produces a more accurate image that may be achieved with the paralleling technique using the XCP film-holding device. Density and contrast are influenced by kVp and mAs.

17. **C.** The periodontal probe is the most reliable method when determining the presence of or current status of the periodontal pocket or gingival sulcus. The radiographic film is rated "fair." Nabor's probe functions to identify furcations, and the dental explorer functions to identify dental caries and other dental defects.

18. **B.** The normal height of this juncture is approximately 1 to 1.5 mm below the CEJ level of the adjacent teeth.

19. **C.** The height of the interseptal crestal bone refers to the horizontal bone between adjacent teeth.

20. **C.** Greater than one third of the tooth exists out of the bone to identify a poor crown-root ratio with a guarded prognosis. Mobility, furcation involvement, and sclerosed alveolar bone are not characteristic identifiers of a poor crown-root ratio.

21. **B.** Going from an 8-inch BID to a 16-inch BID = $^8/_{16} = ^1/_2$; Invert the $^1/_2$ to $^2/_1$; square the $^2/_1 = 4$. The BID was increased in length by a factor of 4; 4 multiplied by 0.5 second = 2 seconds. Going from an 8-inch BID to a 16-inch BID, the intensity decreases and the exposure time increases.

22. **D.** When increasing the BID length (source-to-object distance) is doubled, (8 to 16), the intensity decreases and the exposure time increases. The distance is doubled (from 8 to 16) and the square of 2 = 4. Therefore, we decrease the intensity by 4.

23. **C.** When the BID length (source-to-object distance) is decreased, the intensity increases and the exposure time decreases. The inverse of 3 is $^1/_3$, and the square of $^1/_3$ is $^1/_9$.

24. **B.** When the BID length is decreased, the intensity increases and the exposure time decreases. $^8/_2 = 4$ and the inverse of 4 is $^1/_4$. The BID length is decreased by a factor of 4. Now square $^1/_4 = ^1/_{16}$, and multiply by 4 seconds (exposure time of the 8-inch BID) = $^1/_4 = 0.25$ second.

25. **C.** From an 8-inch BID to a 2-inch BID, the intensity increases and the exposure time decreases. $^8/_2 = 4$, and the square of 4 is 16.

26. **B.** When the source-to-film distance is doubled, the intensity decreases and the exposure time increases. $^8/_{16} = ^1/_2$; the inverse of $^1/_2 = 2$; 2 squared = 4; 4 times $^1/_2 = 2$ seconds.

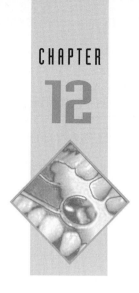

CHAPTER

12

Planning and Managing Dental Hygiene Care

CAROL A. SPEAR, BSDH, MSDH   CHRISTINA B. DeBIASE, BSDH, MA, EdD
MARGARET SIX, BS, MSDH

 INFECTION CONTROL

The clinical practice of dental hygiene involves the potential for exposure to infectious agents transmitted through body fluids, such as blood and saliva. It is essential, therefore, for dental care providers to protect themselves from infection by utilizing **infection control** (methods that decrease the spread of infection) and following **universal precautions**. Following universal precautions means that all patients and contaminated materials must be treated as being potentially infectious and that the same infection control procedures for any given dental procedure must be followed for each patient. In December 1991, the Occupational Safety and Health Administration (**OSHA**) issued the Standard for Occupational Exposure to Bloodborne Pathogens, Final Rule, in the Federal Register. This document lists rules and regulations that must be followed for the prevention of occupational exposure to potentially infectious material and mandates the practice of universal precautions.

Personal Protective Equipment

Personal protective equipment (PPE), which is clothing or equipment provided by the employer and worn by the employee, serves as a physical barrier between the body and the source of potential contamination. OSHA mandates that the dental care provider wear appropriate gloves, mask, eye protection, and clothing during patient care involving contact with blood and saliva.

Available glove types include single-use sterile, nonsterile examination and overgloves, and utility gloves. The selection of glove worn depends on the invasiveness of the procedure for which the glove is worn. Treatment gloves are available with or without powder and are made from natural latex or synthetic materials (e.g., vinyl, nitrile, tactylon).

Individually wrapped **sterile gloves**, which are often called **surgeon's gloves**, are recommended for use during invasive procedures such as surgery and periodontal débridement. This type of treatment glove is of a higher quality than are the other types and is available in various sizes. **Nonsterile examination gloves** may be worn for noninvasive procedures or when handling contaminated objects. These gloves are not available in specific sizes but rather as small, medium, etc. Both sterile and nonsterile treatment gloves must be changed for each patient; the gloves are changed more often if they are torn or if the texture changes during use.

Overgloves are thin plastic gloves that may be worn over nonsterile examination gloves when it is necessary to touch nondisinfected or nonsterile objects (e.g., the patient's chart) outside of the oral cavity during the patient's treatment. Overgloves must not be worn over sterile gloves. To avoid cross-contamination, a better alternative to wearing overgloves is to remove treatment gloves before touching contaminated objects outside of the oral cavity and replace them with new gloves before resuming treatment.

Utility gloves are heavy nonsterile puncture-resistant gloves that must be worn during cleaning of contaminated instruments and other sharp objects in preparation for sterilization. These gloves must be cleaned and disinfected after use.

The wearing of gloves does not preclude handwashing before and after donning gloves. Hands should be washed and dried thoroughly. Rings should not be worn, because they contribute to tears in the gloves and they may harbor bacteria or moisture that can lead to skin irritation.

Because of the increased use of latex gloves and other products containing latex, there has been an increased occurrence of hypersensitivity to latex products. This may involve the dental operator or the patient. Individuals at high risk of developing latex allergy include health care professionals and individuals with spina bifida, those susceptible to allergies (**atopy**), and those who have had multiple surgeries at an early age. In addition, individuals who are allergic to any of the following may react to latex: **apple, avocado, chestnut, banana, celery, figs, kiwis, peach, pear, pineapple,** and **tomato.**

Latex hypersensitivity can be initiated by protein, which is a natural component of latex, by chemical additives, or by a combination of the two. Adverse reactions to latex-containing products may be one of three types: (1) **irritant contact dermatitis (nonallergic)**, (2) **delayed type IV hypersensitivity (allergic contact dermatitis)**, and (3) **immediate type I hypersensitivity**.

Contact dermatitis and type IV hypersensitivity may exhibit similar symptoms. Acute symptoms include redness, itching, burning, edema, and dryness. Chronic symptoms include cracks, fissures, crusting, peeling, scabbing scores, and open lesions. The area affected in contact dermatitis is confined to the area of the glove or other latex product, whereas the affected area in type IV hypersensitivity may move beyond the area touched or covered by the latex products. The onset of contact dermatitis occurs within minutes or hours after exposure, whereas that of type IV hypersensitivity may be delayed for 6 to 48 hours after. Because symptoms of these two reactions are similar, a true diagnosis must be made by a patch test conducted by an allergist.

These reactions may be induced by chemical additives to the latex gloves or by glove powder. Other contributing factors include improper hand washing and drying before donning gloves, hand-cleansing agents, poor-fitting gloves, and chapped skin.

Type I hypersensitivity is the most severe allergic reaction and is attributed to the naturally occurring proteins in the latex. Symptoms may occur within seconds to 1 hour after exposure and range from mild localized hives (**urticaria**) and itching to systemic reactions that include rhinitis, wheezing, anaphylactic shock, and even death.

Dental personnel or patients who are allergic to latex must avoid contact with all latex products (**Table 12-1**). Various synthetic gloves (e.g., vinyl, nitrile, and neoprene) are available. If a staff member is allergic to latex, nonpowder gloves should be worn by other staff members in the treatment area because glove proteins can migrate to the powder and become airborne. For treatment of a known latex allergic patient, schedule the patient early in the day to minimize airborne latex powder, and avoid the use of latex-containing items during treatment. Avoidance of unexpected latex allergies in patients can be accomplished by questioning the patient during the medical history review before beginning any treatment.

A **facemask** must be worn by the dental operator during any intraoral treatment in which splatter or aerosol is generated. It is suggested that the mask be changed for treatment of each patient. However, it must be changed if it becomes wet and ceases to act as a filter.

Standard masks will filter out at least 95% of small particles that contact their surface and are not designed to protect the wearer against inhalation of highly infectious aerosols such as those containing *Mycobacterium tuberculosis*. **High-efficiency particulate air (HEPA)** filter masks must be worn in these situations. A complete facial shield may be worn to protect against splatter to the face and eyes; however, a mask must be worn under the shield for protection from aerosol that may be sucked up under the shield.

Protective eyewear must be worn by the dental care provider during any treatment in which aerosol, splatter, or projectiles may be generated. This includes splatter from potentially infectious material and chemicals. Acceptable types of protective eyewear are safety glasses or goggles with side shields and full facial shields. Although not mandated by OSHA, it is beneficial for the patient to wear protective eyewear during dental treatment. The patient is exposed to infectious and chemical splatter and aerosol and often the potential for objects dropped onto the face.

Protective attire is the garment worn over regular clothing. This outerwear should have a high neck, long sleeves, and sufficient length to cover exposed street clothes and may be disposable or reusable. Reusable attire must be laundered at the office or by a professional laundry service. All protective attire should be changed daily, or more often if it becomes visibly soiled, and should be worn only in the treatment area.

Instrument Sterilization and Surface Disinfection

The prevention of **cross-contamination** or the spread of microorganisms from one source to another (i.e., from patient to patient, patient to object, or object to patient) is of primary concern in the practice of dentistry. This is accomplished by a combination of sanitization, disinfection, and sterilization. **Sanitization** is synonymous with cleaning or reducing the level of organic and inorganic contaminants from a surface. **Disinfection** is a process that destroys microorganisms but may not kill spores. **Sterilization** is a process by which all forms of life, including bacterial spores, are destroyed.

To determine the method of sterilization or disinfection that must be used to decontaminate instruments or equipment, one must determine if the item is critical, semicritical, or noncritical according to Spalding's Classification of Inanimate Objects (**Table 12-2**).

TABLE 12-1 Common Dental Latex Products

Gloves	Orthodontic elastics
Ear loops on facial masks	Ambubags
Elastic waist/wrist bands	Inhalation masks ($N_2O - O_2$)
Rubber dams	Stethoscopes
Prophy caps	Blood pressure cuffs

TABLE 12–2 Classification of Inanimate Objects

SURFACE CATEGORY	DEFINITION	STERILIZATION/ DISINFECTION	EXAMPLES
Critical	Penetrate soft tissue or bone	Sterilize or disposable	Needles Curets Explorers Probes
Semicritical	Touch intact mucous membrane, oral fluids	Sterilize after each use	Radiographic biteblock Ultrasonic handpiece
	Does not penetrate	High level disinfection when sterilization cannot be used	Amalgam condenser Mirror
Noncritical	Do not touch mucous membranes (only contact unbroken epithelium)	Cleaning and tuberculocidal intermediate-level disinfection	Light handles Certain x-ray machine parts Safety eyewear
Environmental surfaces	No contact with patient (or only intact skin)	Cleaning and intermediate to low disinfection	Counter tops Equipment surfaces Housekeeping surface

From Wilkins E: Clinical Practice of the Dental Hygienist, 8th ed. Philadelphia, Lippincott Williams & Wilkins, 1999, p 67.

Methods of sterilization include **moist heat** (steam under pressure), **dry heat, chemical vapor,** and **ethylene oxide (Table 12-3).** Steam under pressure is the most common and economical method of sterilization, and it can be used for sterilizing a wide variety of items. Corrosion, however, may occur with carbon steel or geared or hinged objects, and the moisture contributes to dulling of cutting edges.

Dry heat is suitable for sterilizing items that cannot be subjected to steam under pressure. However, the long exposure time is a disadvantage. Chemical vapor sterilization does not cause corrosion of carbon steel instruments and occurs in a short time period; however, adequate ventilation is needed for operation. Ethylene oxide sterilization is gaseous sterilization. Almost all types of materials and items can be sterilized with this method. However, it is not commonly used in small offices because of the lengthy time of operation, need for appropriate ventilation, and gas absorption requiring airing of plastic, rubber, and cloth items.

Chemical disinfectants are categorized as **high level, intermediate level,** or **low level.** High level disinfectants include **glutaraldehyde** and **hydrogen peroxide.** Items must be immersed in these disinfectants for **20 to 30 minutes for disinfection or 6 to 10 hours for sterilization** to occur. High level disinfectants are not recommended because of the long sterilization time, the problem in maintaining sterility of items during storage, and the potential for corrosion.

Intermediate level disinfectants should be utilized for disinfection of noncritical objects or surfaces and are commonly called **surface disinfectants.** Acceptable surface disinfectants are those that are **Environmental Protection Agency (EPA) registered, tuberculocidal, lipophilic,** and **hydrophilic.** Hydrophilic viruses have a protein coating and are much more difficult to kill than are lipid-enveloped viruses. Surface disinfectants that exhibit the aforementioned properties include **synthetic phenols, chlorines, iodophors, quaternaries,**

sodium bromide, and **chlorine.** However, not all commercial brands of these chemicals exhibit a hydrophilic virus kill **(Table 12-4).** The procedure for **surface disinfection** involves three steps: **spray, wipe, and spray.** For the initial spray, a disinfectant that contains a detergent or a cleaning agent may be used. Next, the surface is wiped (cleaned) with a paper towel. Finally, the surface is sprayed with the surface disinfectant and allowed to air dry for 10 minutes.

It is important to note that neither disinfection nor sterilization can occur unless the object or surface is first cleaned of bioburden.

Protective Barriers

An effective way to maintain disinfection of surfaces is to cover them with a barrier immediately after the disinfection process. Surface covers are usually plastic and include wrap,

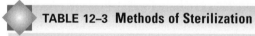

TABLE 12–3 Methods of Sterilization

METHOD	STERILIZING REQUIREMENT		
	TIME	TEMPERATURE	PRESSURE
Moist heat Steam under pressure (steam autoclave)	15–30 min	250°F 121°C	15 psi
Dry heat oven	120 min	320°F 160°C	
Unsaturated chemical vapor	20 min	270°F 132°C	20–40 psi
Ethylene oxide gas	10–16 hr	75°F 25°C	

From Wilkins E: Clinical Practice of the Dental Hygienist, 8th ed. Philadelphia, Lippincott Williams & Wilkins, 1999, p 61.

TABLE 12–4 Chemical Agents for Surface Disinfection Reference Chart

	ADVANTAGES	DISADVANTAGES	NAME	EPA REG #	DILUTION	HYDROPHILIC VIRUS KILL	FOR MORE INFORMATION CONTACT
Alcohols	Do not use for environmental surface disinfection. Rapid evaporation rate. Diminished activity with bioburden.						
Chlorines	Rapid acting;	Discard diluted	Clorox	5813-1	1:100	Yes	Clorox
	Broad spectrum;	solutions daily;	Dispatch	56392-7	None	Yes	Caltech
	Economical	Diminished activity	(0.55%)				
		by organic matter;					
		Corrosive					
Iodophors	Broad spectrum;	Unstable at high	IodoFive	4959-16	1:213	Yes	Cottrell, Ltd
	Few reactions;	temperatures;					
	Residual biocidal	Dilution & contact	Biocide	" "	" "	" "	Biotrol
	activity	time critical;					
		Discard daily;	Iodophor Disinfect.	" "	" "	" "	Smart Practice
		Discoloration of some surfaces;					
		Inactivated by hard water					
Synthetic Phenolics	Broad spectrum;	Discard daily for most diluted solutions;	Omni II	46851-1	1:32	Yes	Cottrell
			ProPhene	" "	" "	" "	Cottrell
	Residual biocidal activity	Degrades certain plastic over time;	Vital Defense -D	" "	" "	" "	Block
		Difficult to rinse;	ProSpray	46851-5	None	Yes	Cottrell
		Film accumulation	Birex$_{5e}$	1043-92	1:256	No	Biotrol
			Dual Phenol Germicidal Cleaner	67813-3	1:256	No	Smart Practice
			BiArrest-2	67813-1	1:256	No	Infection Control Technology
			Tri-Cide	11725-7	1:256	Yes	HealthSonics
			Dencide	63281-4	1:256	Yes	Dentsply
			Asetiphene 128	303-223	1:128	Yes	Huntington
			PUMP				
			CoeSpray	334-417	None	Yes	GC America
			Aseptiphene RTU	" "	" "	" "	Huntington
			AEROSOL				
			Lysol IC Disinfect.	777-53	None	Yes	Sultan
			AseptiSteryl	706-69	None	Yes	Huntington
			Discide Disinf Spray	" "	" "	" "	Palmero
			Citrace	56392-2	None	Yes	Caltech
			Medicide/ ADC Disinfect. Deodor	334-214	None	No	ADC

(Continues)

bags, or tubing. The use of protective barriers does not preclude surface disinfection but is used in combination with it.

Other Methods for Preventing Cross-Contamination

Packaging of materials or supplies in individual packets as a unit dose for individual patients is an effective way to avoid contamination of bulk items. The use of disposable items is another effective method for reducing cross-contamination. Examples of **disposables** include saliva ejectors, air/water syringes, impression trays, and prophy angles. **Any nondisposable item with a small lumen, such as an air/water syringe must be properly cleaned before sterilization can occur**. This involves cleaning the lumen, in addition to the outer surfaces. If the lumen is not cleaned

TABLE 12–4 Chemical Agents for Surface Disinfection Reference Chart (Continued)

	ADVANTAGES	DISADVANTAGES	NAME	EPA REG #	DILUTION	HYDROPHILIC VIRUS KILL	FOR MORE INFORMATION CONTACT
Dual or Synergized Quaternaries	Broad spectrum Contains detergent for cleaning Few reactions	Easily inactivated by anionic detergents and organic matter Deleterious to some materials	Cavicide DisCide TB Precise QTB GC SprayCide SaniTex Plus Asepticare ⁺II	46781-6 1839-83 " " 1130-15 " " 1130-13	None None " " None " " None	Yes Yes " " Yes " " Yes	Kerr Palmero Caltech GC America CrossTex Huntington
Sodium Bromide and Chlorine	Broad spectrum; Reduced storage	May not be used for immersion Chlorine smell	Microstat 2	70369-1	2 tablets per quart	Yes	Septodont

Total time for surface disinfection is 10 minutes for all, except Dispatch (2 minutes) and Microstat 2 (5 minutes).
IMPORTANT INFORMATION
All products to be used as disinfectants on precleaned surfaces must be EPA-registered. Listing does not imply endorsement, recommendation, or warranty. Other products available. Purchasers are legally required to consult the package insert for changes in formulation and recommended product uses. Check compatibility of material before use on dental/medical equipment.
This chart is a publication of the Organization for Safety & Asepsis Procedures (OSAP). OSAP assumes no liability for actions taken based on the information herein. This resource was amended and reprinted with permission of OSAP. OSAP is a nonprofit organization which provides information and education on dental infection control and office safety. For more information, please call 1-800-298-6727.
Organization for Safety & Asepsis Procedures (OSAP)
P.O. Box 6297·Annapolis, MD 21401·www·osap·org·410-571-0003·Fax: 410-571-0028·Email:osap@clark.net
©OSAP October 1998. All rights reserved.

properly, bioburden collects; corrosion occurs; and microorganisms grow and colonize in these areas protected from the effects of sterilization.

Aerosol and **splatter** created during dental procedures create the potential of microbial cross-contamination between the patient and the operator or adjacent environmental surfaces. This can be reduced by providing the patient with a **pretreatment ADA-approved mouthrinse** containing chlorhexidine gluconate or essential oils or **having the patient brush before treatment**, **using rubber dams** whenever possible and **utilizing high-speed evacuation**.

Any dental impression or appliance must be rinsed and then placed in a sealed plastic bag containing an intermediate disinfectant or sprayed with the disinfectant and sealed in a bag for 10 to 15 minutes before sending it to a laboratory. Likewise, any appliance that the laboratory returns to the patient must be disinfected in the same manner. When operating the dental lathe in the laboratory, wear protective eyewear and a mask. Use sterile rag wheels, stones, and fresh pumice and pan liners for each patient's appliance.

Because of the potential for infection through cross-contamination to the dental health care provider, the following practices are prohibited. Do not eat or drink, store food or drink, handle contact lenses, or apply make-up or lip balm in the treatment, sterilizing, or x-ray processing areas or in the laboratory. Do not store food in refrigerators where dental products or potentially infectious materials are stored. Keep separately designated areas in the laboratory for receiving contaminated items and for handling clean or sterile items. All infectious waste, including chemicals, must be disposed of according to local, state, and federal regulations and may vary from locale to locale. Generally speaking, blood-soaked items and hard and soft tissue are considered regulated waste and must be placed in appropriate biohazard infectious waste containers and disposed of by specified agencies.

Safe handling of sharp items during treatment and disposal is very important to the operator. **Sharp items include scaling and surgical instruments, anesthetic and irrigation needles, and orthodontic wire.** Disposable sharp items must be placed into hard "sharps" containers. Needles should be recapped by a one-handed scoop technique or by use of a barrier cap holding device. Disposable self-sheathing "safe" syringes may be used rather than autoclavable syringes.

Biofilm in Dental Unit Waterlines

Biofilm is a consortia of microbes (bacteria, fungi, and protozoa) in an acellular nutrient matrix or plaque that forms on all surfaces over which water flows. **Dental unit waterlines (DUWLS)** provide for the growth of biofilm because of the small-diameter long tubing that provides for a large surface area for biofilm attachment. Biofilm pathogens include *Staphylococcus aureus, Pseudomonas, Legionella,* and fungi (see Chapter 7).

Currently, the best control of biofilm in DUWLS has not been determined. Research is ongoing in this area. Three types of controls presently available are: (1) a **separate** sterile water supply, (2) continuous or intermittent **chemical disinfection** (e.g., sodium hypochlorite, hydrogen peroxide, iodine, or citric acid preparations), and (3) **filtration**. **Purging water lines for 2 to 3 minutes before the start of each day and for 30 seconds between each patient** has been recommended. This procedure flushes out some loose biofilm from the lines, but it does not eliminate or destroy the attached biofilm.

Material Safety Data Sheets and Labeling

A dental care provider must maintain and file a **material safety data sheet (MSDS)** for every product utilized in the dental facility. An MSDS is provided by the manufacturer of each dental product. An MSDS lists hazards of the material, precautions for handling, and procedures to follow in emergencies occurring from the use or handling of the product.

Exposure Control Plan

The OSHA Bloodborne Pathogen Standard requires that each dental office or facility have a written **Exposure Control Plan** that describes procedures that must be followed for eliminating or minimizing occupational exposure to bloodborne pathogens. The following must be included in the Exposure Control Plan: classification of employees according to occupational exposure, employee training and education, engineering controls and work practices with emphasis on safer medical devices and PPE, housekeeping and decontamination, required immunizations, and post-exposure management protocol. This plan must be updated and edited and reviewed by all employees annually.

RECOGNITION AND MANAGEMENT OF EMERGENCY SITUATIONS

Dental hygienists are employed in numerous settings, and they treat patients who exhibit numerous and complicated medical or dental histories. Furthermore, dental hygienists are educated to treat patients who may exhibit systemic disease, compromised immune systems, or syndromes that may affect the provision of dental hygiene care. Health professionals feel competent and comfortable providing the services for which they are educated to perform and do so on a daily basis. The occurrence of a medical emergency may be approached with trepidation due to the infrequency with which emergencies are encountered. Therefore, it is very important that the dental hygienist review emergencies that may occur in the dental office and rehearse, within the office setting, the recognition and management of these emergency situations. The preparedness of the dental team may make the difference between life and death.

 PREVENTION

Many emergencies can be prevented through a careful assessment of the patient prior to the provision of dental care. A thorough and concise collection and analysis of the patient's medical and dental history data are necessary before each appointment. Information collected and careful observation of the patient may reveal problems that require further investigation. This investigation may be the clarifying measure that is needed to recognize and prevent a potential emergency situation. Current medications and conditions being monitored by the patient's physician warrant special attention.

 VITAL SIGNS

The collection of **vital signs** is an important part of the patient assessment procedure. Blood pressure, pulse, respiration, and temperature are signs that are quick and easy to collect and directly reflect a person's health. Signs such as age, height, and weight should be documented on the permanent record and updated regularly.

Blood pressure is measured in millimeters of mercury (mm Hg) using a **sphygmomanometer** and a stethoscope. The first audible sound is recorded as the **systolic pressure,** which represents the force of blood on the vessel walls during ventricular contraction. **Diastolic pressure,** the final audible sound, is the measurement recorded during ventricular relaxation. Blood pressure is recorded in the form of a fraction with the higher pressure (**systolic**) recorded on top and the lower pressure (**diastolic**) on the bottom. Normal systolic pressure is is <130 mm Hg, whereas normal diastolic pressure is <85 mm Hg. A baseline blood pressure is important for comparison during an emergency situation. It is important to identify the patient with **hypertension** (elevated blood pressure) prior to dental treatment. Stress or anxiety associated with dental treatment may exacerbate the blood pressure of the hypertensive patient. Local anesthetics with vasoconstrictors could place the undiagnosed hypertensive patient into an emergency situation. Recognition and referral of the undiagnosed hypertensive patient and the appropriate management of those patients previously diagnosed will help to prevent a medical emergency. **Hypotension** (low blood pressure) is associated with emergency situations such as syncope, diabetic coma, shock, and adrenal crisis.

The **pulse** should be recorded as a routine vital sign and recorded with notations concerning irregularities of rhythm or strength. The pulse is felt as a result of the pulsation of blood passing through an artery in response to the contraction of the heart. The pulse rate corresponds to the number of heartbeats per minute. The **radial pulse** is felt on the radial artery located on the ventral, thumb-side of the wrist (**Figure 12-1**). The **carotid pulse** located in the neck is

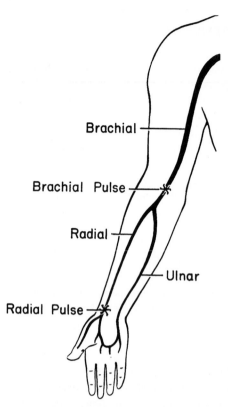

Figure 12-1. Arteries of the arm. Note the location of the radial pulse. The brachial pulse may be felt just before the brachial artery branches into the radial and ulnar arteries. (From Wilkins E: Clinical Practice of the Dental Hygienist, 8th ed. Philadelphia, Lippincott Williams & Wilkins, 1999, p 110.)

monitored during cardiopulmonary resuscitation (CPR). The normal adult pulse rate is equal to 60 to 100 beats/min. **Tachycardia** (pulse rate >100 beats/min) is associated with anxiety or stress, hyperglycemia, and cortisol deficiency.

Bradycardia (a pulse rate <50 beats/min) may be observed in patients who are fasting or taking depressants or those who are in a compromised state of health.

Respiration is counted as one cycle of breath being inhaled and exhaled. Normal adult respiration is between 14 and 20 per minute. **Tachypnea** (increased respiration) is observed in the patient who is hyperventilating. **Hyperventilation** (25-30 respirations/min) may occur as a response to anxiety or fear related to dental treatment. When the dental patient hyperventilates, the dental procedure should be terminated and efforts should be made to calm the patient. Instruct the patient to breathe slowly (7-10 breaths/min), which helps to restore the decreased blood carbon dioxide level to normal. The patient's hands may be cupped over the nose and mouth to facilitate the inspiration of carbon dioxide. The patient experiencing a hyperventilation episode is deficient in carbon dioxide; therefore, oxygen should never be administered in this situation. **Bradypnea** (decreased respiration) may be observed during sleep, stroke, and respiratory failure.

Pyrexia (temperature elevated above 99.5°F) in the dental patient may be an indication of infection or disease. Normal oral temperature falls between 96°F and 99.5°F (35.5°C-37.5°C). If the dental patient is found to be pyretic, elective dental procedures should be postponed and rescheduled. Adult vital signs are represented in **Table 12-5A & B.**

 EMERGENCY EQUIPMENT AND APPROPRIATE TRAINING

Every dental office should be equipped with the basic equipment necessary for the management of a variety of possible medical emergencies. Readiness of the dental team to respond to an emergency efficiently and effectively requires

 TABLE 12–5A. Adult BP and Oral Care Modifications

CATEGORY	SYSTOLIC PRESSURE (MM HG)	DIASTOLIC PRESSURE (MM HG)	ORAL CARE PROCEDURES
Normal	<130	<85	No modified oral care
High Normal	130–139	85–89	No modified oral care
Hypertension			
Stage I	140–159	90–99	No modified oral care, medical referral, inform patient
Stage II	160–179	100–109	Selective oral care,* medical referral
Stage III	180–209	110–119	Emergent nonstressful procedures (ENP),** immediate medical referral/consultation
Stage IV	≥210	≥120	Emergent nonstressful procedures (ENP),** immediate medical referral

*May include, but not limited to, oral prophylaxis, nonsurgical periodontal therapy, restorative procedures, and nonsurgical endodontic therapy.
**May include, but not limited to, oral procedures to alleviate pain, infection or masticatory dysfunction with limited physiological and psychological effects. Example: simple incision and drainage of an intraoral fluctuant dental abscess. Medical benefits of ENP in stage III and IV hypertensive patients should outweigh the risk of complications secondary to the patient's hypertensive state.

Modified from Fifth Report of the Joint National Committee on Detection, Evaluation and Treatment of High Blood Pressure. Arch Intern Med 1993;153:154–83, Muzyka BC and Glick M: The hypertensive dental patient. JADA 128(8):1109–1120, 1997, and Martin C et al: Electronic Blood Pressure Screening: fast, easy and essential. Access 12(1):33–37, 1998.

appropriate training and equipment. Equipment must be monitored regularly to ensure that it is working effectively.

Telephone numbers for emergency medical service (EMS) systems (dial 911), fire department, poison control center, and local police should be posted at all telephone extensions. Every dental office should maintain a well-equipped drug kit. A list of recommended drugs and their indication for use are found in **Table 12-6**.

Other essential emergency equipment includes a portable oxygen tank (**green** E series), Ambu bag, tourniquet, syringes, suction tips, Magill forceps, blood pressure equipment, a first aid kit, and an eyewash station. Ammonia vaporoles are easily taped to the back of a dental chair for quick retrieval. Cricothyrotomy equipment and a cardiac defibrillator should be included in offices in which personnel have advanced training in emergency procedures.

Appropriate training requires that all dental office personnel be educated in emergency procedures. Each office should develop a protocol for managing the unexpected situation, and personnel should practice through mock drills and role-play. All health care providers should be certified in **CPR**. Cardiac defibrillators are now being placed in many areas that serve the public. **Automated external defibrillators (AEDs)** provide computer-analyzed defibrillation to the patient in cardiac arrest. It is recommended that dental personnel receive education and training in the use of the AED.

RECOGNITION AND MANAGEMENT

Whereas many medical emergencies can be prevented through careful assessment of the dental patient, the possibility remains that an unexpected situation may arise during the course of a normal workday. In this event, recognition, critical thinking to determine the appropriate course of action, and management of the situation are paramount.

Syncope

When a patient loses consciousness in the dental operatory, the dental hygienist must assess the situation quickly and

TABLE 12–6 Basic Drug Kit

CATEGORY	CONDITION	SUGGESTIONS
Catecholamine	Anaphylaxis	Epinephrine (Adrenalin) EpiPen
Antihistamine	Allergic reaction	Chlorpheniramine (Chlor-Trimeton) Diphenhydramine (Benadryl)
Vasodilator	Angina	Nitroglycerin (Nitrostat, nitrolingual spray) Amyl nitrite
Antihypoglycemic	Insulin shock/diabetic patient Hypoglycemia/non-diabetic patient	Fruit juice or Gluco-Stat
Antiplatelet	Myocardial infarction	Aspirin
Bronchodilators	Asthma	Albuterol (Proventil, Ventolin) Metaproterenol (Alupent)

determine the course of action for the provision of care. Loss of consciousness may be something as benign as syncope or the result of a more serious condition such as myocardial infarction or airway obstruction. **Syncope** (fainting) can be defined as a sudden, temporary loss of consciousness owing to a drop in blood pressure, resulting in impaired blood flow to the brain. Dental fears and phobias may prompt an episode of syncope. Adolescents and young adults are more likely to experience syncope as a result of anxiety or stress related to a dental procedure. Patients in the dental operatory may express a feeling of faintness, nausea, dizziness, and the need for fresh air before fainting. Physical signs include pallor, dilated pupils, perspiration, and an increase in respiration and pulse rate, leading to the loss of consciousness. Utilizing the **Trendelenburg position** (i.e., the heart and feet raised higher than the head) to recline the patient in the dental chair normally elicits immediate recovery from the syncope episode. It is recommended that the pregnant patient be instructed to lie on her side left while elevating her legs. This position prevents the additional weight of the fetus from pressing on the inferior vena cava, which would decrease blood flow. Wafting an ammonia vaporole under the patient's nose will also prompt an immediate response. The dental hygienist should continue to monitor vital signs until the patient has recovered and reschedule dental treatment for a later date. **Orthostatic hypotension**, also referred to as postural hypotension, is a sudden decrease in systolic pressure, which results in syncope when a patient sits or stands to an upright position after reclining for a period of time. Treatment includes reclining the patient to a supine position until the patient regains consciousness and recovers. The patient should then be slowly returned to an upright position.

TABLE 12–5B Adult Vital Signs

VITAL SIGN	VALUES OF SIGNIFICANCE IN DENTAL AND DENTAL HYGIENE APPOINTMENTS
Body temperature (oral)	Normal 37.0°C (98.6°F) Normal range 35.5°C to 37.5°C (96°F to 99.5°F)
Pulse Rate	Normal range 60 to 100 per minute
Respiration	Normal range 14 to 20 per minute

E. Wilkins, Clinical Practice of the Dental Hygienist, 8th ed. LWW, 1999, p. 107.

Hypoglycemia/Hyperglycemia

Alterations in blood glucose levels can pose a significant risk to the dental patient. Patients who present with a diagnosis of **type I** or **type II diabetes mellitus** require particular attention and careful assessment by the dental hygienist. As a metabolic disorder, **diabetes mellitus** is characterized by faulty insulin production resulting in the decreased metabolism of carbohydrates. When collecting or updating the medical history for the diabetic patient, additional questions regarding the prescribed regimen of insulin or oral hypoglycemic drugs, meal times, and blood glucose levels should be considered. Type I [formerly known as insulin-dependent diabetes mellitus (IDDM)] diabetes requires that the patient supply insulin to the body on a regular basis in response to the blood glucose levels. Careful monitoring and diet control are required to attain the proper balance. During times of illness, stress, and decreased food intake, insulin requirements may change. Failure to adjust the insulin dosage may result in a hypoglycemic or hyperglycemic state**.** Review and management of these conditions are found in **Table 12-7.**

Seizure Disorders

When a medical history reveals a history of seizure activity, additional questions are required. Identification of anticonvulsant medications and dosage regimen should be documented. The history of seizure type, duration, and frequency should be ascertained to provide helpful information in the event that a seizure occurs during the dental appointment. Although nothing can be done to stop the seizure, measures to help ensure patient safety are indicated. **Partial (simple or complex)** and **absence (petit mal) seizures** are of relative short duration and are not convulsive. **Generalized tonic-clonic seizures** result in a loss of consciousness and

may require emergency care. Recognition and management of the generalized tonic-clonic seizure are displayed in **Table 12-8**.

Stroke

Interference in the normal blood supply to the brain as a result of hemorrhage, ischemia, or thrombosis is defined as a **cerebrovascular accident (CVA)** or **stroke**. A severe CVA may result in death or render the patient severely disabled. The patient who suffers from a less severe stroke may experience transient disabilities in which the patient may recover with physical therapy. Effects of a stroke may include paralysis, memory loss, speech disturbance, and personality changes. **Transient ischemic attack (TIA or ministroke)** is a momentary decrease in the blood flow to the brain and may provide a warning sign before the occurrence of a more serious CVA. Symptoms of a stroke include weakness on one side of the body, paralysis, speech disturbances, dizziness, and severe headache. When a stroke is suspected, the EMS should be contacted immediately (dial 911). For the patient who is conscious, monitor vital signs; provide oxygen; and provide comfort and reassurance until the EMS arrives. For the unconscious patient, basic life support and CPR are provided as necessary until the EMS arrives.

Cardiac Emergencies

Angina pectoris is a condition of severe chest pain resulting from a decrease in normal blood supply to the heart. The patient previously diagnosed with angina will normally self-administer prescribed nitroglycerin to relieve the symptoms. When pain persists after three doses within a 15-minute period, **myocardial infarction** (i.e., heart attack) may be pos-

TABLE 12–7 Recognition and Management of Diabetic Emergencies

	INSULIN SHOCK	DIABETIC COMA
Lab findings	↑Insulin	↓Insulin
	↓Blood glucose	↑Blood glucose
Symptoms	• Rapid onset	• Slow onset
	• Confusion/erratic behavior	• Acetone breath (sweet smelling)
	• Hunger and headache	• Polydipsia
	• Moist skin	• Polyuria
	• Pallor	• Weak/rapid pulse
	• Dilated pupils	• Dry flushed skin
	• Increased pulse rate	• Kussmaul breathing
Treatment	Administer sugar	Activate the EMS
	• Fruit drink	Monitor vital signs
	• Gluco-Stat	Administer oxygen
		Initiate basic life support as necessary

TABLE 12–8 Generalized Tonic/Clonic Seizure

OBSERVATION	MANAGEMENT
Aura • Change in taste, smell, or hearing	If recognized, provide safety for the patient
Patient loses consciousness	Activate the EMS
Tonic/clonic spasms (1-3 minutes)	Provide protection
• Epileptic cry	• Cushion the head
• Tonic rigidity followed by clonic muscle spasms	• Remove objects that could harm the patient if struck
• Cyanosis	• Assess the airway
Consciousness returns	• Monitor vital signs
• Incontinence possible	Provide comfort and support for the patient
• Confusion	• Suction with Hi-Vac to remove excess saliva or vomitus
• Disoriented	Provide assistance to the EMS
Post convulsive period	Document the seizure episode
• Headache	• Duration
• Muscle aches	• Complications/injuries
• Deep sleep	

sible. Myocardial infarction is the result of diminished or complete loss of blood supply to the heart owing to coronary artery occlusion or thrombosis. Symptoms, which include radiating chest pain, nausea, perspiration, and labored breathing, are indicative of a heart attack. The absence of pulse, respiration, and heartbeat in an unconscious patient indicates **cardiac arrest**. The EMS should be activated immediately with basic life support, and CPR measures should be initiated. Aspirin and oxygen may be administered to the patient experiencing symptoms of a heart attack.

Many states require that licensed dental hygienists obtain and maintain type C health care provider certification from the American Heart Association in CPR. In the dental office, various medical emergencies may result in loss of consciousness, cessation of breathing, and ultimately cardiac arrest. The provision of **CPR** may maintain a patient's breathing and circulation until the EMS arrives to provide advanced care. **Table 12-9** outlines the steps followed for the delivery of CPR by one person.

When two persons are available to assist in performing CPR, one person assumes responsibility for ventilation and the other person completes cardiac compressions. When the pulse is not detected after the delivery of the first two ventilations, begin with **5 compressions followed by 1 ventilation**. Reassess after 1 minute, and continue a 5:1 cycle until the EMS arrives. The ratios for child and infant CPR are displayed in **Table 12-10**.

Airway Obstruction

Airway obstructions may be partial or complete and represent a serious medical situation prompting immediate atten-

tion. The patient exhibiting partial airway obstruction should be encouraged to cough and should be assisted if breathing becomes impaired. The universal sign of a patient grasping the neck aids in the recognition of an airway obstruction. Failure to remove the obstruction expeditiously results in lack of oxygen, cyanosis, and loss of consciousness. The **Heimlich maneuver** is used to remove foreign objects blocking the airway. Perform the maneuver by standing behind the choking patient with arms wrapped around the patient's midsection. Placing the fists between the naval and the sternum, give abdominal thrusts, which are directed inward and upward. Continue abdominal thrusts until the foreign object is dislodged. If the maneuver is unsuccessful and the victim loses consciousness, activate the EMS and continue performing abdominal thrusts until successful or help arrives. The management of an obstructed airway in children older than 8 years of age is performed the same as that for an adult. **Table 12-11** outlines the management of an airway obstruction in an adult.

A few modifications in the management of an airway obstruction in children (<8 years of age) and infants (<12 months) are necessary. Performing a blind fingersweep is contraindicated in young children and infants. This is because of the risk of accidentally forcing the foreign object deeper into the airway when blindly sweeping the oral cavity with a hooked finger. The fingersweep should only be used when the foreign object is visible. For an infant, back blows are delivered between the shoulder blades in addition to the chest thrusts, to assist in the removal of the foreign object. Management of airway obstruction in children (1-8 years) and infants (<12 months) is found in **Table 12-12.**

Respiratory Conditions

Asthma is a respiratory disease characterized by breathing difficulties, dyspnea, tightness of the chest, wheezing, and coughing due to bronchospasm. Asthma attacks may be prompted by allergens, viral respiratory tract infection, stress, or exercise. When treating the asthmatic patient, information concerning medication, frequency, and factors that are known to prompt an attack should be documented. When an asthma attack occurs, the patient will normally self-administer the bronchodilator prescribed by the physician. It is important for the dental patient who suffers from asthma to keep an inhaler in a convenient location for quick delivery if necessary. Position the patient in a manner in which the patient feels most comfortable and monitor the patient's recovery. If the prescribed dosage of medication does not provide relief for the patient who is having a severe attack, oxygen may be administered and the EMS should be activated.

Allergic reactions are the body's response to specific allergens. It is important to document and update regularly all known allergies in the patient's record. In the dental office, allergic reactions to commonly prescribed antibiotics and latex sensitivity are frequently noted. Although allergic reactions to local anesthetics utilized in the dental office are

TABLE 12–9 CPR: One Person

ASSESSMENT	RESPONSE AND MANAGEMENT
1. Establish consciousness	Are you OK?
2. Patient unconscious	Activate the EMS-Call 911
3. Open airway	Tilt the head back-lift the mandible
4. Assess airway	Look, listen, and feel for respiration
• No respiration	Ventilate-give 2 breaths
5. Check the carotid pulse	Locate the Adam's apple; slide the fingers laterally
6. Detectable pulse	Rescue breathing 12 breaths/min
7. Pulse undetectable	Begin cardiac compressions
	• Interlocking hands, place the heel of one hand on the lower part of the sternum
	• Compression depth: 1½-2 inches
	• 15 compressions (80-100 per minute) followed by 2 ventilations
8. Reassess for a pulse	Complete 4 cycles
• Pulse undetectable	• 15 compressions:2 ventilations
9. If the pulse resumes	Perform rescue breathing
	• 1 breath every 5 seconds
10. No pulse	Continue CPR until the EMS arrives

TABLE 12–10 Child and Infant CPR Protocol

CPR	CHILD (1-8 YEARS)	INFANT <12 MONTHS
Assessment	**Response and Management**	**Response and Management**
1. Establish consciousness	Are you OK?	Try to illicit a response by touch
2. Unconscious	Yell for help	Yell for help
3. Open the airway	Head tilt/lift mandible	Head tilt/lift mandible
4. Assess the airway	Look, listen, and feel for respiration	Look, listen, and feel for respiration
5. No respiration	Deliver 2 rescue breaths 1½ -2 seconds per breath	Deliver two small rescue breaths (puffs)
6. Check the pulse	Carotid pulse	Brachial pulse
7. No pulse	Begin compressions • Place the heel of one hand on the lower part of the sternum • 5 compressions:1 breath • Compression depth: 1 ½-2 inches • Complete 20 cycles 5:1	Begin compressions • Two fingers placed below the nipple line • 5 compressions:1 breath • Compression depth: ½-1 inch • Complete 20 cycles 5:1
8. Activate EMS after 1 minute of CPR	Call 911	Call 911
9. Assess pulse	Carotid	Brachial
• No pulse	Continue CPR	Continue CPR
• Pulse detected	Rescue breathing 1 every 3 seconds	Rescue breathing 1 every 3 seconds

rare, preparation for the management of this emergency is necessary.

Anaphylaxis is a severe, immediate allergic reaction with life-threatening complications, which necessitates emergency care. Symptoms immediately apparent include uti-

TABLE 12–11 Management of Airway Obstruction in Adults

FOREIGN BODY AIRWAY OBSTRUCTION	ADULTS AND CHILDREN OLDER THAN 8 YEARS OF AGE
1. Determine if the patient is choking	• Are you choking? • Look for the universal sign
2. The patient is choking	Begin the Heimlich maneuver • Stand behind the victim and wrap your arms around the waist • Place the fists above the naval • Give 5 abdominal thrusts
3. Repeat step 2 until successful or the victim becomes unconscious	Activate the EMS-Call 911
4. Unconscious victim	• Finger sweep the oral cavity to attempt removal of the foreign object • Open the airway and give 2 breaths • Reposition and try again
5. Ventilation is unsuccessful	• Straddle the victim • With the hands interlocked, place the heel of one hand between the naval and the xiphoid process • Perform 5 abdominal thrusts
6. Repeat steps 4 and 5	Continue until successful or the EMS arrives

caria (hives), nausea, angioedema, laryngeal edema, respiratory distress, wheezing, dyspnea, and ultimately failure of the cardiovascular system. Management of this emergency includes activation of the EMS, administration of epinephrine, basic life support, and CPR administered when necessary. A mild allergic reaction is characterized by a delayed response and may manifest with symptoms such as a rash, rhinitis, hives, or localized swelling. Treatment includes the administration of an oral antihistamine such as chlorpheniramine or diphenhydramine and careful monitoring to ensure that the reaction does not progress. Referral to a physician for a complete evaluation is recommended.

Shock

Shock is a state that occurs in response to the lack of oxygenated blood to cells of the brain and the body. This state may occur as a result of myocardial infarction, anaphylaxis, hemorrhage, or severe infection. Symptoms include hypotension, pallor, moist skin, tachycardia, weakness, and polydipsia. The EMS should be activated immediately to provide advanced care for the condition of the victim in a state of shock. Interim care consists of placing the patient in the Trendelenburg position, providing comfort and warmth, monitoring vital signs, maintaining the airway, and administering oxygen.

 OTHER EMERGENCIES

Eye Injuries

Eye injuries can be avoided in the dental office by ensuring that operators and patients wear **safety glasses** at all times. The body's natural response to a foreign object in the eye is the

TABLE 12–12 Management of Airway Obstruction in Children

FOREIGN BODY AIRWAY OBSTRUCTION	CHILDREN 1-8 YEARS	INFANT <12 MONTHS
1. Determine if patient is choking	Are you choking?	Obvious breathing difficulties Absence of crying
2. The patient is choking	Begin the Heimlich maneuver • Stand behind the victim and wrap your arms around the waist • Place your fists above the naval • Give 5 abdominal thrusts	Begin the Heimlich maneuver • Give 5 back blows • Place the infant face down; with the heel of one hand, direct blows between the shoulder blades • Follow by five chest thrusts
3. Repeat step 2 until successful or the victim becomes unconscious 4. Unconscious victim	If a second rescuer is available, he or she should call 911 • Finger sweep only if the object is visible • Open the airway; give 2 breaths • Reposition and try again	If a second rescuer is available, he or she should call 911 • Finger sweep only if the object is visible • Open the airway; give 2 breaths • Reposition and try again
5. Ventilation is unsuccessful 6. Repeat steps 4 and 5	Give 5 abdominal thrusts Activate the EMS after 1 minute	5 back blows followed by 5 chest thrusts. Activate the EMS after 1 minute

production of excess tears in an effort to wash and cleanse the eye. Rubbing or wiping the eye should be avoided to prevent further injury from the foreign object. Lifting the upper lid out and over the lower lid may facilitate the movement of the object to the lower lid for easy removal with a cotton-tipped applicator. Rinsing the eye with water utilizing an eyecup may eliminate the foreign object. When unable to remove the object, cover the eye with a gauze square and refer the patient for medical attention. When caustic solutions are splashed into the eye, generously flush with clear water utilizing an eyecup or the **eyewash station** for 15 to 20 minutes and refer the patient for medical attention.

Hemorrhage

Hemorrhage is defined as excessive and prolonged bleeding from any part of the body. **Arterial bleeding** is characterized by blood spurting each time the heart contracts, whereas **venous bleeding** is described as oozing. The general rule for severe hemorrhage, as a result of trauma, is to apply pressure to the wound, activate the EMS, and observe the patient for signs of shock. In the dental office, modifications may be needed for the patient taking anticoagulants to prevent excessive bleeding during dental treatment. To control bleeding following extraction, the patient is instructed to bite down on sterile gauze that has been placed over the socket. For prolonged bleeding, the patient may be instructed to bite on a dampened teabag for 10 minutes. Vigorous rinsing, carbonated beverages, and smoking should be avoided to prevent dislodging the clot.

Pinching the nostrils for a few minutes can most often control a **nosebleed**. Instruct the patient to lean forward and breathe through the mouth. When these measures fail to control the bleeding, medical attention may be necessary to cauterize the bleeding vessel.

Poisoning

The **poison control center** is the best resource to determine treatment for an accidental poisoning. If poisoning is suspected, evidence of the substance ingested is needed to assist in providing the correct antidote. **Syrup of ipecac** may be administered to induce vomiting, and water or milk may be used to dilute the poison and reduce rapid absorption. When a caustic substance is ingested, vomiting should not be induced to prevent additional damage to the pharynx and esophagus.

Burns

Skin burns are categorized as first, second, or third degree. **First-degree burns** are painful, red, and swollen, whereas **second-degree burns** have the addition of blisters. Treatment of first- and second-degree burns includes cleansing with cool water and application of an antiseptic and a dressing applied with a sterile bandage. **Third-degree burns** are serious and involve all layers of the skin. Medical assistance is required, and the EMS should be activated promptly. The patient should be monitored for signs of shock and basic life support measures should be initiated if necessary.

Dental Emergencies

Traumatic injuries to the head and neck often occur during participation in various contact sports. Wearing appropriate protective equipment such as a helmet or mouth guard may prevent many injuries. An **avulsed tooth** is one that has been removed from the socket by traumatic force. Immediate emergency care is required to implant the avulsed tooth back into the socket. If possible, the tooth should be rinsed gently and placed directly into the socket. Emergency dental care is required for assessment and provision of definitive treatment. If excess trauma prevents replacing the tooth into the socket, instruct the patient to hold the tooth in the oral cavity or place in a cup of milk to keep the tooth moist while traveling to the dental office for implantation.

Emergency dental treatment is required for the patient who has fractured a facial bone or dislocated his or her mandible. **Facial fractures** may require oral and maxillofacial surgery. The patient should be transported to an appropriate facility. A **dislocation** renders the patient unable to close the mouth and is a very uncomfortable, painful condition. Treatment for a dislocated mandible is described in **Figure 12-2.**

PERSONAL PLAQUE CONTROL

Disclosing Agents

A **disclosing agent** is a liquid or tablet preparation that contains a dye that is used to identify supragingival plaque on tooth surfaces. The staining of otherwise colorless bacterial plaque allows the patient and dental care provider to easily see these deposits. This provides a visual aid for patient instruction and for self-assessment by the patient. Common disclosing agents available are: **erythrosine** (D & C Red

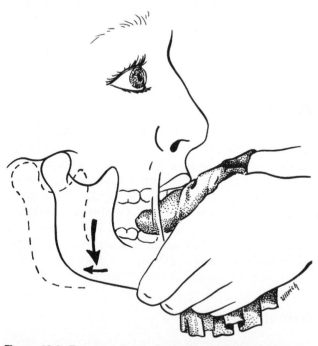

Figure 12-2. Treatment for a dislocated mandible. With thumbs wrapped in toweling and placed on the buccal cusps of the mandibular teeth, the fingers are curved under the body of the mandible. The jaw is pressed down and back with the thumbs while pulling up and forward with the fingers to permit the condyle to pass over the articular eminence into its normal position in the glenoid fossa. As the jaw slips into place, the thumbs must be moved quickly aside. (From Wilkins E: Clinical Practice of the Dental Hygienist, 8th ed. Philadelphia, Lippincott Williams & Wilkins, 1999, p 909.)

No. 28), **two-tone** (FD & C Blue No. 1 and D & C Red No. 28), which stains mature plaque blue and new plaque red, and **fluorescein** (FD & C yellow No. 8), which is visible only with an ultraviolet light source. Other less commonly used disclosants include **iodine, mercurochrome,** and **merbromin** preparations and **Bismarck Brown**.

It must be emphasized that disclosing agents reveal only supragingival plaque and are not a true indicator of the patient's oral hygiene practices. Gingival health is the true indicator of the patient's oral hygiene practices in plaque removal.

Mechanical Plaque Removal

Research studies have shown that a toothbrush can reach 1 to 2 mm below the gingival line. Proper brushing and flossing can remove **zone 1** (supragingival) and part of **zone 2** (subgingival) plaque. Supragingival and subgingival irrigation devices can disrupt zone 1 and **zone 3** (subgingival unattached) plaque. If the irrigant is an antimicrobial agent with substantivity, zone 2 plaque may also be disrupted (see Chapter 13).

Mechanical plaque removal may be accomplished through the use of a wide variety of devices. These devices include **manual and powered toothbrushes,** which vary in shape, size, and function; **interdental brushes; floss; flossing aids; wood wedges; plastic** and **wood picks; yarn; gauze; tongue scrapers;** and **irrigators**. The oral condition, dexterity, and motivation of each individual must be considered before recommending a device for use for mechanical plaque removal.

A toothbrush consists of a head on which bristles are attached, a handle, and a shank that connects the handle and head. The head can vary in size and contains **tufts** (groups) of **nylon** or **natural bristles**. Nylon bristles are preferred because natural bristle tips are irregular and not standardized, which can attribute to trauma to the teeth and soft tissue. In addition, natural bristles are hollow; harbor microorganisms; and do not dry as quickly as do nylon bristles.

Bristle stiffness is primarily related to the size of the bristle diameter. Stiffness increases as the diameter increases. The **bristle diameter** determines whether a brush is soft, medium, or hard and ranges from **0.007 to 0.015 inches**. Those bristles with diameters ranging from 0.007 to 0.009 inches are considered soft.

The filaments on a brush head are grouped together in small bundles or tufts, and a brush head may have a few tufts (**tufted**) or several tufts (**multitufted**). In addition, the ends of the bristles may be cut flat or rounded and polished.

Various bristle planes range from flat planes with filaments of equal lengths to planes of variable lengths. Handles also vary in size and shape.

It is recommended that one use a soft nylon brush with end-polished bristle tips. The size of the head, bristle plane, and size and shape of the handle should be determined on an individual basis. As long as the brush head is small enough for the individual patient's oral cavity and effective plaque removal is accomplished without harm to the oral hard and soft tissues, any shape of toothbrush may be used.

Automatic or powered toothbrushes were designed originally with one of three types of brushing motions: **reciprocating** (back and forth), **arcuate** (up and down), or a **combination** of these two movements. A second generation of power brushes evolved that includes brush heads with **counter-rotating bristle tufts, one-directional rotary round bristle heads, counter-rotating (oscillating) round heads,** and **counter-rotating (oscillating)/pulsating round bristle heads**. The oscillating/pulsating brush head moves up to a speed of 3800 strokes per minute. The use of these powered brushes has been shown to be safe and effective in plaque removal.

The latest generation of powered toothbrushes includes sonic and ultrasonic brushes. The brush heads of both are similar in design to that of a manual toothbrush. The **sonic** brush head vibrates at 31,000 brush strokes per minute (520 per second), which creates low-frequency acoustic energy (200 Hz) and cavitation. The **ultrasonic** brush head operates at a high frequency range of 1.6 MHz. Research shows that cavitation as well as rapid fluid streaming, which are created at the bristle ends, are effective in stain removal, damage of bacterial cell wall fimbriae, and removal of plaque bacteria up to 4 mm beyond the bristle tips. Manual toothbrushes are limited in their cleaning potential, because contact must be made between the bristle tips and the dental plaque. Sonic and ultrasonic bristles can remove plaque without direct bristle contact with the plaque, which is beneficial in interproximal and subgingival areas.

The use of powered toothbrushes has been shown to be effective in plaque removal, especially for patients with minimal dexterity. Optimum effects result, however, when they are used correctly. Generally, this requires instruction from the dental professional.

Several different toothbrushing methods with manual brushes exist **(Table 12-13)**. The **method of choice depends** on the **specific patient's oral condition, dexterity, and motivation**. In addition, individualized instruction is essential and involves **active participation** by the patient in his or her own oral cavity. It is often difficult for a patient to transfer a technique demonstrated on a dentoform to utilizing the technique in his or her own oral cavity. A **specific sequence for brushing all surfaces** of **all teeth** must be followed. In addition, each group of teeth should be brushed for approximately 10 counts before moving the brush to the next group of teeth. Lastly, the tongue must be brushed by gently brushing from the posterior dorsum of the tongue to the tip.

Some toothbrushing methods are more efficient and beneficial than are others. Currently, the Bass and scrub brush methods are the most often recommended. The Bass method of brushing engages not only the facial, lingual, and proximal supragingival surfaces of a tooth but also the subgingival surfaces of a tooth **(Figure 12-3)**. It is suggested that the roll stroke not be incorporated with the Bass method, because there is a tendency to direct more attention to rolling the brush rather than sulcular cleaning. Too vigorous use of

TABLE 12-13 Toothbrushing Methods

METHOD	TECHNIQUE	INDICATION
Bass (Sulcular)	Bristles directed apically at 45 degrees to the tooth Bristles nearest the gingival margin inserted into the sulcus; remaining bristles on the facial/lingual crown	Subgingival and supragingival cleaning of facial, lingual, and limited proximal surfaces
Scrub brush	Vibratory horizontal strokes generated without removing he bristle ends from the sulcus.	Children and mentally or physically impaired
Stillman	Bristles moved in a horizontal scrubbing motion	Supragingival cleaning of the crown and gingival stimulation
Charters	Bristles directed **apically** at 45 degrees to the tooth Bristles placed partly on the facial/lingual crown and partly on the adjacent gingiva. Back and forth strokes applied.	Cleaning of the apical portion of the orthodontic bracket and fixed bridges
Modified Bass or Stillman	Bristles directed **occlusally/ incisally** at 45 degrees to the tooth Bristles placed on the facial/lingual crown and pointed away from the gingival margin Back and forth strokes applied Same bristle placement and stroke as the Bass or Stillman, but add a roll stroke toward the occlusal/incisal surface	Cleaning of the entire supragingival facial/lingual surfaces
Roll stroke	Bristles pointed apically and rolled occlusally/incisally	Cleaning of the entire supragingival facial/lingual surfaces
Fone (circular)	Bristles activated in a circular motion	Young children and mentally or physically impaired
Leonard	With teeth edge-to-edge, bristles are directed at 90 degrees to the long axis of the teeth Vertical (up and down) strokes applied from the gingival margin of the maxillary teeth to that of the mandibular teeth	Not recommended

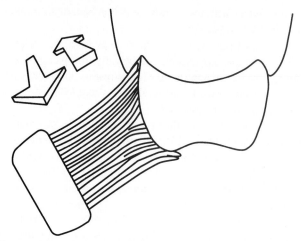

Figure 12-3. Bass (sulcular) brushing. Bristles are directed apically at 45 degrees to the tooth. Bristle tips nearest gingival margins are inserted into the sulcus, whereas the remaining bristle ends are on the facial/lingual of the tooth crown. Vibrating horizontal strokes are generated without moving the bristle ends from the sulcus.

any toothbrushing method can result in detrimental effects, such as gingival and tooth abrasion.

Total oral cleanliness includes cleaning the tongue. Microorganisms attach to the teeth, dental appliances, and oral soft tissue. **Tongue cleaning** is beneficial to reduce halitosis and is especially beneficial for patients with fissured tongues. Cleaning the dorsum of the tongue can be accomplished by drawing a toothbrush forward from the posterior to the tip or by lightly drawing a tongue scraper made of plastic or flexible metal over the tongue.

Generally, one must utilize other adjuncts besides toothbrushes for adequate plaque removal and gingival and periodontal health.

Dental floss is recommended for cleaning the proximal surface of teeth that are in contact with adjacent teeth. Floss is available **waxed or unwaxed** and in the shape of a **round** thread, **twisted yarn** or **flat ribbon (tape).** It comes also in various flavors. Any type may be used as long as it is used correctly. The floss is gently guided with a see-saw motion between two adjacent teeth until it passes the contact point. It is then wrapped around one proximal surface to form a "C" so that it touches the facial and lingual proximals of the tooth. Next, it is moved with pressure against the tooth up and down along one side of the papilla. Without removing it from between the contact, it is then wrapped in a "C" shape around the adjacent proximal surface and moved up and down against that surface along the other side of the papilla.

Flossing under pontics and proximals of abutment teeth of fixed bridges and flossing teeth with orthodontic arch wires attached can be accomplished with the use of **floss threaders** and **tufted dental floss.** Floss threaders are needle-like; they are usually plastic and have a large eye through which floss is threaded. The needle is used to pull the floss under the pontic or contact point. Tufted floss has

a stiffened end followed by a tufted portion and then plain floss. The stiffened end allows for easy insertion of the floss under pontics or contact points.

For cleaning proximals of teeth with open contacts, **yarn** or strips of **gauze** may be used against the proximal surface in a shoe-shine motion. Proximal surfaces adjacent to open gingival embrasures between adjacent teeth that come into contact are easily cleaned with **conical-shaped interdental brushes** or **end-tufted brushes** that have only a few bristles at the end of a brush head.

Other adjuncts that may be used for cleaning proximal surfaces are **wood wedges** and **wood or plastic picks.** Care, however, must be taken when using these objects, because they can easily abrade the interdental papilla. Floss or dental tape, when used correctly, is the safest adjunct for cleaning proximal surfaces between which the interdental papilla fills the gingival embrasure.

Traditionally, patient compliance with flossing is poor. This has led to the development of various **floss-holding devices,** along with the aforementioned proximal cleaners. An **electrically powered interdental cleaning device** has been developed. It consists of a fine filament that **extrudes** from a tip attached to a handle. The tip is placed on the interdental space. When it is activated, a fine filament **extrudes** and elliptically rotates to disrupt plaque attached to interproximal surfaces.

Rubber tips that are often attached to toothbrush handles were once recommended for **gingival stimulation.** Research, however, has indicated that gingival stimulation is **not recommended.** More important, removal of plaque from tooth surfaces that touch the gingiva results in gingival health.

Oral irrigators are most commonly available as power-driven devices that deliver a **pulsating/intermittent jet of liquid** from a tip. The tip is usually conical and may be hard plastic or rubber. It is attached to a hose, which connects to a reservoir that holds water or a chemotherapeutic agent. **Single-stream (monojet) plastic tips** are held slightly away from the tooth and directed at 90 degrees to the gingival third of the tooth and moved along the facial/lingual and proximal areas. **Tips with soft rubber points** on their ends are used for subgingival irrigation and are inserted up to 2 mm into the sulcus. **Tapered plastic tips** can be directed apically at the gingival margin.

Oral irrigators may be recommended for patients with gingival inflammation, inflamed pockets, and orthodontic appliances. Oral irrigators, as well as other unique adjuncts, often have a novelty effect that results in short-term use by the patient.

If the patient's tissue is healthy, he or she should continue doing whatever he or she normally does when utilizing oral hygiene adjuncts for plaque removal. It may not be necessary to totally change a patient's oral hygiene practices but simply to alter them. Before demonstrating a technique or suggesting the use of an oral hygiene adjunct, ask the patient what he or she uses and have the patient demonstrate brushing and flossing techniques. Suggestions can then be made for changes.

Dentifrices

Dentifrices are marketed as toothpastes, gels, powders, or liquids and may be classified as cosmetic or therapeutic. **Cosmetic features** include cleaning, polishing, and breath freshening. To be classified as **therapeutic**, a dentifrice must reduce caries, gingivitis, plaque and calculus formation, or dentinal sensitivity or enhance tooth whitening. Dentifrice ingredients are divided into **active ingredients** that have a therapeutic effect and **inactive components** that have no therapeutic effects (**Tables 12-14 and 12-15**).

The **American Dental Association (ADA) Seal of Acceptance** is awarded to drugs and chemicals that meet the ADA Council on Scientific Affairs' standards for use in diagnosis, treatment, and prevention of oral diseases. The seal is awarded for dentifrices in four categories: (**1**) **anticavity**; (**2**) **anticavity, antiplaque/gingivitis, tartar control**; (**3**) **anticavity, desensitizing**; and (**4**) **anticavity, tartar control**.

Chewing Gum

Immediately after the teeth are exposed to sugar, the oral pH drops because of acid production by *Streptococcus mutans*. **If sugar-free or sugar-containing gum is chewed imme-diately after the sugar exposure for at least 20 minutes, saliva is increased and the acid environment is neutral-ized.** With the increase in saliva, there is an increase in naturally occurring calcium and phosphate ions. This results in remineralization of any demineralized sites on the enamel resulting from the sugar exposure. Sugar-free (artificially sweetened) gum should be used if it is chewed at times other than immediately after exposure to sugar. Studies indicate that gum sweetened with **xylitol** appears to have greater cariostatic effect than that sweetened with sorbitol.

Mouthrinses

Mouthrinses may be categorized as either **therapeutic** or **cosmetic**. Those with no therapeutic effect are not considered for acceptance by the ADA Council on Scientific Affairs. Cosmetic mouthrinses are used primarily for rinsing the mouth of loose debris and for imparting a temporarily pleasant taste.

Water is a naturally occurring mouthrinse. Other self-prepared mouthrinses can be mixed and include saline and sodium bicarbonate solutions. Hypertonic solutions reduce edema by drawing fluid out of body cells through the process of osmosis (**Table 12-16**).

Basic ingredients for cosmetic and therapeutic mouthrinses include water, ethyl alcohol, flavoring, coloring, sweetening agent, and one or more active ingredients (**Table 12-17**).

Currently, only three commercially prepared mouthrinses are accepted by the ADA. They are the over-the-counter fluoride and essential oil rinses and the prescription chlorhexidine gluconate mouthrinse.

Fluoride mouthrinses are recommended for individuals who exhibit high caries' risk or dentinal hypersensitivity, whereas essential oil and chlorhexidine rinses are suggested for individuals who present with gingival and periodontal inflammation. Chlorhexidine gluconate is rapidly absorbed by the oral tissues and slowly released over a long time. This property of **substantivity** prolongs its antibacterial effect. Both essential oil and chlorhexidine preparations can be utilized as pretreatment rinses to reduce the microbial content both orally and in any generated aerosol.

For optimal benefits, a 1-minute rinse is indicated for fluorides, and a 30-second rinse is used for essential oils or chlorhexidine gluconate preparations. Eating, drinking, and smoking must be avoided for at least 30 minutes after rinsing with any of these three rinses.

Before advising patients in the use of a dental product, one should scrutinize product labels and claims. Once a product is suggested, clear directions for its use must be explained to the patient. Optimum beneficial effects from a dental product depend on the correct usage and an awareness of the shelf-life of the product so that its working potential is at 100%.

Bristles are directed apically at 45 degrees to the tooth. Bristle tips nearest the gingival margin are inserted into the

TABLE 12–14 Therapeutic Dentifrice Ingredients

ACTIVE INGREDIENT	PURPOSE
Fluoride (Na or Sn)	Antimicrobial Promotes remineralization
Potassium nitrate Sodium citrate Strontium chloride	Relieves dentinal hypersensitivity
Triclosan (non-ionic phenol) with a PVM/MA copolymer (polyvinylmethyl ether maleic acid)	Antibacterial Reduces plaque, calculus, and gingivitis
Essential oils (thymol eucalyptol, menthol, methylsalicylate) Zinc citrate	Reduces plaque
Tetrasodium pyrophosphate Disodium dihydrogen Pyrophosphate Sodium tripolyphosphate Zinc citrate	Anticalculus
Chlorine dioxide Essential oils with zinc chloride	Antihalitosis
Peroxides Sodium bicarbonate	Whitening by stain reduction
Fluoride, calcium, and phosphate salts	Remineralization of enamel

TABLE 12–15 Inactive Dentifrice Ingredients

INACTIVE INGREDIENT	EXAMPLE	PURPOSE
Cleaning agent	Calcium carbonate	Removes stain
	Dicalcium carbonate	Polishes
	Silica	
	Aluminum oxide	
Humectant	Glycerin	Maintains moisture and prevents drying
	Glycerin	
	Sorbitol	
	Propylene glycol	
Coloring	Vegetable dyes	Enhance appearance
Sweetener	Artificial sweeteners	Imparts pleasant flavor and patient acceptance
	Sorbitol	
	Glycerin	
Preservatives	Alcohols	Prevents deterioration and prolongs shelf-life
	Benzoates	
Flavoring	Essential oils (peppermint, wintergreen, clove, cinnamon)	Enhances appeal and patient acceptance
	Menthol	
	Artificial sweeteners	
Foaming agent (surfactant)	Sodium laural sulfate	Lowers surface tension
Binder (thickening agent)	Alginates, colloids, cellulose	Stabilizer
		Prevents separation of liquid and solid ingredients
Buffering agent	Sodium hydroxide	Stabilizes pH
Water		Adds moisture

sulcus, whereas the remaining bristle ends are on the facial/lingual of the tooth crown. Vibrating horizontal strokes are generated without moving the bristle ends from the sulcus.

DIETARY COUNSELING

Prevention of oral disease is the primary role of the dental hygienist. This includes the assessment of a patient's diet, nutritional counseling, and identification of patients in need of referral to a dietitian. Often, a dietary analysis is performed by the hygienist when a patient exhibits a high risk of caries. Because all nutrients (e.g., carbohydrates, protein, fat, vitamins, minerals, and water) have a role in growth, maintenance, and repair of all body tissues, an imbalance of these nutrients can be a factor in tissue integrity and the immune response. Therefore, patients with inflammatory diseases such as chronic gingivitis, periodontitis, or acute necrotizing ulcerative gingivitis would benefit from an adequate balance of nutrients to hasten tissue healing and repair. If periodontal surgery is indicated for a patient, an assessment of the patient's nutritional status is indicated before the surgery so that, if needed, diet modifications can be made. This optimizes postoperative healing and minimizes infection. The nutritional status of medically compromised patients, such as diabetics or alcoholics, may best be determined by a dietitian with whom the dental hygienist can work to provide continuity of care.

Whether a dietary analysis is made because of caries' potential or for other disease manifestations, the same basic procedure is followed. A working knowledge of the Food Guide Pyramid is essential for the hygienist when conducting a dietary assessment and counseling (see Chapter 6).

For a meaningful evaluation of a patient's diet and effective counseling, **comprehensive data** must be collected. These data include **health, social,** and **dental histories** and also a **clinical evaluation** and **dietary intake evaluation**. A health history provides information on diseases and medications that could interfere with the nutritional status of an individual. The social history of an individual can identify the factors that influence food intake and include economic resources, ethnic or religious practices, frequency of dining out, motivation and education level, and physical and mental challenges. The dental history includes oral hygiene practices, fluoride intake, oral habits, previous dental treatment, and dental complaints (see Chapter 10). Clinical evaluation of the patient includes an appraisal of posture, gait, weight loss or gain, and an intraoral assessment of the patient's teeth and soft tissues.

TABLE 12–16 Self-Prepared Mouthrinses

RINSE	PREPARATION
Isotonic sodium chloride	$^{1}/_{2}$ tsp salt to 8 oz water
Hypertonic sodium chloride	$^{1}/_{2}$ tsp salt to 4 oz water
Sodium bicarbonate	$^{1}/_{2}$ tsp salt to 8 oz water
Sodium chloride with sodium bicarbonate	$^{1}/_{2}$ tsp sodium chloride with $^{1}/_{4}$ tsp sodium bicarbonate mixed with 8 oz water

TABLE 12–17 Categories of Active Mouthrinse Ingredients

COMPOUND	EXAMPLES	ACTION
Oxygenating	Hydrogen peroxide Sodium perborate	Cleaning Antimicrobial
Phenolic (essential oils)	Mixture of thymol, eucalyptol, menthol, and methylsalicylate	Antimicrobial activity; reduces plaque
Bisbiguanides	0.12% Chlorhexidine gluconate	Antibacterial activity; reduces plaque
Quaternary ammonium	0.5% Cetylpyridinium Domiphen bromide	Reduces plaque
Herbal extract	Sanguinarine Echinacea Goldenseal Calendula Bloodroot Grapefruit seed Extract Aloe vera gel	Possible antimicrobial, anti-inflammatory, analgesic
Fluoride	Sodium fluoride Stannous fluoride	Antimicrobial Promotes remineralization
Anticalculus	Tetrasodium pyrophosphate Disodium dihydrogen pyrophosphate	Inhibits crystal growth and retards calculus formation
Surfactant pre-brushing rinse	Sodium benzoate	No statistical proof of reduction of plaque or inflammation

Data on dietary intake can be obtained in three ways: (1) **a food frequency questionnaire**, (2) **a 24-hour diet recall**, and (3) **a 3- to 7-day food diary**.

A food frequency questionnaire is a list of foods that are given to the patient with instructions to check the number of times per day, week, or month that a food is eaten. The questionnaire can be completed in a short time; however, it is not specific enough to allow for evaluation of nutritional content and relies on the patient's memory. It allows only for an overview of the patient's food consumption and carbohydrate intake.

A record of food eaten during the previous 24 hours can be obtained by interviewing the patient. This may be utilized along with the frequency questionnaire to increase the reliability of the food intake data collected.

A more reliable method of accounting for an individual's food intake is to ask the patient to write down his or her food and drink intake for a 3- to 7-day period. Most often this is a **5-day diary**, which includes a weekend. Requesting that the patient records a diary intake for too many days may decrease compliance. The patient should be instructed to record the **time when the food is eaten and the amount, the type of food, and how the food is prepared each day** (Table 12-18). It is a good idea to assist the patient by having him or her recall all that was eaten 24 hours previously and then recording it on the first day of the diary. This gives the patient a better understanding of how the diary should be recorded.

An appointment should be made for reviewing the patient's diary as soon as possible after it has been completed. At this time, the hygienist can begin to analyze the patient's diet for its cariogenicity and nutritional status. The number of servings of each food group is recorded for each day, and then the daily average for each food group is calculated. This can be compared with the suggested amount recommended by the USDA Food Pyramid for an individual of the same sex, age, and activity level, and deficiencies or excesses are noted. When making suggestions for diet modification, prescribe a diet that varies as little as possible from the patient's usual diet and take into consideration the patient's likes and dislikes.

The cariogenicity of the diet is evaluated by circling foods that contain refined and natural sugars (**Table 12-19**). Active participation by the patient is advocated and can be accomplished by asking the patient to circle items that he or she thinks contain sugar. After this activity, the hygienist can verify the sugar-containing foods and discuss foods that contain hidden sugar (**Table 12-20**).

TABLE 12–18 Instructions for Recording a Food Diary

1. Record foods and drink as soon as possible after consuming.
2. Record all meals and snacks eaten each day, including on the weekend.
3. Do not record days when you are sick or dieting.
4. Record, as closely as possible, all amounts of foods or drink consumed (e.g., 1 cup whole milk, 4 oz ground beef, 1 tsp sugar).
5. Indicate how a food is prepared (e.g., baked, broiled, fried, grilled, raw).
6. Record the time when a meal or snack is eaten.
7. List added sugar, cream, sauces, and condiments.
8. For combination foods such as soups, stews, casseroles, or pizza, record all the ingredients and amounts as accurately as possible.
9. Record the brand names of foods.
10. List all miscellaneous items, such as cough lozenges, gum, and breath mints.

TABLE 12–19 Carbohydrates of Similar Cariogenicity

Sucrose	Honey
Fructose	Brown sugar
Glucose (corn syrup)	
Molasses	
Maltose	

Starches are less cariogenic than all sugars. Although the cariogenicity of fructose is similar to that of sucrose, fresh fruits are low in this because of their low percentage of fructose and high percentage of water. In addition, **firm fresh fruits**, such as apples, actually stimulate salivary flow, which helps to neutralize acid. Dried or sticky fruits (e.g., raisins, apricots), on the other hand, are more cariogenic. Lactose is the least cariogenic sugar; however, if left in the oral cavity for long periods, it also has a cariogenic potential.

Once the sugars have been identified in the food diary, the number of exposures is calculated. Sugars eaten at the same time are calculated as one exposure, whereas those eaten 10 or more minutes apart are recorded as separate exposures. The factor of 20 represents the approximate number of minutes that the plaque pH remains at tooth demineralization potential (pH of <5.5) when sugar in liquid form is metabolized as acid by plaque bacteria. If sugar is in solid retentive form, the number of minutes of acid production may be doubled to 40. The number of liquid sugar exposures is multiplied by 20, and the number of solid exposures by 40. These two sums are added to derive at the total minutes of sugar exposure in the oral cavity for the 3- to 7-day intake of food.

Once the tooth acid exposure for the evaluated food intake has been determined, dietary recommendations can be made. The physical form of food, frequency of intake, and time eaten influences potential cariogenicity. The following are recommendations for reducing caries' potential of a diet:

- Eat fermentable carbohydrates at mealtime. When eaten with meals, protective foods such as fat and protein serve as buffers to neutralize plaque acid.
- Snack on raw hard fruits or vegetables that require chewing. Chewing stimulates salivary flow, which neutralizes acid.
- Use products that contain artificial sweeteners such as xylitol, especially in gum and soft drinks.
- Avoid sticky, retentive foods.
- Avoid natural sugars (e.g., honey) and refined sugars.

TABLE 12–20 Foods Containing Hidden Sugars

Mayonnaise	Sausage	Fruit drinks
Salad dressing	Peanut butter	Cereals
Ketchup	Cough drops/syrup	Powdered creamers
Luncheon meats	Canned soups	Soft drinks
Bacon	Canned vegetables	Breads
Wieners	Canned fruits	Breath mints

- Brush after a sugar exposure, or chew gum for at least 20 minutes to stimulate increased salivary flow.

ANXIETY AND PAIN CONTROL

Pain and anxiety are commonly experienced symptoms during a dental appointment. The dual nature of pain includes the transmission of an impulse to the central nervous system (CNS), which consists of pain perception and the individual's pain reaction. Anxiety is the negative response to an anticipated event. Methods that can be utilized to overcome pain and anxiety during a dental procedure include the use of **topical anesthesia, local anesthesia, dentinal desensitizers, and nitrous-oxide oxygen (N_2O-O_2) analgesia.**

Nitrous-Oxide Oxygen Analgesia

Nitrous oxide in combination with oxygen (nitrous-oxide oxygen/N_2O-O_2 analgesia) can be delivered to a patient through the process of inhalation to produce **conscious sedation**. During conscious sedation, the patient is in the **analgesic stage (stage I)** of the four stages of anesthesia. In this stage, the patient is awake, relaxed, responsive to commands, and able to cooperate and experiences some analgesia and a high threshold of pain. Stage II is the delirium or excitement stage; stage III is surgical anesthesia; and stage IV is surgical anesthesia with respiratory paralysis. N_2O-O_2 can be administered as the sole sedative during dental treatment to relax patients who are mildly apprehensive, or it can be administered along with local anesthesia.

The **equipment** for N_2O-O_2 sedation consists of a **blue cylinder of nitrous oxide gas** and **a green cylinder of oxygen**; a **gas delivery machine** with **yokes** that hold the cylinders in contact with the gas machine **control valves; flow meters** that indicate rate of gas flow, **pressure gauges, reservoir bag**, and a **gas hose**; and a **nasal mask with or without a scavenger system**. A **nasal scavenging mask** consists of an inner and slightly larger outer mask. The patient receives the nitrous oxide-oxygen combination via hoses connected to the inner mask. A relief-valve is attached to the inner mask to release exhaled nitrous oxide into the outer mask. These gases are vented from the outer mask through two hoses, which connect to a high-speed evacuation system. The evacuation system vents the gas outside of the building away from windows and air intakes.

Chronic exposure to N_2O by dental personnel has potential health risks. These risks include reduced fertility; spontaneous abortion; increased rate of neurologic, renal, and liver disease; and impaired mental performance, manual dexterity, and audiovisual acuity.

A scavenger system, good work practices by the dental professional, maintenance of equipment, and regular monitoring of environmental nitrous oxide (N_2O) can control chronic exposure of nitrous oxide to the dental personnel.

Work practices include selecting the right size of nasal mask for a good fit and seal around the nose, flushing the unit with oxygen after N_2O-O_2 administration, and instructing the patient to avoid mouth breathing during N_2O-O_2 administration. Routine inspection and maintenance of equipment will reduce the possibility of N_2O leaks and efficient performance of scavenger equipment.

N_2O-O_2 sedation is **indicated** for the following situations or patients:

- Mild anxiety
- Hypersensitive gag reflex
- Inability to sit comfortably because of back pain
- Medically compromised who would benefit from more oxygen (e.g., cardiovascular disease, hypertension, asthma)
- Cerebral palsy and mental retardation

There are no absolute contraindications to the use of nitrous oxide, because it is nonirritating to mucous membranes and it is eliminated, almost unchanged, from the body through the lungs. However, the following are **relative contraindications** that may make it less than an optimum choice for patient management: **pregnancy, nasal obstruction, chronic pulmonary disease** (emphysema, bronchitis), **emotional instability, epilepsy,** and **patients** who **do not like** the feeling of **losing control.**

The following are the procedures for nitrous oxide-oxygen analgesia:

1. Assess the patient's **medical status** and **record vital signs**.
2. **Explain** the procedure to the patient.
3. Select the **appropriate size of nasal mask** for the patient.
4. **Start oxygen flow** at an estimated tidal volume of 6 to 8 L/min, which is the amount of air that an individual needs for one respiration cycle.
5. **Place the nasal mask** on the patient and adjust the mask for comfort.
6. **Adjust** the volume of oxygen (**tidal volume**) by asking the patient if he has enough oxygen to breathe comfortably.
7. Once the tidal volume is established, **titrate** or introduce nitrous oxide at a rate of 1 L/min. while decreasing the oxygen at the same rate with a 1- to 2-minute pause between each adjustment until the **baseline** is reached. The baseline is the level of sedation at which the patient is awake but drowsy and relaxed.
8. **Monitor** the patient and proceed with dental treatment. If the patient demonstrates any signs of oversedation, such as hyperresponsiveness to stimuli or loss of consciousness, discontinue the nitrous oxide and give 100% oxygen.
9. Near the end of the dental procedure, **discontinue the flow** of **nitrous oxide** and **increase** the **oxygen** flow to **100%** for 3 to 5 minutes or until the patient has fully recovered.

Dentinal hypersensitivity is a brief sharp pain in the tooth that occurs in **response** to **thermal, tactile, chemical, or acid stimuli**. Examples of these stimuli are hot or cold temperatures; touch with metal instruments; or exposure to salt, sugar, or acids. The facial cervical area of a root is the most common area of root exposure. Abrasion or erosion from toothbrushing, scaling, and acidic foods can contribute to removal of cementum and exposure of dentinal tubules.

The exact mechanism of pain transmission from the tooth surface to the pulp is not known, but the **hydrodynamic theory** is the most widely accepted. To understand this theory, one must review the anatomy of the tooth. The dentin consists of millions of dentinal tubules. Each tubule is filled with fluid and contains a cytoplasmic cell process that extends from the odontoblast cell body at the edge of the pulp. **Nerves (A-delta fibers)** in the pulp are in close proximity to the odontoblasts. The tubules are wider at their pulpal end (2.5 μm) than they are at their dentinoenamel end (0.8 μm).

A stimulus at the dentinoenamel end of the dentinal tubule initiates fluid movement, which elicits movement of the odontoblastic processes and results in stimulation of the adjacent A-delta nerve fibers. This is interpreted as pain.

Various chemical and physical agents are available to treat dentinal hypersensitivity. These agents are available as **self-applied over-the-counter** or **prescription dentifrices, gels,** or **pastes,** or as **professionally applied** products. See **Table 12-21** for a listing of commonly applied desensitizing agents. The effects that these products produce include **intratubular protein precipitants or obtundents, interruption of nerve transmission, stimulation of secondary dentin,** or **physical sealing of open tubules. Iontophoresis** is a method, not commonly used today, for transferring fluoride ions into the ends of dentinal tubules. This is done by

TABLE 12–21 Common Desensitizing Agents

AGENT	ACTIVE INGREDIENT
Self-Applied:	
Over-the-Counter Dentifrices	Potassium nitrate
	Strontium chloride
	Dibasic sodium citrate
	(All in combination with fluoride)
Prescription gels or paste	0.4% Stannous fluoride
	1.1% Sodium fluoride
Professionally Applied:	
Fluoride gels, pastes, liquid	Sodium fluoride
	Stannous and acidulated fluoride combination
	Sodium silico fluoride
Oxalates	Monohydrogen-monopotassium
	Ferric
Varnishes	Sodium fluoride varnish
Restorations*	N/A

*This aggressive treatment may be done if hypersensitivity is severe and other methods fail.

TABLE 12–22 Topical Anesthetic Agents

AGENTS:	CLASSIFICATION:	ANESTHESIA DURATION:	TOXICITY:
Benzocaine	Ester	5-15 minutes	Minimal
Tetracaine	Ester	20-60 minutes	Extreme
Lidocaine	Amide	15 minutes (gel, ointment)	Minimal
		45 minutes (transoral patch)	
Dyclonine hydrochloride	Ketone	30 minutes	Minimal

applying NaF to an exposed dentin surface and then administering a low-voltage current via a handpiece to the tooth.

Patient management of dentinal hypersensitivity includes the following: (1) differential diagnosis to determine that tooth pain is actually a result of dentinal hypersensitivity; (2) control of etiologic factors such as plaque, improper toothbrushing, and diet high in fermentable carbohydrates; (3) patient home care, and (4) professional application of desensitizing agents.

Topical Anesthesia

A **topical anesthetic** is a drug that is applied to the surfaces of the mucous membrane to produce desensitization. This occurs by **anesthetizing the terminal nerve endings**. The degree of anesthesia produced is related to the amount of absorption of the drug by the tissue. Thick keratinized tissue absorbs a topical anesthetic more slowly than does thin nonkeratinized tissue.

A topical anesthetic can be used for superficial anesthesia to an area that is to be injected with a local anesthetic; to prevent gagging during radiographic exposures or impression taking; for relief of temporary gingival discomfort during probing or scaling and suture removal; and to soothe pain from oral ulcers or laceration.

Topical anesthetics are available in various forms (e.g., **ointment, gel, liquid, spray,** and **transoral patch**) and in both **ester** and **amide** preparations **(Table 12-22).** A transoral patch is an adhesive patch that is impregnated with an anesthetic. The patch is placed directly on the gingiva and provides profound soft tissue anesthesia; it may produce minimal pulpal anesthesia. Ointment, gels, and sprays produce anesthesia only to soft tissue. Maximum effectiveness occurs after a 1- to 2-minute application of the topical solution and after 15 minutes when the transoral patch is applied.

Local Anesthesia

Local anesthesia is the loss of sensation in a circumscribed area of the body as a result of depression or inhibition of the propagation of nerve impulses in peripheral nerves. Because the impulse does not reach the brain, pain is not perceived by the patient. Familiarity with the physiology of nerve con-

duction allows for an understanding of the mode of action of a local anesthetic **(Table 12-23).**

The rapid sequence of **depolarization** and **repolarization** of a nerve cell is its **action potential**. When the action potential occurs in one segment of the nerves, it begins a chain reaction that continues along the nerve fiber to the CNS, where it is perceived as pain. A local anesthetic reduces permeability of the cell membrane to sodium ions (Na^+) when a stimulus is introduced. This prevents depolarization and, thus, blocks the transmission of an impulse along a nerve fiber to the CNS.

Chemically, the structure of an injectable local anesthetic consists of a **lipophilic part** and a **hydrophilic part** joined by an **intermediate chain**. The lipophilic part is aromatic in structure, which enables the anesthetic agent to penetrate the lipid-rich nerve cell membrane and block impulse conduc-

TABLE 12–23 Physiology of Nerve Conduction

I. **Resting State (Potential) of a Nerve**
   A. Positively charges **sodium ions (Na^+)** are forced **outside the cell membrane** by the sodium pump located within the cell membrane, which creates a negative charge within the cell.
   B. Cell membrane becomes impermeable to Na^+.
   C. **Potassium ions (K^+)** remain **inside** nerve cell because of the negative charge of the nerve membrane, even though the nerve membrane is freely permeable to K^+.
   D. The nerve is **polarized.**

II. **Depolarization of a Nerve**
   A. A chemical, thermal, mechanical, or electrical stimulus produces excitation of the nerve fiber.
   B. Nerve membrane becomes **permeable to Na^+.**
   C. Na^+ moves inside the nerve cell; K^+ moves outside.
   D. **Inside** the nerve becomes **positively charged** and **outside** becomes **negatively charged.**

III. **Repolarization of a Nerve**
   A. Immediately, the sodium pump forces Na^+ out of the cell.
   B. Cell membrane becomes impermeable to Na^+.
   C. K^+ diffuses back inside the nerve cell.

IV. **Propagation of the Impulse**
   A. When depolarization occurs, current flows to an adjacent resting segment of the nerve.
   B. **Depolarization** begins in one segment of the nerve and **continues** through the entire length of the nerve fiber to the **central nervous system,** where it is perceived as pain.

tion. The hydrophilic part is a derivative of ethyl alcohol or acetic acid and allows the anesthetic to diffuse through interstitial fluid in tissue to reach the nerve. Anesthetics that have no hydrophilic part are not suitable for injection. The nature of the intermediate chain determines whether the anesthetic is classified as an **ester** or an **amide** (**Table 12-24**).

The mean difference between an ester and an amide is the manner in which each is metabolized. **Ester anesthetics** are hydrolyzed primarily in the plasma and activated by the enzyme pseudocholinesterase. Individuals with the genetic condition of atypical plasma cholinesterase cannot adequately inactivate esters, and this increases the potential for toxicity. In addition, a higher incidence of allergic reactions occurs with ester anesthetics.

Amide anesthetics are metabolized in the liver. Toxicity may occur in individuals with impaired liver function, because they are unable to metabolize these anesthetics adequately.

Currently, all local anesthetics used in dentistry produce vasodilation upon injection. This results in increased blood flow to the injection site; rapid absorption of the anesthetic into the bloodstream, which increases risk of overdose; decreased duration of action; and increased bleeding at the injection site. To counteract these vasodilating actions, vasoconstrictors are added to local anesthetics (**Table 12-25**).

Selection of the type of anesthetic agent to use depends upon several factors that include:

1. Duration of action of the agent
2. Length of time anesthesia/pain control needed
3. Health status of the patient
4. Medications taken by the patient
5. Allergy to a local anesthetic

The duration of action of an anesthetic agent varies according to the amount and type of anesthetic agent and the presence and amount of vasoconstrictor (**Table 12-26**). Short-duration agents provide palpal anesthesia for approximately 30 minutes or less; intermediate-duration agents

provide for approximately 60 minutes; and agents of long duration for more than 90 minutes.

Other factors can influence the duration of action of an anesthetic agent. Individuals may vary in their response to an anesthetic. Inflamed or infected soft tissue at the site of injection results in shorter duration of anesthesia because of increased vascularity in the area. The accuracy of the dental clinician in administering the injection can affect the duration simply due to lack of deposition of the agent near the nerve. Lastly, nerve blocks produce longer periods of anesthesia than do infiltrations.

A patient's health status and medications taken may influence the amount or use of local anesthetics for dental treatment. Not only anesthetics with epinephrine but also elective dental treatment should be avoided in patients with some health conditions or who are taking some medications (**Table 12-27**). Generally, vasoconstrictors are considered safe for patients with mild-to-moderate cardiovascular disease, except for those indicated in Table 12-27, because the amount of anesthetic vasoconstrictor is considerably less

TABLE 12-25 Dental Local Anesthetic Vasoconstrictors

GENERIC NAME	PROPRIETARY NAME	CONCENTRATIONS
Epinephrine	Adrenalin	1:50,000; 1:100,000*; 1:200,000
Levonordefrin	Neo-Cobefrin	1:20,000
Norepinephrine	Levophed	1:30,000

*Most commonly used.

TABLE 12-26 Duration of Action of Local Anesthetic Agents

AGENT	PULPAL	SOFT TISSUE
Short Duration:		
Lidocaine 2%	5-10	60-120
Prilocaine 4% (infiltration)	5-10	90-120
Mepivacaine 3%	20-40	120-180
Intermediate Duration:		
Lidocaine 2% with epinephrine 1:100,000	60	180-240
Mepivacaine 2% with levonordefrin 1:20,000	60	180-240
Prilocaine 4% (nerve block)	60	120-240
Prilocaine 4% with epinephrine 1:200,000	60-90	120-240
Long Duration:		
Bupivacaine 0.5% with epinephrine 1:200,000	>90	240-540
Etidocaine 1.5% with epinephrine 1:200,000 (nerve block)	>90	240-540

TABLE 12-24 Types of Local Anesthetic Agents

CATEGORY	GENERIC NAME	PROPRIETARY NAME
Esters	Procaine*	Novocain
	Propoxycaine*	Ravocaine
	Procaine/propoxycaine	Novocain/Ravocaine
Amides	Bupivacaine	Marcaine
	Etidocaine	Duranest
	Lidocaine	Xylocaine, Alphacaine, Octocaine
	Mepivacaine	Carbocaine, Arestocaine, Isocaine, Polocaine
	Prilocaine	Citanest

*No longer available for use.

TABLE 12–27 Health Conditions/Medications that Indicate Avoidance of Elective Dental Care and Vasoconstrictors

- Uncontrolled hypertension (>200 systolic or >115 diastolic)
- Uncontrolled hyperthyroidism
- Myocardial infarction within 6 months
- Cerebrovascular accident within 6 months
- Unstable angina
- Uncontrolled cardiac dysrhythmias
- Coronary bypass surgery within 6 months
- Nonspecific β-blockers
- Monoamine oxidize inhibitors
- Tricyclic antidepressants
- Sodium bisulfite allergy

than that produced by the body's own sympathetic nervous system when activated by anxiety or pain.

A true allergy to a local anesthetic is rare. Allergic reactions to ester local anesthetics are more common than those to amides. Individuals who are allergic to one type are rarely allergic to the other. More often, these allergic reactions are a response to **para-aminobenzoic acid (PABA)**, a breakdown product of an ester anesthetic, rather than to the anesthetic agent itself. Individuals who are allergic to sodium bisulfite should not be given anesthetics that contain epinephrine, because sodium bisulfite is incorporated in anesthetic solution as a preservative for epinephrine.

The **armamentarium** necessary for the administration of local anesthesia includes a syringe, needle, anesthetic cartridge, topical anesthetic, and cotton-tipped applicators and also a hemostat, forceps, or cotton pliers.

The **syringe** holds the anesthetic cartridge and needle. Types of anesthetic syringes include **reusable (autoclavable)** metal and **disposable** syringes (**Table 12-28**). The autoclavable **aspirating and self-aspirating syringes** are the most common types used in dentistry. However, OSHA has mandated that dental care providers evaluate for use **disposable self-sheathing "safe" needles.** This is an effort to help prevent needlestick exposures to the operator during patient care.

Aspirating and self-aspirating syringes allow for aspiration during an injection. **Aspiration** is the negative pressure applied during an injection, which results in drawing of blood into the anesthetic cartridge if the needle lumen rests

TABLE 12–28 Types of Anesthetic Syringes

I. Reusable (autoclavable)
  A. Breech-loading, metallic, cartridge type
    1. Aspirating
    2. Self-aspirating
    3. Nonaspirating
  B. Pressure type
  C. Jet injector
II. Disposable Self-Sheathing Safe Syringes

in a blood vessel. If this occurs, the needle must be withdrawn, the anesthetic cartridge replaced, and the procedure repeated. Injection of an anesthetic solution directly into the bloodstream is contraindicated.

A barbed **harpoon** located at the end of the plunger of an **aspirating syringe** engages the rubber stopper of an anesthetic cartridge and allows the exertion of negative pressure on the thumb ring of the syringe during an injection. There is no harpoon on a **self-aspirating syringe.** Instead, there is a **metal projection** at the needle end of the syringe that rests against the rubber diaphragm of the cartridge.

Aspiration with a self-aspirating syringe is achieved by exerting pressure on the thumb disc or ring, which increases pressure within the cartridge. When the pressure is released, negative pressure is produced and aspiration occurs.

Anesthetic **needles** consist of an angled point or **bevel** that is directed into the tissues, a **hub** at the other end that attaches to the syringe, and the length or **shank** between the bevel and hub. Sterile needles are packaged in plastic encasements. The gauge of a needle is the diameter of its lumen. Commonly used **needle gauges** in dentistry are **25-, 27-,** and **30-** gauge. The diameter of the lumen decreases as the number increases. The 25-gauge needle is recommended for most injections, because its rigidity allows for injecting with minimal deviation of the needle, there is less chance of needle breakage, and aspiration is achieved more easily through a wider lumen.

Two **needle lengths** are utilized in dentistry. A **short** needle is approximately 1 inch in length, and a **long** needle is approximately $1^{5}/_{8}$ inches in length. The choice of needle length depends on the type of injection administered.

An anesthetic **cartridge** consists of a **glass cylinder** that contains the anesthetic, a **rubber plunger** on one end of the cylinder into which the harpoon of an aspirating syringe is embedded, a **diaphragm** on the other end of the cylinder in which the needle penetrates, and an **aluminum cap** that secures the diaphragm. A cartridge contains **1.8 ml** of solution composed of the **anesthetic agent;** a **vasoconstrictor;** a **preservative (sodium bisulfite); sodium chloride,** which makes the solution isotonic with body tissues; and **distilled water.**

Cotton-tipped applicators are used for applying topical anesthetic to the mucous membrane before an injection. **Gauze is** used to wipe the injection site prior to application of the topical anesthetic and before the needle is inserted. A **hemostat, forceps, or pliers** should be available for retrieving a broken needle from the soft tissue if this unlikely event were to occur.

On each anesthetic cartridge is imprinted the percentage and type of anesthetic agent and the ratio of vasoconstrictor, along with the manufacturer's name. Calculation of the amount of anesthetic agent in a cartridge is important when trying to determine the **maximum recommended or safe dose (MRD)** of anesthetic that can be administered to individual patients (**Table 12-29**). The maximum safe dose of a local anesthetic is the maximal amount of the drug that can be safely administered to a healthy individual (**Table 12-30**)

TABLE 12–29 Calculation of the Amount of Anesthetic Agent and Vasoconstrictor in a Cartridge

Example: 1 cartridge of 2% Lidocaine HCL and Epinephrine 1:100,000
1. Amount of local anesthetic
   a. A 2% solution of anesthetic contains 20 mg/ml.
   b. There are 1.8 ml of total solution in one local anesthetic cartridge.
   c. 20 mg × 1.8 ml = 36 mg of lidocaine in this 2% solution.
2. Amount of vasoconstrictor
   a. 1:100,000 concentration of epinephrine = 0.01 mg/ml.
   b. One anesthetic cartridge contains 1.8 ml of solution.
   c. 0.01 mg/ml (1:100,000) of epinephrine × 1.8 ml = 0.018 mg of epinephrine in one cartridge.

TABLE 12–31 Maximum Recommended (Safe) Dose of Vasoconstrictors for Healthy and Cardiac Patients

| | | MAXIMUM DOSE IN NUMBER CARTRIDGES | |
AGENT	CONCENTRATION	HEALTHY ADULT	CARDIAC PATIENT
Epinephrine	1:50,000	5	1
Epinephrine	1:100,000	10	2
Epinephrine	1:200,000	20	4
Levonordefrin	1:20,000	10	2
Norepinephrine	1:30,000	5	2

The maximum safe dose of an anesthetic solution may also be determined by the vasoconstricting agent. In some cases, the maximum safe dose of an anesthetic may be reached before the maximum safe dose of the vasoconstrictor in the same cartridge of solution, and vice versa. **See Table 12-31** for a comparison of the maximum recommended safe dose of vasoconstrictors between a healthy adult and a cardiac patient.

To determine the MRD of an anesthetic agent, one must consider the patient's age, physical status, and body weight. The milligrams per pound of body weight for each anesthetic have been predetermined. The MRD for each of three commonly utilized local anesthetics in dentistry is indicated in Table 12-30.

The **trigeminal nerve** is the **fifth** of the 12 **cranial nerves** and is broken into **three divisions: maxillary, mandibular, and ophthalmic.** Only the maxillary and mandibular divisions are pertinent to intraoral local anesthesia. The nerves of the maxillary division are entirely sensory, whereas the mandibular division contains both sensory and motor roots **(Table 12-32).**

Three **types of injections** are used to obtain local anesthesia: local infiltration, field block, and nerve block. **A local infiltration** involves deposition of the anesthetic close to the terminal endings of the nerve fibers in the immediate area to be treated. An example of this would be injection into an interproximal papilla. A **field block** involves injecting the solution near large terminal nerve branches and results in anesthesia to one tooth and surrounding tissues. Deposition of solution is usually at a tooth apex and away from the area to be treated. **A field block is often incorrectly referred to as a local infiltration.** A **nerve block** involves deposition of anesthetic solution close to a main nerve trunk and away from the treatment area. This often includes a larger area of anesthesia than does a field block. Determination of what type of injection to administer depends on the area in which treatment is to be rendered and whether or not the teeth, soft tissue, or both need to be anesthetized. A working knowledge of the anatomy and innervation of the nerves of the maxillary and mandibular division of the trigeminal nerve is necessary for

TABLE 12–30 Maximum Recommended Doses of Commonly Used Local Anesthetics in Dentistry

LOCAL ANESTHETIC	MRD
2% (20 mg/ml) Lidocaine with/without vasoconstrictor	2 mg/lb, or 300 mg max
2% (20 mg/ml) or 3% (30 mg/ml) Mepivacaine	2 mg/lb, or 300 mg max
4% (40 mg/ml) Prilocaine with/without vasoconstrictor	2.7 mg/lb, or 400 mg max

Example: Calculate the MRD or 2% lidocaine for a person weighing 100 lb.
1. MRD for 1 lb = 2 mg
2. MRD for 100 lb is 200 mg (100 lb × 2 mg)
3. If 1 cartridge contains 36 mg of lidocaine, 200 mg of lidocaine equals 5.56 cartridges (200 × 36).
4. MRD for this person is 5.56 cartridges.

TABLE 12–32 Nerves of the Maxillary and Mandibular Division of the Trigeminal Nerve

DIVISION	NERVES
Maxillary	Greater (anterior) palatine
	Nasopalatine
	Posterior superior alveolar
	Middle superior alveolar
	Anterior superior alveolar
Mandibular	Inferior alveolar
	Lingual
	Buccal
	Incisive
	Mental

the successful administration of local anesthesia in the oral cavity (**Table 12-33 and Figure 12-4**).

Administration of a successful anesthetic injection involves assessing the health history of the patient, taking vital signs, explaining the procedure to the patient in a non-threatening way, preparing the syringe with an appropriate anesthetic cartridge and needle, visualizing and palpating to locate the penetration site, and applying topical anesthetic for 1 to 2 minutes. A short needle is used for all injections listed in Table 12-33, except for the inferior alveolar and lingual nerve block and infraorbital nerve block. Using a handrest and with the bevel oriented toward the bone, gently insert the needle into the mucosa until the bevel is completely under the mucosa. Deposit a few drops of solution, and pause for 5 seconds. Slowly advance the needle to the target site while injecting anesthetic solution drop by drop in front of the needle until the end of the needle reaches the target area. Do not insert the needle all the way to the hub. Aspirate, and then slowly deposit the solution in the area. Deposition of solution at a rate of 1 ml/min or 2 minutes for a full cartridge is recommended. Slowly withdraw the needle. Recap the needle with a **one-handed scoop technique** or by using a **needle barrier**. Rinse the patient's mouth, and observe the patient. Review with the patient what to expect from the anesthesia and record in the patient's chart the area anesthetized, the type and amount of anesthetic used, and the patient's reaction.

As with the administration of any drug, care must be taken to carefully observe the patient for any signs of **drug overdose or allergy**. Common causes of local anesthetic overdose include the administration of an excessive dose of the agent (over the MRD) or absorption into the circulation because of using an anesthetic with no vasoconstrictor or injecting directly into a blood vessel. Reactions to an **overdose of local anesthetic** may range from mild to moderate or severe (**Table 12-34**). Depending on the reaction, management can range from monitoring of vital signs and administering oxygen to basic life support and transportation of the patient to a hospital.

Overdose reactions to vasoconstrictors occur more often with epinephrine than with other vasoconstrictors, because this drug is more commonly used. An **epinephrine overdose** is more likely to occur if concentrations greater than 1:00,000

TABLE 12–33 Common Local Anesthetic Injections

INJECTION	INJECTION SITE	AREAS ANESTHETIZED
Infiltration (field block)	Mucofacial fold above the tooth apex	Pulp of the tooth, facial periosteum, and facial mucous membrane
Posterior superior alveolar (PSA) nerve block	Mucobuccal fold at distal portion of the second molar, just behind the zygomatic arch	Pulp and overlying bone and facial mucosa of the Mx third, second, and first molars, except for the mesial-buccal root of the Mx first molar
Middle superior alveolar (MSA) nerve block	Mucobuccal fold above the Mx second premolar	Pulp and overlying bone and facial mucosa of the mesial-buccal root of the Mx first molar and the first and second Mx premolars
Anterior superior alveolar (ASA) nerve block	Mucobuccal fold slightly mesial to the canine eminence	Pulp and overlying bone and facial mucosa of the Mx central incisor, lateral incisor, and canine
Infraorbital	Above the Mx first premolar at the mucobuccal fold toward the infraorbital foramen	Pulp and overlying bone and facial mucosa of the Mx central incisor, lateral incisor, canine, first and second premolars, mesial-buccal root of the first molar, lower eyelid, lateral aspect of nose, and upper lip
Greater palatine nerve block	Slightly anterior to the greater palatine foramen on the palate distal to the Mx second molar	Hard palate and overlying mucosa from the Mx third molar through the first premolar on the side injected
Nasopalatine nerve block	Lateral to and at the base of the incisive papilla	Hard palate and overlying mucosa of all Mx canines and incisors
Inferior alveolar and lingual nerve block (mandibular block)	Middle of the pterygomandibular triangle at the height of the coronoid notch	Inferior alveolar nerve block: Md teeth (pulp) to the midline, body of the mandible and inferior portion of the ramus, facial mucosa from the Md second premolar to the midline, and lower lip on the side injected Lingual nerve block: All lingual gingival tissue to the midline, anterior two thirds of the tongue, and sublingual mucosa on the side injected
Buccal nerve block	Mucous membrane distal and buccal to the most posterior Md molars and parallel to the occlusal plane	Soft tissue buccal to the Md molars
Mental nerve block	Mucobuccal fold directly over the mental foramen (near the Md second premolar)	Facial mucosa from the mental foramen to the midline, including the lower lip and skin of the chin on the side of injection
Incisive nerve block	Same as for the mental nerve block, except massage the injection site with a finger for 1-2 minutes	Same soft tissue as in the mental nerve block, and pulp of the Md first and second premolars, canine, lateral incisor and central incisor on the side of the injection

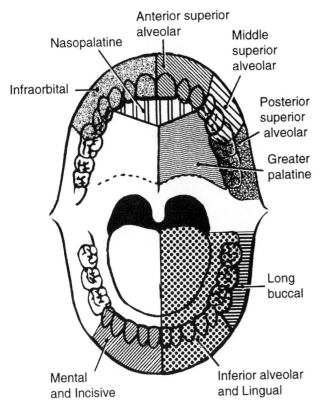

Figure 12-4. Diagrammatic representation of teeth and soft tissues anesthetized by common dental injections. (From Wilkins E: Clinical Practice of the Dental Hygienist, 8th ed. Philadelphia, Lippincott Williams & Wilkins, 1999, p 506.)

TABLE 12–34   Clinical Signs and Symptoms of Local Anesthetic Overdose

MILD REACTIONS:

Confusion	Chills
Dizziness	Sweating
Tinnitus (ringing in ears)	Vomiting
Headache	Disorientation
Slurred Speech	Elevated blood pressure
Muscular tremor	Elevated heart rate
Numbness of perioral tissues	Elevated respiratory rate
Flushing of skin	Loss of consciousness

SEVERE REACTIONS:

Tonic-clonic seizures
CNS depression
Depressed blood pressure, heart rate, and respiratory rate

sue, remove it with forceps or a hemostat. If the needle fragment is not visible, inform the patient and reassure him or her. Then, refer the patient to an oral maxillofacial surgeon.

Pain during injection may occur from a dull or barbed needle or from rapidly injecting the anesthetic. To avoid pain, use sharp needles, apply topical anesthetic prior to injecting, inject slowly, and store the anesthetic cartridges at room temperature.

A burning sensation, usually short in duration, may be the result of various situations. These include use of contaminated anesthetic solution from improper storage, overheated cartridges, use of solutions whose shelf-life has expired, and rapid injection of solution. Avoid this situation by storing cartridges in their original containers and not in a disinfectant or cartridge warmer, by discarding solutions with expired dates, and by injecting solution slowly.

A hematoma may occur if there is inadvertent puncture of a blood vessel, particularly an artery, during injection. Attention to correct injection sites and minimizing the number of needle insertions can prevent this. Application of ice to the area as soon as the hematoma begins to form will minimize this manifestation.

Facial nerve paralysis occurs usually during the administration of an inferior alveolar nerve block when local anesthetic solution is inadvertently deposited within the parotid gland. Loss of motor function of the muscles of facial ex-

are administered and in patients with cardiovascular disease. Clinically, the signs or symptoms of a vasoconstrictor overdose are similar to the "fight or fight" response **(Table 12-35).** Management of these reactions ranges from reassuring the patient and monitoring vital signs to administering oxygen and obtaining medical assistance.

Allergic reactions to local anesthetics occur most commonly to ester anesthetic agents and are rare with amide anesthetics. Allergic reactions may occur to components of the anesthetic cartridge as discussed earlier. Reactions may be **immediate or delayed** and should be managed as described in the section on Emergencies. Management may range from monitoring vital signs and administering an antihistamine to administering oxygen, basic life support, and transport to a hospital.

Local complications from administration of local anesthesia may also occur. These complications include **needle breakage, pain during injection, burning during injection, hematoma, facial nerve paralysis, paresthesia, trismus, tissue sloughing, edema,** and **intraoral lesions.**

Needle breakage can be prevented by following basic guidelines. Use large-gauge needles (25 vs 27 or 30); never bend the needle; advance the needle slowly; never force it against resistance or redirect it while it is completely within the tissues; and do not insert it all the way to the hub. If breakage occurs and the needle fragment is protruding from the tis-

TABLE 12–35   Signs and Symptoms of Vasoconstrictor Overdose

Anxiety	Pallor
Tenseness	Respiratory difficulty
Restlessness	Palpitations
Headache	Sharp elevation in systolic blood pressure
Tremor	Elevated heart rate
Weakness	Cardiac dysrhythmias
Dizziness	

pression is temporary and lasts only a few hours. This can be prevented if the proper technique is followed during injection. Reassure the patient, and explain that the paralysis lasts for only a short time.

Paresthesia is prolonged anesthesia for hours or days to the area anesthetized. This may result from nerve irritation from a contaminated anesthetic agent, or from trauma to the nerve during injection. Proper storage of cartridges and proper injection technique will aid in preventing this. Although paresthesia usually resolves within 2 months, it may last longer. Examine the patient every 2 months, and refer the patient to an oral maxillofacial surgeon if it continues.

Trismus is spasm of the muscles of mastication that results in soreness and difficulty in opening the mouth. This can be caused by multiple needle insertions, administering a contaminated solution, or insertion of a large amount of solution into a restricted area. Store cartridges properly; use sharp needles; inject minimal amounts of solution; and deposit the solution slowly. Adhere to recommended techniques for injection. Apply moist heat immediately for 20 minutes every hour. Analgesics may be recommended. Instruct the patient to open and close the mouth for 5 minutes every 3 to 4 hours. If trismus persists for more than 48 hours, infection may exist and antibiotics may be recommended. If this continues, refer the patient to an oral maxillofacial surgeon.

Infection may occur from use of a contaminated needle or anesthetic solution or improper preparation of soft tissue prior to injecting. Care must be taken to follow proper infection control procedures when unsheathing or sheathing the needle or when handling or storing the cartridge. Initially, infection is not obvious, and pain may be similar to that of trismus. Therefore, immediate treatment is the same as that for trismus. If the patient does not respond within 3 days, infection is likely and antibiotic therapy should be started.

Tissue sloughing may be the result of irritation from the lengthy application of topical anesthetic or from sensitivity to the local anesthetic or vasoconstrictor. To prevent this, apply topical anesthetics for only 1 to 2 minutes, and avoid using high concentrations of vasoconstrictors. Analgesics may be recommended for discomfort, and the condition usually resolves in a few days.

Edema may be caused by trauma during injection, hemorrhage, infection, allergy, or contaminated anesthetic solution. Manage the edema by managing the cause. To prevent edema, follow proper infection control protocol and injection administration techniques and conduct a medical assessment before administration of the anesthetic.

Intraoral lesions may be caused by the patient inadvertently biting the tongue, lips, or mucosa while anesthetized or as a result of trauma to the tissue from the injection. Aphthous ulcers or herpetic lesions often develop after trauma. Topical anesthetic pastes may provide relief, and the lesions usually subside in 7 to 10 days. The patient should be instructed to avoid eating or chewing while anesthesia is present, and the operator should use caution during injection of the anesthetic.

Complications, whether local or systemic, may occur during the administration of local anesthesia even when precautions and preventive measures are taken. Therefore, the dental operator must be prepared to manage complications if they do occur.

 ## PATIENTS WITH SPECIAL NEEDS

Although numerous conditions requiring special patient management have been presented here, this section is by no means complete. The dental hygienist must endeavor to treat each patient as an individual with unique needs that may require modifications, additions, or deletions to the standard of care.

Sensory Impairments

Visual Impairment/Blindness

Legal blindness is defined as a visual acuity of 20/200 (a person sees at 20 feet what a person with normal vision sees at 200 feet) or less after the best optical correction. In addition, the peripheral vision or the widest diameter of visual field is no wider than 20 degrees. **Vision impairment** refers to sight no better than 20/70 after optical correction or some loss of peripheral vision. The leading causes of blindness are macular degeneration (loss of central vision), diabetic retinopathy, senile cataracts, glaucoma, vascular disease, trauma, and infections. The goal of treatment is to improve sight and halt the progression of the impairment by corrective surgery, drug therapy, corrective lenses, regular eye visits, and educational programs (e.g., Braille) designed on the basis of the age of onset of the disability.

A thorough medical history is essential and aids in the development of creative oral hygiene instructions. An appeal to the other senses is usually the best approach. Referring to a patient's memory when describing oral recommendations is only helpful if the individual has acquired blindness. Certain guidelines should be followed when working with the vision impaired:

- Lead the patient by standing slightly in front; the patient will hold onto your bent arm near the elbow for guidance.
- Indicate changes in the floor, and prepare a path to the dental chair that is free of obstacles
- If the patient has a guide dog, allow the dog to stay in the corner of the operatory; do not distract or be playful with the guide dog while he is working.
- Avoid loud noises.
- Notify the patient if you are going to leave the room, and speak to the patient before touching him or her.
- Always describe procedures to the patient in a step-by-step fashion, using the patient's own mouth to provide instructions.

- If the patient is partially sighted, avoid the glare of light into the eyes.

Hearing Impairment/Deafness

Deafness is defined as defective/functional hearing with or without the assistance of a hearing aid. Deafness is the inability to understand speech even with use of a hearing device. The hearing loss may be associated with outer, middle, or inner ear mechanisms. Deafness can be attributed to heredity, prenatal infection of the mother (e.g., rubella and birth trauma), chronic ear infections, infectious diseases (meningitis), trauma, or toxic effects of drugs.

There are four types of hearing loss:

1. **Conductive hearing loss:** involves the outer/middle ear pathways
2. **Sensorineural hearing loss:** consists of damage to sensory hair cells of the inner ear or nerves that supply the inner ear
3. **Mixed hearing loss**: includes a combination of conductive and sensorineural loss
4. **Central hearing loss:** involves damage to the nerves or nuclei of the CNS in the brain or pathways to the brain

Decibel Loss can be categorized as:

- **Slight-**15-25 decibels
- **Partial-**25-65 decibels
- **Severe-**65-95 decibels
- **Profound-**95 decibels and higher

Management of hearing loss can include surgery, hearing aids, and education to enhance communication skills through lip reading; sign language; and telecommunication devices. When communicating with the deaf the following recommendations are advised:

- Face the patient, remove your mask, and speak normally. Pause more frequently than usual, because many patients rely on lip reading. Avoid sitting in front of a window or bright light that may cast a shadow on your face.
- Use a pencil and paper to communicate oral care recommendations, if necessary.
- Avoid background noise. Ask the patient to turn off a hearing aid when using high-pitched powered scaling and toothbrush devices.
- Become familiar with common signs that may be helpful during the appointment, such as open, close, and rinse.
- Tell, show, and do all procedures to reinforce them and enhance the patient's understanding.

Developmental Disorders

Mental Retardation

Mental retardation (MR) is defined as significant subaverage intellectual functioning that exists concurrently with deficits in adaptive behavior and is manifested during the **developmental period** (younger than age 18). MR is classified based on the **intelligence quotient (IQ).**

- **Mild-**IQ = 51-70/89% of the retardate population. The level of functioning is usually third to sixth grade level and is referred to as **educable.**
- **Moderate-**IQ = 36-50/6% of the retardate population. The level of functioning is about first- or second-grade level.
- **Severe-**IQ = 20-35/3.5% of the retardate population. An individual with an IQ in the range of 25 to 49 is referred to as **trainable** and is usually employed in a sheltered workshop doing small manual labor tasks.
- **Profound-**IQ below 20/1.5% of the retardate population. An individual in the severe or profound category is usually institutionalized and dependent on a caregiver to perform the daily living tasks.

The etiology of MR may include some form of brain damage incurred prenatally, perinatally, or postnatally during the developmental period. MR rarely exists as an entity in and of itself. The retardate population as a whole has a higher frequency of emotional disturbances, sensory defects, language disorders, neuromuscular impairments, seizures, leukemia, hepatitis, and congenital heart disease. One of the more distinctive syndromes exhibiting MR is **Down syndrome** or **trisomy 21.** This individual is usually small in stature with a stocky build, has a short wide neck and waddling gait, has microcephaly (a small head shape), an underdeveloped nose, epicanthic folds at the angle of eyes-commonly experiencing nearsightedness and cataracts, and hands that are small with stubby fingers and a simian crease. Oral complications associated with Down syndrome include caries and periodontal disease (primarily due to dental neglect), macroglossia, gingival hyperplasia, short constricted palate and an underdeveloped maxilla leading to Class III malocclusion, posterior crossbite and anterior openbite, delayed and unsequential exfoliation of teeth, small cone-shaped teeth with hypoplastic enamel, premature loss of permanent teeth due to defective neutrophil chemotaxis, elevations in parotid enzyme activity, and a metabolic block in collagen maturation.

Persons with MR also exhibit destructive oral habits such as bruxism, tongue-thrusting, clenching, drooling, and self-injurious behavior (e.g., head banging, biting, and scratching of the face or hands). **Pica** (i.e., a craving for non-food substances) is also common in MR. Working with the caregiver to establish routine oral hygiene and develop toothbrush modifications suitable for the patient or caregiver is advised. Dietary modifications to prevent caries are essential as persons with MR (particularly those institutionalized) are often given a diet and/or behavioral reinforcers that are highly cariogenic. Tender, loving care (TLC) is usually the best motivator for the patient with mental retardation.

Autism

Autism is a pervasive behavioral developmental disability manifested by limited ability to understand and communicate. Autism affects males three to four times more than females. The etiology is unknown, but it is theorized that autism may be due to inappropriate child-rearing and environmental stimuli, heredity, or organic disturbances related to the brain. The IQ is usually below 70, but **autistic savants** may exhibit unusually high IQ levels.

The signs and symptoms of autism may be apparent by the first year of life. They may include problems with social interaction (associate better with inanimate objects than people, social/emotional detachment, and stereotypic, ritualistic, repetitious play); limited range of speech (**aphasia**-no speech or **echolalia**-meaningless repetition of words); cognitive abnormalities, and self-injurious behaviors. Many persons with autism are also mentally retarded, and approximately one third of these patients may also have epilepsy. Medical treatment is not specific and may consist of psychotherapy, behavior modification, medications (e.g., psychotropic drugs, hormones, megavitamins), special education (structured learning environment), or speech therapy. Autism is rarely cured.

Because manual dexterity can be affected, dental intervention may include the use of oral hygiene modifications. In addition, the dental management of caries is significant because caries risk is associated with food retention due to poor tongue coordination; a preference for soft, sweet tasting foods; and drug-induced xerostomia. Drug-induced gingival hyperplasia is also a possibility in those persons taking anticonvulsant agents. Strategies for communicating oral hygiene instructions to the person with autism include:

- Rehearsals: caregiver practice with the patient
- Eye contact: give praise and rewards
- Constant repetition of dental procedures
- Consistency
- Avoid loud voices and bright lights, because they may upset the patient
- Use of 50% nitrous oxide: 50% oxygen analgesia for extensive dental needs

Epilepsy

Epilepsy is a variable symptom complex that is characterized by recurrent paroxysmal attacks of unconsciousness or impaired consciousness, usually accompanied by tonic or clonic spasms. **Seizures** can occur as a result of trauma at any time from conception to death. Examples of traumatic events include physical injury, infectious diseases, toxins, and cerebral degenerative diseases. Epilepsy can be classified into two basic types:

1. **Partial seizures** begin locally and are subdivided into **simple** (without loss of consciousness), **complex** (involving impaired loss of consciousness), and **those evolving into generalized tonic-clonic seizures.**
2. Generalized seizures are bilaterally symmetric without local onset and may be nonconvulsive or convulsive. **Grand mal** is the most common convulsive form; usu-

ally preceded by an **aura**; loss of consciousness; tonic-clonic seizures of 1 to 3 minutes' duration; and a confused, disoriented, and fatigued recovery.

Common anticonvulsant medications used in the treatment of seizures include phenytoin; carbamazepine; valproic acid; phenobarbital sodium, and primidone. Because psychological stress can increase seizures, psychological or psychiatric support therapy is also considered to be an effective form of treatment.

Dental intervention for a person with a known seizure disorder should involve assessment and management of drug-induced gingival hyperplasia **(see Chapter 13).** Although gingival overgrowth may occur despite meticulous oral hygiene measures, routine dental visits are recommended to assess the severity of the hyperplasia and manage any complications related to the condition. In addition, knowledge of emergency measures should a seizure occur are essential. The following considerations should be taken to prevent a dental emergency:

- Ask your patient if prescribed medications have been taken; when was the last seizure, what type of seizure occurred; was there an aura; how often do the seizures occur; and what events precipitate a seizure?
- Schedule short appointments in the morning; avoid anxiety or stress-provoking situations, and keep a calm atmosphere.

Cerebral Palsy

Cerebral palsy (CP) is a nonprogressive neuromuscular disorder that results from an injury to the brain. Injury to the brain at any age can result in paralysis or disruption of motor function. Possible etiologic factors occurring during pregnancy or delivery include anoxia, maternal infection (rubella), blood type incompatibility, severe malnutrition, or maternal diabetes. Infectious diseases (e.g., meningitis, encephalitis), lead poisoning, or direct trauma after birth may cause cerebral palsy.

The signs and symptoms of the disorder can include:

- Tense, contracted muscles, uncontrolled movements of limbs, eyes, or head; poor coordination; muscle spasms; and a lack of manual dexterity
- Hearing, speech, and visual impairments
- Mental retardation
- Seizure disorders

The types of CP are based on the parts of the brain affected and the physical characteristics that result. The six classifications of CP are:

1. **Spasticity**: the most common form; the cerebral cortex is affected; involves hyperirritability of muscles, poor head control, and an inability to use the arms and legs
2. **Athetosis**: the basal ganglia is affected; involves involuntary muscle contractions, twisting, contorted movements, poor balance

3. **Ataxia**: the cerebellum is affected; characterized by partial contractions of muscles, impaired balance and coordination, and difficulty grasping objects
4. **Rigidity**: muscles rigid and stiff
5. **Flaccidity**: involuntary muscle quivering throughout the body
6. **Mixed**: combination of two or more areas

Medical management of CP consists of surgical and orthopedic intervention and physical, speech, and occupational therapy as needed. Counseling may be helpful, because many persons with CP have normal or exceptional intelligence and become frustrated with communication and public acceptance of them based on their appearance.

Orofacial manifestations of CP include:

- Enamel hypoplasia
- Caries and periodontal disease related to numerous factors such as poor manual dexterity, neglect, impaired self-cleansing due to poor oral musculature control resulting in food and plaque retention, and consumption of a semi-soft high-carbohydrate (cariogenic) diet because of dysphasia (difficulty swallowing) and difficulty chewing
- Medication-induced gingival hyperplasia
- Facial contortions and drooling due to abnormal functioning of the tongue, lips, and cheeks
- Oral habits such as tongue-thrusting, mouth breathing, and bruxism leading to severe attrition
- Class II malocclusion with a high narrow palatal vault
- Tooth fractures due to unstable ambulation

Minor movement of the head from left to right or forward and back may elicit exaggerated contractions of the arms and legs. Scheduling the patient for morning appointments, knowledge of wheelchair transfers, head and arm restraining devices, mouth props, and suitable oral hygiene adjuncts are recommended. In addition, the patient may benefit from a daily fluoride gel.

Oral Clefts

Clefts of the lip or palate are caused by a failure of normal fusion of the embryonic processes during development in the first trimester of pregnancy. Predisposing factors include genetics, environment, smoking, folic acid deficiencies, substance abuse, and infectious diseases (see Chapters 4, 6, and 8). Clefts can be subdivided into seven classifications:

- **Class 1** = Cleft of the tip of the uvula
- **Class 2** = Cleft of the uvula (bifid uvula)
- **Class 3** = Cleft of the soft palate
- **Class 4** = Cleft of the soft and hard palates
- **Class 5** = Cleft of the soft and hard palates continuing through the alveolar ridge on one side and usually associated with a cleft of the lip on the same side
- **Class 6** = Cleft of the soft and hard palates continuing through the alveolar ridge on both sides resulting in a

"floating" premaxilla; usually associated with a bilateral cleft of the lip
- **Class 7** = Submucous cleft of the soft palate caused by an absence of muscle union above the mucosa of the soft palate.

Males experience clefts about twice as often as do females, except for isolated clefts of the palate. If a cleft is unilateral, the left side is more commonly affected. In addition to the facial deformities, these individuals experience feeding problems (particularly as infants), hearing loss, middle ear and upper respiratory infections, and speech abnormalities.

When treating the patient with an oral cleft, identify the type of cleft and how the cleft has been closed (e.g., by surgery or by an **obturator**, which is a removable appliance fabricated to fill the void created by a carcinoma or a developmental cleft). Frequently there will be teeth in a cleft, missing teeth, or hypoplastic teeth, or the patient will be wearing orthodontic appliances to align the teeth properly. Meticulous oral hygiene and regular fluoride treatments, obturator care, and nutritional counseling are necessary to reduce the risk of dental disease. If the patient wears an obturator, keep it in place for the majority of the appointment after the soft tissues have been examined and the maxillary teeth have been débrided, so that the patient can comfortably rinse and communicate with you. Suction well, and keep the patient in a semiupright position when an oral cleft is exposed to prevent fluids from entering the nasal cavity.

Head and Neck Cancer

Cancer involving the oral cavity, pharynx, and thyroid account for slightly more than 4% of all new cancers in the United States for 2001 (see Chapter 8) The major cause of oral cancer is the combination of excessive smoking and drinking behaviors. The effective management of head and neck cancers requires a team approach that frequently involves maxillofacial reconstructive and cosmetic surgery and prosthetics, radiation, chemotherapy, and psychiatric and general dental and dental hygiene treatment modalities. Radiation therapy given as a localized form of treatment destroys the nucleus of the cancer cell terminating its growth, maturation, and replication. Normal cells in the field of radiation may also be damaged; however, **fractionating** the dose of radiation gives normal tissue the opportunity to recover and repair itself. Common oral complications associated with radiation therapy and measures to prevent or manage these conditions include:

- **Mucositis**: saline, sodium bicarbonate, or chlorhexidine rinses, topical steroids, topical anesthetics (**Clark solution** = $1/3$ antihistamine + $1/3$ viscous liquid anesthetic + $1/3$ liquid antacid); avoid alcohol and tobacco; eat a well-balanced soft diet; maintain hydration
- **Xerostomia**: sugarless gum and candies, frequent sips of water or ice chips, water and a few drops of glycerin in a

aerosol spray, no commercial mouthwashes due to alcohol content, salivary substitutes, saliva stimulant drugs (Pilocarpine)

- **Radiation caries** (rapid breakdown around the cervical third of the tooth) and **tooth sensitivity**: daily custom fluoride trays or brush-on gels, meticulous oral hygiene
- **Osteoradionecrosis (ORN)**: avoid trauma to the mucosa; perform oral/periodontal surgeries, extractions, root canals, etc., before radiation therapy and, if required, after radiation, then **hyperbaric oxygen** is needed to promote healing; practice meticulous oral hygiene; and antibiotics are given to control an infection before ORN develops
- **Secondary infections**: culture and treat accordingly (e.g., antibiotics, antifungals, or antivirals)
- **Trismus** (fibrosis of the muscles of mastication): exercises and stretching appliances
- **Dysgeusia** (taste disturbances): zinc supplements
- **Dysphagia**: soft nutritious diet (moist and blended foods), drink plenty of liquids with meals

Blood Disorders

Leukemia

Leukemia is a malignant proliferation of immature white blood cells (WBCs). The disease is characterized by abnormally large numbers of specific types of leukocytes and their precursors **(blast cells)** located within the circulating blood and bone marrow and infiltrated into other body tissues and organs. These blast cells become predominant in the bone marrow, thus reducing the numbers of normal WBCs, red blood cells (RBCs), and platelets. There are four main types of leukemia based on the onset and the type of WBCs affected:

1. **Acute lymphocytic leukemia (lymphoblastic) (ALL)**
2. **Chronic lymphocytic leukemia (CLL)**
3. **Acute myeloid leukemia (AML) (myeloblastic)**
4. **Chronic myeloid leukemia (CML)**

The etiology of leukemia is unknown. Some factors believed to be linked with the disease include genetics, ionizing radiation, and environmental chemical agents. The estimated number of new cases of leukemia in the U.S. is approximately 2.5% of all cancer cases for 2001. Initial symptoms include fever and lymphadenopathy due to the **leukopenia**, fatigue and pallor due to **erythrocytopenia**, and ecchymosis of skin and bleeding from the nose and gingiva owing to **thrombocytopenia (see Chapters 4 and 8).**

Chemotherapy is the treatment of a disease with chemical agents. Chemotherapeutic drugs work by destroying cancer cells. In an effort to kill the malignant cells, normal cells with the same rapidly dividing characteristics are also affected. Locations of cells with a high mitotic index include the bone marrow, hair, alimentary tract (including the oral cavity), and the genitourinary tract. Consequently, patients suffer from side effects of the chemotherapy such as bleeding, infection, **alopecia** (hair loss), **mucositis** (sloughing and ulcerations of the oral soft tissues), nausea, vomiting, and diarrhea.

Oral management of the patient undergoing chemotherapy, particularly for leukemia, requires routine assessment of blood counts. Medical consultation is advised. Typically, dental procedures can be performed safely if the neutrophil count is ≥1000 cu/mm and the platelet count is ≥50,000 cu/mm. Antibiotic premedication before dental treatment may be warranted, particularly if the patient has a low neutrophil count or an **indwelling catheter** in place. Oral management procedures, particularly during episodes of mucositis, may include chlorhexidine rinsing; gentle débridement with a supersoft toothbrush; oral infection management with the appropriate antifungals, antivirals, or antibiotics; topical anesthetic ointments, sprays, or rinses (Clark solution) for pain control; and topical thrombin agents for hemostasis. Management in most cases is only palliative. Continued therapy may involve a bone marrow transplant. Oral assessment prior to transplant and maintenance during the recovery phase are paramount to decrease the risk of a life-threatening infection. Routine dental care is advised during periods of disease remission.

Hemophilia

Hemophilia is a congenital disorder of the blood clotting mechanism. There are four common forms of hemophilia:

1. **Hemophilia A** is a factor VIII deficiency; it is the most common form.
2. **Hemophilia B** or **Christmas disease** is a deficiency in factor IX.
3. **Hemophilia C** is a deficiency in factor XI.
4. **von Willebrand disease** is characterized by a reduction in factor VIII, prolonged bleeding times, and poor platelet adhesion.

Hemophilia A and B are inherited by males through the x-linked recessive trait carried by females. von Willebrand disease is transmitted by an autosomal codominant trait, thus affecting both males and females.

The normal concentration of clotting factors is between 50% and 150%. Mild hemophilia is defined by a factor range of 5% to 50%, and bleeding occurs only after severe injury. **Moderate hemophilia** consists of a clotting factor of 2% to 5% with infrequent spontaneous bleeding after minor trauma. **Severe hemophilia** results when the clotting factor is less than 1%. Spontaneous, prolonged bleeding into muscles, joints **(hemarthrosis)**, and soft tissues occurs after any emotional or physical trauma.

Medical management consists of venous injections of clotting factor. Mild forms of hemophilia are treated with fresh frozen plasma containing the factor. Severe forms are treated with one of two types of plasma extracts:

1. **Cryoprecipitate**-freeze-dried clotting factor from a large number of donors, stored at room temperature for 6 months, or refrigerated for up to 2 years
2. **Concentrate**-factor prepared fresh from a single blood donation and stored in freezer

A thorough health history is essential for proper oral management of the patient with hemophilia. Always consult with a physician before the appointment. Blocks and infiltration anesthesia should be used with caution owing to the risk of creating a dissecting hematoma that could obstruct the airway. Care should also be taken to avoid trauma by the placement of a radiograph packet, impression tray, saliva evacuation tips, dental instruments, and orthodontic brackets. Débridement procedures should be completed in one appointment, if possible, and replacement factor should be at least 30%. For surgical procedures, the replacement factor should be at least 50%. Local and systemic hemostatic agents (Amicar, Gelfoam, and Surgicel) may be indicated postoperatively.

Efforts should be made to teach parents measures to prevent mouth injuries. Aspirin and nonsteroidal anti-inflammatory drugs (NSAIDs) commonly prescribed for joint pain should be avoided. If the patient with hemophilia has undergone joint replacement, assess the patient for the need for antibiotic prophylaxis before dental treatment.

Anemias

Sickle Cell Disease

Sickle cell trait is heterozygous state in which the affected individual carries one gene for hemoglobin S. The RBCs become sickle-shaped when they become deoxygenated, reducing the flow of oxygenated blood to the extremities and thus increasing the risk of bone necrosis. This condition is common among African Americans and white populations of Mediterranean origin.

The signs and symptoms include fatigue, shortness of breath, nausea, abdominal pain, bone pain, tingling of the fingers and toes, muscular weakness, and widening of the marrow spaces in the skull exhibiting a **"sun ray" appearance,** because the bony trabeculae radiate outward. Symptoms may also include blindness; jaundice; pallor; cracking, splitting, and spooning of fingernails; increased size of heart, liver, and spleen; lymphadenopathy; low hematocrit, and blood in the stools. Intraorally, patients also exhibit:

- Loss of trabeculation of the alveolar bone on a radiograph because the marrow spaces are large and irregular
- Increased probing depths
- Gingival pallor
- Infection
- Bleeding
- A sore, smooth, red tongue
- Loss of taste

Pernicious Anemia

Pernicious anemia is a deficiency of **intrinsic factor** resulting in the impaired absorption of B_{12} and folic acid by the body. Older adults are often affected; they may experience chronic atrophic gastritis and may have increased risk for gastric carcinoma, myxedema, or rheumatoid arthritis. Loss of taste and a red, sore, smooth tongue are characteristic signs of this condition.

Vitamin B_{12} injections are the only treatment necessary in the initial stages of this disorder.

Iron Deficiency Anemia

Microcytic or **iron deficiency anemia** is caused by excessive blood loss from menses or bleeding from GI tract, gastrectomy, or a malabsorption syndrome that reduces absorption of iron from GI tract. This condition is common in children with poor diets. Weakness and fatigue are common symptoms of this disorder. Depending on the severity and the cause, iron supplementation, transfusions, or hormone therapy may be indicated.

From a dental standpoint, iron supplements cause staining of the teeth and routine débridement becomes necessary **(see Chapter 10).**

Metabolic Conditions

Diabetes

Diabetes mellitus is a metabolic disease characterized by a reduction in carbohydrate metabolism and an increase in lipid and protein metabolism caused by a deficiency in insulin produced by the pancreas. Hyperglycemia is the result **(see the section on Emergencies).** The etiology of diabetes is often unknown but can be caused by pancreatic cancer, inflammation or surgery, an endocrine imbalance from hyperpituitarism, hyperthyroidism, pregnancy, or the administration of steroids.

Diabetes mellitus is subdivided into two types:

Type 1: (IDDM) Sudden onset, usually affecting persons younger than 40 years of age. There is an absolute insulin deficiency, and the individual is dependent on exogenous insulin to sustain life and prevent acidosis. The initial signs and symptoms of IDDM include **polyuria, polydipsia, and polyphagia.**

Type 2: (NIDDM) The most common of the two types of diabetes mellitus. Slow onset of symptoms affect obese persons older than 40 years of age(referred to as the adult form). Pancreatic insulin secretion may be low, normal, or high, but patients exhibit an insulin resistance that impairs the use of insulin secreted. Oral hypoglycemic agents or diet may be used to treat the disease.

Blood glucose levels are directly proportional to blood pressure, weight, tobacco use, and alcohol consumption. Glycemic control is imperative to prevent systemic complications such as eye, kidney, heart, and periodontal diseases. Unstable diabetes can exacerbate periodontal disease and periodontal disease can cause blood glucose levels to rise **(see Chapter 13).**

Assess for glycemic control by asking questions about the patient's lifestyle, such as how often the blood glucose level is monitored and by whom; what forms of treatment have been prescribed and the level of compliance; what dietary habits are practiced; and the condition of the oral soft tissues. Dry cracked lips, xerostomia, parotid gland enlargement, burning inflamed mucosa, gingival edema and bleeding, poor wound healing, candidiasis, periodontal abscesses, significant probing depths, and neuropathy are consistent with uncontrolled diabetes. The patient with uncontrolled diabetes may require premedication with an antibiotic before dental treatment.

Pregnancy

Maintaining good oral hygiene to prevent hormonal-induced gingival changes such as pregnancy gingivitis and pregnancy tumor are essential. In addition, recent studies link periodontal disease to preterm low-birthweight babies. Nutritional counseling and oral hygiene instructions (OHIs) to reduce the risk of caries associated with morning sickness, gagging when toothbrushing, and a craving for sweets are also recommended. The administration of analgesic drugs for dental pain should be considered carefully.

First Trimester

Meticulous plaque control, and OHI, diet counseling are paramount during this period. Elective dental treatment radiographs and local anesthesia should be avoided. Urgent care only is advised.

Second Trimester

This is the safest period for dental treatment. Routine dental care is advised, and radiographs can be exposed, if necessary.

Third Trimester

Routine dental care is permitted. Avoid placing the patient in a supine position for long periods, because blood return from the inferior vena cava may become impeded and the patient may become faint. Turn the patient to the left side if she begins to feel faint or uncomfortable.

Muscle Disorders

Muscular Dystrophy

Muscular dystrophy refers to a group of genetic myopathies characterized by progressive skeletal muscle atrophy and weakness. There are three types of MD:

1. **Duchenne muscular dystrophy** is present at birth and primarily affects males younger than 10 years of age. The condition is transmitted by a sex-linked recessive factor (mothers are the carriers). The signs and symptoms involve:
   - Progressive muscle wasting and weakness beginning with the hips, spine, pelvis, and abdomen, eventually involving the extremities, and the need for a wheelchair
   - Waddling gait and **lordosis** (curvature of the spine)
   - Enlargement of the calf muscles
   - Tripoding when rising from a prone position (**Gower sign**)
   - Respiratory complications
2. **Facioscapulohumeral muscular dystrophy** affects males and females, and the onset is usually between 10 and 18 years of age. As the name implies, the signs and symptoms consist of impairment of the muscles of facial expression (e.g., difficulty whistling, frowning, closing the eyes), prominent scapulas, weak shoulder muscles, and difficulty raising arms. This form is autosomal dominant.
3. **Limb-girdle dystrophy** affects the pelvic girdle first, followed by weakness in the shoulders. It is an autosomal recessive trait and usually affects persons in their 20s.

The etiology is for muscular dystrophy is unknown, but prenatal diagnosis, carrier detection, and genetic counseling are beneficial in preventing its occurrence. Modifications to treatment include:

- Adaptive oral hygiene aids to manage the increased risk for periodontal disease and caries associated with the patient's poor oral musculature control, limited manual dexterity, and need for a soft diet due to loss of strength of the muscles of mastication and a decreased biting force
- Wheelchair transfer
- Mouth propping devices

Persons with muscular dystrophy often exhibit retained primary teeth, hypoplastic teeth, and xerostomia from the inability to keep the lips together

Myasthenia Gravis

Myasthenia gravis (MG) is an autoimmune neuromuscular disease characterized by fluctuating weakness of symmetric voluntary muscles, especially the oculofacial and proximal limb muscles. The autoimmune process results in defective nerve impulse transmission at the neuromuscular junctions. The onset of MG is at approximately 20 years of age; MG affects females twice as often as males. Later in adult life, more men are affected than are women.

Early signs and symptoms include weakness of eye movement with double vision and drooping eyelids; difficulty swallowing; lack of facial expression; disturbed speech and expression; and a weak voice (muffled and tired). The patient may need to support the chin with one hand while talking. Progressive symptoms affect the muscles used during breathing, and serious respiratory complications can result. Anticholinesterase agents, steroids, and immunosuppressive medications are used in the treatment of MG.

Short, frequent dental appointments are advised due to weakness. Eliminate infection or a stressful situation, such as dental surgery, that may exacerbate the condition. Maintain good suction during procedures, and assess for oral side effects of medications. Monitor daily steroid dosage, and evaluate the need for steroid supplementation to alleviate the risk of adrenal crisis.

Disorders of Central Nervous System

Multiple Sclerosis

Multiple sclerosis (MS) is a chronic degenerative disease of the white matter or **myelin** tissue of the CNS. These areas of destruction are replaced with sclerotic tissue (plaques) at scattered sites (mainly spinal cord and optic nerves). Plaques accumulate until the nerve becomes permanently damaged and the conduction of nerve impulses is disrupted, causing widespread and varied symptoms with periods of exacerbation and remission.

The patient with MS will experience:

- Vision impairment
- Coordination difficulty, tremors, fatigue, weakness, and numbness of body parts
- Speech disorders
- Urinary frequency, urgency, and later incontinence
- Susceptibility to upper respiratory infections, in particular

Medical management entails rest, physical therapy, occupational therapy, psychological counseling, and immunosuppressive drugs. Oral management considerations include: prednisone assessment for dose-associated risks; possible trigeminal neuralgia and facial weakness; wheelchair transfers; oral hygiene adaptations to accommodate impaired dexterity; short appointments; reducing the risk of periodontal and periapical infection that might exacerbate the condition; mouth propping devices; good suction; and chair adjustments to make the patient comfortable.

Bell Palsy

Bell palsy is the paralysis of facial muscles innervated by the facial nerve (cranial nerve VII). The etiology is unknown, but bacterial/viral infections, trauma from tooth extraction, and surgery of parotid gland area have been implicated.

The signs and symptoms include:

- Weakness or paralysis of the facial muscles→ no pain
- Corner of the mouth droops→ excessive salivation/drooling
- Eyelids do not close→ watering and lower lid infections
- Speech and mastication difficulties

Patients usually return to normal within 1 month. Many recover spontaneously, but in some cases residual effects persist. Steroids are usually all that is needed; however, in cases of permanent damage, surgical procedures to repair cranial nerve VII are performed to improve appearance. Because the eyelid may not close on the affected side, protective eyewear must be worn by the patient at all times. The pocketing of food on the affected side may require the use of a powered toothbrush and a daily fluoride gel.

Parkinson Disease

Parkinsonism is a progressive disorder of the CNS characterized by a loss of postural stability, slowness of spontaneous movement, resting tremor, and muscle rigidity. The condition is caused by a deficiency in the neurotransmitters dopamine and norepinephrine and an overproduction of cholinergic neurotransmitter substance.

Signs and symptoms involve:

- Tremors, rigidity, and loss of motor function
- Shuffling gait with flexed arms and knees, forward tilt of the body
- Mask-like appearance → a delay in responsiveness
- Dysphagia → excessive drooling

Physical and occupational therapy, drug therapy to replenish the shortage of dopamine, and psychological counseling to deal with depression is paramount in managing the disease.

Oral management of drug-induced xerostomia and its complications regarding caries, denture fit, diet counseling to suggest nutritious foods that are easily swallowed, and use of powered toothbrushing devices to assist with dexterity issues are advised.

Spinal Cord Injury

Impairment of spinal cord function from external traumatic force may result in paralysis. Damage to the spinal cord at the level of the cervical vertebrae results in **quadriplegia.** Injury at the thoracic, lumbar, or sacral level causes **paraplegia.** Rehabilitation requires a team approach. Occupational, recreational, physical, and psychological therapies are essential. Sometimes respiratory therapy, dietary counseling, and assistance with bladder (catheter) and bowel (colostomy) care are needed. Treatment for spasticity and seizures include exercise and drug therapy.

Oral intervention may include assessment and management of drug-induced xerostomia and gingival hyperplasia; **task analysis** to determine the patient's skill level; oral hygiene adaptive aids based on abilities; oral care and dietary recommendations for a jaw fracture and immobilization, if associated with the spinal cord injury; chlorhexidine and fluoride rinses; caregiver instructions; wheelchair transfer and catheter placement (tubes straight and below the level of the bladder); dental chair adjustments to promote patient comfort; and perhaps the fabrication of a **bitestick appliance** to assist with daily functions.

Spina Bifida

Spina bifida is a congenital defect resulting in failure of one or more vertebral arches to fuse and manifests as an opening in the spinal column. A portion of the spinal cord may protrude through the opening with the meninges (**myelomeningocele**) or without the meninges (**myelocele**). A deficiency in folic acid during gestation has been implicated as a cause of this condition (**see Chapter 6**).

Signs and symptoms may include a deformity from protrusion of the cord; bone deformities (e.g., clubfoot, spinal curvatures, dislocation of hip); **hydrocephaly**, and sensation loss. Neurosurgery is performed to close the defect and place a **cerebrospinal fluid (CSF) shunt** to drain the excess fluid from the ventricles of the brain. Multiple orthopedic surgeries may be needed to correct the bone deformities. Dental treatment modifications may require oral hygiene adjuncts; assessment and management of drug-induced gingival hyperplasia; antibiotic coverage for a CSF shunt (ventriculoatrial shunts require premedication; lumboperitoneal and venticuloperitoneal shunts do not appear to cause an increased risk for infection, but the need for antibiotic prophylaxis can be established through medical consultation); and wheelchair transfer.

Respiratory Conditions

Cystic Fibrosis

Cystic fibrosis (CF) is an inherited disorder that is transmitted by a mendelian autosomal recessive gene. The condition affects the exocrine glands, which are responsible for mucus, sweat, and saliva secretions. These secretions are very viscous and impede the function of the lungs and pancreas. Therefore, secretions accumulate in the lungs making breathing, particularly exhaling, difficult. Thick secretions block the pancreatic duct and result in inadequate secretions of pancreatic enzymes into the duodenum for digestion. Persons with CF are susceptible to bronchitis, pneumonia, and emphysema.

The signs and symptoms include: barrel-chested appearance; failure to gain weight; frequent bulky, foul, fatty stools; enlarged submandibular and sublingual glands; viscous, sticky saliva and increased calculus deposition; chronic productive cough; clubbing of fingers and toes; salty perspiration (high excretion of sodium and potassium in sweat); dehydration; and, in advanced cases, diabetes, cirrhosis of the liver, and male sterility.

Diagnosis is usually made using a **sweat test.** Parents often remark that their child's skin tastes salty when kissed. In fact, after perspiring a cap of salt crystals can be seen on the head. Persons with CF are frequently prescribed antibiotics for lung infections, aerosol inhalants to expand bronchial tubes and hydrate mucus, mist tents to promote hydration, and **postural drainage** exercises to break up the mucus secretions. Dietary recommendations include consumption of a high calorie/protein diet that limits fat intake,

and increased salt and fluid intake, particularly during the summer to avoid dehydration.

Oral management requires:

- Placing the individual in a more upright position
- Bleaching may be indicated if tetracycline was one of the antibiotics given as a child
- Frequent recall appointments to remove calculus
- Scheduling during temperate months to avoid extremes of hot or cold
- Assessing for caries related to xerostomia (no watery secretions)
- Providing diet counseling to avoid high fermentable carbohydrates

Mouth breathing may also contribute to xerostomia and gingival inflammation.

Asthma

There are two types of asthma:

1. **Extrinsic:** family history of allergies with bronchospasms triggered by smoke, pet hair, exercise, and climate. Histamine is produced causing bronchial secretions, airway inflammation, and edema. The smooth muscle surrounding the airway narrows and airflow is disturbed.
2. **Intrinsic:** occurs in middle-aged adults and is associated with upper respiratory infections.

The signs and symptoms of asthma are wheezing, coughing, tightness in chest, and dyspnea. Emotional disturbances, once believed to be an etiologic factor, are now considered to initiate hyperventilation that is then responsible for triggering the asthmatic episode.

Management consists of bronchodilators from the β-adrenergic, anticholinergic, and corticosteroid categories. Oral management involves creating a relaxed, climate-controlled environment; assessment of steroid dosage risk; and a thorough health history documenting the last asthma attack, age of onset, triggers, and so forth. Ask patients to bring their inhalers with them, and place them in an easily accessible location in case of an attack. Aspirin and NSAIDs should be avoided because of their allergic potential, and erythromycin is contraindicated because it inhibits the clearance of many drugs such as theophylline, thus potentiating its effects.

Emphysema

Emphysema is an abnormal condition of the pulmonary system that features both overinflation and destructive changes in alveolar walls, resulting in loss of lung elasticity and decreased $CO_2 \leftrightarrow O_2$ exchange from the reduction in surface area. As the alveoli lose their elasticity and tear, air spaces are created that resist airflow and breathing becomes labored. Chronic emphysema usually accompanies chronic bronchitis and can also be associated with asthma and tuberculosis (TB).

The primary preventable etiology is cigarette smoking, but occupational risks also occur. Signs and symptoms include a barrel-chested appearance; wheezing and coughing; and cyanosis of the lips and fingertips because of a reduced level of oxygen-rich blood in circulation. The workload of the heart increases as it attempts to oxygenate the tissues and can lead eventually to congestive heart failure (CHF).

Postural drainage of mucus is one form of medical management. The patient with emphysema must also consume 2000 to 3000 ml of fluid daily. Bronchodilators, antibiotics, corticosteroids, and expectorants are prescribed, and exposure to low concentration oxygen with humidification for several minutes hourly is advised.

During a dental appointment, the patient needs to have time to cough and not feel rushed. Keep the patient in the upright position; assess the steroid dosage risk; and avoid the use of narcotics, barbiturates, and high oxygen concentrations that are usually used with nitrous oxide analgesia. Long waits in the reception area are contraindicated due to exposure to potential infections. Afternoon appointments in warmer weather are preferable.

Tuberculosis

TB is a communicable disease that is transmitted by inhaling droplets containing *Mycobacterium tuberculosis.* The anatomic lesion is the **tubercle.** Signs and symptoms consist of a low-grade fever, lymphadenopathy, loss of appetite, fatigue, persistent cough, and night sweats.

Antituberculosis drugs are prescribed over a 6-month period (i.e., isoniazid, pyrazinamide and rifampin). Infectivity is usually decreased a few weeks after therapy.

Oral management advises not to treat the patient if he or she has active TB, unless it is an emergency. In emergency cases, use a facility with a special ventilation system and an isolated operatory that is isolated from other patients. The practitioner should wear the highest level of filtration mask. Medications may cause myelosuppression, resulting in delayed healing, infection, and gingival bleeding. Monitor blood counts and caution the patient to use a soft toothbrush. Always consult with the physician and refer the patient when unsure of the patient's medical status. Persons with a past or present history of TB, drug regimen compliance, and three negative cultures can be treated as normal.

Inflammatory/Autoimmune

Crohn Disease

Crohn disease is a chronic granulomatous inflammatory disease of the alimentary tract characterized by segmental distribution of intestinal ulcers (including oral ulcers) with intervening mucosal edema giving this disease a **classic "cobblestone" appearance.** The etiology is unknown. Most cases affect males and females in their 20s.

The signs and symptoms involve recurrent and persistent diarrhea (without blood), abdominal pain in the right lower quadrant, an abdominal mass, unexplained fever, malaise, and weight loss. In children, arthritis, anemia, and impaired growth may present.

Medical management consists of corticosteroids, anti-inflammatory drugs, antibiotics, nutritional supplements, bedrest, and surgery to remove segments of diseased bowel. An ileostomy is sometimes necessary.

Oral management might consist of flexible scheduling due to a disease flare-up, monitoring steroid dosage risk, and the treatment of oral ulcerations.

Lupus Erythematosus

Lupus erythematosus is an inflammatory connective tissue disorder of unknown etiology that occurs predominantly in young women. The clinical signs vary, but at least four signs must be present to diagnose the condition. Signs and symptoms of lupus include:

- Malar butterfly rash pattern across the bridge of the nose that is aggravated by sunlight
- Intraoral ulcerations and petechiae
- Alopecia
- Mottled erythema on the sides of the palms and fingers
- Thrombocytopenia and hemorrhage under the nailbeds
- Photosensitivity
- Arthralgias, with or without joint deformity
- Renal involvement
- Immunosuppression and generalized adenopathy
- Recurrent pleurisy, bacterial or viral pneumonia
- Pericarditis, murmur, and valvular dysfunction

Involvement of the CNS can cause personality changes and seizures.

Treatment depends on the current clinical conditions but usually consists of aspirin, NSAIDs, antimalarial agents, immunosuppressants, and corticosteroids. The elimination of stress, exposure to sunlight, and physical fatigue are also advised.

Oral intervention involves monitoring the blood counts and the steroid dosage risk; assessing for oral bleeding, petechiae, and temporomandibular joint (TMJ) pain; adjusting the dental chair for patient comfort and the light to reduce glare; and managing lichenoid-like ulcerations. Clark's solution may prove helpful. Antibiotic premedication before dental procedures may be necessary.

Arthritis

Arthritis is a general term used to describe a group of disorders characterized by inflammation of the joints with associated pain. Possible etiologies include infection, insufficient blood supply, impaired immune response, traumatic disorders, endocrine abnormalities, tumors, allergy and drug reactions, and inherited or congenital conditions. The two major types of arthritis are:

1. **Rheumatoid**: Chronic, bilateral inflammation of the **small peripheral joints** affecting the fingers, hands, elbows, wrists, feet, and TMJ. It affects women usually between the ages of 25 and 55 years. Treatment involves aspirin, NSAIDs, adrenocortical steroids, and immunosuppressive agents such as methotrexate. Surgery to restore function to deformed joints or for joint replacement may be required.
2. **Osteoarthritis: Noninflammatory type** of joint destruction; unilateral, affecting one or more **large joints** (e.g., knees, hips, TMJ, and cervical and lower lumbar vertebrae). Younger men and older women are usually affected, and the condition seems to become more pai370   Dental Hygiene in Reviewnful with physical activity. Signs and symptoms include swelling of cartilage covering diseased bone causing a cracking sound when the joint is flexed; bone spurs due to loss of cartilage and end-to-end bone contact; and dull aching, limited movements. Treatment may range from simple monitoring without treatment to NSAIDs, hot/cold compresses, periods of rest and exercise, and walking aids or braces to artificial joints. Steroids do not benefit this patient.

Oral management includes assessment of manual dexterity and the need for oral hygiene adaptive aids; adjusting and padding the dental chair to ensure comfort; moist heat and mouth props for TMJ pain; and scheduling short appointments. TMJ pain may lead to limited oral opening, decreased mobility, and an anterior openbite caused by the destruction of the condyles and loss of condylar height. Assess the patient for bleeding, ulcers, exogenous steroid risk for adrenal crisis, and the need for premedication with an antibiotic. **Prosthetic joints require antibiotic coverage** before dental treatment if the replacement occurred 2 years ago or less or if the patient has uncontrolled IDDM, hemophilia, rheumatoid arthritis, lupus, or any other immunocompromising condition with a reduced capacity to resist infection. Pins, screws, and plates do not require premedication.

Scleroderma (Progressive Systemic Sclerosis)

Scleroderma is an autoimmune disease of connective tissue characterized by an overproduction of collagen. The etiology is unknown, but irregularities in collagen synthesis associated with immunologic disorders and microvascular abnormalities have been postulated. Signs and symptoms include muscle weakness and joint pain; immobility and rigidity of skin (mask-like face); and dysphagia owing to esophageal and peptic strictures that also affect the lungs, heart, and kidneys. Death can occur from renal failure, cardiac failure, pulmonary insufficiency, or intestinal malabsorption.

Oral signs consist of thin, rigid lips; thin intraoral lining mucosa with poor healing capacity; pale, firm gingiva; mobile teeth; and tongue immobility. There is no specific treatment, but corticosteroids, antacids, antibiotics, and physical therapy are often employed.

A limited oral opening is observed and may restrict the wearing of dentures and other oral appliances. Patients are sensitive to cold, dampness, stress, and fatigue. Appointments should be short, and the dental chair should be placed in a semiupright position and padded for the patient's comfort. Dietary counseling should occur to ensure that a low cariogenic nutritious soft diet is consumed. Assess the patient for steroid dosage risk.

Mental Conditions

Alcoholism (Dependency)

Alcoholism is a dependency on alcohol developed after long periods of abuse. The signs and symptoms involve:

- Inability to stop drinking or limit drinks before intoxication
- Amnesia during periods of intoxication;
- Increased tolerance
- Withdrawal symptoms, such as shakes with relief from more use of alcohol

Successful medical management involves:

1. Early intervention
2. Detoxification
3. Rehabilitation (e.g., group therapy, counseling, psychiatry)

Oral signs and symptoms may include xerostomia; coated tongue; glossitis due to vitamin deficiency; poor oral hygiene; bleeding upon probing; alcohol breath; and erosion of enamel from vomiting. Oral hygiene instructions and a home fluoride rinse or gel are advised. Mouth rinses that contain alcohol should be avoided. Metronidazole, which is used in the treatment of periodontal disease, has an Antabuse effect and will elicit vomiting when combined with alcohol.

Schizophrenia

Schizophrenia is a complex, chronic mental disorder. It is a major psychotic illness characterized by delusions of persecution, hallucinations, disorganized thinking, incoherence, alcohol and drug abuse, social isolation, peculiar behavior, and odd beliefs.

The etiology may be a complex interaction between inherited and environmental factors, manifesting between the ages of 15 and 35 years.

The medical treatment for schizophrenia includes psychosocial therapy and antipsychotic agents (e.g., phenothiazines, butyrophenones, thioxanthenes). Reactions to medications can occur, particularly in the elderly, and there is a risk of agranulocytosis.

Oral intervention involves assessment and management of drug-induced xerostomia. Because there is also a risk of drug-induced leukopenia, the WBC count should be checked before treatment. Oral ulcerations may also occur from the agranulocytosis and require palliative support therapy. Drug/alcohol abuse may be evident from the patient's pupils, breath, and overall demeanor. Only treat the patient when symptoms of the disorder are controlled. Keep the routine simple, and never argue with the patient.

Depression

Depression is a disturbance marked by apathy, fear, sadness, loss of mobility, and energy. Causes for depression might include unforeseen tragic events, illness, death, or disappointment with one's career or personal plans. Patients with depression often exhibit antisocial behavior; they lack motivation and initiative; and they possess feelings of isolation.

Medical management includes correction of sleep disturbances; improvement of diet and eating patterns; exercise; antidepressants; and psychotherapy with or without hospitalization.

Oral intervention consists of assessment and management of drug-induced xerostomia, motivating the patient to perform daily oral care, and TLC. Provide positive reinforcement and show a genuine interest in the patient.

Anxiety

Anxiety is a disorder that is characterized by apprehension, tension, or dread that results from anticipation of danger or harm. The person's being, self-esteem, or identity feel threatened. The four major forms of anxiety are:

1. **Panic attack**: unexpected or cued by a specific trigger (social or specific phobias)
2. **Panic disorder**: recurrent panic attacks; sometimes coincides with agoraphobia
3. **Phobias**: afraid of specific substance or event (flying)
4. **Obsessive-compulsive**: repetitive thought or impulse that preoccupies the day; compulsions are repetitive acts that the person performs against his or her wishes or standards (e.g., frequent handwashing)

The medical management for anxiety includes the elimination of caffeine, alcohol, and drugs; assessment for depression; cognitive behavioral therapy exercises; psychotherapy; and antianxiety agents (e.g., benzodiazepines) and antidepressant medications.

Oral intervention consists of diet counseling; assessment and management of tooth hypersensitivity and drug-induced xerostomia; and measures of support to motivate and help the patient feel more secure.

Alzheimer Disease

Alzheimer disease is defined as a presenile dementia of unknown cause. This disease begins in middle age, affects nerve cells of the frontal and temporal lobes of the cerebrum, and leads to speech defects and progressive loss of mental faculties. More than half of the cases are diagnosed in persons older than 65 years of age.

The signs and symptoms of Alzheimer disease are categorized into four stages:

1. **Early**: forgetfulness, personality changes, social withdrawal, apathy, and personal hygiene neglect
2. **Middle**: disorientation, loss of coordination, anxiety, language difficulty, sleep pattern disturbance, progressive memory loss, and pacing
3. **Advanced**: profound comprehension difficulty, gait disturbances, bladder and bowel incontinence, seizures, and aggression
4. **Terminal**: physical immobility, dysphagia, mutism, pathologic reflexes, unawareness of environment, and total helplessness

Tranquilizers and antipsychotic agents have been prescribed to manage aggressive or uncooperative behavior.

Oral intervention must take place early in the disease. Drug-induced **tardive dyskinesia** (CNS disorder causing facial distortions) may make oral hygiene treatment challenging. Drug-induced xerostomia must be assessed routinely and managed with daily fluoride gel to prevent rapid cervical and root decay.

Cardiovascular Disease

Cerebrovascular Accident [(CVA) or Stroke]

A CVA involves a sudden development of focal neurologic deficits resulting from an interference in cerebral blood flow. The patient is often disabled by changes in motor, communication, and perceptual function. Risk factors for stroke include previous strokes, hypertension, atherosclerosis (particularly carotid vessel calcifications), cardiac abnormalities, diabetes mellitus, elevated blood lipids, periodontal disease, smoking, drug and alcohol use, stress, and inactivity.

The four possible etiologies of stroke follow:

1. **Thrombosis**: stationary clot within a blood vessel of the brain or neck that shuts off oxygen supply to a portion of the brain tissue resulting in a cerebral infarction
2. **Intracerebral embolism**: blood vessel blocked by a clot or other material carried through the circulation from one part of the body to another
3. **Ischemia**: blood flow reduced to an area of the brain. A transient ischemic attack (TIA) is the most common manifestation; has a short duration
4. **Intracerebral hemorrhage**: escape of blood through ruptured or unruptured vessel walls

The warning signs of stroke depend on the magnitude of injury to the brain and the degree of cerebral vessel involvement. The patient usually experiences unilateral weakness of the face or extremity, aphasia or dysarthria, temporary dimness or a loss of vision, and dizziness or unstable ambulation.

Medical management may consist of surgery, physical and occupational therapy, and medications (e.g., anticoagulants, antihypertensives, thrombolytics, vasodilators, and steroids). As dental patients, numerous issues and needs should be considered. **Hemiplegia** may lead to food pocketing, drooling, dysphagia, and impaired dexterity; therefore, powered toothbrushes may have merit. Anticoagulant therapy may initiate oral bleeding and requires monitoring of a recent **prothrombin time** (should not treat if exceeds $1^1/_2$-2 times the normal range of 11-15 seconds) or the **international normalized ratio** (**INR**-should not be treated if exceeds 3.0). Blood pressure should also be monitored, and drug-induced xerostomia should be assessed and managed. Avoid vasoconstrictors in dental anesthetics. Caution should be taken if pain relievers or antibiotics (e.g., aspirin, NSAIDs, herbs, erythromycin, or metronidazole) are being prescribed for dental procedures or conditions, because these agents are known to potentiate the effect of the anticoagulant drugs. Impaired mental function leads to slowness, poor memory, loss of initiative, speech difficulty, visual impairment, and an increased sensitivity to pain and touch. Personal factors such as fear, dependency, anxiety, and depression will be a challenge when trying to motivate this patient. Brief appointments, scheduled in the morning, are recommended.

Heart Valve Disease

The signs and symptoms of valvular heart disease include dyspnea, cyanosis, ruddy complexion, polycythemia, clubbing of fingers and toes, murmurs, CHF, distention of neck veins, ascites, weakness, hepatomegaly, dizziness, syncope, and coma.

Medical management of valvular heart disease usually includes surgery to close the defect(s) or replace a valve. Surgically repaired defects normally close within 1 to 3 weeks postoperatively. Nevertheless, antibiotic premedication is warranted for closed defects without residual leaks for 6 months or less after surgery. Surgically constructed systemic pulmonary shunts or extracardiac conduits that contain replacement valves also require antibiotic premedication prior to dental procedures. Consult with the most recent AHA guidelines or the patient's cardiologist to determine risk levels if unsure (**see Chapter 7**).

Congenital heart disease refers to defects of the anatomic structure of heart or major blood vessels occurring during the first 9 weeks in utero. Common causes of congenital heart disease include heredity, vitamin deficiencies, drugs and alcohol, infections, excessive radiation, and chromosomal aberrations. Types of congenital cardiac defects include:

- Atrial and ventricular septal defects
- Patent ductus arteriosus
- Transposition of great vessels
- Tetralogy of Fallot
- Pulmonary stenosis
- Coarctation of the aorta

Acquired heart disease refers to a heart condition or abnormality that is not inherited. Common causes of acquired heart disease include bacteria, viruses, rheumatic fever, and infective endocarditis.

Rheumatic fever can develop 2 to 3 weeks after a **group A β-hemolytic streptococcal pharyngeal infection** and can result in rheumatic heart disease, if unsuccessfully treated. The diagnosis of rheumatic fever is an elevated antibody titer. This **antigen-antibody response** causes tissue necrosis and inflammation consistent with **rheumatic heart disease.** The aortic or mitral valve is usually damaged. The scarring and calcifications that form in and around the affected valve may result in **stenosis** or **regurgitation.** Subsequent symptoms of rheumatic heart disease include shortness of breath, murmur, angina pectoris, CHF, elevation of diastolic BP, enlarged heart, and blood in the sputum. **Antibiotic coverage prior to dental procedures is required for all patients with rheumatic heart disease.** As much treatment as possible should be rendered during each coverage period, and at least 9 days to 2 weeks should elapse between subsequent visits. Excellent oral hygiene should be maintained to reduce the patient's dental needs.

Failure to premedicate could result in infective **endocarditis** from the **bacteremia** associated with periodontal débridement, oral surgeries, and so forth. The risk for infective endocarditis is high to moderate for patients with acquired and congenital heart diseases. Initial symptoms of endocarditis may be flu-like with signs involving petechiae, fingernail and retinal hemorrhages, and murmur. Secondary symptoms may include paralysis; blindness; chest, abdominal, and bone pain; confusion, and stroke. Persons with a previous history of endocarditis should receive antibiotic premedication before dental procedures.

Hypertension

Hypertension refers to an abnormal elevation of blood pressure and serves as a contributing risk factor for many vascular diseases. Only about 10% of cases can be attributed to some known etiology such as renal disease, pheochromocytoma, or taking oral contraceptives. This is called **secondary hypertension.** The remaining 90% of hypertensive cases have an unknown etiology. This type is defined as **primary hypertension.** Primary risk factors include heredity, obesity, race (higher in African Americans), climate (reduced for tropics), excess sodium in diet, gender and age (men younger than 45 years and women older than 45 years of age), oral contraceptive use, environment, and smoking. (**The stages of hypertension are outlined in the Emergency section of this chapter.**)

Signs and symptoms consist of headaches, dizziness, shortness of breath, and difficulty in concentration. Long-term effects of the disease include occipital headache, blurred vision, dyspnea, and chest pains.

The medical management of hypertension involves:

1. Reduction of sodium intake and weight
2. Cessation of smoking
3. Reduction of stress
4. Use of antihypertensive drugs [e.g., diuretics, vasodilators, adrenergic blocking agents, calcium channel blockers, angiotensin converting enzyme (ACE) inhibitors, and sedatives]

Always check the patient's BP, and refer a patient with stage II, III, or IV hypertension to a physician. If, for example, stress is associated with the dental visit, it should be addressed and managed with medication or hypnosis. In addition, assisting the patient with smoking cessation is an important function of the dental health care provider. No dental hygiene treatment should be rendered for the patient exhibiting stage IV hypertension. Strong vasopressors in dental anesthetics should be avoided. Long-term administration of NSAIDs is known to decrease the activity of many antihypertensive drugs, and thus NSAIDs are likewise contraindicated. The patient should be assessed and managed for drug-induced xerostomia and gingival hyperplasia.

Angina Pectoris

Angina refers to a discomfort in the chest and adjacent areas that results from transient and reversible myocardial oxygen deficiency. Cardiac pain is often precipitated by exertion or exercise, strong emotions, or a large meal.

The signs and symptoms of angina include chest pain of sudden onset and brief duration (1-3 minutes); pain that radiates down the left arm and up to the mandible; and nausea and vomiting; palpitations, pallor, faintness, sweating, anxiety, fear, and dyspnea.

Medical treatment usually involves the administration of drugs such as the nitrates (nitroglycerin sublingually), β-adrenergic blockers, or calcium channel blockers; weight control; a low-fat diet, cholesterol, and sodium; exercise; and smoking cessation.

Dental care should include:

- Asking the patient what precipitates an angina attack and how often an attack generally occurs
- Scheduling short morning appointments
- Providing a calm atmosphere to reduce anxiety or stress
- Keeping the patient in a comfortable semisupine position
- Having nitroglycerin available
- Avoiding the use of a strong vasoconstrictor or anticholinergic drugs
- Discontinuing treatment if the patient begins to appear fatigued or has a change in heart rate or rhythm

Myocardial Infarction

Acute myocardial infarction (AMI) is the most extreme manifestation of ischemic heart disease, resulting from a sudden reduction or arrest of coronary blood flow caused by thrombosis or an artery narrowed by atherosclerosis. Prolonged myocardial ischemia results in irreversible damage to the heart muscle.

Persons experiencing an AMI have a feeling of indigestion, pressing or crushing sensation in the middle to upper sternum, cold sweats, weakness, nausea, lowered BP, and shortness of breath. **The difference between an AMI and angina is the intensity and the duration of the pain. Infarct pain is not relieved by nitrates.**

Medical management of an AMI includes oxygen; the prescription of pain relief medications, sedatives, anticoagulants, β-adrenergic blockers, and antiarrhythmic drugs; and an evaluation for coronary artery bypass surgery.

For dental management, follow the same precautions as those outlined for the patient with angina. In addition, monitor the PT or INR if the patient is on anticoagulant therapy. It has been recommended to avoid elective dental care for at least 6 months after an AMI. Antibiotic premedication is not required for a history of angina, AMI, bypass surgery, or the placement of cardiac stents.

Congestive Heart Failure

CHF is an abnormality of cardiac function responsible for inability or failure of the heart to pump blood at a rate necessary to meet the needs of the body tissues. The etiologies of CHF are coronary artery disease, hypertension, cardiomyopathy, valvular heart disease, infective endocarditis, or a pulmonary embolism. Normally, the left ventricle is affected first, resulting in a backup of blood into the lungs and **pulmonary edema.** The patient exhibits difficulty breathing. This is often followed by a failure of the right ventricle leading to a back flow of blood into the systemic circulation, causing **systemic or pitting edema.** This may be observed as a swelling of the ankles, distended neck veins, hepatomegaly, and ascites. Clubbing of the fingers may also be observed.

Additional signs or symptoms may include severe headache, mental confusion, dizziness, fatigue, dyspnea/**Cheyne-Stokes respirations** (periods of hyperventilation alternated with apnea), chest pain, and cyanosis.

Medical management includes diet control, reduced sodium intake, and weight reduction; limited activity; and drugs such as ACE inhibitors, diuretics, glycosides, vasodilators, and long-acting nitrates.

Dental interventions should involve short appointments in a relaxed, calm atmosphere; monitoring of vital signs; assessing the level of physical limitation exhibited by the patient; positioning the patient semisupine or higher to ensure comfort and avoid repositioning the chair quickly to prevent **orthostatic hypotension;** use vasoconstrictors cautiously, and assess and manage drug-induced xerostomia, oral ulcerations/lichenoid reactions, gag reflex, and cough.

Cardiac Arrhythmias

A **cardiac arrhythmia** is any variation in normal rhythm of heartbeat ranging from **bradycardia** to **tachycardia** to **fib-**

rillation. General causes include cardiovascular disease, pulmonary disorders, systemic diseases (e.g., fever, infection, anemia, hypothyroidism), electrolyte imbalances, and drug side effects.

Signs and symptoms may include an abnormally slow, fast, or irregular heart rate, with symptoms such as dizziness, fatigue, palpitations, syncope, CHF, angina, or cardiac arrest.

The medical management of arrhythmias usually involves the glycosides (e.g., digitalis, digoxin), quinidine, procainamide, β-blockers, calcium channel blockers, lidocaine, and Coumadin. In addition, treatment includes surgery, cardioversion (defibrillators), and the placement of implanted pacemakers. **Pacemakers** are electronic stimulators used to send a specified electrical current to the myocardium to control or maintain minimum heart rate. There are two types:

1. **Demand**: stimulates heart only when rate varies from a predetermined norm
2. **Fixed rate**: electrical stimuli provided independent of natural heart activity when the natural beat is too slow

The dental management of patients with arrhythmias involves monitoring the heart rate; assessing the cause of the patient's arrhythmias (if the cause is related to rheumatic heart disease, the patient will require antibiotic premedication); assessing the existence of a pacemaker; and if taking Coumadin, obtaining a current PT or INR. When a patient has a cardiac pacemaker, electrosurgical units, magnetorestrictive ultrasonic scalers, or ultrasonic bath cleaners should not be used on or near the patient to prevent interference. Appointments should be short and relaxed, and the use of strong vasopressors should be avoided.

Renal Disease

End-stage renal disease (ESRD) begins as renal insufficiency and can only be detected by slight laboratory abnormalities, such as a lowered glomerular filtration rate. As the disease progresses, functioning nephrons are damaged, limiting the kidneys' ability to perform their excretory, endocrine, and metabolic functions. This condition is referred to as **uremia (see Chapter 5)**. Signs and symptoms of uremia include anemia; hypertension; dilute urine excretion; hyperkalemia, sodium depletion, and other electrolyte disturbances; an accumulation of urea (azotemia) and other waste products in the blood due to poor filtration; changes in bone formation leading to bone fractures (renal osteodystrophy) and osteomalacia of the mandible; bleeding tendencies owing to a factor III deficiency and abnormalities in platelet aggregation; coronary artery disease; GI disturbances; whitish coating of the arms and trunk from perspiration (uremic frost); hyperpigmentation of the skin (and staining and hypoplasia of the teeth, if uremia was present during tooth development); increased calculus formation; oral ulcerations and candidiasis (seen in transplant cases); parotitis resulting in an ammonia-like breath; a metal taste in the mouth from urea in the saliva; depression; and convulsions.

Medical management can range from drug therapy and diet modifications to dialysis and transplant in ESRD. **Dialysis** involves the surgical implantation of a peritoneal shunt or an **arteriovenous (AV) fistula.** The latter technique, also referred to as hemodialysis, allows repeated access to the patient's circulation without needle punctures. The blood leaves the body from the shunt or fistula site; it is filtered through a machine and is returned to the patient. Heparin is administered to prevent clotting at the site. Dialysis is performed two to three times per week for 3 to 5 hours a day. The patient is at risk for developing muscle tetany associated with calcium depletion, Hepatitis B and C, HIV infection, or a localized infection at the access site. The major risk associated with transplant is organ rejection. Despite advances in tissue typing and antirejection therapy, most organ recipients experience infection.

Dental management requires consultation with the patient's physician to assess the patient's disease stage and his or her level of control, as well as the need for antibiotic premedication. Drugs that are excreted by the kidneys should be avoided, such as aspirin, NSAIDs, acyclovir, and ketoconazole. The patient's infectious disease status and platelet count should be assessed; the BP should be monitored and if an AV fistula is present in the arm, the opposite arm should be used to take the BP as well administer any intravenous drugs; and the patient should be appointed on the day between dialysis appointments.

In renal transplant cases, or any type of **organ transplant** for that matter, all potentially infectious teeth should be restored or extracted, and all areas of periodontal involvement should be managed with surgical/nonsurgical therapy before the transplant, based on need and time factors. Because of the intensive immunosuppressive (and sometimes myelosuppressive) agents (e.g., cyclosporine, prednisone) that are administered to prevent antirejection, the patient may experience oral infections such as candida and herpes; oral ulcerations; gingival hyperplasia, and bleeding. Antibiotic premedication and steroid supplementation before dental procedures may be necessary.

Adrenocortical Insufficiency

Adrenocortical insufficiency (AI) refers to hypofunction of the adrenal glands caused by atrophy of the adrenal cortex (primary) or deficiency of adrenocorticotropic hormone (ACTH) caused by the therapeutic administration of corticosteroids for a medical condition (secondary). Medical conditions that may require exogenous steroid therapy are rheumatoid arthritis, asthma, lupus, pemphigus, dermatologic conditions, ocular disorders, neoplasms, intestinal problems, hematologic disorders, and organ transplants.

When a patient takes exogenous steroids over a period of time (20 mg of hydrocortisone or equivalent for at least 2 weeks within the past 1-2 years; different sources list 1 or 2 years, but currently no formal consensus has been made, the plasma levels of cortisol increase and the adrenal glands suppress their production of ACTH. Therefore, in a stressful situation (i.e., oral surgery) when the adrenal glands are called upon to produce additional cortisol, they cannot because a deficiency of ACTH exists. This inability to physiologically handle the stress makes the patient vulnerable to adrenal crisis. Consequently, when persons are given oral steroids, the drugs are usually given in a dose pack; the dosage is gradually decreased over time to wean the patient off of the drug, thus triggering the adrenal glands to begin functioning.

Signs and symptoms of primary AI or Addison disease are weakness, fatigue, abnormal mucous membrane and skin pigmentation, weight loss, and hypotension. The manifestations of secondary AI include weight gain, round moon-shaped face, "buffalo hump" on the back (cushingoid), delayed healing, increased susceptibility to infection, oropharyngeal candidiasis, alveolar osteoporosis, acne, hypertension, and abdominal striae.

Dental management of stressful situations may require sedation to control anxiety, corticosteroid supplementation, and prophylactic antibiotics for procedures producing bacteremia.

Liver Disease

Two common diseases involving the liver include **hepatitis** and **alcoholism.** The liver functions by secreting bile that is needed for fat absorption, converting sugar to glycogen, and the excretion of bilirubin. Poor liver function can cause impairments in protein, lipid, carbohydrate, and drug metabolism and altered synthesis of coagulation factors. Hepatitis can result from infectious and noninfectious causes **(see Chapter 7).**

Most cases of viral hepatitis, particularly types **A** and **E,** resolve without complications. Types **B, C,** and **D** replicate in the liver and may pose a persistent infection or **carrier state.** The carrier state may cause permanent liver disease by progressing into chronic active hepatitis. Treatment of viral hepatitis involves early postexposure **immune globulins** or hepatitis B vaccine.

Patients with active hepatitis have signs and symptoms that include jaundice (e.g., eyes, skin, oral mucosa), nausea and vomiting, fever, fatigue, arthralgia, hepatomegaly, and splenomegaly. These individuals should not receive elective dental treatment. Dental management of the patient with liver disease should include recent monitoring of platelet count and PT, assessment and management of oral bleeding, determination of hepatitis status, and avoidance of drugs metabolized by the liver (e.g., many local anesthetics, analgesics, sedatives, and antibiotics used in dentistry).

Patients with alcohol-related habits (e.g., chronic ingestion of large amounts of ethanol) often exhibit extraoral signs of the alcoholism that include alcoholic breath; hand, tongue, and eyelid tremors; red eyes and puffy eyelids; red skin and angiomas of forehead, cheeks, and nose; ascites; and parotid gland enlargement. Intraoral manifestations include high rates of periodontal disease, caries, and oral can-

cer (particularly if the patient is also a smoker); glossitis, candidiasis, and angular cheilosis; gingival bleeding, ecchymoses, and petechiae; bruxism and attrition; and xerostomia. The quantity and duration of alcohol consumption necessary to produce cirrhosis of the liver is unclear. In addition, prolonged ingestion of alcohol leads to sensory and motor impairments; malnutrition (folic acid deficiency); immune dysfunction; bleeding tendencies; jaundice; and anemia. Motivating this patient to improve his or her oral condition after a lifestyle of oral neglect is a challenge. If this patient is undergoing treatment for alcoholism with Antabuse, alcohol-based mouthwashes are contraindicated.

HIV/AIDS

More than 1.5 million Americans are estimated to have been exposed to the **AIDS virus.** Individuals infected with the virus usually exhibit the antigen in 2 to 6 weeks and develop antibodies within 6 to 12 weeks **(seroconversion).** The mean incubation period is between 10 and 12 years **(see Chapter 7).** Because the virus destroys the **CD4 lymphocytes,** the symptomatic patient (CD4 (400) usually exhibits fever, malaise, night sweats, weight loss, oral candidiasis, lymphadenopathy, diarrhea, and opportunistic infections. A CD4 count of less than 200 may involve Kaposi sarcoma, lymphoma, pneumonia, wasting, carcinoma of the cervix or rectum, opportunistic infections, and encephalopathy.

Medical management includes the use of antiretroviral agents and the prevention and treatment of opportunistic infections and other disease-associated conditions. Oral lesions associated with HIV disease are discussed in Chapter 8. The patient should be educated about the oral manifestations of the disease, because an oral change may be the first indication of AIDS and may represent an infection that must be managed quickly in an individual with an impaired immune response. Recent blood counts and the need for antibiotic premedication must be assessed prior to dental treatment. Meticulous home care and periodontal débridement in conjunction with chlorhexidine or Betadine subgingival irrigation are recommended for the management of aggressive periodontal complications. Other oral signs and their management include radiation/chemotherapy to treat Kaposi sarcoma; antifungal agents for candida; antiviral agents for herpes; anesthetic rinses, ointments, or steroids for recurrent aphthous ulcerations; chlorhexidine and tongue brushing for hairy leukoplakia; and artificial salivas and fluoride for xerostomia.

Oral Habits and Fads

Oral Piercings

Oral piercings are becoming a common practice among young people. The tongue is the most common site. Complications resulting from oral piercings include:

- Hemorrhage
- Nerve damage

- HIV, hepatitis, tetanus, and other communicable diseases
- Localized inflammation and infection with potential for Ludwig angina (regional spread of infection) or a systemic bacteremia
- Trauma to the lingual gingiva due to the jewelry rubbing against the tissues
- Tissue hyperplasia at the piercing site
- Dehiscence if jewelry rubs against the facial gingiva
- Cracked and fractured teeth
- Aspiration or ingestion of the jewelry itself

Dental intervention includes instructing the patient interested in obtaining a piercing about the complications associated with oral piercing; the need for careful evaluation of the piercer's credentials and infection control procedures; the need for quality jewelry and keeping the site clean to prevent infection because swelling that occurs during the first 3 to 4 weeks after the piercing will affect eating and speaking. The jewelry should be removed when exposing intraoral radiographs and during and after procedures that require local anesthesia.

Smoking Cessation

The dental hygienist can play an active role in helping patients to quit smoking. One suggested program of intervention involves **4 As**: (1) **Ask** them about their smoking behaviors once you have obtained their trust; (2) **Advise** them about the risks of smoking and the benefits of stopping; be empathetic about what motivates them to smoke personally, and urge them to stop; (3) **Assist** them by setting a quitting date, providing helpful hints for success such as avoiding situations or people whom they associate with smoking and also encouraging the use of drugs, gum, patches, and inhalers that aid in cessation and enlisting the help of family and friends; and (4) **Arrange** follow-up by contacting them on the quit date agreed upon, praising them along the way, and acting as a support system if they feel an urge to relapse.

Infant/Toddler Dental Issues

Behaviors such as teething and digit sucking are issues that must be dealt with early to prevent oral complications as the child grows. **Teething** is a natural process and is not an illness. Normal manifestations of teething include drooling, irritability, disturbed eating and sleeping patterns, a desire to chew, and a slight elevation in body temperature. Recommended treatment is palliative and should include keeping the area clean and free of food debris; acetaminophen for discomfort or slight fever of short duration; a smooth chewable object large enough that it cannot be broken off or aspirated; and an approved topical anesthetic to relieve localized irritation and discomfort. **For eruption patterns see the Dental Anatomy section in Chapter 4.**

Non-nutritive sucking is usually not a dental concern, unless it persists into the mixed dentition stage. Potential clinical manifestations of digit sucking or pacifier use include:

- Anterior openbite and overjet
- Labial flare of the maxillary anterior teeth
- High palatal vault
- Posterior crossbite
- Lingual inclination of the mandibular anterior teeth

Secondary oral habits such as lip-sucking, mouth breathing, tongue thrusting, and speech problems may also result. In order to correct the habit, it is important to know the cause. Corrective appliances, the use of an orthodontic pacifier and bottle nipple, counseling, and behavior modification that includes a reward system are often very effective management strategies.

Suggested Sources

Infection Control

Andrews N: Dental unit waterline contamination. J Pract Hygiene 3:11, 1994.

Bednarsh HS, Eklund KJ: New postexposure prophylaxis guidelines stress immediate intervention. Access 12(6):42-51, 1998.

Bednarsh HS, Eklund KJ: OSHA issues new compliance directive. Access 14(3):35-40, 2000.

Cottone JA, Terezhalmy GT, Molinari JA: Practical Infection Control in Dentistry, 2nd ed. Baltimore, Williams & Wilkins, 1996.

Gladwin M, Bagby M: Clinical Aspects of Dental Materials. Philadelphia, Lippincott, Williams & Wilkins, 2000, pp 201-217, 279-283.

OSAP: Dental Unit Waterlines. Monthly OSAP Focus No. 12, 1999.

OSAP: Infection Control in Dentistry Guidelines. Annapolis: OSAP, 1997, pp 1-8.

OSHA: Occupational Exposure to Bloodborne Pathogens; Final Rule, Federal Register, 56(235):64175-64182, 1991.

OSAP: OSAP Update on Needle-Safety Legislation. Monthly OSAP Focus No. 1, 2000.

OSAP: Preprocedural Mouthrinses. Monthly OSAP Focus, No. 8, 1999.

Sprouls LS: An irritation or an allergy? Dental Teamwork 9:24, 1996.

Wilkins EM: Clinical Practice of the Dental Hygienist. Philadelphia, Lippincott, Williams & Wilkins, 1999, pp 42-53, 55-71.

Emergency Situations

American Heart Association: Heartsaver Plus, 1997-1999.

Little JW, et al: Dental Management of the Medically Compromised Patient, 5th ed. St. Louis, CV Mosby, 1997.

Malamed SF: Medical Emergencies in the Dental Office, 5th ed. St. Louis, CV Mosby, 2000.

Nunn P: Medical emergencies in the oral health care setting. J Dent Hygiene 74 (II), 2000.

Wilkins E: Clinical Practice of the Dental Hygienist, 8th ed, Lippincott Williams & Wilkins, 1999.

CPR/Defibrillation

http://www.americanheart.org/
http://www.proed.net/ecc/

Heart Disease/Heart Health

http://www.curiousheart.com
http://www.heartnews.org
http://heartinfo.org
http://www.women.americanheart.org/index2.html

Blood Pressure/Pulse

http://heartofthematter.org/html/healthnews/heartrate.html

Stroke

http://www.nemahealth.org
http://www.strokeassociation.org

Diabetes

http://www.diabetes.org
http://www.niddk.nih.gov/health/diabetes/diabtes.htm

Asthma and Emphysema

http://www.lungusa.org
http://www.mayohealth.org

Epilepsy

http://www.efa.org/education/firstaid.html
http://www.seizure-ed.com

Online Textbooks of Emergency Care

http://www.emedicine.com

Personal Plaque Control

Barnes CM: Powered toothbrushes: A focus on the evidence. Compend Cont Educ Oral Hyg 7(2):3, 2000.

Darby ML, Walsh MM: Dental Hygiene Theory and Practice. Philadelphia, WB Saunders, 1995, pp 437-455.

Edgar WM: A role for sugar-free gum in oral health. J Clin Dent 10(2):89, 1999.

Emling RC, Yankell SL: The application of sonic technology to oral hygiene: the third generation of powered toothbrushes. J Clin Dent 8(1):1, 1997.

Gordon JM, Frascela JA, Reardon RC: A clinical study of the safety and efficacy of a novel electric interdental cleaning device. J Clin Dent 7(3):70, 1996.

Harris NO, Christen AG: Primary Preventive Dentistry, 3rd ed. E. Norwalk, Appleton & Lange, 1991, pp 79-161.

Isaacs RL, Beiswanger BB, Rosenfield ST, et al: A crossover clinical investigation of the safety and efficacy of a new oscillating/rotating electric toothbrush and a high frequency electric toothbrush. Am J Dent 11:7, 1998.

Kashket S: Historical review of remineralization research. J Clin Dent 10(2):56, 1999.

Lyle DM: The role of pharmacotherapeutics in the reduction of plaque and gingivitis. J Pract Hyg 9:46, 2000.

McInnes C, Engel D, Martin RW: Fimbria damage and removal of adherent bacteria after exposure to acoustic energy. Oral Microbiol Immunol 8:277, 1993.

McInnes C, Johnson B, Emling RC, Yankell SL: Clinical and computer-assisted evaluations of the stain removal ability of the Sonicare electronic toothbrush. J Clin Dent 5(1):13, 1994.

Parrott PB: The building blocks of dentifrices. J Pract Hyg 8:48, 1999.

Stanford CM: Efficacy of the Sonicare toothbrush fluid dynamic action on the removal of human supragingival plaque. J Clin Dent 8(1):10, 1997.

Volpe AR, Petrone ME, DeVizio W, et al: A review of plaque gingivitis, calculus, and caries clinical efficacy studies with a fluoride dentifrice containing Triclosan and PVM/MA Copolymer, Internat. J Appl Dent Res 7(Suppl):S1, 1996.

Wilkins EM: Clinical Practice of the Dental Hygienist, 8th ed. Philadelphia, Lippincott Williams, & Wilkins, 1999, pp 350-415.

Wu-Yuan CD, McInnes C: Ability of the Sonicare electronic toothbrush to generate dynamic fluid activity that removes bacteria. J Clin Dent 5(3):89, 1994.

Zammitti S: Use of environmental scanning electron microscopy to evaluate dental stain removal. J Clin Dent 8(1):20, 1997.

Dietary Counseling

Darby ML, Walsh MM: Dental Hygiene Theory and Practice. Philadelphia, WB Saunders, 1995, pp 576-587.

Davis JR, Stegeman CA: The Dental Hygienist's Guide to Nutritional Care. Philadelphia, WB Saunders, 1998, pp 54-58, 199-217, 365-423.

Nizel AE, Papas AS: Nutritional in Clinical Dentistry, 3rd ed. Philadelphia, WB Saunders, 1989, pp 277-365.

Olson LS: The Nutrition Balancing Act. Access 13:22, 1999.

Smith C: Sweet nothings: The scoop on sugar consumption in America. Access 14:20, 2000.

Wilkins EM: Clinical Practice of the Dental Hygienist, 8th ed. Philadelphia, Lippincott Williams & Williams, 1999, pp 441-453.

Anxiety and Pain Control

Darby ML, Walsh MM: Dental Hygiene Theory and Practice. Philadelphia, WB Saunders, 1995, pp 466-467, 651-721, 723-739.

Hargreaves KM: Etiology and Nature of Dentinal Hypersensitivity, Dentinal Hypersensitivity: A Clinical Discussion of Etiology and Nature, Diagnosis, and Treatment. Newton, Dental Learning Systems, 1994, pp 2-6.

Malamed SF: Handbook of Local Anesthesia, 4th ed. St. Louis, CV Mosby, 1997, pp 2-310.

McGlothlin JD, Crouch KG, Michelsen RL: Control of Nitrous Oxide in Dental Operatories; Technical Report. Cincinnati, CDC, NIOSH, 1994, pp. 1-85.

Paarmann C, Herzog A: Achieving reliable anesthesia with the inferior alveolar injection. J Pract Hyg 4:11, 1995.

Rees TD: Treatment of Dentinal Hypersensitivity, Dentinal Hypersensitivity: A Clinical Discussion of Etiology and Nature, Diagnosis and Treatment. Newton, Dental Learning Systems, 1994, pp 11-16.

Wilkins EM: Clinical Practice of the Dental Hygienist, 8th ed. Philadelphia, Lippincott, Williams & Wilkins, 1999, pp 492-511, 595-601.

Patients with Special Needs

Dajani AS, et al: Prevention of bacterial endocarditis. JAMA 277 (22): June 11, 1997, pp1794-1801.

DeBiase CB: Dental Health Education: Theory and Practice. Philadelphia, Lea & Febiger, 1991.

Little JW, et al: Dental Management of the Medically Compromised Patient, 5th ed. St. Louis, CV Mosby, 1997.

Malamed SF: Medical Emergencies in the Dental Office, 5th ed. St. Louis, CV Mosby, 2000.

Wilkins EM: Clinical Practice of the Dental Hygienist, 8th ed. Philadelphia, Lippincott Williams & Wilkins, 1999, pp 492-511, 595-601.

http://www.dentalcare.com
http://www.dentalsite.com
http://www.adha.org
http://www.aerie.com/nohicweb
http://jeffline.tju.edu/DHNet
*http://*www.hivdent.org
http://www.perio.org/links/links.html

Questions and Answers

Questions

Infection Control

1. OSHA mandates that the dental care provider wear appropriate PPE (i.e., gloves, mask, eye protection, and clothing) during patient care involving contact with blood and saliva. This PPE should be worn only in the clinical treatment area.
   A. Both statements are TRUE.
   B. Both statements are FALSE.
   C. The first statement is TRUE, and the second one is FALSE.
   D. The first statement is FALSE, and the second one is TRUE.

2. Which type of protective glove should be worn when cleaning (scrubbing) contaminated instruments prior to sterilization?
   A. Sterile surgeon's gloves
   B. Examination gloves
   C. Overgloves
   D. Utility gloves

3. Latex hypersensitivity may be exhibited as one of three types of reactions. Which one of the following is an allergic contact dermatitis?
   A. Irritant contact dermatitis
   B. Delayed type IV hypersensitivity
   C. Immediate type V hypersensitivity
   D. Immediate type I hypersensitivity

4. After a known HIV-positive patient has been treated, dental instruments should be
   A. processed in the same manner as instruments used on all other patients.
   B. soaked in a disinfectant before sterilizing.
   C. handled with double-gloved hands.
   D. sterilized twice as long as instruments used on all other patients.

5. An acceptable surface disinfectant must be tuberculocidal and kill hydrophilic and lipophilic viruses. Lipophilic viruses include HBV and HIV and are much harder to kill than are hydrophilic viruses.
   A. Both statements are TRUE.
   B. Both statements are FALSE.
   C. The first statement is TRUE; the second is FALSE.
   D. The first statement is FALSE; the second is TRUE.

6. All of the following chemicals are acceptable surface disinfectants EXCEPT one. Which one is the EXCEPTION?
   A. Phenols
   B. Iodophors
   C. Chlorine
   D. Quaternaries
   E. Glutaraldehydes

7. Anesthetic needles, orthodontic wire, irrigation needles and anesthetic carpules must not be disposed of in the regular trash. They must be disposed of in infectious waste boxes or in plastic bags.
   A. Both statements are TRUE.
   B. Both statements are FALSE.
   C. The first statement is TRUE; the second is FALSE.
   D. The first statement is FALSE; the second is TRUE.

8. Which method of heat sterilization would contribute to dulling cutting edges?
   A. Steam under pressure
   B. Dry heat
   C. Chemical vapor
   D. Ethylene oxide

9. According to Spalding's Classification of Inanimate Objects, critical items are those items that penetrate or touch skin or mucous membrane. These items must be sterilized by heat or by a high level of disinfection.
   A. The first statement is TRUE, and the second is FALSE.
   B. The first statement is FALSE, and the second is TRUE.
   C. Both statements are TRUE.
   D. Both statements are FALSE.

10. Surface disinfection occurs after an intermediate-level disinfectant is sprayed onto a surface and allowed to air dry for at least 10 minutes. This procedure is not effective unless the surface is first cleaned.
    A. Both statements are TRUE.
    B. Both statements are FALSE.
    C. The first statement is TRUE, and the second is FALSE.
    D. The first statement is FALSE, and the second is TRUE.

Emergency

11. The administration of oxygen is indicated for the management of all of the following medical emergencies except one. Which one is the exception?
    A. Myocardial infarction
    B. Angina pectoris
    C. Hyperventilation
    D. Stroke

12. The ratio of chest compressions to ventilations for one person performing CPR is which of the following?
    A. 5 compressions to 2 ventilations
    B. 15 compressions to 2 ventilations
    C. 2 compressions to 5 ventilations
    D. 15 compressions to 1 ventilation

13. Which of the following symptoms may help to differentiate between angina pectoris and myocardial infarction?
    A. Respiratory distress
    B. Excessive perspiration and apprehension
    C. Duration of chest pain after the administration of a vasodilator
    D. Radiating chest pain

14. When only one person is available to perform CPR for an infant or a child younger than 8 years of age, when is it appropriate to activate the EMS?
    A. Immediately
    B. After 20 cycles of 5 compressions to 1 ventilation
    C. After 2 rescue breaths are delivered
    D. After the victim has been unconscious for 2 minutes

15. Which of the following observations is not indicative of hypoglycemia?
    A. Dry flushed skin
    B. Shakiness, weakness
    C. Elevated pulse rate
    D. Hunger
    E. Confusion

16. A healthy 15-year-old girl complains of being dizzy and "feeling weird" as the dental hygienist is explaining the procedures that are planned for today's dental treatment. She suddenly looks very pale, begins to perspire, and feels nauseated. Which of the following suggestions would be appropriate in the management of this patient's symptoms?
    A. Administer oral carbohydrates.
    B. Dismiss the patient and refer to the physician.
    C. Realize that she is probably tired and ignore the symptoms.
    D. Recline the patient in the dental chair to a supine position.

17. Mr. Smith is a 40-year-old man whose medical history reveals a history of epilepsy. Tegretol is the only medication that he is currently taking and his dental health is excellent. During his dental hygiene appointment, Mr. Smith complains of a strange taste and odor. Soon after, he begins a series of convulsive movements. What type of seizure is Mr. Smith experiencing?
    A. Petit mal seizure
    B. Simple partial seizure
    C. Generalized tonic/clonic seizure
    D. Complex partial seizure

18. For the management of Mr. Smith's seizure, which of the following choices is recommended?
    A. Restrain Mr. Smith in an attempt to halt the convulsions.
    B. Place a tongue depressor in Mr. Smith's mouth to prevent him from swallowing his tongue.
    C. Recline and lower the dental chair, remove any equipment near him, assess the airway, and monitor vital signs.
    D. Call 911 and begin CPR

19. Mary is 62 years of age and faithfully visits the dental office every 3 months for the maintenance phase of her periodontal condition. Her patient record reveals treatment for angina pectoris and type II diabetes. Medications include glucophage, Nitrostat, and a multivitamin taken daily. As the hygienist completes periodontal débridement, Mary asks for a break and reaches for her purse to retrieve her Nitrostat. Fifteen minutes after taking her medication, Mary is confused because the pain normally subsides quickly after taking two to three doses of her prescribed medication. Hearing this complaint, the appropriate management of this patient would be which of the following choices?

A. Administer an additional vasodilator that is found in the office drug kit.
B. Consider myocardial infarction as a possibility and activate the EMS; provide oxygen; and monitor vital signs.
C. Dismiss Mary to go home or to her physician, whichever she prefers.
D. Give Mary a glass of orange juice that you keep available for your patient's with diabetes.

20. Gary, who is 45 years old, is a new patient to the dental practice. He has not been to the dentist in 5 years and complains of numerous dental problems. Gary is 5'9" tall and weighs 250 lb. He describes his job as a stockbroker as very stressful and admits that he smokes too much. The dental hygienist collects Gary's medical history, which reveals a family history of diabetes and cancer. Gary has not seen his family doctor in 2 years and is not currently taking any medication. Gary's vital signs are as follows: BP 180/112, pulse 90 per minute, and respirations 16 per minute. Which of the following choices would be the appropriate management of this patient?
    A. Gary's vital signs are within normal limits, proceed with dental treatment.
    B. Complete the dental treatments planned for today and ask Gary if he is interested in a smoking cessation program.
    C. Inform Gary that his blood pressure falls into the stage 3 hypertension category and refer him to a physician for evaluation.
    D. Explain to Gary the important connection between smoking and periodontal disease.

Personal Plaque Control

21. Two-tone disclosing solution contains FD & C Blue No. 1 and D & C Red No. 28. It stains new plaque blue and mature plaque red.
    A. Both statements are TRUE.
    B. Both statements are FALSE.
    C. The first statement is TRUE, and the second is FALSE.
    D. The first statement is FALSE, and the second is TRUE.

22. All of the following are acceptable features of a toothbrush, EXCEPT one. Which one is the EXCEPTION?
    A. Angled handle
    B. Straight handle
    C. Natural bristles
    D. Nylon bristles
    E. Soft bristles

23. The brushing method in which the bristle head is directed at 45 degrees to the facial/lingual tooth surface and the row of bristles nearest the marginal gingival directed into the sulcus and then vibrated back and forth:
    A. Scrub brush
    B. Charters'
    C. Modified Stillman
    D. Modified Bass

24. Which of the following would you recommend for cleaning proximal tooth surfaces of a person who has tight contacts and overhanging margins of restorations?
    A. Waxed floss
    B. Unwaxed floss

C. Wood wedges
D. Interproximal brush

25. Which adjunct works best for cleaning proximals of teeth with open contacts?
    A. Unwaxed floss
    B. Waxed floss
    C. Wood wedges
    D. Yarn
    E. Rubber tips

26. Gingival stimulation is recommended for maintenance of gingival health. Rubber tips are the suggested adjunct for accomplishing this.
    A. Both statements are TRUE.
    B. Both statements are FALSE.
    C. The first statement is TRUE, and the second is FALSE.
    D. The first statement is FALSE, and the second is TRUE.

27. Which type of powered toothbrush removes plaque up to 4 mm beyond the bristle tips without actual contact of the bristles to the tooth?
    A. One directional rotary round head
    B. Counter-rotating round head
    C. Counter-rotating pulsating round head
    D. Sonic brush head

28. Which active dentifrice ingredient is an anticalculus agent?
    A. Fluoride
    B. Sodium citrate
    C. Essential oils
    D. Sodium bicarbonate
    E. Tetrasodium pyrophosphate

29. Which active ingredient is most commonly found in a desensitizing dentifrice?
    A. Zinc citrate
    B. Potassium nitrate
    C. Peroxide
    D. Chlorine dioxide
    E. Triclosan

30. Which type of fluoride is **not** found in a dentifrice?
    A. Sodium
    B. Stannous
    C. Acidulated phosphate fluoride

31. What feature determines the hardness of the bristles on the head of a toothbrush?
    A. Diameter of bristles
    B. Length of bristles
    C. Number of bristles
    D. Number of tufts

32. Disclosing solution is a valuable aid in patient education because it can be used to detect supra- and subgingival plaque.
    A. Both the statement and reason are correct and related.
    B. Both the statement and reason are correct but are NOT related.
    C. The statement is correct, but the reason is NOT correct.
    D. The statement is NOT correct, but the reason is correct.
    E. Neither the statement NOR the reason is correct.

33. Commercially available mouthrinses that are accepted by the ADA Council on Scientific Affairs include all of the following EXCEPT one. Which one is that EXCEPTION?
    A. Essential oils
    B. Tetrasodium pyrophosphate
    C. Sodium fluoride
    D. Chlorhexidine gluconate

34. Which of the following agents found in mouthrinses has the property of substantivity?
    A. Essential oils
    B. Hydrogen peroxide
    C. Chlorhexidine gluconate
    D. Cetylpyridinium domiphen bromide
    E. Tetrasodium pyrophosphate

Dietary Counseling

35. All of the following are carbohydrates of similar cariogenicity EXCEPT one. Which one is the EXCEPTION?
    A. Sucrose
    B. Fructose
    C. Glucose
    D. Lactose
    E. Maltose

36. Which of the following would least likely contain hidden sugar?
    A. Mayonnaise
    B. Ketchup
    C. Sour cream
    D. Bacon
    E. Fruit drinks

37. Upon analyzing your patient's food diary, you find that your patient has eaten 12 sucrose-containing foods on a given day. Of these 12 foods, 2 are eaten at breakfast, 2 are eaten together at noon, 3 are eaten together at dinner, and 2 are eaten together at 10 PM. The remaining foods are eaten during the day at more than 20-minute intervals. What is the patient's total number of sugar *exposures* during this given day?
    A. 7
    B. 9
    C. 10
    D. 12

38. All of the following practices are practical suggestions for the patient who has a high caries' risk, EXCEPT one. Which one is the EXCEPTION?
    A. Chew gum (sugar or sugar-free) for at least 20 minutes after a sugar exposure.
    B. Decrease intake of fermentable carbohydrates.
    C. Eliminate all CHOs from one's diet.
    D. Limit excessive snacking.

39. Although fructose has the same cariogenic potential as that of sucrose, firm fresh fruits (e.g., apples) are less cariogenic because they stimulate salivary flow, which helps to neutralize plaque acid.
    A. Both the statement and the reason are correct and related.
    B. Both the statement and the reason are correct but are NOT related.

C. The statement is correct, but the reason is NOT correct.

D. The statement is NOT correct, but the reason is correct.

E. NEITHER the statement NOR the reason is correct.

40. Natural or refined sugars eaten with a meal are less cariogenic than when eaten alone because food such as fat and protein buffer or neutralize plaque acid.

A. Both statement and reason are correct and related.

B. Both the statement and the reason are correct but are NOT related.

C. The statement is correct, but the reason is NOT correct.

D. The statement is NOT correct, but the reason is correct.

E. NEITHER the statement NOR the reason is correct.

Anxiety and Pain Control

41. Nitrous-oxide oxygen analgesia is utilized in dentistry to produce conscious sedation. During conscious sedation, the patient is in the analgesic stage (stage 1) of anesthesia.

A. Both statements are TRUE.

B. Both statements are FALSE.

C. The first statement is TRUE; the second is FALSE.

D. The first statement is FALSE; the second is TRUE.

42. What is the designated color of a tank of nitrous oxide?

A. White

B. Green

C. Blue

D. Red

43. Chronic exposure to N_2O from leakage around the nasal mask, patient's oral cavity or faulty hose connection to the machine is a potential health risk to the dental operator. This exposure can be minimized by utilization of a scavenger system.

A. Both statements are TRUE.

B. Both statements are FALSE.

C. The first statement is TRUE; the second is FALSE.

D. The first statement is FALSE; the second is TRUE.

44. All of the following conditions are relative contraindications for administration of N_2O-O_2 analgesia EXCEPT one. Which one is the EXCEPTION?

A. Pregnancy

B. Nasal obstruction

C. Emphysema

D. Upper respiratory infection

E. Mild anxiety

45. What procedure should be followed if the patient exhibits signs of N_2O-O_2 overdose?

A. Continue administration of N_2O, but increase the O_2

B. Monitor the patient, and continue the same dosage.

C. Discontinue the flow of N_2O and O_2 immediately.

D. Discontinue the flow of N_2O, and increase the oxygen flow to 100%.

46. According to the hydrodynamic theory, dentinal nerve stimulation that leads to dentinal hypersensitivity is initiated by:

A. uncalcified dentinal tubule endings that expose nerve endings.

B. exposure of nerve endings to the oral environment.

C. movement of dentinal tubule fluid around odontoblastic processes.

47. Which of the following agents would be an active component of a self-applied prescription desensitizing paste?

A. Potassium nitrate

B. Sodium fluoride

C. Strontium chloride

D. Ferric oxalate

48. Topical anesthetics are available in gels, liquid, sprays, and transoral patches. All forms of this type of anesthetic produce profound soft tissue anesthesia and minimal pulpal anesthesia.

A. Both statements are TRUE.

B. Both statements are FALSE.

C. The first statement is TRUE; the second is FALSE.

D. The first statement is FALSE; the second is TRUE.

49. Which of the following topical anesthetics is classified as an amide?

A. Benzocaine

B. Tetracaine

C. Lidocaine

D. Dyclonine hydrochloride

50. Which part of the structure of a local anesthetic determines whether it is classified as an ester or an amide?

A. Lipophilic

B. Intermediate chain

C. Hydrophilic

51. Which one of the following local anesthetics is metabolized in the plasma?

A. Procaine

B. Bupivacaine

C. Lidocaine

D. Mepivacaine

E. Prilocaine

52. Upon injection of an anesthetic containing a vasoconstrictor, all of the following situations occur, EXCEPT one. Which one is the EXCEPTION?

A. Decreased blood flow to the injection site

B. Slow absorption of anesthetic into the bloodstream

C. Decreased duration of anesthesia

D. Decreased bleeding at the injection site

53. Which of the following anesthetics has the longest duration of action?

A. Lidocaine

B. Bupivacaine

C. Prilocaine

D. Mepivacaine

54. Gingival health can affect the duration of action of a local anesthetic. Inflamed tissue at the site of injection results in shorter duration of anesthesia.

A. Both statements are TRUE.

B. Both statements are FALSE.

C. The first statement is TRUE; the second is FALSE.

D. The first statement is FALSE; the second is TRUE.

55. Which of the following components of an anesthetic cartridge is the preservative for the vasoconstrictor?
    A. Distilled water
    B. Epinephrine
    C. Norepinephrine
    D. Sodium chloride
    E. Sodium bisulfite

56. A 25-gauge needle is recommended over 27-gauge needles for most dental injections because there is less chance of needle breakage and aspiration is achieved more easily.
    A. Both statement and reason are correct and related.
    B. Both statement and reason are correct but NOT related.
    C. The statement is correct, but the reason is NOT correct.
    D. The statement is NOT correct, but the reason is correct.
    E. Neither the statement NOR the reason is correct.

57. How many milligrams of a local anesthetic are in one carpule containing 2% lidocaine HCl and epinephrine 1:100,000?
    A. 1.8
    B. 2.0
    C. 18
    D. 20
    E. 36

58. Extensive periodontal débridement must be performed on all surfaces of the maxillary right first molar and both premolars. Which injections must be administered if the patient exhibits sensitive roots and gingival tissue around root surfaces?
    A. Posterior superior alveolar and middle superior alveolar nerve blocks
    B. Posterior superior alveolar nerve block and infiltration over the premolars
    C. Middle superior alveolar and nasopalatine nerve blocks
    D. Posterior and middle superior alveolar nerve blocks and greater palatine nerve block
    E. Posterior, middle, and anterior superior alveolar nerve blocks

59. All of the following are nerves of the mandibular division of the trigeminal nerve EXCEPT one. Which one is that EXCEPTION?
    A. Posterior superior alveolar
    B. Inferior alveolar
    C. Buccal
    D. Lingual
    E. Mental

60. Which of the following nerve blocks must be administered along with an inferior alveolar and lingual nerve block in order to achieve anesthesia of all the molars and premolars and their surrounding facial and lingual gingival tissue?
    A. Infraorbital
    B. Buccal
    C. Mental
    D. Incisive

Patients with Special Needs

61. You encounter a patient who has a past history of tuberculosis. The patient cannot remember the course of treatment that he received. How should you proceed?
    A. Treat the patient as normal.
    B. Treat the patient only if the procedure is elective.

C. Refer the patient to a hospital-based practitioner
D. Defer treatment until a medical consult has been obtained.

62. Which of the following disorders is characterized by patchy ulcerations of the alimentary tract that may lead to GI obstructions?
    A. Crohn disease
    B. Sickle cell disease
    C. Lupus erythematosus
    D. Rheumatoid arthritis

63. Which condition is characterized by large joint destruction and typically affects younger men and older women?
    A. Osteoporosis
    B. Osteoarthritis
    C. Rheumatoid arthritis
    D. Ankylosing spondylitis

64. Which of the following signs and symptoms is **not** characteristic of cystic fibrosis?
    A. Heavy calculus deposits
    B. Frequent bulky, foul, fatty stool
    C. Enlarged submaxillary and sublingual salivary glands
    D. Dehydration, particularly during exercise and warm weather
    E. Perspiration exhibiting excessive levels of calcium and phosphorus

65. All of the following are signs of Lupus except one. The EXCEPTION is?
    A. Malar rash
    B. Arthralgias
    C. Joint deformities
    D. Photosensitivity

66. Which of the following drugs is contraindicated for the asthmatic patient taking theophylline?
    A. Acetaminophen
    B. Clindamycin
    C. Erythromycin
    D. Prednisone

67. An ammonia-like breath is characteristic of which of the following conditions?
    A. Diabetes
    B. Liver disease
    C. Renal disease
    D. Leukemia

68. All of the following drugs are used in the treatment of tuberculosis except one. The EXCEPTION is?
    A. Azathioprine
    B. Pyrazinamide
    C. Isoniazid
    D. Rifampin

69. Class III malocclusions are most commonly exhibited in the patient with:
    A. cerebral palsy.
    B. Down syndrome.
    C. cystic fibrosis.
    D. epilepsy.

70. Which of the following types of hearing loss results from a disease or injury that interferes with the normal movement of the bones of the middle ear affecting the transmission of sound waves through the outer and middle ear?
    A. Conductive
    B. Sensorineural
    C. Cochlear
    D. Senile

71. A person is considered to be legally blind if, after the best optical correction, the visual acuity in the best eye is no better than _____.
    A. 20/200
    B. 20/170
    C. 20/100
    D. 20/70

72. Which of the following statements is false regarding patients with cleft palates?
    A. Males are afflicted more than females.
    B. If a cleft is unilateral, the right side is most common.
    C. Upper respiratory infections usually accompany the condition.
    D. Cleft lip and palate affect about 1:800 live births in the U.S.

73. Hyperbaric oxygen treatments are typically administered to:
    A. increase carbon dioxide in the tissues.
    B. increase the growth of aerobic organisms.
    C. improve tissue oxygenation and optimize healing.
    D. dilate blood vessels and promote blood flow to the heart.

74. A maternal deficiency in which of the following vitamins increases the risk of neural tube defects in the newborn?
    A. C
    B. E
    C. Pantothenic acid
    D. Folic acid

75. Alopecia refers to which of the following side effects of chemotherapy?
    A. Taste disturbances
    B. Immune suppression
    C. Nausea and vomiting
    D. Dry, flaky skin
    E. Hair loss

ANSWERS

Infection Control

1. **A.** PPE should not be worn out of the treatment area, because it is contaminated and is a source of infection.

2. **D.** Utility gloves are heavy and more puncture resistant than the others and should be worn if instruments are cleaned by hand scrubbing.

3. **B.** Allergic contact dermatitis is synonymous with delayed type IV hypersensitivity. Irritant contact dermatitis is nonallergic.

4. **A.** These instruments should be handled and processed in the same manner as those used on any patient because any patient could be HIV positive. This would include cleaning the instruments and then running them through one sterilization cycle in a heat sterilizer. If double gloving is done, it must be done on **all** patients.

5. **C.** The entire statement is true, except that lipophilic viruses are easier to kill than are hydrophilic viruses.

6. **E.** Glutaraldehydes are high level disinfectants in which items must be immersed.

7. **C.** Sharp objects must be disposed of by placing them in hard puncture-resistant containers and not in cardboard boxes or plastic bags.

8. **A.** Moisture contributes to dulling of cutting edges, whereas dry heat and gases do not.

9. **D.** Critical items are those that penetrate skin or mucous membrane, and these must be heat sterilized. An item that touches but does not penetrate tissue may be sterilized by immersion in a high-level disinfectant.

10. **A.** Neither disinfection nor sterilization will take place if an item is not first cleaned of bioburden.

11. **C.** Hyperventilation is treated by the administration of CO_2.

12. **B.** The American Heart Association guidelines recommend 5 compressions to one ventilation for 2-person CPR.

13. **C.** With myocardial infarction, there is no relief of pain following the administration of a vasodilator.

14. **B.** It is important to assess the situation and begin CPR immediately. When a child or infant is found to be unresponsive, it is often due to an airway obstruction and with appropriate attention, the condition may be reversed within a short time.

15. **A.** Persons exhibiting hypoglycemia or insulin shock have moist, pale skin. Dry flushed skin is a symptom of ketoacidosis, hyperglycemia, hypoinsulinism, and diabetic coma.

16. **D.** Because the patient appears to have become apprehensive about the dental procedures planned for her during the appointment. Fainting is not an uncommon response to stress or anxiety and may be experienced by a fearful dental patient. Syncope may be suspect when these signs and symptoms present in an adolescent or young adult patient with an unremarkable medical history.

17. **C.** The patient described is experiencing an aura before losing consciousness, and starting convulsions.

18. **C.** Never attempt to restrain the patient or put anything in the patient's mouth. The patient does not actually swallow his tongue, but it could roll back against the pharyngeal wall, blocking his airway. Opening the airway is best accomplished by performing a head tilt-mandible lift. Activation of the EMS would be indicated if the tonic-clonic seizure continued for more than 5 minutes.

19. **B.** You should suspect an AMI when a patient does not respond to nitroglycerin.

20. **C.** It is true that the patient has several risk factors for cardiovascular disease and that he could benefit from smoking cessation, diet counseling, periodontal treatment,

and intensive plaque control measures, but the severity of his hypertension requires an immediate referral and treatment before proceeding with his dental needs. Smoking cessation information would be important for Gary to receive at subsequent appointments, after his hypertension is under control.

21. **C.** A two-tone disclosant does contain FD & C Blue #1 and D & C Red #28, but it stains mature plaque blue and new (freshly deposited) plaque red.

22. **C.** The size and shape of the handle should be determined on an individual basis according to the individual's preference. Toothbrush bristles, however, should be soft in order to prevent toothbrush abrasion and recession. Natural bristles, unlike nylon, are irregular and can attribute to hard and soft tissue trauma. Likewise, natural bristles do not dry readily and they harbor bacteria.

23. **E.** Bass brushing is the only toothbrush method that involves directing the row of bristles nearest the gingival margin into the sulcus and vibrating back and forth. Modified Bass is the same technique but concludes with a roll stroke.

24. **A.** Wood wedge and interdental brushes are not recommended for cleaning proximal surfaces of teeth in tight contact. Waxed floss glides more easily between tight contacts than does unwaxed floss, which shreds readily.

25. **D.** Floss works best when proximal surfaces are in contact and wood wedges and rubber tips when teeth are in contact with an open gingival embrasure. Yarn can be used in a shoe shine method on proximal surfaces of teeth with no adjacent tooth in contact.

26. **B.** Gingival stimulation is not recommended. Removal of plaque from the teeth is the primary function that results in gingival health

27. **D.** All other powered manual toothbrush bristles must touch dental plaque in order to remove it.

28. **E.** Fluoride and essential oils are antimicrobial; sodium citrate relieves hypersensitivity; and sodium bicarbonate whitens teeth.

29. **B.** Zinc citrate and Triclosan are antibacterial, whereas chlorine dioxide is antihalitosis agent and peroxide reduces stain.

30. **C.** Only sodium and stannous fluorides are incorporated into dentifrices.

31. **A.** Bristle stiffness or hardness is determined by the bristle diameter with stiffness increasing with diameter size.

32. **C.** Disclosing solution does not reach subgingival plaque and, therefore, cannot be used to detect it.

33. **B.** Tetrasodium pyrophosphate is an anticalculus agent and is not currently accepted by the ADA.

34. **C.** Chlorhexidine gluconate is the only ingredient with substantivity, which means that is absorbed by the tissues and slowly released over a long period of time.

35. **D.** Lactose, found in milk, is the least cariogenic sugar.

36. **C.** Most condiments, processed meats, and fruit drinks contain sugar. Sour cream contains none.

37. **A.** Foods eaten at the same time are calculated as one exposure, whereas those eaten 10 minutes or more apart are separate exposures.

38. **C.** Carbohydrates provide energy for the body, and many are high in nutrition. It would be unwise to eliminate all carbohydrates from the diet.

39. **A.** Eating fresh fruit requires chewing, which stimulates salivary flow. The increased salivary flow neutralizes acid that may be produced by the action of plaque bacteria on the fructose.

40. **A.** Although natural and refined sugars are utilized by plaque bacteria, which then produce acid, the acid is neutralized by the buffering action of protein or fat.

Anxiety and Pain Control

41. **A.** The purpose of the use of N_2O-O_2 in dentistry is for relaxation of the patient, which is attained in stage 1 of the four stages of anesthesia. Stages beyond this result in excitement and surgical anesthesia.

42. **C.** Blue is the standard color designated for nitrous oxide.

43. **A.** Chronic exposure of N_2O to the dental care provider can potentially cause reduced fertility; spontaneous abortion; increased neurologic, renal, and liver disease; and impaired mental performance, manual dexterity and audiovisual ability. A scavenger system is equipment that enables venting of any expelled N_2O from the patient to the outside air.

44. **E.** Administration of N_2O-O_2 to an anxious patient would be indicated, because it would relax the patient. Nasal obstruction, emphysema, and upper respiratory infections may inhibit inhalation of gases, and no elective medication should be administered during pregnancy.

45. **D.** N_2O flow must be stopped and flushed from the body by increasing the flow of oxygen to 100% for 3 to 5 minutes or until full recovery is achieved.

46. **C.** A stimulus at the dentinoenamel end of the dentinal tubule initiates fluid movement, which in turn elicits movement of odontoblastic processes that leads to stimulation of adjacent nerve fibers in the pulp.

47. **B.** Potassium nitrate and strontium chloride are active desensitizing agents that are available for self-application in over-the-counter dentifrices. Ferric oxalate preparations are available only as professionally applied agents. A 1.1% sodium fluoride prescription paste is available for home use.

48. **C.** Gel, liquid, and spray topical anesthetics anesthetize only soft tissue; the transoral patch, however, produces profound anesthesia to the soft tissue and minimal pulpal anesthesia.

49. **C.** Benzocaine and tetracaine are esters and dyclonine hydrochloride is a ketone.

50. **B.** The lipophilic part enables the anesthetic to penetrate the lipid nerve fibers, and the hydrophilic part allows the anesthetic to diffuse through interstitial fluid in tissue to reach the nerve.

51. **A.** Ester-type anesthetics are metabolized in the plasma. Procaine is the only ester listed. All the others are amides which are metabolized in the liver.

52. **C.** A vasoconstrictor increases the duration of anesthesia, because it constricts blood vessels and keeps the agent in the area of the nerve.

53. **B.** Bupivacaine is the only anesthetic listed that has a duration of greater than 90 minutes.

54. **A.** Anesthesia is of a shorter duration in inflamed tissue, because of increased vascularity at the site.

55. **E.** Sodium bisulfite is the only preservative currently utilized for vasoconstrictors in local anesthetics.

56. **A.** A 25-gauge needle is more rigid than a 27- or 30-gauge needle and would break less easily, and it has a wider lumen through which aspiration is more easily achieved.

57. **E.** A 2% solution of lidocaine contains 20 mg/ml, and there are 1.8 ml of total solution in one anesthetic cartridge. To determine the milligrams of local anesthetic in one cartridge, multiply 1.8 by 20 which is 36 mg.

58. **D.** The posterior superior alveolar nerve block anesthetizes the pulp and overlying bone and facial mucosa of the Mx first molar, except for its mesial buccal root. The middle superior alveolar nerve block anesthetizes the pulp and overlying bone and facial mucosa of the mesial buccal root of the Mx first molar and all of the Mx first and second premolars. The greater palatine nerve block is necessary to anesthetize the lingual gingival around these teeth.

59. **A.** The posterior superior alveolar nerve is a branch of the maxillary division of the trigeminal nerve.

60. **B.** The buccal nerve block anesthetizes the buccal gingival of the mandibular molars.

61. **D.** The patient should be treated only if it is an emergency. If the procedure is elective, defer treatment until the patient's medical status has been confirmed.

62. **A.** This description is a classic sign of Crohn disease.

63. **B.** Rheumatoid arthritis affects the smaller joints. Ankylosing spondylitis affects the spine. Osteoporosis is a disorder of decreased bone mass.

64. **E.** Persons with CF have two to five times the normal levels of sodium and potassium in their perspiration.

65. **C.** Joint pain is a characteristic of lupus, but joint deformity is not.

66. **C.** Erythromycin potentiates the effects of many drugs by inhibiting their clearance from the body.

67. **C.** Urea in the saliva is responsible for ammonia-like breath. Experiencing a diabetic coma may elicit an acetone breath in a person with diabetes.

68. **A.** Azathioprine is a drug used to prevent organ rejection in transplant patients. It causes myelosuppression and immunosuppression.

69. **B.** Persons with Down syndrome have a midfacial defect. Persons with CP (and often CF) exhibit class II malocclusion.

70. **A.** Sensorineural hearing loss results when the cochlea or cochlear nerves of the inner ear become damaged, inhibiting the transmission of the heard message to the brain.

71. **A.** 20/70 is considered vision impairment.

72. **B.** Unilateral clefts usually affect the left side.

73. **C.** Hyperbaric oxygen is required before an extraction, for example, to improve healing of irradiated tissues.

74. **D.** Maternal folic acid deficiencies have been implicated in conditions such as spina bifida.

75. **E.** Hair loss is a side effect of chemotherapy, because the hair follicles are rapidly dividing cells. In an effort to destroy rapidly dividing cancer cells, the drugs destroy normal cells with a similar mitotic index.

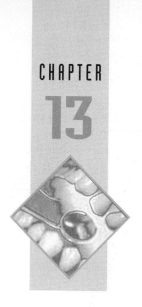

Performing Periodontal Procedures

LOUISE T. VESELICKY, DDS, MDS, MEᴅ   CATHRYN L. FRERE, BSDH, MEᴅ
CAROL A. SPEAR, BSDH, MSDH

 ## ETIOLOGY AND PATHOGENESIS OF PERIODONTAL DISEASES

Bacterial Plaque

When looking at the etiology of periodontal disease, **plaque** is always considered to be the primary factor involved. Plaque tends to form on surfaces of the teeth. Initially, plaque, called **supragingival plaque,** forms above the gingival line. This plaque contains numerous gram-positive cocci and rods. As plaque matures, it tends to form **subgingivally** and attaches to the tooth. This plaque consists of filamentous forms and cocci that appear as corncob-like structures under a microscope. There is also subgingival plaque, which forms under the gingiva, but it is not attached to the gingiva. This plaque, which is referred to as **nonadherent** or **unattached plaque,** consists of spirochetes, motile organisms, and anaerobes (see Chapter 7 to review the types of bacteria associated with health and disease). Bacterial plaques, also called **biofilms,** contain up to 1 to 2×10^{11} bacteria/g at or below the gingival margin. For many years, the belief was that the pathogenic bacteria in the plaque initiated periodontal destruction due mainly to the direct bacterial damage from the toxic products released from specific bacteria. This theory is still true; however, there are more factors leading to tissue destruction in periodontal disease. The immune system plays a vital role. The host response protects the host by mounting an immune response to the bacterial plaque. The initial response to bacterial plaque involves the release of neutrophils from engorged blood vessels. The host response to periodontal biofilms results in the local release of **cytokines**-biologic mediators including **interleukins, tumor necrosis factor, prostaglandins,** and also enzymes such as **elastases** and **collagenases.** The host response is amplified by these biologic mediators. This results in increased local periodontal destruction. There is also

a systemic immune response, which results in the induction of **serum antibodies.** A patient may also have an **immune system disease** that results in a hypofunctional immune response, which can lead to more periodontal breakdown.

Risk Factors

When determining a patient's response to the etiologic plaque, it is important to look at host risk factors. **Risk factors** in reference to periodontal disease are considered to be environmental conditions, habits, or diseases that increase or decrease a patient's susceptibility to periodontal infection. Certain diseases and the presence of certain bacteria may place a patient at greater risk for developing periodontal disease. **Diabetes, neutrophil disorders, osteopenia, stress,** and **smoking** have been shown to be some of the risk factors for developing periodontal disease.

Smoking is a major risk factor for developing periodontal disease. It is not the primary cause of the disease but rather a powerful modifier. The actual pathogenesis of periodontal disease in the smoker is not clearly understood. However, studies suggest that smoking may affect neutrophil function, cease serum antibody response to periodontal pathogens, and affect fibroblast function. *Bacteroides forsythus* has been found to be a prevalent periodontal pathogen in the pockets of smokers with periodontal disease. The gingiva in smokers is usually **fibrotic with rolled margins.** Minor gingival redness and edema are usually present compared with the severity of the disease. Numerous studies have shown that approximately 86% to 90% of **refractory periodontitis** cases (i.e., cases that do not respond to treatment) are associated with smoking. Thus, smoking greatly decreases the host's response to periodontal therapy. In addition, when a patient quits smoking, there is evidence that the periodontal condition improves. Thus, **smoking cessation programs** are becoming part of dental practice. Dental hygienists should be actively involved in these programs (see Chapter 12).

The patient who undergoes **organ transplant surgery** must be free of overt periodontal disease before the surgery. Patients who have had a transplant are at an increased risk for developing an infection and should, therefore, be monitored more closely to control and prevent further progression of periodontal disease.

In addition, recent evidence has suggested a positive association between the presence of periodontal infection and **cardiovascular disease (CVD)/stroke.** Patients with periodontal disease have a 1.5- to 2-fold greater risk of incurring fatal CVD than do patients without periodontal disease. Dental infections appear to increase the risk for developing coronary artery disease similar to other risk factors such as hypertension, diabetes, age, smoking, and elevated serum triglycerides. The exact mechanism for this association is presently unclear. However, a few proposed mechanisms should be mentioned. **Bacterial products,** such as the lipopolysaccharide endotoxins from gram-negative bacteria, **stimulate the release of inflammatory cells.** The inflammatory response characteristic of periodontal disease, marked by high levels of inflammatory mediators, appears to exacerbate the process of atherogenesis.

Another proposed mechanism is that certain oral bacterial strains of *Streptococcus sanguis* as well as *Porphyromonas gingivalis* **induce the aggregation of platelets,** which may increase the risk for thromboembolic events.

Evidence is mounting that pregnant women who have periodontal disease may be seven times more likely to have a **preterm, low-birthweight baby. Prostaglandins** and **tumor necrosis factor-α,** which are present during a normal pregnancy, may be **raised to an abnormally high level.** This rise, in the presence of periodontal disease, may induce early labor. Women who are contemplating pregnancy should have a complete oral examination to rule out or treat periodontal disease, if present. This should be an integral part of prenatal care.

Periodontal health is clearly a significant factor that contributes to the overall health of the whole person as well as to the health of the individual's teeth.

Gingivitis/Periodontitis

As early as 1976, Page and Schroeder described **periodontitis** as a chronic inflammatory disease of microbial origin. They histopathologically analyzed periodontal disease by looking at cellular inflammatory markers and loss of collagen. The disease initiated with plaque accumulation on the teeth and progressed from gingivitis to periodontitis. In order for periodontitis to be present, gingivitis must precede it. However, all cases of gingivitis do not lead to periodontitis. Other factors must affect the progression of the disease to the irreversible stage.

The **initial lesion** develops after **2 to 4 days** of plaque accumulation. **Vasculitis is also** associated with the vessels near the junctional epithelium. There is an **increase in fluid** in the gingival sulcus. The number of **leukocytes (neutrophils)** also increase. There is also up to a 5% to 10% **loss of collagen** surrounding the vessels close to the junctional epithelium. Clinically, no evidence exists of any pathologic changes in the gingival tissues.

The **early lesion** develops within **4 to 7 days** of plaque accumulation. All of the features of the initial lesion are present and magnified. An accumulation of **T lymphocytes** is present at the site of the acute inflammation near the junctional epithelium in the gingival connective tissue. There is a **further loss of collagen** near the junctional epithelium. Within the site of the acute inflammation, the collagen loss may be 60% to 70%.

The **established lesion** develops within **14 to 21 days** of plaque accumulation. **B lymphocytes** and the **plasma cell** are the predominant cell types in the inflammatory infiltrate. All of the features of the previous lesions are present in the established lesion. **Immunoglobulins** are present in the gingival connective tissue and epithelial tissue-especially the tissues immediately surrounding the blood vessels involved. There is some **proliferation and apical migration of the junctional epithelium.** Some pocket formation may or may not occur. **The initial, early, and established lesions are all reversible.** They are defined clinically as **gingivitis.**

Gingivitis is considered to be a disease characterized by inflammation of the gingiva. Changes may occur in the color, contour, consistency, position, or surface texture of the gingiva. There is usually bleeding or an exudate upon probing. Gingivitis may be localized, generalized, marginal, papillary, or diffuse. Gingivitis does not involve loss of bone or permanent connective tissue attachment loss (see Chapter 10).

The **advanced lesion** is characterized by the presence of **attachment loss.** Thus, this lesion is defined as **periodontitis.** The features of the established lesion are still present. However, the inflammatory process extends to the alveolar bone and periodontal ligament and results in **loss of bone and tissue. Periodontal pockets are present.**

Periodontitis involves a progression of the inflammatory process deeper into the tissues that surround the teeth, including the periodontal ligament, cementum, and alveolar bone. The continued presence of gingival inflammation leads to disruption in the free gingival fibers, then apical migration of the junctional epithelium, finally leading to loss of periodontal ligament fibers and alveolar bone loss.

Periodontitis, in general, has different stages of active disease. For many years, it was thought that the disease progresses slowly over time. However, observations of patients followed over time have shown that attachment loss can occur rather rapidly in episodic bursts of periodontal disease activity. In addition, loss of attachment can occur at a slow rate over long periods. Recent evidence shows that the disease is site specific. Different patients or the same patient may have sites with slow progression of the disease as well as sites with rapid bursts at different points in time.

Classification Systems

At the **1999 International Workshop for a Classification of Periodontal Disease and Conditions,** a new classification system was developed for classifying periodontal disease and conditions. The new system for classifying gingivitis is more comprehensive than the old one. For the sake of completeness, both the old and new systems are presented in outline form. However, the written descriptions of the different diseases are formatted in the old classification system with reference to the new classification system when appropriate. Gingivitis may be classified into two categories: the old system of classification (**Figure 13-1A**) and the new classification system (**Figure 13-1B**).

Dental Plaque-Induced Gingival Diseases

Gingivitis associated with dental plaque only is the most common of all periodontal diseases. It is present in people of all ages. It is characterized clinically by **redness, gingival bleeding, edema or enlargement, smooth surface texture, and bulbous papillae.** There is no connective tissue attachment loss or bone loss. The amount of gingival inflammation is usually directly related to the amount of plaque present. A direct causative effect of supragingival plaque on gingivitis was clearly established in a study by Loe, Theilade, and Jensen in 1965. Patients did not perform personal oral hygiene for 21 days. Samples of plaque were taken at intervals and analyzed by darkfield microscopy. Simple coccal flora and small rods were seen for the first few days of plaque formation on a clean tooth surface. Filaments and fusobacteria (corncob structures) appeared after 3 days. Vibrios and spirochetes appeared at 5 days of plaque accumulation. After beginning personal oral hygiene, the vibrios and spirochetes disappeared, first followed by the filaments and fusobacteria. Gingival inflammation resolved in about 1 week. This study was associated with the **nonspecific plaque hypothesis**. This hypothesis stated that supragingival plaque was associated with gingival inflammation-the more plaque, the more inflammation is present. Plaque removal could control or eliminate the gingival inflammation. As theories on the etiology of periodontal diseases developed over the years, a **specific plaque hypothesis** was formulated; this hypothesis stated that specific organisms are associated with health versus disease. Up to 20 or more different bacteria may be capable of causing different forms of periodontal disease. The theory of bacterial succession states that certain oral bacteria are present in biofilms in the mouth. As periodontal disease progresses, the bacteria change into more and more virulent species (see Chapter 7).

Plaque-induced gingivitis may also occur in a mouth that has previously undergone active periodontal disease. There is evidence of previous bone and attachment loss. The gingivitis is the same but is on a reduced periodontium.

Contributing Factors to Periodontal Disease

Local

Even though plaque is the primary etiologic factor in the development of periodontal disease, some local or contribut-

ing factors should be addressed. These factors allow plaque to accumulate more heavily on the surfaces of the teeth. Some of these factors contribute to plaque accumulation by making it more difficult for the patient to remove the plaque. These factors include **iatrogenic** dentistry such as overhanging margins and poorly contoured restorations, including crowns, bridges, amalgams, gold, and tooth-colored restorations. Some teeth have improper contours and open contacts that allow food to impact in these areas along with plaque. **Brackets** and **wires** placed on the teeth during orthodontic therapy can contribute to plaque retention. The **anatomy of the teeth/roots** can affect the accumulation of plaque. Teeth such as the maxillary lateral incisors have developmental grooves that sometimes extend onto the root surface. Plaque tends to accumulate in these deep grooves and can result in a localized defect in these areas. The mesial surface of the maxillary first bicuspids has deep developmental depressions that can also be traps for plaque. **Mouth breathing** is a factor that contributes to periodontal disease. A patient's own saliva consists of protective antibodies that contribute to the immune response of protecting the periodontium. When a patient is a mouthbreather, the tissues dry out and gingivitis or periodontitis can develop more easily.

Systemic

Gingival diseases can be modified by systemic factors associated with the **endocrine system, such as puberty-associated gingivitis, menstrual cycle-associated gingivitis,** and **pregnancy-associated gingivitis.**

Hormone-influenced gingivitis has been seen during puberty, fluctuations in the menstrual cycle, pregnancy, and steroid therapy. Subgingival growth of some gram-negative anaerobes, especially *Prevotella intermedia,* has increased. This form of gingivitis is characterized by an exaggerated response to plaque. It is not necessarily the amount of plaque present that results in these conditions, but the response to this plaque. There is usually intense inflammation and redness, edema, and enlargement of the gingiva. In severe cases of hormone-influenced gingivitis, the inflamed site may progress to a **pyogenic granuloma (pregnancy tumor).** This presents clinically as a painless protuberance from the gingival margin and interproximal space. It is important to emphasize oral hygiene and the significance of attaining and maintaining healthy gingival tissues to patients who are about to experience puberty as well as to female patients contemplating pregnancy.

Patients who have **uncontrolled diabetes** (have a difficult time controlling blood glucose levels) are at an increased risk for periodontal disease. In addition, diabetic patients with periodontal disease have a more difficult time controlling their blood glucose levels. The incidence of periodontal disease in the diabetic population increases as the patient goes through puberty and ages. Periodontal disease has also been shown to be more frequent and severe in diabetic patients who have advanced systemic complications.

I. Gingival Disease
  A. Plaque-associated gingivitis
    1. Chronic gingivitis
    2. Acute necrotizing ulcerative gingivitis
    3. Gingivitis associated with systemic conditions or medications
       a. hormone-influenced gingivitis
       b. drug-induced gingivitis
       c. HIV gingivitis

  B. Gingival manifestations of systemic diseases and mucocutaneous lesions
    1. Bacterial, viral, or fungal
    2. Blood dyscrasias
    3. Mucocutaneous diseases
  C. Other gingival changes

Figure 13-1. *A,* Classification of gingival disease. (From the American Academy of Periodontology: Current Procedural Terminology for Periodontics and Insurance Reporting Manual. Chicago, AAP News, 1992.)

I. Gingival Disease
  A. Dental plaque-induced gingival diseases*
    1. Gingivitis associated with dental plaque only
       a. without other local contributing factors
       b. with local contributing factors (See VIII A)
    2. Gingivitis diseases modified by systemic factors
       a. associated with the endocrine system
          1) puberty-associated gingivitis
          2) menstrual cycle-associated gingivitis
          3) pregnancy-associated
             a) gingivitis
             b) pyogenic granuloma
          3). diabetes mellitus-associated gingivitis
       b. associated with blood dyscrasias
          1) leukemia-associated gingivitis
          2) other
    3. Gingival diseases modified by medications
       a. drug-influenced gingival diseases
          1) drug-influenced gingival enlargements
          2) drug-influenced gingivitis
             a) oral contraceptive-associated gingivitis
             b) other
    4. Gingival diseases modified by malnutrition
       a. ascorbic acid-deficiency gingivitis
       b. other
  B. Non-plaque-induced gingival lesions*
    1. Gingivitis diseases of specific bacterial origin
       a. *Neisseria gonorrhea*-associated lesions
       b. *Treponema pallidum*-associated lesions
       c. streptococcal species-associated lesions
       d. other
    2. Gingival diseases of viral origin
       a. herpesvirus infections
          1) primary herpetic gingivostomatitis
          2) recurrent oral herpes
          3) varicella-zoster infections
       b. other

    3. Gingival diseases of fungal origin
       a. *Candida*-species infections
          1) generalized gingival candidosis
       b. linear gingival erythema
       c. histoplasmosis
       d. other
    4. Gingival lesions of genetic origin
       a. heredity gingival fibromatosis
       b. other
    5. Gingival manifestations of systemic conditions
       a. mucocutaneous disorders
          1) lichen planus
          2) pemphigoid
          3) pemphigus vulgaris
          4) erythema multiforme
          5) lupus erythematosus
          6) drug-induced
          7) other
       b. allergic reactions
          1) dental restorative materials
             a) mercury
             b) nickel
             c) acrylic
             d) other
          2) reactions attributable to
             a) toothpastes/dentifrices
             b) mouthrinses/mouthwashes
             c) chewing gum additives
             d) foods and additives
          3) other
    6. Traumatic lesions (factitious, iatrogenic, accidental)
       a. chemical injury
       b. physical injury
       c. thermal injury
    7. Foriegn body reactions
    8. Not otherwise specified (NOS)

Figure 13-1. *B,* Classification of periodontal diseases and conditions. (*Can occur on a periodontium with no attachment loss or on a pericardium with attachment loss that is not progressing.) [*B,* From the International Workshop for a Classification of Periodontal Diseases and Conditions. Ann Periodontol 4 (1):2, 1999.]

The increased incidence of periodontal disease in the diabetic population does not coincide with increased plaque and calculus levels. Epidemiologic studies have shown that patients with periodontal disease are at an increased risk of developing diabetes. Patients who exhibit only a family history of diabetes may have a polymorphonuclear neutrophil (PMN) chemotactic defect.

Gingivitis associated with **leukemias** and **other blood dyscrasias** usually consists of swollen, glazed, and spongy tissues. The color changes are usually evident from red to deep purple. Gingival bleeding is usually present due to local (plaque) and systemic factors (low platelets).

Medication-influenced gingival overgrowth or gingival hyperplasia is associated with an increase in the size of a tissue and produced by an increase in the number of its cell components (see Chapter 9). Three types of medications are associated with gingival overgrowth. The first type is **phenytoin** or **dilantin**. Phenytoin is an anticonvulsant agent used to treat seizure disorders. Usually, a 50% incidence of gingival hyperplasia is associated with this medication. The incidence rises to 80% up to 100% if the patient is taking other antiseizure medications. This gingival overgrowth may occur with or without plaque control and is usually not dose dependent. It may disappear spontaneously within a few months after the drug is discontinued.

Cyclosporine is an immunosuppressive agent used to prevent organ transplant rejection and to treat several diseases of autoimmune origin. The reported incidence of gingival hyperplasia due to cyclosporine is approximately 35%. The amount of gingival overgrowth is usually related to the dose of the drug.

Calcium channel blockers that are used to treat hypertension fall into the third category of medications that result in gingival overgrowth. Some examples of these medications include: nifedipine (Procardia), verapamil (Isoptin), diltiazem (Cardizem), and amlodipine (Norvasc). Because many calcium channel blockers are currently on the market, it is a good idea to use a drug reference book to identify the patient's drugs and become familiar with their mode of action. The incidence of gingival hyperplasia related to calcium channel blockers has been shown to be up to 29%. Neither the dose nor the duration of the drug has been reported to have a significant contribution regarding whether the patient developed gingival hyperplasia. It has also been suggested that presence of gingival inflammation and dental plaque is not essential for the onset of gingival overgrowth, but that it may play a role in its severity. The severity of gingival overgrowth in patients taking both cyclosporine and a calcium channel blocker is greater than in patients taking either drug alone. A possible mechanism of action of both cyclosporine and calcium channel blockers in producing gingival hyperplasia is that the drugs inhibit calcium-dependent collagenase production.

Overgrown gingiva should be removed surgically when it interferes with speech, function, aesthetics, or oral hygiene. In a study on the effects of periodontal treatment of patients with cyclosporine- and calcium channel blocker-induced gingival hyperplasia, patients who actively participated in supportive periodontal therapy (maintenance) at regular intervals and had good oral hygiene greatly reduced the recurrence of drug-induced gingival overgrowth.

Gingivitis, which is also associated with the use of **oral contraceptives,** may appear clinically as overgrown or hyperplastic tissue. Gingivitis may also appear as that seen in the endocrine-related gingival disease changes. Quite a lot of inflammation may be present compared with the amount of plaque.

Systemic conditions are also associated with gingival overgrowth, such as that associated with the regional enteritis of **Crohn disease**, **idiopathic gingival fibromatosis,** and **Hurler syndrome** (see Chapter 8).

Nutritional deficiencies, especially **vitamin C (ascorbic acid) deficiency,** can manifest itself in the gingival tissues by being red, swollen, and bleeding easily (see Chapter 6).

The **non-plaque-induced gingival lesions** are described in more detail in Chapter 8. The clinical manifestation of the non-plaque-induced gingival lesions may be the **classic acutely inflamed gingiva, desquamative gingivitis, localized gingival enlargement,** or **ulcerations.** In desquamative gingivitis, the gingiva sloughs off and leaves an intensely red surface.

It is unclear how prevalent periodontal disease is in the HIV-positive population. Studies have found an incidence of 1% to >50%. **HIV gingival disease** may be one of the first signs of HIV infection and thus may help to identify the HIV-positive patient. Thorough periodontal débridement, 1- to 3-month supportive periodontal therapy visits, and chlorhexidine rinses are all used to treat HIV-related periodontal diseases.

Periodontal Case Types

The American Dental Association (ADA) and American Academy of Periodontics (AAP) have developed a classification system for periodontal disease that includes case types I, II, III, IV, and V.

Case type I is given a **diagnosis** of **GINGIVITIS.** As previously mentioned, gingivitis is inflammation of the gingiva characterized clinically by changes in color, gingival form, position, surface appearance and presence of bleeding, and exudate. No evidence of bone resorption or apical migration of the epithelial attachment is seen.

Case type II is defined as **EARLY OR SLIGHT PERIODONTITIS.** The progression of the gingival inflammation has gone into the deeper periodontal structures and alveolar bone crest, with slight bone loss. Usually, a slight loss of connective tissue attachment and alveolar bone occurs with moderate pocket depths of 4 to 5 mm.

Case type III is defined as **MODERATE PERIODONTITIS.** This is a more advanced stage of the condition, with increased destruction of the periodontal structures and noticeable loss of bone support, which is possibly accompanied by an increase in tooth mobility. There may be furcation involvement in multirooted teeth. Up to one third of the bone has been lost around the root. Moderate-to-deep pockets up to 6 mm are present.

Case type IV is defined as **ADVANCED PERIODONTITIS.** There is a further progression of periodontitis with major loss of alveolar bone support, which is usually accompanied by increased tooth mobility. Furcation involvement in multirooted teeth is likely. More than one third of the bone around the tooth has been lost. Pocket depths are >6 mm.

Case type V is defined as **REFRACTORY PERIODONTITIS.** This type includes patients with multiple disease sites that continue to demonstrate attachment loss after appropriate therapy. These sites presumably continue to be infected by periodontal pathogens no matter how thorough or frequent the treatment provided. This case type also includes patients with recurrent disease at single or multiple sites.

Traditionally, the diagnosis of periodontitis was further subdivided based on age of onset, sex ratio, familial background, abnormalities in the host defense, local etiologic factors, rate, distribution, and severity of periodontal destruction. This classification scheme was defined in the 1989 World Workshop in Periodontics. The 1999 International Workshop for a Classification of Periodontal Disease and Conditions revised the 1989 Workshop classification. Both are presented here for completeness (**Figure 13-2A and B**).

Adult Periodontitis

Adult periodontitis affects patients older than 35 years of age, usually 55 years of age or older. There is usually no sexual predilection for the disease. The AAP case type classifications are similar to the mild, moderate, and severe forms of adult periodontitis. Destruction is usually related more to the mass of deposits present. With increasing age, a slight increase in bone loss usually occurs. However, the immune response in adult periodontitis is not clearly understood. One study looking for a potential genetic link in adult periodontitis found that patients with severe periodontal destruction tested positive for one of the genetic forms (alleles) of the IL-1A gene plus one of the Il-1B alleles compared with patients who did not have such severe periodontal disease. Heredity may play a part in adult periodontitis. The fact that the disease goes through periods of bursts and periods of quiescence most likely reflects the local immune response.

The bacteria associated with adult periodontitis include: *P. gingivalis, P. intermedia, B. forsythus, Fusobacterium nucleatum, Eikenella corrodens, Campylobacter rectus*, and *Treponema denticola*. The spirochetes can be characterized by their size as small, intermediate, or large. In a disease state, the proportion of intermediate spirochetes is high.

In the new classification scheme, the term adult periodontitis has been replaced with the term **chronic peri-**

odontitis. The age-dependent aspects of "adult" periodontitis were removed. Patients with this disease can have localized or generalized forms.

Early Onset Periodontal Diseases

The **early onset forms of periodontal (EOP) diseases** are more aggressive forms of the disease. These patients are younger than 35 years of age. The disease is characterized by rapid bone and attachment loss, which is fairly resistant to conventional therapy. A patient with EOP may lose as much as 4 to 5 μm of attachment per day or 1.8 mm/yr, which is three to four times the rate of attachment loss found in adult periodontitis. A defective host response may allow plaque to grow faster and accelerate the production of toxic products. Functional abnormalities are present in the PMNs and monocytes. It is important to do some form of full-mouth periodontal probing on all patients, especially on patients who have EOP, because the appearance of the tissue and the amount of deposits may be deceiving. When a patient has been identified as having early onset disease, it is important to do a complete periodontal evaluation of the entire family. Studies have noted a genetic predisposition to develop EOP. The dental hygienist should also be involved in the longitudinal monitoring of children of patients with EOP who may not show signs of the disease. The three general forms of EOP are: prepubertal, juvenile, and rapidly progressive periodontitis.

Prepubertal periodontitis affects children anywhere from the time between eruption of the primary dentition and puberty. Prepubertal periodontitis may be **localized (L-PP)** or **generalized (G-PP).** There is usually severe gingival inflammation with rapid bone loss, mobility, and early tooth loss. It may affect only the primary dentition or the primary and permanent dentition. Even though a complete radiographic series is most ideal for diagnosis, panographs are sometimes necessary for prepubertal cases due to the difficulty in managing younger children. Radiographs usually reveal early bone loss around primary teeth with no evidence of root reabsorption. A low caries rate is usually seen. There are minimal deposits of plaque and calculus. Prepubertal periodontitis, which was first described in 1983, is a rare disease. There are usually abnormalities in host defense (PMN and mononuclear leukocyte defect). Children affected with the G-PP are usually affected by some other systemic condition that reduces their resistance to bacterial infections. These conditions include **leukocyte adherence deficiency, congenital primary immunodeficiency, hypophosphatasia, chronic neutrophil defects,** or **cyclic neutropenia**. In the new classification system, this set of diseases is classified under **Periodontitis as a Manifestation of Systemic Disease.** Any child younger than 12 years of age with periodontal disease needs an immunologic/medical evaluation by a physician to rule out diseases with a host deficit. Prepubertal children with periodontitis who do not have a systemic disorder, depending on the features of their

II. Periodontics
   A. Adult periodontitis
   B. Early-onset periodontitis
      1. Pre-pubertal periodontitis
      2. juvenile periodontitis
      3. Rapidly progressive periodontitis
   C. Periodontics associated with systemic disease
   D. Necrotizing ulcerative periodontitis
   E. Refractory periodontitis

III. Mucogingival conditions
IV. Occlusal trauma
   A. Primary occlusal trauma
   B. Secondary occlusal trauma

Figure 13-2. *A,* Classification of gingival disease. (From American Academy of Periodontology: Current Procedural Terminology for Periodontics and Insurance Reporting Manual. Chicago, AAP News, 1992.)

II. Chronic Periodontitis
   A. Localized
   B. Generalized
III. Aggressive Periodontitis
   A. Localized
   B. Generalized
IV. Periodontitis as a Manifestation of Systemic Diseases
   A. Associated with hematological disorders
      1. Acquired neutropenia
      2. Leukemias
      3. Other
   B. Associated with genetics disorders
      1. Familial and cyclic neutropenia
      2. Down syndrome
      3. Leukocyte adhesion deficiency syndromes
      4. Papillon-Lefèvre syndrome
      5. Chediak-Higashi syndrome
      6. Histiocytosis syndromes
      7. Glycogen storage disease
      8. Infantile genetic agranulocytosis
      9. Cohen syndrome
     10. Ehlers-Danlos syndrome (Types IV and VIII)
     11. Hypophosphatasia
     12. Other
   C. Not otherwise specified (NOS)
V. Necrotizing Periodontal Diseases
   A. Necrotizing ulcerative gingivitis (NUG)
   B. Necrotizing ulcerative periodontitis (NUP)
VI. Abscesses of the Periodontium
   A. Gingival abscess
   B. Periodontal abscess
   C. Pericoronal abscess
VII. Periodontitis Associated With Endodontic Lesions
   A. Combined periodontic-endodontic lesions

VIII. Developmental or Acquired Deformities and Conditions
   A. Localized tooth-related factors that modify or predispose to plaque-induced gingival diseases/periodontitis
      1. Tooth anatomic factors
      2. Dental restorations/appliances
      3. Root fractures
      4. Cervical root resorption and cemental tears
   B. Mucogingival deformities and conditions around teeth
      1. Gingival/soft tissue recession
        a. facial or lingual surfaces
        b. interproximal (papillary)
      2. Lack of keratinized gingiva
      3. Decreased vestibular depth
      4. Aberrant frenum/muscle position
      5. Gingival excess
        a. pseudopocket
        b. inconsistent gingival margin
        c. excessive gingival display
        d. gingival enlargement (See I.A.4. and I.B.4)
      6. Abnormal Color
   C. Mucogingival deformities and conditions on edentulous ridges
      1. Vertical and/or horizontal ridge deficiency
      2. Lack of gingiva/keratinized tissue
      3. Gingival/soft tissue enlargement
      4. Aberrant frenum/muscle position
      5. Decreased vestibular depth
      6. Abnormal Color
   C. Occlusal trauma
      1. Primary occlusal trauma
      2. Secondary occlusal trauma

Figure 13-2. *B,* Classification of periodontal diseases and conditions. [†Can be further classified on the basis of extent and severity. As a general guide, extent can be characterized as localized = ≤30% of sites involved and generalized = >30% of sites involved. Severity can be characterized on the basis of the amount of clinical attachment loss (CAL) as follows: slight = 1 or 2 mm CAL; moderate = 3 or 4 mm CAL; and severe = ≥5 mm CAL.] [*B,* From the International Workshop for a Classification of Periodontal Diseases and Conditions. Ann Periodontol 4(1):3, 1999.]

periodontal disease, would be categorized as having **aggressive periodontitis** or **chronic periodontitis** in the new classification system.

The treatment for prepubertal periodontitis usually involves the use of amoxicillin and periodontal débridement. Tetracyclines are not used on this age group due to the danger of severe staining of the permanent teeth that are still developing. Patients with prepubertal periodontitis who have an underlying systemic condition need to have the disease under control to prevent the loss of teeth due to the periodontal disease. These patients must be on a strict maintenance schedule (as much as four to six times per year depending on their oral hygiene). Space maintenance should be provided when needed for teeth lost early.

Juvenile periodontitis tends to occur around the circumpubertal period. The age of onset is from 12 to 26 years of age. Thus, teenagers and those in their early 20s are affected. Females are usually affected more than males by 3:1. Approximately one half of the patients affected with prepubertal periodontitis later manifest signs of juvenile periodontitis. Juvenile periodontitis is characterized by severe angular bone defects in the permanent first molars or incisors. The bone has a moth-eaten appearance. Usually, minimal plaque and calculus are present. African Americans seem to be affected more than are Caucasians. Attachment loss is three to five times greater than that found in adult periodontitis. These patients have elevated serum antibody levels to *Actinobacillus actinomycetemcomitans*. Approximately 70% of patients with juvenile periodontitis have a neutrophil chemotactic defect. Juvenile periodontitis may be localized or generalized. The localized form has the severe angular, **moth-eaten appearance of the bone defects limited to the permanent first molars or incisors**. The generalized form is usually seen in patients post puberty. At least 14 teeth or more are affected. The affected permanent teeth are variable and greater in number than those found in the localized form, but they include the first molars and incisors. Treatment recommendations are periodontal débridement with the use of systemic antibiotics. Systemic tetracycline and doxycyclines have been used in the treatment of juvenile periodontitis. The earlier the disease is treated, the more chance there is of saving the affected teeth and controlling the disease process. Regenerative surgical procedures with the use of systemic antibiotics have also been used in the treatment of juvenile periodontitis.

Rapidly progressive periodontitis (RPP) is another early onset disease with rapid loss of attachment and alveolar bone support. The age of onset is usually in the late 20s or 30s. The clinical appearance of this disease is similar to generalized juvenile periodontitis, except that the distribution and severity are relatively random and first molars and incisors are no more severely affected than are other teeth. Plaque-associated materials range from minimal in early stages to moderate in advanced stages of RPP. Females tend to be affected more than males by a ratio of 2:1 or 3:1.

RPP is associated with an immune dysfunction in the neutrophil. A definitive method of diagnosing RPP is to have a sequence of radiographs showing the **rapid progression of bone loss in a short time**. Treatment includes periodontal débridement with systemic antibiotics as well as periodontal surgery where indicated. *A. actinomycetemcomitans* is not usually the offending organism in cases of RPP. It appears to be more the gram-negative anaerobes, *Bacteroides* species, and spirochetes. Thus, metronidazole is often used with periodontal débridement. Case reports in the literature have illustrated the usefulness of bacterial and antibiotic sensitivity testing in special patient populations. These populations include, but are not limited to, patients with refractory periodontitis, patients who are medically compromised, and patients with EOP and RPP.

The highly destructive periodontal diseases just described are now called **aggressive periodontitis** in the new classification system. Patients who meet the criteria for LJP are now classified as having **localized aggressive periodontitis**. Patients presenting with generalized juvenile periodontitis or RPP are now classified as **generalized aggressive periodontitis**. Setting age limits tends to cause some major problems in truly determining how to diagnose the disease, because patients with the same etiology and presenting symptoms may be older than 35 years of age.

PERIODONTITIS ASSOCIATED WITH SYSTEMIC DISEASE

Periodontitis associated with systemic disease includes a wide range of disorders. Some of these disorders have already been mentioned under prepubertal periodontitis. They include but are not limited to: those associated with hematologic disorders such as **acquired neutropenia, leukemias;** those associated with **genetic disorders such as familial and cyclic neutropenia, Down syndrome, leukocyte adhesion deficiency syndromes, Papillon-Lefévre syndrome, Chédiak-Higashi syndrome, histiocytosis syndrome, glycogen storage disease, infantile genetic agranulocytosis, Cohen syndrome, Ehlers-Danlos syndrome (types IV and VIII), and hypophosphatasia.** These diseases appear to have **impaired neutrophil function** in common. This seems to underscore, again, the importance of a properly functioning neutrophil in the pathogenesis of periodontal disease. The clinical presentations may defer by the specific disease as well as by control of the disease. More research is being done to study each of these disease entities and to look at how they initiate or potentiate periodontal disease.

HIV infection may manifest itself in the gingival tissues. This form of periodontal disease is seen in HIV-positive patients. In HIV infection, the disease is very aggressive. There is extensive tissue necrosis with severe loss of periodontal attachment and bone. Spontaneous bleeding and nocturnal bleeding also occur. Patients who present with the HIV form of periodontal disease usually have severe pain deep in the bone. The clinical manifestations of this disease resemble **necrotizing ulcerative periodontitis (NUP)**. Treatment for **HIV periodontal disease, which resembles NUP,** usually involves local débridement with the topical use of irrigation with povidone-iodine. Systemic antibiotics are used if fever, severe necrosis of the tissue, or bone exposure is present. The systemic antibiotic of choice is usually metronidazole. It is important to warn patients not to use alcohol while taking this medication owing to a severe disulfiram reaction. Patients should also be told to rinse twice a day with 0.12% chlorhexidine gluconate. HIV gingival disease has also been called **linear gingival erythema**. The amount of erythema is usually disproportionate to the amount of visible supragingival plaque. It usually fails to completely resolve after good plaque control therapy. These lesions have the appearance of established marginal gingivitis with petechiae-like or diffuse red lesions of the attached gingiva or oral mucosa. The linear band tends to bleed. *Candida* has consistently been isolated in the subgingival plaque of HIV-positive patients. This suggests that plaque may serve as a continuous reservoir for oral candida infections. Plaque may play a role in the petechiae and red lesions seen in HIV gingival disease in that treatment of HIV patients with topical antifungal agents results in some resolution of the gingivitis. The microflora of HIV gingival disease are qualitatively similar to the microflora of HIV periodontal disease. The microflora of conventional periodontitis is similar to the microflora of HIV periodontal disease.

Patients who have had radiation therapy for cancer treatment tend to develop dental problems from the drying effect of the radiation treatments. Salivary glands are often damaged with radiation treatment. Patients tend to develop caries as well as periodontal disease due to the lack of protective saliva.

Necrotizing ulcerative gingivitis (NUG) is an acute, often recurrent gingival infection of complex etiology. **NUP** is a term used for a severe, necrotizing, often recurrent, ulcerative infection of the gingival tissues that also includes connective tissue and bone destruction. It is uncertain as to whether these two diseases are part of a single condition or if they are separate diseases. Thus in the new classification system, the term **necrotizing periodontal disease** is used and includes the clinical manifestations and conditions of NUG and NUP. The clinical appearance of the gingiva is that of necrosis of the tips of the papillae with **punched out crater-like depressions at the crest of the interdental papilla**. The surface of the craters is covered by a **gray, pseudomembranous sloughing tissue**. The patient has **pain, spontaneous bleeding,** and a **fetid breath odor**. The patient may also have an elevation in temperature or **local lymphadenopathy**. The clinical features of the necrotizing periodontal diseases are usually diagnostic. Microscopically, the connective tissue is invaded by spirochetes and fusiforms. *P. intermedia* and *F. nucleatum* appear more frequently. These diseases are related to **smoking, stress, immunosuppression, systemic diseases, malnutrition,** and

significant life changes. Listgarten described **four zones in the NUG lesion**: **Zone 1** is the bacterial zone, which is the most superficial and contains varied bacteria and few spirochetes of small, medium, or large types. **Zone 2** is the neutrophil-rich zone, which contains many leukocytes that are mainly neutrophils and also numerous bacteria. **Zone 3** is the necrotic zone, which consists of disintegrated tissue cells, fibrillar material, collagen fiber remnants, and many intermediate and large spirochetes with few other organisms. **Zone 4** is the zone of spirochetal infiltration, which consists of well-preserved tissue infiltrated with intermediate and large spirochetes with no other organisms.

Treatment for the necrotizing periodontal diseases usually consists of local débridement. A 0.12% chlorhexidine gluconate rinse may also be prescribed. Systemic antibiotics may be indicated, especially if the patient has an elevated temperature or lymphadenopathy.

Refractory Periodontitis

Refractory periodontitis is a disease that presents with multiple periodontal sites that continue to demonstrate attachment loss even after appropriate comprehensive therapy. This category includes patients who do not respond to any treatment provided no matter how thorough or frequent and also includes patients with recurrent disease at few or many sites. The disease affects 4.5% of patients (usually 1 in 20 patients in a periodontal practice). Patients are usually 30 years of age or older. It may or may not be associated with abnormalities in the host defense. Patients who smoke are more likely to develop refractory periodontitis than are those who do not smoke. The microflora includes elevated subgingival levels of *B. forsythus, A. actinomycetemcomitans, F. nucleatum, S. intermedius, E. corrodens,* and *P. gingivalis*. There is also an appearance of nontypical microflora such as *Pseudomonas* and *Candida* species in refractory cases that further complicates the understanding of this complex etiology. Treatment should include some form of bacterial culturing and antibiotic sensitivity testing. A wide variety of systemic antibiotics have been used such as tetracyclines, amoxicillin, metronidazole, ciprofloxacin, and clindamycin. There may also be a potential for use of a local delivery agent such as doxycycline or chlorhexidine gluconate, which are both available now and are discussed in more detail under treatment.

Proposed mechanisms for the increased incidence of refractory periodontal disease in smokers include: alterations of the periodontal tissue vasculature, direct effects on the bacterial microflora, inhibitory effects on immunoglobulin levels, and antibody responses to plaque bacteria.

In the new classification system, the separate disease category for refractory periodontitis was eliminated. Because some multifactorial clinical conditions and treatments for periodontal disease do not respond to therapy, the term refractory is still defined as described here. However, this term may be used when proper therapy fails to control the condition for any of the forms of periodontal disease (e.g., **refractory aggressive periodontitis, refractory chronic periodontitis, refractory periodontitis associated with systemic disease**).

Abscesses of the Periodontium

A separate category exists for **abscesses of the periodontium**, which are either gingival, periodontal, or pericoronal. A **gingival abscess** is a localized, painful, rapidly expanding lesion that is usually acute; it is confined to the marginal gingival or interdental papilla, and it may be fluctuant with purulent exudate. The abscess may be caused by the presence of a foreign object, such as a toothbrush bristle or popcorn kernel that is forced into the gingiva. Treatment involves local incision and drainage and curettage of the area. Systemic antibiotic therapy is used if lymphadenopathy or elevated temperature is present. However, thorough débridement is the key to successful treatment.

The **periodontal abscess** is a localized purulent infection within the tissues adjacent to the periodontal pocket. This abscess may lead to the destruction of periodontal ligament and alveolar bone. The treatment is the same as that used for a gingival abscess. In addition, a surgical procedure may be indicated to gain better access for débriding the periodontal site. It may be caused from inadequate periodontal débridement in a deep and tortuous periodontal pocket. Patients with moderate to advanced periodontal disease are susceptible to developing periodontal abscesses. Patients with furcation involvement, diabetes, and other root anomalies may develop periodontal abscesses. Sometimes, these abscesses develop after use of systemic antibiotics for non-oral infections in patients with untreated periodontal diseases.

A **pericoronal abscess (pericoronitis)** is an inflammation of the gingiva in relation to the crown of an incompletely erupted tooth. This abscess is usually seen around third molars. A flap of tissue lies over the area, called the operculum, under which bacteria and food debris accumulate. Treatment includes cleaning and irrigation of the area. Systemic antibiotic therapy is also used. The impacted tooth is later removed.

A **periodontal pocket/lesion originates at the crest of the bone**. As it progresses, the bone and tissue destruction may progress all the way to the apex of the tooth. **An endodontic lesion usually results in bone being lost initially at the apex.** As the lesion becomes more advanced, the bone destruction progresses toward the crest of the bone. The two lesions are sometimes present on the same tooth. They may be independent of each other, or they may be connected. The main consideration in treatment is that the endodontic therapy is usually recommended first. Successful endodontic treatment will often completely resolve the lesion. The longer an endodontic-periodontic lesion is left untreated, the greater is the need for endodontic as well as periodontal therapy to resolve the lesion.

An isolated very narrow deep pocket may be found on a tooth. This may be due to an endodontic problem or a peri-odontal problem. This type of lesion may sometimes be indicative of a vertical root fracture, and the prognosis of this type of fracture is poor.

PRESCRIBED PERIODONTAL THERAPY

It has been clearly established that periodontal disease is a result of a bacterial infection. Thus, the **goals of periodontal therapy are to control infection and regenerate the periodontium**. Periodontal therapy should resolve inflammation, arrest disease progression, maintain esthetics, maximize patient comfort, regenerate lost periodontium, and create an environment that discourages recurrent disease. Control of infection involves **proper home care, periodontal débridement, surgical treatment,** and **adjunctive use of topical, local delivery,** and **systemic antibiotics**. The dental hygienist plays a major role as the healthcare provider in helping patients to control periodontal "infection." Regeneration of the periodontium involves surgical treatments of **bone grafting, guided tissue regeneration, connective tissue grafting,** and **root surface treatments**. Another aspect to regeneration is the potential to use some type of modifiers of the immune system to regenerate tissue such as **growth factors, cytokines/cytokine antagonists, anti-inflammatory drugs,** or **antibodies**. A low-dose doxycycline, **Periostat**, has been approved by the Food and Drug Administration (FDA). Periostat works by altering the tissue **collagenases** released as part of the host response to the bacterial plaque challenge on the periodontium. Other chemically modified tetracyclines, which have no antimicrobial effect but do affect the overactive immune response, are currently being developed and tested for efficacy.

After a thorough case evaluation and periodontal diagnosis has been made, a periodontal treatment plan should be developed. This **treatment plan** should include the periodontal procedures to be performed as well as a list of people who will be performing these procedures. If any restorative treatment needs to be performed, the outline for restorative procedures should be included in the treatment plan. The plan of treatment should be presented to the patient and should also be accepted by the patient.

PERIODONTAL INFECTION CONTROL

The first method of controlling infection is by **personal plaque control** (see Chapter 12). The next element in the control of infection is thorough periodontal débridement. **Scaling** has been defined as instrumentation of the crown and root surfaces of the teeth to remove plaque, calculus, and stain from these surfaces. **Root planning** has been defined as a definitive treatment procedure designed to remove cementum or surface dentin that is rough, impregnated with calculus, or contaminated with toxins or microorganisms. Root planing involves the removal of calculus and aggressive smoothing of a root to form a hard glassy surface. Although it results in healing, it can lead to root reduction, hypersensitivity, and operator and patient fatigue. The new term, **periodontal débridement,** refers to the treatment of gingival and periodontal inflammation through mechanical removal of tooth and root surface irritants (i.e., plaque, calculus, and endotoxins) without aggressive removal of cementum to the extent that the adjacent soft tissues return to a healthy, noninflamed state.

The indications for periodontal débridement are teeth with periodontally involved sites that show signs of inflammation, elevated levels of periodontal pathogens, progressive attachment, and alveolar bone loss.

The objectives for periodontal débridement are to suppress or eliminate periodontal pathogenic bacteria and replace them with a flora that is conducive to gingival health for that patient; to convert inflamed, bleeding, or suppurative site pockets to healthy gingival tissue; to shrink deepened pathologic pockets to shallow, healthy gingival sulci that is easier for the patient to maintain; and to provide a root surface compatible with the re-establishment of a healthy connective tissue and epithelial attachment. The roots of teeth that are affected with periodontal disease contain an **endotoxin [a lipopolysaccharide (LPS)]** on their surfaces. This endotoxin is derived from the cell walls of gram-negative bacteria. It is currently thought that the endotoxin adheres to the thin smear layer of the surface of the cementum rather than penetrating into the cementum. In addition, most of the residual endotoxin that remains on the root surface is believed to be associated with residual plaque and calculus rather than being absorbed into the cementum. Because it is superficial, it can be removed easier than was previously thought. Thus, extensive, aggressive periodontal débridement of the root surface is not necessary to ensure a root that is relatively free of bacterial endotoxins.

Before the clinician attempts to perform periodontal débridement, he or she must assess the severity of the condition by clinical examination, radiographs, and instrumentation. The following is a description of some of the factors that affect the effectiveness of periodontal débridement. One factor is the anatomy of the roots. Some teeth have root concavities in them, such as the mesial of the maxillary first bicuspids and the distal surface of the maxillary canines. Other teeth, especially maxillary lateral incisors, may have a palatal groove on the lingual aspect that tends to accumulate plaque and result in a localized periodontal defect. Many anomalies are associated with the crowns or roots of third molars, which may be present and functional in the patient's mouth. Early recognition and documentation of potential problem areas associated with root anomalies will contribute to consistent and comprehensive periodontal care. Another factor is the depth of the pockets. Studies have shown that once a pocket presents as ≥5 mm, the ability to thoroughly clean the area is decreased. The position of the teeth in the arch may affect the operator's ability to adequately access these sites. If instruments are dull or inappropriate for the area being scaled, efficiency decreases. The area in the mouth being treated is also a factor. The maxillary anterior teeth are usually easier to débride than is the distal of a second or third molar. The size of the mouth, cheek elasticity, and range of opening are all factors that may affect the results of the patient's treatment. The operator's dexterity is also important.

It is important to realize that osseous defects around the teeth, especially if they are deep, are difficult if not impossible to access during periodontal débridement. When teeth have furcation involvement, the furcations can prove to be quite difficult to clean thoroughly. Most hand-scaling instruments are too wide to even access the entrance to furcations. Studies have shown that sonics and ultrasonics with fine tips are more effective than is hand scaling in débriding furcations due to this problem.

In order to assess oneself at the time of periodontal débridement, one should use visual cues such as the mouth mirror, compressed air, and optimum lighting to check for deposits, which may still be present. An explorer should be used to check for remaining calculus and assess the smoothness of the root surface.

 ## INSTRUMENTS AND INSTRUMENTATION

Examination instruments include mouth mirrors, periodontal probes, and explorers. Utilization of these instruments is essential in the process of assessing the patient's periodontal status and determining a treatment plan (see Chapter 10).

Scaling instruments include curets (universal and area-specific), sickles, hoes, and files. All consist of a handle, shank, and blade with one or more cutting edges. During successful removal of calculus with any of the scaling instruments, a series of steps is required. This involves exploring with a light grasp to feel the calculus, adapting the cutting edge against the tooth, tightening the grasp on the handle, activating a laterally pressured vertical or oblique short work stroke, and relaxing the grasp on the handle before repeating the series of steps (i.e., **explore, adapt, tighten, stroke, relax**).

Universal Curet

A universal curet is designed so that one double-ended paired instrument can be used to scale any tooth surface in the oral cavity. Its curved blade consists of two cutting edges that meet at a rounded toe (tip). Each cutting edge is formed by the junction of the facial surface and one lateral surface. The rounded back surface and curved blade are prime features for root surface adaptation (**Figure 13-3).**

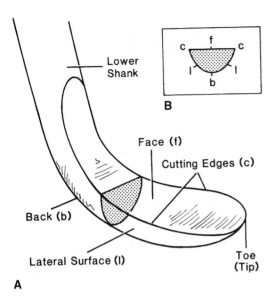

Figure 13-3. Parts of a curet. *A,* Curet with parts labeled. The lower shank is also called the terminal shank. The curet has a round toe, whereas the scaler has a pointed tip. *B,* Cross-section of a curet labeled *f* (face), *c* (cutting edges), *l* (lateral surfaces), and *b* (back). (From Wilkins E: Clinical Practice of the Dental Hygienist, 8th ed. Philadelphia, Lippincott Williams & Wilkins, 1999, p 516.)

Each blade on a universal curet is a mirror image of the other. The blade is honed so that the terminal shank is 90 degrees to the terminal shank and the internal angle of each cutting edge is 70 to 80 degrees. To properly position a cutting edge against a tooth surface, the **lower shank (i.e., the section of shank closest to the blade) must be tilted toward the tooth surface.** Thus, the **angle formed between the tooth surface and the face of the curet blade is >45 degrees and <90 degrees (Figure 13-4).**

A double-ended universal curet may be utilized in two ways. One method is to scale the facial or lingual and mesial

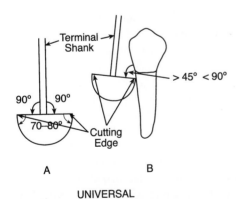

Figure 13-4. Universal curet design and tooth adaptation. *A,* Cross-section of a universal curet blade. The blade is positioned so that the face of the blade is 90 degrees to the terminal shank. Note the 70- to 80-degree internal angle and two cutting edges. *B,* Placement of one cutting edge against a tooth. Note that the terminal shank must be tilted toward the tooth so that the appropriate working angle (>45 degrees and <90 degrees) is formed between the face of the blade and the tooth surface.

surfaces with one cutting edge on one blade; then, the instrument is flipped and one cutting edge on the other blade is used to scale the distal surface on the same tooth. In this method, the handle of the instrument must be parallel with the proximal surface being scaled. Therefore, in order to scale the entire facial or lingual aspect of a tooth, the instrument must be flipped over. This "twirling" can lead to an insecure grasp on the instrument and possible dropping of the instrument or accidental trauma to the patient. In addition, it is very difficult to attain a parallel handle position for scaling distal surfaces of posterior teeth.

The second method for utilizing the universal curet is to scale the facial/lingual and mesial surfaces of a tooth with one cutting edge on a blade and the distal surface of the same tooth with the opposite cutting edge on the same blade. In this method, the distal, facial, and mesial surfaces of one quadrant are scaled with one end of a paired instrument; then, the instrument is flipped and the other end of the curet is used to scale the distal, lingual, and mesial surfaces of the same quadrant. This method involves less "twirling" of the instrument. It requires a change in handle position when scaling distal surfaces as opposed to facial/lingual and mesial surfaces. To scale the facial/lingual and mesial surface of a tooth, the handle is held vertically; to scale the distal surfaces of the same tooth, the handle is positioned more perpendicularly to the long axis of the tooth and the opposite cutting edge of the same blade is adapted to the distal surface.

Gracey Curets

Gracey curets are curets designed so that each blade is adapted to a specific area of the mouth. Because each "**area-specific**" curet may be utilized only in any one particular area of the mouth, more than one Gracey curet is necessary to débride a full complement of teeth. **Each curet** is usually designed with mirror image working ends or blades for accessing specific areas of the teeth (**Table 13-1**).

Gracey curets designed for scaling proximals of posterior teeth may also be designed so that the mesial and distal blades that adapt to the buccal or lingual aspect of a tooth are on one handle. These combinations of blades may be manufactured as follows: 11/14 and 12/13; 13/16 and 14/15; or, 15/18 and 16/17 (**Table 13-2**).

 TABLE 13–1 Mirror Image Gracey Combinations

GRACEY CURET	AREA OF USE
1/2, 3/4	Anterior teeth: all surfaces
5/6	Anterior teeth and premolars: all surfaces
7/8, 9/10	Posterior teeth: buccal and lingual surfaces
11/12, 15/16	Posterior teeth: mesial surfaces, and mesial surface of each root
13/14, 17/18	Posterior teeth: distal surfaces, and distal surface of each root

TABLE 13–2 Mesial-Distal Gracey Combinations

GRACEY CURET	MESIAL AND DISTAL AREAS OF USE
11/14, 14/15, 15/18	Buccal MdR
	Lingual MdL
	Buccal MxL
	Lingual MxR
12/13, 13/16, 16/17	Lingual MdR
	Buccal MdL
	Lingual MxL
	Buccal MxR

The curved blade of a Gracey curet, like that of a universal curet, has a rounded toe and two lateral surfaces that meet with a flat facial surface and rounded back surface. Unlike the universal curet, however, the blade of a Gracey curet has only one usable cutting edge, and the face is **offset** or honed at 70 degrees to its terminal shank. If the terminal shank of the Gracey curet is held parallel to the surface of the tooth to be scaled, the lower cutting edge is the correct cutting edge for scaling that tooth surface. This visual cue is important for correct adaptation of the instrument. When the terminal shank is positioned parallel to (but not touching) the tooth surface, the lower cutting edge will be properly positioned against the tooth surface. The angle formed by the face of the blade to the tooth will be >45 degrees and <90 degrees: this same angle must also be achieved with a universal curet (**Figure 13-5**).

Various shank design features of Gracey curets allow for different areas of use, periodontal pocket access, and calculus removal. The shanks may be straight or have multiple bends. Those with multiple bends allow for easier access to the posterior teeth. Flexible small-diameter shanks allow for tactile sensitivity and removal of light calculus, whereas shanks with a rigid larger diameter allow for moderate-to-heavy removal of calculus.

For access to pockets of 5 mm or greater or sulci of teeth with long clinical crowns, **After Five Graceys** have been designed with shanks 3 mm longer than the original Gracey curets. These curets are available in all of the Gracey numbers and with flexible or rigid shanks. Mini Five Graceys have the same longer shank length as do After Fives, but the blade is thinner and half the length of the After Five or Standard Gracey. The short blade and long shank allow for access to narrow areas of recession or clefts.

Calculus removal is achieved with Gracey curets by following the same basic steps as with the universal curet. With a light exploratory stroke, insert the blade of the Gracey curet apically to the depth of the sulcus or pocket (coronal edge of the junctional epithelium) just under any calculus. Once the calculus has been detected, adapt the cutting edge against the tooth by positioning the terminal shank parallel

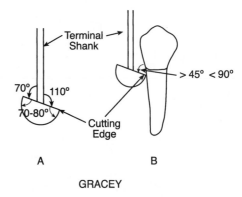

Figure 13-5. Gracey curet design and tooth adaptation. *A,* Cross-section of a Gracey curet blade. Blade is offset at 70 (110 , opposite angle) to the terminal shank. Note the 70- to 80-degree internal angle of blade and cutting edge. *B,* Placement of Gracey cutting edge against tooth. Note the angle (>45-degree and <90-degree) formed by the face of the blade and the tooth surface and the parallel position of the terminal shank to the tooth surface.

to the tooth surface and rotate the instrument handle until only the lower third of the cutting edge engages the tooth. Tighten your grasp on the instrument, and apply lateral pressure against the tooth as the blade is pulled coronally in a short work stroke. Relax your grasp, and repeat this series of steps as you progress along the tooth surface.

If débridement of *only* subgingival plaque or sheet calculus must be accomplished, the blade should be lightly inserted to the depth of the pocket as discussed earlier. To prevent gouging, however, a little more than the lower third of the cutting edge is adapted to the tooth, and a series of overlapping multidirectional "shaving" strokes is administered until the root surface is clean. Care must be taken to avoid overzealous smoothing of the root surface.

Sickle Scalers

The blades of a **sickle scaler** may be straight or curved with **two cutting edges** formed by the junction of one facial and two lateral surfaces. The lateral surfaces converge to form a sharp point at the tip and a sharp back surface. This design gives the blade a triangular cross-section with the face positioned at 90 degrees to the terminal shank (**Figure 13-6**).

Both **curved** or **straight** sickles (**jacquette scalers**) are available with straight or angled (**contra-angled/modified**) shanks. Straight sickles are best adapted to anterior teeth because their shank, blade, and handle are in the same plane. Sickles with contra-angled shanks enable instrumentation of posterior teeth, along with anterior teeth. These modified sickles are designed with paired mirror image blades on one handle.

Because of the triangular design of the blade, sickles are recommended for removal of supragingival calculus primarily on proximal tooth surfaces. The pointed tip allows for removal of calculus from just under the contact point of two teeth. It is contraindicated to use sickle scalers subgingivally

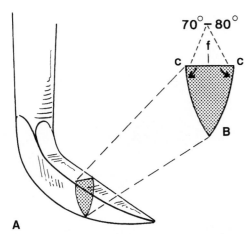

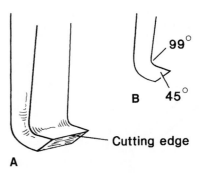

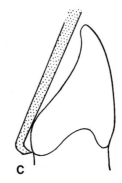

Figure 13-6. Straight sickle scaler. *A,* The straight blade converges to a point where the two cutting edges meet at the tip. *B,* Cross-section of the scaler shows the face *(f),* the two cutting edges *(c),* and the 70- to 80-degree internal angles. This type of sickle scaler is also known as the Jacquette scaler. (From Wilkins E: Clinical Practice of the Dental Hygienist, 8th ed. Philadelphia, Lippincott Williams & Wilkins, 1999, p 518.)

Figure 13-8. Hoe scaler. *A,* The hoe has a single cutting edge. *B,* The blade is turned at an angle of 99 degrees to the shank, and the cutting edge is beveled at a 45-degree angle. *C,* Adaptation to a tooth for removal of calculus is with a two-point contact where possible. (From Wilkins E: Clinical Practice of the Dental Hygienist, 8th ed. Philadelphia, Lippincott Williams & Wilkins, 1999, p 519.)

because of the pointed tip, sharp back surface, and straight cutting edges that do not adapt well to curved root surfaces.

In utilization of the sickle scaler, one cutting edge is used to scale the distal aspect of a tooth and the opposite cutting edge on the same blade is used to scale the mesial aspect of the same tooth. Only the lower third of the cutting edge nearest the point is placed against the tooth surface (see Figure 10-1). The shank should be tilted toward the tooth surface so that the face of the blade is >45 degrees but <90 degrees to the tooth surface. Once the cutting edge is adapted, a short prying stroke is activated to remove calculus **(Figure 13-7).** For calculus removal under the contact

point of two teeth, insert the blade apically between one tooth surface and the interdental papilla and ensure that the side of the point remains on the tooth surface. If the blade is inserted horizontally, the tip may lacerate the gingival crest of tissue.

When a double-ended contra-angled sickle is used, one cutting edge on a blade adapts to distal surfaces on the facial aspect of a quadrant and the opposite cutting edge of the same blade adapts to the mesial surface of the facial aspect of the same teeth. The other blade on the instrument is utilized on the lingual aspect of the same quadrant.

Hoe Scalers

Hoe scalers are designed with one straight cutting edge on a blade that is about 100 degrees to the shank **(Figure 13-8).** These scalers are used to remove large amounts of supragingival calculus. Because of the blade design, they are not recommended for use subgingivally on a curved root.

Chisel Scalers

Chisel scalers consist of a single straight cutting edge on a blade that is continuous with a slightly curved shank **(Figure 13-9).** These instruments are suited to remove supragingival proximal calculus, when there is spacing and no interdental papilla between two adjacent teeth.

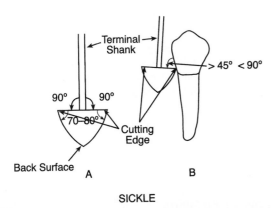

SICKLE

Figure 13-7. Sickle curet design and tooth adaptation. *A,* Cross-section of a sickle scaler. The blade is positioned so that the face of the blade is 90 degrees to the terminal shank. Note the 70- to 80-degree internal angle, two cutting edges, and sharp back surface. *B,* Placement of one cutting edge against a tooth. Note that the terminal shank must be tilted toward the tooth so that the appropriate working angle (>45 degrees and <90 degrees) is formed between the face of the blade and the tooth surface.

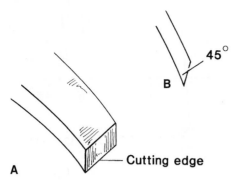

Figure 13-9. Chisel scaler. *A*, A chisel scaler has a single cutting edge, and the blade is continuous with a slightly curved shank. *B*, A 45-degree bevel is at the cutting edge. (From Wilkins E: Clinical Practice of the Dental Hygienist, 8th ed. Philadelphia, Lippincott Williams & Wilkins, 1999, p 519.)

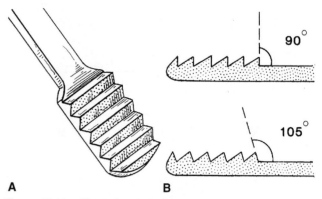

Figure 13-10. File scaler. *A*, A file has multiple cutting edges. *B*, Each blade is at a 90-degree or a 105-degree angle with the shank. (From Wilkins E: Clinical Practice of the Dental Hygienist, 8th ed. Philadelphia, Lippincott Williams & Wilkins, 1999, p 520.)

File Scalers

A **file scaler** consists of multiple blades. Each blade has one straight cutting edge **(Figure 13-10)**. This instrument can be utilized for crushing calculus, smoothing root surfaces in pockets when other bulkier instruments are inaccessible, or for smoothing overhanging proximal restorations. The entire working surface of the blade must be placed against the tooth and then activated by a pull stroke.

Because of the continued development of curets, sickles, and power scaling devices, hygienists rarely use hoes, chisels, and files today.

Maintenance and Sharpening

Proper maintenance of examination and periodontal scaling instruments directly affects their life and function. All instruments must be first cleaned by hand scrubbing with heavy utility gloves or, preferably, in an ultrasonic unit. After cleaning, the instruments must be wrapped or placed in an appropriate cassette and sterilized using heat.

Instrumentation results in dulling of cutting edges; therefore, instrument cutting edges must be inspected routinely and sharpened accordingly. Sharp instruments reduce operator fatigue because of less pressure, strokes, and time needed to remove calculus or stain; decrease burnishing of calculus; improve tactile sensitivity; and result in less patient discomfort and fatigue.

To avoid cross-contamination and potential exposure from an accidental instrument stick, instruments should be sharpened while they are sterile. After sharpening, clean and re-sterilize the instruments for later use. It is safe to sharpen with a sterile stone dull sterile instruments prior to use at the chairside. However, care must be taken to avoid contamination of the instruments just before use.

It is imperative to understand the design of the blade of an instrument in order to sharpen it correctly. A cutting edge on any scaling instrument is the junction or line where two surfaces meet-usually the facial and lateral surface of a blade.

When the cutting edge is pressed against the tooth, it becomes rounded or dull and does not engage calculus on a tooth. Because a dull cutting edge is rounded, it has thickness and will reflect light. Sharpness can also be checked by applying the cutting edge against a small plastic rod at the correct angle for scaling. If the edge does not catch without pressure, it is dull.

The objectives of sharpening are to produce a sharp cutting edge and to maintain the original shape of the blade. Therefore, the overall size of the blade becomes smaller, but the original shape does not change.

When sharpening a Gracey curet, universal curet, or sickle scaler, the stone should be placed against the lateral surface of the instrument (or instrument against the stone) so that the angle formed between the face of the instrument and the stone is approximately 110 degrees. This angulation ensures maintenance of the 70-degree internal angle of the blade **(Figure 13-11)**. Whether the instrument is held stationary and the stone moved, or the stone is placed flat and stationary and the instrument moved, this 110-degree angle must be maintained during the sharpening process.

Chisels, hoes, and files are sharpened by placing the flat beveled surface of the cutting edge against a sharpening stone or file. To sharpen an explorer, draw the side of the point of the tip against the stone in a circular fashion in order to create a sharp point.

Sharpening stones may be made of natural stone, such as the Arkansas stone, or from artificial materials. Artificial stones include the following: ruby, carborundum, and ceramic stones.

Air Powder Polishing

Air powder polishing systems employ the mixture of air, water, and sodium bicarbonate that is delivered as a spray to the tooth surface in order to remove stain and plaque. These systems are comprised of a unit containing the power source and reservoir for the sodium bicarbonate, hoses for water and air that attach to the corresponding dental unit, recepta-

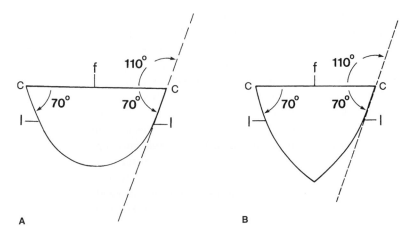

Figure 13-11. Angulation for sharpening. Cross-sections of a curet *(A)* and a sickle scaler *(B)* show correct angulation of the face of the blade with the flat sharpening stone *(broken line)* to reproduce the internal angle of the instrument at 70 degrees. Note the cutting edges *(c)* and the lateral surfaces *(l)*. (From Wilkins E: Clinical Practice of the Dental Hygienist, 8th ed. Philadelphia, Lippincott Williams & Wilkins, 1999, p 536.)

cles for water and air, and a handpiece and spray nozzle through which the sodium bicarbonate mixture is propelled. Proper utilization of an air powder polishing system involves keeping the nozzle tip 4 to 5 mm away from the tooth surface, directing it at the enamel at the appropriate angle, and moving it in a circular motion **(Figure 13-12).**

Air polishing requires less time and energy for the clinician, generates no heat, and removes stain effectively without removal of enamel. However, this system has its disadvantages. Significant aerosol is generated, and precautions must be taken to prevent cross-contamination. Abrasion of the mucosa or cementum may occur if the spray is not directed specifically at the enamel. If soft tissue is abraded, the potential exists for uptake of sodium bicarbonate in the bloodstream; therefore, it is contraindicated for hypertensive patients. Nonmetallic restorations may be pitted if contact is made with the generated spray.

Aerosol can be minimized by using a commercial aerosol reduction device. This device consists of a disposable cup and clear tube extension that is attached directly to the air polisher nozzle and tubing that attaches to a saliva ejector or evacuation system.

Because of the potential negative consequences, the clinician must consider the individual patient before incorporating the use of an air powder polisher into the treatment plan.

Ultrasonic and Sonic Scaling

Ultrasonic scaling devices were first introduced in the 1950s. These powered scaling devices convert high-frequency electrical energy into high-frequency sound waves, which produce mechanical energy as rapid vibrations in the scaling tips (i.e., inserts). **Cavitation**, or the creation of bubbles that collapse and release energy, is created when water flowing through the ultrasonic insert meets the vibrating tip of the insert. The mechanical vibrations remove calculus from the tooth, and the cavitation removes plaque endotoxins from the root surface.

Ultrasonic tips were historically bulky and designed primarily for accessing and removing supragingival calculus. Now, thinner and longer tips are available and can be utilized safely to débride subgingival calculus and plaque. In addition, water lavage flushes debris from the subgingival areas, and cavitation destroys or disrupts the cell walls of

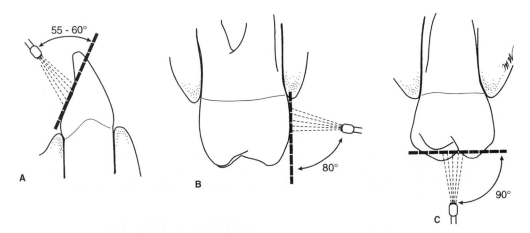

Figure 13-12. Air-powder polishing. Direct the aerosolized spray for *(A)* the anterior teeth at a 60-degree angle, *(B)* the posterior teeth facial and lingual or palatal at an 80-degree angle, and *(C)* the occlusal surfaces at a 90-degree angle to the occlusal plane. (From Wilkins E: Clinical Practice of the Dental Hygienist, 8th ed. Philadelphia, Lippincott Williams & Wilkins, 1999, p 614.)

plaque bacteria. The addition of chemotherapeutic agents to some ultrasonic units permits delivery of these agents to the periodontal sites during ultrasonic instrumentation. Periodontal débridement through the use of powered scaling instruments not only results in removal of endotoxins but also less root reduction and patient and operator fatigue.

The two types of powered scaling devices are ultrasonic and sonic scalers. **Ultrasonic scaling devices** consist of an electric generator, foot control and handpiece assembly separate from the dental unit, and scaling tip inserts. **Sonic scaling devices** consist of a handpiece, which attaches directly to the dental unit and is activated by the dental unit handpiece control and various styles of scaling tips (**Table 13-3**).

The various designs of ultrasonic and sonic inserts include bulkier inserts for removal of supragingival calculus or subgingival calculus that is easily accessible and more slender, longer inserts for subgingival débridement. The water delivery system may be either through the tip or through a hollow thin metal attachment that empties a fine water spray onto the insert tip.

Before attaching an insert to an ultrasonic or sonic handpiece, purge the water lines of the unit. Use a saliva ejector or preferably high-speed evacuation to prevent or reduce the production of aerosol. Once the powered scaler is "tuned" according to the manufacturer's specifications, a fine mist of water or chemotherapeutic agent will spray from the insert tip. The operator should activate the insert tip by pressing on the foot pedal. During instrumentation, use a light erasing motion with the side of the insert tip against the tooth. Never use the point of the insert against the tooth.

Traditionally designed ultrasonic or sonic inserts are adapted to the tooth similarly to their hand instrument counterparts. Longer slim inserts designed specifically for sub-

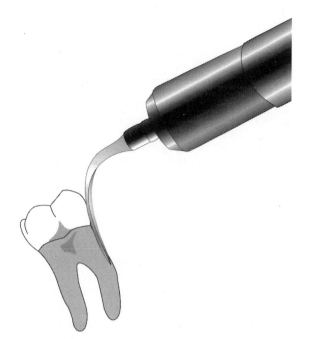

Figure 13-13. Adaptation of a slim ultrasonic insert. The insert tip is directed apically with the entire length of the insert against the root surface. Adaptation is similar to that of a periodontal probe. (Courtesy of Janet Bee, BA, MSDH: Knowledge and Utilization of Ultrasonic/Sonic Scaling Instruments: A Survey of West Virginia Dental Hygienists. Master's Thesis, Morgantown, West Virginia University, 1999.)

gingival débridement are inserted and adapted very similar to that of a periodontal probe. Upon insertion, the insert tip is directed apically with the entire length of the insert against the root surface (**Figure 13-13**).

Avoid use of ultrasonic or sonic scalers on implant abutments. Also, the operator should be cognizant of potential pulpal damage through heat production, hearing damage from the high-pitched noise that these devices produce, and the potential for infection through aerosolization of generated water spray. Immunocompromised patients, therefore, should not be treated in the same room or nearby area immediately after utilization of a power scaling device on previous patients. Some manufactured ultrasonic devices are contraindicated for use near persons with pacemakers because of the electromagnetic interference that they create. An exact safe distance has not been established.

Powered scaling inserts must be maintained properly for maximum efficiency. Follow the manufacturer's directions for replacing o-rings and cleaning and sterilizing. It is important to check the insert tips for wear, because worn-down insert tips lose their efficiency. Some manufacturers provide indicators for checking the wear of ultrasonic tips.

Subgingival Irrigation

In-office professional **subgingival irrigation** is an adjunctive therapy to root débridement. It is usually performed as a single treatment after periodontal débridement. Irrigation

TABLE 13–3 Types of Powered Scaling Devices

ULTRASONIC SCALERS
Operate at a frequency range between 25,000 and 50,000 cycles/sec

Types
Magnetostrictive
• Creates a magnetic field and produces vibrations by expansion and contraction of a stack of metal strips or rods
• Potential for interfering with activity of pacemakers worn by the patient or operator
• Elliptical or 360-degree rotation in all planes produces activity on all sides of the tip inserts.

Piezoelectric
• Activated by dimensional changes in quartz or metal alloy crystal transducers in the handpiece that create no magnetic field
• Linear movement is produced on only two sides of the tip insert.

Sonic Scalers
• Operate at a frequency range between 2500 and 7000 cycles/sec
• Driven by compressed air from dental unit-not electrical energy
• Elliptical movement producing activity on all sides of the tip
• Pressure sensitive; increased pressure of the tip against a tooth results in inactivation

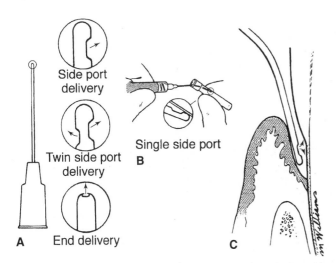

Figure 13-14. Professional irrigation. *A,* Types of cannula tips with side-port or end-delivery openings. *B,* Prepare the cannula for use by bending the sterile tip within the encasement to make the insertion easier. *C,* With knowledge of each probing depth, insert the cannula gently to near the bottom of a pocket. No force should be used. (From Wilkins E: *Clinical Practice of the Dental Hygienist,* 8th ed. Philadelphia, Lippincott Williams & Wilkins, 1999, p 568.)

is accomplished by administering an antimicrobial agent into periodontal pockets via a disposable hand syringe, a jet irrigator with cannula, or an ultrasonic unit **(Figure 13-14).** Several antimicrobial agents have been utilized for subgingival irrigation, although little research data exist on most. These agents include **chlorhexidine gluconate, povidone-iodine, stannous fluoride, essential oils, sanguanarine, tetracycline, hydrogen peroxide, sodium bicarbonate,** and **salt solutions.** The lack of **substantivity** of many of these agents is a key factor in their ineffective antimicrobial activity. The quick turnover rate of crevicular fluid inhibits retention of these agents. Nonsubstantive agents, therefore, would have little time to provide much bactericidal effect. Of all these available agents, the most utilized for subgingival irrigation is chlorhexidine gluconate **(Table 13-4).**

Factors that may affect the subgingival delivery and antimicrobial effect of chemotherapeutic agents include the presence of calculus, irrigator tip design, irrigation force, agent substantivity, and crevicular fluid. Calculus can impede penetration of the agent in deep pockets, and increased protein levels in crevicular fluid inhibit antimicrobial action of some agents (e.g., chlorhexidine).

Currently, professional in-office subgingival irrigation remains a controversial treatment in periodontal therapy. The

long-term benefit of a single procedure of subgingival irrigation following root débridement is not proved. The development of subgingival fibers or gels containing antimicrobial agents that are placed and held in periodontal pockets for several days show promise as adjunctive aids in periodontal therapy.

REASSESSMENT

After allowing at least 4 to 6 weeks for adequate healing following periodontal débridement, the patient should be seen for a complete periodontal examination. Following periodontal débridement, the healing usually results histologically by the formation of a long junctional epithelium. The color, contour, consistency, and surface texture of the gingiva should be that which is consistent with health. This should result in a reduction in probing depths. After the gingival tissues shrink, some residual calculus may be seen. This should be removed. Studies have shown that after periodontal débridement, residual calculus is most often seen just apical to the cementoenamel junction. No bleeding or suppuration should occur upon probing. If the periodontal condition does not improve after periodontal débridement procedures, further investigations should be performed. An evaluation of the patient's medical status may be warranted. Some form of **bacterial culturing** may be done to determine what periodontal pathogens may still be present in high concentrations in the gingival pockets. Consideration should be given to use some form of systemic antibiotic, and the periodontal débridement procedure should be repeated. The results of the bacterial culturing, if antibiotic sensitivity testing was also done, can be used to help determine which antibiotic to use. Osseous defects may be present that would be an indication to perform some form of periodontal regenerative surgery in a particular site or sites.

Studies have shown that 42 days after a single session of periodontal débridement, subgingival spirochetes return to baseline levels. Periodontal débridement, which has been shown to consistently eliminate *P. gingivalis,* is referred to as initial nonsurgical periodontal therapy. After the initial therapy, if all parameters re-evaluated are consistent with gingival health, the patient should be placed on a periodontal maintenance schedule. **Periodontal maintenance** is referred to as supportive periodontal therapy (SPT). It is essential to reinforce home care procedures throughout all phases of initial therapy (see Chapter 12). A reliable predic-

TABLE 13-4 Common Antimicrobial Agents Utilized in Subgingival Irrigation

AGENT	% CONCENTRATION	SUBSTANTIVITY	STAINING
Chlorhexidine	Full strength (.12)-.02	Yes	Yes
Povidone-iodine	50, 5	–	Yes
Stannous fluoride	1.64, .4	Yes	Yes

tor of the patient's oral hygiene compliance and plaque control is based on the patient's plaque control performance at the post-initial therapy phase of treatment.

ADJUNCTIVE NONSURGICAL THERAPY

Local delivery agents have been used in the management of periodontal disease. Currently, **tetracycline fibers, doxycycline polymer, minocycline powder,** and **chlorhexidine chips** are available for use in the United States. To date, **metronidazole** and **minocycline gels** are being considered by the FDA for approval. In general, local delivery appears to be as effective as periodontal débridement with regard to reducing signs of periodontal inflammation, including pocket depth and loss of clinical attachment. However, they have not proved to be more beneficial than periodontal débridement alone. Local delivery may be an adjunct treatment for refractory sites or sites that have difficult access for thorough periodontal débridement. The issue of bacterial resistance developing after use of local delivery agents has not been totally resolved. There is currently no definitive evidence that one local delivery system is significantly better than another. It is also unclear as to whether local delivery agents will prevent further periodontal disease progression and whether local delivery agents are effective against organisms that invade tissue.

Another method of using antibiotics in the treatment of periodontal disease is the use of **systemic antibiotics** in conjunction with periodontal débridement. Systemic antibiotics such as amoxicillin are **not** recommended for routine use in the treatment of adult periodontitis or chronic periodontitis. In addition, these drugs are **not** recommended for use at routine maintenance (supportive periodontal therapy) sessions other than for prophylactic premedication, which may have been indicated in the patient's medical history. There is a concern about the overuse of systemic antibiotics, which can lead to **bacterial resistance**. Systemic antibiotics are recommended for use in the treatment of the **aggressive periodontal diseases** such as the old category of early onset periodontal diseases including prepubertal periodontitis, juvenile periodontitis, and rapidly progressive periodontitis; any form of refractory periodontitis; and also some forms of acute NUG and NUP. Systemic antibiotics may also be used in the treatment of patients who have a systemic disease associated with periodontitis. Some of the antibiotics commonly used in the treatment of periodontitis are tetracyclines, including minocycline (Minocin) and doxycycline; metronidazole plus amoxicillin; clindamycin; amoxicillin; and ciprofloxacin. In some of these cases, it may be beneficial to use a microbiologic laboratory and sample some of the deeper pockets and sites that bleed upon probing. Some culturing techniques may be able to check for antibiotic sensitivity and allow the operator to choose the most efficacious antibiotic.

One study was done to evaluate the tissue distribution of the new macrolide antibiotic azithromycin in patients subjected to oral surgery for chronic inflammatory diseases of the periodontium. There was a marked penetration of azithromycin into both normal and pathologic periodontal tissues, which suggests that azithromycin therapy represents a promising option when treating chronic inflammatory periodontal diseases.

PERIODONTAL SURGICAL PROCEDURES

At this point, a discussion of **osseous defects** in the alveolar bone is warranted. There are two defects in the cortical alveolar bone-a dehiscence and a fenestration. A **dehiscence** is a cleft-like absence of alveolar cortical plate that usually results in a denuded root surface. An alveolar **fenestration** is a circumscribed defect in the cortical plate that exposes a facial or lingual root surface **(Figure 13-15)**.

When the base of a periodontal pocket is located coronal to the crest of the alveolar bone, it is called a **suprabony pocket**. When the base of the pocket is located apical to the crest of the alveolar bone, it is called an **infrabony pocket**. The defect that results from a pocket base being apical to the crest of the bone is referred to as an infrabony defect. Infrabony defects are classified according to the number of remaining osseous walls.

Figures 13-16 and 13-17 illustrate a **three-wall infrabony defect**, which occurs most frequently in the region illustrated. The remaining walls of bone are the facial, lingual, and proximal. A three-wall defect may also occur as a trough-like defect on the facial or lingual aspect. A three-wall defect may wrap around the tooth and involve two or more adjacent root surfaces. These are called circumferential defects. A three-wall defect can be described as being narrow, wide, shallow, or deep.

A **two-wall defect** is the most prevalent defect. It has been called a crater or an interdental crater. The two-wall defect is found interproximally. It has a facial and lingual wall. A two-wall defect can also occur with facial and proximal or lingual and proximal walls present **(Figure 13-18)**.

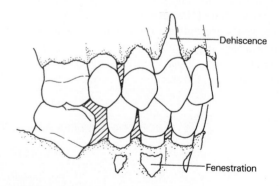

Figure 13-15. Fenestration. (From Fedi PF, Vernino AR, Gray JL: The Periodontic Syllabus, 4th ed. Philadelphia, Lippincott Williams & Wilkins, 2000, p 12.)

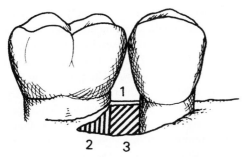

Figure 13-16. Three-wall defect. (From Fedi PF, Vernino AR, Gray JL: The Periodontic Syllabus, 4th ed. Philadelphia, Lippincott Williams & Wilkins, 2000, p 161.)

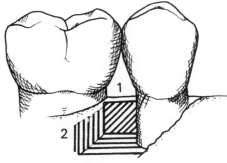

Figure 13-18. Two-wall defect. (From Fedi PF, Vernino AR, Gray JL: The Periodontic Syllabus, 4th ed. Philadelphia, Lippincott Williams & Wilkins, 2000, p 162.)

A **one-wall defect** usually occurs interdentally. The remaining wall may be proximal or facial or lingual. It is important to note that osseous defects may have sites with a combination of one-, two-, and three-wall lesions (**Figure 13-19**).

In terms of treating these periodontal osseous defects, a three-wall defect has the best periodontal prognosis. Depending on the topography of the defect, regeneration may be attempted, osseous resection may be done; roots may be amputated; repeated sessions of periodontal débridement may be performed; or the tooth may be extracted. **Periodontal surgical procedures** may be indicated for some patients. The indications for surgery are usually infrabony defects that may be amenable to hard tissue grafts, removal of excess gingival tissue, mucogingival defects, or any areas in which a surgical procedure may result in a gain in hard tissue supporting structures. In general, periodontal surgical procedures are considered to be resective or regenerative. Resective periodontal surgical procedures involve a **gin-**

givectomy, which is the removal of excess gingival tissues, or **gingivoplasty,** which is the recontouring of existing gingival tissues. These procedures may be indicated when extra gingival tissue is present with no infrabony defects. Some mucogingival flap procedures include the removal of excess gingival tissues, lining of the diseased pocket/sulcular epithelium, or marginal tissues. Bone recontouring or **osteoplasty** as well as bone removal or **ostectomy** are the resective procedures that may be performed on the bone.

Regenerative periodontal procedures include all procedures that result in reconstruction and regeneration of the **mucosal, gingival, osseous,** and **aesthetic defects**. Many materials are available for regenerative procedures, which include membranes (reabsorbable and nonreabsorbable), human and synthetic bone grafts, dermal matrices, and bovine bone matrix proteins that contribute to more predictable results in regenerative periodontal surgical procedures. The concept of guided tissue regeneration involves use of techniques and materials that allow cells from the periodontal ligament to get to the healing periodontal surgical site first. In the usual healing response, epithelial cells reach the wound first. Thus, healing takes place by repair forming a long junctional epithelium. If gingival connective tissue cells get to the healing site first, root reabsorption can occur. If osseous cells reach the wound site first, ankylosis can occur. However, if periodontal ligament cells get to the healing site first, regeneration will occur. Guided tissue regeneration involves placement of a barrier over the osseous defects; this action prevents epithelial, gingival connective tissue, and osseous cells from getting to the wound site first.

Sutures are placed to provide wound closure, position the tissues, aid in the control of hemorrhage, and help reduce postoperative pain. Suture materials are absorbable and nonabsorbable. Some sutures are made from black, braided silk. Other sutures are made from synthetic fibers such as nylon monofilament, polyviolene-polyester, polypropylene, and polyglycolic acid. There are sutures made from animal intestines called gut. They come in plain and chromic. The plain and chromic gut sutures are absorbable as well as the polyglycolic acid. There is no single suture material that is ideal for every situation. In general, in periodontics nonabsorbable silk, black braided sutures are used. However, for

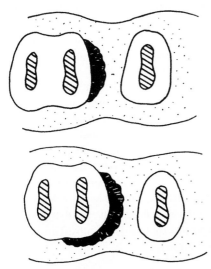

Figure 13-17. A three-wall defect may also occur as a trough-like defect on the facial or lingual aspect. Occasionally, a three-wall defect may wrap around the tooth and involve two or more contiguous root surfaces. These are referred to as a **circumferential defect**. (From Fedi PF, Vernino AR, Gray JL: The Periodontic Syllabus, 4th ed. Philadelphia, Lippincott Williams & Wilkins, 2000, p 161.)

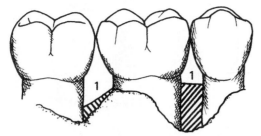

Figure 13-19. One-wall defect. (From Fedi PF, Vernino AR, Gray JL: The Periodontic Syllabus, 4th ed. Philadelphia, Lippincott Williams & Wilkins, 2000, p 162.)

some of the regenerative procedures, gut or Vicryl sutures are also used.

After surgery, a periodontal dressing is sometimes placed over the wound site. **Periodontal dressings** are used to protect the wound, to enhance patient comfort for the initial period after surgery, to help hold the flap in the desired place, and to maintain the initial blood clot by protecting the wound from being disturbed. Several dressings are available for use. The most common are the eugenol and non-eugenol. Currently, the non-eugenol dressings are the most frequently used. The dressing is smooth and pleasant tasting and is usually well tolerated by patients. Dressings are placed, post-surgically, after the initial clot has formed. It is important to place the dressing **over** the flap and prevent it from flowing in between the teeth and the bone.

Dressings are usually placed with a lubricated glove or with sterile saline on a gloved hand to keep the material from sticking to the glove. The dressing is placed over the surgical site up to the cervical third of the tooth to prevent the dressing from interfering with occlusion. The dressing should extend apically to cover the wound but should not overextend into the vestibule, floor of the mouth, or near frena attachments. Some clinicians do not use a periodontal dressing post surgically. They believe that after a few days, the dressing can become a plaque trap and thus make the surgical site difficult to keep clean. A compromise would be to place a dressing for a few days and then to have the patient make an appointment to remove the dressing and allow for easier plaque removal.

The dental hygienist may also be involved in presenting **postoperative care instructions** to the patient. The instructions should be given orally and also in writing. The most important aspect for the initial postoperative period is to protect the blood clot, which usually involves no eating or drinking hot foods or alcohol for up to 4 hours. However, the patient must maintain a nutritious diet during the postsurgical phase of therapy. The patient should be advised to spend minimal time talking, and he or she is usually told to go home and rest. Cold packs can be applied to the surgical site to aid in hemorrhage control as well as prevent swelling. The patient should be told that it is not unusual for the pillow to be lightly tinged with blood after surgery. However, if profuse bleeding is noted, the patient should call and be examined immediately. The patient can apply gauze pressure to the site. He or she should avoid mouthwashes, constant spitting or rinsing, and strenuous exercise for the first 24 hours. It is important to have the patient start on the prescribed pain medication as soon as possible. The patient can be given a prescription or over-the-counter pain medication depending on the extent of the surgery. The patient should be warned that the teeth may be sensitive, especially to hot and cold if the dressing is removed or dislodged. This sensitivity usually decreases by itself if the teeth are kept clean. The teeth should not be brushed or flossed on the day of surgery. (It is a good idea to have the patient brush and floss the entire mouth immediately before surgery.) The day after surgery, the teeth may be brushed and flossed; care should be taken not to dislodge the dressing if one is present. If a dressing is not present, the surgical site can be gently swabbed with a cotton-tipped applicator. The patient may use warm salt water to rinse. It is also common to prescribe an antimicrobial rinse such as chlorhexidine gluconate to be started 24 hours after surgery. The success of the surgery depends, to a large extent, on the patient's ability to keep the site clean for the first few months after surgery. This is another important area in which the dental hygienist plays a vital role.

The **postoperative appointment** is usually scheduled within 7 to 14 days after the surgery. If periodontal dressing was placed, and is still present, it is gently removed by placing a fairly blunted instrument under the dressing and lifting it up. There is usually plaque present under the dressing. The surgical site should be lightly débrided supragingivally with an instrument. An antimicrobial rinse such as chlorhexidine gluconate should be used. The sutures should be wiped with a tissue dipped in chlorhexidine gluconate. If the healing appears to be within normal limits, and there is no evidence of infection or swelling, the sutures should be removed. The suture is gently lifted up at the knotted end with cotton pliers and cut with scissors. Gently pull the knotted suture so that the remainder of the suture material will pass through the tissue and be removed. The number of sutures removed should coincide with the number of sutures placed. Some minor hemorrhage may be present with the suture removal that can be controlled by gentle gauze pressure. The site should be gently débrided and flossed. The patient should be given home care instructions and arrange follow-up appointments at 2- to 4-week intervals to monitor the postoperative healing processes. Studies have shown that the level of personal plaque control post surgically has a positive correlation with the success of the surgery. Various types of regenerative surgical materials dictate that postsurgical areas may not be probed for 6 to 12 months. This interval depends on the material used.

MAINTENANCE

Longitudinal studies have shown that patients who have been treated successfully for periodontal disease should be placed on a **3-month recall**. Supportive periodontal therapy (maintenance) appointments include:

- Review of medical and dental history
- Oral hygiene instruction/patient education
- Radiographs as needed
- Hard and soft tissue examination
- Complete periodontal examination
- Periodontal débridement as needed
- Plaque removal and fluoride treatment, if indicated

The hygienist needs to enforce with the patient the importance of compliance to set recall intervals. The hygienist plays an essential role in the maintenance of the periodontal health of the patient.

 # IMPLANTS

Since ancient Chinese civilizations, humans have attempted, with little success, to develop an effective replacement for missing teeth using dental implants. It was not until 1978, when Branemark, a Swedish orthopedic surgeon, introduced a sound, scientifically based osseointegrated oral implant system to North America, that implants became a successful replacement for missing teeth. For many people who have difficulty with removable oral prostheses, the dental implant provides prosthesis stability and increases the efficiency of eating and speaking. Elimination of removable, soft tissue borne prostheses relieves the wearer of a source of tissue irritation. Furthermore, implants provide force-bearing bone to retain alveolar bone mass in the absence of natural teeth, and the implant can support a prosthesis made to restore a patient's facial aesthetics in many cases. Any of these benefits can, in turn, have the additional benefit of bolstering the patient's self-esteem and confidence.

New strides in **implantology** have brought dental implants from a "last resort" treatment modality to a common treatment option. The predictability of implant retention, the development of various treatment options, and the increased awareness by the public of this treatment option has brought implant treatment to an increasing number of dental offices. Other dental offices inherit new patients who already have dental implants, thus making knowledge of implant evaluation and maintenance an imperative for all dentists and dental hygienists.

Categories of Dental Implants

Currently, three implant categories may be encountered. The **transosteal implant** (also referred to as the staple implant) passes through the alveolar bone and penetrates both cortical plates. A stabilizing bone plate is placed through a submental incision into the inferior border of the mandible. Retaining posts are attached to the bone plate, which pass through the mandible to the alveolar crest and through the mucosa **(Figure 13-20).** These posts, which were introduced in 1975, are limited to the atrophied mandible to support a removable full arch prosthesis. Although these posts have attained a high 10-year success rate, they are no longer frequently placed due to the current success of osseointegrated root-form implants (see later).

Subperiosteal implants (Figure 13-21) date back to the 1940s. Also used with the moderately to severely atrophied alveolus, these implants are placed under the periosteum and on the bone rather than in or through it. They are constructed to conform to the topography of the bone, determined by either direct bone impressions or from computer tomography (CT) images, and placed beneath a full-thickness periosteal flap directly onto the bone. These support partial and complete removable prostheses.

The 1960s marked the development of **endosteal implants** (place through the gingiva into the bone) with the introduction of the **blade** implant **(Figure 13-22).** This thin band of metal, designed in various materials and numerous shapes, could be used in a narrow alveolar ridge to replace a single tooth or to support partial or complete arch prostheses. Suitable for both the maxilla and the mandible, the dental implant was used frequently. These implants require the

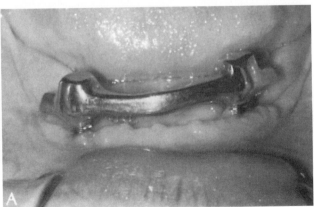
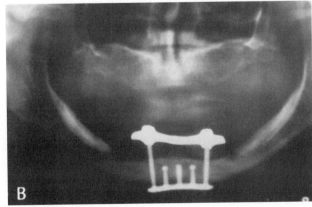

Figure 13-20. *A,* Mandibular transosteal (staple type) implant as it appears clinically. *B,* Radiographic view of the staple implant. (Courtesy of HJ Bianco, Jr, DDS, MS, West Virginia University, Morgantown, WV. From DeBiase CB: Dental Health Education: Theory and Practice. Philadelphia, Lea & Febiger, 1991, p 147.)

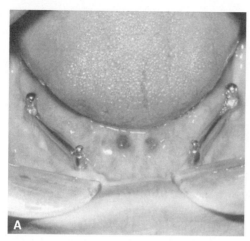
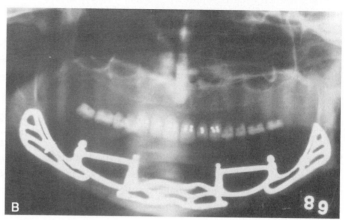

Figure 13-21. *A,* Clinical view of a mandibular subperiosteal implant. *B,* A radiographic view. (Courtesy of HJ Bianco, Jr, DDS, MS, West Virginia University, Morgantown, WV. From DeBiase CB: Dental Health Education: Theory and Practice. Philadelphia, Lea & Febiger, 1991, p 147.)

shared support, however, of natural teeth to replace a single tooth or support a partial prosthesis. In the case of a full arch prosthesis, support is required from the rami.

The introduction of Brânemark's **osseointegrated root-form implants (Figure 13-23),** backed by up to 30 years of well-documented clinical trials with evidence of long-standing survival, the ability to stand alone, maintenance of alveolar bone, and low risk in comparison with all other forms of dental implants, has made this type the most frequently placed. Previously reported endosteal implants obtained only connective tissue anchorage of which a high percentage eventually failed. Brânemark's scientifically sound implant system, dependent on direct mechanical bone anchorage for strength during functioning, has achieved a high success rate of 97%.

Contraindications for Dental Implants

Pretreatment evaluation of an implant candidate, as with other patients who require oral and maxillofacial surgery, includes medical and psychological elements. In general, a person must be able to cope physically and mentally with the surgical procedures and the prosthetic end-product.

Some medical conditions, however, automatically exclude dental patients from implant treatment. These conditions include systemic diseases that compromise healing and the immune response such as AIDS, cancer, blood dyscrasias, and uncontrolled diabetes. Recent and anticipated radiation therapy to the head and neck are also contraindications. The dental hygienist can counsel smokers regarding the deleterious effects of the habit on postsurgical healing.

Endosteal Root-Form Implants

Since the acceptance of Brânemark's endosteal dental implant system, many other root-form modalities have come onto the market. Brânemark's **two-stage** system is a characterized by a pure titanium, screw-type implant **body** (the bone anchoring component) with threads **(Figure 13-24).** Some of the new forms are **one-stage** cylinder-shaped bod-

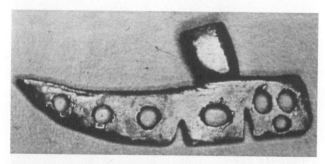

Figure 13-22. The blade type of endosteal implant. (Courtesy of HJ Bianco, Jr, DDS, MS, West Virginia University, Morgantown, WV. From DeBiase CB: Dental Health Education: Theory and Practice. Philadelphia, Lea & Febiger, 1991, p 148.)

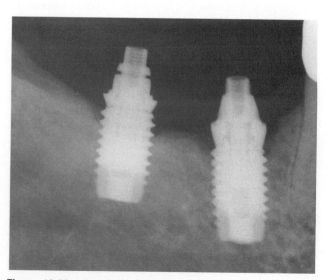

Figure 13-23. A radiographic view of a root-form endosteal implant. (Courtesy of Mark W. Richards, DDS, MS, West Virginia University, Morgantown, WV.)

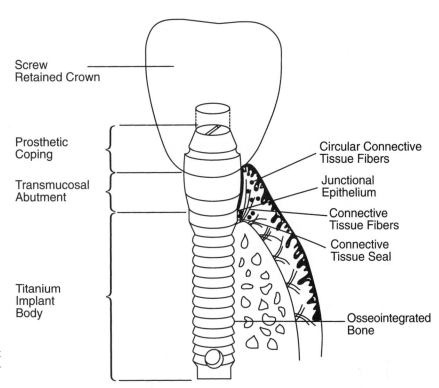

Screw
Retained Crown

Prosthetic
Coping

Transmucosal
Abutment

Titanium
Implant
Body

Circular Connective
Tissue Fibers

Junctional
Epithelium

Connective
Tissue Fibers

Connective
Tissue Seal

Osseointegrated
Bone

Figure 13-24. Components and periimplant tissues of a two-stage threaded, root-form endosteal implant system.

ies without threads; others have a hollow basket design. The implant body surfaces can be highly polished, matte finished, or coated with a rough titanium plasma spray (TPS). Hydroxyapatite (HA) or tricalcium phosphate (TCP) coatings are also used. The manufacturers claim that the different shapes and surface coatings promote more rapid and higher quality of osseointegration or **biointegration** (i.e., direct bonding with the bone as with ankylosed teeth).

In the first stage of surgery in a two-stage system, the implant body is placed into a drilled receptor site, covered, and allowed to osseointegrate for 4 months for mandibular implants and 6 months for maxillary implants. At the second stage of surgery, the implant body head is exposed, and a **transmucosal abutment** is added. The tissue is again allowed to heal for several weeks. During the prosthodontic phase of treatment, a **superstructure** is attached to the abutment, and either a fixed or removable restorative prosthesis is delivered.

Although the submerged, two-stage integrated dental implants are the most common dental implants in service today, one-stage implants, first developed by the International Team for Oral Implantology (ITI), are being placed and studied. Several manufacturers now provide a nonsubmerged implant to be installed in a single-stage surgical procedure, which allows the superstructure to be attached directly to the transmucosal implant body head. Prosthesis fabrication and placement is completed soon after the soft tissue has healed.

The most commonly used biomaterials for the endosteal dental implant fixture are commercially pure (CP) titanium and titanium-aluminum-vanadium alloy; however, one may

encounter ceramic, carbon, and composite materials. CP titanium is a low-density, high-strength metal that is highly biocompatible because it spontaneously forms an anticorrosion oxide film on its surface when exposed to air, water, or body fluids. This highly active titanium oxide film is responsible for osseointegration.

Implant Restorations

Depending on the clinical, functional, aesthetic, and psychological needs of the patient, the end-restoration can be fixed or removable, and constructed of porcelain, metal, or acrylic resin. The fixed restorations can have single or multiple units. Single tooth restorations can be permanently cemented, whereas multiple units are more often retained with screws. These implant-supported fixed prostheses are called retrievable because the restorative unit can be unscrewed and removed by the dental clinician when needed. The screw heads are either exposed or recessed in a "chimney" and covered with a composite material.

Full-arch prostheses can be either fully implant supported (removable or fixed) or partially soft tissue supported (removable). Removable implant overdentures are retained either mechanically (i.e., with clipbar and clips or ball and o-ring) or by use of a keeper and magnets **(Figure 13-25).**

Periimplant Environment

Like that of the natural tooth, the periimplant sulcus is lined with nonkeratinized sulcular epithelium (see Figure 13-25) at the base of which is junctional epithelial cells attached to

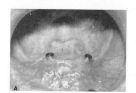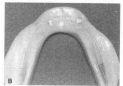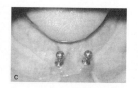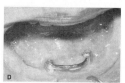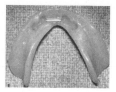

Figure 13-25. *A,* Two cylinder implants are magnetized to support a complete prosthesis as shown in *B. C,* Ball abutments can improve denture retention. *D,* Two cylinder implants can be used to support a bar. *E,* The prosthesis is made with a clip that attaches to the bar for retention. (Courtesy of HJ Bianco, Jr, DDS, MS, West Virginia University, Morgantown, WV. From DeBiase CB: Dental Health Education: Theory and Practice. Philadelphia, Lea & Febiger, 1991, pp 150 and 151.)

the implant surface by hemidesmosomes. It is the function of this "**biologic seal**" functions to protect the periimplant tissues from the potentially harmful oral environment. This mucosal seal must be maintained by thorough oral hygiene procedures by the patient and prophylactic treatment by the dental clinician.

The depth of the healthy submerged (two-stage) implant sulcus is determined by the thickness of the mucosa covering the alveolar ridge and, therefore, by the length of the transmucosal abutment. Because the microgap created by the junction of the fixture and abutment contains bacteria and cellular debris, the base of the junctional epithelium is always located apical to the microgap, making it possible to have a 2- to 6-mm depth of sulcus in healthy periimplant tissues. With the one-stage system, the lack of a fixture-abutment junction results in a 1- to 2-mm sulcus depth.

Apical to the junctional epithelium and coronal to the bone crest is a zone of connective tissue (>1 mm wide) that faces the implant. Investigations have shown that the histologic structure and composition of the periimplant connective tissue are significantly different from that of natural teeth. These differences have an impact on the tissues' defense and reaction to local microbial irritants. First, due to the lack of cementum on the implant surface, there are no dentoalveolar or dentogingival fiber bundles to attach the implant to the soft tissues. Holding these soft tissues close to the implant are circular collagen fibers running parallel to the bone surface and collagen fibers originating from the bone running to the gingival margin parallel to the implant.

Second, an examination of the connective tissue surrounding implants shows that the healthy periimplant soft tissues have a higher collagen content (85% vs 65%) and fewer fibroblasts (1%-3% vs 5%-15%) than that of healthy tissue surrounding teeth, equating the supracrestal tissue of the implant to scar tissue.

Finally, supracrestal tissues of teeth have a rich vascular supply from the supraperiosteal blood vessels and the vascular plexus of the periodontal ligament, whereas the vascular supply of the periimplant soft tissues is limited to those vessels originating from the supraperiosteal blood vessels. These findings have supported the speculation that periimplant tissues have an impaired defense against microflora irritants and magnify the importance of maintaining the integrity of the permucosal seal.

Research has demonstrated that microbial establishment and colonization on teeth and titanium implants follow the same patterns and that the compositions and volumes are similar in early (3-week) plaque formation. Longer exposure (3 months) was shown to produce more advanced mucosal lesions in the implant sites. In the natural teeth sites, the lesions were limited to the connective tissue, but the lesions around the implants involved both connective tissue and bone, leading investigators to think that the periimplant mucosa, with lower fibroblast content, was not as able to contain the plaque-associated lesion as with natural teeth. The shift from the early microflora to that associated with disease is the same for that found in the natural dentition and implant sites (**periimplantitis**), with the pocket flora characterized by gram-negative, anaerobic bacteria (e.g., *P. gingivalis, P. intermedia, A. actinomycetemcomitans, B. forsythus, C. rectus,* and spirochetes).

Dental Hygienist's Role in Implant Therapy

As a member of the dental team, the dental hygienist plays an important role in the care of patients who require implant therapy. In the pretreatment phase, the dental hygienist educates the patient about the proposed treatment plan; he or she used pictures and diagrams, videos and written material, and understandable terminology. The need for a commitment to good oral hygiene is emphasized, because the success of long-term dental implant therapy depends not only on good surgical and restorative techniques but also on meticulous plaque control. Plaque control efficiency should be 85% or better.

When the prosthesis is delivered, the hygienist helps to teach the patient about new measures to maintain the specific prosthesis and surrounding tissues. After receiving the prosthesis, the patient with a dental implant should be given maintenance treatment for 1 month for necessary débridement, baseline data collection, and review of oral hygiene. After this baseline is established, the implant health should be monitored and hygiene services should be provided as with a patient on "periodontal maintenance" treatment every 3 or 4 months. The intervals between visits should be determined by the patient's dexterity, rate of accumulation of deposit, health of the soft tissue, design of the prosthesis, and systemic considerations.

Baseline charting should include the implant modality and location of the dental implant (a subperiosteal implant may have a soft tissue reaction distant from an abutment), the type of prosthesis, and the screwdriver type for retrievable structures.

Attachment levels relative to a fixed reference point should be done at baseline. In some cases, this can be performed only when the superstructure is not in place. As mentioned earlier, abutment and tissue height may result in a reading greater than what would be considered "healthy" in the natural dentition; however, with dental implants, the actual reading in millimeters is not as critical as are changes in that measurement over time.

Routine probing is controversial. Because the probe does not stop at the epithelial attachment and penetrates deep into the connective tissue zone with average probing forces, thus disturbing the biologic seal, many clinicians recommend that probing be done only when pathology is suspected. Also, some fixed restorations will not allow probing with the long axis of the implant body due to a bulbous crown and narrow abutment. When probing is performed, only a plastic probe should be used with very light pressure.

As with all periodontal record keeping, one should routinely record the contour, consistency, and color of the soft tissues related to the implant; the presence of bleeding upon probing; and evidence of exudate. Lack of keratinized gingiva does not indicate the integrity of the implant is in jeopardy, but the soft tissues may be sensitive to oral hygiene procedures performed by the patient. A plaque record should be recorded.

At each maintenance appointment, the mobility of implants should be tested and noted. Because a healthy implant is firmly osseointegrated without the presence of a periodontal ligament, one would expect zero mobility. The patient should be asked about any discomfort or strange taste in the mouth, giving an indication of implant integrity and abutment or superstructure stability. If mobility is noted, the hygienist must be determine if the mobility is the result of loss of osseintegration, screw failure, or loss of a cement bond. Evidence of percolation of fluids or bubbles at the body-abutment or abutment-superstructure junctions may give a clue. Light percussion is another test for discomfort due to loss of osseointegration.

Because mobility testing does not detect early stages of periimplant pathology, the radiographic survey is a leading tool to test for the integrity of the implant. Recommendations suggest that radiographs of the implants be taken at baseline (i.e., when the restoration is delivered), at 6 months, then annually for the first 3 years. Thereafter, the patient can be monitored radiographically biannually, unless pathology is suspected. Use of a long cone paralleling technique with a position-indicating device produces a consistent image. Bone loss can also be "measured" by comparing bone level in relation to the threads of the implant. In addition to monitoring the bone level, radiographs can be used to detect periimplant radiolucencies and gaps between implant components.

The aim of débridement is to produce a clean surface without roughening, pitting, or altering the implant surface material. It is important to be familiar with the manufacturer's guidelines regarding the patient's implant system. Factors such as the surface texture of the fixture, the presence and extent of HA or plasma sprayed coating, and the location of the fixture and abutment junction must all be considered when submarginal roughness is encountered to determine if the roughness is calculus, residual cement, or natural implant structure.

Scratching of the implant surface promotes subsequent accumulation of deposits; it makes home care more difficult to manage and should be avoided during instrumentation. Damage to the HA or TPS surface may affect its biocompatability. Therefore, plastic, nylon, or graphite instruments are recommended for scaling hard deposits; the lightest pressure is necessary for removal of the deposit. Metal instruments and metal, sonic, and ultrasonic tips result in alteration of surface structure and may cause galvanic action, which leads to corrosion. These instruments are totally unacceptable for use on implants. Use of the air powder abrasive system can reach some areas that are inaccessible with plastic instruments and has been suggested for work on implants, except those with HA-coated fixtures. To avoid pitting, the system should be used cautiously at the lowest power setting and at a 45-degree angle to the implant. Air should be used to check the structures for complete removal of calculus.

Soft deposits are preferably removed with a toothbrush or other manual aids. Polishing should be done on a selective basis with a tin oxide or aluminum oxide paste and a highly flexible rubber cup or soft brush, using light pressure.

Severe etching of titanium implant surfaces has been demonstrated after 1 minute of exposure to acidic fluoride preparations. Thus sodium fluoride agents with a neutral pH should be used on patients who have titanium implants.

Retrievable prostheses, which create areas difficult for the patient to perform oral hygiene procedures (**Figure 13-26**), should be removed every 6 months to 1 year for evaluation of soft tissues and thorough débridement of abutment and superstructures. While in use, the small screwdriver should be ligated for safety. The prosthesis is maintained as with any prosthesis of the same materials.

Patient education can be a real challenge because many of these patients have had a history of a plaque-related disease, and some patients are under the misconception that dental implants are an easy, permanent solution for tooth loss. Totally edentulous patients may not have performed hygiene procedures around oral structures for some time. Other patients fear that they may harm the implant and are hesitant to perform necessary procedures. Patient education begins before the implant is placed and continues after placement at each maintenance appointment by identifying areas of need and positively reinforcing proper plaque control techniques. An in-the-mouth demonstration and patient practice along with written instructions and pictures is helpful in patient education.

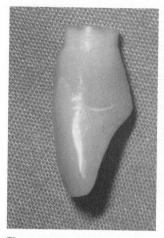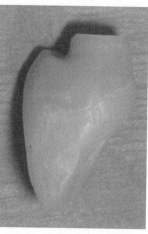

Figure 13-26. Two interim crowns from two different implant patients. Because of the lingual placement of the implant for the case on the right, aesthetics required a ridge lap on the facial of the crown, creating a plaque trap for the patient. (Courtesy of Mark W. Richards, DDS, MS, West Virginia University, Morgantown, WV.)

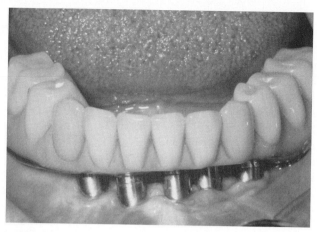

Figure 13-27. This hybrid "high-rise" denture is fully implant supported. Note the long exposed abutments. (Courtesy of Mark W. Richards, DDS, MS, West Virginia University, Morgantown, WV.)

When deciding which of the numerous home care products available to recommend, it is important to consider the patient's level of dexterity and motivation, along with abutment and prosthesis design. Brushing twice and flossing once daily is recommended, using the Bass brushing method around the soft tissue and Charter's brushing method for the underside of the fixed superstructure.

In addition to the standard toothbrush and floss, an interdental brush with plastic-coated inner wire can be used for open embrasures. The patient should be instructed to replace this brush before the covered wires become exposed. End tuft brushes and electric rotary brushes can effectively reach areas such as the tissue side of the hybrid, "high-rise" prosthesis **(Figure 13-27)**. The rotary brush is suitable for the patient with low dexterity and may help other patients to comply. The wooden point is another aid for hard-to-reach areas that is compatible with titanium dental implants. In addition to household yarn and shoelaces, ribbon gauze, sponge-type flosses, and special implant flosses are available on the market. These flosses are bulkier than the standard floss and are suitable for open embrasures and long, exposed abutments. Some are designed with an insertion tip, but a floss threader or crochet hook can help with placement. To cover the broad area of an abutment, the filament can be criss-crossed on the facial side and the abutment shoe-shined or buffed while moving the aid upward and downward. To ensure low abrasivity, an ADA-approved dentifrice is recommended.

For areas inaccessible to mechanical cleaning aids, such as tissues under a long flange or a ridge overlap restoration, daily antimicrobial application can help maintain soft tissue health. To keep staining of natural dentition and prostheses to a minimum, specific areas can be targeted by a brush, floss, cotton swab, or interdental sponge tip saturated with 0.12% chlorhexidine solution or with an irriga-tion device set at the lowest setting using a 0.06% chlorhexidine solution.

Implant Failure

Although well-placed endosseous dental implants have a high success rate, one occasionally fails (i.e., due to loose bone support). Investigation into these failures has shown that the two most common causes for dental implant failure after second-stage surgery are: (1) bacterial insult resulting in periimplantitis, and (2) excessive occlusal stress, or a combination of the two. Three signs of the failing implant are mobility, periimplant radiolucency, and pain on percussion or function. Those failing for bacterial-related causes are also characterized by pronounced gingival inflammation, heavy plaque, bleeding upon gentle probing, suppuration, and increased probing depths. Lack of periimplant radiolucency does not confirm adequate osseointegration, however, and one must evaluate the health of the implant by clinical observations.

Suggested Sources

Pathogenesis of Periodontal Disease

Altman LC, Page RC, Vandesteen GE, et al: Abnormalities of leukocyte chemotaxis in patients with various forms of periodontitis. J Periodontol Res 20:553-563, 1985.

Annals of Periodontology: International Workshop for a Classification of Periodontal Diseases and Conditions. Am Acad Periodontol 4:2-3, 53, 1999.

Beck JD, Garcia RI, Heiss G, et al: Periodontal disease and cardiovascular disease. J Periodontol 67:1123-1137, 1996.

Bergstrom J, Blomlof L: Tobacco smoking as a major risk factor associated with refractory periodontal disease (abstract). J Dent Res 71:297, 1992.

Blandizzi C, et al: Periodontal tissue disposition of azithromycin in patients affected by chronic inflammatory periodontal diseases. J Periodontol 70:960-966, 1999.

Carranza FA, Newman MG: Clinical Periodontology, 8th ed. Philadelphia, WB Saunders, 1996, pp 60, 91-92, 132, 218-223, 235-237, 251, 458-459.

Clemons GP, Reynolds, MA, Agarwal S, et al: Current concepts in the diagnosis and classification of periodontitis. California Dent Assoc J 18:33-38, 1990.

Fedi PF, Vernino AR, Gray JL: The Periodontic Syllabus, 4th ed. Philadelphia, Lippincott Williams & Wilkins, 2000, pp 12, 160-162.

Fleszar TJ, et al: Tooth mobility and periodontal therapy. J Clin Periodontol 7:495, 1980.

Genco RJ: Assessment of risk of periodontal disease. Compend Contin Educ Dent Suppl 18:S678-S683, 1994.

Gibbs CH, Hirschfield JW, et al: Description and clinical evaluation of a new computerized periodontal probe: The Florida Probe. J Clin Periodontol 15:137-144, 1988.

Glossary of Periodontal Terms of the American Academy of Periodontology. Chicago, American Academy of Periodontology, 1986.

Greenstein G, Polson A: The role of local drug delivery in the management of periodontal diseases: A comprehensive review. J Periodontol 69:507-520, 1998.

Haber J, Wattles J, Crowley M, et al: Evidence for cigarette smoking as a major risk factor for periodontitis. J Periodontol 64:16-23, 1993.

Haffajee AD, Socransky SS, et al: Clinical, microbiological, and immunological features of subjects with refractory periodontal diseases. J Clin Periodontol 15:390, 1988.

Hall EE: Prevention and treatment considerations in patients with drug-induced gingival enlargement. Curr Opin Periodontol 4:59-63, 1997.

Hart TCL: Genetic considerations of risk in human periodontal disease. Curr Opin Periodontol 2:3-11, 1994.

Hart TCL: Genetic risk factors for early onset periodontitis. J Periodontol 67:355-366, 1996.

Hughes FJ, Smales FC: Investigation of the distribution of cementum associated lipopolysaccharides in periodontal disease by scanning electron microscope immunohistochemistry. J Periodont Res 23:100, 1988.

Ilgenli T, Atilla G, Baylas H: Effectiveness of periodontal therapy in patients with drug-induced gingival overgrowth: Long-term results. J Periodontol 70:967-972, 1999.

Informational Paper on the Pathogenesis of Periodontal Diseases. The Research, Science, and Therapy Committee of the American Academy of Periodontology. J Periodontol 70:457-470, 1999.

Ismail II, Burt BA, Eklund SA: Epidemiologic patterns of smoking and periodontal disease in the United States. J Am Dent Assoc 106:617-623, 1983.

Jeffcoat MK, McGuire M, Newman MG: Evidence-based periodontal treatment: Highlights from the 1996 World Workshop in Periodontics. J Am Dent Assoc 128:713-724, 1997.

Jeffcoat MK, Reddy MS: Progression of probing attachment loss in adult periodontitis. J Periodontol 62:185-189, 1991.

Leon LE, Vogel RI: A comparison of the effectiveness of hand instrumentation and ultrasonic débridement in furcations as evaluated by differential darkfield microscopy. J Periodontol 58:86-94, 1987.

Loesche WJ, Syed SA, et al: The bacteriology of acute necrotizing ulcerative gingivitis. J Periodontol 53:223, 1982.

MacFarlane GD, Herzberg MC, Wolff LF, et al: Refractory periodontitis associated with abnormal polymorphonuclear leukocyte phagocytosis and cigarette smoking. J Periodontol 63:908-913, 1992.

McKechnie LB: Root morphology in periodontal therapy. Dent Hygienists News 6:3-6, 1993.

McMullen JA, VanDyke TE, Horoszewicz HU, Genco RJ: Neutrophil chemotaxis in individuals with advanced periodontal disease and a genetic predisposition to diabetes mellitus. J Periodontol 52:167-173, 1981.

Michalowicz BS: Genetic and heritable risk factors in periodontal disease. J Periodontol 65:479-488, 1994.

Michalowicz BS: Genetic risk factors for the periodontal diseases. Compend Contin Educ Dent 15(8):1036-1050, 1994.

Murray PA: HIV Disease as a risk factor for periodontal disease. Compend Contin Educ Dent 15(8):1052-1063, 1994.

Nakib NM, Bissadu N, Simmerlink J: Endotoxin penetration into root cementum of periodontally healthy and diseased human teeth. J Periodontol 53:368, 1982.

Offenbacher S, Katz VL, Fertik GS, et al: Periodontal infection as a risk factor for preterm low birthweight. J Periodontol 67:1103-1113, 1996.

O'Leary TJ: Tooth mobility. Dent Clin North Am 3:567, 1969.

Position Paper of the American Academy of Periodontology. Diabetes and Periodontal Diseases. J Periodontol 70:935-949, 1999.

Position Paper on Periodontal Disease as a Potential Risk Factor for Systemic Diseases. Committee on Research, Science and Therapy of the American Academy of Periodontology. J Periodontol 69:841-850, 1998.

Proceedings of the World Workshop in Clinical Periodontics. From the American Academy of Periodontology, Chicago, 1989.

Ramfjord SP, Ash MM: Periodontology and Periodontics. Philadelphia, WB Saunders, 1979.

Shaffer WG, Hine MK, Levy BM: A Textbook of Oral Pathology. Philadelphia, WB Saunders, 1983, pp 629, 782, 784-785.

Socransky SS, Goodson JM, Kung RT: Sulcular temperature and future attachment loss. J Dent Res 70:135, 1991.

Socransky SS, Haffajee AD, Goodson JM, Lindhe J: New concepts of destructive periodontal disease. J Clin Periodontol 11:21-32, 1984.

Sofaer JA: Genetic approaches in the study of periodontal disease. J Clin Periodontol 17:401-408, 1990.

Tavassoli S, Yamalik N, et al: The clinical effects of nifedipine on periodontal status. J Periodontol 69:108-112, 1998.

Tupta-Veselicky L, et al: A clinical study of an electronic constant force periodontal probe. J Periodontol 65:616-622, 1994.

Woodall I, Young NS, O'Heir TE: Periodontal Débridement: Comprehensive Dental Hygiene Care, 4th ed. St. Louis, CV Mosby, 1993, pp 533-570.

Periodontal Instrumentation and Subgingival Irrigation

American Academy of Periodontology: The Role of Supra- and Subgingival Irrigation in the Treatment of Periodontal Diseases. Chicago, AAP, 1995, pp 1-12.

Bee JL: Knowledge and Utilization of Ultrasonic/Sonic Scaling Instruments: A Survey of West Virginia Dental Hygienists. Thesis. Morgantown, WV, West Virginia University, 2000, pp 18-20.

Bray KK: Reaching Consensus on Power-Driven Instrumentation: Proceedings from the 1996 World Workshop in Periodontics. Access 12:26, 1998.

Carr M: Ultrasonics. Access Special Suppl, May-June 1999, pp 2-8.

Fong C: Dispelling air polishing myths. J Pract Hygiene 9:25, 2000.

Gladwin M, Bagby M: Clinical Aspects of Dental Materials. Philadelphia, Lippincott Williams & Wilkins, 2000, pp 193-198.

Greenstein G: Supragingival and subgingival irrigation: Practical application in the treatment of periodontal diseases. Compend Contin Educ Dent 13:1098, 1992.

Guignon AN: Expanding the role of ultrasonic scaling in clinical practical. J Pract Hygiene 9:30, 2000.

Jorgensen MG, Slots J: Practical antimicrobial periodontal therapy. Compend Contin Educ 21:111, 2000.

Keselyak N: Incorporating ultrasonics into clinical practice. Compend Contin Educ Suppl 7(3):7-10, 2000.

Low SB: Technology and ultrasonic débridement. Compend Contin Educ Oral Hygiene Suppl 7(3):3-5, 2000.

Lyle DM: Pharmacotherapeutics: The use of povidone-iodine in dentistry. J Pract Hygiene 9:57, 2000.

Miller CS, Leonelli FM, Latham E: Selective interference with pacemaker activity by electrical dental devices. Oral Surg Oral Med Oral Pathol Oral Radiol Endod 85:33-36, 1998.

Nield-Gehrig JS, Houseman GA: Fundamentals of Periodontal Instrumentation, 3rd ed. Philadelphia, Williams & Williams, 1996, pp xiii, 504.

Pattison AM, Pattison GL: Periodontal Instrumentation, 2nd ed. San Mateo, Appleton & Lange, 1992, pp viii, 485.

Perry DA, Beemsterboer P, Carranza FA: Techniques and Theory of Periodontal Instrumentation. Philadelphia, WB Saunders, 1990, pp ix, 388.

Schoen DH, Dean MC: Contemporary Periodontal Instrumentation. Philadelphia, WB Saunders, 1996, pp x, 246.

Wilkins EM: Clinical Practice of the Hygienist. Philadelphia, Lippincott Williams & Wilkins, 1999, pp 201-217, 295-297, 512-541, 544-563, 566-569, 603-616.

Young NA: Periodontal débridement: Re-examining non-surgical instrumentation. I: A new perspective on the objectives of instrumentation. Semin Dent Hygiene 4:1, 1994.

Young NA: Periodontal débridement: Re-examining non-surgical instrumentation. II: Expanding the role of ultrasonic and sonic instrumentation. Semin Dent Hygiene 5:1, 1995.

Implants

Adell R, Lekholm U, Rockler B, Branemark PI: A 15 year study of osseointegrated implants in the treatment of the edentulous jaw. Int J Oral Surg 10:387-416, 1981.

Assael LA: The nonsubmerged osseointegrated dental implant. Dent Clin North Am 42:203-223, 1998.

Augthun M, Tinschert J, Huber A: In vitro studies on the effect of cleaning methods on different implant surfaces. J Periodontol 69:857-864, 1998.

Berglundh T, Lindhe J: Dimension of the periimplant mucosa: Biological width revisited. J Clin Periodontol 23:971-973, 1996.

Berglundh T, Lindhe J, Ericsson I, et al: The soft tissue barrier at implants and teeth. Clin Oral Implants Res 2:81-90, 1991.

Berglundh T, Lindhe J, Jonsson K, Ericsson I: The topography of the vascular systems in the periodontal and periimplant tissues of dog. J Clin Periodontol 21:189-193, 1994.

Block MS, Kent JN, Guerra LR: Implants in Dentistry: Essentials of Endosseous Implants for Maxillofacial Reconstruction. Philadelphia, WB Saunders, 1997, pp 19, 260-261, 263, 269-270.

Buser D, Weber HP, Donath K, et al: Soft tissue reactions to nonsubmerged unloaded titanium implants in beagle dogs. J Periodontol 63:226-236, 1992.

Felo A, Shibly O, Ciancio SG, et al: Effects of subgingival chlorhexidine irrigation on periimplant maintenance. Am J Dent 10:107-110, 1997.

Koutsonikos A, Federico J, Yukna RA: Implant maintenance. J Pract Hygiene 5:11-15, 1996.

Leonhardt Å, Berglundh T, Ericsson I, Dahlén G: Putative periodontal pathogens on titanium implants and teeth in experimental gingivitis and periodontitis in beagle dogs. Clin Oral Implants Res 3:112-119, 1992.

Lindhe J, Karring T, Lang NP (eds): Clinical Periodontology and Implant Dentistry. Munksgaard, Munksgaard, 1997, pp 870-871.

Meffert RM, Langer B, Fritz ME: Dental implants: A review. J Periodontol 63:859-870, 1992.

Misch CE: Contemporary Implant Dentistry. St. Louis, CV Mosby, 1999, pp 245-248, 652-653.

Misch CE: Endosteal implants for posterior single tooth replacement: Alternatives, indications, contraindications, and limitations. J Oral Implantol 25:80-94, 1999.

Pontoriero R, Tonelli MP, Carnevale G, et al: Experimentally induced peri-implant mucositis: A clinical study in humans. Clin Oral Implants Res 5:254-259, 1994.

Pröbster L, Lin W, Höttemann H: Effect of fluoride prophylactic agents on titanium surfaces. Int J Oral Maxillofac Implants 7:390-394, 1992.

Steele DL, Orton GS: Hygiene/maintenance guidelines. In Fredrickson EJ, Stevens PJ, Gress ML: Implant Prosthodontics: Clinical and Laboratory Procedures. St. Louis, CV Mosby, 1995, pp 163-173.

Thomson ND, Evans G, Meffert R, Davenport WD: Effects of various prophylactic treatments on titanium, sapphire and hydroxyapatite-coated implants: An SEM study. Int J Periodontol Restor Dent 9:301-311, 1989.

Websites

www.dentalcare.com
www.jeffline.tju.edu/DHNet/cases/oralb/index.html
www.odont.lu.se/depts/par/virtual.html
www.perio.org

Questions and Answers

Questions

Periodontal Disease

1. The predominant oral flora seen in localized aggressive periodontitis (juvenile periodontitis) is:
   A. *Porphyromonas gingivalis*
   B. Spirochetes
   C. *Actinobacillus actinomycetemcomitans*
   D. *Eikenella corrodens*

2. A differential diagnosis between necrotizing ulcerative gingivitis (NUG) and acute herpetic gingivostomatitis is important because:
   A. NUG is considered contagious.
   B. Acute herpetic gingivostomatitis is considered contagious.
   C. NUG, if untreated, leads to erosive lichen planus.
   D. A and B.
   E. A and C.

3. When considering the prognosis of an infrabony pocket, which type of defect has the *best* prognosis?
   A. Three-wall
   B. Two-wall
   C. One-wall
   D. All with a similar prognosis

4. A healthy 14-year-old, African American, female patient presents to your dental practice. Her chief complaint is "loose teeth." The supervising dentist requests complete periodontal probing measurements. Measurements indicate >6 mm of attachment loss around the incisor and first molars. Based on the child's age and pocket distribution, your preliminary analysis would suggest that this patient is affected by:
   A. prepubertal periodontitis (i.e., periodontitis as a manifestation of systemic disease).
   B. localized juvenile periodontitis (i.e., localized aggressive periodontitis).
   C. generalized juvenile periodontitis (i.e., generalized aggressive periodontitis).
   D. chronic periodontitis.

5. The primary etiologic factor in gingivitis is:
   A. elevated steroid hormone levels.
   B. mouth breathing.
   C. bacterial plaque.
   D. nutritional deficiencies.

6. Which of the following statement is false?
   A. Bleeding on probing may be a clinical sign that the epithelial lining of the gingival sulcus of is ulcerated.
   B. Probing depths increase in gingivitis because the junctional epithelium and dentogingival connective tissue attachment has migrated apically.
   C. Inflamed gingival tissue contains gingival fibers that have been destroyed and increased fluid (edema) exists in the tissues.
   D. Inflamed gingival tissue may appear blue because of venous stagnation and anoxia in the tissues.

7. All of the following statements regarding gingival inflammation are true except one. What is the exception?
   A. The primary causative factor is dental calculus.
   B. No loss of gingival attachment or bone is seen in gingivitis.
   C. It is the most common form of periodontal disease.
   D. Contributing factors may include mouth breathing, or systemic factors such as pregnancy, oral contraceptives, or nutritional deficiencies.

8. Which of the follow statements best defines periodontitis?
   A. Periodontitis is an inflammation of the gingiva.
   B. Periodontitis is an inflammation of gingiva characterized by increased probing depths.
   C. Periodontitis is an inflammation of the periodontium, which is characterized by apical migration of the junctional epithelium with associated loss of attachment and crestal alveolar bone.
   D. Periodontitis is an inflammation of the periodontium characterized by increased probing depths and no loss of attachment or crestal alveolar bone.

9. A suprabony periodontal pocket is one in which the base of the sulcus and epithelial attachment are coronal to the crest of the alveolar bone. Is this statement correct?
   A. True
   B. False

10. Which of the following limit the effectiveness of nonsurgical periodontal periodontal débridement procedures?
    A. Probing depths >5 mm
    B. Probing depths in conjunction with furcations
    C. Limited access to the posterior teeth
    D. Dull instruments
    E. All of the above

11. The significance of an amalgam overhang as an etiologic agent in chronic periodontal disease has to do mainly with its role as a(an):
    A. mechanical irritant.
    B. plaque-retaining area.
    C. nondeflecting tooth surface.

D. overcontoured tooth surface.
E. method of impingement on interproximal gingival fibers.

12. Which of the following medications is **not** associated with gingival overgrowth?
    A. Carbamazepine
    B. Cyclosporine
    C. Nifedipine
    D. Phenytoin
    E. Verapamil

13. The transition from gingivitis to periodontitis is **BEST** associated with:
    A. increasing age of the patient.
    B. changes in the nutritional status of the patient.
    C. the presence of occlusal traumatism.
    D. changes in the composition of the bacterial plaque.
    E. the number of overhangs and overcontoured restorations.

14. Severe attachment loss is often associated with all of the following diseases except one. The EXCEPTION is

    _____.
    A. cyclic neutropenia.
    B. uncontrolled diabetes.
    C. hypophosphatasia.
    D. hyperparathyroidism.

15. A differential diagnosis of generalized destruction of alveolar bone in a 6-year-old child would include all of the following except one. The EXCEPTION is _____.
    A. prepubertal periodontitis (periodontitis as a manifestation of systemic disease).
    B. cystic fibrosis.
    C. Down syndrome.
    D. Chédiak-Higashi syndrome.

16. Which of the following parameters are accurate predictors of periodontal breakdown?
    A. Bleeding on probing
    B. Gram-negative anaerobic bacteria
    C. Probing depths
    D. All of the above
    E. None of the above

17. The severity of gingival overgrowth in patients taking phenytoin plus other antiseizure medications such as valproic acid is_____ patients taking phenytoin alone.
    A. less than
    B. greater than
    C. similar to

18. All of the following are objectives of nonsurgical periodontal débridement except one? The EXCEPTION is

    _____.
    A. provide a root surface free of endotoxin.
    B. promote shrinkage of probing depths.
    C. resolve bone defects.
    D. reduce or eliminate the amount of bleeding upon probing.

Periodontal Instruments, Instrumentation, Débridement Irrigation, and Air-Powder Polishing

19. Where does the work stroke with a scaler during periodontal débridement begin?
    A. In connective tissue
    B. On the surface of the calculus
    C. In the junctional epithelium
    D. At the apical edge of the junctional epithelium
    E. At the coronal edge of the junctional epithelium

20. The patient has a 5-mm probing depth on the mesial of the distal root of tooth No. 30 on which there is 3 mm of recession. Which of the following instruments would best access this root for periodontal débridement?
    A. 1/2 Gracey
    B. 11/12 Gracey
    C. 13/14 Gracey
    D. 11/12 After Five Gracey
    E. 13/14 After Five Gracey

21. The goal of periodontal débridement is to produce a periodontal environment free of infection. This is accomplished by smoothing the roots to a hard glassy surface in order to remove endotoxins.
    A. Both statements are TRUE.
    B. Both statements are FALSE.
    C. The first statement is TRUE; the second one is FALSE.
    D. The first statement is FALSE; the second one is TRUE.

22. All of the following instruments have two usable cutting edges on one blade EXCEPT one. Which one is the exception?
    A. Sickle scaler
    B. Jaquette scale
    C. Universal curet
    D. Gracey curet

23. When a universal curet, Gracey curet, or sickle scaler is properly adapted for the work stroke in calculus removal, the angle formed by the facial surface of the blade to the tooth surface is:
    A. 0 degrees.
    B. 45 degrees.
    C. >0 degrees <45 degrees.
    D. >45 degrees <90degrees.
    E. >90 degrees <110 degrees.

24. Which visual cue indicates proper working angulation of a Gracey curet?
    A. Terminal shank perpendicular to the tooth
    B. Terminal shank parallel to the tooth surface
    C. Terminal shank parallel to the long axis of the tooth
    D. Handle parallel to the tooth
    E. Handle perpendicular to the long axis of the tooth

25. A cutting edge on a universal or Gracey curet is formed by the junction of
    A. two lateral surfaces.
    B. the facial and back surfaces.
    C. one lateral surface and the facial surface.
    D. one lateral surface and the back surface.

26. The universal curet is designed so that the angle of the face of the curet blade to the terminal shank of the instrument is
    A. 0 degrees.
    B. 45 degrees.
    C. 70 degrees.
    D. 90 degrees.
    E. 110 degrees.

27. Along what area of the blade of a universal curet, Gracey curet, or sickle scaler should a sharpening stone be moved during sharpening of an instrument?
    A. Back surface
    B. Lateral surface
    C. Junction of the facial and lateral surfaces
    D. Junction of the back and lateral surfaces

28. Which of the following instruments is best suited for scaling a root surface?
    A. Curet
    B. Sickle
    C. File
    D. Hoe
    E. Chisel

29. Power-scaling devices include ultrasonic and sonic scalers. Both of these power-scaling devices can be used successfully in periodontal débridement.
    A. Both statements are TRUE.
    B. Both statements are FALSE.
    C. The first statement is TRUE; the second one is FALSE.
    D. The first statement is FALSE; the second one is TRUE.

30. Piezoelectric ultrasonic scalers may interfere with the function of a pacemaker worn by a patient, BECAUSE they produce a magnetic field.
    A. Both the statement and the reason are correct and related.
    B. Both the statement and the reason are correct and NOT related.
    C. The statement is correct, but the reason is incorrect.
    D. The statement is NOT correct, but the reason is correct.
    E. NEITHER the statement NOR the reason is correct.

31. All of the following are true concerning the use of the longer slim ultrasonic inserts designed for subgingival débridement EXCEPT one. Which one is the exception?
    A. Heat production may cause pulpal damage.
    B. Avoid use on implants.
    C. Adapt to the tooth surface similar to the hand instrument counterpart.
    D. Adapt to the tooth surface similar to that of a periodontal probe.

32. The quick turnover rate of crevicular fluid inhibits retention of a single procedure of subgingival irrigation. Therefore, to achieve any bactericidal effect, an agent exhibiting substantivity is recommended for subgingival irrigation.
    A. Both statements are TRUE.
    B. Both statements are FALSE.
    C. The first statement is TRUE; the second one is FALSE.
    D. The first statement is FALSE; the second one is TRUE.

33. Which antimicrobial agent has NOT been used for subgingival irrigation?
    A. Stannous fluoride
    B. Acidulated phosphate fluoride
    C. Povidone-iodine
    D. Chlorhexidine gluconate
    E. Tetracycline

34. Air powder polishing is contraindicated for all of the following EXCEPT one. Which one is the exception?
    A. Hypertensive patients
    B. Metallic restorations
    C. Nonmetallic restorations

Implants

35. During the examination of a patient, you notice mobility of a two-stage implant. Percussion of the implant does not cause discomfort for the patient. Gentle probing of the implant yields 4- to 5-mm probing depths, consistent with baseline records. The tissues have a normal contour and color, and there is no bleeding on provocation or suppuration. The radiograph shows no periimplant radiolucency or crestal bone loss. Clinical observations indicate:
    A. signs of periimplantitis.
    B. the implant is failing.
    C. a loose abutment.
    D. excessive occlusal forces.

36. To remove light calculus covering implant abutments,
    A. scale with high carbon steel instruments, using very light pressure.
    B. scale with a sonic instrument, because it has a lower frequency than the ultrasonic instrument.
    C. polishing with a course abrasive paste is all that is needed.
    D. plastic, nylon, or graphite instruments are the instruments of choice.

37. The interface between the soft tissues and the implant head can best be described as
    A. a firm chemical adhesion by hemidesmosomes.
    B. similar to that found between the soft tissues and natural teeth.
    C. a fragile seal dependent on hemidesmosomes and close adaptation of circular fibers.
    D. a direct adhesion called biointegration.

38. Investigations comparing the periimplant soft tissues with the periodontal tissues surrounding the natural tooth indicate that the periimplant soft tissues have
    A. greater defense against microbial attack because of their rich vascular supply.
    B. greater defense against microbial attack because of the firm connective tissue barrier formed with the implant.
    C. impaired defense against microbial attack because of their lower collagen content.
    D. impaired defense because of their lower fibroblast content.

ANSWERS

Periodontal Disease

1. **C.** *Actinobacillus actinomycetemcomitans* has been found to predominate in the localized aggressive periodontitis (juvenile periodontitis) lesion. The other organisms are also seen in chronic and aggressive periodontitis.

2. **B.** Acute herpetic gingivostomatitis is considered contagious. It is of the herpes viral origin. Although NUG is not contagious and is of bacterial etiology, NUG can be a manifestation of an underlying systemic condition (e.g., HIV infection). It can also be caused by smoking or stress.

3. **A.** The more walls that are present, the better is the prognosis of the defect. Thus, a three-wall defect has the best prognosis.

4. **B.** This patient appears to have localized juvenile periodontitis (localized aggressive periodontitis). It is localized because it affects only the incisors and molars. It is considered to be aggressive due to the age of the patient.

5. **C.** Plaque is ALWAYS considered to be the primary etiologic factor in periodontal disease.

6. **B.** There is no apical migration of the connective tissue attachment in gingivitis. Gingivitis involves no loss of connective tissue attachment or bone.

7. **A.** This statement is false, because calculus is NEVER considered to be a primary etiologic factor in the development of gingival disease. It is actually the plaque that forms on the surface of the calculus.

8. **C.** Gingivitis involves inflammation of the free and attached gingival tissues. There may even be pseudo-pockets present if the gingivitis involves hyperplasia. There is no loss of attachment or crestal bone.

9. **A.** This statement is true. An infrabony periodontal pocket is one in which the pocket bottom is apical to the epithelial attachment and crest of the alveolar bone. It is located within the bone.

10. **E.** All of the above are factors that can limit the effectiveness of nonsurgical periodontal débridement procedures.

11. **B.** The significance of any iatrogenic restoration is that it becomes a plaque retention area.

12. **A.** The medications that have been associated with gingival hyperplasia are the calcium channel blockers: verapamil and nifedipine; the antirejection drug cyclosporine; and the anti-seizure medication phenytoin. The antiseizure medication carbamazepine has NOT been associated with gingival hyperplasia.

13. **D.** The most documented change from gingivitis to periodontitis occurs when the bacterial plaque changes from gram-positive cocci to vibrios, spirochetes, gram-negative rods, anaerobes, and motile bacteria.

14. **D.** Hyperparathyroidism is not usually associated with periodontal disease.

15. **B.** Cystic fibrosis is not usually associated with periodontal disease.

16. **E.** There are currently NO accurate predictors of periodontal disease. The only way to determine whether active disease (connective tissue attachment and bone loss) has occurred is to monitor attachment levels over time.

17. **B.** Phenytoin is the only antiseizure medication that has been associated with gingival overgrowth. However, when it is taken in combination with ANY other antiseizure medication, the overgrowth is greater than with phenytoin alone.

18. **C.** Nonsurgical periodontal débridement alone cannot resolve bone defects.

Periodontal Instruments, Instrumentation, Débridement Irrigation, and Air-Powder Polishing

19. **E.** The coronal edge is the base of the pocket or sulcus. As long as the work stroke is activated at this point, all subgingival plaque and calculus should be removed.

20. **D.** A mesial Gracey curet should be used on the mesial surface of any root whether or not the tooth is a single or multirooted tooth. In addition, the total attachment loss around this tooth is 8 mm; therefore, an After Five Gracey should be used because its shank is 3 mm longer than that of a traditional Gracey curet.

21. **C.** The goal of periodontal débridement is to produce an environment free of infection. Research has shown, however, that endotoxins that cause the infection adhere only loosely to the root surface and can be removed without excessive smoothing of the root.

22. **D.** There is only one usable cutting edge on a Gracey curet. Each of the other three choices has two usable cutting edges on a blade.

23. **D.** Any angle less than 45 degrees would place the face of the instrument against the tooth and could burnish calculus. An angle equal to or greater than 90 degrees would place a lateral surface against the tooth and the opposite cutting edge against the sulcular lining. This would result in burnishing of calculus and laceration of the sulcular lining.

24. **B.** A Gracey curet is designed with the blade offset to the terminal shank so that when the terminal shank is parallel to the surface being scaled and the cutting edge is properly positioned against the tooth. The long axis of the tooth may not always be parallel with the surface of the tooth being scaled. The position of the handle of a Gracey curet has nothing to do with correct adaptation of a Gracey cutting edge.

25. **C.** Two lateral surfaces do not junction on a blade, nor do a facial and back surface. The lateral surface is continuous with the back surface and forms a round half-moon shape with no formation of an angle.

26. **D.** The only angles formed by the face of the blade to the terminal shank are 90 degrees for a universal curet and sickle curet and 110 degrees (70 degrees opposite the angle) for a Gracey curet.

27. **B.** Placing the stone against the junction of the facial and lateral surface would dull the instrument blade, because the stone would be against the cutting edge. The object of sharpening is to remove either the lateral or facial surface until the two surfaces (facial and lateral) junction.

28. **A.** A curet has a curved blade that better adapts to a rounded root. The other choices have sharp angular blades that can gouge a round root.

29. **A.** Sonic and ultrasonic scalers are power driven and have been shown to successfully débride root surfaces of endotoxin without excessive removal of the root surface.

30. **E.** Piezoelectric ultrasonic scalers produce no magnetic field and, therefore, do not interfere with the function of a pacemaker.

31. **C.** Slimline inserts must be adapted with the entire length of the insert tip against the tooth. Placement of the instrument against the tooth as one would place a hand instrument blade would displace the gingiva and would not sufficiently reach the pocket depth.

32. **A.** The property of substantivity allows the agent to remain in the area for a while and would enhance the action of a chemotherapeutic agent during a single application.

33. **C.** Acidulated phosphate fluoride is used only to prevent caries.

34. **B.** The baking soda used in an air powder polisher can enter the bloodstream and is contraindicated for hypertensive patients. The salt can also create pitting of nonmetallic restorations.

Implants

35. **C.** Mobility of an implant may be due to failure of retention at implant component junctions (i.e., screw failure or loss of a cement bond).

36. **D.** Investigations have shown that plastic, nylon and graphite instruments produce the least damage to implant parts when compared with other scaling modalities.

37. **C.** The adhesion provided by the hemidesmosomes of the junctional epithelium is fragile and easily disturbed by mechanical forces and microbial byproducts. Implants lack a surface analogous to the cementum of the natural tooth that provides for insertion of connective tissue fibers.

38. **D.** As with scar tissue, there is a lower fibroblast content, which may compromise the tissues' ability to repair damage done by the microbial byproducts.

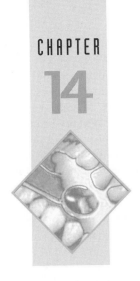

Dental Caries/Utilizing Preventive Agents

JACK S. YORTY, DDS

Dental caries is a dietobacterial disease of the hard dental structures. It represents a potential continuum from microscopic changes on a tooth surface and subsurface to complete destruction of the entire coronal portion of a tooth. The presence of dental caries has been noted throughout history and has continued to plague people, especially in newly industrialized countries. The availability of refined sugars and fermentable carbohydrates has allowed this disease to reach epidemic proportions during the 17th, 18th, and 19th centuries. Only recently has its complex nature become better understood, and measures to halt its progress have come into common practice. Although a great deal has been learned about caries etiology and epidemiology, most of the emphasis during the 20th century has been on repairing the damage caused by caries disease and not on its scientific management.

This chapter addresses the current concepts of evidence-based care and medical model management of dental caries disease. The 21st century will undoubtedly bring better methods for prevention, earlier detection, and reversal of initial caries lesions. The dental profession must be ready to utilize new scientifically based knowledge and combine it with current proven management techniques to best serve the public's needs and expectations.

ORAL ECOSYSTEM

Saliva

Proper management of caries disease begins with an understanding of the oral cavity's ecosystem. Although the oral cavity is unique for each individual, it has many common characteristics. One of the most important of these characteristics is saliva. **Saliva** is formed primarily from the major and minor salivary glands and is secreted into the mouth, where

it is mixed with crevicular fluid to form a proteinaceous film that coats all surfaces of the oral cavity. An average adult produces about 0.5 to 1.0 L of saliva every day and 1 to 2 ml/min when at rest. Production of saliva varies based on the time of day and with stimulation. Human saliva contains many components. Inorganic minerals such as calcium and phosphates aid in remineralization of damaged hydroxyapatite, which is the primary structure of tooth enamel crystals. Microorganisms are found in abundance in saliva. Approximately 200 to 300 species of bacteria, yeast, and protozoa have been identified in the human oral cavity. If the ecologic balance of these microorganisms is altered, colonization of high numbers of pathogenic species may occur, resulting in the development of caries or periodontal disease. Secretory antibodies from an individual's immune system, which are also found in saliva, may help to keep the pathogenic microorganisms in check. The dynamic nature of bacterial colonization, which is perhaps influenced by diet, poor hygiene, or other factors, could overwhelm any immune response. This can result in a destructive disease process, either localized or generalized. The changes that occur on the tooth surface may cause such varying alterations in the microscopic environments that either **demineralization** or **remineralization** may occur. Many factors influence the surface dynamics. As a key factor in this process, saliva:

- Enhances the clearance of food-derived carbohydrates
- Reduces and dilutes harmful metabolic products (acids)
- Provides a protective coating that may prevent adhesion of cariogenic bacteria
- Has immunoglobulins, agglutinins, and proteolytic enzymes that may be bactericidal
- Allows for buffering of pH after sugar challenges
- Contains calcium, fluoride, phosphate, and other minerals that enhance remineralization and resistance against cariogenic agents[1]

If the metabolic activity of the microorganisms in plaque is increased (e.g., by a sucrose challenge), enough acid byproducts could be generated to adversely affect the delicate equilibrium on the tooth surface and result in loss of minerals. The loss may progress enough to cause a wide variety of changes, ranging from white spots to cavitation and ultimately to pulp exposure.

Microorganisms

Colonization of microorganisms on the tooth surfaces usually begins with *Streptococcus sanguis* and *Streptococcus mitis*. *Streptococcus mutans* arrives later in large enough numbers to cause harm, only if conditions are right. High and frequent doses of sucrose in the host's diet can promote this change in flora. Colonization of bacteria is a complex process that involves interactions among all oral microorganisms and their environment. All organisms must have a favorable environment for growth and must survive competition from other bacterial strains. Each population occupies an **ecologic niche** (a special combination of food and shelter) within the host community. When the niche becomes saturated, only very competitive microorganisms can displace indigenous bacteria. Environmental changes can occur that may be harmful to bacteria. These would include oral hygiene procedures or antimicrobial therapy that might suppress normal flora and allow yeasts to overgrow and become dominant. Unrestricted growth of plaque produces local environmental conditions that may selectively promote the accumulation of pathogenic bacterial species. The earliest bacteria to colonize tooth surfaces are grampositive cocci and rods. As the community becomes more complex, anaerobic bacteria begin to establish themselves. After 14 days, the undisturbed plaque reaches a very complex composition. The composition of the oral flora is dependent on the oral environment and is influenced by three main factors: the host, factors external to the host, and factors associated with the bacterial community. After treatment, isolated reservoirs of bacteria (e.g., the tongue, periodontal pockets, tonsillar pillars) can serve as seed areas that may recolonize other host sites or other individuals. Colonization is complex and may be site specific. Saliva (the host factor) plays a significant role in maintaining balance with the ecosystem on tooth surfaces. Saliva helps to maintain control over the oral flora through its antibacterial components (e.g., IgA, IgG, and IgM), cleansing activity, nutrients, and pH buffering capacity. Diet, an external factor, can influence the microflora in several ways. Fibrous foods can physically cleanse the tooth, and foods with fermentable carbohydrates can be metabolized by bacteria in plaque to produce organic acids.

Plaque

Bacteria adhere to the tooth surface by becoming incorporated with the proteinaceous salivary coating called the **pellicle.** Bacterial colonies, pellicle, and debris make up the film called **dental plaque**. Plaque is a soft, translucent, and tenaciously adherent material that accumulates on tooth surfaces. It consists mainly of bacteria and their products. Microorganisms make up the bulk of the mass of dental plaque. Dr. Walter Loesche proposed the **specific plaque theory** in the 1970s. His idea was that not all components of dental plaque are pathogenic. Management of either caries or periodontal disease should be directed toward the specific harmful microorganisms. This is the basis of the **medical model** approach for treating all types of diseases. Plaque is deemed pathogenic only when signs of associated disease are present. The general activity of plaque growth and maturation is predictable and of therapeutic importance. The goal of therapy is to suppress cariogenic plaque and replace it with pathogen-free plaque. Mechanical débridement and chemical agents applied to achieve short periods of sterility on the tooth surface can reduce the number of colonies of *S. mutans* and allow them to be replaced with less harmful colonies of *S. sanguis* and *S. mitis*.[2]

Because dental caries may occur throughout life, it is important to make an early, accurate diagnosis and begin treatment (remineralization) as soon as possible. The goal of early treatment is to reduce all unfavorable conditions in order to prevent cavitation. Safe alteration of the oral environment in order to control pathogenic bacteria and still maintain a well-balanced symbiosis among all oral microorganisms and the host is the preferred outcome. The medical model of caries disease management is designed to achieve this outcome. A brief description of this approach is shown in **Table 14-1.**

Acid Challenge (Stephan Curve)

Organic acids cause a drop in local environmental pH. The drop in pH can be seen over time as challenges occur from the sugar availability. This is shown in the **Stephan curve (Figure 14-1).** This curve measures changes in pH in vivo with an antimony electrode following a glucose rinse. Curve I depicts caries-free individuals. Curve II shows caries-inactive subjects. Curve III represents the response for slight caries-active subjects. Curve IV shows the response for

TABLE 14–1 Medical Model

Etiology	*Streptococcus mutans* infection
Symptoms	Demineralization of tissue in tooth
Treatment, symptomatic	Restoration of cavitated lesions
Treatment, therapeutic	Elimination of *S. mutans* infection
Symptomatic post-treatment Assessment	Examine teeth for new lesions
Therapeutic post-treatment Assessment	Bacteriological testing for *S. mutans*

From Sturdevant CM: The Art and Science of Operative Dentistry, 2nd ed. St. Louis, CV Mosby, 1995, p 64.

marked caries-active subjects. Curve V depicts extreme caries-active subjects.

Acid production from caries-active plaque can overcome the buffering capacity of saliva and cause a local drop in pH that is sufficient to dissolve tooth minerals. Continuous acid attack on the tooth may occur from 20 to 50 minutes after exposure to sucrose. At a pH of 5.5, the enamel surface minerals remain intact, but subsurface mineral is being lost.

Enamel Surface Dynamics

The pathologic process can be reversed, prevented, or delayed by removing or changing adverse environmental factors **(Figure 14-2)**. This should be done without any long-term impact on resident (normal) microflora through:

1. **Diet modification:** reduction of sucrose, glucose, and fructose and increased use of sugar-free (artificial sweeteners) or sugar alcohols such as xylitol, sorbitol, and mannitol.
2. **Fluorides:** the number of fluoride ions diffusing into plaque increase as the pH drops. This reduces the bacterial cell metabolism and results in decreased acid production.
3. **Antimicrobials:** the bisbiguanides (e.g., chlorhexidine) are effective against yeasts and most bacteria. They are both bacteriostatic and bactericidal; they interfere with bacterial membrane function, including substrate trans-

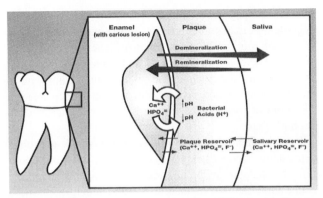

Figure 14-2. Enamel surface dynamics. (From Winston AE, Bhaskar SN: Caries prevention in the 21st century. J Am Dent Assoc 129:1580, 1998.)

port and maintenance of ion gradients. Biguanides are released slowly and have good **substantivity**. No resistant strains have been developed, which makes it suitable for long-term therapy.[1]

Loesche describes the tooth surface dynamics in the following statement. "A state of equilibrium sets in when the acid produced by the endogenous catabolism of the reserve polymers is neutralized by the salivary buffers and the exiting tooth mineral. As the pH returns to neutrality, the net flux of calcium and phosphate from the tooth is balanced by the diffusion of these ions into the tooth from the supersaturated plaque fluid and saliva. The equilibrium condition reflects a transitional period and gives way to a remineralization phase. In this remineralization phase, the plaque acid production is minimal or nonexistent, so that conditions favor the continued diffusion of calcium and phosphate ions into the tooth. The fluoride ions, which are found invariably in low levels in the plaque, migrate with the calcium and phosphate ions and enhance the formation of hydroxyapatite and fluorapatite in the superficial enamel layer. Successive cycles of demineralization-remineralization lead to a fortification of the superficial enamel layer with fluorapatite, which gives this layer added resistance to acid demineralization. If the remineralization periods are in excess of the demineralization episodes, the subsurface lesion will mineralize, and the caries lesion will arrest. However, if the frequency of sucrose consumption is great, and if *S. mutans* or *Lactobacilli* come to dominate in the plaque flora, the repair process associated with remineralization is overwhelmed and cavitation occurs."[2]

S. mutans are more closely associated with initial caries than are *Lactobacilli*. Resident normal flora such as *S. mitis* and *S. sanguis* can produce sufficient acid to demineralize enamel, but only in unusual circumstances. Bacterial succession to an acid environment shows that *S. mutans* may cause early demineralization and that *Lactobacilli* will colonize demineralized white spot enamel lesions subsequent to *S. mutans*.

Infected dentin has a low pH and hosts a less diverse bacterial community. Dentin collagen becomes degraded, and

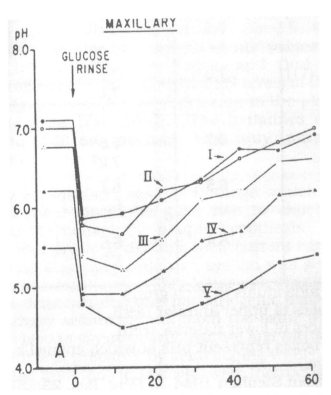

Figure 14-1. Stephan curve. (From Loesche WJ: Dental caries: A treatable infection. Grand Haven, MI, ADD, 1995, p 213.)

minerals are dissolved. This process favors bacteria that can degrade and metabolize proteins and peptides. Demineralization of root surfaces occurs at a higher pH level than enamel. Therefore, less aciduric and acidogenic strains of *Streptococcus* and *Actinomyces viscosus* may contribute to the development and progression of root surface lesions. The flora of root surface lesions is similar to that of deep dentin lesions.

Dental plaque consists of numerous small microbial ecosystems, which each consist of a unique microflora. Significant changes to the environment of any isolated site could allow the development of a pathogenic group whose acid-producing metabolism dominates the ecosystem, thus leading to demineralization.[1]

Various oral bacteria form extracellular polysaccharides. These bacteria make up part of the acellular matrix of dental plaque and enable it to resist cleansing forces. Oral environments that are deficient in saliva support a mainly acidogenic and aciduric flora with high numbers of *S. mutans* and *Lactobacilli.* This is most clearly seen in patients with **xerostomia** (extremely dry mouth). Saliva substitutes do not provide the buffers, cleansing action, and remineralization functions that adequate amounts of whole, natural saliva can provide.

Oral bacteria are nourished by the saliva bath in which they live. Glucose, pyruvate, lactic acid, urea, glycoprotein, and vitamins have been measured in human saliva. Food consumption by the host results in an explosion of nutrients that can overwhelm oral bacteria. Most oral bacteria grow in a pH range of 6 to 8, but some are aciduric and grow at lower pH values. Such lower pH values are reached when a large or continuous intake of sugar occurs. Dietary sucrose provides a selective advantage to establishment of *S. mutans* and greatly increases their prevalence in plaque.

Sugars contribute in at least two ways to the pathogenesis of dental caries. Polymers are produced as byproducts that form an intermicrobial matrix that binds the bacteria to the teeth. Metabolic end-products are excreted, thus causing a drop in the pH of dental plaque.

The acidity of the tooth environment is not only influenced by the number and species of bacteria present but also by the buffering capacity of saliva and plaque fluid, the flow rate and viscosity of saliva, the diffusion characteristics of plaque, the presence of fluoride in enamel and plaque, the type of diet ingested, and the frequency of sugar intake. When the pH of plaque drops below a critical value, calcium phosphates in enamel hydroxyapatite become soluble and tooth materials are lost. **Lactic acid** is the main acid produced upon exposure of plaque to sugars, and this is the major cause of the drop in pH.

Pellicle forms within minutes after a tooth surface is cleaned. It reaches a thickness of 0.01 to 1 mm within 24 hours (uncolonized). Major constituents of pellicle include salivary glycoproteins, phosphoproteins, lipids, and gingival sulcular fluid. At 4 hours, there are very few bacteria in pellicle. At 8 to 12 hours, a coating of bacteria is present. Coc-coid bacteria and a few filamentous bacteria can be identified at 24 hours. At 48 hours, the composition consists mainly of filamentous organisms. *S. mutans* comprises only about 2% of the initial streptococcus microflora. This is thought to be due to its low concentration in saliva.[1] A shift occurs between 24 and 36 hours to a plaque dominated by *Actinomyces.* Anaerobic organisms such as *Corynebacterium* predominate after 9 days. Calculus may be detected in fissures and pits of caries-inactive individuals in as early as 7 days. Various acids (e.g., acetate, lactate, formate, and butyrate) can be produced in resting saliva. When fermentable carbohydrate is available to plaque, a rapid shift to lactate occurs, which corresponds to a drop in pH. It gradually increases to approach normal (pH 6.0-7.0) in 30 to 60 minutes (Stephan curve). The buffering capacity of plaque is 10 times higher than that of saliva.[1]

LESION DEVELOPMENT

Dental caries is a chronic disease that progresses very slowly. It is seldom self-limiting and can progress until the whole tooth is destroyed. The **lesion** is the localized area of destruction and is the sign of the disease. It represents a continuum that ranges from microscopic mineral loss to total tooth devastation. The tooth surface is unique in that it is not covered with surface shedding epithelium. The enamel is a microporous solid that consists of tightly packed crystals (hydroxyapatite). Demineralized enamel is more porous than healthy enamel. This can make measurement of mineral loss possible. Enamel's optical properties change with porosity. Enamel lesions become less translucent and appear as white/opaque spots. Mineral loss can be equated with the porosity of enamel. Drying the tooth, polarized light, and x-rays are methods used to estimate porosity or mineral loss.

Oral bacteria tend to colonize and grow in areas of the dentition where they are protected against intraoral mechanical disturbances. These areas are called **retention sites** or **stagnation areas.**[1] The most common retention sites are the occlusal pits and fissures, proximal surfaces below contact areas, smooth surfaces below the height of contour, and root surfaces, respectively. After 14 days of undisturbed plaque formation, the enamel changes become macroscopically visible after air-drying. After 3 to 4 weeks with undisturbed plaque formation, the outermost microsurface exhibits complete dissolution with subsurface layer developmental irregularities. At this stage, it is possible to identify the classical zones of a **white spot** enamel lesion **(Figure 14-3).** The **surface zone** is a virtually unaffected area. It is wedge-shaped with its base at the enamel surface. The **translucent zone** is a structureless area about 5 to 100 μm in width, which is the advancing front of the lesion. The **dark zone** is located between the translucent zone and the body of the lesion. It is seen 90% to 95% of the time.[3]

Because the enamel is a microporous solid, it allows stimuli from the oral cavity to pass through it into the pulpo-

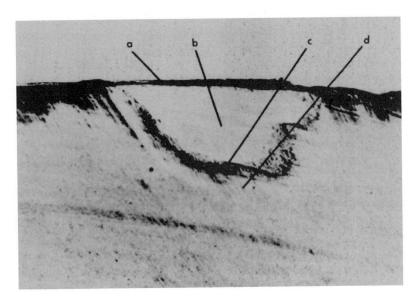

Figure 14-3. Incipient lesion zones. [From Silverston LM, et al (eds): Dental Caries. London and Basingstoke, Macmillan, 1981. In Sturdevant CM: The Art and Science of Operative Dentistry, 3rd ed. CV Mosby, 1995, p 93.]

dentinal organ system. The most common reaction to stimulation is **tubular sclerosis.** This sclerosis occurs before the front edge of the enamel lesion reaches the dentinoenamel junction. Dentinal changes represent a continuum of pulpodentinal reactions to variations in acid challenge at the enamel surface. Bacterial invasion into the dentinal tubules is merely a sign of lesion progression. Dentin begins to decompose due to acid action and proteolytic enzymes. **Dead tracts** may be produced if bacterial invasion is rapid. These tracts are odontoblastic processes that are destroyed without the production of **sclerotic dentin.**[1] Brown discoloration at the dentinoenamel junction occurs as a result of the biochemical changes of collagenous dentin due to the demineralization and incorporation of exogenous pigments.

When the demineralization of the dentin approaches the pulp at a distance of between 0.5 and 1 mm, inflammatory reactions may be seen in the subodontoblastic region. There is no infection of the pulp as yet, and inflammation is the result of bacterial products.[1]

On root surfaces, active lesions are well defined and show a yellowish or light brown discoloration. They are usually covered with plaque containing large numbers of *A. viscosus* and have a soft/leathery consistency. Inactive lesions appear in a well-defined black or dark brown with a smooth, hard, and shiny surface. Mineral loss occurs deep to the surface, and most active lesions are covered by a well-mineralized surface layer.

Tooth habitat plays a crucial role in the development of caries lesions. The stage of eruption, functional usage, and tooth-specific anatomy are key elements of occlusal (i.e., pit and fissure) caries, which offer excellent mechanical shelter for microorganisms. These lesions begin in the lateral walls of fissures. Demineralization occurs through the enamel rods to the dentinoenamel junction. Discoloration and opacification of enamel adjacent to the fissure appear. Remineralization can occur and make progression more difficult

to detect. Extensive cavitation of dentin and undermining of enamel will darken the occlusal surface.

Smooth surface lesions are slightly less numerous than are pit and fissure caries. However, the proximal contacting surfaces of teeth offer an excellent shelter for pathogenic bacteria. Poor soft tissue form can stimulate plaque growth just beneath the contact area, making this location highly susceptible to caries activity. The facial and lingual smooth surface areas, below the height of contour, can also be a sheltered area if oral hygiene is inadequate. Caries in this location are usually indicative of a highly caries-active mouth.

Root surface lesions are more common in elderly patients due to niche availability, decreased salivary flow, poor oral hygiene from decreased dexterity, and reduced motivation. These can be rapid in progression, asymptomatic, close to the pulp, and difficult to restore.

 PHYSICAL CHARACTERISTICS AND PREVALENCE OF CARIES

Caries progression from microscopic changes to visible cavitation should be regarded as the culmination of a long series of alternate dissolutions at a low pH and a partial re-precipitation when pH rises. Eventually, after repeated cariogenic challenges, a clinically detectable "white spot" lesion appears in the enamel. This lesion is the result of chemical dissolution of tooth substance caused by bacterial byproducts. There is a subsurface demineralization covered by a well-mineralized surface layer. Diffusion of fluid through the porous surface layer into the body of an enamel lesion is very slow. Lesion fluid under a surface zone is a well sealed off pool in which diffusion occurs much faster than it does through the surface layer. Once the surface layer is broken, lesion fluid exchanges material and ions much faster. Root lesions allow rapid diffusion into and out of the

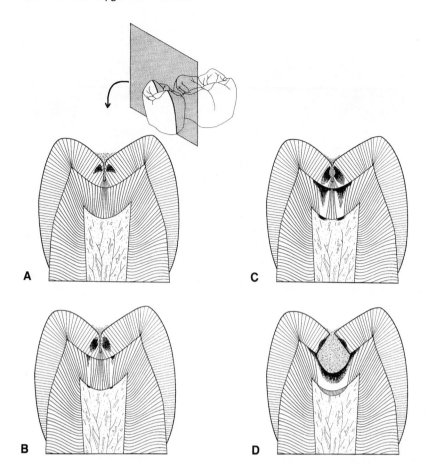

Figure 14-4. *A-D,* Pit and fissure lesion morphology. (From Sturdevant CM: The Art and Science of Operative Dentistry, 3rd ed. St. Louis, CV Mosby, 1995, p 80.)

porous surface layer. When a low pH has been established in a lesion, recovery to normal values is slow. Acid production from caries-active plaque can overcome the buffering capacity of saliva and plaque and cause a local pH drop that is sufficient to further dissolve tooth minerals.

If remineralization occurs before cavitation, there may be a brownish discoloration from exogenous pigments. The remaining exposed surface becomes harder and dark brown or black. This condition is called **arrested caries** and may be more resistant to future cariogenic challenge than undisturbed enamel. **Incipient** primary caries is a lesion in enamel characterized by a virtually intact surface, but it has a porous subsurface. It appears chalky white when dried. These lesions are reversible.

Cavitation occurs when the subsurface demineralization is so extensive that the tooth structure subsurface collapses. A cavitated lesion is **not** reversible. After cavitation, Lactobacilli are likely to become well established. Tooth destruction becomes more rapid, and symptoms such as sensitivity and pain may occur.

Most Common Sites for Caries Lesions

The three most common sites for caries lesions are pits and fissures on the occlusal surfaces of posterior teeth, proximal surfaces just below the contact area, and root surfaces. The

shapes of these lesions vary somewhat due to their morphologic surroundings. **Pit and fissure lesions** begin on the walls of the fissure and affect a greater area of the dentinoenamel junction than does a comparable smooth surface lesion. Their shape is an inverted "V" with a narrow entrance and a progressively wider expansion as it approaches the dentinoenamel junction (**Figure 14-4**).

Smooth surface lesions are broad at their area of origin (just below the contact point) and conical or pointed as they extend toward the dentinoenamel junction. This gives them a V-shaped appearance with a wide base, and the apex of the V is directed toward the dentinoenamel junction (**Figure 14-5**). **Root surface** lesions are less well-defined and U-shaped, and they progress more rapidly due to the absence of or thinness of cementum.[3]

The color of a lesion may also be a useful aid. Actively progressing caries show little discoloration but are softer in texture. Generally, the darker the discoloration, the greater is the remineralization. In advanced lesions, diseased dentin can be categorized as **necrotic dentin**, **infected dentin**, and **affected dentin**. Necrotic dentin is a wet, mushy, easily removable mass that is structureless and teeming with bacteria. Infected dentin is softened and contaminated with bacteria. It is often leathery in texture and appearance. Both infected and necrotic dentin contain irreversibly denatured collagen.[3] **Caries-disclosing agents** such as a 0.5% basic fuschin in propylene glycol solution, a 1% acid red dye in propylene glycol, an 8%

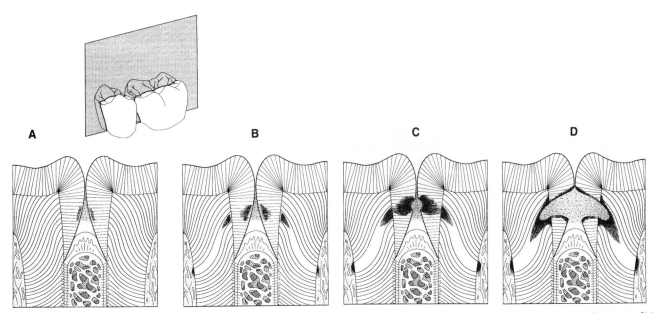

Figure 14-5. *A-D*, Smooth surface lesion shape. (From Sturdevant CM: The Art and Science of Operative Dentistry, 3rd ed. St. Louis, CV Mosby, 1995, p 90.)

povidone-iodine in water solution, or numerous commercial preparations will stain this collagen, thus making it possible to distinguish between dentin that must be removed from a lesion from that which can remain. The simple technique to be followed is to stain the tooth for 10 seconds, rinse with water, remove brightly stained red tissue, and then repeat the process until all brightly stained material is removed. Affected dentin is softened and demineralized but minimally invaded by bacteria. It does not stain and may remain during cavity preparation. Stained dentin contains an average of 550,000 CFU/mg. Unstained dentin contains less than 10,000 CFU/mg. This distinction is clinically important.[4]

There are five identifiable zones of dentinal caries. They are described as follows:

Zone 1: Normal dentin, no bacteria or other changes are present.

Zone 2: Subtransparent dentin, there is demineralization of intertubular dentin and deposition of fine crystals in the lumen of the tubule.

Zone 3: Transparent dentin, this dentin is softer than normal dentin. It shows a loss of minerals from intertubular dentin and many large crystals in the tubule lumens. No bacteria are present. The collagen is intact. The lesion can still be remineralized.

Zone 4: Turbid dentin, bacteria have invaded this zone. Very little mineral is left. Tubules are filled with bacteria. Collagen is irreversibly denatured. Remineralization cannot occur, and the tissue must be removed before restoration.

Zone 5: Infected dentin, the outermost layer consists of decomposed dentin. It is saturated with bacteria. No structure remains (collagen or minerals). The tissue must be removed before restoring the dentin.[4]

Nursing/Bottle Caries

Bottle caries is a dental condition that can destroy the teeth of an infant or young child. Bottle caries is caused by the frequent exposure of an infant or child's teeth for long periods of time to liquids that contain sugars, such as milk, formula, fruit juice, and other sweetened liquids. Each time that a child drinks a liquid that contains sugars, bacterial acids attack the teeth for about **20 minutes**. The frequency and the length of time that the teeth are exposed to acid attack are critical to the nursing or baby bottle caries equation. Other contributing factors include a reduction in swallowing and saliva production during sleep, more viscous saliva in children, and a warm oral environment during sleep, which provides a culture medium for bacterial growth. With repeated attacks, cavitated dental lesions can occur. Using the bottle containing these liquids as a pacifier or during sleep can result in destruction of the maxillary anterior teeth primarily, because the tongue lies over the mandibular teeth during feeding and protects them to some extent from repeated acid attacks **(Figure 14-6).** If the condition is allowed to progress, posterior teeth may become involved. First molars are affected more commonly than are canines, because they erupt earlier. This phenomenon can also occur in breast-fed children if at-will feeding or prolonged nursing takes place.

Prevention of bottle caries can be achieved by taking precautions, such as wiping the child's teeth and gums with a damp washcloth or gauze pad after feedings. Begin brushing the child's teeth as soon as the first tooth erupts. Flossing should begin when multiple teeth are present. Never allow a child to fall asleep with a bottle containing sweetened liquids. Water is acceptable. Never give a child a pacifier dipped in a sweet liquid. Replace the bottle with a cup at age 1. Be sure that adequate fluoride is available to aid in making

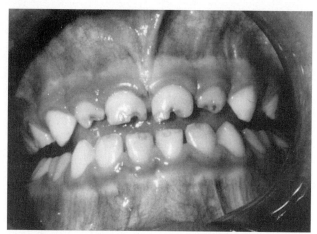

Figure 14-6. Nursing bottle caries. (From DeBiase CB: Dental Health Education: Theory and Practice. Philadelphia, Lea & Febiger, 1991, p 63.)

teeth more resistant to caries. Initiate regular dental visits for children between 6 and 12 years of age.[5]

Black's Caries Lesion Classification

In the late 19th century, Black astutely observed the incidence and location of dental caries lesions in his practice. He developed a classification system for these lesions that is still in common use today.[6]

Class I: Cavitated lesions occurring in the pit and fissure defects in the occlusal surfaces of the bicuspids and molars, the lingual surfaces of upper incisors, and the buccal and lingual grooves that are found occasionally on the occlusal surfaces of molars **(Figure 14-7)**

Class II: Cavitated lesions in the proximal surfaces of premolars and molars **(Figure 14-8)**

Class III: Cavitated lesions in the proximal surfaces of the incisors and canines that do not require removal and restoration of the incisal angle **(Figure 14-9)**

Class IV: Cavitated lesions in the proximal surfaces of incisors and canines that require removal and restoration of the incisa angle (see Figure 14-9)

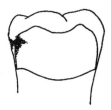

Figure 14-8. Dental caries, class II: Cavities in proximal surfaces of premolars and molars. (From Wilkins EM: Clinical Practice of the Dental Hygienist, 8th ed. Philadelphia, JB Lippincott, 1993, p 241.)

Class V: Cavitated lesions in the gingival one third of teeth (not in pits) and below the height of contour on the labial, buccal, and lingual surfaces of the teeth **(Figure 14-10)**

Class VI: Cavitated lesions in the incisal edges and cusp tips [This description is not included in Black's Classification system **(Figure 14-11)**

Caries Epidemiology

Dental caries has traditionally been reported as an index of DMF-T (diseased), M (missing), and F (filled) teeth or surfaces (see Chapter 17). The index makes a statement about the total caries experience of an individual. Dental caries disease is difficult to evaluate, because it is a chronic disease characterized by active and inactive phases. There are no current clinical methods to diagnose when these phases begin or end. When a caries lesion has been diagnosed, it is not possible to know when it was established, how long it has been present, if it is arrested, or if active demineralization is occurring. Even with these inherent problems, knowledge gained from epidemiologic studies about causal factors can be used to develop control and preventive therapies.[7]

In the 20th century, caries can be viewed on a global basis as having three general areas. The first area covers rural China, Africa, and South America. In this area, the prevalence and severity of dental caries are usually higher in more urbanized regions compared with lower socioeconomic groups living in rural communities. The second area consists of newly industrialized countries such as Taiwan, India, Chile, Uganda, and Thailand. An increased caries rate is

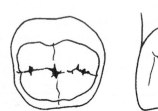

Figure 14-7. Dental caries, class I: Cavities in pits or fissures: occlusal surfaces of premolars and molars; facial and lingual surfaces of molars; and lingual surfaces of maxillary incisors. (From Wilkins EM: Clinical Practice of the Dental Hygienist, 8th ed. Philadelphia, JB Lippincott, 1993, p 241.)

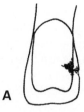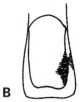

Figure 14-9. *A,* Dental caries, class III: Cavities in proximal surfaces of incisors and canines do not involve the incisal angle. B, Dental caries, class IV: Cavities in proximal surfaces of incisors or canines that involve the incisal angle. (From Wilkins EM: Clinical Practice of the Dental Hygienist, 8th ed. Philadelphia, JB Lippincott, 1993, p 241.)

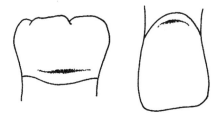

Figure 14-10. Dental caries, class V: Cavities in the cervical third of facial and lingual surfaces (not pit or fissure). (From Wilkins EM: Clinical Practice of the Dental Hygienist, 8th ed. Philadelphia, JB Lippincott, 1993, p 241.)

seen in children and adults with more edentulousness in the elderly. Socioeconomic status and increases in refined carbohydrates and sugars are directly linked to the higher incidence of caries. The third area is found in North America, Australia, Europe, and Japan. Here, a decrease is seen in the caries rate of children, and the number of retained teeth in adults is increasing. This seems to be related to the implementation of the prevention concept and topical fluorides. Common factors in industrialized countries that have declining caries rates include:

1. Increased dental resources (manpower)
2. Increased availability of fluoride (toothpaste and water supply)
3. Increased demand for dental care
4. Implementation of a preventive approach by dentists

Several high caries risk groups exist even in industrialized societies. These groups include the developmentally disabled, mentally retarded, some immigrant groups, individuals who are human immunodeficiency virus-positive, people in low socioeconomic groups, and frail older adults.

Caries incidence in children in the United States has been declining since the 1960s. This decline has been greater on interproximal and smooth surfaces compared with the fissured or occlusal surfaces of teeth. Lesion progression rate has also been slowed significantly. Again, the widespread use of fluoride is given credit for this effect. Among children in the United States, 50% of all carious teeth appear in 12% of the population. Greater than 75% of all carious teeth occur in 25% of the population.[7] Children who are at risk come from families in the low socioeconomic levels, iso-

lated rural areas, or central urban areas. Families with single parents or families who have recently immigrated to the United States are at highest risk.

Caries lesions in adults can be either coronal or root caries. People older than 65 years of age have more surfaces at risk due to gingival recession. The highest coronal caries rates have been found in frail older adults who have been institutionalized. As shown in the N-Hanes III Study of 1988 to 1991,[8] women had the lowest percentage of untreated caries at 6.6% compared with men at 10.4%. African-Americans had the highest percentage of untreated caries at 27.7%.

Root surface caries incidence depends upon the following:

1. The amount and virulence of acidogenic bacteria present in the mouth
2. The acidogenic potential of the diet and the number of times per day that a person eats
3. The inherent or acquired resistance of the teeth to demineralization[7]

The older the patient, the more likely he or she is to have teeth at risk; therefore, that person is more likely to have root caries. For people who have lived all of their lives in a fluoridated area, the risk is halved. For individuals taking xerostomia-inducing medications or who are physically or medically frail or institutionalized, the risk increases significantly because they are unable to maintain oral hygiene at an adequate level.

In the industrialized world, caries is a specific problem in several at-risk groups as well as in lower educational and socioeconomic groups. Currently, the group with the greatest treatment needs is that of older adults. They have more treatment needs than do children younger than 14 years of age living in a nonfluoridated area.[7]

 PREVENTION

Oral Hygiene

Cleaning of the teeth does not kill the oral microorganisms but removes them from tooth surfaces. Sufficient numbers remain to recolonize the teeth. Tooth brushing has a negative relation to caries development in that the daily application of a fluoridated dentifrice has been shown to be an effective caries reduction technique. Flossing, when performed effectively, has a caries-preventive effect on the proximal tooth surfaces. The quality rather than the frequency of plaque removal is much more important.[1] It is of obvious benefit to the host to favor the establishment of *S. sanguis* versus S. *mutans*. Simple oral hygiene procedures help to achieve this by disrupting plaque succession. This frequent disruption, which is achieved by thorough plaque control and a diet low in sucrose, favors the growth of *S. sanguis*. The success of a treatment strategy aimed at controlling caries progression without restorative treatment, depends mainly on the provider's knowledge of dental caries

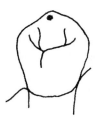

Figure 14-11. Dental caries, class VI: Cavities on incisal edges of anterior teeth and cusp tips of posterior teeth. (From Wilkins EM: Clinical Practice of the Dental Hygienist, 8th ed. Philadelphia, JB Lippincott, 1993, p 241.)

and how this information is transmitted for the benefit of the individual patient. Total arrest of caries progression on an individual basis can be achieved only by adequate control of the local environment.

Fluoride

In 1901, McKay noted an unusual permanent stain or "mottled enamel" on the teeth of many of his patients. He was able to determine that something in the community water supply was responsible and that these teeth seemed less susceptible to dental caries. It was not until 1930 that fluoride was identified as the agent responsible for the enamel mottling and reduced caries susceptibility. Trendley Dean, the first director of the Dental Hygiene Unit at the National Institutes of Health, used the term **fluorosis** to describe this condition. Dental fluorosis can result from excessive long-term fluoride ingestion during tooth development in the late enamel secretion and early enamel maturation stages. It is characterized by a deficiency in the mineral content, hypocalcification, on the surface and in particular the subsurface enamel, causing enamel to appear opaque. Studies showed very mild or mild signs of fluorosis in 22% of children in the United States with an increased prevalence of fluorosis during the last half of the 20th century. Dietary fluoride supplements, prolonged use of infant formula beyond 1 year of age, and tooth brushing with a fluoride dentifrice before 2 years of age have been shown to be increased risk factors in dental fluorosis.[9] Fluorosis is **not** a necessary side effect of caries prevention and treatment.

Very mild fluorosis was characterized by Dr. Dean as small opaque "paper white" areas affecting less than or equal to 25% of the tooth surface; **mild fluorosis** affected 26% to 50% of the tooth surface. In **moderate dental fluorosis**, all enamel surfaces were involved and susceptible to moderate brown staining. **Severe fluorosis** was characterized by pitting of the enamel, widespread brown stains, and a "corroded" appearance[9] **(Figure 14-12)**.

Dean also made the connection between fluoride and reduced caries prevalence. In 1945, field studies were started

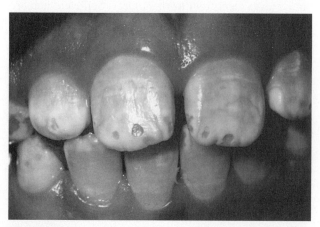

Figure 14-12. Mottled enamel-fluorosis. (Photograph courtesy of Dr. C.B. DeBiase.)

in four pairs of cities. It was found after 13 to 15 years of study that caries incidence was reduced 50% to 70% among children in the communities with fluoridated (1-1.2 ppm) water supplies. This prompted the adoption of community water fluoridation as the cornerstone for dental caries reduction throughout the United States.[9] Currently, approximately 62% of the United States population using public water supplies or about 56% of the total population receives tap water with optimum fluoridation.[10] Sodium silicofluoride is usually the type of fluoride added to municipal water supplies.

Recently, the prevalence of dental caries in both fluoridated and nonfluoridated communities has declined. This trend is attributed to the spread of fluoridated water to areas without fluoridation through bottling and processing of foods and beverages and the widespread use of fluoride toothpaste.

Fluoride affects teeth pre-eruptively by its incorporation into the developing enamel and posteruptively by topical action. Fluoride prevents dental caries predominantly after eruption of the tooth. Its three main actions are primarily topical for both adults and children by: **inhibition of demineralization, enhancement of remineralization,** and **inhibition of bacterial activity in dental plaque.**[9] A slight, but significant increase in the fluoride content of saliva from various sources produces an increased beneficial effect on the outermost layers of enamel during the enamel maturation period, resulting in improved remineralization and reduced demineralization during acid challenge. Fluoride found in solution at low levels becomes concentrated in dental plaque, where it substantially inhibits dissolution of tooth mineral by acid. "Fluoride enhances remineralization by adsorbing to the tooth surface and attracting calcium ions present in saliva. Fluoride also acts to bring the calcium and phosphate ions together and is included in the chemical reaction that takes place, producing a crystal surface that is much less soluble in acid than the original tooth mineral."[9] The amount of mineral loss during demineralization is a function of both pH and fluoride concentration. Fluoride from topical sources such as drinking water is taken up by cariogenic bacteria when they produce acid. Once inside, fluoride interferes with the internal metabolism of the cell. Bacterial acid production is reduced, which reduces the dissolution rate of the tooth minerals.

Recent studies show that high fluoride content in the hard dental tissue is less important than a moderate increase in the daily fluoride concentration of oral fluids. Enamel is primarily made up of **apatite** $[Ca_{10}(PO_4)_6(OH)_2]$. Apatite consists of 37% calcium, 52% phosphate, and 3% hydroxyl. Many foreign ions (e.g., fluoride, strontium, selenium, barium) may become incorporated into its crystalline structure and may affect its solubility. Each crystal is surrounded by a layer of firmly bound water or a **hydration shell.** Crystals are densely packed and arranged in rods. Water makes up 4% by weight and 11% by volume. Fluoride can be permanently bound into the apatite lattice, when formed, as **fluo-**

rapatite.[1] The solubility of enamel, once erupted, is pH dependent. Below a pH of 5.5, the enamel tooth minerals can start to dissolve. When the pH recovers above 5.5, mineral starts to re-precipitate onto the remaining apatite crystallites. If fluoride is incorporated into the crystallite structure, the resultant mineral is less soluble to acid attack. This cycle is an essential part of the post-eruption maturation process of enamel. This explains why unerupted (immature) enamel is more soluble.

Fluoride concentrations in whole saliva are generally higher than in duct saliva. The increased levels in whole saliva arise from fluoride trapped in the oral cavity when direct contact is made with oral tissues and plaque by fluoride in drinking water, rinses, toothpaste, and diet. Plaque fluoride is found mainly in the bound form. Only a small percentage is in the ionized form. Bound fluoride may be released by weak acids formed during sugar fermentation. Fluoride concentration in whole saliva can be closely related to the fluoridated toothpaste used. Regular repeated use of fluoridated toothpaste provides elevated baseline fluoride ion concentrations in saliva and plaque with a dose-response relationship to the fluoride concentration of the toothpaste. Oral soft tissue plays a significant role as a reservoir for fluoride after topical application.

Calcium fluoride is the major product of the reaction between fluoride and dental apatite. It acts as a reservoir where fluoride is released into the liquid environment. Saliva is unsaturated with respect to calcium fluoride. The rate of dissolution of calcium fluoride increases with decreasing pH levels. The precipitation of calcium fluoride in early caries lesions with subsequent release of fluoride is believed to be a key mechanism for the caries-reducing effect of concentrated topical fluorides.[1]

When fluoride is present in the aqueous phase around the tooth, in saliva and in plaque fluid, enamel solubility is low, which tends to prevent its demineralization. The amount of enamel dissolved in aqueous media is decreased significantly when the solution contains fluoride of concentrations near 1 ppm. A discontinuation of the fluoride supply leaves the enamel open to renewed demineralization; therefore, fluoride should be provided throughout life for full prevention. The interference with enamel dissolution (fluoride's topical effects) is by far the most important factor in caries prevention.[1] Teeth do not develop a lasting resistance toward caries. Because the predominant loss of teeth up to 60 years of age is due to dental caries, constant exposure throughout life is necessary.

Plaque fluid contains acids from plaque bacteria and dissolved tooth minerals. Calcium and phosphate are transported through the plaque fluid to the mineral crystals. Fluoride must be available in plaque fluid to influence these processes. Fluoride is available from saliva, crevicular fluid, and the mineral surfaces of teeth. The concentration may change dramatically with the application of topical fluorides. Concentrations return to baseline levels within 3 to 6 hours. Differences may also be affected by clearance rates.

Rinsing after tooth brushing can have a significant effect on the fluoride concentrations of saliva and plaque fluid. Heavy rinsing reduces the amount of fluoride of people brushing twice daily or more to amounts equal to those brushing once daily or less.[11]

Remineralization of enamel occurs when mineral is deposited as calcium hydroxyapatite. Its deposition is crystalline and the result of regrowth of crystallites affected by the caries process. The new crystals are randomly aligned, which explains the porosity of arrested lesions. Fluoride enhances remineralization by becoming incorporated into the crystal lattice as **fluorhydroxyapatite** and aiding in the diffusion of mineral ions through pores in the enamel surface. Dentin lesions can also be remineralized with the help of fluoride. Therefore, caries extending past the dentinoenamel junction can still be remineralized. Systemic/topical fluorides are available via several different delivery systems **(Table 14-2)**.

Several fluoridation strategies are available to enhance the topical effects. These include fluoridated salt, fluoride rinses, fluoridated milk, and pediatric fluoride supplements. Fluoride supplements, however, can be a significant risk factor in the development of dental fluorosis due to prescription errors related to improper dosages. The American Dental Association (ADA)'s Council on Dental Therapeutics reduced the recommended fluoride dose for **pediatric fluoride supplements** in 1994 **(Table 14-3)**.

Compliance is a significant problem. Patient compliance, regarding proper use of fluoride by a particular individual, may be more important for caries prevention than the effectiveness of the fluoride concentration. Compliance combined with increased fluoride in infant diets raises questions about the continued use of supplemental fluoride for infants. Caution should be exercised with respect to fluoride exposures in baby food and toothpaste when supplements are also taken. Supplements are available in drops, tablets, lozenges, rinses, and vitamins. Drops are ideal for very

TABLE 14–2 Fluoride Delivery Systems

	FLUORIDE CONCENTRATION	FREQUENCY OF APPLICATION
Water Fluoridation	Optimal 1 ppm	Continuously
Fluoride Toothpaste	500–1500 ppm	Twice daily
Fluoride Tablets	0.25–1 mg/tablet	Daily
Fluoride Drops	1000–2000 ppm	Daily
Rinsing Solutions	250–1000 ppm	Daily, weekly
Salt Fluoridation	250–350 ppm	Continuously
Milk Fluoridation	7.5 ppm	At school
Concentrated Solutions	10,000 ppm	Biannual
Concentrated Gels	4000–12,300 ppm	Biannual
Foams	9040–12,000 ppm	Biannual
Lacquers (Varnishes)	1000–22,600 ppm	Biannual

Modified from ten Cate, et al: Fluoride mechanisms DCNA 43(4):735, 1999.

TABLE 14–3 Current ADA/CDT Guidelines of Pediatric Supplement Dosages

	CONCENTRATION OF FLUORIDE (PPM) IN THE WATER SUPPLY		
AGE	<0.3	0.3–0.6	>0.6
0–6 months	0	0	0
6 months–3 years	0.25 mg	0	0
3 years–6 years	0.50 mg	0.25 mg	0
6 years to at least 16 years	1 mg	0.50 mg	0

Modified from Stookey GK: Caries prevention JDE 62(10):805, 1998.

young children, because they can be dispensed directly on the teeth or in juice or water. It is not recommended to combine fluoride drops with milk, because milk binds with fluoride and reduces its effectiveness. Tablets should be chewed (not swallowed) to enhance the topical effects.

Recent studies support the use of **professionally applied topical fluoride treatments** for patients with evidence of modest caries activity or caries risk. Fluoride systems approved by the Food and Drug Administration (FDA) include solutions and gels with 2% sodium fluoride, 8% stannous fluoride, and 1.23% acidulated phosphate fluoride (APF). Stannous fluoride is used less frequently for caries control due to its lack of stability and shelf-life and poor acceptance due to taste and enamel pigmentation. All three systems impart significant benefits with a 28% to 32% reduction in caries incidence.[12] Although APF gels are the treatment of choice for recalls, neutral sodium fluoride is a recommended alternative when porcelain and composite restorations are present. Neutral sodium fluoride is clinically proved to be most effective when used as a four-visit protocol.

Because most children are at high risk for caries between 6 and 14 years of age, professionally applied fluoride is an appropriate preventive measure for that group. The time when teeth are most susceptible to caries formation is during the first 2 years after eruption. High concentrations of fluoride in the outer layers of enamel are thought to occur primarily posteruptively and are considered to be the reason for the increased resistance of the enamel to caries.[12]

It is now recognized that it is not necessary to perform a scale and polish before topical fluoride treatments. Results of recent clinical trials indicate that the benefits of topical APF treatments were not influenced by the presence or absence of dental prophylaxis.[9]

The treatment procedure should use FDA-approved products and minimize swallowing of fluoride gel or solution.[12]

1. Seat the patient upright with the head tilted slightly forward, and instruct the patient not to swallow.
2. Dry the teeth to prevent dilution of the fluoride, and reduce the action of saliva as a barrier to fluoride penetration.
3. Use only enough gel, foam, or solution to treat all tooth surfaces. Gels or foams are usually placed in trays, and

solutions are continuously painted on the teeth. The paint-on system is also ideal for exposed root surfaces or when an isolated number of teeth require fluoride. Patients should be instructed to gently chew to force the fluoride interproximally when using the tray method.

4. Have an adequate saliva evacuation system, and ask the patient to expectorate thoroughly for 1 to 2 minutes after treatment.
5. Tooth surfaces should be treated for 4 minutes to achieve maximum benefit. Some companies recommend 1-minute gels, because approximately 75% of fluoride uptake occurs in the first minute and some patients may be unable to tolerate the full 4 minutes. These products are no different in composition from the 4-minute gels.
6. Patients should be advised not to eat, drink, or rinse the mouth for 30 minutes following a topical fluoride treatment.

The optimal number of applications of fluoride or treatment frequency has never been established. However, it is recommended that patients with high caries activity and caries risk have a series of four to five topical treatments within a period of 4 to 6 weeks to help arrest incipient lesions. It is further recommended that topical fluoride treatments be considered for all patients who have evidence of caries activity regardless of age and for all children between the ages of 6 and 14 years who appear to be at risk of developing caries. The number and frequency of applications should be dictated by professional judgment related primarily to risk of caries.[12]

Fluoride lacquers or varnishes became available for use in the United States in 1994. The product is a 5% sodium fluoride (2.26% fluoride) varnish with the trade name of *Duraphat*. Its caries prevention potential is essentially equivalent to that of professionally applied topical fluoride systems. Its use in children has actually been shown to be more beneficial than similar applications of APF gels. Data for fluoride varnish met the ADA Council on Scientific Affairs criteria for claims of being "at least as good as" the topical fluoride gels. The varnish also demonstrates a strong desensitizing effect when applied to exposed dentin (see Chapter 13). The recommended technique for placement is[12]:

1. Prior to application of the varnish, the teeth are brushed with a dentifrice to remove plaque and debris.
2. The varnish is then applied to the tooth surface with a soft brush, cotton swabs, or a probe. Although drying the tooth surface with air or gauze is not essential, it is recommended. The amber color promotes visual control of the varnish.
3. The varnish should be painted on tooth surfaces and drawn through interproximal areas rapidly before it hardens.
4. No drying of the varnish is necessary, and the patient can leave promptly after the application.
5. The patient should be instructed to avoid eating hard foods or brushing teeth for a minimum of 2 hours after the application.
6. Re-applications are recommended at 4- to 6-month intervals.

Because the varnish is less than 1 mm thick and is lost from the teeth over a 24- to 48-hour period, the amount ingested is 3 to 6 mg per application. Safety, therefore, is not a practical concern, and its use is often recommended in children instead of traditional fluoride gels.

Fluoride dentifrices (toothpastes) have been recognized as the primary reason for the decline in caries observed in many parts of the world during the last 2 decades. Its frequency of use has been shown to be related to the amount of benefit received. Brushing three times daily can result in about 45% fewer caries lesions. Brushing once per day can result in a 21% reduction in caries incidence. Reports indicate that the use of sodium fluoride results in a significantly greater efficacy than similar use of any other fluoride salt. This form of fluoride provides more fluoride ions in an aqueous environment.

Over-the-counter (OTC) mouth rinses contain 0.05% (225 ppm) sodium fluoride and are intended for use once daily in patients older than 6 years of age. **School-based fluoride rinse programs** utilize 0.2% sodium fluoride once a week. **Self-applied prescription gels** for daily use typically contain either 0.4% stannous fluoride (1000 ppm fluoride), 1.1% sodium fluoride (5000 ppm fluoride), or 0.5% APF. Stannous fluoride gels are approved by both the FDA and the ADA Council. In general, fluoride rinses and gels are recommended as adjunctive measures for use in addition to professional fluoride treatments and fluoride dentifrices in special clinical situations where dental caries or caries risk is a major problem (e.g., orthodontic appliances, physical disabilities, condition or treatment-induced xerostomia such as that experienced by patients undergoing head and neck radiation therapy).

Convincing evidence exists to show the merits of fluorides in the reduction of root caries. Community water fluoridation and professionally applied fluoride have shown benefits. Semiannual APF gel applications or daily use of a 0.05% sodium fluoride rinse were very effective. Sodium fluoride gels or varnishes as professional treatments to prevent or arrest root surface caries is recommended. Fluoride dentifrices have been shown to reduce the incidence of root caries by 67%.[12]

Fluoride-releasing restorative materials increase resistance of the adjacent enamel to acid demineralization, thus lowering the rate of secondary caries. Glass ionomer cements offer the highest fluoride release. This occurs during the first weeks after placement. Sustained release is due to a recharging of the restoration during topical fluoride application and brushing with a fluoride dentifrice. Applications of stannous fluoride solution to the walls of cavity preparations for 15 seconds in amalgam restorations resulted in a decrease of secondary caries of approximately 65% during a 2-year study.[12]

Fluoride ingestion poses a risk for **fluorosis or toxicity**. Systemic intake of fluoride must be monitored closely. Optimal levels of fluoride intake in terms of amounts ingested per unit of body weight is 0.05 to 0.07 mg fluoride per kilo-gram of body weight.[10] Considerable variation exists, but this is often exceeded in some children. Because most commercially available toothpaste contains 1000 to 1100 ppm fluoride and 2- to 3-year-old children ingest about 0.3 g (~60%-65% of the dentifrice on a toothbrush), a small pea-sized quantity of toothpaste should be used with pre-school-aged children. Mouth rinses contain 0.05% fluoride (230 ppm) in over-the-counter preparations and 0.2% fluoride (920 ppm) in prescription form. Gels vary from 1000 to 5000 ppm by prescription or 10,000 to 12,300 ppm in office applied doses. Dietary supplements, which are meant to be ingested, mimic the effects of water supply fluoridation. They are dispensed in dosages ranging from 0.25 to 1 mg fluoride (see Table 14-3). Proper dosage and compliance are common problems, and supplemental use has been identified as a risk factor for fluorosis. The optimal water fluoridation concentration is about 1 ppm.

Fluoride concentrations are variable and can be adjusted higher in colder climates and lower in warmer climates. Daily ingestion of 4 to 4.5 ppm is the maximum level and is used only in cold climates. It can be elevated to that level for school water supplies in areas with no public water fluoridation. This is possible because of the low water consumption associated with cold climates. Home-filtering systems can remove up to 90% of the fluoride in water. Individual water sources must be tested for fluoride content before prescribing supplements or other fluoride products for young children. Considerable variation also exists among bottled waters. Infant formula may contain varying amounts of fluoride. Soy-based products have higher fluoride levels than do milk-based products. Human breast milk and cow's milk contain little fluoride. Fruit juices and soft drinks have fluoride concentrations that are closely linked to the water content in the area of their respective bottling plants. Tea contains a naturally high fluoride concentration in the 1.33 to 2.56 ppm range.[10]

Mean dietary fluoride ingestion ranges from 0.05 mg/day among 2-month-old infants living in nonfluoridated areas to quantities of 1 mg or more for children 4 to 8 years of age living in fluoridated communities. Acute fluoride toxicity may occur from ingestion of high amounts of fluoride over a short time span. The **toxic dose** is 8 mg of fluoride per kilogram of body weight. The **lethal dose** is 32 to 64 mg of fluoride per kilogram of body weight. Acute fatal fluoride poisoning would occur after ingestion of 5 to 10 g for a 70-kg adult and 320 mg for 2-year-old children who weigh about 10 kg. Examples of a lethal dose for a 10-kg child would require that the child consumes the entire contents of a large tube of 1100 ppm dentifrice, 26 ml of a 1.23% APF topical gel, or 1 L of 0.05% fluoride rinse. A toxic dose (5-8 mg of fluoride/kg of body weight) would require a 10-kg child to ingest about 1 oz of toothpaste or 6 to 8 oz of fluoride rinse.[10]

Signs and symptoms of acute toxic doses of fluoride can begin within 30 minutes of ingestion and may last for as long as 24 hours. **Gastrointestinal tract** involvement occurs when fluoride in the stomach reacts with hydrochloric acid to form hydrofluoric acid, which is an irritant to the stomach lining. Symptoms include nausea, vomiting, diarrhea, abdominal pain, increased salivation, and thirst. **Systemic involvement** can be found in the **blood** where calcium may be bound to circulating fluoride, causing symptoms of hypocalcemia; **central nervous system** demonstrating hyperreflexia, convulsions, and paresthesias; and the **cardiovascular respiratory systems** resulting in depression, which may lead to cardiac failure or respiratory paralysis if untreated.

Emergency treatment of toxic ingestion of fluoride begins with induction of vomiting by either mechanical (digital stimulation of the tongue or back of the throat) or drug (Ipecac syrup) methods. Emergency medical services should be notified at once, and the patient should be transported to a hospital. Basic life support must be maintained throughout treatment. Fluoride-binding liquids such as milk or lime water can be administered when the patient is not vomiting.

Additional beneficial measures that can be administered at the hospital include administration of calcium gluconate for muscle tremors; gastric lavage; cardiac monitoring; endotrachial intubation; monitoring of blood pH and calcium, magnesium, and potassium levels; and intervenous nourishment to restore proper blood volume and calcium levels.[13]

Dietary Factors

Severe dietary deficiencies (malnutrition) in children may result in restricted organ development, including the salivary glands. Adults may have diminished cell function. Deficiencies of calcium, phosphate, and vitamins A, D, and C can affect tooth tissue formation. Enamel hypoplasia due to vitamin D deficiency can lead to a higher caries incidence. Saliva composition responds to changes in diet. Impairments in saliva secretion and composition occur during severe short-term starvation. Studies are ongoing to clarify the various types and degrees of nutritional imbalances on caries susceptibility and on factors having an impact on actual caries development.

Although the nutrients contained in whole saliva are sufficient to sustain the viability of most oral microorganisms, frequent consumption of fermentable carbohydrates is associated with a high incidence of dental caries. Development varies widely among individuals. Systemic effects, tooth development, and saliva secretion may influence the progress of the disease.

All common dietary sugars (e.g., sucrose, glucose, fructose and lactose) are used in energy metabolism of many plaque bacteria. Fermentation of carbohydrates during anaerobic metabolism of the bacteria causes an increase in the concentration of organic acids, (lactic acid, in plaque and caries lesions). An increase in caries is seen when a modern diet with a high sugar content and ready-to-eat sweet snacks are available. Availability of less than 50 g of sugar per person per day is associated with a DMFT (i.e., diseased, missing, filled teeth) score of less than three.[1]

All of the dietary sugars can be fermented to acids by the plaque bacteria and may influence the microbial growth on teeth. Sucrose favors colonization of pathogenic oral microorganisms and increases the stickiness of the plaque. Starch is a polysaccharide of glucose. The most highly cariogenic foods may be those that contain both starch and sucrose. These foods include sweetened breakfast cereals, sweet biscuits, cakes, pies, and cookies. Some foods may actually protect the teeth from caries initiation and include cheeses, fats, and phosphate- and fluoride-containing products.

The length and frequency of sugar exposure can be more important factors in cariogenicity than the physical form of the sugar and polysaccharide starch. The oral carbohydrate concentrations and the length of time that carbohydrates remain in the mouth during and after eating are critical. **Clearance** times may be prolonged by retentive factors in the dentition (e.g., cavities, poor restorations) or low secretion rate or high viscosity of saliva. Slow clearance increases the risk of caries. Fresh fruits, vegetables, and various drinks are eliminated in about 5 minutes. Chewing gum, caramels, toffees, bon bons, chocolates, and lozenges in about 20 to 40 minutes. Food intake causes salivary stimulation, which has mechanical rinsing effects and increases the buffering capacity. Clearance can also be enhanced by tooth brushing. Sugar-free chewing gum accelerates clearance. Sugar substitutes, noncaloric sweeteners, such as cyclamate, saccharin, and aspartame, are not metabolized to acids by oral microorganisms. Caloric sweeteners, such as the sugar alcohols (e.g., sorbitol, xylitol), satiate the oral microorganisms, leaving no room for absorption of other sugars.

Diet counseling may be necessary for some individuals to reduce the amount and frequency of sugars and fermentable carbohydrates. This starts with an assessment of dietary habits. Taking a very specific diet history at 1- to 2-hour intervals for 24 hours is a method used to determine the number, frequency, stickiness, and amounts of fermentable carbohydrates ingested. This information can give the counselor a good picture of the patient's cariogenic food risk potential. Also, the number and types of foods with nutritive potential value should be recorded. Recommended guidelines for daily energy intake include carbohydrate; 55% to 60% of the total energy; fat, 20% to 30%; and protein; 10% to 15%. Sucrose intake should be a maximum of 10% of the total energy intake.[1] (See Chapter 6)

Changing dietary habits may be a difficult process. Psychological and social aspects of dietary modifications should be considered. Some individuals are in diet-related risk groups. People who suffer from long-term illnesses can be malnourished. Hospitalized patients may receive medications that contain sucrose, such as nystatin and cough suppressants. Other institutionalized individuals may be reinforced for appropriate behaviors with soft drinks, candy, or sugar-coated cereal. Drug addicts sometimes crave sweets. People such as food samplers, bakery workers, and those with irregular work schedules may be more likely to ingest large amounts of sweets. Maintenance of proper oral hygiene, nutrition, and low sugar intake during pregnancy can prove difficult for some women.

A trained professional staff member should interview patients and advise them on how to complete the diet diary. A review of the information recorded for the previous 24-hour period is next conducted. A record of the food intake for 4 to 7 days will give a more accurate representation of the patient's specific eating habits. Evaluation and counseling may indicate the need for a significant modification in the patient's diet to reduce cariogenic potential and increase nutritive value.[1]

Changes in basic behavior are often difficult to achieve and may require incremental steps with constant reinforcement and encouragement for a successful outcome. Any dietary advice should be given in complete compliance with the patient's overall health requirements.

Chemoprophylactic Agents

Chemoprophylactic agents include any compound that interferes with metabolic activity or adhesion of dental plaque bacteria. These agents are used as noninvasive treatment modalities for early caries and periodontal disease. The clinical efficacy of a chemoprophylactic agent depends on its potency and its **substantivity.** Substantivity is an agent's ability to bind or adsorb to oral surfaces. Both the binding and release rates of the agent are critical.

"The mode of action of chemoprophylactic agents include:

1. Inhibition of bacterial colonization
2. Disruption of mature plaque
3. Inhibition of bacterial growth or metabolism
4. Modification of plaque biochemistry and ecology"[1]

Delivery systems for chemoprophylactic agents should possess:

1. Compatibility between the agent and constituents of the vehicle
2. Bioavailability of the agent at the site of action
3. Patient compliance"[1]

Types of chemoprophylactic agents include mouth rinses, dentifrices, gels, varnishes, chewing gums, and lozenges. The active agents that are most potent are cationic. **Chlorhexidine** is a frequently used agent. It is a **bisbiguanide,** which is very effective against gram-positive bacteria. *S. mutans* are particularly sensitive. Chlorhexidine is both bactericidal and bacteriostatic. It binds to the bacterial cell wall and interferes with cell function and leakage of cell contents. There is an immediate antimicrobial effect with chlorhexidine after mouth rinsing. Plaque and salivary bacterial flora are reduced by 80% to 95% with a 0.2% solution. Chlorhexidine offers good substantivity and retention of antimicrobial action. Oral bacteria have not been shown to develop resistant strains against it. Possible side effects include tooth discoloration, desquama-

tion and soreness of the oral mucosa, and taste disturbances. The recommended dosage calls for 15 ml of a 0.12% solution taken twice daily.

Sanguinaria extract is another antimicrobial agent that is effective against both gram-positive and gram-negative bacteria. This agent interferes with the synthesis of the bacterial cell wall and septum, and it has lipophilic properties. Metal ions, such as copper, tin, and zinc, also have some bacteriostatic effect.[1]

 # CARIES RISK ASSESSMENT

Purpose

The *purpose* of a caries risk assessment for an individual would include:

1. Explanations for the reasons behind ongoing caries disease in order to define a relevant treatment program, targeting the most important etiologic factors
2. Determination of the effect of causal treatment and guidance on when further measures are necessary
3. Provision of information that the clinician can use to predict caries disease or the continuation of disease[1]

Risk Profile

The management of caries disease should be based on solid scientific evidence and not on chance or beliefs. A series of tests and clinical examinations combined with a skilled operator's interpretation will best determine an individual's **risk profile.** No single test can give an absolute assessment of a patient's caries risk.

Examples of a high-risk *clinical profile* would be a patient with several of the following conditions present:

1. High *S. mutans* and *Lactobacillus* counts after initial antimicrobial therapy
2. Two or more new, active incipient lesions
3. Orthodontic treatment in progress
4. Extensive restorative treatment required
5. Poor dietary habits
6. Low salivary flow
7. Poor general health
8. High DMFT
9. Low fluoride exposure[3]

Rationale

The *rationale* for a caries risk assessment for large groups is related to four major goals:

1. *Targeting those in need.* Accurate and practical caries prediction will successfully identify children at high risk for disease. Such a result would permit preventive dental services to be targeted to those individuals who need them most.

2. *Greater effectiveness of preventive procedures.* By targeting those children who are most susceptible to caries, more intensive preventive services can be employed that may have a significantly greater impact in preventing tooth decay.

3. *Appropriate levels of care.* By successfully identifying the high-risk group, the larger low caries group is also defined. Analogous to the more intensive care for the high-risk group, preventive care for the low-risk group can be scaled down to a level commensurate with the lower expected disease pattern.

4. *Economic efficiency.* By appropriately matching preventive care to the assessed risk status of each individual, it may be possible to achieve economic benefits in private or public health care settings. For high-risk individuals, the major impact would be to increase the net benefit from preventive services. For the low caries risk individuals, the major outcome would be savings in expenditures by avoiding preventive dental services that would demonstrate only marginal effects.[14]

Evaluation Methods

Tests usually begin by measuring the amount of *S. mutans* in saliva as related to the number of colonized tooth surfaces. A high saliva count means that many tooth surfaces are subjected to increased risk of caries. Low-risk individuals have salivary counts of **10^5 CFU/ml** or less. High-risk individuals have salivary counts of **10^6 CFU/ml** or above. Some interesting observations show that most individuals with high caries activity have high *S. mutans* scores. Few individuals with low *S. mutans* scores have high caries activity, and caries-free individuals may be found in both *S. mutans* classes. High *S. mutans* levels can be found in populations with low sugar intake. Therefore, one must make a distinction between risk and activity. They do not always occur simultaneously.

The chairside method of testing begins with adding a bacitracin disk to a tube of high sucrose-containing broth medium 15 minutes before adding the test strip. The patient is instructed to chew a piece of paraffin wax to stimulate salivary flow and mix the bacteria with the saliva. The test strip is contaminated with the patient's saliva in the mouth and then removed through the patient's closed lips. The strip and tube are then incubated for 48 hours. The strip is compared with a chart to give the approximate number of colonies. High risk is equal to or greater than 10^6 CFU/ml.

The chairside method of testing for *Lactobacillus* is to collect saliva and drip it over both sides of a selective agar strip. The strip is incubated for 4 days at 35°C to 37°C in a Rogosa SL-agar medium. The strip is then compared with test strips to determine the number of colony-forming units per milliliter. Below **10^3 CFU/ml** is considered to be a low risk. Above **10^5 CFU/ml** is considered to be a high risk. If high levels remain after caries lesions and other retention sites have been corrected, the individual probably has a diet rich in carbohydrates. *Lactobacillus* is highly influenced by dietary carbohydrate intake and is also significantly correlated to root caries.

Flow rate of saliva is a very important factor in determining an individual's risk of caries. A severe decrease in flow rate, as is seen in xerostomia, may result in extreme increases in caries risk. Flow rate can be measured at rest or when stimulated. A resting rate, when measured over a 5- to 15-minute period, of less than 0.1 ml/min is considered to be a high risk to the patient. A stimulated rate (i.e., by chewing paraffin wax for 5 minutes) of 1 to 3 ml/min is considered normal. A rate of **0.7 ml/min** or less is considered a high risk. Xerostomia or dry mouth is not a specific disease but may be related to various local or systemic conditions. Many factors can contribute to a low flow rate. Excessive smoking or alcohol intake, normal aging, altered psychic states, medications, autoimmune diseases, post-irradiation therapy, and dehydration are among the most common causes. Local factors may include congenital absence of salivary glands, glandular hyperplasia, sialolithiasis and sialadenitis, and neoplasias. Systemic conditions with secondary effects on salivary glands include diabetes mellitus, Sjögren syndrome, lupus erythematosus, scleroderma, and polydermatomyositis. Post-irradiation therapy of the head and neck may lead to severe forms of the condition. Medications from several drug categories such as hypnotics, antispasmodics, decongestants, diuretics, antihistamines, amphetamines, tranquilizers, and neoplastic inhibitors have all been implicated in xerostomia. Chronic xerostomia may result in painful oral soft tissue problems, a high incidence of caries, and poor retention of dental prostheses. Buffering capacity of the saliva is reduced, resulting in a more acid oral environment and high risk of caries. Treatment options include medication dose adjustments, artificial saliva substitutes, and topical fluorides.[15]

Salivary buffering capacity is closely related to combined levels of *Streptococci* and *Lactobacilli*. Below a threshold value of **pH less than 4,** the caries process seems to be facilitated. The chairside test method includes placing a drop of stimulated saliva on a test strip containing an acid and a pH indicator. The color of the strip is then compared with a chart to determine the final pH.[1]

A distinction must be made between "risk" and "activity." Caries activity occurs when whenever a plaque deposit on a tooth surface causes demineralization in the underlying enamel. Caries risk is defined as the probability that the patient will develop new caries lesions within a defined time period. There is only one certain way to assess the activity dynamics of individual lesions; that is, by longitudinal observation and recorded representations of the status of the lesion. During an oral examination, clinical data should be collected to evaluate both risk and activity These co-indicators may greatly affect the course of treatment for each patient and lesion.[16]

Host Resistance

An important, yet difficult to define factor in risk assessment is that of host caries resistance. The immune system's role in caries resistance is very complex. Nonspecific immune factors include lysozyme, lactoperoxidase, lactoferrin, high molecular weight glycoproteins, and bacterial agglutinins. These factors may interact with salivary immunoglobulins to amplify the beneficial immune response. IgA is the most prominent salivary immunoglobulin. It is actively secreted into the oral cavity through crevicular fluid transudate. IgG, IgM, complement factors, and phagocytic cells are also found in crevicular fluid. Serum IgA differs from salivary IgA with respect to molecular structure. Secretory IgA is produced in both major and minor salivary glands and is more resistant to proteolytic enzymes from bacteria such as *S. mutans* than from serum IgA, IgG, or IgM. Increased antibody levels to *S. mutans*, either secretory IgA or IgG, can enhance the elimination of *S. mutans* from the oral cavity and interfere with its cariogenic activities. Antibodies can act by various methods to block bacterial surface adhesions that are important for interaction with oral surfaces or that interfere with important cell-bound or extracellular enzymes. IgG can activate the **complement system** (a group of proteins found in the serum of many animals in the inactive form) and facilitate bacterial phagocytosis and killing. Experiences with dental caries does not lead to acquired immunity. Titers of antibodies detected at random moments cannot determine, and do not reflect, a cumulative caries experience of many years. Even in studies of patients with immunodeficiencies compared with normal individuals, no clear-cut effect on caries prevalence was found.

In order to develop a vaccine against dental caries, the responsible microorganism must be identified; an antigen must be produced that has maximum immunogenic activity; and there must be minimal undesirable side effects. An ideal vaccine would produce antibodies that limit the colonization of the cariogenic organisms in dental plaque and affect production of acids and polysaccharides to a level that does not result in caries. As of yet, no human trials have been carried out on a caries vaccine. Safety must outweigh any potential reduction in a non-life-threatening disease such as dental caries. Also, would the reduction in caries activity be any less than that of daily ingestion of topical fluorides?

To best determine the caries risk of an individual, the more relevant the data, the better. Finding the previous caries experience (DMFS or DMFT), intake frequency and type of carbohydrates, fluoride exposure, dental plaque amounts and formation rates, bacteria counts from microbiologic tests, salivary flow rate, salivary buffering capacity, immunologic factors, social habits, and current medications and medical health will give the most accurate risk assessment and best approach to the management of caries disease. Caries tests should not be seen as a replacement for a thorough clinical examination or for sound judgment. Each individual case must be evaluated separately in order to select the most effective treatment. Continuous re-assessment is also an essential part of proper care.[1]

Caries Identification and Diagnosis

Caries diagnosis and management is a process involving multiple criteria that must be adjusted according to the patients overall caries risk. Diagnosis is needed to:

1. Establish the presence of caries in tooth surfaces.
2. Determine the extent of the caries lesion.
3. Select the treatment with the best long-term prognosis.
4. Monitor behavior of caries lesions over time to evaluate treatment efficacy.
5. Screen a large population for caries.
6. Screen populations for risk factors.[1]

The word **diagnosis** comes from the Greek roots *through/knowledge.* Information gathered from diagnostic methods must be combined with basic knowledge to produce a diagnosis. Because caries is a disease process, a continuum from submicroscopic levels to coronal destruction, early diagnosis may be difficult. Lesions that can be treated by nonsurgical methods must be separated from those in need of operative treatment. The main clinical purpose of diagnostic procedures is to affect health outcome. This can only be achieved if subsequent treatment decisions can differ from those reached if the procedure was not applied. Threshold values must be established. Some diagnostic information must be judged subjectively. Clinical examination can be very subjective.[1] Armamentaria used in clinical examinations vary in sensitivity. **Visual inspection** under adequate lighting or **fiber-optic transillumination,** a dry field, and magnification is most commonly used to identify caries lesions. With the routine use of magnification, occlusal caries detection has increased dramatically. Visual evidence of cavitation, surface roughness, opacification, and discoloration are all signs of caries activity. Separation of the teeth in order to gain visual access is another option when encountering questionable lesions.[17] **Tactile evidence** of surface roughness and softness are also clinical signs. Use of sharp explorers is discouraged. If used improperly, one runs the risk of iatrogenic promotion of disease initiation or progression by causing cavitation or inoculation of cariogenic organisms[18] **(Figure 14-13).**

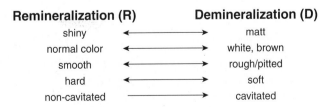

Figure 14-13. Physical appearance of the tooth surface as a possible indicator of lesion activity. [From Benn DK, Dankel DD, et al: Standardized data collection and decision making with an expert system. J Dent Educ 61 (11):885, 1997.]

Radiographic Interpretation

Radiographic imagery can be a valuable diagnostic aid. It makes examination of early lesions in inaccessible areas possible. Lesion penetration depth can be evaluated by radiographs. They are noninvasive and provide a lasting record of the lesion at a moment in time that can be used to measure disease activity in the future. Mineral loss within the dental hard tissues creates the basis for radiographic detection. Once exposed, a radiograph can be produced that shows a higher contrast between sound and demineralized dental hard tissues. Bitewing films, which are correctly exposed and processed, will in most cases provide radiographs of sufficient quality. However, many subsurface lesions in approximal surfaces are radiographically undetectable. One can be certain that caries is present if the result of a radiographic examination is positive, but one cannot be certain that caries is not present if the result of the examination is negative. Proximal radiographic radiolucencies should be examined visually and tactilely whenever possible, because not all radiolucencies are associated with cavitation. After remineralization, arrested caries lesions are found routinely on proximal surfaces and are visible clinically as discolored hard spots. Often, radiographically visible proximal lesions that have penetrated half-way through the dentin are noncavitated and can be treated nonsurgically. Lesions that extend beyond half-way are associated with cavitation over 60% of cases.[18] Caries risk status also plays an important role in determining the type of treatment needed for each individual. A high-risk individual may prompt earlier surgical intervention than will a low-risk individual. Estimates of progression risk are needed as a basis for treatment decisions. In premolars and molars, the average time for a lesion to progress through enamel is estimated at 4 years. Even dentin caries may progress slowly. Large variation exists.[19]

When determining the appropriate time to restore an approximal lesion, certain factors must be considered:

1. The probability is high that the lesion will progress over a given period of time despite nonsurgical efforts to arrest it.
2. The consequences of restoring a lesion that otherwise would have progressed
3. The consequences of not restoring a lesion that progresses
4. The probability that the lesion will not progress
5. The consequences of restoring a lesion that would not have progressed given proper nonsurgical care
6. The values and costs of arresting a lesion through nonsurgical care[1]

Certain radiologic factors must also be considered. These include:

1. The quality of the radiograph is important.
2. The earliest stages of caries lesions cannot be revealed.
3. No unequivocal distinctions exist between approximal surfaces that are sound, have subsurface lesions, or are cavitated.
4. Radiographs usually underestimate the extent of demineralization but may also overestimate it. The earliest depth radiographically detectable is 400 (m.
5. Interpretation is subject to a variation within and between observers.
6. Radiography only provides part of the information needed to make appropriate treatment decisions.[3]

Progression of an approximal lesion into dentine is not considered to be a valid indication for restorative treatment in children who have a low prevalence of caries, because a rapid progression is unlikely and the probability of cavitation, which impairs the prognosis by plaque accumulation, is quite low.[20]

When an early lesion is detected, there appears to be adequate time to use suitable preventive methods so that subclinical lesions never progress to a stage where they are clinically visible. Although the average lesion takes at least 4 years to progress through the enamel of permanent teeth, progression is usually slower for older individuals, particularly those with long-term exposure to fluoride. Restorative treatment can be restrained in favor of preventive measures for about 3 years.

Other, more sensitive, diagnostic techniques may be available soon. These techniques include quantitative light-induced or laser-induced fluorescence, electrical conductivity, and ultrasound.[21] As more sensitive and measurable techniques become practical, earlier detection and monitoring of progression or regression of lesions over time will make caries management a more exact science. Until then, risk assessment and conventional diagnostic aids along with provider acumen will determine how caries are managed.

Caries activity is a difficult to predict. Risk is defined as the probability that an individual will develop at least a certain number of caries lesions and reach a given stage of disease progression in a specified time, conditional upon his or her exposure status remaining stable during the period in question. To date, information based on clinical examinations provided the only statistically highly significant predictors, and that of microbiologic predictors did not contribute significantly to the power of the models. The predicting power of even the best screening measures that are currently available is modest. Each treatment decision must be made individually by a dental professional.

 ## CARIES MANAGEMENT

Caries Control

As discussed earlier, management of patients and individual lesions depends on numerous factors. Because the medical model approach to disease treatment is becoming more widely accepted as the method of choice, the nature of its process can be seen in **Figure 14-14.**

Once lesions have been identified, the patient's risk status has been determined, and an approach to management has been agreed upon by both the provider and the patient, the

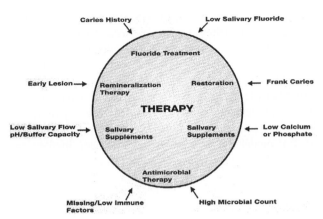

Figure 14-14. Risk assessment, diagnostic information, and therapy. (From Winston AE, Bhaskar SN: Caries prevention in the 21st century. J Am Dent Assoc 129:1584, 1998.)

surgical or nonsurgical treatment regimen should commence. The goal is to preserve as much healthy tooth structure as possible. The "medical model" for disease management should be the preferred method. Risk reduction measures and remineralization therapy are initiated for non-cavitated lesions.

Conservative operative dentistry should be performed on cavitated lesions. When open cavitated lesions are present, the infected dentin should be clinically removed; and an intermediate restoration should be placed to remove the nidus of infection and seeding of cariogenic microorganisms. Glass ionomer or resin modified glass ionomer materials that release fluoride make excellent intermediate restorations. Multiple teeth with acute threatening lesions are treated by the quadrant or the entire mouth as quickly as possible. This stabilizes the caries process for each lesion and limits further spread of infecting organisms. Once the caries lesions have been sealed, antimicrobial therapy, plaque control, and diet modification measures will become more effective. Re-evaluation of the clinical status of the patient must be made, and a lower risk level must be achieved before definitive restorative treatment is initiated. The indications for caries control measures are when:

1. Caries is extensive enough that adverse pulpal sequelae are likely to occur.
2. The goal of treatment is to remove the nidus of caries infection.
3. A tooth has extensive caries involvement that cannot or should not be finally restored because of questionable pulpal prognosis.[3]

When ready for final, definitive restorations, conservative and hygienic dentistry is essential. Cavity preparations should be extended only far enough to gain access to the infected dentin and remove unsupported tooth structure for adequate resistance and retention form and finishing. The choice of restorative materials must also be carefully selected. Pit and fissure sealants should be the preferred treatment for shallow occlusal enamel lesions. **Box only prepa-**

rations can suffice for approximal lesions with⋯ occlusal involvement. **Slot preparations** are adequate ⋯en proximal lesions are accessible on root surfaces. Ac⋯ to proximal lesions by use of tooth separation techni⋯ ⋯ ⋯ay also be feasible. Minimization of loss of tooth str⋯ ⋯ should be the goal in all cases.

When diagnosing recurrent caries or repla⋯ ⋯ent of old restorations, making sure that a restoration really needs to be replaced is imperative. Slowing the re-restore cycle will help to increase a tooth's serviceability. As much as 71% of a general dentist's practice may involve the replacement of existing restorations.[19] Old amalgams should not be routinely replaced because of questionable margins. The patient's caries risk status and the self-sealing properties of amalgam restorations are important factors to consider. In the case of restoration replacement, additional trauma and tooth removal are inevitable. The decision not to re-treat patients who constitute a low caries risk is likely to be the correct one. Periodic monitoring of teeth at risk of recurrent caries is the prudent course of action.[22]

Sealants

Among the most conservative and most successful of the posterior restorations are the **occlusal sealants.** Sealant materials may vary from unfilled resins to filled resins, light-cured to chemically cured resins, and fluoride-releasing to non-fluoride-releasing resins. No matter what material is used, case selection and meticulous attention to technical details are essential. In all sealant placements, moisture control is the key to success. Saliva contamination of the etched enamel surface will result in precipitation of salivary glycoproteins that prevent the sealant from bonding. It is best to remove soft caries with a small round bur or air-abrasion device, because a sealant will not adhere to organic debris. Teeth with large lesions should be restored with a preventive resin or metallic material. The average success rate for a properly placed sealant varies from 50% to 90% for first-time placements. The highest period for re-treatment is at 6 months, when typically 17% of sealants need repairs or replacements.[23] Sealants have been shown to be effective in occlusal caries reduction for 5 to 7 years. Their effectiveness in caries-active patients can be seen in the prevention of caries in newly erupted teeth, incipient caries arrest, prevention of pathologic bacterial growth in sealed fissures, and prevention of cross-infection at other susceptible sites. A placement technique for light-cured sealants follows:

Step 1. Teeth with heavy debris and plaque should be cleaned using dry flour of pumice, water, and a prophy cup or brush. Avoid prophy pastes that contain glycerin or fluorides. Teeth that are relatively clean may be treated with a 3% hydrogen peroxide solution on a bristle brush.

Step 2. Using a small round bur or air-abrasion device, remove any organic debris or stains present in deep grooves, pits, or fissures. A drop of disclosing solution can be used to determine if all the organic debris has been removed.

Step 3. After adequate isolation (well-sealed rubber dam preferred), etch the enamel surfaces with an appropriate etching gel/solution (usually 37% phosphoric acid) for 20 to 30 seconds. Be sure to carry the etchant 2 mm up the cusp inclines. Liquid etchants are placed with a sable brush, whereas gel etchants are placed with a tuberculin or diabetic syringe. When possible, liquids are preferred because of their ability to better penetrate pits and fissures.

Step 4. Trace the grooves with an explorer tip to ensure that air bubbles do not prevent the etchant from reaching the deepest portions of grooved or pitted areas. Immediately after use, wipe off the etching solution from the explorer to avoid acid damage to the instrument.

Step 5. Wash the tooth for 30 seconds up to 1 minute with water. If the pits and fissures are unusually deep, longer rinsing times (1 minute) are recommended.

Step 6. Dry the tooth, using the air syringe and high-speed evacuation for a minimum of 15 seconds. If disclosing solution was used, none should remain in the pits and fissures. Repeat steps 3, 4, 5, and 6 if the enamel does not appear uniformly frosted. A second etch may be applied for 30 seconds rather than 60 seconds if only a slight improvement in the etched appearance is required.

Step 7. For unfilled sealants, place the sealant into the etched grooves with the manufacturer's applicator, brush, explorer, or ball burnisher. For filled sealants, apply and light cure a bonding agent before placing the sealant.

Step 8. Trace the sealant through the grooves and pits with an explorer tip to remove any entrapped air bubbles.

Step 9. For unfilled sealants, remove the excess sealant with a dry cotton pellet. For filled sealants, remove the excess material with a dry plastic brush. In either case, a thin line of sealant should remain in the deepest part of the grooves.

Step 10. Cure the light activated sealant for a minimum of 40 seconds. If the occlusal surface is wider than the diameter of the curing tip, repeat the curing by overlapping the mesial and distal portions of the tooth.

Step 11. Remove the rubber dam and check the occlusion. If using a filled sealant, adjustments are usually necessary. Fine diamonds or finishing burs are the instruments of choice for this procedure.

Recall

Recall frequency of patients to assess caries risk levels and to re-evaluate health and treatment should be customized for every individual. It should be independent of periodontal disease criteria or insurance coverage. The frequency must be determined by the need. Those at high risk require shorter intervals for examination and reinforcement of behavioral changes. Those at low risk may be seen at longer intervals and require less oversight to maintain adequate oral health.

Although dental caries disease has affected humans since ancient times, its total eradication has as yet escaped us. Scientific knowledge and technologic improvements now exist that can prevent an individual from suffering its painful and destructive consequences. By applying the principles of the medical model and evidence-based treatment, humans can now enjoy a lifetime free from advanced caries disease.

Sources

1. Thylstrup A, Fejerskov O: Textbook of Clinical Cariology, 2nd ed. Copenhagen, Denmark, Munksgaard Publisher, 1994, pp 17-411.
2. Loesche WJ: Dental Caries, A Treatable Infection. Grand Haven, MI, ADD, 1994, pp 213, 231, 319.
3. Sturdevant CM: The Art and Science of Operative Dentistry, 3rd ed. St. Louis, CV Mosby, 1995, pp 60-128.
4. Starr CB, Langenderfer WR: Use of a caries-disclosing agent to improve dental residents' ability to detect caries. Oper Dent 18:110-114, 1993.
5. American Dental Association Pamphlet: Baby Bottle Tooth Decay. Chicago, American Dental Association, 1989.
6. Gilmore WH, Lund MR, Bales DJ, Vernetti J: Operative Dentistry. St. Louis, CV Mosby, 1977, p 49.
7. Ettinger RL: Epidemiology of dental caries. Dent Clin North Am 43:679-694, 1999.
8. Brown LJ, Winn DM, White RA: Dental caries restoration and tooth conditions in U.S. adults, 1988-1991: Selected findings from the Third National Health and Nutrition Examination Survey. J Am Dent Assoc 127:1315-1325, 1996.
9. Division of Oral Health, National Center for Chronic Disease Prevention and Health Promotion: Achievements in Public Health, Atlanta, CDC, 1900-1999. Atlanta, CDC, 1999, pp 1-8. http://www.cdc.gov/epo/mmwr/preview/mmwrhtml/mm4841al.htm
10. Warren JJ, Levy SM: Systemic fluoride, sources, amounts, and effects of ingestion. Dent Clin North Am 43:695-711, 1999.
11. ten Cate JM, van Loveren C: Fluoride mechanisms. Dent Clin North Am 43:713-742, 1999.
12. Stookey GK: Caries prevention. J Dent Educ 62 (10):803-811, 1998.
13. Wilkins EM: Clinical Practice of the Dental Hygienist, 8th ed. Philadelphia, JB Lippincott, 1993, pp 473-474.
14. Bowen WH, Tabak LA: Cariology for the Nineties. Rochester, NY, University of Rochester Press, 1993, p 211.
15. Konzelman JL, Terezhalmy GT: Xerostomia Diagnosis and Treatment. U. S. Navy Medicine, November-December, 1983, pp 16-18.
16. Suddick RP, Dodds MWJ: Caries activity estimates and implications: Insights into risk versus activity. J Dent Educ 61:876-884, 1997.
17. Liebenberg WH: Direct access to equivocal approximal carious lesions. Quintessence Int 27(9):607-616, 1996.
18. ten Cate JM, van Amerongen JP: Caries Diagnosis, Conventional Methods. Indiana Conference, 1996, pp 27-37.
19. Benn DK: Practical Evidence-based management of the initial caries lesion. J Dent Educ 61 (11):853-854, 1997.
20. Verdonschot EH, Angmar-Mansson B, ten Bosch JJ, et al: Developments in caries diagnosis and their relationship to treatment decisions and quality of care. Caries Res 33:32-40, 1999.
21. Winston AE, Bhaskar SN: Caries prevention in the 21st century. J Am Dent Assoc 129:1579-1587, 1998.
22. Anusauvice KJ: Treatment regimens in preventive and restorative dentistry. J Am Dent Assoc 126:730-731, 1995.
23. Dennison JB, et al: A clinical comparison of sealant and amalgam in the treatment of pits and fissures. 2. Clinical application and maintenance during an 18-month period. Pediatr Dent 22 (3):176-183, 1980.

Questions and Answers

Questions

1. An average adult will produce about _____ liters of saliva per day.
   A. 0.5-1 L.
   B. 1-1.5 L.
   C. 1.5-2 L.
   D. 2-2.5 L.

2. The earliest bacteria to colonize a clean tooth surface are _____ and _____.
   A. *S. mutans* and *Lactobacillus.*
   B. *Actinomyces* and *Corynebacterium.*
   C. *Streptococcus sanguis* and *Streptococcus mitis.*
   D. *Pseudomonas* and *Haemophilus.*

3. When the salivary and plaque pH drops below _____ demineralization of the enamel is likely to occur.
   A. 7.0
   B. 6.3
   C. 6.0
   D. 5.3

4. "White spot" caries lesions may be visualized by drying the tooth in question. These lesions may be remineralized.
   A. The first statement is true, and the second statement is false.
   B. The second statement is true, and the first statement is false.
   C. Both statements are true.
   D. Both statements are false.

5. The shape of a smooth surface enamel caries lesion appears as a/an _____.
   A. broad area of origin and a conical or pointed extension toward the dentinoenamel junction.
   B. inverted V-shaped area of origin with the apex of the V directed toward the surface.
   C. "v-shaped" and poorly defined extension into the dentinoenamel junction.
   D. inverted "v-shaped" area with a narrow entrance and a progressively wider area closer to the dentinoenamel junction.

6. In advanced caries lesions, infected dentin is decomposed, saturated with bacteria, and has no recognizable structure left. It must be removed before restoring the tooth.
   A. Both statements are false.
   B. Both statements are true.
   C. The first statement is true, and the second statement is false.
   D. The first statement is false, and the second statement is true.

7. The major part of fluoride's caries inhibition can be attributed to its topical posteruptive effects.
   A. True
   B. False

8. The chemoprophylactic agent chlorhexidine is a bisbiguanide that is cationic, bactericidal, and bacteriostatic. It possesses good substantivity, is most effective against gram-negative bacteria, and bacteria do not develop resistance against it.
   A. Both statements are true.
   B. Both statements are false.
   C. The first statement is true, and the second statement is false.
   D. The first statement is false, and the second statement is true.

9. A stimulated salivary flow rate below _____ ml/min is considered at high risk.
   A. 1-3 ml/min.
   B. 1-1.5 ml/min.
   C. 0.7-1 ml/min.
   D. 0.7 ml/min.

10. A premise of the "specific plaque theory" is that plaque is pathogenic only when signs of associated disease are present.
    A. True
    B. False

11. The most frequently seen site of a primary caries lesion is the _____.
    A. root surface.
    B. occlusal surface.
    C. proximal surface.
    D. lingual surface

12. When placing a sealant on a posterior tooth, there is no need to remove debris from the deepest portions of the pits and fissures. Bonding in these areas will be enhanced by the presence of moisture and organic material.
    A. Both statements are true.
    B. Both statements are false.
    C. The first statement is true, and the second is false.
    D. The first statement is false, and the second statement is true.

13. Dental fluorosis is a result of short exposure to topical fluorides and is a necessary consequence of caries prevention.
    A. True
    B. False

14. When measuring the salivary pH changes during a sugar challenge, the **Stephan curve** shows that caries active subjects take _____ for the pH to return to normal as do caries inactive subjects.
    A. the same time.
    B. a shorter time.
    C. a longer time.

15. The cariogenicity of foods is related to

    _____.
    1. the content of various sugars.
    2. the content of polysaccharide starch.
    3. the frequency of intake.
    4. the stickiness.
        A. 1, 2, and 3.
        B. 1, 2, and 4.
        C. 2, 3, and 4.
        D. all of the above

16. Fluoride's primary beneficial effects are derived from its

    _____.
    A. systemic, pre-eruptive effects on enamel.
    B. topical, post-eruptive effects on enamel.
    C. reduction of acid production in bacterial cells.
    D. all of the above.

17. Local factors that may influence xerostomia include all of the following except _____.
    A. glandular hyperplasia.
    B. neoplasias.
    C. diabetes mellitus.
    D. congenital absence of salivary glands.
    E. sialolithiasis.

18. Currently, the population group with the greatest dental caries treatment needs in industrialized societies is

    _____.
    A. infants.
    B. children aged 4 to 14 years.
    C. adult women.
    D. older adults.

19. Fluoride dentifrices have been recognized as the primary reason for the decline in dental caries during the past 2 decades. Frequency of brushing is related to the amount of benefit received.
    A. Both statements are true.
    B. Both statements are false.
    C. The first statement is true, but the second statement is false.
    D. The first statement is false, but the second statement is true.

20. The lethal dose of fluoride is 32 to 64 mg of fluoride per kilogram of body weight.
    A. True
    B. False

ANSWERS

1. **A.** 0.5-1 L/day. Saliva is the fluid produced by the salivary glands in a total volume of 0.5 to 1 L/ day. (From Thylstrup A, Fejerskov O: Textbook of Clinical Cariology, 2nd ed. Copenhagen, Denmark, Munksgaard Publisher, 1994, p 17.)

2. **C.** *Streptococcus sanguis* and *Streptococcus mitis*. Initial colonizers constitute a highly selected part of the oral microflora, mainly *Streptococcus sanguis* and *Streptococcus mitis*. (From Thylstrup A, Fejerskov O: Textbook of Clinical Cariology, 2nd ed. Copenhagen, Denmark, Munksgaard Publishers, 1994, p 90.)

3. **D.** 5.3. Once the pH falls below 5.5, tooth mineral is dissolved. (From Sturdevant CM: The Art and Science of Operative Dentistry, 3rd ed. St. Louis, CV Mosby, 1995, p. 88.)

4. **C.** Both statements are true. On clean, dry teeth, the earliest clinical evidence of caries on the smooth enamel surface of a crown is a white spot. It has been shown experimentally and clinically that incipient caries of enamel can remineralize. (From Sturdevant CM: The Art and Science of Operative Dentistry, 3rd ed. St. Louis, CV Mosby, 1995, p 92.)

5. **A.** Broad area of origin and a conical or pointed extension toward the dentinoenamel junction. A cross-section of the enamel portion of a smooth surface lesion shows a V-shape with a wide area of origin and the apex of the V directed toward the dentinoenamel junction. (From Sturdevant CM: The Art and Science of Operative Dentistry, 3rd ed. St. Louis, CV Mosby, 1995, p 90.)

6. **B.** Both statements are true. Infected dentin is both softened and contaminated with bacteria. Affected dentin is softened and demineralized dentin that is not yet invaded by bacteria. Infected dentin must be removed. Affected dentin may remain. (From Sturdevant CM: The Art and Science of Operative Dentistry, 3rd ed. St. Louis, CV Mosby, 1995, p 99.)

7. **A.** True. Fluoride's predominant mechanism of action occurs after tooth eruption. The data from studies during the last 2 decades have shown significant benefits from fluoridated water when ingestion begins after tooth eruption. [From Stookey GK, Caries prevention. J Dent Educ 62 (10):805, 1998.]

8. **C.** The first statement is true, and the second statement is false. Chlorhexidine is a bisbiguanide. It is generally more effective against gram-positive bacteria than against gram-negative bacteria. It readily binds to negatively charged bacterial cell walls. At high concentrations, chlorhexidine is bactericidal. The effect is bacteriostatic at lower concentrations. Its efficacy has been ascribed to its substantive properties and antimicrobial effects even when adsorbed to tooth surfaces. No known resistant strains against it have been identified. (From Thylstrup A, Fejerskov O: Textbook of Clinical Cariology, 2nd ed. Copenhagen, Denmark, Munksgaard Publishers, 1994, pp 316-318.)

9. **D.** 0.7 ml/min. There is a threshold value for increased caries risk at around 0.7 ml/min for the stimulated secretion rate. (From Thylstrup A, Fejerskov O: Textbook of Clinical Cariology, 2nd ed. Copenhagen, Denmark, Munksgaard Publishers, 1994, p 345.)

10. **A.** True. The nonspecific plaque theory based its premise on the idea that all plaque was bad. The specific plaque theory is based on the premise that plaque is pathogenic only when signs of associated disease are present. Plaque can facilitate remineralization by having high concentrations of fluoride, calcium, and phosphate ions. Certain nonpathogenic bacteria can prevent the establishment of pathogenic strains. (From Loesche WJ: Dental Caries: A Treatable Infection. Grand Haven, MI, ADD, 1994, p 319.)

11. **B.** Occlusal surface. Pit and fissure (occlusal surfaces) caries have the highest prevalence of all dental caries. (From Sturdevant CM: The Art and Science of Operative Dentistry, 3rd ed. St. Louis, CV Mosby, 1995, p 78.)

12. **B.** Both statements are false. When placing pit and fissure sealants, control of moisture and saliva is very important. Removal of debris will allow for bonding to the intact tooth structure. Sealants will not adhere to organic debris. [From Dennison JB, et al: A clinical comparison of sealant and amalgam in the treatment of pits and fissures. 2: Clinical application and

maintenance during an 18 month period. Pediatr Dent 22 (3):176-183, 1980.]

13. **B.** False. Dental fluorosis can result from excessive long-term ingestion of fluoride during tooth development. Fluorosis is not a necessary side effect of caries prevention and treatment. (From Division of Oral Health, National Center for Chronic Disease Prevention and Health Promotion, CDC: Achievements in Public Health, 1900-1999. Atlanta, CDC, 1999, pp 1-8. http://www.cdc.gov/epo/mmwr/preview/mmwrhtml/mm4841al. htm

14. **C.** A longer time. Caries-active subjects have a high count of acidogenic bacteria. These bacteria continue to produce acids in higher amounts and for longer periods than in caries inactive individuals with low bacteria counts. (From Loesche WJ: Dental Caries: A Treatable Infection. Grand Haven, MI, ADD, 1994, pp 213, 231, and 319.)

15. **D.** All of the above. The cariogenic potential of foods is related to the content of various sugars, polysaccharide starches, their frequency of intake, and their consistency (stickiness).

    The Vipeholm study in Sweden from 1946 to 1951 showed that the length, frequency, and to a lesser extent the form of sugar exposure were critical factors in cariogenicity of foods. (From Thylstrup A, Fejerskov O: Textbook of Clinical Cariology, 2nd ed. Copenhagen, Denmark, Munksgaard Publishers, 1994, pp 288-294.)

16. **B.** Topical, posteruptive effects on enamel. Fluoride may reduce the incidence and severity of dental caries by its systemic, pre-eruptive effects omenamel development and by its effects on cariogenic bacteria, but its most important effect is through its posteruptive effects on the enamel surface. [From Stookey GK, Caries prevention. J Dent Educ 62 (10):805, 1998.]

17. **C.** Diabetes mellitus. Local factors that may cause or contribute to xerostomia include rare absence or aplasia of major salivary glands, glandular hyperplasia seen in mumps, sialolithiasis, sialadenitis, and neoplasias. Systemic conditions associated with xerostomia include diabetes mellitus and Sjögren syndrome. The most dramatic form of xerostomia is seen secondary to external irradiation of the head and neck. (From Konzelman JL, Terezhalmy GT: Xerostomia: Diagnosis and treatment. U. S. Navy Med Nov-Dec, 1983, pp 16-18.)

18. **D.** Older adults. As the population ages, more people aged 60 years or older will have intact dentitions than ever before. Thus, more teeth than ever will be at risk for caries among persons of that age group. (From Division of Oral Health, National Center for Chronic Disease Prevention and Health Promotion, CDC: Achievements in Public Health, 1900-1999. Atlanta, CDC, 1999, p 5.)

    http://www.cdc.gov/epo/mmwr/preview/mmwrhtml/mm4841al. htm

19. **A.** Both statements are true. The extensive use of fluoridated dentifrices has been a primary reason for the decline in caries observed in many parts of the world during the past 2 decades. It is important to note that the frequency of use of fluoride dentifrices is related to the magnitude of the benefit to the patient. [From Stookey GK: Caries prevention. J Dent Educ 62(10):808, 1998.]

20. **A.** True. The certain lethal dose of fluoride is in the range of 32 to 64 mg F/kg of body weight. Acute fatal fluoride poisoning would occur after ingestion of 5 to 10 g for 70-kg adults and 320 mg for 2-year-olds weighing about 10 kg. [From Warren JJ, Levy SM: Systemic fluoride, sources, amounts, and effects of ingestion. Dent Clin North Am 43 (4):703, 1999.]

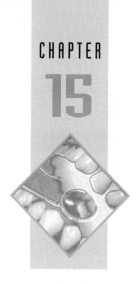

CHAPTER

15

Providing Supportive Treatment Services

MICHAEL BAGBY, DDS, PHD   MARCIA GLADWIN, RDH, EDD

 ## PROPERTIES AND MANIPULATION

The proper use of all dental materials is fundamental to the art and science of dentistry. Materials used in the practice of dental hygiene include therapeutic agents, dental biomaterials, and instruments made from common industrial materials. An understanding of the physical, chemical, and mechanical properties of materials is important, because this knowledge influences their handling. Proper handling of dental materials is a primary factor in their success or failure. Furthermore, the proper care and maintenance of instruments (e.g., prevention of corrosion) will affect their longevity.

Whether a material is used for preventive or restorative purposes, the oral environment places great restrictions on which materials can be used and the manner in which they are used. Both teeth and dental materials must withstand biting forces, degradation by acids, and temperature changes while meeting the biocompatibility and esthetic needs of the patient.

Standards and Selection of Dental Materials

In the United States, standards and guidelines for evaluating dental products are developed and administered by the Council on Scientific Affairs of the American Dental Association (ADA). If a product is shown to be safe and effective, it can be awarded the Seal of Acceptance. The Acceptance Program of the ADA is voluntary. Manufacturers are not required to have the ADA's seal to market dental products in the United States, but these products must be approved for sale by the Food and Drug Administration (FDA).

Classification of Dental Materials

Like oral tissues, dental materials serve various functions. Some materials replace lost tooth structure and restore the function of the teeth. These materials must withstand biting forces and, therefore, have strength and wear resistance. Other materials are used to make impressions of oral tissues from which replicas are made. In dentistry, as with other disciplines, the use of a material must be matched to the properties of that material. Use or function is often used to classify dental materials.

Phases

Materials are commonly classified into one of three phases: **solid, liquid,** or **gas.** The atomic bonds between gas molecules are very weak and easily broken by the normal microscopic vibrations of the thermal energy of the material at room temperature. Liquids have greater attraction between molecules compared with gases, but liquids are not strong enough to carry a load or maintain a shape without support. Solids exhibit the strongest attraction between atoms and molecules. The atomic bonds of solids maintain the shape of objects and resist external forces placed on them.

Materials and Their Atomic Bonds

Atoms of a material and the manner in which they are bonded together determine the properties of that material. Weak bonds make for weak materials and vice versa. Materials can be classified into three categories based on their primary atomic bonds: **metals, ceramics,** and **polymers.** A fourth category is **composites.** Composites are "mixtures" of two materials from two different categories. Dental composites are a combination of a ceramic with a polymeric material.

Primary Bonds

Primary bonds are the strong bonds between atoms of materials. These bonds involve the transfer or sharing of electrons between atoms. All bonds are a result of the electromagnetic force and the distribution of positive and negative charges of atoms and molecules. **Ionic bonds** are the result of an electron being given up by one atom and being accepted by another, thus forming oppositely charged ions. The opposite electrical charges of these ions attract one another, and the result is a **ceramic material**. Ceramic materials are very strong when they are compressed, because the atoms are forced together. However, ceramic materials are weak and brittle when atoms are pulled apart.

Covalent bonds are the result of sharing a pair of electrons between two atoms. Covalent bonds are strong and directed between the atoms of the bond. Polymers are long chains of covalently bonded carbon atoms. The chains are strong but sometimes the materials are not, because their properties are determined by how the long chains are bonded to each other. Examples of polymers include manmade plastics and rubbers as well as many biologic macromolecules such as proteins and DNA.

Metals

Metals have characteristic properties that allow us to easily determine if a material is a metal. Metals are typically dense, heavy materials. They are good conductors of both electricity and heat. These properties of metals are a result of the **metallic bond**. The metallic bond is similar to the covalent bond in that valence electrons are shared among atoms. The difference is that the electrons in a metal object are not shared by two atoms but are shared by all the atoms that make up that object. Metals can be thought of as positive cores in a cloud of negative mobile valence electrons. A weak primary bond in all directions results. The enormous number of bonds in a metal results in a strong material. The nondirectional nature of the metallic bond has an important effect on the properties and use of metals. Metals are **ductile**; they can easily be bent without breaking, yet they retain their strength. The ease with which metals can be bent and shaped enables the manufacture of strong tools that are tough and fracture resistant.

Secondary Bonds

Secondary bonds or **van der Waals forces** are the result of partial charges due to an uneven distribution of electrons around an atom or molecule. The partial charges can be temporary or permanent or very weak or somewhat strong. Secondary bonds are important when determining the properties of polymers, because they determine the interaction of the polymer chains and, therefore, the properties of the polymer. **Hydrogen bonds** are a special type of secondary bond. The hydrogen atom contains only one electron. When this single electron is pulled away from the hydrogen nucleus by an electronegative atom, such as oxygen, the nucleus is left partially unshielded to a much greater extent than other elements with multiple electrons. The resultant hydrogen bond between molecules is much stronger than are the other secondary bonds.

Polymers

Polymers consist of long chains of covalently bonded repeating units. The chains are thousands of units long and consist of carbon, hydrogen, and other elements. The variety of bonds between polymer chains results in a wide diversity of polymeric materials. If weak secondary bonds between chains are easily broken, the chains slide by one another very easily at room temperature. These materials, which are soft, weak, and flexible, are called **plastics**. Stronger secondary bonds, such as the hydrogen bond, cause the chain-to-chain interaction to greatly increase. Such polymeric materials are stronger, stiffer, and more brittle.

Polymers have been developed which incorporate primary atomic bonds between the chains in their polymeric structure. These polymers have cross-links between the chains, which prevent the chains from sliding by each other. A stiff, strong material results. Another important group has widely spaced cross-links. They can be stretched out a great deal, and they return to their original shape. They are called **rubber materials**.

Composites

Composites are materials made of two or more different materials. Common composites are mixtures of a polymer and ceramic, such as fiberglass. Each material that makes up a composite is called a **phase**. Materials or phases are chosen and combined so that the resultant composite has better properties than either material. A composite can be thought of as a team of materials, usually on a microscopic level. Teeth and bones are made of composite materials. Enamel is a composite of apatite (i.e., a type of ceramic material) and protein, which is a polymer.

Colloids

Colloids are also two phase materials. Colloids are mixtures of gases, liquids, or solids at the microscopic level. Colloids are not true solutions of one material dissolved in another, such as salt water. Colloids are suspensions of one material in another, such as fog. Properties of composite materials are a result of properties of the component materials. Properties of colloids, on the other hand, are a result of the properties of the components, but they are also greatly affected by the properties of the surfaces of the component phases. The large amount of surface area around the very small particles gives colloids their properties. Common colloids are gelatin, foam, milk, smoke, and emulsions. Several colloids are used in dentistry as impression materials.

Properties of Dental Materials

Determination of what is required and what will best meet the clinical situation is a very complex question. Typically, there is a compromise between the numerous characteristics of dental materials. A material's characteristics can be divided into three categories: physical, chemical, and biologic properties. **Physical properties** are based on the laws of physics that describe mass, energy, force, light, heat, electricity, and other physical phenomena. Examples are color, density, and thermal conductivity. **Mechanical properties** constitute a subgroup of physical properties that describe a material's ability to resist forces. Mechanical properties depend on the amount of material and the size and shape of the object. Examples are strength and stiffness of a material. **Chemical properties** of materials describe the setting reactions of materials and the corrosion, decay, or degradation of materials. **Biologic properties** of materials are the effects that the materials have on living tissues.

Physical Properties

Physical properties include the density of a material, the boiling and melting points, and the vapor pressure. Thermal conductivity, heat capacity, heat of fusion, heat of vaporization, and coefficient of thermal expansion are physical properties that are also called **thermal properties**.

Coefficient of Thermal Expansion

Most materials expand when they are heated. The **coefficient of thermal expansion** is a measurement of this change in size. A polymeric material such as polymethylmethacrylate (an obsolete tooth-colored restorative material) shrinks and expands seven times more than does the tooth structure. The process of heating and cooling and the accompanying opening and closing of the gap is called **percolation**. Percolation results in tooth sensitivity and recurrent decay.

Miscellaneous Physical Properties

The **viscosity** of a material is its ability to flow. Thick or viscous liquids flow poorly, whereas thin liquids flow easily. Viscosity is a very temperature-dependent property; liquids flow much better when they are warm. A low viscosity and the ability to wet a surface are very important in the use of many dental materials. **Wetting** a surface with an adhesive material such as a pit and fissure sealant brings the material into intimate contact with that surface. Chemical and micromechanical bonding can occur. Wetting is measured by determining the contact angle of a liquid on a solid. A low contact angle such as a drop of water on ice indicates good wetting. A high contact angle such as water on most plastics indicates poor wetting.

Enamel is the hardest biologic tissue in the human body. **Hardness** is a property measured by scientific instruments that press a tip (made of a very hard material such as steel or diamond) into the surface of a material. The size of the resultant indentation created in the surface by the tip is measured. Hardness is calculated based on the size of the indentation. Some materials are quite soft. A different kind of

hardness test is used, because these materials are "spongy" and an indentation is not left behind in the material. A durometer measures how deep into a material a loaded steel ball sinks. **Durometers** are used to measure the hardness of rubber materials, such as impression putties.

Harder materials tend to be more **resistant to abrasion** than are softer ones. The abrasion resistance, or wear resistance, of dental restorations by food and opposing teeth and the wear of restorations on opposing teeth are important factors to know when choosing a restorative material. If a material is too hard, it will wear opposing teeth at an unacceptable, accelerated pace.

As materials function in the oral cavity, they are exposed to various aqueous fluids. **Solubility** is the amount of material that dissolves in a liquid in a given time. Excessive solubility of dental cement leads to a loss of material and increases the risk of recurrent decay. Some materials absorb water and swell. This property is called **water sorption**. Polymers absorb microscopic amounts of water.

The appearance of a restoration can be an important factor. **Color** is a complex phenomenon that is a psychological response to a physical stimulus. The physical stimulus is light reaching the rods and cones of the eye. The processing of those stimuli by the brain is a psychological phenomenon that makes the perception of color vary among individuals. Two people may agree that two objects match in color, whereas a third person may disagree. In addition, the color of objects depends on the light in which the object is viewed. Matching restorative materials to a patient's adjacent teeth can be a difficult task. In dentistry, esthetic materials have their own set of color samples called shade guides.

Some materials are **radiolucent** and are not seen in radiographs. Examples are some ceramic materials and denture acrylic resin. Other materials are **radiopaque** and are evident on radiographs, such as a metal restoration (**Figure 15-1;** see Chapter 11). Some dental restorative materials have been formulated by the manufacturer to match the radiopacity of enamel. The purpose is to facilitate the diagnosis of recurrent decay.

Mechanical Properties

Because teeth are used to tear and grind food, they must be strong; the materials used to replace missing tooth structure must also be strong. Engineers have studied the strength and stiffness of materials. If a rubber band is stretched, it increases in length. As the amount of stretch increases, the accompanying force or pull of the rubber band increases. The atomic bonds of the rubber band are stretched and oppose the applied force. If the pull on the rubber band is released, the band returns to its original length. The atomic bonds that were stretched return to their original length. This phenomenon is called **elasticity**.

When a force is placed on an object, such as hanging a weight (load) from a rubber band, the force affects the object. Inside the object (the rubber band), an equal and opposite force

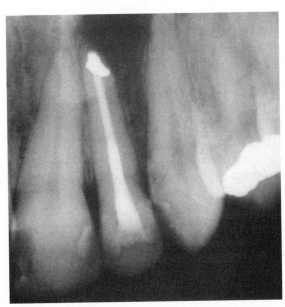

Figure 15-1. Radiograph of teeth, bone, composite restorations, liners, gutta percha (root canal filling material), amalgam retrofill, and amalgam restorations. (Courtesy of Dr. C. Russell Jackson, Morgantown, WV. From Gladwin M, Bagby MD: Clinical Aspects of Dental Materials. Philadelphia, Lippincott Williams & Wilkins, 2000, p 176.)

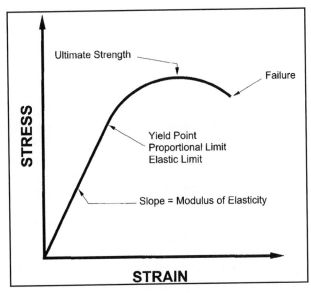

Figure 15-2. Typical stress-strain plot. (From Gladwin M, Bagby MD: Clinical Aspects of Dental Materials. Philadelphia, Lippincott Williams & Wilkins, 2000, p 38.)

or stress develops that resists the load. The force or stress that develops in the object is from the stretching of atomic bonds. As a greater load is placed on the object, the bonds are stretched more and a greater stress occurs in the object.

The change in shape of a loaded object is quantified in terms of the fractional change in length. **Strain** is the change in length divided by the original length. The units of strain are seen as fractions (e.g., 0.02) or percentages (e.g., 2%). As mentioned earlier, the force that develops in a loaded object is called stress. The **stress** is proportional to the load. The stress is also related to the size of the object. Stress is the load divided by the cross-sectional area of the object:

$$\text{Stress} = \text{load/area}$$

The units of stress are pounds per square inch (psi). In the metric system, the units used are pascals (or megapascals).

It turns out that the load and the change in length, or stress and strain, are proportional. The proportionality constant or the slope of a graph of stress and strain is called the **modulus of elasticity** or Young's modulus:

$$\text{Modulus of elasticity} = \text{stress/strain}$$

The modulus of elasticity is characteristic of a material. The higher the modulus of elasticity, the stiffer is the material. Enamel has a high modulus of elasticity, whereas a rubber band has a low modulus. The units of modulus are the same as those of stress; that is, pounds per square inch or megapascals.

When strain increases, stress also increases **(Figure 15-2)**. The slope of the line is equal to the modulus. If the strain continues to increase, at some point the line on the graph begins to curve. Stress is no longer proportional to strain. At this point, if the stress is released, the object does *not* return

to its original length. It has become permanently deformed, and this is called **plastic deformation**. The point where the line starts to curve is called the **elastic limit**, the **proportional limit**, or the **yield point**. If loading is continued, at some point the object breaks. Failure occurs. The stress at that point is called the **ultimate strength**. The load on the object has caused a force to develop that is greater than the strength of the atomic bonds holding the material together; the object then breaks.

Combinations of several kinds of stresses are most common. **Compression** is a pushing or crushing stress. **Tension** is a pulling stress. **Shear (slip) stress** occurs when parts of an object slide by one another. **Torsion stress** is a twisting force. **Bending** is a combination of compressive, tensile, and shear.

Mechanical Properties of Dental Materials

In order to properly function, a restoration must be hard (hardness), strong (yield strength), and stiff (modulus) enough to withstand the forces of mastication. The yield strength is more important than the ultimate strength for many uses of materials. If a restoration yields or plastically deforms, it is no longer the same shape and is unlikely to precisely fit the cavity preparation.

Most of the time, a restoration or impression should not **plastically (permanently distort)** deform when force is applied. The restoration and the teeth should **elastically deform** and return to their original shape when the biting force is removed. The same is true for impressions. Impressions should return to their original shape after they have been removed from the mouth.

The ability to absorb energy and not deform is called **resilience**. Resilience is measured as the area under the stress-strain curve up to the yield point. The energy absorbed up to the failure point on the stress-strain diagram is the **toughness** of the material. Plastics in general have high resilience and toughness values.

Certain dental materials change too slowly to be easily observed but quickly enough to affect the use of the material and the resultant patient care. Two of these changes are creep and stress relaxation. **Creep** is the resultant small change in shape when an object is continuously compressed. Creep can be thought of as extremely slow flow. Stress relaxation is a slow decrease in force over time. If a rubber band is stretched to a constant length, over a period of time the pull of the rubber decreases or relaxes. The loss of pull (i.e., the decrease in stress or force) by the rubber band over time is called **stress relaxation**. Both creep and stress relaxation depend greatly on temperature.

It is very difficult to make objects without holes, scratches, cracks, bubbles (voids), or other defects. Stress is concentrated greatly around defects. This phenomenon is called **stress concentration**. Fracture becomes more likely as cracks develop near defects and spread throughout the object. Controlling defects in objects is important in order to reduce stress concentration and produce stronger products. In dentistry, it is important to mix and handle materials properly to reduce the occurrence of voids and defects.

Adhesion or Bonding

Adhesion or bonding is the joining of two objects together using an adhesive or cement. Adhesion or bonding is also important when a protective layer is applied to an object, such as painting a metal surface to prevent rust or using pit and fissure sealants to prevent decay. Whereas true adhesion involves chemical bonds between materials being joined, not all bonding to tooth structures is truly adhesive. **Micromechanical** bonding of dental materials to tooth structure is common. This type of bonding uses surface irregularities that are smaller than can be seen with the naked eye or felt with a dental explorer.

Macromechanical bonding is used for cementing (luting) crowns and bridges to teeth with "nonadhesive" cements. Macromechanical bonding uses surface irregularities that can be seen by the naked eye and felt with a dental explorer. Such dental cements fill in the roughness on the surface of the tooth and inside of the crown. The crown is luted or glued in place in the same manner as two pieces of wood are glued together.

Uses of Adhesive Materials in Dentistry

Adhesion is commonly used to retain restorations in place. Undercuts and other mechanical locks are unnecessary when adhesive materials are used. Adhesion is also used to attach orthodontic brackets and other appliances to teeth. Adhesion reduces or eliminates microleakage of restorations. As a result, postoperative sensitivity is reduced. Post-

operative sensitivity and recurrent decay are caused by fluids and bacteria moving in and out of the small space (margin) between a restoration and the tooth. The pulp is irritated by the movement of fluid, and the result is pain. Adhesion also reduces the staining of margins of esthetic materials.

Surface Factors

When applying an adhesive to an object, the surface must be clean. Adhesives will not bond to the surface irregularities if they are filled or covered by debris. If the surface and the adhesive are not somewhat chemically compatible, the adhesive will not **wet** the surface adequately; the adhesive will not flow into the irregularities; and bonding will be poor. Whether the bonding is macromechanical, micromechanical, or truly adhesive (chemical), the surface must be clean to allow intimate association of the adhesive (bonding material) and the adherend (the surface).

Acid Etching Process

Acid etching was initially conceived by Buonocore in the 1950s to seal pits and fissures. An acid, typically **37% phosphoric acid**, is applied to enamel for 15 to 30 seconds and the surface is etched (i.e., chemically roughened). The surface is rinsed with water and dried. The etched surface is "porous," and a low viscosity polymer flows into the irregularities and cures (or sets). The polymer is locked into the surface irregularities and forms a strong bond. Acid etching is a micromechanical bonding technique that was first used to retain pit and fissure sealants. Later, when dental composite restorations were developed in the 1960s, acid etching techniques were included to reduce leakage and staining of margins. In addition, acid etching can be used to bond composites to teeth to correct fractures, rotations, or other defects.

A correctly etched enamel surface is shown in **Figure 15-3**. Primary teeth need to be etched for a longer time than do permanent teeth, because the enamel rods are less regularly arranged. The results of acid etching primary teeth are less reliable than are those of permanent teeth.

Dentinal Bonding

Current dentinal bonding systems function by way of micromechanical bonding and secondary atomic bonds. Dentinal bonding systems constitute an extension of the acid etch technique. Dentinal bonding systems bond to both enamel and dentin.

When dentin is cut or prepared by dental instruments, a layer of debris called the **smear layer** is produced on the surface. The smear layer on dentin also extends a short distance into the dental tubules. The smear layer is ground dentin that weakly adheres to the cut dentin surface. Enamel, on the other hand, cuts more cleanly because it is a more highly calcified tissue.

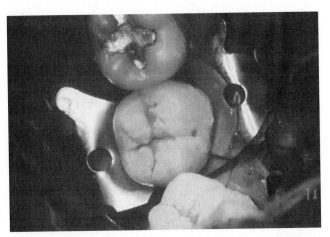

Figure 15-3. Photograph of etched enamel. Note the chalky appearance. (Courtesy of Dr. Ronald House, Morgantown, WV. From Gladwin M, Bagby MD: Clinical Aspects of Dental Materials. Philadelphia, Lippincott Williams & Wilkins, 2000, p 45.)

Three-Step Dentinal Bonding Systems

1. Both dentin and enamel are cleaned and etched in the same manner as is the acid etch technique. Typically, 37% orthophosphoric acid is used. Etching dentin removes the smear layer from the surface of the dentin. Etching also decalcifies a layer of dentin that is several microns thick. Collagen fibers, which constitute a major organic component of dentin, are left on this decalcified surface. After etching, the surface is rinsed with water as with acid etching, but the surface is only slightly dried and is not desiccated.

2. The primer is applied. **Primers** are low-viscosity hydrophilic resins. The primer often contains a volatile solvent such as acetone to thin the organic chemicals and improve the wetting of the etched surface. The primer flows into the surface irregularities of etched enamel and into the open tubules of etched dentin. The primer also flows around the collagen fibers that were exposed when the dentin was etched.

3. The "adhesive" material is applied. This material is a low viscosity resin much like that used for the acid etching technique. The difference is that the dentin bonding adhesive may contain some hydrophilic chemicals. The dentin bonding adhesive sets, or polymerizes, in the same manner as does the enamel bonding resin.

After the dentinal bonding system has been placed, the composite material is placed. The composite material bonds to the dentinal bonding material and reacts with the air-inhibited layer of the adhesive. The result is retention of the restoration and reduced microleakage. Newer dentinal bonding systems have reduced the number of steps to only two.

Materials Based on Polyacrylic Acid

Glass ionomer materials and polycarboxylate cements are adhesive materials based on polyacrylic acid. Polyacrylic acid is a long chain molecule with acid (carboxyl) groups hanging off the side. The acid groups react with the powder component of the cement when the material sets to form a solid mass. The acid groups can also react with the tooth structure and chemically bond to dentin and enamel. Bonding glass ionomer materials and polycarboxylate cements to enamel and dentin is simple compared with dentinal bonding systems and composites. In other words, no separate adhesive is placed and then followed by the restorative material. The material itself is chemically adhesive. The material is mixed and is then applied to the tooth. In addition to chemical adhesion, micromechanical retention is possible if the surface has microscopic irregularities such as partially open dentinal tubules.

Bonding and Dentistry

Depending on the clinical situation, the dentist will choose among a variety of adhesive materials. Acid etching of enamel is still used to place pit and fissure sealants and bond orthodontic brackets. Dentinal bonding systems are the norm when composite restorations are placed. Dentinal bonding systems are used to reduce sensitivity of exposed root surfaces of teeth. Glass ionomer materials are the materials of choice for many clinicians for restoring cervical lesions and cementing metallic crowns. All adhesive materials require proper handling and a clean surface for maximum bonding.

DENTAL POLYMERS

Polymers are materials that are made of very long molecules. They are formed by chemically linking molecular building blocks called **monomers**. The chemical reactions that produce such macromolecules are called **polymerization** reactions. Acrylic resins are used in dentistry for various devices and prostheses. Dental acrylic resin is the same polymer as that used in Plexiglas. This tough plastic is used as a glass substitute in windows. Acrylic resins and composite materials such as restorative materials, cements, sealants, and adhesives all set via addition polymerization. The first step in an **addition polymerization reaction** is the formation of a free radical. A free radical can be formed by several methods: by heat, light, or a chemical reaction. The "set on demand" nature of light-activated materials has made them very popular. Several dental materials have both chemical and light activation (cure) capabilities. They are called dual-cured materials.

After the free radical is formed, it reacts with the C=C of a monomer molecule and starts to grow a polymer chain. A new C-C bond is formed between the free radical and one of the carbons atoms of the C=C. A free radical, located on the other carbon atom of the previous C=C, is also formed. The polymer chain continues to grow by reacting with thousands of additional monomer molecules.

Problems with Dental Restorative Resins

Polymerization reactions make a few very large polymer molecules from very many small monomer molecules. Atoms and molecules become packed much closer together when they are polymerized, and shrinkage is the result. In dentistry, polymeric restorative materials shrink when they set and have the potential to open gaps at margins. Also, polymeric materials have coefficients of thermal expansion 2 to 10 times greater than those of the tooth structure. Thermal expansion and contraction of polymeric restorative materials increase the risk of recurrent caries.

Composite Materials

Over the years, dental polymers have been improved by several modifications. Fillers and coupling agents were added. Stronger polymers were developed. All were used to manufacture **dental composites**. Dental composites come in a variety of shades (colors) and handling characteristics. Their use continues to expand and replace other materials. Detection of a well-placed composite restoration can be a difficult task. Whereas a good shade match and excellent margins may make a composite restoration almost invisible, they feel slightly softer to a sharp explorer. Composite restorations may appear radiopaque or radiolucent on radiographs depending on the filler in the product (see Chapter 11).

Components of a Dental Composite

The **matrix** of dental composites is a polymer that is chemically similar to enamel and dentin adhesives. The monomer is bifunctional and has two C=C groups. Bifunctional monomers result in cross-linked polymer chains and greatly improve the strength of the resultant material. The matrix of a dental composite polymerizes via addition polymerization. Polymerization is activated via a chemical reaction (**chemical cure**) or light activation (**light cure**). Light-cured materials are the most commonly used dental composite materials. Composites chemically bond to primers and adhesives of dental bonding systems because both have C=C functional groups and both set via addition polymerization.

Filler particles constitute a strong second phase that is added to improve the physical properties of dental composites. Fillers are ceramic materials that are formulated to have the proper strength, hardness, and chemical and optical properties for use in dental composites. Fillers have a low coefficient of thermal expansion. The filler particles are ground to have the proper size particle and are **silanated**. Silanated particles chemically bond to the polymer of the composite. The silanated filler is mixed with monomers, diluents, coloring agents, and other chemicals to form a paste. With the exception of proper handling, the percent filler is the most important determinant of physical properties of dental composites. As the filler content increases, the

resin content decreases. Polymerization shrinkage decreases. The coefficient of thermal expansion becomes more like that of tooth structure. Hardness and abrasion resistance increase. Manufacturers attempt to maximize the filler content of their dental composites.

To obtain the maximum benefit of the addition of filler particles, the matrix is bonded to the filler particle with a **coupling agent**. Silane coupling agents are long molecules that react with the polymer matrix at one end, whereas the other end reacts with the ceramic filler. The coupling agent couples or transfers stress from the relatively weak matrix to the relatively strong filler.

The size of the filler in a dental composite determines surface smoothness of the resultant restoration. Larger particles result in a rougher surface. Composites are most often classified by the size of their filler particles. This chapter discusses three categories of dental composites: macrofill, microfill, and hybrid (blends).

Properties of Dental Composites

Light-cured materials are convenient to use; however, the curing light can only penetrate through several millimeters of composite or tooth structure. As a result, dental composites are placed in layers or increments and cured after each layer is placed. Incremental addition allows the first layer to set and shrink before additional layers are added.

When composite materials are placed in increments, each increment chemically bonds to the previous increment. Chemical bonding occurs because addition polymerization is inhibited by atmospheric oxygen. This inhibition of the reaction results in a thin layer of unreacted material on the surface of a newly set composite (if the surface was exposed to air when it set). The thin air-inhibited layer does not cure whether the material is light-cured or chemical-cured. When a second layer is added, oxygen is excluded and the first air-inhibited layer and the new material are chemically bonded together when the second layer is cured.

Not all C=C bonds react when a dental composite sets. Typically, only about 50% of the C=C bonds react. Therefore, it is possible to repair or add to a composite restoration by cleaning the surface of debris and properly adding new material. Some of the unreacted C=C bonds in the old material will react with the setting matrix of the new material.

Types of Dental Composites and Their Properties

Macrofilled Composites

The first dental composites developed in the 1960s are now called **macrofilled** composites. The filler is a quartz material with particles that are 10 to 25 μm. Filler content is 70% to 80% by weight. The large size of the filler particles in macrofilled composites results in a restoration that feels rough to the dental explorer and can appear rough to the eye.

The typical macrofilled composite will turn slightly gray when rubbed with an instrument. Macrofills have little clinical importance at this time, except that some orthodontists still use them. The rough feel and easy detection is an advantage when removing bonded orthodontic brackets or appliances and the accompanying bonding material.

Microfilled Composites

In the late 1970s, **microfilled composites** were marketed. The particle size is much smaller than that of macrofill composites (i.e., 0.03-0.5 μm). Microfill composites polish very smooth and lustrous. The surface appearance is very similar to that of enamel. The very small filler particles typically consist of fused silica. The problem with microfilled composites is the low percentage of filler (i.e., 40%-50%). The surface area of the very small filler particles requires much more resin to wet the surface of the filler particles. The high resin content results in an increased coefficient of thermal expansion and lower strength. Currently, microfilled composites are used when esthetics are the dominant concern.

Hybrid Composites

Hybrid composites were developed in the late 1980s; these composites are strong and polish well. Their filler content is 75% to 80% by weight. The average size of the filler particles is 0.5 to 1 μm, but these particles have a wider range of sizes-0.1 to 3 μm. They are called hybrids or blended composites, because they have a range of particle sizes. Hybrid composites are very popular because their strength and abrasion resistance are acceptable for small- to medium-sized class I and class II restorations. Their surface finish is almost as good as that of microfills, and thus they are used for class III and class IV restorations. A summary of the properties of the three types of dental composite materials is listed in **Table 15-1**.

New Composite Materials

Two new types of composite materials have been developed. **Flowable composites** flow into the cavity preparation due to their low viscosity. Manufacturers have decreased the filler content of the material to reduce the viscosity and increase flow. **Condensable composites** have a filler particle feature that inhibits the sliding of the filler particles by one another. The result is a thicker stiffer feel, and the manufacturers call these products condensable.

Pit and Fissure Sealants

Pit and fissure caries continue to be common despite the preventive efforts of modern dentistry. Pit and fissure sealants are effective in reducing caries and the need to restore teeth. The goal is to fill susceptible pits and fissures with a polymeric material and deprive cariogenic bacteria of

TABLE 15–1 Types of Dental Composites

PROPERTY	MICROFILL	MACROFILL	HYBRID
Filler size	0.03-0.5	10-25	0.5-1
Filler (wt %)	40-50	70-75	75-80
Strength	Low	Fair	Good
Abrasion resistance	Good	Poor	Very good
Thermal expansion	Poor	Fair	Good
Current uses	Classes III, IV, V, and veneers	Few	Classes I, II, III, and IV

From Gladwin M, Bagby MD: *Clinical Aspects of Dental Materials.* Philadelphia, Lippincott Williams & Wilkins, 2000, p 63.

a niche to colonize. Sealant materials are usually an unfilled resin and polymerize by chemical activation (chemical cure) or light activation (light cure). Pit and fissure sealants are discussed in greater detail in Chapter 14.

Composite Cements

Composite cements or composite luting materials have the same structure as do other dental composites-a resin matrix reinforced with silanated filler. Composite cements have a greater percentage of resin to increase flow and smaller sized particles for a lower film thickness. One advantage of composite cements is their ability to bond restorations to tooth structure. Composite cements are the luting materials of choice for ceramic restorations. They are also used when retention of a restoration is a problem.

Glass Ionomer Materials

The first glass ionomer products developed set via an acid-base chemical reaction. These are sometimes called chemical-cured glass ionomers. Glass ionomer restorations are "tooth colored" but opaque in appearance. Glass ionomer restorative materials are supplied as powder/liquid systems. The liquid is a solution of polyacrylic acid and results in an adhesive material. The powder consists of ground fluoride, which contains glass. The set material slowly leaches fluoride, some of which is absorbed by the surrounding tooth structure. Correct mixing and placement of this material are critical. The proper powder-liquid ratio is mixed, and a viscous material results. Success with placement of chemical-cured glass ionomer restorations depends on the technique used. If mixing is too slow or placement is delayed, the adhesive property of the material is lost. In addition, glass ionomer materials are susceptible to dehydration during the initial setting of the material as well as during finishing of the restoration. If the material is not protected from dehydration, surface crazing occurs. **Crazing** is the formation of many shallow surface cracks. Chemical-cured glass ionomer materials have a high initial solubility in oral fluids, but solubility is low after the setting reaction is complete.

Although the advantages of adhesion and fluoride release make chemical-cured glass ionomers useful materials, their shortcomings have limited their clinical use. Chemical-cured glass ionomer restorative materials are brittle. Glass ionomer products are very popular for use as luting cements and as restorative materials in low stress areas of teeth. The fluoride release properties of glass ionomer restorative materials makes them the materials of choice for class V lesions for patients with a high risk for caries.

Light-Cured Glass Ionomer Products

Light-cured glass ionomer products were developed in the late 1980s. They are also called **resin-modified glass ionomers**. They still have an acid-base setting reaction, in addition to free radical polymerization. As a result, these products set when exposed to the same curing light that is used for composites. Light-cured products are popular because of their cure-on-demand setting reaction. They are still adhesive and release fluoride. Light-cured glass ionomers are easier to place and finish. When compared with chemical-cured glass ionomers, light-cured materials are stronger and tougher and not as sensitive to dehydration. Light-cured glass ionomers are quite popular.

Compomers

Due to the popularity of glass ionomer materials and composite/dentinal bonding systems, a combination of the two materials has been developed. The **compomer** label is used to describe materials that bond and set like dentinal bonding/composite systems but reportedly release some fluoride similar to glass ionomers. A few of these products are somewhat like glass ionomers, but most are very much like composites. Compomers typically use the same dentinal bonding systems as do composites. Some initial release of fluoride occurs. The promise of fluoride release and good handling characteristics has resulted in a large number of compomer products on the market.

 # DENTAL AMALGAM

Dental amalgam is a very old but still a widely used restorative material. The popularity of dental amalgam is due to its cost effectiveness and ease of use. Probably more than half of the single tooth restorations currently placed in posterior teeth are amalgam restorations. Dental amalgam is used in all surfaces of posterior teeth.

Dental amalgam is made by mixing approximately equal parts (by weight) of a powdered metal with liquid mercury. The powdered metal is called an **amalgam alloy** and is predominantly silver (Ag) and tin (Sn). The process of mixing the alloy with mercury is called **trituration**. A mechanical device called a **triturator** "shakes" the capsule that contains the alloy powder and mercury at high speed. The triturated material is then condensed into the cavity preparation. The cavity preparation is overfilled, and the excess is removed (carved).

The particles of the amalgam alloy may be formed by two methods. The first method is to grind an ingot of metal to produce rough irregular fillings. Such amalgam alloys are called **lathe-cut alloys**. A second method used to produce dental amalgam particles is to spray molten metal into an inert atmosphere. The droplets cool as they fall and produce round particles called spherical alloys. Spherical alloys pack together better and require less mercury. Spherical amalgams set faster than lathe-cut amalgams. Some products are a mixture of both lathe-cut and spherical particles.

Advantages of Using Dental Amalgam

Amalgam is a long-lasting, cost-effective restorative material because of its toughness and wear resistance. In addition, amalgam has the ability to seal its margins during function. As the amalgam corrodes at the tooth/restoration interface, the corrosion products fill in gaps and reduce microleakage. In some patients, the margins of a dental amalgam may look broken down but are actually well sealed just below the surface. Amalgam is the least technique sensitive, permanent, restorative material available to the dentist. Based on clinical research, the average life expectancy for a conservative class I amalgam is 15 to 18 years. A class II amalgam should last for 12 to 15 years.

Low Copper Dental Amalgam

Low copper amalgams are included for historical perspective. Today, high copper amalgams are state of the art and dominate the market. Composition of a low copper or "conventional" amalgam alloy is based on GV Black's composition, which is approximately 65% silver (Ag), 25% tin (Sn), 5% copper (Cu), and sometimes 1% zinc (Zn). The setting reaction is:

$$\text{Excess Ag}_3\text{Sn} (\gamma) + \text{Hg} \rightarrow \text{unreacted Ag}_3\text{Sn} (\gamma)$$
$$+ \text{Ag}_2\text{Hg}_3 (\gamma_1) + \text{Sn}_8\text{Hg} (\gamma_2)$$

When the liquid mercury is mixed with the amalgam alloy, the mercury is both absorbed by the particles and dissolves the surface of these particles. The liquid mercury becomes saturated with silver and tin. Precipitation of γ_1 and γ_2 phases begins and continues until the mercury is consumed and a solid mass results. The setting reaction may take as long as 24 hours to complete and for strength to reach a maximum.

High Copper Dental Amalgams

Starting in the 1960s, various high copper dental amalgams were developed. The clinical performance of many but not all of these amalgams is superior to that of the best low copper amalgams. High copper amalgams can be categorized into several groups. "Blended," "admix," or "dispersion" alloys are a mixture of lathe-cut and spherical particles. Lathe-cut particles have the same composition as do low copper amalgam alloys-predominantly silver and tin. The other particles are spherical and contain copper and silver. The notable feature of high copper amalgams is the lack of a tin-mercury product, which is the weakest and most corrosion-prone phase. Instead, tin reacts with copper to form several CuSn reaction products, thus eliminating the tin-mercury product, which is detrimental to the life of the restoration.

Factors That Affect Handling and Performance

Manufacturers supply amalgam alloy in several forms. Pre-proportioned disposable capsules containing both the alloy powder and mercury are the most popular.

Mixing and handling by the dentist and the auxiliaries affect properties of the set amalgam. The speed and time of trituration are set to obtain the proper consistency of the mixture. Overtrituration and undertrituration affect the setting time and physical properties of amalgam. The composition of the set dental amalgam depends on several factors. The **mercury-alloy ratio** is the amount of mercury mixed with the amalgam alloy. Use of more mercury increases the mercury-containing reaction products, which tend to be the weaker phases. Use of less mercury results in less of the mercury-containing reaction products. Proper trituration and condensation techniques can also reduce the mercury content of the set amalgam. The liquid mercury must wet all alloy particles and condense into a dense mass without voids. An inadequate mercury-alloy ratio results in voids and poor restorations. Proper condensation techniques reduce or eliminate voids.

Amalgam Properties

Minimal dimensional change after condensation is important to prevent leakage or expansion. Many factors affect dimensional change, such as mercury-alloy ratio, trituration, and condensation techniques. The best results are obtained by following the manufacturer's recommendations.

The strength of amalgam restorations must resist the biting forces of occlusion. The 1-hour strength of spherical alloys is much greater than that of lathe-cut or admix amalgams. Strength differences between types of amalgams are much less after 24 hours. Dental amalgam has a high compressive strength, but the tensile and shear strengths are comparatively low. Therefore, amalgam should be supported by tooth structure for long-term clinical success, which is approximately 10 to 20 years. Also, amalgam needs sufficient bulk. A thickness of 1.5 mm or more is necessary to withstand occlusal forces.

Creep is a slow change in shape that is caused by continuous compression. When high copper amalgams were developed, creep became less of a predictor of clinical failure.

Amalgam corrodes in much the same way that iron rusts. **Galvanic corrosion** occurs when two dissimilar metals exist in a wet environment. An electrical current flows between the two metals, and corrosion (oxidation) of one metal occurs. The likelihood of galvanic corrosion increases if two phases are present in a metal. Dental amalgams always have more than two phases, and they also exist in a corrosive environment (i.e., the oral cavity). Therefore amalgams corrode and eventually fail. The clinical problem is that often corrosion occurs below the surface of the restoration. An assessment of the status of an amalgam restoration for marginal breakdown and internal corrosion is beyond current clinical diagnostic techniques. Instead, alleged recurrent decay is the dominant reason for replacing amalgam restorations. An acidic environment promotes galvanic corrosion. Poor oral hygiene and a cariogenic diet will expose both teeth and restorative materials to a destructive environment. The same factors that promote caries will accelerate corrosion. Therefore, patient behavior can affect the longevity of amalgam and other restorations.

Mercury Toxicity

Mercury and its chemical compounds are toxic to the kidneys and the central nervous system. Proper handling of mercury will prevent harm to all dental care providers. The most significant danger is from mercury vapor. Mercury has a high vapor pressure and evaporates at room temperature. The mercury vapor is inhaled by the lungs during normal breathing. It is important that the ADA recommendations for mercury hygiene are followed. They include proper handling and storage along with prompt clean-up of all mercury spills.

Mercury toxicity is not a problem for patients. Numerous governmental and nongovernmental scientific panels have rebuffed claims of mercury toxicity in patients. The only exception is in the case of patients who are allergic to mercury. Very few (<0.1%) cases of mercury allergy have been reported in the scientific literature.

Finishing and Polishing

The goal of finishing an amalgam restoration is to produce margins that are continuous with the adjoining tooth structure and to produce proper contours. Polishing produces a smooth and lustrous surface that reduces the likelihood of corrosion and reduces the ability of plaque to adhere to the surface. Polishing lathe-cut and admix amalgams should be delayed for 24 hours to allow the amalgam to set and become hard enough to withstand the polishing procedure. Spherical amalgams set much faster. Some can be polished 20 minutes after being placed. Appropriate finishing and polishing of amalgam restorations improve their appearance and function.

 DENTAL CEMENTS

Dental cements are used to cement or **lute** inlays, crowns, bridges, and other restorations and appliances to the tooth structure. In addition, dental cements are used for pulpal protection. The term "cement" implies that the material will be used to glue or lute things together. Most dental cements retain restorations in place with mechanical retention. Some dental cements are adhesive by way of true chemical bonds. Luting cements have the most demanding requirements of any dental material. During the setting reaction, they must change from a fluid liquid to a rock-hard solid in a few minutes. The resultant material must be biocompatible and insoluble in oral fluids. The set material is almost insoluble in water. Therefore, it is important that instruments are cleaned after mixing and before the material sets. If one delays clean-up, the set material is very difficult to remove from instruments.

Dental cements are also used as an intermediate base or liner when the remaining dentin does not have adequate thickness to protect the pulp from thermal changes. A base or liner is placed on dentin between the pulp and the restorative material. Because the solubility of dental cements is much greater than the overlying restorative material, bases and liners must not be applied on margins. A **liner** is used to protect the pulp from chemical irritation. A liner may also stimulate dentin formation or release fluoride. Liners are too thin (<0.5 mm) to provide thermal insulation. They are also too weak to support a restorative material or resist amalgam condensation forces. A **base** is stronger and thicker than a liner. Bases provide thermal insulation, support the restorative material, and may release fluoride. Previously, the distinction between bases and liners was clear-cut. Today, liner materials are much stronger and the distinction between bases and liners is quite blurred.

Some dental cements may also be used as a temporary filling material. For some cements, the material is mixed to a thicker consistency than that used for luting. The cement is chosen based on the particular clinical requirements of the situation. A temporary restoration (filling) may be placed as an emergency procedure when time restraints prevent a more complex treatment. **Table 15-2** summarizes the uses of dental cements.

Chemistry of Dental Cements

With the exception of composite cements, dental cements are brittle ceramic materials. Their chemistry is a simple acid-base reaction. The resultant product is insoluble in water and oral fluids. Dental cements are typically powder-liquid systems; the liquid is an acid and the powder is a base. The powder must be insoluble in oral fluids but reactive with the acid. If one understands the properties of the components of a dental cement, then one will be able to predict the properties of the resultant set material:

ACID + excess BASE → residual base + insoluble SALT

In terms of the components of the dental cement:

Liquid + excess powder → residual powder + matrix

The residual powder and the matrix must be insoluble in oral fluids. The chemistry of composite cements is the same as that of acrylics and composites.

Zinc oxide and eugenol cements are commonly called ZOE cements. Reinforced ZOE products are used for temporary restorations and intermediate bases. Reinforcing additives include alumina, rosin, and polymethylmethacrylate resin. ZOE is obtundent and, therefore, very effective when used for pulpal protection or as a sedative filling. ZOE products, including reinforced ZOE, do not have adequate strength and are too soluble for use as a permanent cement. Its use as a base has declined greatly, because cements that

TABLE 15–2 Reference Guide for Liners, Bases, and Cements

CEMENT	USE TECHNIQUE	MIXING TIME*	MIXING OF A PROPER MIX	CHARACTERISTICS TIME*	SETTING
Calcium hydroxide	Cavity liner	Mix quickly in a small area of the pad	10 sec	Uniform color	2–3 min
Zinc phosphate	Luting agent	Add divided increments in the specified time using a large slab area	1–1½ min	Mix will stretch 1 inch between the slab and the spatula	5½ min
	Base	Same as luting agent (above)	1–1½ min	Thick, putty-like (non-sticking) consistency	5½ min
Glass ionomer	Luting agent	Add the powder to the liquid in one portion	30–45 sec	Use while glossy	7 min
	Base	Same as the luting agent (above)	30–45 sec	Use while glossy	7 min
ZOE	Base and temporary restoration	Add half-scoop increments using a small mixing area	1½ min	Thick, putty-like (almost crumbly) consistency	2½–3½ min
Temporary cement	Temporary luting agent	Equal lengths; mix all at once	30 sec	Uniform color	2 min

From Gladwin M, Bagby MD: Clinical Aspects of Dental Materials. Philadelphia, Lippincott Williams & Wilkins, 2000, p 245.

release fluoride have become accepted. Temporary cement formulations are still popular. The biocompatibility is very good, because ZOE seals margins very well.

Most temporary ZOE cements are paste or paste products. They are dispensed in equal lengths on a paper mixing pad. The pastes are supplied in different colors and are swirled together with a cement spatula until a homogenous color is obtained.

ZOE powder or liquid products use a scoop and a dropper to dispense the components. A glass slab or paper pad is used for mixing these materials. The powder is forced into the liquid using a cement spatula. The mixing process first incorporates large increments of powder then smaller increments as further additions of powder become more difficult to add. The mixing process requires time to incorporate enough powder to get acceptable properties. When a luting mixture is desired with a powder/liquid product, mixing is continued until a consistency is obtained that a "1-inch string" of material occurs when the flat surface of the cement spatula is pulled from the mixed material. When a base consistency is desired, mixing is continued until the material has the consistency of pie dough; it can be rolled into a ball with fingers covered with cement powder but is slightly crumbly. Water accelerates the setting reaction of ZOE. Therefore, ZOE materials set faster in the mouth than out of the mouth, which makes them quite useful and popular.

Zinc phosphate cement has been used in dentistry for centuries. At one time it was the strongest and least soluble cement available. Zinc phosphate cement is used for luting inlays, crowns, bridges, orthodontic bands, and other appliances. Zinc phosphate cement is supplied by manufacturers as a ZnO powder and phosphoric acid liquid. The powder and liquid are mixed to a thick or thinner consistency depending on the clinical use. The mixture is thinner (lower powder-liquid ratio) when used for luting and thicker (higher powder-liquid ratio) when used as a base. Proper mixing of this cement is critical. Zinc phosphate cement is difficult to handle and has inferior properties when improperly mixed. Because the mixed cement has a low pH until it has set, zinc phosphate cement is irritating to the pulp. In many cases, when zinc phosphate cement is used as a base, liner, or varnish is applied to the preparation.

The setting reaction is very exothermic. The heat of the reaction accelerates the setting rate. Zinc phosphate cement is mixed slowly and over a large area of a chilled glass slab to dissipate the heat of the setting reaction. The powder is incorporated into the liquid with force. The powder is added first in small increments and then larger ones. The heat of the reaction of the first small increments is dissipated into the glass slab if mixing is slow enough.

When a luting mixture is desired, mixing is continued until a "1-inch string" occurs when tested with the cement spatula. When a base consistency is desired, a higher powder-liquid ratio is used. Mixing is continued until the material has the consistency of putty. If too little powder is used, the mixed mass will be sticky and difficult to handle. A proper base mixture will not stick to instruments and can be pushed or condensed into place. The mixing process for zinc phosphate cement is shown in **Figure 15-4**.

Glass ionomer cements consist of a fluoride-containing glass powder and an aqueous solution of polyacrylic acid. Glass ionomer materials are strongest and least soluble dental cement. They are adhesive; they release fluoride; and they have good biocompatibility. This combination of properties makes them quite popular materials. They bond to stainless steel and other alloys. It is critical that glass ionomer cement is properly mixed and handled. If not mixed and handled properly, a nonadhesive material results. The manufacturer's recommended powder-liquid ratio should be followed, and mixing should be completed in 60 seconds or less. The mixed material must be placed while the cement surface appears glossy. After that time, adhesion is reduced or lost.

Glass ionomer materials have become quite popular as a result of their physical and mechanical properties and clinical performance. Numerous products are on the market. Glass ionomer cement is one of the most popular luting materials. It has been called the material of choice for luting metal crowns and ceramometal crowns.

Glass ionomer restorative materials are popular for treating patients with a high risk for caries. They have the same setting reaction as do luting materials, but they are thicker materials with a much higher film thickness. They are stronger and less soluble. Light-cured glass ionomer liners have adequate strength for use as a base and are quite popular. Dentists often use a glass ionomer restorative material for a temporary restoration or a large base. Resin-reinforced glass ionomer cements have been introduced. They have the usual acid-base reaction, but they also undergo addition polymerization. Addition polymerization can be activated chemically or with light. These glass ionomer products are stronger and tougher than are those that set via an acid-base reaction only.

Polycarboxylate cements consist of a zinc oxide powder and an aqueous solution of polyacrylic acid. They bond to the tooth structure and result in very little leakage. Polycarboxylate cement is not as acidic as some other cements and is very biocompatible. Polycarboxylate cement is used as luting cement and for an intermediate base. Unfortunately, polycarboxylate cement is not very strong and has a moderate solubility. Polycarboxylate cements are mixed and handled in the same manner as are glass ionomer cements.

Composite cements are composite materials with a higher percentage of resin to reduce viscosity. They are sometimes referred to as resin cements. With the use of a dentinal bonding system, they are the materials of choice for luting all ceramic restorations. If the ceramic material is properly etched and silanated, composite cement will bond the restoration to the underlying tooth structure. Composite cements are also useful for recementing poorly fitting crowns when the patient does not wish to have the inadequate crown remade. Composite cements come in various

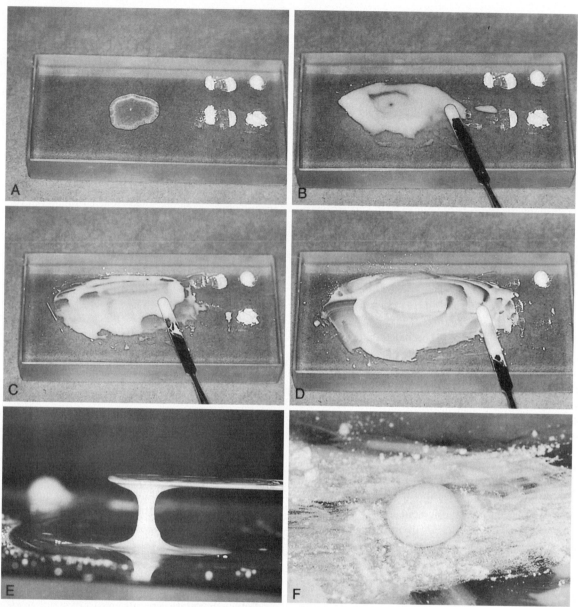

Figure 15-4. The mixing process for zinc phosphate cement is shown. A, Powder and liquid are dispensed on a chilled glass slab. The powder is divided into increments. B, Part of the first increment is mixed into the liquid. C and D, Increments are added to the mixture, using the entire surface of the glass slab. E, When mixed for luting, the cement will "string" 1 inch. F, A mixture for a base can be rolled into a ball. (From Gladwin M, Bagby MD: Clinical Aspects of Dental Materials. Philadelphia, Lippincott Williams & Wilkins, 2000, p 89.)

shades and are also used to cement veneers, orthodontic appliances, and other types of restorations.

Calcium hydroxide liners and bases were once very popular materials. They were placed under most composite restorations. Calcium hydroxide products promote the formation of secondary dentin. They are still recommended when a cavity preparation leaves little dentin covering the pulp. They are the recommended materials for direct pulp-capping procedures. A direct pulp cap is a material that is placed on vital pulp tissue when all of the overlying dentin is removed and the pulp is exposed. Calcium hydroxide materials are paste or paste systems. The oldest calcium hydroxide products were weak and used as liners. Improve-

ments strengthened the material, and now some products are strong enough to be used as a base. With the development of dentinal bonding systems and the current understanding of the biocompatibility of composite materials, the use of calcium hydroxide products has greatly diminished.

Temporary cements are used to retain a temporary restoration while the permanent restoration is being fabricated. Temporary cements are typically paste or paste systems. They consist of a unique group of materials in that both a maximum strength and a minimum strength are required. At one time, temporary cements were ZOE formulations. They mix easily and set quickly in the humidity of the mouth. The set material is brittle, and the excess is easily removed. The obtundent property may even settle down an irritated pulp after it has been insulted by tooth preparation, impression procedures, and the construction of a temporary crown. With the development and use of resin cements, many dentists believe that using ZOE temporary cement will inhibit the setting of a resin cement, because eugenol inhibits free radical polymerization. Temporary cements that do not contain eugenol have been developed. Instead of eugenol, fatty acids and other chemicals are used to react with zinc oxide. These products have similar properties but do not handle as well. They are not brittle, and the excess cement can be difficult to remove.

IMPRESSION MATERIALS

Impression materials are used to make replicas (models or casts) of teeth and other oral tissues. The casts are used to construct restorations and other appliances. The impression must be an accurate duplication of the hard and soft tissues of interest and stable enough to allow disinfection and production of a model. Because impression materials are used for various purposes, there is a wide variety of products with which to make impressions of oral tissues. Some materials are mixed, whereas others are softened or melted. These materials are then loaded into an impression tray; they are placed in the mouth and seated onto the tissues of interest. The tray functions as a carrier and can stabilize the set impression material. Paste or paste impression materials and many other dental materials are supplied in tubes. The orifice of each tube is sized proportionally to provide the proper ratio of the two pastes when equal lengths are dispensed.

Impression materials set by either a chemical reaction or a physical change. Some materials set by chemical reactions to form elastic rubber materials and are called **thermoset**. The chemical reaction involves chain lengthening, cross-linking, or both. Others set by a physical change that occurs when they cool-either solidification or gelation. Impression materials that undergo a physical change when cooled are called **thermoplastic**. Solidification occurs when molten wax cools and changes from a liquid to a solid state. **Gelation** is the process by which gelatin changes from a liquid to a semisolid state when it cools. Thermoplastic materials are not as stable as are thermoset materials. Each impression material has its own advantages and disadvantages for use in dentistry. **Table 15-3** lists the classification and use of impression materials.

Various impression techniques are employed for partial denture construction. Table 15-3 does not address all possible techniques. Use of a custom tray is recommended. Edentulous trays for hydrocolloid use are not common. These materials could be used, but their use is not economical.

Impression Compound

Impression compound is a stiff thermoplastic material. Impression compound is wax; filler is added to improve handling and stability. This compound is stronger and more brittle; when softened, it flows much less. It is melted in a warm water bath and placed in the mouth in a moldable state. When cooled to mouth temperature, the material returns to a rigid state. Many dentists use impression compound for preliminary impressions for full dentures.

Zinc Oxide and Eugenol

ZOE have been formulated for a wide variety of uses in dentistry, one being an impression material. The chemistry of

TABLE 15–3 Classification and Use of Impression Materials

TYPE OF IMPRESSION MATERIAL	ELASTIC VS. INELASTIC	SETTING PROCESS	USED FOR THE CONSTRUCTION OF			
			FULL DENTURE	PARTIAL DENTURE*	INLAY, CROWN, OR BRIDGE	STUDY MODELS
Plaster	Inelastic	Chemical	Preliminary	No	No	No
Wax or impression compound	Inelastic	Physical	Preliminary	No	No	No
ZOE	Inelastic	Chemical	Final†	No	No	No
Reversible hydrocolloid (agar)	Elastic	Physical	Not used‡	Yes	Yes	No
Irreversible hydrocolloid (alginate)	Elastic	Chemical	Preliminary	Yes	No	Yes
Polysulfide	Elastic	Chemical	Final†	Yes	Yes†	No§
Condensation silicone	Elastic	Chemical	Final†	Yes	Yes	No§
Addition silicone	Elastic	Chemical	Final†	Yes	Yes	No§
Polyether	Elastic	Chemical	Final†	Yes	Yes	No§

*There are a variety of impression techniques for partial denture construction. This table does not address all possible techniques.
†Use of a custom tray is recommended.
‡Edentulous trays for hydrocolloid use are not common.
§These materials could be used but their use is not economical.
From Gladwin M, Bagby MD: Clinical Aspects of Dental Materials. Philadelphia, Lippincott Williams & Wilkins, 2000, p 97.

ZOE materials is the same as that of the dental cement. ZOE impression materials are supplied as two pastes. One paste contains eugenol and inert fillers; the other component contains zinc oxide powder mixed with vegetable oil to form a second paste. ZOE impression materials set to a hard and brittle mass; this limits their use to impressions of edentulous ridges for removable dentures and bite registration.

Reversible Hydrocolloid (Agar)

Two hydrocolloid impression materials are used. One sets via a chemical reaction and is called **irreversible hydrocolloid** or **alginate**, whereas the material that gels when cooled to mouth temperature is called **reversible hydrocolloid** or **agar**.

Reversible hydrocolloid is very inexpensive to use and results in a very accurate impression. Reversible hydrocolloid is premixed by the manufacturer and is supplied as a semisolid thermoplastic material in tubes and sticks. Reversible hydrocolloid requires special equipment to use the materials. The rubbery material called the **gel** is boiled to change it to a viscous liquid called the **sol**. The material is cooled to a temperature at which the material is tolerated by oral tissues. At mouth temperature, the material gels and returns to its elastic state.

Irreversible Hydrocolloid (Alginate)

Alginate materials are not as accurate as reversible hydrocolloid materials but are much cheaper and easier to use. Alginate materials are supplied as powders that are mixed with water. The powder is predominantly inert filler. The reaction ingredient in the powder is potassium alginate, which is a carbohydrate polymer that dissolves in water to form the sol. Carboxylate groups react with calcium ions and cross-link the material to form a gel.

The temperature of the water controls the rate of the setting reaction. Warmer water increases the setting rate, whereas cooler water slows the setting reaction. Alginate is supplied by most manufacturers in both regular set and fast set varieties. Mixing the alginate material is an aggressive aerobic activity. First, the powder and water are gently stirred together. Once all the powder has been wetted by the water, the effort should greatly increase. The paste is pushed against the side of the rubber mixing bowl to force the water and powder together. Aggressive spatulation continues until a smooth creamy mix is obtained. The typical mixing time is 1 minute. Removal of the impression is delayed for 2 to 3 minutes after gelation. Strength and elasticity improve during this additional setting time. The impression is removed with a quick motion.

As with irreversible hydrocolloid materials, alginate impressions must be disinfected and poured with care. Gain or loss of water (**imbibition, evaporation, or syneresis**) will affect the accuracy of the resultant cast. Alginate impression material is used for various purposes. It is inexpensive and easy to use but lacks accuracy for the fabrication of precisely fitting restorations. Proper mixing and handling result in acceptable study models and appliances such as mouthguards and fluoride trays.

Polysulfides

Polysulfide impression material was the first nonaqueous elastomeric "rubber" impression material developed for dentistry. Polysulfide materials set by way of a condensation polymerization reaction. Polysulfide impression materials are much more accurate than is alginate. With proper handling, polysulfide impression materials can be used for inlays, crowns, and bridges. However, they are not as accurate as other nonaqueous elastomeric materials; they have an odor; and they will stain clothing.

Condensation Silicones

Condensation silicone impression materials were the next impression materials to be developed for dentistry. They are based on silicone rubber that is commonly used in other industries. They are hydrophobic. The setting process is the result of a condensation reaction. Condensation silicone impressions must be poured without delay. They are not as popular as newer materials that provide better results.

Polyethers

Polyether impression materials are very stiff compared with other elastic materials and set quickly. Most polyether impression materials come in a single viscosity much like the medium viscosity of other types of materials. They are clean materials to use, but they have an unpleasant taste. Polyether impression materials are very accurate and easy to pour with gypsum products. The properties and ease of use of this material make it a very popular material with a large market share.

Addition Silicones

Addition silicones are the most popular type of impression, especially for crown and bridge impressions. They are the most accurate, stable, and expensive impression materials. Addition silicone impression materials are also called vinyl **polysiloxanes** and **polyvinylsiloxanes**. The reactive group is a carbon-carbon double bond ($C=C$), which is called a vinyl group. As expected, polymerization occurs by way of free radicals and addition polymerization. Polymerization involves chain lengthening and cross-linking to create a stable rubber material. No reaction byproduct is formed.

Manufacturers produce addition silicone materials in several viscosities. Putty impression materials are mixed by kneading the two colors together with the fingers. The palms of the hands should not be used, because the materials are slightly heated and working time is decreased. Latex gloves must not be worn when mixing addition silicone putties.

Sulfur in the latex material inhibits the polymerization reaction, possibly preventing proper setting of the material.

GYPSUM MATERIALS

Gypsum products are used mainly for making replicas of oral structures from impressions. Gypsum products are supplied as fine powders that are mixed with water to form a fluid mass, which can be poured and shaped and which subsequently hardens into a rigid, stable mass. Notable properties of gypsum products include accuracy, dimensional stability, ability to reproduce fine detail, strength, abrasion resistance, compatibility with impression materials, and ease of use.

Three types of gypsum products are commonly used in dentistry: plaster, stone, and high strength or improved stone. Chemically, they are all calcium sulfate hemihydrate and are produced as a result of heating gypsum and driving off part of the water of crystallization by a process called **calcination**. Gypsum products differ in terms of the physical characteristics of their powder particles as a result of differing calcination methods; this is responsible for their varied uses and properties. The manufacturers also modify the particles and add other chemicals to improve the properties.

Types of Gypsum Products

Plaster is manufactured by grinding the gypsum rock to a fine powder followed by heating the powder in an open container. The resultant powder consists of porous, irregular particles. Plaster is the weakest and least expensive of the three gypsum products. It is used mainly when strength is not a critical requirement.

Dental stone is made from gypsum by carefully controlled calcination under steam pressure in a closed container. This method of calcination releases the water of crystallization from the crystal slowly so that the resultant powder particle is more regular, more uniform in shape, and less porous compared with the powder particle of plaster. Stone is stronger and more expensive than is plaster. Stone is used mainly for making casts for diagnostic purposes and for complete and partial denture construction when greater strength and surface hardness are desired. Stone is usually buff (light tan) in color. However, stone can be obtained in other colors. It is often referred to as type III stone.

High strength or **improved stone** is made from gypsum by calcining the gypsum in a calcium chloride solution. This method of calcination results in a powder particle that is very dense and cuboidal in shape with a reduced surface area. High strength stone is the strongest and most expensive of the three gypsum products and is used mainly for making casts or dies for inlay and crown fabrication. High strength stone is often referred to as type IV stone, or die stone. Other types of dental gypsum products are produced for special uses.

Setting Reaction of Gypsum Products

When any of the three types of gypsum products (calcium sulfate hemihydrate) is mixed with water, the hemihydrate is changed back to the dihydrate by the process of hydration. Heat is liberated, as shown by the following reaction:

$$CaSO_4 \cdot (\frac{1}{2}H_2O + 1\frac{1}{2}H_2O \rightarrow CaSO_4 \cdot (2H_2O + heat)$$

The calcium sulfate hemihydrate dissolves in the mixing water and the dihydrate precipitates, because it is less soluble than the hemihydrate. As calcium sulfate dihydrate precipitates out of solution, interlocking crystals develop and result in the formation of a hard mass.

Water-Powder Ratio

The relative amounts of water and powder used to make a workable mixture of a particular gypsum product are called the **water-powder ratio**. For dental use, an excess amount of water is always necessary above the theoretically correct amount required for the hydration reaction. The excess is needed to make a workable mixture that can be poured and shaped. This excess water is distributed as free water in the set mass without taking part in the chemical reaction and contributes to subsequent porosity or voids in the set product. The proper water-powder ratio for each product is dependent upon the physical characteristics of the powder particles. Therefore, plaster requires more water to wet and fill the pores and float the irregular porous particles. The dense particles of dental stone require less water to float. The regular shape allows them to roll over one another more easily. High strength stone, because of its very dense and cuboidal type of particle and modifications by the manufacturer, requires even less water than stone. For dental use, the proper water-powder ratio for the average mix of plaster is 45 to 50 ml of water/100 g of plaster or 0.45 to 0.50; for stone, 0.28 to 0 30; and for improved stone, 0.19 to 0.24. It is important to follow the manufacturer's directions. The water-powder ratio has a direct effect on the properties of each gypsum product and must be controlled for optimum results.

Setting Time

The clinician should be made aware of two time intervals during the setting process. **Working time** is the length of time from the start of mixing until the setting mass reaches a semi-hard stage. It represents the available time for manipulating the product. It represents the partial progress of the setting reaction. Working time is generally 3 to 5 minutes. Final **setting time** represents the length of time from the start of the mixing until the setting mass becomes rigid and can be separated from the impression. The final setting time indicates the major completion of the hydration reaction. Usually 30 to 45 minutes is used as a subjective criterion for the time of final set. The setting time of a gypsum product is controlled by the manufacturer's particular formulation. Hence, several gypsum products are available with varying setting characteristics. An increase in the water-powder ratio increases the setting time and vice versa.

Setting Expansion

All gypsum products expand externally upon setting. Plaster exhibits the most expansion: 0.2% to 0.3%; stone: 0.08% to 0.1%; and high strength stone, the least: 0.05% to 0.07%. The growing crystals of the gypsum cause an outward crystal thrust. A minimal setting expansion is desirable for accurate dimensional reproduction for most casts and dies. Most gypsum products that are used for casts and dies have been modified by the manufacturer to provide for minimal expansion by the addition of chemicals, which also control the setting characteristics. Thus, a particular gypsum product has both setting time and expansion characteristics controlled by the manufacturer. An increase in the water-powder ratio decreases the setting expansion.

Strength and Surface Hardness

The strength of the gypsum product is usually measured in terms of crushing or compressive strength. As expected from the setting reaction, strength develops rapidly during the first 30 to 45 minutes as the hydration is completed. The strength is dependent upon the porosity of the set material, which is related to the water-powder ratio necessary to make a workable mixture. Plaster (which requires the most water to make a fluid mixture) has the weakest 1-hour compression strength (1500 psi); improved stone has the strongest 1-hour compression strength (5000 psi); and stone is intermediate in strength (3000 psi).

Casts and dies should be allowed to set for 1 to 2 hours or preferably longer before beginning subsequent laboratory procedures. Surface hardness is related to the compressive strength but reaches its maximum more rapidly because the surface is the first to dry. The greatest surface hardness occurs when the product reaches its dry strength. The dry strength may be two or more times greater than the wet strength.

Use of Gypsum Products

The technical use of gypsum products is relatively simple, requiring only a mixing bowl, mixing spatula, water at room-temperature, and the respective gypsum product. Water and powder must be proportioned accurately for optimum properties. Powder is weighed, and water is measured by volume. Hand mixing is usually done in a flexible plastic or rubber bowl with a stiff-bladed spatula to combine the powder and water into a smooth, homogenous, workable mixture that is free of air bubbles. A minimum of air inclusion in the mixed product is desirable to prevent surface and internal defects caused by air voids. Mixing is continued until a smooth, homogenous mixture is obtained (in ~1 minute). Mixing can also be done mechanically with a vacuum mixing machine. This provides a gypsum mixture that is free of air bubbles and homogenous in consistency.

When filling the impression, the gypsum mixture needs to flow slowly "ahead of itself" to prevent the entrapment of air. This is usually accomplished with a dental vibrator. Vibrating the mixture after mixing can also be used to bring air bubbles to the surface. Manipulation of gypsum products, although relatively simple, requires careful attention to detail for accurate results.

RESTORATIVE MATERIALS FOR FIXED RESTORATIONS

Indirect Fixed Restorations

Many types of fixed indirect restorations can be found. **Indirect restorations** are those restorations constructed outside the mouth. **Fixed restorations** cannot be removed from the oral cavity; they are luted (cemented) in place, such as **inlays, crowns, and bridges**. Three types of dental materials are used for most indirect restorations: **metallic, ceramic, and ceramometal materials**. Most metallic indirect restorations are made by a casting procedure. Metals are very tough and work very well in high-stress situations, but their esthetics are poor. Ceramic materials are used when esthetics are important. Ceramic materials can simulate the natural colors and translucency of teeth. Various materials and processing techniques are utilized to construct ceramic restorations. Ceramic materials lack the toughness and fracture resistance required by bridges. Eventually, a metal-ceramic combination was developed to meet these functional requirements. The tough strong metal supports the weak esthetic ceramic material. The result is called a ceramometal restoration (or porcelain bonded to metal, or porcelain fused to metal) and serves as an important "workhorse" in modern restorative dentistry.

Casting Process

Dentistry has used the "**lost wax casting technique**" for almost 1 century to make metal restorations. The restoration is first made in wax. This is known as the **wax pattern**. The casting process requires a mold space into which the molten metal flows. The mold space is made by embedding the wax pattern in an investment material. The invested pattern is heated; the wax is melted and burned away. This "burn-out" procedure results in a mold space into which the molten metal is cast. **Figure 15-5A and B** shows a wax pattern and the resultant casting.

The most common **investment materials** are gypsum-based products. The same handling variables discussed for gypsum products apply to gypsum bonded investments. A sil-

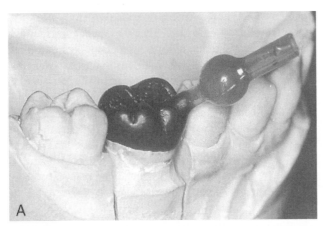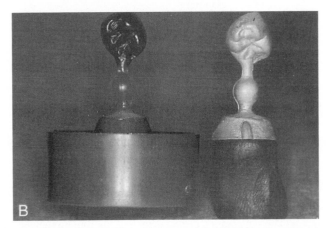

Figure 15-5. A wax pattern (A) and the completed casting (B). (From Gladwin M, Bagby MD: Clinical Aspects of Dental Materials. Philadelphia, Lippincott Williams & Wilkins, 2000, p 119.)

ica material is added to dental stone to produce **gypsum bonded investments**. The silica material is added to improve the investment's resistance to heat and increase thermal expansion of the mold. The mold must be expanded to the amount that exactly compensates for the thermal shrinkage of the solid metal casting as it cools to room temperature.

Several types of equipment are used to make dental castings. Gold casting alloys for all-metal crowns are easily melted with a "blow torch" using compressed air and natural gas (used to heat homes and offices). Higher melting alloys require oxygen or acetylene gas. Other methods to melt casting alloys include electrical resistance heating (e.g., in a toaster) or induction melting. The most common casting machine used to force the molten alloy into the mold is called a centrifugal casting machine. It rapidly spins the mold, crucible, and molten alloy in a circle. It uses centripetal force to force the molten alloy into the mold space.

Casting occurs when the molten alloy flows into the ingate of the casting ring, which was previously occupied by the **sprue**. The liquid metal flows down the channel space into the mold and fills the space previously occupied by the wax pattern with molten metal. When the metal cools, it solidifies and the casting is complete. After cooling, the casting is retrieved from the casting ring by removing the investment. Next, the casting is cleaned. The sprue is cut off, and the casting is finished and polished.

Casting Alloys

Cast metal restorations use alloys rather than pure metals. Alloys are metals that are a combination of several elements. Casting alloys for all-metal restorations have traditionally been gold alloys and thus the name, full gold crown or gold inlay. Gold (~75% by weight) is combined with copper (~5%), silver (~10%), palladium (~2%), zinc (~1%), and other elements to form high noble dental alloys. Percentages of elements vary depending on the type of casting alloy and the manufacturer. Gold alloys are easily cast with gypsum bonded investments and relatively simple equipment.

The properties of dental casting alloys are described in the ADA specification. The specification has no composition requirements but has performance criteria for strength, elongation, tarnish, and biocompatibility. **Elongation** is a measure of the ability to burnish the margins of a restoration. **Burnishing** margins of soft **malleable** gold restorations pushes the metal toward the tooth to close any gap between the tooth and the casting. Less cement is needed to fill in the space. The better the margins "fit" against the tooth preparation, the less chance there will be for marginal breakdown and recurrent caries.

Four types of casting alloys are described in the ADA specification. They are called **types I, II, III, and IV**. The differences are predominantly the strength and elongation of the casting alloy. Type I is the weakest, has the greatest elongation, and is used for inlays. Type IV is the strongest, has the least elongation, and is used for high stress bridges and partial denture frameworks.

Many terms are used to describe metals. Some have precise meaning; others do not. Metals are classified as noble elements based on their lack of chemical reactivity. The **noble metals** include gold, platinum, palladium, and other inert metals. **Precious metals** are classified based on their cost. Precious metals are the noble metals and silver. Alloys with less than 25% noble elements are called predominantly **base metals**. The term "nonprecious" is used to describe alloys that have no noble elements. The gold content of alloys can be described in several ways. **Percent** is the parts per 100. **Carat** is the parts per 24. **Fineness** is parts per 1000.

Alloys for Ceramometal Restorations

The metal substructure or **coping** for ceramometal restorations is waxed and cast much like that of a gold crown. Porcelain is supplied by manufacturers as powders. Porcelain powders are mixed with water and applied (or stacked) in layers. Each layer has esthetic properties to simulate the appearance of both dentin and enamel. Dental porcelains are fired at very high temperatures-850°C to 1100°C (1550°F-

2000°F). Firing porcelain causes the powders to become "sintered" and changes them into a solid. The metal must neither melt nor distort, because it serves to support the porcelain during firing and clinical service.

Ceramic Materials

The shades and translucency of porcelain are unmatched in its ability to simulate the appearance of teeth. The mechanical properties of this brittle material are inadequate for restoring most areas of the mouth. Several techniques have been developed to strengthen ceramic materials. Ceramometal crowns strengthen the porcelain by bonding it to metal. The advantages of metal include its tough mechanical properties and the ability to obtain a precise fit. The disadvantage is that metals are opaque to light even in very thin layers. Light is not transmitted through the restoration as it is through a tooth. Therefore, a ceramometal restoration is not as natural or life-like in appearance when compared with a porcelain jacket crown.

Laboratory Processed Composite Materials

Laboratory-processed composites, very similar to direct restorative materials, are used for inlays, onlays, and crowns. Composite materials are processed in dental laboratories using pressure and heat to improve the density and polymerization. The major advantage is that polymerization shrinkage gaps are filled by cement when the restoration is luted.

 # RESTORATIVE MATERIALS FOR REMOVABLE PROSTHESIES

As with a fixed bridge, a **removable full or partial denture** is a prosthesis; it replaces missing teeth. Alloys used for partial denture frameworks are very similar to those presented earlier. Acrylic resins were developed in the 1930s and were first used in dentistry in the 1940s. They quickly replaced other materials that were previously used in the construction of dentures. They have been adapted for many other uses in dentistry.

Acrylic Resins

Acrylic resins are hard, brittle, glassy polymers. The commercial plastic called Plexiglas is an acrylic resin product. Acrylic resin is clear and colorless and can be easily colored. The most common acrylic monomer is **methylmethacrylate**. Acrylic resin systems set via addition polymerization in the same manner as do dental composites. The same terms for activation are used for classification.

Cold-cured or **chemical-cured** acrylic resin systems are supplied as a powder and a liquid. The same materials are used for the "brush-bead" build-up technique for artificial fingernails. The powder consists predominantly of poly-methylmethacrylate resin beads with the addition of colorants and benzoyl peroxide. When the powder and liquid of an acrylic resin system are mixed, several stages in the setting process take effect. The liquid methylmethacrylate dissolves the polymethylmethacrylate resin. This important property has a significant effect on the handling properties of acrylic resin systems. In the initial stages, the changes are physical. The mixed powder and liquid feel grainy or sandy. The powder and liquid are separate phases. As some powder dissolves, the mixed material becomes thicker and less "runny." As more powder is dissolved, the material reaches the dough stage. At this point, the material is easy to handle and mold. Up to this point, the changes are mainly physical. The doughy material then becomes thicker and stiffer as the material polymerizes. The reaction generates heat, and the material becomes first warm and then hot. The material becomes rigid and solid as polymerization reaches completion.

Heat-cured acrylic resin systems are very similar to chemical-cured systems. The major exception is that a chemical activator is not present in the liquid. Heat-cured systems are also available as powder/liquid systems. When they are mixed, they go through the same initial stages of the setting process. Because of the absence of a chemical activator, the mixed material stays in the dough stage for an extended time. After the material is formed into the desired shape, the material is heated in a water bath. Polymerization begins, and the dough changes to a rigid material. Products that are properly heat-cured are slightly stronger and tougher than are cold-cured acrylic resins.

Methylmethacrylate and other monomers evaporate easily at room temperature. If a monomer evaporates during handling or processing, the resultant material will be porous. Porosity weakens the material. Also, the denture is likely to collect debris in the pores and become foul smelling. Considerable effort is made to prevent porosity when acrylic resins are processed. Pressure and temperature controls are used to minimize porosity.

Full Dentures

A **complete denture** or full denture replaces an entire arch of missing teeth. A full denture also replaces alveolar bone that is reabsorbed when teeth are missing. Dentures are made with acrylic materials colored to simulate the missing tissues. A complete denture has two major components: the denture teeth and the denture base. Denture teeth are purchased from a manufacturer and are most commonly made of acrylic resin. The denture base is made in the dental laboratory following the dentist's prescription. The denture base is made on the master stone cast, which is a positive reproduction of the patient's alveolar ridge.

Partial Dentures

Many patients are partially edentulous. The remaining teeth are frequently used to support and retain the prosthesis. If the prosthesis can be removed by the patient, it is called a **removable partial denture** or simply a partial denture. Most partial dentures are supported by both natural teeth and the alveolar ridge. A lower partial denture with just a few remaining natural teeth to secure the partial denture functions much better than does a complete lower denture. Most partial dentures utilize a cast metal "framework" for retention. The **framework** consists of clasps, connectors, and mesh. The framework has clasps that rest on and go around the natural abutment teeth. The clasps are metal, which can be bent to adjust the fit. The framework also has an area of mesh that the acrylic resin flows into and around when the partial denture is processed. The result is that the denture base and teeth are mechanically attached to the framework. The denture base is constructed and utilized in much the same way as a complete denture, except that the mesh areas of the partial denture framework are embedded in acrylic resin.

At one time, the frameworks of partial dentures were made with gold alloys. The large amount of metal necessary to construct a framework makes using gold alloys quite expensive. Nickel-chromium and cobalt-chromium alloys that are now used in dentistry were adapted from similar alloys common in the aerospace industry. The high melting temperatures of these alloys require slightly different casting techniques and investment materials. Silicate and phosphate bonded investments are used to cast high melting partial denture framework alloys and ceramometal alloys. They can withstand much higher burnout temperatures compared with gypsum-bonded investments, but they are more difficult to use.

Repairing Acrylic Prostheses or Appliances

It is not unusual for a denture or other acrylic prostheses or appliances to fracture. Repairs are made using additional cold-cured acrylic material as glue to repair the fracture. The process involves several steps. The surfaces to be repaired are first cleaned and are often ground to remove a thin layer of material and any contaminants. Monomer is applied to the clean surfaces to dissolve some of the set material. The acrylic material is mixed, applied to the surface, and then sets. The same process is used to "chemically" bond acrylic denture teeth to the denture base during denture processing. The repaired prosthesis is finished and polished using acrylic burs and a pumice wheel, much like that used to polish a complete denture.

Handling Acrylic Devices

It is important that patients regularly clean their dentures. They should be instructed to brush their prostheses with a denture cleaner and a denture brush or use other denture cleaning procedures. It is usually recommended that patients should not sleep with dentures in the mouth. Therefore, pa-tients should store their dentures in cool water at night. During dental appointments, it is important to store acrylic devices in water so that they do not warp. This applies not only to dentures but also to acrylic orthodontic retainers, athletic mouth guards, and occlusal splints.

DENTAL IMPLANTS

The typical **dental implant** penetrates through the oral mucosa (See Chapter 13). The interface of the surface of the implant with the body is a portal of entry for bacteria and other microorganisms and is susceptible to infection.

POLISHING NATURAL AND RESTORED TEETH

Finishing and Polishing Amalgam Restorations

Finished and polished amalgams are less prone to plaque retention, have a greater resistance to tarnish and corrosion, contribute to healthier surrounding tissue, and have greater longevity than unpolished amalgams. Traditionally, finishing and polishing should be performed at least 24 hours after amalgam placement. This allows the amalgam alloy to set completely before being exposed to abrasives within the oral cavity. For previously placed amalgams, finishing and polishing may be started as soon as the procedure is indicated.

Purpose of Finishing and Polishing

Finishing and polishing amalgams are achieved by properly smoothing the **cavosurface** margins (the area formed by the cavity wall and the external tooth surface), reconstructing functional anatomy, and creating an amalgam surface that is smooth and free of voids. It is necessary to obtain a smooth surface and achieve a high gloss. If only a high gloss is achieved through the polishing sequence, the remaining scratches tend to corrode faster than does a smooth surface. Ultimately, this will not prolong the life of the restoration.

Indications for Finishing and Polishing

Previously existing as well as new amalgam restorations should be finished and polished to correct various problems or conditions incurred during placement. These problems are often a result of incorrect condensing, poor carving, moisture contamination, natural expansion, or wear. In all of these cases, plaque has a greater chance of accumulating on the restoration surface, which creates a higher risk for recurrent caries.

It is important during patient assessment that all amalgam restorations be carefully evaluated to determine if amalgam finishing or polishing is indicated (**Table 15-4).**

TABLE 15–4 Determining Factors for Finishing and Polishing Versus Replacement

FINISH AND POLISH	REPLACE RESTORATION
A. Overhangs	A. Open contact
B. Lack of functional anatomy	B. Excessive corrosion
C. Tarnish	C. Amalgam fracture
D. Overextension	D. Open margin
E. Premature occlusal contacts	E. Recurrent decay

From Gladwin M, Bagby MD: Clinical Aspects of Dental Materials. Philadelphia, Lippincott Williams & Wilkins, 2000, p 229.

TABLE 15–5 Evaluation Criteria for Amalgam Finishing

A. Excessive amalgam has been removed from the cavosurface margins.
B. Amalgam appears to be smooth.
C. Occlusion registers properly with articulating paper.
D. Occlusal and marginal anatomy is better defined.
E. Porosity and pits are removed.
F. Contour of the restoration approximates the original contour of the tooth.
G. Adjacent tooth structure is left undamaged.

From Gladwin M, Bagby MD: Clinical Aspects of Dental Materials. Philadelphia, Lippincott Williams & Wilkins, 2000, p 233.

Amalgam Finishing and Polishing Considerations

Amalgam finishing and polishing can be considered as two separate procedures or steps in a single process. During the **amalgam finishing**, marginal irregularities are removed, and all areas of roughness are smoothed. During **amalgam polishing**, the surface is smoothed to a high luster using a sequence of abrasives from fine to most fine. Whenever an amalgam restoration is finished, polishing is then performed; but for those restorations not indicated for finishing, polishing may be done alone. The abrasives used during finishing are coarser than are the milder abrasives used during polishing.

During the finishing and polishing procedures, it is essential to avoid generating any heat at the amalgam restoration. Because of the high thermal conductivity of amalgam, excess heat could injure the pulp and cause pain. When heat is generated above 140°F (60°C), mercury may be released from the restoration to its surface, resulting in a dull cloudy appearance. Excessive heat generation may also result in an increased susceptibility to breakdown and corrosion. Water is often used as a coolant during these procedures. After each step, when burs or abrasives are changed, it is recommended that the area be thoroughly rinsed, dried, and evaluated.

Table 15-5 lists the evaluation criteria for amalgam finishing. Do not proceed to the polishing procedure until these criteria have been met. Polishing will not accomplish a smooth surface unless each step during the finishing process has been successfully accomplished.

Amalgams can be polished in two ways:

1. A rubber cup, polishing brushes, and polishing strips with slurries of pumice and tin oxide are used. The liquid used in the polishing slurries may be water, mouthwash, glycerin, or alcohol. The abrasive agents do the polishing; the cups and brushes only deliver and move the agents around on the tooth surface. It is critical that tooth surfaces are thoroughly rinsed and that cups and brushes are changed before the next agent is used to prevent contamination of more abrasive particles with finer ones. When a large abrasive particle is mixed inadvertently in with a finer one, the purpose of using a finer abrasive is then defeated.

2. A rubber cup and points impregnated with abrasive particles are used. They are supplied in colors of brown, green, and a yellow-banded green. Each color denotes a different degree of abrasiveness. They are often referred to as "brownies," "greenies," and "super greenies." They should be used with a low-speed handpiece at a slow rate, along with light intermittent strokes.

The advantages of polishing using this method are rapid results and less mess compared with the two abrasive slurries. One disadvantage is that the cups and points wear quickly from use and autoclaving. Eventually, a metal shank is exposed that will scratch the amalgam surface. The greatest disadvantage, however, is heat production. The amalgam surface MUST NOT be heated above 140° by the polishing procedure. Heat is generated rapidly with the use of abrasive-impregnated rubber cups and points. The evaluation criteria for amalgam polishing are listed in **Table 15-6**.

DETECTION AND MANAGEMENT OF RESTORATIVE MATERIALS DURING SCALING AND POLISHING

Detection of Tooth Structure and Restorative Materials

Many areas of tooth structure and types of restorative materials are easily identified. There will be times, however, during an examination or scaling when it will be difficult to distinguish between exposed dentin and a recent, well-placed composite resin restoration. In such cases, the restorations are overlooked and an inappropriate polishing procedure may result.

TABLE 15–6 Evaluation Criteria for Amalgam Polishing

1. Amalgam is void of scratches and appears smooth.
2. Amalgam has a high polish and lustrous shine.
3. There is no damage to adjacent tooth structure.
4. Time utilization is satisfactory.

From Gladwin M, Bagby MD: Clinical Aspects of Dental Materials. Philadelphia, Lippincott Williams & Wilkins, 2000, p 235.

For example, to distinguish between dentin and a glass ionomer restoration, several statements may be made. Both appear radiopaque. Dentin feels smooth to the explorer, whereas glass ionomer feels rough. A detectable margin also differentiates between these two materials. If a sharp explorer were to pass over these two surfaces, a variance in sound would be noted, with the dull sound being indicative of glass ionomer. The sound referred to as sharp or dull is slight and in all probability is a combination of auditory and tactile sensations perceived by the operator. Another way of explaining this concept is to state that most clinicians would agree that enamel possesses a certain hardness and smoothness, whereas restorations may have a different texture and feel. Scaling from the dentin surface of the tooth (in an area of gingival recession) onto the composite with heavy pressure could damage the restoration. A careful analysis of a patient's restorative materials must be carried out before initiating any form of treatment.

Criteria used to aid in the identification and differentiation between tooth structure and restorations are **radiographic characteristics, surface smoothness, sound/touch, and location.**

Radiographic Characteristics

The shades of gray between the extremes of radiolucency and radiopacity in radiographs become an aid to the trained clinician in identifying structure. Tooth enamel is the only natural material in the oral cavity that is translucent to visible light. In recent years, considerable efforts have been made to develop tooth-colored restorative materials that have light transfer characteristics similar to tooth structure. These characteristics are evident in both porcelain and resin; the restorations made from these materials are difficult to detect by casual observation (see Chapter 11).

Surface Smoothness

When a surface is smooth, it is free of irregularities. An explorer passed over this type of surface will glide freely with the change in contour and will not meet with resistance.

One of the goals is to produce smooth surfaces on both the natural tooth structure and restorative materials. Less plaque and debris accumulate on smooth surfaces.

Sound and Touch

The criteria of sound and touch with the use of a sharp explorer can provide the most helpful diagnostic tools. The passage of the tip of the explorer at right angles to the surface with minimal pressure and force transmits **tactile and auditory** sensations.

The tactile sensation refers to the character of the surface; it is either smooth (e.g., as in tooth enamel) or rough (e.g., as in a worn composite restoration).

Sound also plays a part in the diagnosis. The **tine** (sharp point) of the explorer is silent on smooth enamel but scratchy or noisy on rough tooth surfaces, worn composite restorations, or residual orthodontic bonding resin. When the tine passes over faulty or worn margins of restorations, it produces a "ping" sound.

Some restorations are so well matched to tooth structure that, without the "sound-feel" difference, they may go undetected. The ideal margin of all restorative materials is undetectable to the passage of the explorer from tooth to restoration or from restoration to tooth. The tine of the explorer serves as an aid, not in the identification of the material, but in the determination of the condition of the restoration at the cavosurface margin.

Location

The location of the restoration is important when identifying tooth-colored restorations. In most cases, the restoration involves restoring a proximal or facial surface. Depending on the material used and the age and marginal integrity of the restoration, the junction of the enamel and restorative material is often visually undiscernible. For this reason, proper **transillumination** with the mouth mirror to identify the exact location of the restoration before using any instrument is critical.

Managing Restorations During Scaling and Polishing

Smooth surfaces on tooth structure and restorative materials are less receptive to bacterial colonization and dental plaque formation. Coronal polishing, which may take place after scaling and root planing, must be accomplished in a way that is not damaging to the tooth and restorative materials. Fairly common examples of detrimental procedures include the production of excess heat during polishing, excessive use of abrasives, damage to margins of cast restorations, and use of high-speed instrumentation.

Production of Excessive Heat During Polishing

As stated earlier, temperatures of 140°F or above will alter the surface characteristics of an amalgam restoration due to a release of mercury. This results in accelerated corrosion and marginal breakdown. otating a bristle brush, rubber cup, or rubber wheel on a thumbnail readily demonstrates how quickly excessive heat can be generated by speed or by pressure. The addition of mouthwash, water, or glycerin to make a slurry when using abrasives such as Silex or tin oxide will decrease the amount of heat produced.

Excessive Use of Abrasives

Excessive use of abrasives can be injurious to patients in several respects. Improper use of an abrasive agent and a rubber cup at the gingival margin can cause trauma to or removal of the surface epithelium in that area.

As discussed in the previous section, abrasive agents can be harmful because of the following factors:

- Particle size of the polishing agent
- Number of particles applied per unit of time
- Speed of the application
- Amount of pressure applied

It is for these reasons that **selective polishing** has become an accepted alternative treatment to polishing with abrasives.

For cast gold restorations, such as inlays, onlays, or crowns, the final polish applied in the dental laboratory provides the smoothest surface that these restorations will receive during patient service. Many polishing agents can create fine scratches in several types of restorations because of speed, pressure, and particle size. Use of a paste that contains the smallest abrasive particle that will remove surface stain and plaque is advised.

Damage to Margins of a Cast Restoration

A third way in which damage could be incurred on a restored surface during scaling is by the opening of a margin of a cemented casting. This particular type of restoration is likely to have a detectable margin. More so than gold foil or amalgam restorations, cemented castings (i.e., inlays, onlays, and crowns) will have a "cement line" margin. A properly mixed cement should have a film thickness of less than 40 μm. The margins of cast restorations are delicate and have been adapted to the preparation by the operator **marginating**, with hand instruments, from cast metal to tooth structure. Because the longevity of the cast restoration de-

pends in part on the condition of the margin, it is critical that it is identified. When scaling in the area of a cast restoration, scaling technique should be altered so as not to jeopardize the margin of any cemented casting.

Figure 15-6A illustrates the casting in place and a thin, fragile gold edge over the **beveled margin** (the sloping or angled edge of the preparation) of the tooth. A potential position of a curet scaler is shown in Figure 15-6B. Figure 15-6C depicts the results of an applied working stroke. Note the destruction of the marginal integrity that will lead to recurrent decay (see Figure 15-6D).

To prevent this damage, exploring with an explorer or a scaling instrument is necessary to locate the margin of the casting. Once the margin is identified, the working stroke must be kept within an area below the margin. On the facial or lingual surface, a more oblique or horizontal stroke should be employed rather than a vertical stroke, still keeping in mind the location of the margin of the casting.

Application of Fluoride

Some restorative materials may be altered or damaged by the application of topical fluorides. Tooth-colored restorations and the enamel margins adjacent to the restoration may discolor with the application of **stannous fluoride**. Application of **acidulated phosphate fluoride** may cause deleterious effects to porcelain, composite, and glass ionomer restorations. A 4-minute application may create a loss of reflection or may dull the appearance of these restorations. The fluoride will microscopically "etch" the outer surface of these materials.

Placement of petroleum jelly over the restoration before the application of the acidulated phosphate fluoride is recommended.

Polishing Materials and Abrasion

The cleaning and polishing of patients' teeth and restorations should also include any removable appliances such as full and partial dentures. An abrasive agent chosen to remove tobacco stain from enamel may not be the best choice for polishing a composite resin. It will be easier to discuss the topic of polishing materials and abrasion if basic terms that are involved in these procedures are first defined.

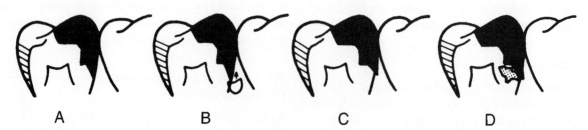

Figure 15-6. The cemented casting. A, Casting cemented into place. B, Curet blade improperly positioned. C, Results of an applied working stroke. D, Recurrent decay resulting from an opened margin. (From Gladwin M, Bagby MD: Clinical Aspects of Dental Materials. Philadelphia, Lippincott Williams & Wilkins, 2000, p 159.)

Cutting is removing material by a shearing-off process. Examples of cutting would be milling, machining, or drilling, and the process results in a somewhat smooth surface. In dentistry, cutting is done with metal burs and hand instruments to create cavity and crown preparations that receive permanent restoration.

Abrasion is the wearing away of a surface and may also be referred to as grinding. Irregular grooves or scratches are produced on a surface as a result of abrasion.

Finishing is the process of producing the final shape and contour of a restoration.

Polishing is the abrasion of a surface to eventually reduce the size of the scratches until the surface appears shiny. This concept not only applies to dentistry in regard to tooth structure and restorative materials but also includes sinks and bathtubs with certain kinds of cleansers that are recommended for those surfaces. This kind of polishing is different from polishing shoes or furniture. The shoe and furniture polish acts as a surface coat, similar to that of car wax.

Abrasives are the materials doing the "wearing" or the abrading. In dentistry, abrasive particles may be bound together onto burs, disks, stones, wheels, or strips or used with liquids to form a paste or slurry.

Types of Abrasives

Many types of abrasives are used in dentistry. The following list includes some of the more common ones that may be used to perform typical clinical or laboratory procedures.

Chalk is a mineral form of calcite. It is also called whiting or calcium carbonate. It is a mild abrasive and is used to polish teeth, gold and amalgam restorations, and plastic materials. In the past, it was the abrasive agent in dentifrices such as Colgate Tooth Powder but it has been replaced by other abrasives.

Pumice is a silica-like volcanic glass that is used as a polishing agent on enamel, gold foil, and dental amalgam and for finishing the acrylic denture bases in the laboratory. It is the abrasive agent in Lava Soap and is used to remove dried or calloused skin in the form of a "pumice stone."

Sand is a form of quartz and may be seen in various colors. Sand particles are rounded or angular. They are typically bonded to paper disks for grinding metals and plastics.

Cuttle is a fine grade of quartz. These particles are also bonded to paper disks and are beige. They are available in coarse, medium, and fine grits. In the past, cuttle was manufactured from the inside shell of a Mediterranean marine mollusk. A "cuttle bone," mounted in a parakeet's cage, is made of the same material.

Garnet refers to several different minerals that have similar properties. These minerals are the silicates of manganese, magnesium, iron, cobalt, and aluminum. This abrasive is usually dark red. Because garnet is very hard, it is a highly effective abrasive. It is found on coated disks and is used for grinding plastics and metal alloys.

Emery is a natural form of aluminum oxide, and it looks like grayish-black sand. This abrasive is sometimes called "corundum." "Emery boards" are used to file fingernails. It is commonly found on arbor bands that attach to a dental lathe for grinding custom trays and acrylic appliances.

Silex, a commercial product, is a silica-like material such as quartz that is used as an abrasive agent in the mouth. It is supplied as a powder and is mixed with various liquids to form a paste or slurry.

Tin oxide, an extremely fine abrasive, is supplied as a white powder and is used as a final polishing agent for teeth and metallic restorations. It is used as a paste or slurry in the same manner as Silex.

Aluminum oxide is a common abrasive used in dentistry. It has essentially replaced emery for several uses. This abrasive is used widely in dentistry in the form of disks and strips. It is also impregnated into rubber wheels and points and is used in the popular "white stones" to adjust enamel or finish metal alloys and ceramic materials.

Bonded and Coated Abrasives Used In Dentistry

To use the abrasives previously discussed, they must be attached to devices that permit an abrasive action. This action is usually rotary-powered; however, in the case of finishing strips, the action is accomplished by hand. Examples of these items include the following.

- **Stones** are available in various shapes, sizes, and grits and are made from various materials.
- **Rubber wheels or points** consist of molded rubber impregnated with an abrasive into a wheel or point shape. The rubber acts as the matrix or binder of the abrasive agent.
- Polishing **disks or strips** are formed from the bonding of abrasive particles to a paper, metal, or plastic backing.
- **Powders** are used in conjunction with other devices, which include:
- **"Vehicles"** such as water, alcohol, glycerin, or mouthwash to make pastes or slurries
- **Brushes, rubber cups, felt cones and wheels, and cloth wheels**

Some are used for laboratory and clinical procedures, whereas others are used only in the laboratory.

Factors That Affect the Rate of Abrasion

Hardness

The hardness of the abrasive particle must be harder than the surface being abraded if an acceptable rate of abrasion is to occur. Otherwise, the abrasive will be worn, and the surface will not be greatly affected. The abrasion rate can be "temperature dependent" (the abrasive heats up during use). The object being abraded could become heated, which may make it softer and affect the rate of abrasion.

Abrasives are usually made of very hard ceramic materials. **Table 15-7** lists the **Knoop hardness number** of several restorative materials, abrasives, and tooth tissues.

Size

Larger abrasive particles produce deeper scratches than do smaller particles. Deeper scratches result in a greater amount of surface material removed. **Grit** is a term that is used to describe the size of the abrasive particle. When a prophy paste is labeled "coarse" or "fine," it refers to the grit or particle size of the abrasive.

Shape

A spherically shaped particle is less abrasive than one that is irregularly shaped. The sharp edges on an irregularly shaped particle tend to dig into the surface rather than roll across it as a rounded abrasive particle would, thus increasing the rate of abrasion.

Pressure

Use of excessive pressure during finishing and polishing procedures causes a higher abrasion rate due to the abrasive particle cutting deeper into the surface. Increased pressure may also result in an increase in temperature of the material being polished. An example of this would be using heavy pressure on an amalgam restoration. A rise in the temperature of the amalgam could release mercury to the surface. This action may increase corrosion and contribute to a marginal breakdown.

TABLE 15–7 Knoop Hardness Values of Restorative Materials, Abrasives, and Tooth Tissues

MATERIAL	HARDNESS
Composite (microfill)	30
Cementum	40
ZOE	40
Composite (hybrid)	55
Dentin	70
Amalgam	90
Gold alloy (type II)	100
Calcite (chalk, whiting)	135
Gold alloy (type IV-hardened)	220
Enamel	340
Pumice	560
Porcelain	590
Sand, quartz, cuttle	800
Garnet	1400
Tungsten carbide	1900
Aluminum oxide, emery	2100
Diamond	7000

Adapted from Handbook of Chemistry and Physics, 64th ed. Boca Raton, FL, CRC Press, 1983.

Speed

This term refers to the rate at which the polishing device is rotating. Like pressure, the speed at which the abrasive is applied also increases the rate of abrasion. Higher speed also results in an increase in temperature. It is important to control the speed of the polishing cup or brush during polishing so that the abrasion rate and increase in temperature are minimized.

Lubrication

The most frequently used lubricant in dentistry is water. It is used with handpieces and burs to cool the tooth when cavity preparations are being made. During finishing and polishing, lubrication is also recommended to carry the heat that is created by the abrasive action away from the surface being abraded. This is done by mixing lubricating agents such as water, mouthwash, glycerin, and alcohol with the abrasive agent, which is usually in powder form. This mixture may be called a "paste" or "**slurry**" depending on the liquid content.

Polishing Process

As discussed earlier, tooth structure and restorative materials are polished for several reasons. These include the following.

Reduce Adhesions. As discussed earlier in this chapter, a smooth surface inhibits adhesion. Plaque, stain, and calculus are less likely to stick to a smooth surface. This is true for both tooth surfaces and restorative materials.

Create a Smooth Surface. Patients expect a smooth surface on any permanent restoration that is placed in their mouths. In addition, they may comment on the smoothness that is produced by polishing during a routine dental hygiene recall appointment.

Increase Esthetics. It is a well-known fact that an unpolished amalgam or gold crown is not as attractive as one that appears smooth and shiny. This also holds true for the tooth surfaces of a heavy cigarette smoker before and after polishing. Esthetics play a very important role in dentistry, and polishing lends itself to help create an attractive detention for the patient.

Reduce Corrosion. When metallic restorations are polished, it reduces the formation of tarnish and corrosion. This, in turn, may extend the lifetime of the restoration.

Polishing Technique

The polishing procedure involves a series of steps. Each step removes a layer of material by abrasion. Using a series of finer and finer abrasives, the scratches become smaller and smaller until they are smaller than the wavelength of visible light, which is less than 0.5 μm. With scratches this size, the surface then appears shiny. The smaller the size of the scratches, the more shiny the surface appears.

If heavy stains are present, a coarse abrasive, which could be a commercial paste or one of powder and liquid mixed at the chair-side, should always be followed by a different abrasive that has a finer grit with a different rubber cup.

Another approach to polishing is to use the same abrasive material in a progression of larger grit to smaller grits to produce smaller and smaller scratches. This technique is more commonly used in finishing and polishing restorations rather than during prophylaxis.

When a polishing sequence is employed, it is important to remember that prophy cups and brushes must be changed before the next, less abrasive agent is used to prevent abrasive contamination. The surfaces being polished should be thoroughly rinsed before the next agent is applied.

The recommended polishing technique is one of slow speed with light, intermittent pressure. Prophy brushes are suggested for areas such as the occlusal surface due to their abrasive nature and possible trauma to soft tissue.

"Selective Polish" Approach

In recent years, it has been determined that it is not necessary to polish all surfaces during every recall appointment because thorough brushing and flossing at home can produce the same effects as polishing. It has been proved that the effects of polishing all teeth may be counterproductive. For this reason, sound professional judgments should be made in deciding when to polish and which teeth to polish. Additional decisions include the appropriate agents to use and the method in which to use them.

It is well established in the literature that portions of the fluoride-rich layer of enamel (usually 3-4 μm in thickness) can be removed during routine polishing with pumice. The uptake of fluoride that the patient has been accumulating between professional polishings from water, dentifrices, and rinses is removed when tooth structure is polished with excessively abrasive agents. It has also been proved that polishing does not improve the uptake of topical fluoride when it is applied professionally.

The purpose of polishing is to produce the smoothest surface possible. Whether it is on the tooth structure or on the restorative material, the purpose is defeated when using coarse abrasive agents, because grooves and scratches are created on the surface that may not have been there previously. This condition serves as a more adhesive surface for the formation of plaque, stain, and calculus more rapidly than before improper polishing.

If a patient insists on rotary polishing, a very mild agent, such as a dentifrice, may easily be dispensed in a dampen dish.

Prophylaxis Pastes

There is a vast assortment of prophylaxis pastes on the market. In recent years, these pastes are marketed not only by companies that make toothbrushes but also by companies that manufacture disposable and autoclavable prophy angles. Prophy pastes are available in bulk, large-volume containers, as well as unit dose cups. These pastes are manufactured in various colors, textures, flavors, grits, and formulations. Prices also vary depending on the brand and quantity purchased.

Abrasive Properties

The abrasive particle used in the paste should not produce a detrimental effect on the surface. A polishing agent should not create deep scratches and grooves, as discussed earlier, but should produce very fine and shallow ones so that light may be reflected and therefore "shine." The agent must, however, remove the stain. An acceptable prophy paste possesses properties of both a high-polish and low-abrasion rate.

When polishing areas of gingival recession, it must be remembered that dentin abrades 25 times faster than enamel. Cementum, which is only temporarily present in areas of recession due to its thin layer and "softness," abrades 35 times faster than enamel. Common practice would dictate that abrasive polishing agents be contraindicated in areas exhibiting significant gingival recession.

Denture Cleansers

Full and partial dentures accumulate plaque, stain, and calculus in the same manner as do natural teeth. Removable appliances should be examined and returned to the patient in a deposit-free condition at the end of the appointment.

The goal in cleaning and polishing dentures, like that of natural teeth and other restorative surfaces, is to remove deposits in a manner that is not detrimental to the surface. Care must be taken so that abrasives, rotary devices, or caustic ultrasonic solutions do not damage the surface of the removable denture appliance.

Dentifrices

As with denture cleansers, dentifrices are discussed in detail in Chapter 12. From a dental material perspective, the most important constituent in a dentifrice is the abrasive agent.

Abrasive Content and ADA Acceptance

One of several types of abrasives may be added to the dentifrice formulation. Several years ago, there were dentifrices on the market that were considered to be very abrasive, such as those recommended for smokers. To reassure the consumer today, the ADA evaluates dentifrices in their Acceptance Program. A dentifrice is **"ADA Accepted"** if it meets the specific requirements set forth by the ADA. Summaries of these requirements are:

- **Abrasivity Level.** The dentifrice must not exceed the abrasivity value of 250. This number is obtained from standardized testing that involves irradiated dentin specimens, brushing them with test and reference dentifrices, and then calculating a ratio from comparing amounts of radioactive phosphorus released by each dentifrice. This number is then multiplied by 1000 to yield an abrasivity score. It would be fairly safe to say that there would be very few, if any, dentifrices on the market today that exceed the abrasivity value of 250.

- **Scientific Data.** The manufacturer of the dentifrice must produce scientific data to support any claims made in advertisements and placed on packaging of the product. These data are usually the result of extensive clinical trials.

Factors That Affect the Abrasion Rate by Dentifrices

Intraoral and extraoral factors influence the rate of abrasion from a dentifrice. Some of the extraoral factors include the type, size, and amount of abrasive in the dentifrice as well as the quantity of dentifrice used. The type of toothbrush, the method of use, the amount of force delivered, and the frequency of brushing are other extraoral factors.

Intraoral factors include xerostomia, saliva consistency and quantity, exposed root surfaces, quality and quantity of deposits, and presence of certain restorative materials.

 # MAKING IMPRESSIONS AND STUDY MODELS

The use of alginate impression material is the most common method for obtaining diagnostic casts. It is pleasant tasting, inexpensive, and easy to manipulate, and it adequately records details of the patient's oral structures. **Study models** or **study casts** are positive reproductions of the patient's dental arches and surrounding tissues. The purpose of taking an alginate impression is to make an accurate reproduction of the maxillary and mandibular arches and adjacent tissues. Study models constructed from alginate impressions can be used for patient treatment planning and also serve as part of the patient's permanent record.

Tray Preparation

Impression trays are usually perforated so that the alginate flows through the perforations when the tray is seated on the dental arch. These perforations act as a retentive mechanism so that the set alginate does not become separated from the tray upon removal.

Impression trays are available in various sizes and materials. Disposable (or single-use) trays are usually made of plastic, and autoclavable (permanent) trays are made of metal. Before taking the impression, the empty tray should be seated in the patient's mouth to determine the correct fit.

After the impression trays have been selected, rope (beading) wax can be molded around the periphery of the tray. This protects the tissues from injury, extends the tray, and may aid in the retention of alginate material in the tray. The maxillary tray may also have rope wax placed in the palatal area of the tray to support the alginate so that an air void does not occur.

Patient Preparation

1. Explain the procedure to the patient if he or she has not had impressions taken in the past. Instruct the patient not to talk, but rather to raise his or her hand to signal any discomfort.
2. Seat the patient in an upright position to minimize the chance of gagging or vomiting.
3. Ask the patient to remove all removable dental appliances, such as full or partial dentures and orthodontic retainers.
4. Cover gingival areas of fixed bridges and other fixed appliances with rope wax to prevent alginate from locking under crowns and pontics, which may cause tearing and distortion upon removal.
5. Ask the patient to rinse with an antibacterial mouth rinse to reduce the amount of bacteria and the amount of saliva, resulting in a more accurate impression.
6. Take the mandibular impression first to familiarize the patient with the procedure, the taste, and consistency of the alginate material.

Alginate Impressions

Alginate material is available in regular-set and fast-set forms. The regular-set material has a **setting time** of approximately 3 to 4 minutes, whereas the fast-set material will set, or gel, in approximately 1 to 2 minutes. The **working time**, or the time that it should take to mix the alginate, is 1 minute.

It is important that the mixture is homogenous-one that has a uniform consistency throughout similar to that of peanut butter.

Taking the Impression

1. Seat the mandibular arch standing at the 7 o'clock position. The patient's chair should be raised, and the occlusal plane should be parallel to the floor.
2. Load the mandibular tray from the posterior, lingual aspect working toward the facial.
3. Press the material into the tray with the spatula to eliminate entrapped air.
4. Using a fingertip moistened with tap water, smooth the alginate material and make a slight indentation in the surface. This helps to place the tray over the teeth correctly and prevent the formation of air bubbles.
5. Retract the patient's cheek using the index finger and thumb of one hand.
6. Rub a small amount of alginate material over the occlusal and interproximal surfaces of the mandibular teeth with the index finger of the other hand.

7. Grasp the handle of the impression tray so that the tray and the alginate are facing downward. Rotate the tray into the mouth by using the front of the tray to retract the near cheek and the free hand to retract the far cheek. Next, straighten it so that the tray handle is in line with the patient's mid-face.

8. Press the tray downward lightly and evenly over the mandibular arch using the index fingers of both hands, until resistance is felt. The lip should flap over the front of the tray, and the alginate should extend into, and fill, the labial periphery.

9. Instruct the patient to breathe normally through the nose. If gagging occurs, seat the patient in the most upright position and ask him or her to lean slightly forward.

10. Keep the tray in place until the alginate is completely set. Because body temperature is higher than room temperature, the alginate material will set faster in the mouth than the remaining alginate in the bowl.

11. Seat the impression on the maxillary arch standing at the 11 o'clock position or behind the patient's head and off to the side.

12. Hold the tray in place until the alginate is completely set, 2 to 3 minutes after the material is no longer tacky.

13. Load the maxillary tray from the posterior aspect working anteriorly; sweeping from the lingual toward the facial. Press the material into the tray with the spatula to eliminate entrapped air. Rub a small amount of alginate on the occlusal and interproximal surfaces of the maxillary teeth, in the same manner as described for the mandibular teeth.

14. With the alginate-filled tray in an upward position, turn the tray slightly to one side and place it in the patient's mouth. Insert by rotating the tray into the mouth as described earlier. Once the tray is inserted, straighten it so that the tray handle is in line with the midface of the patient. Begin to apply light and even pressure upward until resistance is felt. First, seat the impression tray in the posterior region, then seat it toward the anterior, allowing the alginate to flow over the molars. Retract the front of the upper lip as the tray is seated. This allows any excess alginate and air to be expressed through the front of the tray, thus minimizing the chance of air voids and the patient gagging.

15. Instruct the patient to breathe through his or her nose, leaning slightly forward with the head down toward the chest. This helps to minimize the gagging reflex.

Removing the Impression

To remove the mandibular tray, use the fingers of one hand to retract the corner of the mouth and allow air to enter the vestibule. Place the thumb and index finger on the tray handle, using a firm sideways lifting motion. The impression tray should flip free, with the alginate material held securely in the impression tray. The free hand may be used to stabilize the mandibular arch during the tray removal to decrease injury to the temporomandibular joint and the teeth in the opposing arch.

If the tray does not release, a suction seal has been created. To break this seal, place the index finger of one hand under the periphery of the posterior portion of the tray on either the right or left side. The tray should now be easy to remove.

For maxillary tray removal, retract the corner of the mouth with the fingers of one hand to allow air to enter the vestibule. Grasp the tray handle, using a downward sideways flipping motion with the thumb and forefinger. The tray should remove easily, with the set alginate secured in the impression tray. The fingers of the free hand should protect the teeth in the opposing arch during tray removal.

Assess the impression by using the criteria in **Table 15-8**.

Postremoval Procedures

After any impression, ask the patient to rinse with water or mouthwash to remove any excess alginate. Remove any alginate that may be remaining on the teeth or in the interproximal spaces with an explorer or floss. Ask the patient to rinse again. Use a moistened towel to remove any alginate on the face or lips. Be sure to return any removable dental appliances to the patient.

Disinfecting the Impression

Gently rinse the alginate impression under cool tap water to remove any debris that may be remaining in the impression. Gently shake off any excess water. Spray the entire impression (top and bottom) with an OSHA-approved disinfecting solution, and then place the impression in a headrest cover or plastic bag. Disinfection is usually complete in 10 minutes, depending on the disinfectant used. Rinse the impression with water again, shake it dry, and place it in a clean headrest cover or plastic bag. If the impressions cannot be poured immediately, store the impression in an area where there is 100% humidity.

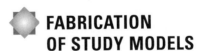 ## FABRICATION OF STUDY MODELS

According to several sources, the terms **diagnostic cast** and **study models** may be used interchangeably. The terms may be technically defined as a "positive replica of the dentition and surrounding structures used as a diagnostic aid and/or base for construction of orthodontic and prosthetic appliances." This procedure is commonly performed in the practice of dentistry to gather information concerning the patient's dentition and to establish an accurate diagnosis.

Construction of a Study Model

Several laboratory techniques are acceptable for fabricating study models. Two techniques include:

TABLE 15–8 Criteria for Evaluating Alginate Impressions

- Lack of voids; free of air bubbles
- No distortion; clear and distinct impression
- Adequately extended; retromolar area is included
- Free of debris; all extraneous material removed
- Adequate detail; recorded all desired structures
- Stable; alginate material attached to tray

From Gladwin M, Bagby MD: Clinical Aspects of Dental Materials. Philadelphia, Lippincott Williams & Wilkins, 2000, p 253.

1. "Double-pour" technique
2. Boxing wax around the impression

"Double-Pour" Technique

The first stage pour is made from a normal mixture of gypsum. The impression sets, face up, on a glass or acrylic slab. The impression is overfilled in all areas by approximately ¼ inch. Two or three small blebs of gypsum material are added to the surface of the poured impression in the shape of small cones to serve as a means of retention. Approximately 10 minutes after the initial pour, and beyond the "loss of gloss" period, the mixture will reach the initial set.

The second stage pour is made of a thicker mixture of gypsum to serve as a base and support for the first pour. A 1-inch thick paddy is made from the gypsum in a rounded shape, approximately the size of the impression tray. It is placed on a flat, smooth glass or acrylic slab or a surface that will not absorb water and stick to the mix.

The poured impression is then inverted onto the paddy. It is important not to apply pressure to the inverted tray or allow it to sink closer than 1/2 inch to the surface.

While the tray is held by the handle, a spatula is used to shape the sides of the stone around the first pour of the impression tray. The two mixes are blended together with the plaster spatula to create a continuous flow and a slight connection of the two mixes. The handle of the impression tray and occlusal surface of the teeth are parallel with the slab to promote a base of uniform thickness. A cross-section of the

base and impression are illustrated in **Figure 15-7**. Note how the additional small mounds of gypsum added to the first pour "interlock" into the base to provide a stronger finished product.

Before the initial set of the second pour, the excess gypsum is trimmed with a laboratory knife to minimize the use of the model trimmer. The cast is separated 45 to 60 minutes from the beginning of the second pour with a laboratory knife. The knife is inserted at the periphery and slightly twisted to release the gypsum from the adhering alginate. The cast is then trimmed.

Boxing Wax Technique

The boxing wax completely encircles the impression tray and creates a temporary mold to contain the plaster or stone. A base is formed for the study model when the gypsum material has set inside the boxing wax.

After impression is disinfected, the excess alginate is trimmed beyond the posterior border of the maxillary and mandibular impression with the laboratory knife. Trimming should be done conservatively. The removal of excess alginate helps to box the impression for the second pour and to maintain the anatomic landmarks on the final cast.

A piece of beading (rope) wax is applied to the periphery of the impression above the handle, so that the entire impression tray is encircled. A warm wax spatula is used to affix the wax approximately 2 to 3 mm down from the peripheral roll of the impression to the impression tray. The boxing wax is then added around the entire impression and should extend and overlap 1/2 inch beyond the vestibular edge of the tray.

The boxed impression is vibrated with a small amount of gypsum on the spatula until it is filled one-half full. It is then set on a flat surface and filled completely with the remaining gypsum product. After 45 to 60 minutes the boxing and beading wax is removed and the casts are separated from the alginate impression. Evaluation criteria for study models are listed in **Table 15-9**.

 OTHER SUPPORTIVE SERVICES

Tooth Bleaching

Teeth that are discolored or have become stained can be treated with a bleaching agent. Depending on the cause of the discoloration or the type of stain, one of several bleaching techniques may be used. The bleaching procedure is often referred to as a **tooth whitening** or **tooth bleaching** treatment.

A **nonvital tooth** is treated differently than a vital tooth. A nonvital tooth is one in which the pulp tissue is necrotic (not living) or missing. The terminology used when vital teeth are treated is **vital tooth bleaching**. **Vital teeth** (i.e., teeth with living pulp tissue) can be bleached in the dental

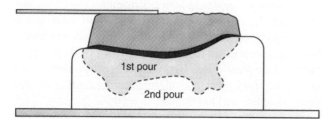

Figure 15-7. Cross-section of the poured alginate impression inverted onto the gypsum paddy. (From Gladwin M, Bagby MD: Clinical Aspects of Dental Materials. Philadelphia, Lippincott Williams & Wilkins, 2000, p 267.)

TABLE 15–9 Criteria for Evaluation of Study Models (Casts)

- Models are free of excessive voids and fractures.
- Models are smooth and hard.
- Casts have appropriate outline form.
- Anatomic structures of casts are not damaged.
- Casts have adequate bases.
- Casts remain occluded when positioned on the posterior border heel cuts.

From Gladwin M, Bagby MD: Clinical Aspects of Dental Materials. Philadelphia, Lippincott Williams & Wilkins, 2000, p 270.

office or at home by the patient. When the patient does the bleaching treatment at home, **night guard bleaching** is the term often applied, because the bleaching agent is applied to the teeth in a custom tray that resembles a night guard appliance.

No tooth structure is sacrificed in the preparation of vital teeth for bleaching. In the treatment of nonvital teeth, an opening into the pulp chamber, from the lingual surface of anterior teeth or from the occlusal surface of posterior teeth, is necessary. Multiple variables affect the outcome of the bleaching procedure. The success of the bleaching procedure is dependent upon the following factors:

- Cause or type of discoloration or stain
- Degree or intensity of the discoloration or stain
- Bleaching agent selected
- Strength of the bleaching agent
- Length of exposure of the tooth to the bleaching agent
- Bleaching technique
- Vitality of the tooth
- Presence of cracks in the surface of the tooth
- Presence of any restoration in the tooth

Causes of Tooth Discoloration

Nonvital Teeth

A tooth with a necrotic pulp or one that has been treated endodontically tends to darken with time. Significantly darkened teeth should be noted during the clinical examination, and the cause of the darkening should be investigated. When a tooth with a necrotic pulp is discovered, endodontic therapy and bleaching reduce the likelihood of an abscess and improve the appearance of the smile.

An injury to a tooth may cause the pulp tissue to become necrotic, with no symptom or sign of necrosis other than a noticeable darkening of the tooth. The decomposition of the pulp tissues, especially the hemoglobin of the red blood cells, produces a dark stain that penetrates the dentinal tubules. After a tooth has been diagnosed as nonvital, appropriate endodontic treatment must be performed. The most common endodontic procedure is root canal therapy. The contents of the pulp cavity, including both the root

canals and the coronal pulp chamber, are removed. The pulp chamber and root canals are then filled with an inert material such as **gutta percha**, which is a natural resin. The entire procedure is performed under aseptic conditions and usually requires multiple treatment appointments. After a nonvital tooth has been successfully treated, a full crown may be recommended to strengthen the tooth. If a root canal treated tooth is not crowned, a bleaching treatment may be performed to lighten the color (shade) of the darkened tooth.

Vital Teeth

Teeth are naturally white with a translucence that contributes to their brightness. However, teeth vary in color or shade from person to person and, as teeth age, they darken. The appearance of teeth due to their shade or color, whether as a result of natural shading or from the aging process, may not be esthetically acceptable to the patient. Bleaching may be an effective treatment option for the esthetic improvement of healthy natural teeth.

Stain

Both vital and nonvital teeth are subject to staining. Two types or classifications of stain are **extrinsic stain** and **intrinsic stain**. These have been discussed in detail in Chapter 10. Some extrinsic stain may be removed by the patient with over-the-counter agents. Dental professionals may remove more tenacious extrinsic stains with scaling, prophylaxis pastes, and various forms of abrasive agents. Extrinsic stains that are resistant to complete removal by scaling and polishing are effectively removed by bleaching treatments. The bleaching process is more effective against extrinsic stains than intrinsic stains.

Intrinsic stain may be classified as either **posteruptive** or **pre-eruptive stain**. Posteruptive stain occurs after the tooth erupts, and examples include amalgam restorations, caries, and endodontic treatment. The stains caused by silver amalgam cannot be successfully bleached. Caries should be removed and the tooth restored before bleaching is attempted. Stains resulting from endodontic treatment can be successfully bleached.

Pre-eruptive stains occur while the teeth are in the calcification stage. These stains are caused by **tetracycline, fluorosis, dentinogenesis imperfecta, and amelogenesis imperfecta**. Mild cases of tetracycline staining and fluorosis have a higher success rate with bleaching than do moderate to severe cases. Bleaching does not significantly improve the appearance of teeth that are affected by dentinogenesis or amelogenesis imperfecta (see Chapter 8).

Contraindications

Teeth stained as a result of caries, pulpal necrosis, or endodontic therapy are not good candidates for patient-applied bleaching. Teeth with sensitive dentin root surfaces should not be bleached aggressively because of the potential for increased tooth sensitivity. A few patients may be sensitive or allergic to a component in the bleaching agent. Some patients may not exhibit the degree of cooperation necessary for successful treatment.

Before bleaching treatments are prescribed, the medical history should be thoroughly reviewed. The procedure is contraindicated in the following patients:

- Pregnant or lactating women
- Children younger than 18 years of age
- Heavy smokers
- Excessive alcohol users

Bleaching Agents

Hydrogen peroxide, H_2O_2, is a strong oxidizing agent that readily decomposes into water and oxygen. The process of decomposition of hydrogen peroxide releases free radicals of oxygen that react with pigments in both extrinsic and intrinsic stains, thus producing the bleaching effect. Free radicals of oxygen contain an unpaired electron and are, therefore, highly reactive.

Hydrogen peroxide can penetrate enamel and dentin and may produce a **reversible pulpitis**, which is a temporary inflammation of the pulp tissue. Tooth sensitivity resulting from pulpitis is the most frequently reported side effect of the bleaching process. Precautions must be taken to protect the patient's eyes, face, intraoral soft tissues (i.e., lips, cheeks, tongue), and clothes from hydrogen peroxide solutions. Hydrogen peroxide is applied to the teeth in either liquid or gel form and in strengths that vary from 5% to 35%.

Carbamide peroxide, $CH_6N_2O_3$, is a weaker oxidizing agent and is more stable than is hydrogen peroxide. It is applied to the teeth in either a liquid or gel form and in strengths that vary from 10% to 15%. Carbamide peroxide decomposes into hydrogen peroxide, which then degrades into water and oxygen. A 10% carbamide peroxide solution is equivalent to 3% hydrogen peroxide, whereas a 15% solution is equivalent to 5% hydrogen peroxide. Most carbamide peroxide bleaching gels contain Carbopol (BF Goodrich, Richfield, OH), a thickening agent that increases adhesion of the gel to the tooth, thus prolonging exposure to the bleaching agent.

Sodium perborate is another weak oxidizing agent. It is sometimes used together with hydrogen peroxide to bleach nonvital teeth. Sodium perborate is the active ingredient in many household fabric bleaches that are designated as being safe for use with colors.

Bleaching Techniques

Nonvital Bleaching

When a nonvital tooth needs bleaching, the root canals must be filled before the bleaching procedure is performed. The bleaching agent is applied to the unfilled pulp chamber (coronal pulp cavity) until the desired shade of the crown is obtained. The pulp chamber and the external opening into the chamber are then filled with a permanent filling mater-

ial, either glass ionomer or composite. When a restored, endodontically treated tooth is bleached, the permanent filling material must be completely removed from the pulp chamber and the external opening into the chamber. The bleaching agent is then applied to the pulp chamber.

The bleaching agent is applied to the pulp chamber in the same manner for a restored endodontically treated tooth as for a tooth not yet permanently restored. A cotton ball saturated with 35% hydrogen peroxide (Superoxol: Moyco Union Broach, York, PA) is inserted into the pulp chamber, and a heated instrument is applied to the cotton ball to accelerate the release of oxygen. When the desired bleaching effect has been achieved, the pulp chamber and access opening are filled with a permanent filling material, either composite or glass ionomer.

Vital Bleaching

In 1989, with the introduction of an effective patient-applied technique, bleaching has grown rapidly in popularity. Two techniques are often used: **a professionally applied, in-office technique**, and **a patient-applied** (at home) **professionally supervised technique**. Over-the-counter products are available to the public, but they are generally ineffective and are not recommended because of the lack of professional supervision in the selection and application of the bleaching agent.

Professionally Applied In-Office Bleaching

The professionally applied technique uses 30% or 35% hydrogen peroxide. The teeth that are to be bleached are isolated with a rubber dam, and the gingiva, tongue, and facial mucosa are protected with a coat of lubricant. The patient's eyes are protected with appropriate eyewear. Hydrogen peroxide is applied to the teeth either in gel form or with a gauze soaked in liquid hydrogen peroxide. The hydrogen peroxide is then activated with a heat source, using either an incandescent lamp or a resin-curing light. To avoid damage to the vital pulp, care must be taken not to apply too much heat to the teeth. The teeth must not be anesthetized with local anesthesia. This would prevent the patient from responding to painful stimulation produced by an excess of heat. The latest innovation in the professionally applied technique is **laser bleaching**. A laser beam, either argon or carbon dioxide, is applied to the teeth to activate the bleaching agent. In addition to activating the bleaching agent, the argon laser interacts directly with dark stains but becomes less effective as the tooth whitens. The effectiveness of the carbon dioxide laser is not related to the lightness of the tooth. Caution must be exercised, in the form of special eyewear, to protect the eyes of both the patient and the dental personnel from the energy of the laser beam.

Patient-Applied, Professionally Supervised Bleaching

Either hydrogen peroxide or carbamide peroxide may be used in the patient-applied, professionally supervised technique.

Results of patient-applied bleaching depend on the strength of the bleaching agent and the length of the treatment.

When hydrogen peroxide gels are used, strengths of 2%, 5%, or 10% are dispensed by the patient into custom-made resin trays. The trays are worn over the teeth for multiple treatment sessions, each lasting for 30 minutes.

The other agent used in this technique is carbamide peroxide. It is dispensed as a 10% or 15% gel into custom-made resin trays. The trays are worn during the day for multiple treatment sessions of 2 hours each. The patient may prefer to wear the trays for 8 hours while he or she is sleeping. **Table 15-10** lists indications and contraindications for the use of patient-applied, professionally supervised vital bleaching.

DEBONDING ORTHODONTIC RESINS

Debonding is the mechanical removal of the orthodontic bracket and the residual bonding resin with the least amount of damage to the tooth structure. It is accomplished in three steps: (1) removal of the bracket, (2) elimination or reduction of the resin, and (3) restoration of the tooth surface to pretreatment characteristics.

The goal of bracket removal is to create a fracture within the bonding resin or between the bracket and resin. Removal of the bracket at this location leaves the enamel surface intact. It is important not to twist the orthodontic pliers when attempting to remove brackets. This action may cause pain, fracture the enamel, or damage the periodontal ligament.

It is important to identify the residual resin before engaging any instrumentation. Rough resin surfaces may be reported by the patient. The clinician may also detect them both visually and tactilely. The use of loupes for magnification may be useful to the clinician. The tine of an explorer may detect the margins of the remaining resin. Once identified, the resin is removed with a tapered, plain-cut finishing bur on a low-speed handpiece. A smooth, brush-like stroke should be used in one direction. The removed resin should appear as fine white shavings. Examine the area frequently to avoid over-instrumentation. This is done by rinsing the

area and air drying it thoroughly. Residual resin will appear opaque compared with the translucent enamel.

To restore the enamel to the pretreatment condition, use a slurry of pumice and a rubber cup after thoroughly examining the surface both visually and tactilely. Aluminum oxide points, disks, and cups may be used for a final polish. Professionally applied fluoride is also recommended at this time because the enamel rich layer was removed during bonding and debonding.

Suggested Sources

http://www.ada.org/p&s/stands/tc-stand.html
http://www.lib.umich.edu/dentlib/Dental_tables/

Properties and Manipulation

ADA Council on Scientific Affairs: Dental mercury hygiene recommendations. JAMA 130:1125-1126, 1999.

Berg JH: The continuum of restorative materials in pediatric dentistry: A review of the clinician. Pediatr Dent 20(2):93-100, 1998.

Christensen GJ: Longevity vs esthetics in restorative dentistry. J Am Dent Assoc 129(7):1023-1024, 1998.

Christensen GJ: What category of impression material is best for your practice? J Am Dent Assoc 128:1026-1028, 1997.

Chu CS, Smales RJ, Wei SHY: Requirements of an impression material for fixed prostheses. Gen Dent 45:548-555, 1997.

Cox CF, Suzuki S, Suzuki SH: Biocompatibilty of dental adhesives. J California Dent Assoc 23(8):35-41, 1995.

Feigal RJ: Sealants and preventive restorations: Review of effectiveness and clinical changes for improvements. Pediatr Dent 20(2):85-92, 1998.

Ferracane JL: Current trends in dental composites. Crit Rev Oral Biol Med 6(4):302-318, 1995.

Gladwin M, Bagby MD: Clinical Aspects of Dental Materials. Philadelphia, Lippincott Williams & Wilkins, 2000.

Greener EH: Amalgam-yesterday, today, and tomorrow. Oper Dent 4:24-35, 1979.

Hilton TJ: Cavity sealers, liners and bases: Current philosophies and indications for use. Oper Dent 21:134-146, 1996.

Leinfelder KF: Changing restorative traditions: The use of bases and liners. J Am Dent Assoc 125:65-67, 1994.

Marshall SJ, Marshall GW Jr: Dental amalgam: The materials. Adv Dent Res 6:94-99, 1992.

Rapley JW, Swan RH, Hallmon WW, Mills MP: The surface characteristics produced by various oral hygiene instruments and materials on titanium implant abutments. Int J Oral Maxillofac Implants 5:47-52, 1990.

Swift EJ: Bonding systems for restorative materials: A comprehensive review. Pediatr Dent 20(2):80-84, 1998.

Van Meerbeek B, Perdigao J, Lambrechts P, Vanherle G: The Clinical performance of adhesives. J Dent 26(1):1-20, 1998.

Polishing Natural and Restored Teeth

Darby ML, Walsh MM: Dental Hygiene Theory and Practice. Philadelphia, WB Saunders, 1995.

Krouse M, Gladwin SC: Identification and management of restorative dental materials during patient prophylaxis. Dent Hyg 58:456, 1984.

Wilkins EM: Clinical Practice of the Dental Hygienist. 8th ed. Baltimore, Williams & Wilkins, 1999.

Making Impressions and Study Models

Boucher CO: Current Clinical Dental Terminology, 2nd ed. St. Louis, CV Mosby, 1974.

TABLE 15-10 Patient-Applied, Professionally Supervised Bleaching

INDICATIONS	CONTRAINDICATIONS
Vital teeth	Nonvital teeth
Extrinsic stain	Severe intrinsic stain
Light to moderate intrinsic stain	Sensitive root/dentin
Cooperative/compliant patient	Sensitivity to components of bleach
	Unreasonable expectations

From Gladwin M, Bagby MD: Clinical Aspects of Dental Materials. Philadelphia, Lippincott Williams & Wilkins, 2000, p 274.

Ehrlich A, Torres HO: Essentials of Dental Assisting. Philadelphia, WB Saunders, 1992, pp 283-293; 470-486.

Wilkins EM: Clinical Practice of the Dental Hygienist, 7th ed. Baltimore, Williams & Wilkins, 1994, pp 164-179.

Woodall IR: Comprehensive Dental Hygiene Care, 4th ed. St. Louis, CV Mosby, 1993, pp 312-335.

Other Supportive Services

Gutmann ME: Composite adhesive resin removal following orthodontic treatment. J Pract Hyg 5:16, 1996.

Wilkins EM: Clinical Practice of the Dental Hygienist, 8th ed. Philadelphia, JB Lippincott, Williams & Wilkins, 1999, pp 636-646.

Questions and Answers

Questions

1. You have been requested to mix alginate and then take an impression. While obtaining the water, you got involved in conversation and did not notice the water was quite warm. Which of the following alterations will occur due to this oversight?
   A. Make the mixture unusable
   B. Lengthen the gelation time
   C. Not affect the gelation time
   D. Shorten the gelation time

2. The modulus of elasticity is a measure of the:
   A. viscosity of a material.
   B. energy absorption without deformation.
   C. ability to stress a material without being deformed.
   D. rigidity or stiffness of a material.

3. The gypsum material known as "high strength stone" may also be referred to as:
   A. plaster.
   B. dental stone.
   C. type III stone.
   D. die stone.

4. Which of the following sets of terms may be used interchangeably to describe a mild abrasive that is used to polish teeth, gold, and amalgam restorations?
   A. Pumice, whiting, and Silex
   B. Calcium carbonate, whiting, and tin oxide
   C. Calcium carbonate, whiting, and chalk
   D. Whiting, Silex, and tin oxide

5. Which of the following terms describes the removal of a material by a shearing off process?
   A. Finishing
   B. Polishing
   C. Cutting
   D. Margination

6. Which of the following properties is directly proportional to a given stress on a material?
   A. Modulus
   B. Strain
   C. Load
   D. Yield point

7. Which of the following dental materials has a setting reaction similar to that of dental composite?
   A. Amalgam
   B. Zinc phosphate cement
   C. Calcium hydroxide liner
   D. Acrylic resin

8. Which type of composite has the smoothest surface when properly polished?
   A. Macrofilled
   B. Microfilled
   C. Hybrid
   D. Condensable composite

9. High-copper amalgams have decreased _____ when compared with low-copper amalgams.
   A. corrosion resistance.
   B. clinical performance.
   C. creep.
   D. compressive strength.

10. Which of the following cements is *not* used to lute permanent restorations?
    A. Zinc phosphate
    B. Zinc oxide-eugenol
    C. Glass ionomer
    D. Polycarboxylate

11. Which of the following elements is used most commonly in the fabrication of dental implants?
    A. Au
    B. Ag
    C. Ti
    D. Pt

12. Percolation of a restoration is related to a mismatch of its _____ with that of tooth structure.
    A. strength.
    B. modulus of elasticity.
    C. corrosion resistance.
    D. thermal expansion.

13. The liquid typically used for acid etching enamel and dentin is:
    A. 5% sulfuric acid.
    B. 37% phosphoric acid.
    C. 10% sodium hypochlorite.
    D. 3% hydrofluoric acid.

14. The filler particles of a dental composite are_____ when compared with the matrix.
    A. stronger
    B. weaker
    C. more flexible
    D. less radiopaque

15. Hybrid composites utilized a range of _____ to maximize filler content.
    A. monomers
    B. particle sizes
    C. particle compositions
    D. surfactants

16. Fluoride is released by _____ materials.
    A. glass ionomers cement
    B. zinc phoshate cements
    C. amalgam
    D. calcium hydroxide levers

17. In the U.S., standards for dental materials are developed and administered by the:
    A. Food and Drug Administration (FDA).
    B. American Dental Association (ADA).
    C. American Association for Dental Research (AADR).
    D. Occupational Safety and Health Administration (OSHA).

18. Which of the following conditions necessitates replacing an amalgam restoration rather than simply polish that restoration?
    A. Tarnish
    B. Overextension
    C. Greater that 10 years old
    D. Fracture

19. Many amalgams last longer than 10 years. Tarnish is corrosive attack that produces a film or layer on the metal surface. An overextension of amalgam beyond the cavosurface of the preparation does not necessitate replacement.Which of the following decreases the rate of abrasion?
    A. Increased hardness of the abrasive particles
    B. Increased hardness of the object being abraded
    C. Increased size of abrasive particles
    D. Increased pressure on the object being abraded

20. Which of the following factors is a contraindication for patient applied bleaching?
    A. Extrinsic stain
    B. Patient compliance
    C. Presence of nonvital teeth
    D. Root surface sensitivity

ANSWERS

1. **D.** The warmer the water, the shorter is the gelation time. Colder water is used to lengthen the gelation time.

2. **D.** The ability to stress a material without it being deformed is elastic deformation. The ability of a material to absorb energy without being deformed is called resilience. The viscosity of a material refers to the ability of a material to flow.

3. **D.** The terms "high strength stone," "die stone," and "type IV" stone may all be used interchangeably.

4. **C.** Whiting, chalk, and calcium carbonate are names for the same mild abrasive agent. Pumice and Silex are more abrasive than whiting.

5. **C.** Examples are milling and drilling. In dentistry, cutting is done with metal burs and handpieces.

6. **B.** Stress and strain are proportional. Modulus is a characteristic of a material that describes stiffness. Yield point (and proportional limit, elastic limit) is the level at which permanent deformation begins to occur.

7. **D.** Both dental composites and acrylic resins set via addition polymerization. The other three materials set by different chemical reactions.

8. **B.** Microfilled composites have the smallest filler particles, thus they will polish to a smoother, shinier surface than will the other composite materials.

9. **C.** Creep is decreased, whereas all the others are increased. Creep is the small change in shape of an object when under continuous compression. Corrosion resistance, compressive strength, and clinical performance are all improved with high copper amalgams.

10. **B.** Zinc oxide and eugenol cements are too weak and soluble for use as a permanent luting material.

11. **C.** Titanium implants are, by far, the most common.

12. **D.** When thermal expansion of a restorative material is mismatched with tooth structure, gaps open and close between the tooth and the material when the temperature changes.

13. **B.** Phosphoric acid is used.

14. **A.** Filler particles are strong stiff materials that typically are radiopaque.

15. **B.** A range of particle sizes is used to fit smaller particles in the spaces in between the larger particles.

16. **A.** Fluoride is leached into the tooth structure from the glass particles during the setting reaction.

17. **B.** The ADA develops and administers standards through the Council on Scientific Affairs.

18. **D.** Fractured amalgams cannot be repaired by polishing procedures.

19. **B.** Harder objects are abraded more slowly. The other choices are factors that increase the rate of abrasion.

20. **D.** Bleaching may increase root surface sensitivity. The other choices are an indication for patient-applied bleaching.

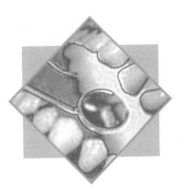

PART IV

Community
Health Activities

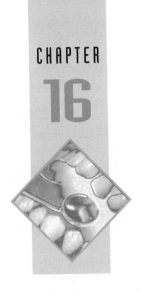

Promoting Health and Preventing Disease Within Groups

PATRICIA S. TATE, BSDH, MEd

A framework is provided within which dental hygienists can maximize community resources to change knowledge, attitudes, values, and behaviors to improve the oral health status of individuals and groups. Learning theories are examined to determine the best instructional approach for a group depending on the individual and composite group learning style. Dental hygienists must possess a fundamental understanding of learning styles, human motivation theories, group dynamics theories, and communications theories to effectively develop oral health promotion and oral disease prevention strategies for groups. In addition, the importance of understanding the influence of social structures on individual and group health behaviors is discussed.

 ## HEALTH PROMOTION CONCEPTS

To begin the study of health promotion, it is useful to define certain terms. **Health** has been described in its simplest form as the absence of disease. However, this definition falls short of the complex nature of health. In 1947, the World Health Organization of the United Nations developed a definition that considers the multifaceted nature of health: "a state of complete physical, mental, and social well-being and not merely the absence of disease and infirmity."[1] This definition has taken on a broader meaning over time by examining the numerous dimensions involved in establishing a healthy individual and a healthy community. Dunn developed the concept of **high-level wellness** or **optimal health.** Dunn defined health as "an integrated method of functioning which is oriented toward maximizing the potential of which the individual is capable. It requires that the individual maintain a continuum of balance and purposeful direction within the environment where he or she is functioning."[2] Dunn suggests that the individual should be proactive, take charge, and be responsible for his or her own health.

The individual must balance all the various components of life in order to achieve a high level of wellness. These components consist of the spiritual, physical, intellectual, social, and emotional aspects of life. By attending to these five areas, an individual will be satisfied and happy with life. Wellness activities such as maintaining a balanced nutritional diet, smoking cessation, using proper oral health regimens, and lowering blood pressure will aid an individual in achieving this status.[3]

When developing educational interventions to help individuals or groups learn new information and behaviors regarding health, the health professional is engaged in health education. The Joint Committee on Health Education Terminology defines **health education** as a combination of learning opportunities "which enables people, as individuals and as members of social structures, to voluntarily make decisions, modify behaviors, and change social conditions in ways which are health enhancing."[4] The concept of **health promotion and disease prevention** assumed a major role in achieving the national oral health objectives for the United States, entitled *Healthy People 2000*[5] and *Healthy People 2010*[6](see Chapter 17). **Health promotion and disease prevention** are defined as "the aggregate of all purposeful activities designed to improve personal and public health through a combination of strategies, including the competent implementation of behavioral change strategies, health education, health protection measures, risk factor detection, health enhancement, and health maintenance."[4] Health education and health promotion are used interchangeably in many cases; however, the differences are significant. As the definitions indicate, health education is primarily the dissemination of information to enhance knowledge and change behaviors. Health promotion and disease prevention involve a systematic process to view individual or group needs and risk factors to ascertain appropriate strategies to use across the community to address health issues and prevent disease. **Figure 16-1** illustrates the components of

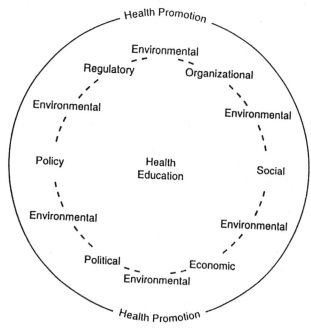

Figure 16-1. Relationship of health education and health promotion. (From McKenzie J, Pinger R: An Introduction to Community Health, 2nd ed. 1997, Jones and Bartlett, Sudbury, MA, p 119. www.jbpub.com. Reprinted with permission.)

health promotion and the relationship between health education and health promotion. An oral health educator should use the full scope of community resources as outlined in Figure 16-1 to most effectively improve the oral health of groups of individuals.

Prevention strategies occur on three levels: *primary, secondary, and tertiary*.[7, 8] Most oral health initiatives are directed at the primary and secondary levels. **Primary prevention** refers to measures that occur when the individual is healthy. The intention is to *block the onset* of disease or injury; this includes the development of school sealant, communal water fluoridation, sports mouthguard, and school-integrated health curriculum initiatives.

Secondary prevention leads to *early diagnosis and treatment* of a disease or condition that will block its development into a disability. Examples of secondary prevention programs include community or school clinical screening and treatment programs for caries and periodontal disease, health fair oral cancer screenings, and education of nursing home staff to perform regular client oral screenings.

Tertiary prevention involves the development of initiatives to *rehabilitate* an individual after a significant disease or injury. Oral cancer rehabilitation efforts are classified as tertiary prevention.

Individuals and groups within society experience many health problems that are based on **risk factors** that the individual may control. Individuals are provided with a free will to make decisions about many of these factors. Each decision will either enhance or diminish the individual's health. Health conditions associated with the use of alcohol, tobacco, careless and reckless driving, inadequate nutrition,

inadequate health care, unprotected sex, and other agents or conditions can be significantly altered when the free will is used to make choices that will positively benefit the individual.

Health educators traditionally provide education to individuals and groups in the hope that the information will effect positive health behaviors. Education alone is ineffective in creating positive oral health behaviors. Some would suggest that it is a waste of community resources to provide educational programming. However, education provides the foundation necessary for making the decisions that will have a positive impact on an individual's oral health. An individual must possess the correct knowledge to make these appropriate decisions and thus attain or maintain a high level of oral health. Therefore, not only is it impractical to suggest that educational initiatives are a waste of resources, but also eliminating the educational component would reduce the effectiveness of the overall program.

LEARNING THEORIES

Human learning is individualistic and occurs through a variety of means. Learning researchers have identified more than 50 different learning theories that are used to describe how people learn facts, concepts, and models; develop reasoning, decision-making, and critical thinking skills; and develop higher level intellectual skills such as analysis, synthesis, and evaluation.[9] **Figure 16-2** lists 10 principles that appear consistently throughout these theories. Health educators or promoters who recognize the value of these principles will succeed in developing educational interventions with higher rates of success. This section focuses on five theories: (1) **operant conditioning,** (2) **social cognition/social learning,** (3) **cognitive learning,** (4) **cognitive dissonance,** and (5) **andragogy.** Researchers have demonstrated that these theories have an impact on the acquisition of oral health knowledge or effect behavioral change.

Operant Conditioning

Skinner did the classical work on the operant conditioning theory.[10] He belonged to a group of psychologists known as behaviorists. Skinner contended that **learning is a function of change in overt behavior and that behavioral changes are an individual's response to events or stimuli in the environment (stimulus-response).** He further stated that the response would continue as long as the response receives **reinforcement.** Positive reinforcement would continue an appropriate behavior, whereas negative reinforcement would stop inappropriate behavior. Skinner is credited with initiating the behavior modification concept that was applied heavily within the dental community during the 60s and 70s. **Behavior modification involves the reinforcement of appropriate dental health behaviors with a reward each time that the behavior is performed.** Rein-

Learning is facilitated if:

1. Several of the senses are used. People retain approximately 10 percent of what they read, 20 percent of what they hear, 30 percent of what they see, 50 percent of what they see and hear, 70 percent of what they say, and 90 percent of what they do and say. Methods that stimulate the widest variety of senses will generally be most effective.

2. The client is actively involved in the process, rather than a passive recipient. Methods that engage and elicit responses from the learner are generally more effective than when the learner is passive. Discussion is basic, and other participative methods usually enhance learning.

3. The client is not distracted by discomfort or extraneous events. Attention to establishing an appropriate learning environment is an important step to take in facilitating learning.

4. The learner is ready to learn. Physical and emotional factors influence readiness. An assessment of readiness makes timing of learning possible and enhances learning.

5. That which is to be learned is relevant to the learner and if that relevance is perceived by the learner. Endeavoring to sense the readiness of the learning and making the connection to existing needs and interests of the client enhances learning.

6. Repetition is used. Reviewing and reinforcing basic concepts several times in a variety of ways enhances learning.

7. The learning encounter is pleasant, if progress occurs that is recognizable by the client, and if that learning is recognized and encouraged. Frequent, positive feedback is important to enhancing learning.

8. Material to be learned starts with what is known and proceeds to the unknown, while concurrently moving from simple to complex concepts. Material to be learned must be organized in ways that make sense to the learner.

9. Application of concepts to several settings occurs, which generalizes the material.

10. It is paced appropriately for the client. Self-pacing of a motivated learner is usually preferable. Attention to the learner's feeling that the pace is too fast or slow will usually enhance learning.

Figure 16-2. General principles of learning. (Modified from Breckon D, Harvey J, Lancaster R: Community Health Education, 4th ed. Gaithersburg, MD, Aspen, 1998, pp 163-164.)

forcement may simply be in the form of praise or encouragement. It has been found that intermittent reinforcement, applied consistently when the appropriate behavior occurs, creates the most long-lasting change.

Social Cognition/Social Learning

Bandura is credited mainly for developing the Social Cognition/Social Learning Theory.[11, 12] Behaviorists who preceded him believed that learning was the result of the individual's experiences, whereas Bandura and other social cognitive theorists expanded the behavioral component of learning to include the environment, the storage of information

tion in learner's memories, and also personal factors (e.g., beliefs and expectations).[13] Bandura contended that **learning occurs through observing and modeling the behaviors, attitudes, and emotional reactions of others.** In addition, he promoted the idea that individuals are more likely to adopt a modeled behavior if the behavior is one that the individual values. Therefore, values play a significant role in the social cognition theory. Reference to this model is found consistently throughout dental behavioral literature.[14-16]

Self-efficacy flows from social cognitive theory and is based on the **concept that an individual is influenced by the behavior of others and that the individual develops**

beliefs that **he or she is** *capable* of performing certain behaviors.[17] Self-efficacy has been used to predict dental behavior in dental research. Correlations have been made between flossing and frequency of dental check-ups with self-efficacy.[16, 18, 19]

Cognitive Model

Behaviorists concentrate on the role of the environment in learning, whereas **cognitive** theorists describe **learning as the changes in internal mental processes that people use to construct their own understanding of the subjects that they study.**[13] Their focus is on the organization of knowledge, information processing, and decision-making.[20, 21] Essentially, cognitive theorists concentrate on the occurrence of mental processes rather than focus on the environment.

Piaget is credited with the development of cognitive learning theory. His decades of study of children revealed patterns of physical and mental action that are related to specific levels of intelligence and correspond to different stages of development in children. These stages move from concrete to abstract thought processes.

A dental hygienist working on health promotion activities with individual clients or with groups should remain cognizant of the implications of each developmental stage to increase the effectiveness of the activity. Children in the **sensorimotor stage (0-2 years)** exhibit motor skill development and hand-to-mouth activity. The professional should teach parents to do mouth care on their child and encourage their children to explore their mouths with a toothbrush. Doing so will facilitate the transition for the child to the next stage. In the **preoperational stage (2-7 years),** children are viewed as concrete, yet intuitive thinkers, who have the ability to understand some symbols but who are unable to work through complex intellectual events. Children should be given concrete opportunities to experience the dental environment using all five senses. This leads to a greater understanding and appreciation of the environment and enhances skill development. The **concrete operational stage (7-11 years)** is the time when the child begins to develop and apply logical approaches to the thought process. However, the child still depends on concrete references to understand and make decisions. During this stage, the child should be engaged in higher level discussions and skill development activities. The professional should furnish the child with basic, concrete references in order to facilitate the learning of new dental health information and development of new skills. During the **formal operations stage (11 years and older),** the child's thought processes involve abstractions. A child is now capable of taking complex intellectual events and thinking through the issues to make decisions without relying on concrete references to solve problems. Within a classroom or other group environment, use of group activities to solve dental health questions will encourage the child to explore the topic and develop answers with a higher level of response. The child is now capable of doing the research necessary to answer the question.[22]

Cognitive theorists encourage the use of teaching methods that will actively involve children and challenge them intellectually. However, the health professional is cautioned to avoid asking children to perform skills that are beyond their cognitive capabilities as outlined earlier.

Cognitive Dissonance

Festinger developed the cognitive dissonance theory to describe the conflict that occurs when an individual experiences inconsistency among his or her cognitions. If an individual's **values and actions (cognitions) are inconsistent (dissonance), the individual will seek ways to bring the values and actions in line with one another.**[23] The desire to make the values, attitudes, beliefs, and behaviors consistent drives the learning process. The desire to reduce or eliminate inconsistency forces the individual to make decisions and solve problems relating to the dissonance factors. The elimination of the dissonance may occur in one of three ways:

1. Reducing the importance of the conflicting value or behavior
2. Acquiring new values, attitudes, or beliefs that change the balance among the cognitions
3. Simply removing the conflicting value, attitude, belief, or behavior

The oral health promoter should determine an individual's set of cognitions to effectively design learning scenarios for appropriate oral health behavior.

Andragogy

Knowles is credited with developing the theory of **andragogy,** which is described as **the theoretical concepts and practices of adult learning.** Most of the previously discussed theories have dealt with **pedagogy,** or **the theory and practice of educating children and youth.** Knowles' research focuses on adults and the differences between adult learning and child learning principles.

The adult learner responds best when the teaching principles are matched with appropriate learning conditions within the teaching-learning interaction. Attending to these principles will increase adult participation in the learning process and make the teaching-learning experience positive for both the adult learner and the oral health educator/promoter. The following is a modified version of Knowles' research in which he suggested pairing the following *learning conditions* with the specific teaching principles to achieve the highest success[24]:

1. *The learner feels a need to learn:* the educator should expose learners to new ways to achieve self-fulfillment; assist learners in clarifying their own desires for improved behavior; aid learners in determining the gap between their desires and their current level of performance; and

help learners to identify the life problems that they experience because of the gaps between their lifestyle and their knowledge.

2. *The learner learns best in an environment that is comfortable, where mutual respect and trust exist and acceptance of differences is encouraged and also where the learner feels a freedom to express opinions:* The educator manages the needs by:

   a. Providing a physical environment that is comfortable by attending to things such as lighting, room temperature, comfortable seating, and appropriate room arrangement so that all participants feel at ease with the interaction

   b. Accepting each learner as a person who should be respected and valued

   c. Building relationships of mutual trust among the learners by encouraging cooperative learning activities and striving to eliminate competition from the learning environment

   d. Disclosing her feelings to an appropriate degree and acting as a facilitator to the learning process

3. *The learner perceives the goals of the learning experience to be his or her own goals:* the educator mutually involves the learner in developing learning goals and objectives simultaneously, including the interests and needs of the sponsoring institution, educator, and subject matter.

4. *The learner develops a commitment to the learning experience by accepting a share of the responsibility for planning and implementing the learning experience:* the educator works with the learner to review the best learning experience options, including methods and materials and jointly determining which option to use.

5. *The learner participates actively in the learning process:* The educator encourages mutual inquiry by the learners by facilitating the organization of learning activities such as group projects, peer learning, and independent studies.

6. *The learning process is **related to** and **makes use of previous learning**:* the educator fosters new learning by gearing her terminology, examples, and so forth to the experience level of the learner; uses discussions, role plays, and case studies to allow learners to utilize their own experiences as resources for the learning; and encourages the learner to integrate new learning into her set of learning experiences to make the learning more meaningful.

7. *The learner has a sense of progress toward the goals:* The educator and the learners mutually develop acceptable criteria and methods to assess achievement toward meeting the learning goals and objectives; and the educator facilitates the development of the learner's self-evaluation skills and application of the skills according to the mutually agreed upon criteria.

Knowles further suggested that it is appropriate to consider applying many of the adult learning principles to the teaching of children. His observations were that as technology and the use of technology expand, children would benefit from the same type of teaching-learning interactions.

Because a significant number of the educational interventions that oral health educators and promoters design will be directed toward adult learners, an understanding of the differences in the learning needs and styles of adults compared with children will make the adult more receptive to the educational message contained within the intervention.

HUMAN MOTIVATION THEORIES

Human **motivation** is the driving force either from within (**intrinsic**) or from outside (**extrinsic**) the individual that moves the individual to action or inaction. For the dental hygienist to effectively *facilitate* motivation to action on oral health matters, an understanding of the principles of human motivation must be developed and applied. The application of the principles comes as a result of the needs assessment stage of the dental hygiene treatment plan process, which is highlighted in Chapters 10 and 12, and the needs assessment stage of the program planning model, which is discussed in Chapter 17. To effectively participate in the motivation of a patient or a group, the dental hygienist must determine the **values, knowledge, attitudes, beliefs,** and **practices** of the individual or the group regarding oral health. Establishing this baseline will enable the dental hygienist to select appropriate motivational strategies that will aid the individual or group in sustaining long-lasting positive oral health behaviors. Long-term behavioral change is difficult to achieve in oral health matters; therefore, failure to include the assessment of values, knowledge, attitudes, beliefs, and practices of the target group will result in noncompliance of the individual or group. Mutually established oral health goals or active involvement of the individual or group in establishing these goals is necessary to ensure **compliance** (i.e., meeting the oral health goals by doing the recommendations provided by the oral health educator/promoter).

Maslow's Hierarchy of Needs

Maslow describes a sociologic human motivational model based upon which need level an individual resides on a hierarchy of needs as shown in **Figure 16-3**. This theory suggests that humans are driven to respond to deficits in their needs at various levels on the pyramid.[25] Until these needs, especially the basic physiologic needs, are met, the individual is unable to move to a higher level of the pyramid. It is important to note that this is not a linear model where the individual moves vertically through the levels. Individuals may move up and down the pyramid, depending on where deficits exist and what circumstances surround the individual's life.

Research indicates that dental needs are more relevant at the safety, social, or ego level.[26] A dental hygienist may identify which need level a person or group is on during the client/group assessment phase by reviewing the responses

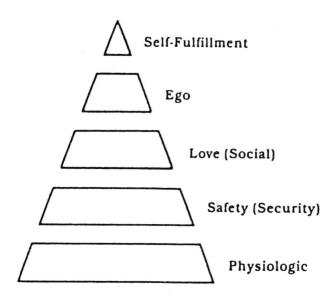

**Psychosocial Needs
Hierarchy Important to Older Generation**

Figure 16-3. Human needs hierarchy. (From Harris N, Christen A: Primary Preventive Dentistry, 4th ed. Stanford, CT, Appleton & Lange, 1995, p 397.)

that individuals provide to questions such as "What is your chief complaint? What concerns do you have regarding your oral health? What personal oral health goals do you have?" In addition, if using an interview assessment tool, the dental hygienist should be cognizant of the body language expressed by the individual. These reactions may demonstrate whether the client or group is at the lower "safety" level or the higher, more self-assured "ego" level. Once it is determined which level the client or group is on, the dental hygienist can develop motivational approaches to match the need levels.[27]

Health Belief Model

The Health Belief model, described by Becker and associates in **Figure 16-4**,[28] provides the basis for most preventive dental education. The model proposes that an individual's decision to assume a health prevention behavior is correlated with that person's perceptions regarding the value of a disease or health condition and the modifying factors relevant to the individual's life. If the individual perceives that the benefits (e.g., healthy gingiva and supporting structures) of the preventive action outweigh the barriers (e.g., cost, inconvenience, and complexity), the individual is more likely to comply with a prevention regimen. The model is a **predictive** tool to suggest whether an individual may be motivated to comply with prevention education.[29, 30]

During the client or group assessment phase, questions should be asked which clearly define the modifying factors

available in the lives of the client or group members. Questions regarding demographics, sociopsychological variables, and structural variables provide clues regarding potential compliance. Research shows ethnicity, social class, and prior knowledge of the disease or condition as predictive factors.[31] In addition, a combination of **perceived susceptibility** (I am likely to get the disease or condition) and **seriousness** (how serious might this disease or condition be to me) accompanied by beliefs about the **benefits** and **importance** or **salience** of preventive dental care have been demonstrated to have a strong correlation with preventive dental care-seeking behavior.[32] Therefore, the perceptions and beliefs of clients or groups should be determined in each of these areas. The model encourages the educator to develop a clear picture of the client or group as related to the various components in order to most effectively design a motivational strategy to enhance the acquisition of preventive dental health behaviors.

Knowledge, Attitudes, and Behavior Theory/Confluence Theory

Confluence theory derives its name from the **flowing or blending together of the individual's cognitive and affective domains to yield behavior.**[33] The cognitive area consists of current knowledge and past experiences; however, the affective area draws on the individual's attitudes, values, and beliefs.

Cognitive + affective = behavior

The theory suggests that humans merge their knowledge of dental health and their dental experiences with all of their attitudes, values, and beliefs regarding dental issues. Consequently, the individual will make appropriate decisions and assume preventive dental health behaviors. Many practitioners relate to their clients using this theory. Frustration results from seeing clients on a regular basis and providing information on the newest preventive methods and technologies only to see the client return with an unimproved oral health status. However, the practitioner feels real elation when he or she sees the client on the next recall appointment and finds that the client has performed all the oral health behaviors taught to her. The question is why do people with the same levels of knowledge and similar values, attitudes, and beliefs behave differently? Some seemingly accept the information and act upon it, at least for a given amount of time, whereas others never act upon the information. Two basic motivational issues are at work when this dissonance occurs. First, how much of a risk-taker is each of the individuals; second, what specific stimuli will trigger a positive behavior for each individual? It is critical to answer both questions in order to affect appropriate preventive oral health behavior. The reality is that just because the dental professional informs clients or groups of the facts regarding oral health, positive behavior does not occur automatically.

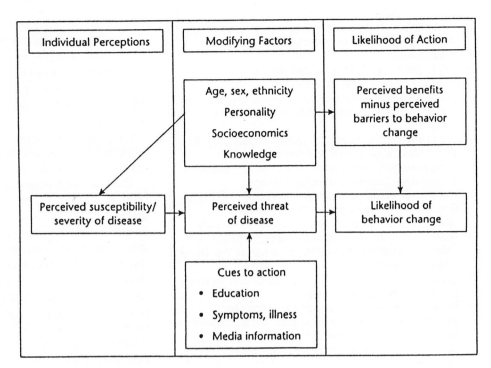

Individual Perceptions	Modifying Factors	Likelihood of Action

Age, sex, ethnicity
Personality
Socioeconomics
Knowledge

Perceived benefits minus perceived barriers to behavior change

Perceived susceptibility/severity of disease

Perceived threat of disease

Likelihood of behavior change

Cues to action
• Education
• Symptoms, illness
• Media information

Figure 16-4. Health belief model. (From Glanz K, Lewis F, Rimers B: Health Behavior and Health Education: Theory, Research, and Practice, 2nd ed. San Francisco, Jossey-Bass, 1997, p 48.)

Associated Issues

Diversity Issues

Anthropologists and sociologists provide health care professionals with evidence that culture has a significant impact on individual and group behavior. Culture establishes the framework for knowledge, attitudes, values, and behaviors of the individuals within the culture. Culture may be defined to include ethnicity, race, religion, gender, socioeconomic status, and regionalism; therefore, dental hygienists should be cognizant of the individual or group status within a given culture to design appropriate strategies to motivate the individual or group to comply with the mutually established oral health goals. People from different cultural groups respond differently to the same dental health promotional initiative. An example would be the dilemma created in a program conducted by a male dental hygienist whose role is to provide hands-on tooth brushing instructions to the participant when the participant's religion forbids the woman to be touched by a man other than her spouse. Therefore, the dental hygienist must appreciate the differences among cultures related to ethnicity, race, domiciliary history habits, customs, economic status, educational level, family history verbal and nonverbal communication, food preferences and restrictions, motivational issues, and health care practices and restrictions.

Darby and Walsh[34] provide guidelines for cross-cultural dental hygiene **(Figure 16-5)** to enable dental hygienists to develop improved skills for meeting the needs of clients and groups of different cultures. Use of these guidelines allows the practitioner or health promoter to identify personal issues that each must grasp before effectively facilitating the acquisition of knowledge and skills by a person of a differ-

ent culture and subsequently improve the person's oral health. Unless sensitivity to the cultural differences exists, the practitioner or health promoter is unable to communicate adequately to meet the education, prevention, and treatment needs of the client or group.

Group Dynamics Issues

Dental hygiene professionals interact in small groups. Examples include: an interdisciplinary professional team to plan, implement, monitor, and evaluate the total care for convalescent hospital clients; an exploratory community committee to seek options to provide dental treatment to children with or without Medicaid support; a biweekly staff to meet in a group dental practice; a legislative group seeking improved funding for adults with disabilities; a school district curriculum committee to revise the elementary health curriculum; or a dental health workshop presented to nursing home staff. Regardless of the purpose or goal of the group, researchers have determined some general principles in place throughout the development and operation of groups. A dental hygienist working in a group setting who grasps these principles will use this knowledge to maximize the work of the group and his or her contributions to the group.

A fundamental need in health promotion and disease prevention within groups is to possess a thorough understanding of how groups function and how behavior is a function of the individual within an environment. Interrelated forces are at play within a group. These forces either support or restrain an individual from achieving a high level of wellness or making decisions that support community wellness. This section presents a compilation of the research conducted on group dynamics, beginning with a definition of "group," identifying the various types of groups, discussing why and

- Approach each client (individual, family, community) as an individual with unique characteristics and life experiences
- Try to get in touch with your own unique characteristics and life experiences. Sensitize yourself on how cultural factors have influenced your personal beliefs, attitudes, behaviors, practices, and values
- Try to identify biases and prejudices in your own life; their origins; their impact on interpersonal communication; their impact on your effectiveness as a healthcare provider, educator, manager, researcher, consumer advocate, and agent of change
- Become a lifelong student of other cultures, particularly the cultures unique to your community
- Assess the culturally related practices, attitudes, values, and beliefs of your clients as part of the dental hygiene process
- Display an accepting, nonjudgmental demeanor when presented with cultural diversity
- Reflect knowledge and recognition of the client's various cultural practices throughout the interaction
- Incorporate culturally relevant variables into the dental hygiene services that will be provided to the client
- Encourage the client to continue cultural health practices that can bring no harm; provide support, understanding, and time when trying to change potentially harmful oral health practice that is culturally determined
- Determine whether the dental hygiene plan of care is in harmony with the client's cultural values; modify dental hygiene plan of care that conflicts with the client's culture
- Recognize special dietary practices of the client; provide nutritional counseling within the framework of the client's culture
- Develop collegial relationships with health professionals from various ethnic and minority groups as a way of promoting cultural exchange that ultimately improves dental hygiene care

Figure 16-5. Guidelines for cross-cultural dental hygiene. (From Darby M, Walsh M: Guidelines for cross-cultural dental hygiene. In Darby M, Walsh M (eds): Dental Hygiene Theory and Practice. Philadelphia, WB Saunders, 1995, p 113.)

how groups form, and concluding with a discussion on what makes a group effective.

A **group** is defined basically as two or more people. However, the literature includes definitions that consist of numerous attributes. Because of the various definitions, Cartwright and Zander compiled the following list of features that characterize group members:

1. Engage in frequent interaction
2. Define themselves as members
3. Are defined by others as belonging to the group
4. Share norms concerning matters of common interest
5. Participate in a system of interlocking roles

6. Identify with one another as a result of having set up the same model-object or ideals in their superego
7. Find the group to be rewarding
8. Pursue interdependent goals
9. Have a collective perception of their unity
10. Tend to act in a unitary manner toward the environment.

Cartwright and Zander suggested that the more features attributed to the group, the closer this collection of people comes to being a "full-fledged" group.[35]

The **types of groups** identified in the literature are developed as a result of one of three circumstances. First, the group may be deliberately formed for a specific purpose. Second, the group may develop spontaneously. Third, the group may have received a designation as a group from some external source. Examples of **groups that form deliberately** include work groups, problem-solving groups, social action groups, legislative groups, or client groups. Generally, these types of groups are very goal oriented with the intention of achieving a specific objective. As the introductory examples presented, these groups are common recipients of dental hygiene disease prevention and health promotion interventions. **Spontaneously developed groups** are ones that evolve because the people in the group believe that they will receive some level of satisfaction from the association. A social group is part of this category. Fraternities, mothers-day-out groups, card groups, and senior citizen travel groups are examples of social groups. The primary characteristic of these groups is that the members like each other; they generally have close contact with each other[36]; and they share similar values and attitudes.[36, 37] **A group that receives its designation from an external source** does so generally because others have categorized the members as belonging to the group. The characteristics possessed by the members vary from one group to the next. Minorities, women, people with disabilities, white men, artists, high school dropouts, and alcoholics are just a few examples of group designations based on singular characteristics. The implication of this designation is that society treats members of these types of groups in specific ways, and the members of these externally assigned groups seek interdependence with individuals within the group because of the distinction given to them by society.[35] If one recognizes why the group exists for which the intervention is directed, this information will lead to the development of appropriate strategies to meet the oral health intervention goal.

Group formation and development is a complex process that has been studied by many researchers. The way that the group forms and the developmental stages through which each group progresses vary among the groups. However, a review of group process studies by Tuchman[38] indicates that certain similarities exist. A representative sequence of stages is found across the studies. The first stage is the **forming** phase in which the group proceeds through an orientation or testing period to determine what the group is all about. This phase is undertaken to define both interpersonal and task behaviors of the group members. The second stage is the **storming** phase, which centers around conflict and polarization on the interpersonal level and which additionally plays out on the task behavior level. If this stage is not resolved, the group usually disbands. The third stage is the **norming** phase, in which the group begins to resolve the conflicts; establishes new standards, roles, and cohesiveness; and develops a group identity. The last stage is the **performing** phase, during which time the group's interpersonal structure enhances the achievement of group goals. Members assume roles that are flexible, and the primary group energy is directed toward completing tasks.[36] Shaw indicates that a group can move up and down the stages and may actually skip a stage without damaging the group process.

What are the characteristics of a strong group? Zander suggests that members **interact freely** and **depend on the action of each other in a strong group.** He further states that the group can grow stronger if **members want to remain as members, because the group is attractive** to them and the **group has the power to influence** those whom it is supposed to guide and to deal with pressures or restraints arising outside its boundaries. An increase in the effects of all four characteristics makes the group stronger.[39]

Group dynamics researchers have examined ways to enhance the effectiveness of groups, and Zander reported their findings as:

1. Choosing clear, challenging, and measurable goals for the group
2. Strengthening the individual group member's desire for group success
3. Improving the process that the group uses to make decisions
4. Establishing effective communication among the group members
5. Establishing group standards that support the individual's customs, goals, and values
6. Encouraging harmony among the group members.

Because the outcome of any group intervention depends on the strength and effectiveness of the group and the willingness of the group to address the intervention topic, the health educator/promoter must utilize whatever strategies are available to increase the effectiveness of the group throughout the intervention. Inasmuch as the efforts of the health educator/promoter are linked to the group's success, the six characteristics should be explored further.

Choosing Clear, Challenging, and Measurable Goals. Group goals that are nonspecific lack the clarity that gives the group direction. Without clarity, the group spends resources counterproductively and still has not fulfilled the aim of the group. Therefore, the group must restate the goal in terms so that the intent is clear to all group members. The goal must also be challenging to provide members with a level of satisfaction of a "job worth doing is worth doing

well." The problem that arises when group goals are developed is that the goal may be written to be either too easy or too difficult. When the goal is too easy, the challenge is missing and the group members may question why they are spending their time, skills, and energies on a goal that fewer people could achieve. If the goal is too difficult, the group will be judged by itself and by external evaluators as being ineffective. Therefore, the group will be judged effective in goal development by both internal and external sources if the goal is stated in reasonable and achievable terms. Finally, the goal must be stated in terms that any internal or external source will be able to determine whether the goal has been attained. The goal should include *what* should change and by *how much*, under *what conditions* should the change occur, and what *data* should be collected to document the level of change.[39]

Strengthening the Desire for Group Success. An individual who views her role as supportive to the group, and her success as secondary to the success of the group, has a strong desire for the group to achieve. If this same attitude permeates throughout all members of the group, the group is said to possess a strong desire for group success. To enhance the desire for group success, members must feel valued, involved, and responsible for how well the group performs. Additionally, the group leader may support this development by emphasizing the importance of teamwork, changing goals determined to be unrealistic, helping the group to overcome barriers to success, and sharing ways to improve individual and group performance. Members who exhibit a desire for group achievement are attracted to moderately difficult goals rather than to easy or difficult ones. They also encourage other members to work hard and be proud of the group's success.[39]

Improving the Decision-Making Process: It is commonly known that decisions made by groups are of higher quality than are those made by individuals alone. The use of a well-established problem-solving process would facilitate quality decision-making by the group. The problem-solving technique that helps groups to develop better decisions includes four stages. First, the group must effectively *describe the problem* so that all members understand what must be resolved. The description should include an understanding of the significance of the problem. Second, the group must discuss the problem and *develop alternative approaches* to solve the problem. This step should start with a well-structured brainstorming session (technique is described in the Teaching Strategies/Learning Activities section) to develop a list of ideas. Third, the group must discuss all merits and disadvantages of each solution and *select the best solution* from all the alternatives. If the problem is complex, the group should break down the problem into workable parts and make decisions about each part independently. The discussion leader should keep the discussion focused on the important issues and should not permit discussion to go on tangents. This can be accomplished by noting when sufficient discussion has occurred, then the discussion leader calls for a vote to select the best decision. However, the best choice is one that does not require a vote but is agreed upon through discussion. All members should feel that they have not lost anything by agreeing to the choice. Each person walks away believing that he or she has been heard, respected, and considered during the decision-making process. This is called a decision by consensus. Fourth, the group must ensure that the *solution is implemented.* Strategies should be developed with appropriate timelines for implementation, and specific individuals or groups should be assigned responsibility for ensuring the completion of specific strategies.

Consider a community planning group that is seeking a positive outcome to a community water fluoridation referendum. The planning group may determine that the biggest *problem* is providing accurate information about water fluoridation to the community. The committee develops a list of all possible ways of delivering the appropriate educational message to the community. After a *discussion* of the advantages and disadvantages of each solution, door-to-door canvassing of the community is selected as the *best solution* to getting the word out. The committee then *designs an implementation plan* and determines which tasks must be performed, who will be responsible for them, when they must occur, and what reporting mechanisms must be in place to ensure that each task has been completed. A group that follows similar steps in the decision-making process will develop decisions that will lead to higher rates of group success.[39]

Communicating Effectively Among Colleagues. Communication is such a significant part of group effectiveness that the next major section is entirely dedicated to the topic.

Establishing Standards that Support Group Customs, Goals, and Values. **Standards** are the clearly understood methods of behavior in a group that are outlined in policies, operating plans, and guidelines. These standards are intended to benefit the group and make it more efficient by attending to issues such as interpersonal relations and goal attainment. As was stated in the cultural diversity section, if the group is closely aligned with individual's personal values, customs, beliefs, and practices, the individual is going to develop a tighter relationship to the group. This close relationship also develops if the standards defined by the group also agree with these same values, customs, beliefs, and practices. In some cases, a group member fails to adhere to the standards. If the person continues to stay out of compliance with the standards after attempts by group members and the group leader to bring the person into alignment, the person can be removed from the group. This fact substantiates the importance of standards to the group process.[38]

Fostering Harmony Among Members. **Harmony** is the condition that exists within a group that brings comfort to both the members and the interactions between the members. Harmony is more prevalent in a group that has

similar goals, values, and aspirations and is stronger with the more group members adhering to those goals, values, and hopes. Knowing this fact, a group organizer may seek members who share similar beliefs just to ensure the possibility that the members will work well together. Group members will sometimes apply pressure to nonconforming members to comply with group standards. One way to achieve compliance is to increase the noncomplying member's commitment to the group by requesting that the member make personal sacrifices for the group. Bringing these members into compliance increases group harmony. Another factor that contributes to group harmony is the size of the group. The fewer members, the more harmonious will be the group. As the size of the group increases, group harmony decreases. This is attributed to the fact that as the group grows, fewer people participate in the decision-making process and attendance decreases. Finally, group cohesiveness is a factor in group harmony. **Cohesiveness** is a group quality that describes the unity within a group. If there is a high degree of group cohesiveness, the result will be greater harmony within the group. This means that the group will work harder at achieving group goals and attending to group needs.[38]

 COMMUNICATION

Health care providers are faced with different communication issues from those faced by most non-health care individuals. Messages delivered to clients must be understood, interpreted, and acted upon to the health benefit of the client. A misunderstanding could result in the individual failing to comply with critical aspects of their home care or treatment. This section defines human communication and describes a communication model that meets the needs of health care providers and clients. There are six contexts or situations within which communication occurs. The contexts are arranged from the fewer number of people involved in the process to the greatest number of people:

1. Intrapersonal
2. Interpersonal
3. Small group
4. Organizational
5. Public
6. Mass

It is important to note that the nature of each context or situation dictates the communication process. Communication research is replete with models that describe the process. This section describes the communication models noted in oral health education literature and concludes with a model of health communication. The health communication model was developed to incorporate the consideration for all types of communication transpiring within the health care arena. Dental hygienists conduct communication not only with clients but also with other health care providers and with groups. The health communication model discusses the impact of communication between the professional and the client, the professional and the professional, and the professional and small groups.

Human communication theories have evolved since the first definitions. Miller stated that "communication means that information is passed from one place to another."[40] This simplistic definition failed to take into account that communication is a complex process and should be defined more specifically. Northouse and Northouse define "**communication** as the **process** of **sharing information through a set of common rules.**"[41] This definition acknowledges that there is a transfer of information within a sharing process between individuals and that the process is governed by a set of rules. These rules may be broadly applied, as in the language that health care providers use between and among each other, or narrowly applied as in the language used in interpersonal relationships within the family structure.

Several communication models are commonly cited in dental literature. Berlo presented a classic model of communication, which described communication as a complex and dynamic process that intertwines the four components of the model: **S**ource, **M**essage, **C**hannel, and **R**eceiver (SMCR).[42] The source or sender of the communication uses communication skills, personal attitudes, knowledge, and a sociocultural system to develop messages. The messages contain specific elements, structure, content, treatment, and codes that are sent through channels using the five senses. The receiver, like the sender, interprets the message using personal attitudes, knowledge, and sociocultural systems. Even though this model clearly delineates the one-directional process, it does not incorporate a feedback component. Therefore, Berlo's model does not allow for interaction between the sender and the receiver; however, when applied, this model can show factors such as a client's knowledge, attitudes, and sociocultural background that lend increased understanding of the communication taking place.

DeBiase[43] reported Brill's **One-To-One Communication** Model to describe the types of interaction that occur during interpersonal communication[44]:

1. The sender has a message to communicate.
2. The sender encodes or transforms the mental information into a series of written or verbal and nonverbal symbols that he or she hopes that the receiver will understand.
3. The message is sent.
4. The receiver reads or listens to and observes the message and decodes it by attaching personal meaning to the information. The receiver's attitudes feelings, or faulty perceptions may interfere with or distort the message at any point in the process.
5. The receiver now responds by providing feedback relevant to how he or she interpreted the message.
6. The original speaker receives and interprets the feedback, and the cycle begins again.

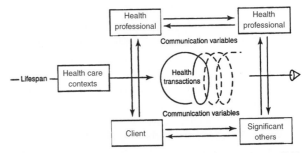

Figure 16-6. Health communication model. (From Northouse P, Northouse L: Health Communication: A Handbook For Health Professionals. Englewood Cliffs, NJ, Prentice Hall, 1998, p 17.)

This model is particularly effective because it incorporates an interactive feedback component in the process. Feedback allows the original sender to evaluate and respond to the receiver's message and restart the process. Consideration of the events taking place in the Brill model is useful for health professionals engaged in professional-to-professional and professional-to-client interpersonal communication.

"Health communication refers specifically to transactions between participants in health care about health-related issues. The **health communication model** takes a broader systems view of communication, and it emphasizes the way in which a series of factors can impact on the interaction in health care settings."[41] This model does not make any less important the factors related to the source, message, channel, and receiver components of traditional models but builds on these by incorporating the three concepts of relationships, transactions, and contexts. This broadens the scope of the model by examining the impact of these three factors on the whole communication process. An understanding of the complexity of the process should help the health professional/educator to develop a communication approach that delivers an appropriate message that is reinforced by the client. **Figure 16-6** outlines the three major factors of the health communication process. The **relationship** factor defines relationships found in all health care settings: professional-to-client, professional-to-significant others of the client, professional-to-other professionals, and the client-to-his or her significant others. The significant others are defined as those within the client's social support system. The **transactions** are defined as any health-related interaction that occurs among those participating in the health communication process. The model shows a continuous feedback loop cycle providing constant interaction among the members. **Contexts** are the situations or settings in which health communication occurs and the systemic properties of the setting. Examples of these settings include a private practice setting, clinic, group setting, or a classroom. The more people involved in the process, the more complex the process becomes.

The model includes a **set of communication variables** that have an impact on the process: *empathy, control, trust, self-disclosure, and confirmation.* When each variable is considered, the sender further enhances the process. **Empathy** is the ability to understand another person; that is, to put yourself in the other person's place and appreciate that person's feelings and concerns. Empathy should not be confused with sympathy, in which the health care professional expresses sadness over the client's condition. A professional who possesses the quality of empathy will try to feel what the client, family member, or other health care professional is feeling and be able to communicate an understanding of the feelings to that individual. In the case of the client, the more empathetic the health care provider is, the more the client feels understood and exhibits a willingness to respond to the health care message.

The **control** variable within health communication considers the issues of *personal* and *relational* control. Both the client and the professional have needs within these two contexts. *Personal control* is the feeling that an individual has that he or she is capable of influencing the events and circumstances in his or her life. It is the sense that the individual is competent. An appreciation of this need is crucial for the health educator/promoter. For a successful interaction between the health promoter and the client, the promoter must make the client perceive that the client is competent and able to manage his or her life events. On the other hand, *relational control* reflects how the individual perceives his or her ability to build and sustain relationships. For effective communication to occur, both the client and the professional must have a sense of shared relational control. If one is perceived to be exerting more influence than the other is, communication lines will be negatively altered. Although sharing relational control is difficult, the health care professional can advance the process by merely recognizing the need and taking personal steps to enhance the client's perception of personal and relational control.

The client demonstrates **trust** when the client feels that he or she can rely on the communication behavior of the health professional. Trust creates the belief that events are predictable and that people are basically sincere, competent, and accepting. This is valued in the communication process, because trust provides a sense of security and connectedness with the health care professional. Another value of trust is that communication becomes easier and more open. Both values significantly improve the communication process. Of the various communication factors, several behaviors encourage trust. A health professional whose communication style includes one or more of the following factors will increase trust in his or her relationship with clients, support group members, and other professionals.[45] Communication should:

1. Be free of value and moral judgements
2. Possess problem-solving orientation, rather than a controlling or blaming orientation
3. Be straightforward, open, and honest rather than full of hidden agenda
4. Be empathetic rather than neutral in tone and content
5. Be perceived by the client to be on an *equal* basis with the professional rather than the professional displaying an air of superiority

6. Encourage the client to be a part of the decision-making process rather than being told that there is only one answer to the problem or question

Self-disclosure is the variable in which a tone is set in any of the possible communication relationship dyads that encourages one to feel comfortable sharing personal information and feelings with the other. It is important for the health care professional to exhibit self-disclosure behavior to the client to demonstrate an appropriate level of care and concern for the client. However, it is not suggested that "full disclosure" be given—only a sufficient amount to foster trust. When the professional is involved in self-disclosure, the focus of the communication must be on the client in order to maintain the professional nature of the interaction. Self-disclosure by the client is especially important during the interview/client assessment process. Clients are more likely to provide sensitive health history information if trust is shared in the client-professional relationship.

The final variable, **confirmation,** is the ability to acknowledge and accept others. Confirming behavior by the professional in client-professional and professional-professional interactions gives the client or other professional the sense that he or she is respected and valued. Increasing a client's or other professional's self-perception of personal respect and value contributes to the confidence level of the relationship. Confirming behaviors are identified as those where the professional uses responses to clients that[46]:

1. Respect the client's feelings, beliefs, and values.
2. Maintain eye contact during an interaction.
3. Use an expressive voice tone.
4. Maintain close proximity to the client while speaking.
5. Maintain a relaxed but energetic manner.
6. Do not include jargon.

Disconfirming behavior is the opposite of these actions during any of the four model relationships. Communication is more effective as confirming behaviors increase and disconfirming behaviors are reduced or eliminated.

The section before "Communication" discussed the importance of addressing diversity issues with clients and groups. Considering that oral health care services and education/promotion interventions address individuals and groups from many different cultures, attending to a common set of rules during the information sharing process can be difficult. What is common to one culture will not be common to another culture. However, before the intervention, the health professional who conducts research on the communication rules of the culture will be more successful in communicating with the client or group. Health care professionals who recognize the communication differences among the participants of different cultures will deliver a message that is more readily responded to by the participants.

There is more to intercultural communication than merely knowledge of the set of common communication rules, communication styles, and needs of the various participants.

Health care professionals may present significant barriers to the communication process by demonstrating any of numerous negative characteristics. The following is a selection of these characteristic barriers:

1. **Ethnocentrism**-an individual's belief that her ethnic group is superior to others. A health care professional who places his or her personal values and beliefs ahead of individuals of other cultures is ethnocentric. For example, an ethnocentric dental health professional might belittle a first-grade Asian child for using of a chewstick to cleanse the teeth, because the health professional thinks that its use demonstrates a lack of understanding of oral health practices and beliefs and is inconsistent with his or her own beliefs and practices.

2. **Prejudice**-a negative view previously developed of another person or group based on incorrect or inadequate information. This characteristic is associated with the practice of **stereotyping** a person or ethnic group by assuming that an individual possesses certain characteristics or traits because that person belongs to a particular group. An example of prejudice occurred when a class of dental hygiene students was given an assignment to research the culture and health practices of several ethnic groups in specific settings. One group reported that Orthodox Jewish senior citizens have no financial restrictions to obtain quality oral health care, because *all* older Jewish people are rich. This line of thinking results in inappropriate oral health information being shared with a client or group if the preset idea is that "money is no object."

3. **Racism**-the belief that certain human characteristics are determined by the individual's race and that one race is superior to another. An example of this type of barrier is a health professional who refuses to provide treatment or have contact with a client or group because of the race of that client or group. A lesser and more insidious example is recommending or performing a lower quality service for a client based on the race of that individual. These actions leave the client or group with a sense of being devalued, humiliated, and angered and a whole array of emotions that lead to the worst possible client-professional relationship**.**

Health care professionals often find it difficult to reconcile their knowledge and beliefs with those held by clients or groups and their accompanying social support system members. Promotion and prevention strategies and treatment modalities that are standards for the traditional United States' dental health culture conflict with various cultures' values, beliefs, and practices. Encouraging an individual or group with a common culture to accept a course of care that conflicts with the culture will result in failure. Not only will the health care provider be frustrated, but also the client/group/social support system members will resist the professional's recommendation. The result will be a poor trust relationship between the client/professional and the professional/significant other.

The dental hygienist in a health promotion role may be responsible for forming groups to study a community oral health issue, developing an oral health initiative, or participating as a member in any type of group. In either case, the dental hygienist should **develop the skill of assessing and analyzing the communication interaction patterns that exist among the group members.** This may be accomplished by observing what communication takes place and between whom and also how often the communication occurs. The results may be mapped to demonstrate what patterns actually exist. With this knowledge, the dental hygienist can do much to increase his or her understanding of the dynamics of the group by determining who the leader is and what role each member plays. This knowledge will help the hygienist to increase group member satisfaction and group effectiveness. In addition, the hygienist may become more aware of which channels are open or closed in a group and, therefore, know best how to effectively deliver information and activate a process within the group.[41]

Verbal and Nonverbal Communication

The process of exchanging information may be either verbal or nonverbal. **Verbal communication** is the primary mode of delivering and receiving messages. However, it is estimated that up to 93% of the meaning of a message is communicated nonverbally.[47] Use of **nonverbal** cues takes the form of body language, such as eye contact, gestures, facial expressions, or even voice intonations or changes. These cues indicate receptivity, agreement, and displeasure with the message being received. The dental hygienist should be cautious to recognize nonverbal cues, acknowledge these signals, and respond to them positively to keep communication open and moving forward in a collaborative manner.

Communication Considerations

To enhance both modes of communication, the sender of the original message should recognize his or her role as more than creating and sending the message. Darby and Walsh[34] reported communication considerations by Potter and Perry[48] that when attended to by the dental hygienist will make the communication more effective:

1. Maintaining *silence* during the communication process allows both sender and receiver the time to gather thoughts and develop appropriate responses. It also permits the sender to view nonverbal cues from the receiver and thus gather more information regarding attitudes, values, and beliefs of the receiver.

2. *Active listening* requires the sender to demonstrate interest in the receiver by really hearing what the person is saying. Within the dominant culture of the United States, active listening is done when the sender uses eye contact; faces the person with arms unfolded; leans

slightly forward; maintains a distance of 3 to 4 feet from the receiver; and avoids any type of distracting behavior (e.g., looking away from the receiver).

3. *Reflective responding* allows the sender to give back to the receiver in summary form what the sender understood the receiver to mean by his or her response to the original message. Here is an example of a receiver response: *Head Start parents will not be able to attend meetings during the evening.* The sender's reflection follows: *It sounds like you think that transportation is going to be a barrier to our evening program.* The receiver may correct a misunderstanding or agree with the sender's reflection. This action opens the communication and enhances decision-making and problem solving.

4. *Conveying acceptance* is important in any communication but is especially critical in a multicultural environment. The sender uses accepting nonverbal cues as well as verbal communication that allow the receiver to freely express him or herself within the context of that particular culture. Negative nonverbal behavior such as heads shaking will demonstrate a judgmental attitude by the sender. This behavior in turn creates a feeling of disapproval and effectively shuts down the communication.

5. *Asking open-ended related questions* will allow the receiver to provide appropriate answers to essential questions as well as provide additional information that will enable the sender to gain more insight into the communication.

6. The sender must listen carefully and analyze the receiver's response in order to *paraphrase* accurately the returning message of the receiver. By restating or summarizing what the receiver says, the sender allows the receiver to correct any misconceptions or misunderstanding of the response.

7. The sender is sometimes unable to ascertain the meaning of the receiver's response. Therefore, the sender must stop the communication and ask the receiver to *clarify* the meaning of the response. Clarification allows the sender and receiver to be on the same communication plane.

8. *Focusing* is a parallel consideration to clarification. Receivers who take the communication on a tangential route must be steered back on course by the sender. This allows the communication to remain on target. Particularly in a group situation, focusing will allow group goals to be attained more efficiently.

9. To increase the likelihood of appropriate decision-making by the receiver(s) of the message, the sender must provide *accurate information* based on sound research data in both one-on-one and group situations.

10. Toward the end of the communication, the sender should *summarize* the key elements of the communication. This allows the receiver(s) to agree, disagree, or provide clarification of the messages within the communication.

MERGING LEARNING AND HUMAN MOTIVATION THEORIES WITH ORAL HEALTH PROMOTION AND DISEASE PREVENTION

Learning theories provide a foundation for the ways in which individuals acquire oral health knowledge and values and develop attitudes and skills. The information provided in the previous sections only highlights the theories. In order to understand the full scope of available theories, the reader should review texts on teaching and learning theories.[49] In order for learning to occur, the learner must be motivated to accept the learning experience. Human motivation theories provide models that teachers use to activate the intrinsic and extrinsic forces that lead an individual to take the action to learn. Addiction studies show that *change* takes place in the individual only when he or she has an intrinsic *desire to change.* This desire may be the result of a life-changing event or may simply be the realization that the time has come to make the change.

The **learning ladder** concept, which is demonstrated as a series of steps on a ladder, describes how **individuals begin in an "unknowing" state and progress through a series of stages to develop a specific "habit" or behavior.**[50] Harris and Christen state that the "first step in applying this concept is to determine which rung of the ladder the individual stands." An individual must go through each step of the ladder to acquire the new habit. If a step is omitted, a long-term habit or behavioral change will not occur. The learner may start at the second or third rung and need to step back to a previous rung for clarification or additional information on the learning topic. However, that person may not entirely skip a step.

The first and lowest step on the ladder is the **unawareness** stage. At this time, the individual has either no information or misinformation regarding the oral health behavior or topic. If a parent has no knowledge of baby bottle caries, he or she does not know to put an infant to bed with a bottle of water rather than formula. **Awareness** occurs when the parent is provided with the information on baby bottle caries during a childbirth class. This is the stage when the individual receives correct information but develops no real sense of personal meaning or desire to act on the information at that time. The **self-interest** stage occurs when the new information becomes meaningful to the individual. An intrinsic drive is activated, and the individual realizes that the information or issue is relevant to him or her. The parent takes the new baby home and realizes the implications of putting the infant to bed with the bottle of formula. DeBiase[43] suggests that **values clarification** may be used during this stage to enhance the development of self-interest. **Figure 16-7** illustrates a values clarification exercise that may be used to aid an individual in reflecting on the importance of oral health to him or her and

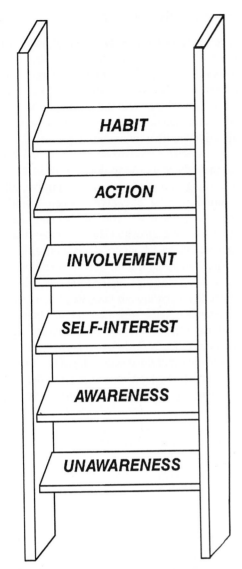

HABIT

ACTION

INVOLVEMENT

SELF-INTEREST

AWARENESS

UNAWARENESS

Figure 16-7. Values clarification exercise. (From DeBiase C: Dental Health Education Theory and Practice. Philadelphia, Lea & Febiger, 1991, p 10.)

discovering how it fits into his or her lifestyle.[51, 52] DeBiase further states that if the individual recognizes that his or her dental health values are not consistent with his or her behavior, that person experiences cognitive dissonance. Because the value is strong but the behavior is missing, the individual develops an inclination to act on the new behavior. This desire for action is the **involvement** stage. Based on the realization of values, the individual moves into the **action** stage to test the new concepts and practices presented by the health promoter. The parent will begin cleaning the child's mouth with a wet cloth and giving the infant water at bedtime. The parent begins to develop a sense of self-satisfaction by providing the child with appropriate home care. The parent is gratified by this action and is then motivated to establish a balance between personal values and behaviors in life by making permanent cognitive and behavioral changes that produce a long-

term **habit**.[18] The result is that the parent develops a daily habit of providing oral care to enhance the child's growth and development.

Learning Styles

Individual learning styles determine the degree and the pace at which learning occurs. The oral health educator should be familiar with learning style options and develop an appreciation for how people learn best. Educators have teaching styles that are not always compatible with a student's learning style. Some people learn best within a group learning environment. Pairing these individuals with an educator who is only comfortable delivering a lecture will result in frustration for both the educator and the learner. Therefore, it is important for the educator to expand his or her teaching style to accommodate the student's learning style to maximize the teaching-learning process.

 ## CREATING LESSON PLANS

Although research indicates that cognitive programs alone are ineffective in creating long-term behavioral change, accurate information must be disseminated to develop awareness. As the Learning Ladder Theory demonstrates, once awareness is established, values and behaviors may be positively affected. Therefore, health promotion initiatives should include an educational intervention to establish the foundation for future attitude and behavioral change. The intervention may occur in various settings and target various population groups, including: a classroom for a group of preschoolers; the school auditorium as part of a teacher in-service; a hospital conference room for nurses performing oral examinations as part of the new patient assessment process; a nursing home for nurses' aides learning techniques for the daily provision of oral health care for clients; and a continuing education workshop for pharmacists for the purpose of expanding their knowledge of oral health products to enhance their abilities to properly inform customers about these products. The types of target population are numerous.

To increase the chances for a successful educational intervention, significant planning is required. The plan must be customized to meet the needs of the target population. The lesson plan should include the following:

1. **Description of the target population** identifying all important characteristics of the group in detail
2. **Needs statement** identifying an understanding of the oral health education needs of the target group,
3. **Goal statement,** which is a broad statement of purpose and target population-specific **lesson objectives** that are clear, concise, measurable, and specific to the target population and lead to outcome assessments
4. **Instructional content** that addresses each objective
5. **Lesson content** that is specific to a target population

6. **Teaching strategies** that relate content to the target population
7. **Teaching aids** that support the content and teaching strategies to the target population
8. **Audiovisual aids/instructional media** to meet the needs of the target population, lesson content, and teaching strategies
9. **Evaluation activities** that measure the learning of the target population as related to the objectives

Needs Assessment/Target Population Description

The **needs assessment** requires the oral health promoter to examine the population in pertinent detail to fully understand the specific needs of the group. This is the most important segment of the educational intervention. An accurate needs assessment provides the foundation for the development of a successful teaching-learning experience. The assessment provides the oral health promoter with the information necessary to **describe the population** demographics (e.g., age range, educational level, socioeconomic level, religious background, ethnicity, gender profile, previous oral health learning experiences, financial resources within the community, political infrastructure within the community, other resources that increase access to care, barriers to health care, and any other characteristics deemed important for the teaching-learning process of the target population). The assessment should also provide information to understand what gaps exist in terms of oral health knowledge, attitudes, values, and practices of the group. In addition, this phase of lesson plan development should examine the physical space where the educational intervention is to be held. A knowledge of space limitations and enhancements will allow the oral health promoter to design appropriate learning strategies, select teaching aids, and perform evaluation activities that will fit the learning environment. All assessment information will allow the planner to design a learning process that focuses on the learner and the gaps rather than on repeating existing knowledge and having insignificant impact on new learning. (See Chapter 17 for details on conducting a needs assessment.)

Goal Statement

The goal statement is a broad statement of purpose specific to the target population that gives direction to the teaching-learning process. This statement is nonspecific, thus setting the stage for all subsequent planning. For example, if the target group is a teachers' in-service involving grades 1 to 3, the goal statement might read: *To enhance the teachers' ability to integrate oral health instruction throughout the health education curriculum.* This statement is broad in scope but indicates that the purpose of the intervention is to lead to incorporation of oral health throughout all aspects of the health curriculum. Stating the goal in these terms clearly sets the foundation for development of the remainder of the lesson plan.

Instructional Objectives

The **instructional objectives** specifically state what the learner is expected to learn or perform at the end of the learning experience. Objectives guide the learning intervention and determine the content, strategies, and evaluation that will be utilized throughout the learning process. Therefore, appropriately designed objectives are crucial to planning an effective learning intervention.

Bloom and associates[53] led the development of a taxonomy of learning that educators use to develop objectives. Bloom separated learning into three domains: **cognitive, affective, and psychomotor.** The cognitive domain identifies the knowledge that one acquires from the learning experience. The affective domain deals with values, attitudes, beliefs, and feelings, whereas the psychomotor domain identifies skill acquisition. Most health education interventions focus on the cognitive domain, because it is easier; however, health educators recognize that even though knowledge is important, behavior will change because of our attitudes, beliefs, and feelings. Therefore, interventions should encourage learners to explore personal values regarding oral health issues.

Each domain is subdivided according to the level of difficulty. For example, the learner who starts at the awareness level of the learning ladder proceeds through the cognitive domain, beginning on the *knowledge* level, and working up to *comprehension* (i.e., an understanding the knowledge learned), *application* (i.e., the ability to apply knowledge), *analysis* (i.e., the ability to break down a topic or issue into its various parts), *synthesis* (i.e., integration of the various components of a topic or problem to bring resolution or create a new product), and ending with the *evaluation* level (based on evidence and criteria, ability to assess the quality of an idea or effort). The *knowledge* level is the lowest and easiest level to meet within the cognitive domain, whereas the evaluation level is reflective of *mastery* and more difficulty and is usually not the level that most objectives address. The goal should be to move to the higher cognitive levels, because at these levels oral health habits become systemic for the client or group.

Similarly, learners move through levels in the affective domain. The five stages the learner transcends from lowest to highest are:

1. *Receiving* (responds to an external stimulus, thus demonstrating an awareness of an idea, situation, or event)
2. *Responding* (reacts to the stimulus by demonstrating an interest in the idea, situation, or event)
3. *Valuing* (places value on a theory, idea, or event and takes action consistent with the value)
4. *Organizing* (places the value among a set of values and integrates the value into the learner's set of values)
5. *Characterizing* (uses the value system to consistently control personal thoughts and actions)[3, 22]

Mager describes a useful objective as one that is specific, meaningful, clear, and measurable.[54] To meet these criteria, the educator should use a format that contains the following components:

1. **Audience**: the individual for whom the learning experience is designed and will perform the behavior
2. **Performance**: action verb used to state what the learner will do
3. **Conditions**: specific conditions under which the performance will occur
4. **Criteria**: standard under which the learner must perform in order to be considered acceptable

An objective statement in the cognitive domain for a senior citizen center group might read:

*Taking a post-test after the oral health presentation on conducting a self-(**condition**) examination; each senior citizen will differentiate between normal and abnormal (**audience; performance**) structures of the tongue to screen for conditions that must be seen immediately by a dentist (**criteria**).*

This objective contains all four components and leaves no question regarding what the educator intends for the audience to be able to do following the educational intervention.

The approach most often used by educators today for objective development comes from Gronlund.[55] His approach to the process differs from Mager's in that he uses only a **general** term to lead the action followed by a **learning outcome** that describes what the learner must perform. In other words, the general terms *know, understand, or comprehend* may be used in the statement and may be followed by what the learner must do to demonstrate that he or she *knows, understands, or comprehends.*

An example of a Gronlund objective in the affective domain for the senior citizens' center group might be:

Displays self-confidence in the self-oral examination by *demonstrating the technique to a* (**general objective**) (**specific learning outcome**) *partner.*

Instructional Content

Content must be designed to reflect the broad goal statement and the instructional objectives. Each objective should be sequenced to permit a logical transition from one objective to another. This logical transition is made most clearly through the development of the intellectual content within the lesson plan. A novice at lesson plan development is best served by writing the content verbatim. Conversely, a seasoned educator may develop content that is a summary of the facts needed to achieve the objectives. Content should demonstrate the following:

1. **Sequential development**: The content should be coherent and move in an orderly fashion.
2. **Movement from the least complex facts and concepts to the more complex:** Make the learning process easy on the student by establishing the foundation of the lesson with the least complex points and build on the foundation until the most complex points are presented.
3. **Logical transition from one objective to the next:** The content should make transitions that are reasonable to the learner and make connections between the objectives.
4. **Accuracy of content:** Careful attention must be paid to facts, details, and resources used to develop the content.
5. **Overall clarity and organization:** The audience should easily understand presentation.
6. **Target population-specific vocabulary and grammar:** All areas identified in the needs assessment related to such variables as age, culture, educational level, and all other demographic factors, as well as values, beliefs, practices of the group, should be considered when selecting vocabulary and making the grammatical presentation.
7. **Sensitivity to learners self-esteem, needs, and interests:** Needs assessment findings on the level of self-esteem and the specific learning needs and interests of the target group should be attended to in order to maintain audience attention and interest.
8. **Level of understandability:** The complexity of the presentation should be based on the previous oral health education experiences of the audience as well as on other factors such as age and educational levels; the presentation should not exceed the ability of the audience to understand the facts, concepts, and skills being taught.

Teaching Strategies/Learning Activities

As the content is designed to achieve the instructional objectives, the planner should be selecting teaching strategies/learning activities that most effectively relate the content to the audience. Strategies and activities are the experiences that assist the learner to internalize content and form concepts, attitudes, and values. They are what give life to the presentation. Part of the needs assessment phase may identify what specific learning activities a cross-section of the group responds to best. Unless appropriate strategies and techniques are chosen, the best-written objectives and content will have minimal impact on the learner. The presenter must feel comfortable with the technique selected but should remember that a comfort level is achieved through continued use. The following are teaching strategies that may be used for almost all participants within a target population; however, some strategies are more appropriate for certain age and skill levels.[3, 22, 56]

1. **Lecture and discussion**: The **lecture** is the most common strategy to relate facts on a subject; generally, it is a form of one-way communication and is most effective in large groups when time is limited. However, the straight lecture format is the least pleasing to learners and results in less learning at the higher levels of the three educational domains. It is generally considered as the most boring strategy, because interaction is limited. The **discussion** is the most common technique applied

in health education. This technique, when applied with the lecture, provides for feedback to teacher and learner on whether facts, concepts, or other complexities are understood and can be appropriately applied. Discussion can be used for problem-solving activities, especially for older children and adults. If a teacher is not a strong or competent facilitator, discussion may become out of control or diverge from the topic. Therefore, it is useful to practice facilitation before introducing the strategy to a classroom. Another difficulty may be that one learner may dominate the discussion and sway others to conform to his or her opinion. The educator should draw the discussion back into focus and keep the interactions on topic.

2. **Demonstrations and experiments:** The purpose of both demonstrations and experiments is to clarify what has been learned. Using demonstrations to show the steps required in a task or behavior allows the learner to clearly see what is necessary to perform to meet the instructional objective. Demonstrations should consistently have the same outcome. On the other hand, an experiment will not have a predicted outcome, because outcomes may vary from one attempt to another. In both cases, the educator needs the skill to perform the demonstration or the experiment and possess finances to pay for the expenses.

3. **Peer instruction:** Peer instruction uses learner-peers to teach the content. This technique requires the peer instructor to know the facts, concepts, and skills to be learned by the fellow learner. Peer learning results in the highest level of learning in all three domains. Learners feel a reduced level of anxiety in the learning process, and the outcomes are the greatest. Because the strategy requires a significant amount of preparation time for the peer teacher, it should be used without creating an undue burden on the peer teacher.

4. **Simulation:** Simulations allow the learner opportunities to try out actions, behaviors, or activities in the security of the classroom that may be re-enacted in another environment at a later date and time. The safe nature of the environment allows the learner to develop the skill without fear of failure. The role of the educator is to describe the simulation activity clearly to the learners and provide constructive feedback on the performance. The disadvantage may be that due to a high level of anxiety on the part of the learner, the experience and outcome may be unsatisfactory.

5. **Dramatization, role-playing, and storytelling:** Plays, skits, and puppet shows are examples of **dramatizations.** These activities are especially useful and fun for elementary and middle school children. In each activity, learners are provided with a script of the part that they are to play. Significant preparation is required in order to make these activities successful. Problems can result if the activity is viewed merely as a fun rather than recognizing the learning inherent in the activity. In a **role-play** situation, the educator gives written information on the role that a learner is to assume, then the learner acts out the part in front of the class. After the role-play, the educator leads the class in a discussion of the topic being role-played. This strategy is especially useful from middle school through adulthood, because higher level educational domains are addressed. Problem analysis and solution development may be an outcome of the role-playing activity. If a learner is not an effective role player, the learning experience may be poor. It is crucial for the educator to know ahead of time if the role player should be effective. **Storytelling** is a strategy that is useful for preschool and early elementary school children. The educator may use a storybook that highlights the learning objectives and read the story to the children. This strategy helps children to recognize positive oral health behaviors and attitudes.

6. **Debate:** The debate allows learners to view two solutions to a problem. Learners volunteer for the support of one solution or the other and must thoroughly research the topic before the actual debate. The educator serves in a support role throughout the development process and conducts the debate. This can be an effective strategy for students in middle school through college. The educator must be a skilled debate facilitator for the activity to be successful and the learning objectives to be met.

7. **Crossword puzzles and games: Crossword puzzles** are useful activities as part of the evaluation process. Words may be answers to questions that test recall and comprehension. This activity is best used with children in third grade and higher. **Games** provide an opportunity to review lesson content and instill fun into the learning process. Educators may develop games that are specific to the topic or use commercially prepared ones that the educator customizes for the lesson. As with dramatizations, if the learner is engrossed in the competitive nature of the game, he or she may lose sight of the learning experience and the activity will be an ineffective learning experience.

8. **Guided discovery:** Guided discovery (guided design) presents a problem to the learner, then the learner works within a small group to list the facts surrounding the problem. The group analyzes and synthesizes the information to develop possible solutions to the problem. This activity addresses the higher level educational domains. Guided discovery can be used for students in elementary grades through college. The problem must be defined at the age and intellectual level of the learning group. The role of the educator is to set the ground rules (i.e., the rules for operation) and facilitate the work of the small group. This includes developing leading questions that will "guide" the learning process through its sequential steps. Guided discovery requires sufficient time for the groups to carry out each step; therefore, time must be available to complete the activity, otherwise the activity will be unsuccessful.

9. **Brainstorming:** The brainstorming strategy is applied when many ideas must be generated in a short time. Learners are given a question or problem and asked to develop possible answers or solutions. The role of the educator is to set the ground rules for the activity and facilitate the process. The educator must ensure that all learners participate, each learner feels safe in offering ideas, all responses are listed, and no evaluation of responses occurs during the brainstorming session. An evaluation of the ideas follows, and ideas of lesser value are eliminated from consideration. Subsequently, the prime ideas remain and discussion and analysis on the merits occur and decisions on the appropriate resolution to the question or solutions to the problem are made. Group skills and decision-making skills are enhanced through the brainstorming process. The technique can be applied to students as young as elementary age through the adult learner.

10. **Case studies:** The case study presents information regarding real life situations that are based on the learning level of the learner. This strategy is used effectively in dental hygiene education to present partial or full histories on clients. The student is required to comprehend, apply, analyze, synthesize, and evaluate the available information on the client and develop and respond to questions with answers that are consistent with the clients' medical and dental histories and current needs. Questions are based on the information provided in the case study narrative and supporting documentation. Case studies may only seek answers to questions on which the student has acquired the knowledge from previous learning experiences. This strategy is valuable because it requires the learner to assimilate the previous learning and apply it to new situations.

11. **Videotaping:** Videotaping may be done while learners are performing a task or behavior and replayed to demonstrate how well the individual performed. The replay may be used to critique the performance and reinforce appropriate technique. The educator serves as a reviewer in the process. This activity is especially useful on the individual level and with elementary grades through adults.

12. **Computer-assisted instruction (CAI):** CAI uses computer software, CD-ROMs, and videodisks to take a learner through various learning situations. These include drill and practice sessions to review new information. Other CAI possibilities include the use of: tutorials to allow learners to proceed at their own pace; demonstrations of tasks or skills to allow students to view the process as often as is necessary to develop confidence in performing the skill; and simulations that give learners the opportunity to view oral health situations that require appropriate decision-making on their part to enable a client to achieve lifelong oral health. The primary advantage to CAI is the interactive quality of the strategy. The student is an active participant in the learning process and must respond both physically and intellectually to the instruction. CAI is a strategy that can be used by people of all ages and learning levels. To be effective, the software must be developed to meet the specific level of the student. The disadvantage is the cost and time required either developing or purchasing the software.

13. **Collaborative learning:** People in small groups work together to develop learning projects. The role of the educator is to provide training in team process and set the ground rules for project development. The learning process is enhanced by the group interaction and feedback provided by the educator. This strategy results in significant learning and increased retention. The disadvantage of collaborative learning is possible conflict among team members that may result in reduced efficiency and poor outcomes for projects. The educator's role is to facilitate team development to prevent or resolve conflict.

14. **Values clarification:** The affective domain is the most important component in changing behaviors. Clients can easily reproduce correct tooth brushing and flossing techniques and answer questions related to any aspect of oral health, but they return for the next recall appointment with the same plaque scores as during the previous visit. The challenge is to help the learner move from knowledge to appropriate oral health behavior. Assisting the learners in clarifying which values are important to them will help them formulate solutions to oral health problems that will enhance their ability to perform these behaviors. The educator's role is to prepare the learners by describing the process in detail and facilitating the discussion or the written activity. The difficulty with the strategy is that it requires the educator to remain neutral in the facilitation role without bringing forward his or her own values.

15. **Problem-based instruction (PBI):** The learner is presented with a real problem in narrative form with data and complex content. The learner must research possible solutions to the problem and decide on the appropriate solution. The educator provides guidelines on the process and serves as a coach and facilitator. The educator does not provide factual information on the problem but guides the learner to resources to *self-discover* the information. PBI differs from the case study approach, because in PBI the learner performs research to learn new information when the need arises to solve the problem; in case studies, however, the learner applies previously learned knowledge. Learners use all levels in the cognitive domain. The disadvantage of PBI is that if other teaching strategies are excluded, the learning can be superficial and lack coherency.

Figure 16-8 uses the psychological developmental stages in cognitive learning to help the educator make appropriate oral health teaching strategy selections.

STAGE-APPROPRIATE TEACHING STRATEGIES

Learner	General Characteristics	Teaching Strategies	Dental Hygiene Interventions
INFANCY-TODDLERHOOD			
Approximate age: Birth–3 yr Cognitive stages (Piaget): Sensorimotor Psychosocial stage(Erikson): Trust vs. mistrust (Birth–12 mo) Autonomy vs. shame and doubt (1–3 yr)	Dependent on environment Needs security Explores self and environment Natural curiosity	Orient teaching to caregiver Use repetition and imitation of information Stimulate all senses Provide physical safety and emotional security Allow play and manipulation of objects	Welcome active involvement Forge alliances Encourage physical closeness Provide detailed information Answer questions and concerns Ask for information on child's strengths/limitations and likes/dislikes
PRESCHOOLER			
Approximate age: 3–6 yr Cognitive stage(Piaget): Preoperational Psychosocial stage(Erikson): Initiative vs. guilt	Egocentric Thinking precausal, concrete literal Believes illness self-caused and punitive Limited sense of time Fears bodily injury Cannot generalize Animistic thinking (objects possess life or human characteristics) Centration (focus is on one characteristic of an object) Separation anxiety Motivated by curiosity Active imagination, prone to fears Play is his/her work	Use warm, calm approach Build trust Use repetition of information Allow manipulation of objects and equipment Give care with explanation Reassure not to blame self Explain procedures simply and briefly Provide safe, secure environment Use positive reinforcement Encourage questions to reveal perceptions/feelings Use simple drawings and stories Use play therapy, with dolls and puppets Stimulate senses: visual, auditory, tactile, motor	Welcome active involvement Forge alliances Encourage physical closeness' Provide detailed information Answer questions and concerns Ask for information on child's strengths/limitations and likes/dislikes

Figure 16-8. Stage-appropriate teaching strategies. (From Bastable S: Nurse As Educator: Principles of Teaching and Learning. 1997, Jones and Bartlett, Sudbury, MA, pp 94-98. www.jbpub.com. Reprinted with permission.)

STAGE-APPROPRIATE TEACHING STRATEGIES

Learner	General Characteristics	Teaching Strategies	Dental Hygiene Interventions
SCHOOL–AGED CHILDHOOD			
Approximate age: 7–11 yr Cognitive stage (Piaget): Concrete operations Psychosocial stage (Erikson): Industry vs. inferiority	More realistic and objective Understands cause and effect Deductive/inductive reasoning Wants concrete information Able to compare objects and events Variable rates of physical growth Reasons syllogistically Understands seriousness and consequences of actions Subject-centered focus Immediate orientation	Encourage independence and active participation Be honest, allay fears Allow time to ask questions Use analogies to make invisible processes real Establish role models Relate care to other children's experiences, compare procedures Use subject-centered focus Use play therapy Provide group activities Use drawings, models, dolls, painting, audio- and video-tapes	Welcome active involvement Forge alliances Encourage physical closeness Provide detailed information Answer questions and concerns Ask for information on child's strengths/limitations and likes/dislikes
ADOLESCENCE			
Approximate age: 12–18 yr Cognitive stage (Piaget): Formal operations Psychosocial stage (Erikson): Identity vs. role confusion	Abstract, hypothetical thinking Can build on past learning Reasons by logic and understands scientific principles Future orientation Motivated by desire for social acceptance Peer group important Intense personal preoccupation, appearance extremely important (imaginary audience) Feels invulnerable, invincible/immune to	Establish trust, authenticity Know their agenda Address fears/concerns about outcomes of oral health Identify control focus Include in plan of care Use peers for support and influence Negotiate changes Focus on details Make information meaningful to life Ensure confidentiality and privacy Arrange group sessions	Explore emotional and financial support Determine goals and expectations Assess stress levels Respect values and norms Determine role responsibilities and relationships Allow for 1:1 teaching without parents present, but with adolescent's permission; inform family of content covered

Figure 16-8. *(Continued)* Stage-appropriate teaching strategies. (From Bastable S: Nurse As Educator: Principles of Teaching and Learning. 1997, Jones and Bartlett, Sudbury, MA, pp 94–98. www.jbpub.com. Reprinted with permission.)

STAGE-APPROPRIATE TEACHING STRATEGIES

Learner	General Characteristics	Teaching Strategies	Dental Hygiene Interventions
	natural laws (personal fable)	Use audiovisuals, role play, contracts, reading materials Provide for experimentation and flexibility	
YOUNG ADULTHOOD Approximate age: 18–40 yr Cognitive stage(Piaget) Formal operations Psychosocial stage(Erikson) Intimacy vs. isolation	Autonomous Self-directed Uses personal experiences to enhance or interfere with learning Intrinsic motivation Able to analyze critically Makes decisions about personal, occupational, and social roles Competency-based learner	Use problem-centered focus Draw on meaningful experiences Focus on immediacy of application Encourage active participation Allow to set own pace, be self-directed Organize material Recognize social role Apply new knowledge through role play and hands-on practice	Explore emotional, financial, and physical support system Assess motivational level for involvement Identify potential obstacles and stressors
MIDDLE-AGED ADULTHOOD Approximate age: 40–65 yr Cognitive stage(Piaget) Formal operations Psychosocial stage(Erikson) Generativity vs. self-absorption and stagnation	Sense of self well–developed Concerned with physical changes At peak in career Explores alternative lifestyles Reflects on contributions to family and society Reexamines goals and values Questions achievements and successes Has confidence in abilities	Focus on maintaining in dependence and reestablishing normal life patterns Assess positive and negative past experiences with learning Assess potential sources of stress due to mid-life crisis issues Provide information to coincide with life concerns	Explore emotional, financial, and physical support system Assess motivational level for involvement Identify potential obstacles and stressors

Figure 16-8. *(Continued)* Stage-appropriate teaching strategies. (From Bastable S: Nurse As Educator: Principles of Teaching and Learning. 1997, Jones and Bartlett, Sudbury, MA, pp 94–98. www.jbpub.com. Reprinted with permission.)

STAGE-APPROPRIATE TEACHING STRATEGIES

Learner	General Characteristics	Teaching Strategies	Dental Hygiene Interventions
	Desires to modify unsatisfactory aspects of life	and problems	
OLDER ADULTHOOD Approximate age: 65 yr and over Cognitive stages(Piaget) Formal operations Psychosocial stage(Erikson) Ego integrity vs. despair	Cognitive changes Decreased ability to think abstractly, process information Decreased short-term memory Increased reaction time Increased test anxiety Stimulus persistence (afterimage) Focuses on past life experiences	Use concrete examples Build on past life experiences Make information relevant and meaningful Present one concept at a time Allow time for processing/response (slow pace) Use repetition and reinforcement of information Avoid written exams Use verbal exchange and coaching Establish retrieval plan (use one or several clues) Encourage active involvement Keep explanations brief use analogies to illustrate abstract information	Involve principal caregivers Encourage participation Assess coping mechanisms Provide written instructions for reinforcement Provide anticipatory problem solving (what happens if . . .)
	Sensory/motor deficits Auditory changes Hearing loss, especially high-pitched tones, consonants (S, Z, T, F, & G), and rapid speech Visual changes Farsighted (needs	Speak slowly, distinctly Use low-pitched tones Face client when speaking Minimize distractions Avoid shouting Use visual aids to supplement verbal instruction Avoid glares, use soft white light Provide sufficient light	

Figure 16-8. *(Continued)* Stage-appropriate teaching strategies. (From Bastable S: Nurse As Educator: Principles of Teaching and Learning. 1997, Jones and Bartlett, Sudbury, MA, pp 94-98. www.jbpub.com. Reprinted with permission.)

STAGE-APPROPRIATE TEACHING STRATEGIES

Learner	General Characteristics	Teaching Strategies	Dental Hygiene Interventions
	glasses to read)	Use white backgrounds and black print	
	Lenses become opaque (glare problem)	Use large letters and well-spaced print	
	Smaller pupil size (decreased visual adaptation to darkness)	Avoid color coding with blues, greens, purples, and yellows	
	Decreased peripheral perception	Increase safety precautions/provide safe environment	
	Yellowing of lenses (distorts low-tone colors: blue, green, violet)	Ensure accessibility and fit of prostheses (i.e., partial and full dentures)	
	Distorted depth perception	Keep sessions short	
	Fatigue/decreased energy levels	Provide for frequent rest periods	
	Pathophysiology (chronic illness)	Allow for extra time to perform	
		Establish realistic short-term goals	
	Psychosocial changes	Give time to reminisce	
	Decreased risk taking	Identify and present pertinent material	
	Selective learning	Use informal teaching sessions	
	Intimidated by formal learning	Demonstrate relevance of information to daily life	
		Assess resources	
		Make learning positive	
		Identify past positive experiences	
		Integrate new behaviors with formerly established ones	

Figure 16-8. *(Continued)* Stage-appropriate teaching strategies. (From Bastable S: Nurse As Educator: Principles of Teaching and Learning. 1997, Jones and Bartlett, Sudbury, MA, pp 94-98. www.jbpub.com. Reprinted with permission.)

Teaching Aids

Teaching aids are devices or objects that are used to enhance the teaching-learning process. Some examples include the use of posters, flipcharts, overheads, handouts, typodonts, toothbrushes, string to simulate floss, pictures, puppets, theaters, samples of dental products, PowerPoint presentation, feltboards, chalkboards, and whiteboards. If presenting an in-service to a nursing home staff, the teaching aids may include a patient, a patient's bed, dentures, denture brushes, denture labeling materials, clasp brush, and a denture storage container. The teaching aids selected must support the content and the intellectual and skill level of the student. The presenter would not use a poster with complex figures and written words if the student is in a Head Start class. Aids would be chosen that are simple to understand, colorful, and interesting to the learner.

Audiovisual Aids/Instructional Media

Instructional media are used both in individual client and group dental health educational interventions. The client may be exposed to audiotapes, videotapes, videodisks, compact disks, CD-ROMs, and other computer-based instructional technologies. Group interventions include these as well as film, filmstrips, opaque projectors, overhead projectors, slides, and multimedia presentations. Films and filmstrips generally are not as current in content, characters' appearance and dress, and quality as are the more recent technologies; therefore, they are either rapidly fading from use or are considered outmoded by many health professionals.

Instructional media are valuable to the learning process for several reasons. First, media can make the content of the educational message more real and immediate for the learner. Live action allows the learner to vicariously become part of the intervention and experience the message in ways that he or she never could in an educational setting alone. Second, the media have the capacity for making communication within the learning process more precise. This is accomplished by standardizing content for all students involved, reducing the time required for delivering the instructional message, and reproducing motions such as tooth brushing, flossing, and other behavioral tasks taught in the intervention, thus enhancing skill acquisition. Third, media can contribute to establishing interest in the content of the message as well as motivating the learner to become self-directed and seek additional information on the message topic. Last, media increases the learner's options to learn and gain information and skills. Differences in the learning environment, the learner's special needs and learning style, and the educator's teaching style may be resolved using selected media. Additionally, instruction can be conducted with selected media when and where the learner desires.

Figure 16-9 lists various audiovisual aids and instructional media options with an accompanying set of recommendations for the use of each. When making decisions about the type of audiovisual aid or instructional media to select, consider the environment where the presentation or activity will be held. Will the facility have the equipment that you desire, or will you have to bring or rent it for the occasion? Will the image produced be visible to all participants? Aids and equipment needs change based on the size of the group. The larger the audience, the larger will be the required image size. If you are using a videotape, several monitors will need to be placed strategically in the facility to accommodate a large crowd.

If audiovisual aids and instructional media are to enhance a presentation, the presenter must attend to several considerations. The presenter must prepare ahead of the presentation and develop as part of the lesson plan how the item will be introduced and what both the presenter and the learner will do during the use of the item. As part of the preparation work, the presenter should use the aid or media item to ensure that he or she is able to operate the item without any problems. Most important, before using the item, the learner must instructed on why the item is being used and told what to do with the information obtained during the use of the aid or media item.[57] This type of preparation should reduce or eliminate any problems associated with the use of the aid or technology and enhance the educational intervention experience.

Evaluation

One purpose of the evaluation is to determine if the instructional objectives were achieved as a result of the teaching-learning experience. The design of the activity depends on the age and the intellectual and skill levels of the audience. In order to assess the extent to which the learner attained the objectives, the educator should collect, analyze, and interpret information on each objective.[58] What were the outcomes of the educational intervention? The lesson plan should specify which type of assessment technique will be utilized.

Evaluation serves a second purpose. The educator uses assessment to determine whether the process was effective in delivering the content and meeting the objectives. This evaluation is usually in the form of a self-assessment of the various components of the plan. Did the presentation meet all of the criteria outlined in the previous "Content" section? How well did the educator execute the teaching activities and use the teaching aids? Did the learners achieve the instructional objectives? Asking these questions leads to revision and improvement of the educational intervention.

Examples of assessment options include:

1. **Pretest**: determines a baseline of knowledge, attitudes, and skills that can be used to compare against a post test to show whether actual increases occurred or the learner already possessed the knowledge, attitude, or skill.
2. **Post test**: multiple choice, true-false, matching, short answer, fill in the blank, or essay questions used to determine if learner acquired new knowledge, attitudes, or skills.

MATERIAL	ADVANTAGES	DISADVANTAGES
AUDIO MEDIA Audiotape Audio LP Disc Audio CD	1. Easy to make original tape. 2. Useful in most subject areas. 3. Equipment cheap, compact, portable & easy to use. 4. Flexible & adaptable in correlation with curriculum. 5. Useful with groups/individuals 6. Duplication cheap & easy. 7. Plentiful commercial software.	1. Tend to overuse. 2. Fixed rate and sequence of info. 3. Hart to update & revise existing tape programs.
COMPUTER BASED (CBI)	1. Can present text, audio and graphic information. 2. Individual student interaction. 3. Keeps records of response. 4. Adapts instruction to needs of learner/learner controlled. 5. Can control other media hardware.	1. Requires computer/programming. 2. Requires essential hardware & software for development & use. 3. Not fully effective for groups. 4. Lots of hardware/software incompatibility problems.
DISPLAY & PRINT **MEDIA** Displays	1. Useful in any location 2. Flexible for presentation change. 3. Easy to prepare and use.	1. Limited to small group use. 2. Requires some showmanship. 3. Not well compared by students with projected media.
Print Media	1. Useful in any location. 2. Wide variety of applications. 3. Quick, easy to prepare if simple.	1. Costly preparation if sophisticated. 2. Requires suitable reading skills.
PROJECTION MEDIA Film 8mm/58mm 16mm	1. Combines motion/audio/visual. 2. Standard projection equipment widely available/easy to use. 3. Useful to describe motion show relationships and provide topic impact. 4. Useful & easy to use with large groups and individuals 5. May utilize special effects. 6. Plentiful commercial software.	1. Need to learn operation of equipment. 2. Impossible to revise. 3. Clothes, hairstyles, etc. may be outdated.
PROJECTION MEDIA Filmstrip 35mm	1. Compact and easy to use. 2. Always in proper sequence. 3. Useful and easy to use with large groups and individuals. 4. Can be supplemented with sound. 5. Plentiful commercial software. 6. Hardware is simple and common. 7. Projection rate may be user controlled.	1. Difficult & costly local prep. 2. Film lab required to make. 3. Permanent sequence/cannot be revised or rearranged easily.
PROJECTION MEDIA Overhead	1. Equipment simple to use with rate controlled by teacher.	1. Media are relatively large. 2. Complex presentations require

Figure 16-9. Audiovisual aids and instructional media. (Adapted from Sanders HM: In-house Publication for Course Audiovisual Equipment and Materials. University of Cincinnati Raymond Walters College, Cincinnati, OH, 1991. By permission of H.M. Sanders.)

	2. Useful with large groups. 3. May face audience in lit room. 4. Info presented in systematic, developmental sequences. 5. Planning/prep not extensive.	skill/special equipment.
PROJECTION MEDIA Slides 35mm	1. Compact and easy to use. 2. Useful & easy to use with large groups and individuals. 3. May be used singularly or in sequence. 4. Easily revised & updated. 5. Easily handled, stored and rearranged for various uses. 6. Can be supplemented with sound. 7. Plentiful commercial software. 8. Hardware is simple and common. 9. Projection rate may be user controlled.	1. Can get out of sequence easily. 2. May be projected incorrectly if slide is used individually.
PROJECTION MEDIA Multimedia	1. Can demand attention & strong emotional impact. 2. Compresses large amounts of info in short presentations.	1. Requires complex equipment, setup and coordination during planning prep and use. 2. Costly production expense.
VIDEO Videocassette Videodisc	1. Combines motion/audio/visual. 2. Standard projection equipment widely available/easy to use. 3. Useful to describe motion show relationships and provide topic impact. 4. Instant replay possible. 5. Videotape is reusable and costs are lower than film. 6. Useful & easy to use with medium groups and individuals. 7. May utilize special effects. 8. Plentiful commercial software.	1. Moderate cost for equipment. 2. Fixed rate & sequence of info. 3. Costly to update and revise.
POWERPOINT	1. Combines motion/audio/Visual. 2. Pace is controlled by speaker 3. Useful and easy to use with all group sizes 4. Easily revised	1. Requires special equipment 2. The use of too many bells and whistles can be distracting to participants. 3. The need to provide equipment at program sites.

Figure 16-9. *(Continued)* Audiovisual aids and instructional media. (Adapted from Sanders HM: In-house Publication for Course Audiovisual Equipment and Materials. University of Cincinnati Raymond Walters College, Cincinnati, OH, 1991. By permission of H.M. Sanders.)

3. **Direct observation** of the demonstration of a new skill: informal viewing of the skill will show how accurately the learner applies the knowledge to the skill.
4. **Reaction paper**: learners respond to open-ended questions regarding objective information presented in the session.

The educator should be creative when designing evaluation activities that not only assess the attainment of objectives but also reinforce the learning. Evaluation does not have to occur only at the end of the learning experience (**summative evaluation**) but may be conducted throughout the presentation to determine if the educator needs to change direction in content and teaching strategies (**normative evaluation**) (see Chapter 18). To continue meeting the learners' needs, it is important to be flexible.

Sources

1. World Health Organization. Constitution of the World Health Organization. Geneva, WHO, 1946, p 3.
2. Dunn H: What high-level wellness means. Achieving High-Level Wellness 1:9-16, 1977.
3. Anspaugh D, Ezell G: Teaching Today's Health in Middle and Secondary Schools. New York, Macmillan College, 1994, pp 1-22.
4. Joint Committee on Health Education Terminology. Report of the 1990 Joint Committee on Health Education Terminology. J Health Educ 22:97-108, 1991.
5. U.S. Department of Health and Human Services. Healthy People 2000: National Health Promotion and Disease Prevention Objectives. DHHS Publication Number (Public Health Service) 91-50212. Washington, D.C., United States Printing Office, 1990.
6. United States Department of Health and Human Services: Healthy People 2010 (Conference edition, Vols 1 and 2). Washington, D.C., United States Printing Office, 2000.
7. Pickett G, Hanlon J: Public Health: Administration and Practice, 9th ed. St. Louis, MO, Times Mirror/Mosby, 1990, pp 83-84.
8. McKenzie J, Smeltzer J: Planning, Implementing and Evaluating Health Promotion Programs: A Primer, 2nd ed. Boston, Allyn & Bacon, 1997, pp 4-6.
9. Greg Hearsley: Explorations in Learning and Instruction: The Theory Into Practice Database. 1999. [www.gwu.edu/~tip/] (12/28/98).
10. Skinner B: Science and Human Behavior. New York, Macmillan, 1953.
11. Bandura A: Social Learning Theory. Upper Saddle River, NJ, Prentice Hall, 1977.
12. Bandura A: Social Foundations of Thought and Action: A Social Cognitive Theory. Upper Saddle River, NJ, Prentice Hall, 1986.
13. Eggen P, Kauchak D: Educational Psychology: Windows on Classrooms, 3rd ed. Upper Saddle River, NJ, Merrill (an imprint of Prentice Hall), 1997, pp 214-231.
14. McCaul K, Glasgow R, O'Neil H: The problem of creating habits: Establishing health-protective dental behaviors. Health Psychol 11:101-110, 1992.
15. Horwitz A: The public's oral health: The gaps between what we know and what we practice. Adv Dent Res 9:91-95, 1995.
16. Ronis D, Antonakos C, Lang C: Usefulness of multiple equations for predicting preventive oral health behaviors. Health Educ Q 23:512-527, 1996.
17. Bandura A: Self-efficacy: toward a unifying theory of behavioral change. Psychol Rev 84:191, 1977.
18. McCaul K, Glasgow R, Gustafson R: Predicting levels of preventive dental behaviors. J Am Dent Assoc 111:601-605, 1985.
19. McCaul K, O'Neil H, Glasgow R: Predicting the performance of dental hygiene behaviors: An examination of the Fishbein and Ajzen model and self-efficacy expectations. J Appl Soc Psychol 18:114-128, 1988.
20. Piaget J: Science of Education and the Psychology of the Child. New York, The Viking Press, 1970.
21. Piaget J: The Principles of Genetic Epistemology. New York, Routledge, 1972.
22. Bastable S: Nurse As Educator: Principles of Teaching and Learning. Sudbury, MA, Jones & Bartlett, 1997, pp 91-108.
23. Festinger L: A Theory of Cognitive Dissonance. Stanford, CA, Stanford University Press, 1957, pp 1-31.
24. Knowles M: Modern Practice of Adult Education: Andragogy vs. Pedagogy. New York, Association Press, 1970, pp 52-53.
25. Maslow A: Motivation and Personality, 2nd ed. New York, Harper & Row, 1970, pp 35-58.
26. Pipe P, Ratcliff P, Walls T, et al: Developing a Plaque Control Program. Berkeley, CA, Praxis Publishing Company, 1972.
27. Gluch-Scranton J: Motivational strategies in dental hygiene care. Semin Dent Hyg 3:1-7, 1991.
28. Becker M et al: A new approach to explaining sick-role behavior in low-income populations. Am J Public Health 64:205-216, 1974.
29. Hochbaum G: Why people seek diagnostic x-rays. Public Health Rep 71:377-380, 1956.
30. Kegeles S: some motives for seeking preventive dental care. J Am Dent Assoc 67:90-98, 1963.
31. Reisine S, Litt M: Social and psychological theories and their use for dental practice. Int Dent J 43:279-287, 1993.
32. Barker T: Role of health beliefs in patient compliance with preventive dental advice. Community Dent Oral Epidemiol 22:327-330, 1994.
33. Brown G: Human Teaching For Human Learning: An Introduction to Confluent Education. New York, Viking Press, 1971, pp 1-25.
34. Darby M, Walsh M: Guidelines for cross-cultural dental hygiene. In Darby M, Walsh M (eds): Dental Hygiene Theory and Practice. Philadelphia, WB Saunders, 1995, pp 103-119.
35. Cartwright D, Zander A: Group Dynamics: Research and Theory, 3rd ed. New York, Harper & Row, 1968, pp 45-61.
36. Newcomb T: The Acquaintance Process. New York, Holt, Reinhart, and Winston, 1961, p 254.
37. Shaw M: Group Dynamics: The Psychology of Small Group Behavior, 3rd ed. New York, McGraw-Hill, 1981, pp 82-104.
38. Tuchman B: Developmental sequence in small groups. Psychol Bull 63:384-399, 1965.
39. Zander A: Making Groups Effective, 2nd ed. San Francisco, Jossey-Bass, 1994, pp 1-11, 15-120.
40. Miller G: Language and Communication. New York, McGraw-Hill, 1951, p 6.
41. Northouse P, Northouse L: Health Communication A Handbook For Health Professionals. Englewood Cliffs, NJ, Prentice Hall, 1998, pp 2-72, 285-310.
42. Berlo D: The Process of Communication: An Introduction to Theory and Practice. New York, Holt, Rhinehart, and Winston, 1960, pp 72-104.
43. DeBiase C: Dental Health Education Theory and Practice. Philadelphia, Lea & Febiger, 1991, pp 9-11, 13-16.
44. Brill N: Working With People: The Helping Process, 2nd ed. Philadelphia, Harper & Row, 1978, p 35.
45. Gibb J: Defensive communication. J Commun 11:141-148, 1961.
46. Drew N: Exclusive and confirmation: A phenomenology of patients' experience with caregivers. Image 18:39-43, 1986.
47. Mehrabian A: Silent Messages. Belmont, CA, Wadsworth, 1971, p 43.
48. Potter P, Perry A: Fundamentals of Nursing: Concepts, Process, and Practice, 3rd ed. St. Louis, CV Mosby, 1993, pp 320-323.
49. Lefrancois G: Theories of Human Learning: Kongers Report, 3rd ed. Monterey, CA, Brooks and Cole, 1995.
50. Harris N, Christen A: Primary Preventive Dentistry, 4th ed. Stanford, CT, Appleton & Lange, 1995, pp 393-394,
51. Horowitz L, Dillenberg J, Rattray J: Self-care motivation: A model of primary preventive oral health behavior change. J Sch Health 57:14-118, 1987.
52. Read D, Simon S, Goodman J: Health Education: The Search For Values. Englewood Cliffs, NJ, Prentice Hall, 1997.
53. Bloom B et al: Taxonomy of Educational Objectives. New York, David McKay, 1956.
54. Mager R: Preparing Instructional Objectives, 2nd rev ed. Belmont, CA, Lake, 1984, pp 19-22.
55. Gronlund N: How to Write and Use Instructional Objectives, 5th ed. Upper Saddle River, NJ, Merrill (an imprint of Prentice Hall), 1995.
56. Fuszard B: Innovative Teaching Strategies in Nursing, 2nd ed. Gaithersburg, MD, Aspen, 1995, pp 26-34, 48-92, 112-163, 181-190.
57. Sanders H: In-house Publication for Course Audiovisual Equipment and Materials. University of Cincinnati Raymond Walters College, Cincinnati, OH, 1991.
58. Gronlund N, Linn R: Measurement and Evaluation in Teaching. New York, Macmillan, 1990.

Questions and Answers

Questions

You are asked by a local cancer support organization to develop an oral health presentation for a group of six people **preparing** to undergo radiation therapy beginning the following week for head or neck cancer. All attendees are treated by the same oncologist and have had no oral health information regarding radiation caries. Answer questions 1 to 6 in response to this information.

1. The social learning theory can be applied to the development of the presentation by using which of the following teaching strategies?
   A. Paired teaching of the use of fluoride trays
   B. Lecture on the subject of radiation therapy
   C. Computerized instruction on flossing methodology
   D. Problem-based instruction on the home-care techniques to maintain teeth throughout radiation therapy

2. Where on the learning ladder do the majority of group members reside in relation to radiation caries?
   A. Unawareness
   B. Interest
   C. Involvement
   E. Action

3. When organizing the lesson plan, which component provides the **foundation** for the presentation?
   A. Objectives
   B. Needs assessment
   C. Teaching strategies
   D. Evaluation process

4. The six people with head or neck cancer will use fluoride trays daily to prevent radiation caries. What component of a useful objective, according to Mager, is **missing** in this objective statement?
   A. Audience
   B. Performance
   C. Condition
   D. Criteria

5. Which of the following **health belief factors** is the most significant factor used to predict whether or not the cancer clients will comply with the educational interventions presented in the lesson plan?
   A. Susceptibility
   B. Seriousness
   C. Cues to action by the oncologist
   D. Time period of the radiation therapy treatment process

6. One of the group members is of a religious affiliation that uses mysticism in the treatment of disease and injury. The person is attending the presentation to increase his knowledge of the disease. What is the oral health presenter's role in this situation?

   A. Maintain a steady course in achieving the goals established for the presentation
   B. Indicate to the person that scientific research does not support his belief, but that he is welcome to hold the belief.
   C. Ignore the person and focus attention on the other five participants.
   D. Ask the person to share more of the belief and discuss prevention strategies that will not conflict with the belief.

7. When designing learning strategies for **adult** learners, a primary adult learning principle is to relate the new learning to previous learning experiences of the individual. How might this learning principle be applied to the cancer group?
   A. Develop teaching strategies based on the presenter's teaching style.
   B. Perform a learning style assessment of the individuals within the group.
   C. Assess the interest level of the group members in the topics under consideration for the presentation.
   D. Perform a pretest of the existing knowledge of the cancer group.

8. Group dynamics researchers indicate that effective communication among group members leads to a more highly functioning group. What is the most fundamental action that an oral health professional may take to enhance communication among group members when they are charged with facilitating the development of an oral health promotion initiative?
   A. Establish opportunities to discuss communication issues among the group members.
   B. Identify and analyze the communication network(s) among the members.
   C. Determine the oral health needs of the group members.
   D. Delegate the task of meeting recorder to a quieter member of the group.

9. The health communication model suggests professional communication relationships with clients, the client's significant others, and other healthcare professionals. The dental hygienist can maximize the communication process in each context by attending to which of the following interpersonal factors?
   A. Attempting to feel what the other person is feeling and communicate an understanding of this feeling.
   B. Maintaining a polite but detached demeanor during the interaction.
   C. Protecting the client from receiving any unpleasant information regarding the individual's oral health status.
   D. Separating the client and family members during the interaction.

10. As a dental hygienist, you are asked to consult with a school district on the development of health promotion activities in the district. What recommendation will you make to produce the best oral health outcomes for the students in the district?
    A. A classroom presentation for each third grade class in the district
    B. Teacher training on appropriate strategies to teach brushing, flossing, and nutrition in the classroom
    C. An integrated health curriculum that incorporates oral health throughout all grades of the district curriculum
    D. A survey of all kindergartners to assess oral health treatment needs

11. Which of the following is the most reasonable expectation for a one-time group oral health education experience?
    A. Act to improve personal oral health
    B. Increase awareness of oral health issues
    C. Reduce caries rates
    D. Select appropriate OPT aids

12. To which level of Maslow's hierarchy would this statement apply? "You really show that you care about yourself by spending time flossing your teeth before bed."
    A. Physiologic
    B. Security
    C. Social
    D. Ego
    E. Self-actualization

13. You are a practicing dental hygienist in a predominately lower-socioeconomic private practice whose patients are from diverse cultures. Patients primarily use English as a second language and exhibit strong cultural practices related to their health. Using the "Guidelines for Cross-Cultural Dental Hygiene," you must do all of the following **except** one to prepare yourself to effectively provide the dental hygiene care needed by your practice population. What is the *EXCEPTION*?
    A. Sensitize yourself on how cultural factors have influenced your personal beliefs, attitudes, and values.
    B. Critique the individual/groups' practices against common standards of oral hygiene care.
    C. Encourage patients to continue to practice cultural health behaviors that bring them no harm.
    D. Assess cultural biases and prejudices in your own life and how they impact on your provision of dental hygiene services.

14. Which of the following represents appropriate characterization of the older adult years?
    A. Decline in all physiologic and sensory systems
    B. Decrease in the ability to learn and practice new skills
    C. Wide range in variability of health, social, and economic factors
    D. Moody, irritable, often confused in the professional surroundings

15. Which of the following is the most important aspect of the Health Belief Model (HBM)?
    A. Identifies how an individual will behave under certain health conditions
    B. Identifies the types of cues necessary to encourage an individual to behave positively to prevent disease
    C. Acknowledges that the individual is in control of his or her own health
    D. Predicts the likelihood of an individual demonstrating positive health prevention behavior

16. As a registered dental hygienist you are asked to lead a community water fluoridation effort. You set about to develop a group of members to successfully produce a victory on the issue. What **GROUP QUALITIES/CHARACTERISTICS** will you endeavor to create to make the group **SUCCESSFUL**?
    A. Effective decision-making process
    B. Uniqueness
    C. Homogeneity of members
    D. Communication through jargon specific to the group and group goals

17. In which stage of development is a group when it is resolving conflicts, members are assuming roles, and the group has an identity?
    A. Forming
    B. Storming
    C. Norming
    D. Performing

18. All of the following strategies are important to enhance communication with the exception of one. Which of the following is an **EXCEPTION** to the list?
    A. Asking close-ended questions
    B. Active listening
    C. Clarifying messages
    D. Summarizing key elements

ANSWERS

1. **A.** A primary principle of social learning is modeling behaviors of others. Therefore, using paired instruction allows for modeling of oral health behaviors demonstrated by a peer.

2. **A.** The description provided on the group stated that the attendees have had no information on radiation caries; therefore, they have no knowledge of the subject. Once knowledge is acquired, they will move through the remaining stages.

3. **B.** The needs assessment provides information that must be considered when developing all other aspects of the lesson plan. Without an accurate needs assessment, all other lesson features may be developed incorrectly and produce poor outcomes.

4. **C.** The audience, the behavior to be observed, and the criteria or standard to measure the behavior against are present. The conditions under which the behavior will occur are missing.

5. **B.** The cancer participant already has the disease; therefore, susceptibility is not an issue. Cues to action are effective only when the perceptions of susceptibility, seriousness, and salience are held by the individual. Once the individual determines that the head or neck cancer is serious to him or her personally, then the individual is likely to comply with the educational intervention.

6. **D.** Encouraging the person to discuss his or her beliefs will allow the presenter to explore appropriate prevention strategies that will "fit" with the person's beliefs and not be detrimental to the health of the individual.

7. **D.** Prior learning is determined through an assessment process such as a pretest. The remaining items are not associated with the principle of prior learning.

8. **B.** Identifying and analyzing communication networks or patterns allows the group leader to tap into the communication strengths of the group members as well as engage the more noncommunicative members of the group. Allows the leader to develop strategies to maximize communication.

9. **A.** If the dental hygienist exhibits an understanding of the feelings of the client (empathy), the client will respond positively to the oral health message. The remaining items are distractors to the "health" communication process.

10. **C.** An integrated health curriculum including oral health for all grades will produce the longest lasting positive oral health benefits within a school district. The remaining options may be strategies to use within the curriculum.

11. **B.** Considering the learning ladder, the first level of an educational process is to increase awareness. The question relates to a group presentation and the most that one should expect is to increase awareness among the group members.

12. **D.** The "ego" or "self-esteem" level reflects caring for personal health issues.

13. **B.** In a cross-cultural environment, the health provider should be aware of the values, attitudes, beliefs, and practices of different cultures being served. Knowledge of these factors will allow the dental hygienist to gauge the individual's or group's practices against cultural standards rather than an arbitrary national standard of care.

14. **C.** Although some decline in systems occurs, there is a wide variability of health, social, and economic factors among older adults that makes it unrealistic to consider that a blanket statement can be applied to describe the population as all systems declining.

15. **D.** The HBM is a predictive tool to determine the likelihood of positive health behavior.

16. **A.** Effective decision-making is a requirement of group behavior to ensure the success of group endeavors.

17. **C.** Of the four options, norming best identifies the description presented.

18. **A.** Communication is enhanced by asking open-ended questions. This allows the responder to provide broad information that the sender may follow up on to clarify and or obtain additional information.

CHAPTER

17

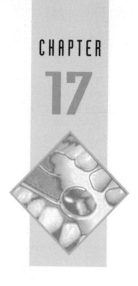

Community Health Activities: Participating in Community Programs

PATRICIA S. TATE, BSDH, MEd

Dental hygienists should be aware of the various components required to effectively participate in community oral health programs. This awareness begins with an understanding of basic community health and oral health concepts and descriptions of the development of community oral health programs in the United States. The criteria for determining community oral health problems and exploration of the concept of change agentry (i.e., how change can be brought about within communities) are reviewed. The principles of community organization, innovation adoption/diffusion, the rates or pace that a community will go through to adopt change, and the characteristics shared by successful community health programs are described. Epidemiologic principles and dental indices currently used in community oral health programs are discussed and outlined. The chapter dedicates significant content to the program planning process by describing three planning models and comparing their features. The role of media in community program planning is discussed. The final section of the chapter discusses the scope of select community groups.

Community Oral Health Concepts

There has been an unresolved controversy for many years over what terms should be used when speaking about the health of the public or community. Should we say "public health" or "community health"? Enough professionals use both terms and often interchangeably that this section will provide definitions for each. **Public** is defined as: of or pertaining to the people as a whole of a community, state, or nation.[1, 2] **Community** is defined as an interactive group of people who live in one area and have common interests.[2] Bell and Newby gave **community** a broader definition by stating that community components include locality; an interdependent social group; interpersonal relationships; and a culture that includes values, norms, and attachments to the community as a whole as well as its parts.[3] The difference

apparently lies in the nature of the groups. The term *public* has a broader scope than does the term *community*. Community has a common thread of location and shared interests and values and norms that binds together the group of people. Thus, communities may be governmental entities such as a city; however, the African-American community, gay and lesbian community, substance abusers, smokers, people with diabetes, people with specific disabilities, senior citizen community, and religious communities are all examples of communities that fit the definitions.[4]

Public health was defined by Winslow as "the science and art of preventing disease, prolonging life, and promoting physical health and efficiency through organized community efforts."[5] Block offers a more expansive definition by stating that "public health is concerned with four broad areas: (1) **lifestyle and behavior**, (2) **the environment**, (3) **human biology**, and (4) **the organization of health programs and systems**. Thus, public health is concerned with keeping people as healthy as possible and controlling or limiting factors that impede health and is the organization and application of public resources to prevent dependency that would otherwise result from disease or injury."[2, 6] McKenzie and Pinger summarize the previous definitions by stating that "public health is the sum of all official (governmental) efforts to promote, protect, and preserve the people's health."[7] **Community health** includes the *efforts of public and private entities* (e.g., individuals, groups, and organizations) in promoting, protecting, and preserving the health of people within a community.[7] The distinction between public and community health is the governmental connection with public health, whereas community health may be provided by either public or private sources.

The American Board of Dental Public Health used Winslow's definition of public health and expanded it to develop the definition of **public dental health:** "the science and art of preventing and controlling dental diseases and promoting dental health through organized community efforts. It is that form of dental practice which serves the *community* as a patient rather than the individual. It is concerned with the dental education of the public, with applied dental research and with the administration of group dental care programs as well as the prevention and control of dental diseases on a community basis."[2, 8] Block suggests that a more contemporary definition of dental public health would be "a concern for and activity directed toward the improvement and promotion of the dental health of the population as a whole, as well as of individuals within that population.[2]" This definition would account for dental public health work that is not an organized community effort and also for activities outside of specific aggregate populations. According to a review of current textbooks on community oral health, **community dental health** is a term that may be used interchangeably with **public dental health**. Two other terms that are used interchangeably are **dental health** and **oral health.** The contrast for some professionals is that dental health refers specifically to teeth, whereas oral health refers to all aspects of the oral cavity. The remainder of this chapter refers to *community oral health* exclusively.

Historical Development of Community Oral Health Programs

Even though community health programs have been in place in the United States since the early 1800s, oral health programs did not exist until the mid-1800s when small clinics were established in New York City, Philadelphia, and Boston. School dental programs began around the World War I era. The need for community oral health programs was highlighted during the enlistment activities for World Wars I and II. During World War I, many recruits were rejected because of poor oral health. Just before World War II, 15% of the recruits were rejected because they could not meet the minimal requirements of three serviceable natural anterior teeth and three opposing posterior teeth in each arch.[9] Other significant events in the development of community oral health included the development of the **Social Security Act in 1935; communal water fluoridation** in Grand Rapids, Michigan, and Newburgh, New York, in **1945;** and **Medicaid and Medicare legislation in 1966.**[10] In addition, the Surgeon General's report *Healthy People* (released in 1979) and the National Health Objectives for 1990 (developed in 1980 and published in *Promoting Health/Preventing Disease: Objectives for the Nation*) provided the foundation for community oral health programs today.[11] The driving force in the development of community oral health programs during the 1990s was the *Healthy People 2000, National Health Promotion and Disease Prevention Objectives for the United States,*[12] which was published in 1990. The plan contained 16 oral health objectives for reducing caries, periodontal disease, oral cancer, and edentulism among Americans of various age groups. In 1995, a mid-course review was conducted, which resulted in the addition of an objective on smokeless tobacco.[13] These objectives were not developed with the highest ideal in mind for the year 2000 outcome. The planning process requested that all objectives be reasonable and achievable. The intent was to build on the 2000 objectives into the future with the hope of achieving the ideal at some point. These objectives established the priorities under which community oral health programs are funded. Therefore, they have been a crucial consideration in the development of program requests. The *Healthy People 2010: Understanding and Improving Health* builds on the preceding initiatives. The overarching purpose is to promote health and prevent illness, disability, and premature death.[14] **Figure 17-1** outlines the oral health objectives designed in the 2010 plan. These objectives should have a similar impact on community oral health program planning as the 2000 objectives.

Oral Health in America: A Report of the Surgeon General, which was published in 2000, is the first report of its nature and the most significant current effort under way to improve the oral health of the public. It relates oral health to general health and well-being. The primary theme of the report is that oral health involves much more than healthy teeth. Achievement of oral health means that an individual is "free of chronic oral-facial pain conditions, oral and pharyngeal cancers, oral soft tissue lesions, birth defects such as cleft lip and palate and disorders that affect the oral, dental, and craniofacial tissues."[15] This new concept of "oral" health merges with caries and periodontal disease to broaden our concerns regarding oral health.

The report identifies eight major findings from an exhaustive scientific review of the nation's oral health[15]:

1. Oral diseases and disorders in and of themselves affect health and well-being.
2. Safe and effective measures exist to prevent the most common dental diseases-caries and periodontal diseases.
3. Lifestyle behaviors, such as tobacco use, excessive alcohol use, and poor dietary choices, affect general health and also oral and craniofacial health.
4. There are profound and consequential oral health disparities within the U.S. population.
5. More information is needed to improve America's oral health and eliminate health disparities.
6. The mouth reflects general health and well-being.
7. Oral diseases and conditions are associated with other health problems.
8. Scientific research is key to further reduction of diseases and disorders that affect the face, mouth, and teeth.

These findings resulted in the development of a National Oral Health plan. The main components follow[15]:

1. **Changing perceptions regarding oral health and disease so that oral health becomes an accepted component of general health requires:**
   a. Changing public perceptions regarding the importance of oral health and the relationship to general health
   b. Changing policymakers' perceptions regarding the inclusion of oral health services in health promotion

Oral Health Goal and Objectives

Goal: Prevent and control oral and craniofacial diseases, conditions, and injuries and improve access to related services.

Objectives:

21-1: Reduce the proportion of children and adolescents who have dental caries experience in their primary or permanent teeth.

21-2: Reduce the proportion of children, adolescents, and adults with untreated dental decay.

21-3: Increase the proportion of adults who have never had a permanent tooth extracted because of dental caries or periodontal disease.

21-4: Reduce the proportion of adults who have had all their natural teeth extracted.

21-5: Reduce periodontal disease.

21-6: Increase the proportion of oral and pharyngeal cancers detected at the earliest stage.

21-7: Increase the proportion of adults who, in the past 12 months, report having had an examination to detect oral and pharyngeal cancer.

21-8: Increase the proportion of children who have received dental sealants on their molar teeth.

21-9: Increase the proportion of the U.S. population served by community water systems with optimally fluoridated water.

21-10: Increase the proportion of children and adults who use the oral health care system each year.

21-11: Increase the proportion long-term care residents who use the oral health care system each year.

21-12: Increase the proportion of children and adolescents under age 19 years at or below 200 percent of the Federal poverty level who received any preventive dental service during the past year.

21-13: (Developmental) Increase the proportion of school-based health centers with an oral health component.

21-14: Increase the proportion of local health departments and community-based health centers, including community, migrant, and homeless health centers, that have an oral health component.

21-15: Increase the number of States and the District of Columbia that have a system for recording and referring infants and children with cleft lips, cleft palates, and other craniofacial anomalies to craniofacial anomaly rehabilitative teams.

21-16: Increase the number of States and the District of Columbia that have an oral and craniofacial health surveillance system.

21-17: (Developmental) Increase the number of Tribal, State (including the District of Columbia), and local health agencies that serve jurisdictions of 250,000 or more persons that have in place an effective public dental health program directed by a dental professional with public health training.

Objectives Related to Oral Health Identified in Other Focus Areas

1. Access to Quality Health Services

1-1. Persons with health insurance

1-2. Health insurance coverage for clinical preventive services

1-3. Counseling about health behaviors

1-4. Source of ongoing care

1-7. Core competencies in health provider training

1-8. Racial and ethnic representation in health professions

1-15. Long-term care services

2. Arthritis, Osteoporosis, and Chronic Back Conditions

2-2. Activity limitations due to arthritis

2-3. Personal care limitations

2-7. Seeing a health care provider

2-8. Arthritis education

3. Cancer

3-1. Cancer deaths

3-6. Oropharyngeal cancer deaths

3-9. Sun exposure

3-10. Provider counseling about preventive measures

3-14. Statewide cancer registries

3-15. Cancer survival rates

5. Diabetes

5-1. Diabetes education

5-2. Prevent diabetes

5-3. Reduce diabetes

5-4. Diagnosis of diabetes

6. Disability and Secondary Conditions

6-13. Surveillance and health promotion programs

7. Educational and Community-Based Programs

7-1. High school completion

7-2. School health education

7-3. Health-risk behavior information for college and university students

7-4. School nurse-to-student ratio

7-5. Worksite health promotion programs

7-6. Participation in employer-sponsored health promotion activities

7-7. Patient and family education

7-10. Community health promotion programs

7-11. Culturally appropriate community health promotion programs

7-12. Older adult participation in community health promotion activities

8. Environmental Health

8-5. Safe drinking water

11. Health Communication

11-1. Households with Internet access

11-2. Health literacy

11-3. Research and evaluation of communication programs

11-4. Quality of Internet health information sources

11-6. Satisfaction with providers' communication skills

12. Heart Disease and Stroke

12-1. Coronary heart disease (CHD) deaths

14. Immunization and Infectious Diseases

14-3. Hepatitis B in adults and high-risk groups

14-9. Hepatitis C

14-10. Identification of persons with chronic hepatitis C

14-28. Hepatitis B vaccination among high-risk groups

15. Injury and Violence Prevention

15-1. Nonfatal head injuries

15-17. Nonfatal motor vehicle injuries

15-19. Safety belts

15-20. Child restraints

15-21. Motorcycle helmet use

15-23. Bicycle helmet use

15-24. Bicycle helmet laws

15-31. Injury protection in school sports

16. Maternal, Infant, and Child Health

16-6. Prenatal care

16-8. Very low birth weight infants born at Level III hospitals

Figure 17-1. Oral health objectives for the year 2010. (From US Department of Health: Healthy People 2010: Understanding and Improving Health. Conference ed. Vols 1 and 2. Washington, DC, US Printing Office, 2000.)

and disease prevention programs, care delivery systems, and reimbursement schedules

c. Changing nondental health providers' perceptions of the significance of oral health to the overall health of clients resulting in increased collaboration with dental professionals in planning and delivering health care

2. **Accelerating the building of the science and evidence base and applying science effectively to improve oral health.** Research is critical for the provision of new knowledge about oral and general health and disease. Increased research in the relationships between chronic oral inflammatory infections (e.g., periodontitis) and diabetes and glycemic control as well as other systemic conditions is required.

3. **Building an effective health infrastructure that meets the oral health needs of all Americans and integrating oral health effectively into overall health.** This calls for expanding our capacity for addressing oral health and integrating it with other public health programs. This infrastructure would facilitate the development of strengthened collaborations with private practitioners, other public programs, and voluntary groups. Additionally, it encourages the recruitment of members of minority groups to positions within the health arena that provides a more equitable geographic distribution of care providers.

4. **Removing known barriers between people and oral health services.** Access to oral health services can be accomplished by providing dental health insurance, both public and private, for groups such as those that live at or below the poverty line, those that lack health insurance, or those reduce that lose insurance at retirement. Other groups that require increased access are children and individuals whose health is physically, mentally, and emotionally compromised.

5. **Using public-private partnerships to improve the oral health of those who still suffer disproportionately from oral diseases.** Communities should seek collaborative opportunities with public health agencies, private industry, social service organizations, community service organizations, educators, faith leaders, health care providers, researchers, the media, community leaders, voluntary health organizations, and consumer groups to eliminate health disparities among all groups of the population. These collaborations enable communities to build and strengthen cross-disciplinary, culturally competent, community-based, and community-wide health promotion and disease prevention initiatives that lead to improved oral and general health.

Criteria for Determining a Community Oral Health Problem

Considering the wide variation in health problems facing a community, it is useful to examine the criteria that are used to help determine the existence of an oral health problem in the community. These criteria[8] are:

1. A condition or situation that is a widespread actual or potential cause of **morbidity** (incidence of disease) or **mortality** (incidence of death)

2. An existing **perception** (understanding or feeling) that the condition is a community health problem on the part of the public, government, or community health authorities

Examples of oral health problems that may be applied to the first criteria are caries activity (morbidity) and deaths due to oral carcinomas (mortality). If surveys are conducted within a community and it is determined that there is a widespread incidence of caries activity among preschool age children, the morbidity rate for caries activity is defined as high for the community. This is evidence of the need for a community-based program to treat current disease and prevent the occurrence of future caries activity in preschool-age children. The second criterion is slightly more difficult to address. Perceptions are not always the reality, but to the holder of the perception, the perception is real. Therefore, if there is a widely held perception within the community that a specific preventable oral health condition exists and the community has the resources to develop a program, the community will **mandate** by vote that a program be developed. In addition to community perception, the second criterion may be met by an **executive order**, whereby a governmental official such as the mayor or governor can identify a program to support and order that money be directed to fund the program.[8] In either case, once the decision is made, funds are allocated or grant requests are developed to design the program.

Differences Between Private Practice and Community Programs

Most textbooks that include sections on community oral health compare private dental practice concerns and community oral health program concerns; however, the approach varies. **Figure 17-2** is a compilation of the comparisons found in a review of current textbooks on community oral health.[2, 8, 9] Clients seeking oral health care in a **private practice setting model** will have their needs determined by an examination that includes information regarding their dental and medical histories, personal accounts of their sociocultural background, and a clinical examination. Given the information from the examination, the practitioner completes a diagnosis of the client's oral condition and develops an appropriate treatment plan that addresses the client's needs and interests. After some negotiation regarding the extent of treatment and financial issues, the client approves the plan and treatment is provided. Upon completion of treatment, the client (usually with the help of a third party dental insurance provider) pays for the services. The treatment is evaluated at the time of service and again at each subsequent visit.

<table>
<tr><td>

Private Dental Practice Model

Purpose: To attend to the oral health needs and interest of individual clients

Work Concentration: Personal oral health care on an individual basis to meet individual needs

Service Methods

1. Examination

2. Diagnosis

3. Treatment plan

4. Treatment

5. Payment

6. Evaluation

</td><td>

Public Oral Health Program Model

Purpose: To improve the oral health status of a given population

Work Concentration: To assess, plan, implement, and evaluate oral health promotion programs and create health services systems to provide a range of dental services

Service Methods

1. Survey/needs assessment

2. Analysis

3. Program plan

4. Program implementation

5. Program funding

6. Program evaluation

</td></tr>
</table>

Figure 17-2. Comparison between the private dental practice model and the public oral health program model.

On the other hand, the **community oral health program model** conducts a survey of the community to determine the community problem and needs. Once the data are collected, this information is analyzed and the results are prioritized to determine which needs must be met. The priorities are used to design a program plan. Once resources for the program are identified and secured, the plan is implemented. Funding for public programs is generally conducted through a local, state, or federal governmental funding source. Community programs may also receive funding from private foundations. Programs are assessed using both **formative/process** (throughout the program) and **summative/outcome** (at the conclusion of the program) evaluations. Each method used in the community oral health program is addressed in detail later in the chapter.

CONCEPT OF CHANGE AGENTRY

Psychological Phases of Innovation Adoption

As an oral health professional, the dental hygienist working in community-based programs can maximize program effectiveness by developing a familiarity with the **process of change**. Program goals are developed which reflect some positive change in oral health behavior. Researchers of behavioral change have found that individuals undergo psychological phases when deciding to adopt or not to adopt an innovation. The **innovation** may be defined as an idea, practice, or object that is perceived to be new by an individual or

other unit of adoption[16]; any of the aforementioned may be a solution to an individual's or a community's oral health problem. These psychological phases include:

1. **Awareness**: The individual becomes aware that a new idea, practice, or object exists or that she has a problem. During this phase, the individual develops a personal need to change; this initiating factor is responsible for the decision to make a change.

2. **Interest arousal**: The individual becomes curious about how the new idea, practice, or object works and what its benefits may be.

3. **Appraisal**: The individual intellectually evaluates the positive and negative aspects of the innovation for herself. She asks the question, "How will this benefit me?"

4. **Trial**: The individual tries the innovation for a short time to determine if it meets her needs.

5. **Adoption/rejection**: The individual decides to continue using the new idea, practice, or object; that is, to make the change or to reject the innovation. Rejection may actually occur any time after the initial awareness phase.[17]

Throughout the planning and implementation phases of a community-based health promotion program, the planner should carefully monitor the progression of community members through each phase. Adoption rates increase significantly when individuals go through each step. The change, if accepted or adopted, becomes more firmly a part of each individual's continued repertoire of knowledge, attitudes, values, or behaviors as a result of this progression through each phase. Failure to undergo each step can easily result in discontinuation of the innovation.

Innovation Diffusion Process

Diffusion is defined as "the process by which an innovation is communicated through certain channels over time among the members of a social system."[16] A **social system** is defined as organized human groups.[18] The aim of diffusion is to maximize the amount of exposure and extend the reach of innovations, strategies, or programs to the community.[19] This may be accomplished by proceeding through the following innovation diffusion stages:

1. **Innovation development:** The important concept to consider during the creation of the innovation is the inclusion of members of the target population in developing the idea, practice, or object and providing information and feedback on its content, design, layout, and presentation. Consideration of promotional strategies during this stage is critical.

2. **Dissemination**: The focus is on taking the new knowledge and transferring it from the developers (i.e., resource system) to the target population (i.e., user system). This requires the identification of communication channels and both formal and informal systems that are best for the diffusion of the innovation to the target population. For example, dissemination of information on a community-based water fluoridation program requires the planning group to use formal channels (e.g., public service announcements and press releases) and informal channels (e.g., community announcements at social, recreational, and church events).

3. **Adoption:** The target population accepts the innovation during this stage. For adoption to occur, the planners must address the issues identified in the next section, *Characteristics of a Successful Community Health Program,* and identify and develop strategies for dealing with any barriers that might impede adoption of the new behavior or a change in existing practices.

4. **Implementation:** This is the first time that the innovation is used by members of the target population. The primary issue at this stage is to enhance the self-efficacy and skills of the adopters and encourage members of the target population to try out the innovation and experience some successes with the innovation.

5. **Maintenance:** During this stage, the adopter is bridging the gap between knowledge of the innovation and the long-term continuation of the innovation. The planner must identify possible sources for discontinuation of the innovation and develop strategies to overcome these problems. Generally, if the innovation is a community-based program, the primary problem is termination of financial support.[19]

Organizational and community-based innovations may be considered successfully diffused if a specific program or service is provided, if changes in policies or regulations occur, or if community members at various levels implement the innovation over the long-term.

Rate of Acceptance of Change

As with clinical clients, it is well understood that not all community members will embrace or even adopt an innovation or new idea. However, those who do adopt the idea will do so at varying rates and will fall within five categorical descriptions[16, 20]:

1. **Innovators (2.5% of population):** more educated; cosmopolitan; eager to take risks; highly active; usually not integrated into the prevailing social structure; attuned to the national media; often viewed as mavericks.

2. **Early adopters (13.5% of population):** active members of the community; respected, knowledgeable opinion leaders within the community; viewed as individuals who can be consulted before a potential adopter will accept a new idea; attuned to the national media; use innovations successfully and discreetly.

3. **Early majority (34% of population):** accept change but are not the first to do so; considered to be followers rather than leaders; above average in age; more educated; experienced within the local community; attend less to the national media and more to the local and regional media; more influenced by interpersonal means than by the media.

4. **Late majority (34% of population):** skeptical members of the community; unwilling to take many risks; cautious about new ideas and innovations but can be convinced as a result of peer persuasion; attend less to national media and more to local media; usually older, less educated, and lower in social status than the early adopters.

5. **Laggards (16% of population):** suspicious of new ideas and innovations; very slow to change on any level; consumed by traditional values; often oriented toward the past and possess a parochial view rather than a cosmopolitan view; usually have little influence and are often isolated or alienated from the prevailing social structure; group that is most likely to be a target for government-sponsored oral health programs; lower socioeconomic status and often feel alienated from society; use media exclusively for entertainment.

There is a final group within a community that does not fall within the adoption curve. This small segment **will not accept an innovation regardless of the strategies applied.** Because this group does not meet any specific set of characteristics, members can be found in any of the descriptions applied to the adopters.

Once the community assessment is done to determine who falls into which category, the planner can use this information to identify the opinion leaders. Inclusion of the opinion leaders in the first phases of the planning process can have long-term positive results for achieving program goals. The planner should provide enough informational resources through print and mass media and conduct face-to-face sessions with opinion leaders to move them from the awareness phase to the adoption phase. When doing so, these individuals will help the planner to promote the program to other community members. Another advantage to determining where community members fall along the adopter bell curve is that it allows planners to determine which types of intervention strategies to use for individuals within a given category. For example, early adopters should respond to cognitively oriented (educational) programs; majority adopters should respond to motivational messages; and, laggards might require assistance to overcome barriers to adoption.[21]

Characteristics of Successful Community Health Programs

To increase the likelihood of success, a community oral health program planner should consider factors that research indicates are necessary for success. The following attributes are critical program components[16, 22]:

1. **Compatibility**: How agreeable are the program goals and other components with the community values, norms, and mores?
2. **Simplicity**: The less complex the program design, the more likely community members are to participate.
3. **Relative advantage:** Do community members view the program goals as creating a personal benefit for them?
4. **Low risk factor:** The lower the personal risk for participation, the higher will be the participation rate.
5. **Trialability:** Can community members participate in a small portion of the program or a pilot program to determine their level of interest?
6. **Divisibility:** Can the program be divided into parts, and can community members select the parts in which they wish to participate?
7. **Observability:** Can the community witness oral health improvements early and often; are program revisions easily observed as a result of community feedback?
8. **High interest:** The greater the appeal of the program across the community, the higher will be the participation rate.
9. **Ownership of program:** If the community members feel a strong sense of ownership in the *development* of program components; then the program belongs to them.
10. **Built-in feedback system:** The program design incorporates a feedback loop that allows community members to easily provide comments for program improvement.
11. **Support of opinion leaders:** The greater and more active the support from community opinion leaders, the higher will be the participation rate.
12. **Easily revised:** Evaluation is continuous, and feedback results in program modification strategies to reflect community input.

If a program is designed with these characteristics in place, program goals are more likely to be achieved and the results will last longer.[23]

Community Organization

Community oral health planners bear in mind community organization principles when they are involved in planning programs for the community. Minkler and Wallerstein define **community organization** as the process by which community groups are helped to identify common problems or goals, mobilize resources, and, in other ways, develop and implement strategies for reaching the goals that they *collectively* set.[24] To achieve the goal in the definition, the planner must utilize the following **fundamental concepts in health education program planning**[24, 25]:

1. **Participation and relevance:** starting where the people are and continue engaging people throughout the process as equals in the process. Participation allows community members to feel a part of the process and also to have ownership in the process.
2. **Personal and community empowerment:** the belief held by members of the community that they have control over their lives and the life of their community. Fostering empowerment in community members may be a struggle for the oral health program planner, because this often requires the planner to relinquish some of his or her own power in the process.
3. **Critical consciousness:** the ability of community members to analyze their social, economic, and health conditions and consequently identify a personal role for changing those conditions. Assuming responsibility for changing personal environmental conditions encourages community members to take leadership roles within the community.
4. **Community competence:** the enhanced problem-solving ability of community members. Cottrell specified that community competence occurs when the various components of a community are able to collaborate effectively in identifying the problems and needs of the community; are able to achieve a working consensus on goals and priorities; are able to agree on ways and means to implement the agreed upon goals; and are able to collaborate effectively in the required action plan.

By combining the community organization principles with the concepts regarding successful community program characteristics, health education principles, and the adoption diffusion process, the community oral health program planner has the tools necessary to design effective community programs.

 EPIDEMIOLOGY

One of the more intriguing aspects of community oral health programming is **epidemiology.** Definitions of epidemiology vary from the study of the distribution (e.g., age, gender, race, geography, time) and determinants (causes) of disease frequency in human populations[26] to the study of health and disease in populations and of how both are influenced by

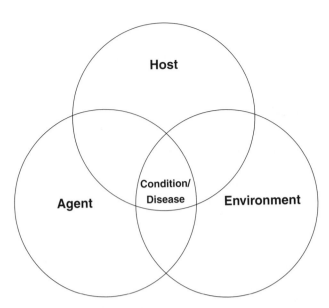

Figure 17-3. Epidemiologic factors.

heredity, biology, physical environment, social environment, and lifestyles.[8] Both discuss disease in populations, whereas one addresses distribution of disease and the other examines the influencing factors related to disease. Both have application to oral epidemiology. For the purpose of this discussion, **oral epidemiology** is defined as the study of oral health and disease in populations and the influencing factors associated with oral health and disease. **Figure 17-3** demonstrates the interactions of the factors under review in an epidemiologic study. These factors are the *host* (the individual or part of the body affected by disease or injury), the *agent* (causative factor of the disease or injury), and the *environment* (conditions under which the host and the agent interact).

When studying the prevalence of dental caries, researches must examine host factors such as the location of caries, age, race, gender, heredity, and emotional status. Environmental factors include the geographic location of residence during tooth formation, nutrition, fluoride, and oral hygiene, and all play a role in determining tooth susceptibility to caries. It is more difficult to perform epidemiologic studies on periodontal disease, because the signs of the disease are much more subjective than are those of caries. When reviewing the host, researchers examine factors such as race, age, gender, systemic disease, emotional disturbances, and intraoral distribution of the disease. Environmental variables, including geographic location, nutrition, antimicrobial agents, and oral hygiene, provide information that sheds light on the study of the periodontal disease process.[27]

Epidemiologic studies are used to[8]:

1. Collect data to **describe normal biologic processes** such as patterns of tooth eruption.
2. Develop an understanding of the **natural development and end of diseases**. This knowledge allows the planner to recognize if a disease or condition requires interven-

tion strategies or if it will terminate due to the fact that it has run its course.

3. Determine the **amount and distribution of oral disease and risk of oral disease** existing within a group. The data establish trends or patterns within the population or subgroups of the general population under investigation. Examination of the data will separate the findings according to demographic factors such as age, gender, race, socioeconomic status, educational status, and religious affiliation. This information allows the researcher to correlate factors with cause and risks.
4. Identify **causal relationships between the factors listed in #3 and the disease or condition**. This knowledge allows the planner to develop intervention strategies to reduce the risk of developing the disease or condition.

The information obtained through any of the aforementioned studies is used to assist the community oral health planner in establishing priorities of need for program development as well as evaluating the quality and effectiveness of a community program.

See Chapter 18 for terminology found in epidemiologic research and reports that should be familiar to the community oral health program planner.

Epidemiologic findings currently indicate the best way to assess each of the following oral conditions is through the associated methods delineated[8, 28]:

1. **Oral cancer:** Use age-adjusted annual incidence rates by gender and race and 5-year survival rates.
2. **Cleft palates:** Review birth certificates.
3. **Human immunodeficiency virus (HIV) oral manifestations:** Use prevalence rates of oral candidiasis, oral hairy leukoplakia, herpes simplex virus, Kaposi sarcoma, and non-Hodgkin lymphoma. The highest rates begin with oral candidiasis, and the remaining conditions are found in descending order of prevalence.

Dental Indices/Indexes

Pendrys defines a **dental index** as a graduated, numeric scale with upper and lower limits and with scores on the scale corresponding to specific criteria.[28] **Indices** have been developed to assess the scope and intensity of almost all oral diseases and conditions. The following list of dental indices is presented because the indices are often used to study the scope and magnitude of oral diseases and conditions existing within a community.[8, 10, 28] The results of these assessments will help the community oral health planner to establish program priorities.

Dental caries can be measured, and the distribution of caries within the population can be determined by using the following indices:

1. *D*ecayed, *m*issing, and *f*illed permanent teeth (**DMF**)
2. *D*ecayed, *m*issing, and *f*illed *s*urfaces of permanent teeth (**DMFS**)

3. Decayed, indicated for *extraction*, *filled* primary teeth **(def)**
4. Decayed, *missing*, and *filled* primary teeth **(dmf)**
5. Root Caries Index **(RCI)**

DMF Index

The **DMF Index** is the most applied and well-known of dental indices today. This index was developed by Klein, Palmer, and Knutson and has been used since the late 1930s; it continues to provide information on community dental caries activity.[29] The index is an irreversible index that is used to identify the number of teeth in the permanent dentition that are currently affected by **decay, missing due to caries, and filled due to caries** activity. It may be identified as the **DMFT,** because the purpose is to look for the **decayed, missing, and filled experience per tooth**. The index is useful for community oral health purposes, because it provides a measure of the number of teeth within the community that have had caries treatment or require treatment for caries.

Process

1. The DMFT is a simple count of all three factors. A tooth is counted once, so recurrent decay is not counted.
2. The examiner uses a mirror, light, and explorer to perform the assessment. No radiographs are secured or used.
3. If there is a question about whether or not a tooth is missing due to decay or other factors, the tooth is *not* counted.
4. An individual score may range from 0 to 32 and is recorded in whole numbers.
5. Group scores are total scores for each community member divided by the number of community members examined. The community score may be recorded in fractional numbers.

DMFS Index

The **DMFS Index** is the same as the DMFT Index, but it examines all **five surfaces of the tooth**. It is a *more* accurate index for assessing dental caries. A tooth scored using the DMFT Index may have several surfaces of decay, but the score will only be one. However, the same tooth in a DMFS survey may have a score of 0 to 5. The result is a more accurate assessment of caries activity per tooth.

Process

The count per individual and per community group is done the same as for the DMFT Index with the exception that all five surfaces of the tooth are examined with a mirror, light, and explorer.

def Index

The **def** is used to examine primary teeth. This index may be used to view caries in a tooth **(deft)** or for all five surfaces

(defs). Because there is confusion over how to assess *e,* some examiners will simply drop the *e* and thus the index becomes *df, dft, or dfs*. As in the DMF Index, the defs and the dfs are more accurate indices compared with the deft and the dft.

Process

1. Use the mirror, light, and explorer to assess active caries and fillings per tooth or per surface.
2. Total the count per child for an individual assessment. The value will be a whole number.
3. Total the counts for all children examined, and divide by the number of children. Again, this may a fractional number.

dmf Index

The **dmf** Index is used as a modification of the def Index. The dmf is used for children who are either too young for teeth to exfoliate or only on the primary molar teeth. Use of the dmf Index will give a more accurate assessment of caries activity in the very young child.

RCI Index

The **RCI Index** was developed by Katz in 1980 to assess the **risk** of an **exposed** root surface to caries.[30]

Process

1. The examiner identifies root lesions and restorations and the number of exposed root surfaces.
2. Data are entered into this formula:

$$\left. \frac{\text{root surfaces: decayed + filled}}{\begin{array}{c}\text{(root surfaces with loss of periodontal attachment:} \\ \text{Decayed + filled + sound)}\end{array}} \right\} \times 100 = \text{RCI}$$

Scores can be derived for individuals, communities, and types of teeth (e.g., anterior, premolars).
3. A score of 23.4% within a given community means that of all the teeth with gingival recession or exposed root surfaces, 23.4% of the teeth were decayed or filled on the root surfaces.

The community oral health planner should remember that assessments of dental caries could be an understatement of the actual amount of carious activity within a community. Inter-rater and intra-rater reliability and other conditions under which the assessments are taken allow for a margin of error. However, the results of the assessment provide a basis for program development, incidence assessment over time, and program evaluation (see Chapter 18).

The etiology of **periodontal disease** is better understood now than when periodontal indices were first developed. It was formerly believed that gingivitis developed into periodontitis. Therefore, it is crucial when selecting an **index** to assess periodontal health that the selection is specific to the condition under study. Periodontal disease can be measured, and the distribution of gingivitis and periodontal disease within the population can be identified using *radiographs or specific indices*. The following indices are selected due to their applicability to community programs:

1. Gingival Index **(GI)**
2. Sulcus Bleeding Index **(SBI)**
3. Modified Gingival Index **(MGI)**
4. Periodontal Index **(PI)**
5. Periodontal Disease Index **(PDI)**
6. Loss of Periodontal Attachment **(LPA)**
7. Community Periodontal Index of Treatment Needs **(CPITN)**

Gingival Index

The **Gingival Index (GI)** developed by Loe and Silness[31] in 1963 is a reversible index that is used to assess the level of inflammation of the gingival tissues.

Process

1. The examiner uses a mirror, light, and probe to circumscribe the tooth.
2. The gingiva on the mesial, distal, facial, and lingual surfaces are assessed.
3. Each surface is given a score from 0 to 3:
   0 = Normal tissue
   1 = Mild inflammation: slight change in color, slight edema; no bleeding upon probing
   2 = Moderate inflammation: redness, edema, and glazing; bleeding upon probing
   3 = Severe inflammation: marked redness and edema; ulceration; tendency to bleed spontaneously
4. The values are averaged to give a score for an individual.

Consideration. The scores provide distinctions between normal and severe gingivitis, but the index is not as sensitive when differentiating between mild and moderate gingivitis.[8]

Modified Gingival Index

The **Modified Gingival Index (MGI)** was created to eliminate the need for gingival bleeding when assessing gingival health.[36] This resulted from the knowledge that bleeding upon probing is an inefficient way to predict future periodontitis.[35, 37] The MGI provides a high degree of visual sensitivity to gingivitis.[8]

Process

The evaluator uses a mirror and light to assess the papillary unit along with the marginal gingiva. This noninvasive assessment focuses on color and form.[32]

The following criteria are applied:

0 = absence of inflammation
1 = mild inflammation; slight change in color, little change in texture of any portion of, but not the entire, marginal or papillary gingival unit

2 = mild inflammation: criteria as earlier but involve the entire marginal or papillary gingival unit
3 = moderate inflammation: glazing, redness, edema, or hypertrophy of the marginal or papillary gingival unit
4 = severe inflammation: marked redness, edema, or hypertrophy of the marginal or papillary gingival unit; spontaneous bleeding, congestion, or ulceration

Consideration. The MGI produces a subjective measure; therefore, calibration is difficult and the process is time-consuming.

Sucular Bleeding Index

The **Sulcular Bleeding Index (SBI)** was designed by Muhlemann and Son in the early 1970s to increase the sensitivity of findings related to gingivitis and the GI.[33]

Process

The examiner uses a mirror, light, and probe to assess four sites on each tooth. The four sites are the *facial* and *lingual* areas of the *marginal gingiva* and the *mesial* and *distal* areas of the *papillary gingiva*.

1. The examiner waits 30 seconds after probing before scoring.
2. Scoring is accomplished using the following criteria[34]:
   a. 0 = Healthy appearance of marginal and papillary gingiva; no bleeding occurs upon probing.
   b. 2 = Marginal and papillary gingiva appear healthy and show no change in color or swelling, but bleeding occurs from the sulcus upon probing.
   c. 2 = Bleeding upon probing and change of color caused by inflammation; no swelling or macroscopic edema is present.
   d. 3 = Bleeding upon probing, change in color, and slight edematous swelling occur.
   e. 4 = (1) Bleeding upon probing, change in color, and obvious swelling occur.
       (2) Bleeding upon probing and obvious swelling occur.
3. The scores for the four areas on each tooth are totaled and divided by 4. The SBI is determined by totaling the scores for all individual teeth and dividing by the number of teeth.

Consideration. The amount of pressure applied during probing to identify sulcular bleeding may vary between 3 and 130 g among different examiners[35]; therefore, the scores may be inconsistent between examiners, and true findings are not reported.

Periodontal Index

The **Periodontal Index (PI)** has been utilized since the mid-1950s when Russell introduced it. This combined index was used to assess both gingivitis and periodontitis and employed only visual assessment without the application of a probe.[38] This index is impractical under the current level of knowledge regarding the development of periodontitis. The PI is mentioned only because of its historical significance.

The **Periodontal Disease Index (PDI)** is a modification of the PI and was developed by Ramfjord in the late 1950s.[39] The important modification was the separation of the assessments of gingivitis and periodontitis. However, owing to the combination of gingivitis and periodontitis, the PDI met a similar fate to that of the PI. Neither the PDI nor the PI is currently used in clinical trial examinations. However, the PDI did provide a method for assessing the loss of periodontal attachment, which is the main concern in the current periodontal clinical trials.

Ramfjord designed the **Loss of Periodontal Attachment (LPA)** assessment as part of the PDI to determine the amount of attachment loss around either all teeth or a selected six teeth.[39] The **six teeth are the maxillary right first molar, left central incisor, left first premolar, mandibular left first molar, right central incisor, and right first premolar.**

Process

Use a millimeter probe to measure pocket depth and loss of periodontal attachment on each of six sites on either each tooth or the six teeth that were selected.

1. Measure from the gingival crest to the base of the pocket (pocket depth) and record the score. (A)
2. Measure from the gingival crest to the cementoenamel junction and record the score. (B)
3. Subtract (B) from (A) to obtain the loss of periodontal attachment value.

Consideration. Although the LPA is currently the most effective method to assess periodontal disease, it has two disadvantages[8]:

1. The length of time that it takes to assess attachment loss during clinical trials. The time frame ranges from 30 to 40 minutes in a fully dentulous mouth.
2. The LPA assesses previous disease activity as opposed to current disease.

Community Periodontal Index of Treatment Needs

The World Health Organization (WHO) developed the **Community Periodontal Index of Treatment Needs (CPITN)** in the early 1980s to establish an index to screen periodontal treatment needs in large groups and provide prevalence and severity data on periodontal conditions.[40, 41] The index combines an assessment of gingival health, pocket depth, and the presence of supragingival and subgingival calculus and reports the findings as one score.[40]

Process

1. Use the CPITN probe: 0.5-mm ball at the tip and marked with black striations between the 3.5-mm and 5.5-mm markings. The ball is intended to provide comfort and prevent the penetration of the base of an inflamed pocket.
2. The mouth is divided into sextants. Participants who are 20 years of age or older are probed around all first and second molars, the maxillary right central incisor, and the mandibular left central incisor. Participants who are 19 years of age or younger will not have the second molars examined.
3. The following codes and criteria[42] are applied:
   0 = healthy gingiva
   1 = bleeding upon gentle probing
   2 = calculus felt during probing but all the black striated area of the probe is visible
   3 = pocket 4 or 5 mm (gingival margin located within the black striated area of the probe
   4 = pocket >6 mm (black area of the probe is not visible)
4. Using the results of the assessment, the most severe code is translated into a **treatment category**[42]:
   0 = no treatment [code 0 (see earlier)]
   I = improved oral hygiene (code 1)
   II = improved oral hygiene and débridement (codes 2 and 3)
   III = Improved oral hygiene, débridement, and complex treatment (code 4)

Considerations. Detractions of the CPITN include concern regarding the combination of calculus, pocket depth, and gingival health. This combination does not reflect the current theory of periodontal disease. Another concern deals with the failure of the CPITN to accurately measure attachment loss.

Plaque and Calculus Index

The primary **plaque and calculus** index used for community program needs assessment is the **Silness and Loe Plaque Index (PLI)**. It is a useful measure of plaque at the gingival margin. Whereas other plaque indices measure plaque on all surfaces, the PLI measures plaque in an area that has more specific implications for oral health.

Process

1. The examiner uses a mirror, light, and explorer to assess the plaque. A disclosing solution may also be used if the examination conditions permit.
2. Four surfaces of each tooth (i.e., mesial, distal, facial, and lingual) are examined for thickness of plaque at the gingival margin.
3. The amount of plaque may be identified only by what may be seen as a probe is moved across the tooth surface or by disclosing solution.
4. Criteria[8, 34, 43]:
   0 = No plaque in the cervical third
   1 = A film of plaque adhering to the free gingival margin and adjacent area of the tooth

2 = Moderate accumulation of soft deposits within the gingival pocket, on the gingival margin, or adjacent tooth surface, which can be seen by the naked eye

3 = Abundance of soft matter within the gingival pocket or on the gingival margin and adjacent tooth surface

5. PLI score is obtained by totaling four plaque scores per tooth. Divide the score by four to obtain the individual tooth PLI. To obtain the PLI score for the person, total the PLI scores for all teeth and divide by the number of teeth examined. The PLI may be determined for a segment or a group of teeth.

6. Interpretation of scores:
0 = Excellent
0.1 - 0.9 = Good
1 - 1.9 = Fair
2 - 3 = Poor

PROGRAM PLANNING PROCESS

Three areas within a community require dental expertise as part of the **community program planning process**:

1. Developing community **health policy** regarding community oral health needs and programs
2. Contributing to community **decision-making**
3. Developing community **oral health programs**

One of the most long-lasting influences that oral health professionals may have on a community is to take an active role in developing health policies. *Policy development* leads to the acquisition of funds and other resources for programs and events. As in the case of community water fluoridation, the community governing body may choose to implement the process in one of two ways: **mandate** (governmental order) or **referendum** (i.e., putting to a vote). The likelihood of successful implementation is greatest when the governing body chooses to adopt the process without putting the question to a vote. Therefore, the role of the oral health planner is to actively work with the governing body to provide the governing body with the information that will support the group in selecting the mandate strategy over the referendum. Planners should also participate with businesses, other employers, and unions to help define employee benefits policies that include appropriate coverage for oral health services for the employee and the employee's dependents.

Communities are faced with various decisions regarding oral health issues. Dental professionals may provide support to groups such as volunteer community agencies or groups, philanthropic foundations, state legislative bodies, and others in the *decision-making* process. Volunteer community agencies such as the United Way provide funding for many different initiatives and services throughout the community. Working with United Way to seek integration of oral health within the planning of different agencies can have a broad-based impact on the community. Philanthropic foundations and organizations seek ways to spend money on what they consider to be important projects. Provision of decision-making support for these groups can lead to more financial assistance within the community. Finally, the active participation of oral health professionals is needed to provide support to state legislative bodies that are reviewing programs for maternal and child health, people with disabilities, senior citizens, and others. This is necessary to ensure that these and other *at-risk* groups receive the oral health services and programs that will help them maintain optimal oral health.

In the case of community oral health program planning, the professional must possess a variety of skills. (Chapter 16 described these skills in detail.) Many different planning models have been used over time and have evolved into the models that are currently in favor. Like the models that preceded them, the current models will change as new theories and approaches are developed. When reviewing various models, consistent components appear throughout. Pickett and Hanlon conducted a review, and they describe the **composite planning process** as a dynamic cyclical process that generally includes the following:

1. Statement of a goal
2. Listing of problems in attaining the goal
3. Definition of objectives
4. Exploration of various methods for meeting the objectives
5. Selection of the method to use during implementation of the program
6. Program implementation
7. Program evaluation

The process usually includes a feedback component that continuously informs the planner of the need to readjust goals and address problems, objectives, methods, and priorities.[6]

This section describes the components of three program planning models: the **PRECEDE/PROCEED Model,** the **Braden-Herban Model,** and the **Jong Model**. The **PRECEDE/PROCEED Model** is the most commonly used model in health promotion and health education planning. The **Braden-Herban Model** is a systems approach and is also the *nursing* model for community planning. This model has components that are especially useful in community oral health planning. The **Jong Model** is also a systems approach to planning community oral health programs. These models have similar components, but they individually provide a process that gives planners a slightly different approach to program planning. Planners of community oral health programs should keep in mind that the community will dictate what planning approach is used. The planner's job is to identify which components from a variety of available models will *fit* the community or are *acceptable* to the community.[4] The task will be to select appropriate planning approaches from various models and merge them into a planning process for the specific community.

PRECEDE/PROCEED Model

This model is a combination of two models that provide a framework with which to apply many of the behavioral change theories presented in Chapter 16 to community-based program planning. The first model PRECEDE is an acronym for *Predisposing, Reinforcing,* and *Enabling Constructs in Educational Diagnosis and Evaluation.* This model is used to assist the planners in diagnosing the educational needs of a community in order to **create behavioral change** in community members. The second model PROCEED is also an acronym that stands for *Policy, Regulatory,* and *Organizational Constructs in Educational and Environmental Development.* This model was added because research demonstrated that educational interventions alone were inadequate in effecting behavioral change. **Figure 17-4** outlines the components of the model, which is a nine-phase process that begins with the hypothesis that health behaviors are complex, multidimensional, and influenced by numerous factors.[44] One of the fundamental concepts of the model is attending to the **community organization principle** of *participation.* The model encourages the participation of community members throughout every phase of planning, implementation, and evaluation.

The first two phases deal with **social and epidemiologic diagnosis.** During these phases, the planners examine the community to learn what the primary health concerns are, which health issues have the highest priorities for members of the community, and how community concerns are related to quality of life issues within the community. This information helps planners to *create relevance* of the program for members of the community, thus increasing the likelihood that the program will be used by the community and that the program will be effective. An oral health problem emerging from the social and epidemiologic diagnosis might be a high caries risk in the adolescent population.

The third phase diagnoses the **behavioral and environmental** components in the community that are risk factors or causes for the problem selected in phases 1 and 2. **Behaviors** are those personal actions of the individual community members, whereas **environment** deals with factors that are external to the individual and may not be under the control of the individual. During this phase, various organizational change theories, community organization theory, and innovation diffusion theory are applied to establish a list of the behavioral and environmental factors. These factors are prioritized, then program intervention objectives are developed for the highest priority factors in order to specify the desired behavioral or environmental change.[45] Using the oral health problem identified during phases 1 and 2, the behavioral factors may be identified as high sucrose diets, whereas the environmental factors may involve a lack of communal water fluoridation, both of which lead to higher rates of caries.

The fourth phase diagnoses the **educational and organizational** factors that are part of the causes of the health problems identified in phase 3. These causes are viewed under three fac-

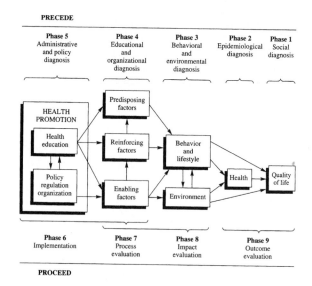

Figure 17-4. The PRECEDE-PROCEED Model for Health Promotion Planning and Evaluation. (From Green L, Kreuter M: Health Promotion Planning: An Educational and Environmental Approach, 2nd ed. Mountain View, CA, Mayfield, 1991, p 24.)

tor categories: *predisposing* (factors that make people **want to engage** in the behavior), *enabling* (factors that make it possible for people to **respond appropriately**), and *reinforcing* (factors that provide **incentives** for the new behavior to continue).[4] Adolescents who are at risk for caries might find that a *predisposing* factor could be a desire to improve their attraction to the opposite sex. Once the desire is identified, an *enabling* factor would be a multidimensional community campaign (e.g., in schools, media, dental offices/clinics) to educate adolescents with regard to the variety of personal oral disease prevention approaches to reduce or eliminate the risk of caries. Establishing a desired friendship with a member of the opposite sex may serve as a *reinforcing* factor for an adolescent.

Phase five is a diagnosis of **administrative and organizational policies,** resources, and circumstances that either enhance or detract from meeting program objectives. Planners should identify intervention strategies by considering the *resources* (e.g., time, people, funding) necessary to implement the strategies, existing *barriers* (e.g., attitudes, access to the program) to implementation and *organizational policies or regulations* (budgetary limitations and special review processes) that could effect implementation strategies. In each case, planners should develop contingency plans for dealing with each problem as well as enhancing the predisposing, enabling, and reinforcing factors identified in phase four.[45]

The PROCEED component of the model appears in phases six through nine. Phase six is the **implementation** phase. Planners must plan for the implementation; that is, to ensure a successful implementation, planners must develop a careful plan on how each intervention strategy is to be implemented and they must identify the "who, what, when, where, and how" of each strategy. Attention to these kinds of details will improve the chance of success.

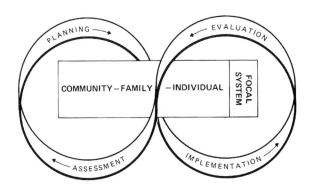

Figure 17-5. Braden-Herban System Decision-Making Planning Model. (From Braden C, Herban N: Community Health: A Systems Approach. New York, Appleton-Century-Crofts, 1976, p 59.)

Phases seven to nine describe the evaluation process. Phase seven performs the **process evaluation** that examines how successfully the plan was implemented according to the plan protocols. **Impact evaluation** occurs during phase eight. This form of evaluation explores the changes (both positive and negative) that the program has on the predisposing, enabling, and reinforcing factors as well as the behavioral, lifestyle, and environmental factors. The final phase performs an **outcomes evaluation** by assessing the effect of the program on health and quality of life indicators within the community.[45]

The PRECEDE-PROCEED Model utilizes all of the change agentry principles discussed in the beginning of the chapter. The planner(s) should have a firm grasp of these principles to effectively utilize the model to address community oral health needs.

Braden-Herban Model

The model that was presented by Braden and Herban (**Figure 17-5**) is known as the **Nursing Model**. It was designed to examine the multiple systems within the community and incorporate the social sciences into the community health planning process. Governmental and voluntary agencies are sometimes known to create a community-based program because funding is available for a specific *type* of program. The program is introduced to the community without involving community members in its development. The results of such programs are poor. The reason for poor results is that the program was *not* built upon the real and perceived needs (social factors) of the community. As has been mentioned earlier, the success of the program depends on involving the community to identify their needs. The Braden-Herban model starts at the *needs assessment* stage and includes the three remaining stages of *planning, implementation, and evaluation.*[46]

Stage I: The *needs assessment* stage requires planners to gather and analyze data on the community.

Stage II: The *planning* stage takes the information from the analysis of the needs assessment

and develops priorities, program goals and objectives, strategies, and solutions to potential problems.

Stage III: The *implementation* stage follows with the actual delivery of the program to the target population.

Stage IV: The *evaluation* stage requires continuous assessment of the program to determine whether or not program goals and objectives are being met.

The details of these stages are addressed more fully later in the chapter.

Figure 17-4 demonstrates the model as a continuous cycle of information feedback and interaction among the components of the process. For example, during the implementation stage of a sports mouthguard program, the planners learn that children are refusing to wear the appliances because they are uncomfortable and the children feel that the mouthguard makes them look "geeky." Along with a group of children, the planners will reassess what adjustment would be required to make the mouthguards more appealing in order for them to be used regularly. The new information is used to revise the program. This example demonstrates how evaluation, needs assessment, and planning can interact during the implementation stage.

The Braden-Herban model required planners to consider five issues as community health planning moves through the four stages.

1. **Costs**: How will the target population pay for services or products? How will the program contain costs to make the program affordable for all members of the community?

2. **Personpower**: Are there adequate types and numbers of personnel to conduct the program? How do we acquire and utilize the needed personnel?

3. **Using prevention to promote health**: Are prevention activities currently in place within the community? If so, what are they and how effective are they? How is prevention incorporated into the program plan?

4. **Access to care**: Can all members of the target population obtain the care necessary to maintain optimal oral health? If not, what are the barriers? How can the barriers be eliminated?

5. **Quality assurance**: How is quality built into the program? How is quality continuously improved throughout all aspects of the program?

If these five issues are kept in mind as the program is planned, implemented, and evaluated, the program will become more comprehensive, efficient, and user-friendly to members of the target population.

Jong Model

The Jong Model in **Figure 17-6** is a flowchart of the components of the planning process. The chart demonstrates the

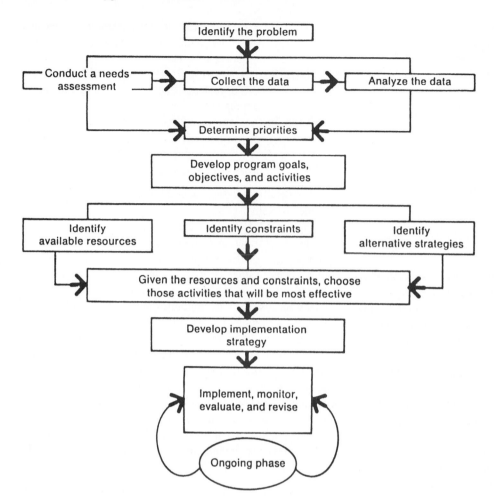

Figure 17-6. Jong Planning Model. (From Mann M: Planning for community dental programs. In Gluck G, Morganstein W (eds): Jong's Community Dental Health. St. Louis, CV Mosby, 1998, p 222.)

interactivity between the parts of the process and clearly displays the need to prepare for contingencies as barriers or constraints arise. The final component of the chart is a cycle of continuous quality improvement. The implementation process is constantly under review in order to find new ways to improve the delivery of the program.

Planning Committee Composition

As in the two previous models, the Jong model incorporates community participation in the earliest stages of plan development. Using the Diffusion/Adoption theory, inclusion of opinion leaders (i.e., members of the community who have credibility with other members of the community and who are generally in the early adopter category) within the initial planning process will help the planner to answer the following questions:

1. How will the natural distrust for something and someone(s) foreign to the community be handled?
2. How will we build support for the program once it is designed?
3. How will we account for failures of previous community health programs and encourage participation in a new program?

4. How will community members be encouraged to participate?
5. How will the assessment be conducted?

This series of questions should be addressed in the initial planning phase; otherwise, the program will be fraught with political, cultural, social, and financial barriers. The primary concern is to include people within the community or target population when defining the oral health problem, establishing priorities, and developing program objectives and strategies.[44]

Using a community organization principle, the planning committee should have representation from all sectors of the community, including oral health and medical professionals, populations with special needs, local government, public and private schools, volunteer agencies, clergy, law enforcement, social service agencies, media, businesses, community service organizations, youth, parents, and senior citizens. This broad representation provides the foundation for thorough:

1. Problem identification as well as serving as a recruiting (diffusion) mechanism for the developed program
2. Prioritization of risks and needs
3. Development of program goals, objectives, and strategies
4. Identification of community resources, program barriers and constraints, and suggestions for alternative strategies
5. Evaluation methodology

Use of Risk and Needs Assessments to Define the Community (Target Population) and Community Oral Health Problems

A planner should know the community well in order to design a successful program. Obtaining an appropriate overview of the community involves examining the community from many different aspects. The first step in defining the community is to **identify the target population.** This is the group within the community for whom the program will be developed to serve. Once the target population is selected, a community risk and needs assessment must be developed and completed. The assessment will have four outcomes[47, 48]:

1. The **problem will be defined,** and the extent and severity of the problem will be identified for the planning group.
2. **Risks** to the oral health of the individual and the community **will be identified** to help planners target members of the community who are at highest risk for oral disease, thus targeting programs that have potential for the highest degree of community impact.
3. A **profile of the community will be developed** so that a clear understanding of the target population is created, then goals, objectives, and strategies are developed that are specific to the community.
4. A **baseline of data is identified** and is used to evaluate the effectiveness of the program.

The risk and needs assessment requires the planner to examine the population in pertinent detail to fully understand the *who, what, when, where, why,* and *how* of the population. This is the most important component of the planning process. An accurate risk and needs assessment provides the foundation for the development of a successful community oral health program. A **risk** is the individual or community characteristic that puts an individual in jeopardy of oral disease or a negative oral condition. For example, youth football players who play without mouthguards could incur in oral injuries, or the lack of communal water fluoridation increases the likelihood of caries in permanent dentitions. **Need** can be defined as a condition that is deemed to be undesirable by public consensus.[49] **Demand,** on the other hand, implies the health-seeking behaviors of a population. Those individuals who have routinely demanded dental care have changed their needs from repair to prevention. Unfortunately, a large segment of the population does not seek dental care and their needs remain unmet.

The assessment provides the planner with the information needed to describe the population (**community profile**) according to age range, educational level, socioeconomic level, religious backgrounds, ethnicity, gender make-up, and any other demographic and sociocultural characteristics deemed important to help the planner understand what will be necessary to create a successful program for the target population.

Demographic information may be obtained from existing records through sources such as the most recent census reports, local chamber of commerce, United Way, library, health department, economic development council, and other local government agencies. The **oral health status** of the community should be assessed either by actual clinical examination; review of client records; or review of local, regional, or national oral health surveys. Additionally, the **assessment** should identify the public and private medical and oral health systems within the community and should provide a description of the patterns, incidence, and distribution of oral disease within the community. The assessment should also provide information to understand what the gaps are in oral health knowledge, attitudes, values and practices and the issues that the program will need to address in order to be successful. The results of this part of the assessment along with information regarding the general health status of the population will provide a **risk appraisal,** demonstrating which part(s) of the population are at greatest risk for oral disease. In addition, the planner should learn what services/programs currently exist, the level of existing participation, and the reason why people do or do not choose to participate. The planner should also find out if the communal water supply is fluoridated; if there is an integrated health education program in the schools; if there is a clinic for low-income residents; and so forth. In addition to services, the planner should discover what health laws or regulations exist within the community. What is the political configuration of the community? How are community decisions made regarding health initiatives? How are funds allocated for community-based programs? What nonpublic funding sources exist within the community? How can the planning committee make use of these funding sources? What resources exist in the community to conduct a program? The planner should also find out what dental facilities (i.e., public and nonpublic) and personnel are available; what dental practitioners participate in Medicaid and Maternal and Child Health Programs; what trained administrative staff are on hand;, and what additional facilities and transportation exist within the community that can support a program. Resource assessment information will aid in the development of the budget for the program. The planners will learn what is available, then they can prioritize the necessary resources.

The review should examine what needs assessments or health programs have taken place in the past and also what the outcomes were. The success or failure of programs should be monitored to determine whether all assessments were followed up after needs were identified and whether the programs were successful. Communities that have a history of needs assessments without programs to follow-up will be less likely to participate in the needs assessment process. The same is true if programs were unsuccessful historically in diffusing the program throughout the community. Program participation rates will be poor.

The assessment should include questions to community members regarding what they believe their oral health needs are as well as questions that identify the community members' perception of their needs. This is a crucial component because the community will *not* participate in the program unless the people think that the program is meeting a their personal needs.

In summary, the **needs assessment** involves an examination of personal attitudes, values, beliefs, and practices; general and oral health status; political structure; religious affiliations and practices; socioeconomic status; cultural composition; employment configuration; safety and welfare issues; transportation options; preschool through higher education options; school health education programs; cost of living; gender, race and ethnicity numbers and ratios; housing situations; income and poverty levels; family and household characteristics; public and non-public health care availability (medical, dental and mental) and accessibility; transportation options; community support for healthcare; current and previous government or privately funded programs; previous experiences and outcomes with community health programs; and political, social and cultural scenes of the community. **All assessment information will allow the planner to design a program that focuses on community characteristics and the primary community oral health risks and needs rather than developing a program based on the planner's perception of the group's needs or a "feel good" program that has little relevance to the community.**

In addition, the planning group should be aware of the results of any previous risks or needs assessments conducted on the target population. These results may be useful in the current assessment. If costs prohibit use of certain assessment tools, the group may seek collaboration with other health care agencies or groups that need population information. This strategy may reduce the costs and provide a more comprehensive review of the community.

Data Collection

Part of the plan should include how the risks and needs assessment is conducted, what data will be collected, who will collect the data, how data will be collected and processed, what costs will be incurred and what funding exists, and how data will be analyzed and reported. The type of data and the manner of collection should be determined well ahead of the data collection step. The assistance of a statistician in this step will clarify the process and reduce the time required to complete the data collection. **Pilot testing** the collection method is useful, because it allows the collection team to see any flaws and make corrections before the actual process begins. Pilot testing eliminates the need to repeat steps to collect missing data or redo the process because incorrect data were collected. However, even in the best-developed plans, when unforeseen information arises, additional data may have to be gathered to clarify the new information. In this case, the collection team will need to follow up on the new information with further data collection efforts.

Data may be either **subjective** or **objective.** *Subjective* data are collected in a manner that may incorporate bias into the process and will not be considered valid or reliable. Data collection usually depends on testing one or more of the five senses. What does the researcher see, hear, smell, taste, or feel about the community that provides the information necessary to create the community profile? *Objective* data are collected using methods that are consistent with scientific research principles and are considered valid and reliable. The results of subjective data are not repeatable, whereas objective data results are repeatable in collection processes of similar groups or when collected on the same subjects by different examiners. Demographic data provided through governmental reports are objective data. Chapter 18 describes these distinctions in more detail.

Tools for Risk and Needs Assessment

To adequately conduct a risk and needs assessment, planners should be aware of the tools and processes available to them to facilitate the collection of data. Data may be collected first hand (*primary data*), or existing data sources (*secondary data*) may be used. The assessment may include only one of the following activities; however, for the best results, the planner should use a combination of activities:

1. **Structured interview** with a sample of the population or with the opinion leader(s) or the supervisor of the population. The process is usually conducted on a one-to-one basis and may be either face-to-face or by telephone. Depending on the design of the interview, this strategy may be either subjective or objective. If different interviewers obtain the same results, it is objective; otherwise, the technique is subjective. **Advantage**: The interviewer is able to obtain significant detail and follow-up on information as it is stated. Technique allows the interviewer to obtain most in-depth information on a target population. **Disadvantage**: Interviews are time consuming; furthermore, if the population is large, increased personnel are required. Therefore, the structured interview is one of the more costly processes. Costs are decreased if the interview is conducted solely with community opinion leaders or the supervisor of the target population (e.g., Director of Nursing in a nursing home). Self-reporting is susceptible to exaggeration and may create overestimation of the positive behaviors of the population. Research indicates that self-reporters often report what they believe the interviewer may want to hear rather than the truth.

2. **Focus groups** conducted with selected community members. The *facilitator* (trained professional experienced in focus group process) of the process is able to use predetermined questions and provide additional questions based on responses. Usually the group size is limited to six to eight members to allow for in-depth discussions on the areas of interest. Group members are encouraged to

elaborate on each other's comments with the intention of developing the best information base. A recorder is used to take notes on the responses of the group members. This allows the facilitator to focus on the group and the process. Structured interview subjectivity and objectivity criteria apply to the focus group. **Advantage:** Results can be exceptional if the process is facilitated appropriately. Process yields in-depth information corroborated by members of the community who possess credible knowledge of the community. **Disadvantage:** Similar to the interview, because the process can be costly. If the group members are selected inappropriately, the results may be less than satisfactory; therefore, group selection is critical to the process. The same is true for selection of the facilitator.

3. **Direct observation** of the behaviors of the target population. The structured interview subjectivity and objectivity criteria apply to the direct observation technique. **Advantage**: The observer is able to determine the actual practices of the population. Technique is especially effective for institutional or school populations. **Disadvantage:** Similar to interview, the technique is time consuming and may be costly.

4. **Questionnaire/survey** distributed to the target population. The structured interview subjectivity and objectivity criteria apply to the questionnaire/survey. Use of standardized questions in the survey will increase the objectivity of the technique. **Advantage:** The planner reaches a greater number of people within the target population at the lowest cost; therefore, a greater amount of information on the population is accumulated. **Disadvantage:** The technique does not allow for follow-up on responses to specific questions, thus the planner does not receive the detail acquired from an interview.

5. **Oral examinations/screenings/epidemiologic surveys** conducted on a sample of the target population. This is an objective data collection technique. **Advantage:** The planner acquires specific information on the oral health status of the target population. **Disadvantage:** Like the interview and direct observation techniques, the oral examination is time consuming, numerous personnel are required, and the project is costly to operate.

6. **Dental histories** collected on the target population. The structured interview subjectivity and objectivity criteria apply to dental histories. **Advantage:** The planner obtains a broad scope of oral health background information on the dental experiences of the target population. **Disadvantage:** The method of obtaining information may be disadvantageous. If the dental history is obtained through a **questionnaire** or **interview**, the same disadvantages apply for each technique (as stated earlier).

As described in Chapter 18, professional personnel should be trained and calibrated in the protocol used to collect dental indices data. The intention is to reduce examiner bias and increase **inter-rater and intra-rater reliability**. Once the dental indices and general assessment data are collected, this information must be organized and categorized in a manner that will enhance the analysis process. Data on risks is separated from that of needs, thus providing clarity throughout the analysis. Appropriate tools such as computer hardware and statistical software should be available to the data collection group. Again, the statistician should provide assistance in determining which software is the best to perform the required tasks. If funding is unavailable, the planning group should include a member from a local college, university, or community organization who may be able to access these systems and reduce or eliminate the cost to the project.

Data Analysis

Once the data are collected, a statistician can help to **interpret the data** and will thus provide the planning group with a means of clarifying all the numbers and facts. The statistician will recommend statistical tests to apply to the data and will offer recommendations on the presentation and interpretation of the data. The purpose is to design the presentation so that the data become an information source and the planning team can then scrutinize the data and make decisions about the nature of the true risks and needs and how to position each on a list of community priorities. A caveat in the analysis stage is to keep in mind what the community members identified as their needs and ensure that these reported needs are attended to somewhere within the program plan.

Data presentation assumes many forms. Data can be placed in graphs, histograms, flow charts, maps of the geographic area displaying associated data, tables of statistics, and so forth. The important point is that the method(s) chosen should be the one(s) that present(s) the information in the clearest, most concise manner. The organization of the data is critical. The data displayed should separate **community demographics** into a section; **medical and oral health status** into another; **community knowledge, attitudes, values, and practices** into another; and, public and nonpublic **systems and access** into another. This allows the planning committee to easily view the data and translate it into the information needed to distinguish risks from needs and thus make decisions. The analysis allows relationships to be defined between and among the variables within the community. Is there a high caries rate, no communal water fluoridation, or no sealant utilization? Is there a high prevalence of oral cancer among teenage smokeless tobacco users? Is there a high prevalence of low-birthweight babies born to mothers with periodontitis? The analysis demonstrates where the problems are and helps the planning group to further target the needs to be addressed in the program.

During this stage, in order to ensure that the program "fits" with the sociocultural aspects of the community, collaboration should be sought with a social scientist when interpreting and analyzing the survey data. This individual will also serve as an excellent resource when designing program objectives and strategies.[10]

The final aspect of analysis is the **development of priorities** for both the needs and the risks. Prioritization is a difficult process because of the complex nature of communities. People hold different viewpoints and have personal agendas that may interfere in the prioritization process. Therefore, the committee must agree on the criteria that will be used to develop the priority list. The planning committee, with strong community representation, examines the list of needs and the related risk factors and makes decisions based on the severity (i.e., morbidity and mortality rates) of the disease or condition across the community. The decision-making goal is three-fold:

1. To reduce or eliminate the risk of dental disease or injury to the target population
2. To meet the oral health needs of the target population
3. To address the oral health objectives in *Healthy People 2010,* when the need exists

The prioritization process can become very sophisticated with the use of formulas to create the list. However, in general, planning committees will examine the following when establishing priorities:

1. Factors that **affect the greatest number of people**
2. Factors that may **contribute to death**
3. The **debilitating quality of the problem**
4. The **degree of risk to a specific population**
5. The **preventability or controllability of the disease** or condition

Community resources (e.g., funding, personnel, facilities) will help to determine the reasonableness of a priority and the extent to which a problem can be addressed in the planning stage.

The results of the analysis are **reported** to several components of the community. Therefore, different reports should be generated and targeted specifically to the group who will receive the report. Members who will fund and implement the program will require a detailed report, whereas those who serve in a supportive role (e.g., local dental or dental hygiene associations and special interest groups who represent the target population) will need summaries of the assessment process.[49]

Finally, the assessment process should be **evaluated** to determine whether the assessment team obtained the necessary data in the appropriate manner, and also whether the team learned what it needed to learn. Changes for future risk and needs assessments should be identified and reported to ensure the best results for future assessments.[49]

Create Program Goals, Objectives, and Activities

Upon completion of the list of priorities, the planning committee must develop program goals and specific objectives in order to meet the goals. This stage establishes the structure that the program will take. Once the priorities are es-

tablished, the planner's task is to work with the planning committee to develop **goals** that are reasonable and achievable for the target population. Goals are described as[7]:

1. Broad statements of purpose
2. More encompassing and global than objectives
3. Written to cover all aspects of a program
4. Providing the overall direction for the program
5. More general in nature than objectives
6. Usually taking longer to complete than objectives
7. More easily measured than objectives

Program **objectives** provide the *specifics on how the program will achieve the goals*. The most important aspect of an objective is that it is measurable. It must also be within the scope of the community (does the community have the resources to meet the objective), must be acceptable to the community (culturally acceptable), and it must be legal.[46] The components of a *program* objective (differs from *learning* objectives described in Chapter 16) include[47]:

1. **What:** the nature of the situation or condition to be achieved
2. **Extent:** the scope and magnitude of the situation or condition to be achieved
3. **Who:** the specific group or segment of the environment in which achievement is desired
4. **Where:** the geographic boundaries of the program
5. **When:** The time frame for achieving the desired situation or condition

If the objective is appropriately structured, it will allow the program staff and the funding agency and other interested parties to determine during the evaluation stages whether or not the program was successful.

The next step is to develop **activities** that will lead to the attainment of the program goals and objectives. In most cases, multiple activities will be necessary to accomplish a single objective. The more methods used to address a single problem, the more likely it is that the problem will be resolved.[7] However, the number of activities will be determined by the length of the program and the availability of resources (e.g., personnel, equipment, facilities, and funding).[27] The actual selection of activities follows a process of brainstorming to develop a list of possibilities. The *Criteria for Successful Programs* should be used as well as the following criteria[6] when evaluating each activity:

1. Compatibility with the culture of the target population and the personnel
2. Budget availability
3. Proven effectiveness
4. Available resources

Mann suggests that resources should be assessed using the following criteria[47]:

1. **Appropriateness:** most suitable resource to get the job done
2. **Adequacy:** the extent or degree to which the resources would complete the job

3. **Effectiveness**: how capable the resources are at completing the job
4. **Efficiency**: the dollar cost and amount of time expended to complete the job

During the selection process, the committee should also identify any **constraints or barriers** to implementing the activity. Within the community, what barriers will prevent this particular activity from being successful in achieving the program objective? These might include conditions such as organizational policies, resource limitations, or community characteristics. Community oral health programs have identified constraints, such as limitations of the state's dental practice act; nonsupportive attitudes of professional organizations; lack of funding; restrictive governmental policies; inadequate transportation systems; personnel shortages; lack of or inadequate facilities; negative community attitudes toward prevention programs or dentistry; community socioeconomic, cultural, and educational status; time limitations for completing the program; lack of a communal fluoridated water supply; and poor oral health status.[47] If the planning committee is unable to diminish or eliminate constraints in order to implement a specific activity, an **alternative activity** with limited or no constraints should be selected.

Once the selection of activities is made, the planning committee should formulate activity statements under each objective. Activities should have three components[47]:

1. What is going to be done?
2. Who is going to do it?
3. When it will be done?

This portion of the plan provides the action steps to be completed, the person or persons accountable for the action, and the time frame to complete the action. The activities become a major portion of the implementation plan that is described later.

The following statements could be developed subsequent to a needs assessment of a community school district:

1. **Problem**: the high caries rate in permanent molars of school children
2. **Priority Statement**: to reduce the caries rate in permanent molars of school children
3. **Goal Statement**: to develop a school sealant program in the highest risk schools across the school district
4. **Objective Statement**: by the end of the third year reduce the caries rate in permanent molars by 50% within the selected schools in school district X (addresses Healthy People 2000 Oral Health Risk Reduction Objective 13.1 and draft Objective 9.9 for 2010)[12, 50]
5. **Activity Statement Number One**: by August 15, 2001, three dentists will be contracted to perform initial diagnosis and follow-up evaluations on 1500 students in the sealant program of school district X.
6. **Activity Statement Number Two**: by August 15, 2001, three dental hygienists and three dental assistants will be hired to apply sealants, which are diagnosed to be appropriate for sealant applications, on the permanent molars of students in school district X.

Program Implementation

The plan is now ready for implementation. As does the planning process, implementation requires strategies. The strategy is the *implementation plan,* which should account for the following: how all of the activities are to be implemented and in what order; which materials, media, methods, and techniques will be used; what specific funds are to be used; and who will monitor the implementation process.[47] To ensure a smooth-flowing implementation, it is useful to conduct a pilot test of the program at least once and sometimes more than once.[51] This trial run of the program gives the implementation coordinator the opportunity to try out the program on a few individuals or at least on a small scale to obtain feedback on how successful the different strategies are going to be. Improvements can be made as a result of the pilot test before the program is implemented on a community-wide basis. The coordinator may learn that different resources are needed, more or different training is required for personnel, or different educational strategies need to be used. If these changes are minor, adjustments can be made without testing the strategy again. However, if major changes take place, pilot testing would be advisable to determine whether it will run smoothly on a larger scale.

Program Evaluation

How well has the program met the individual and community needs or reduced the risks for oral disease and injury? This question and many others are part of the program evaluation process. **Evaluation** is conducted to *ensure the funding agents* that their money is being spent wisely and to *improve* the program. Program improvement is critical to the life of any program. Programs should be dynamic and should continue to address the issues that are relevant to the community; otherwise, these programs become stagnant and die from non-use.

The evaluation process should be *nonthreatening* to program personnel, *timely* in its implementation, and *ethical* in its process. If the evaluation process is incorporated at the start of the program and it is known as an integral part of the program, personnel are more likely to accept it. If personnel see improvement resulting from the process, evaluation is not as likely to be viewed as threatening. If the evaluation is conducted in a timely manner it provides information that may be used to improve the process before significant damage is done to the program. Some program directors may feel pressure from political arenas to demonstrate positive evaluations and may be urged to develop an evaluation process that examines only the positive aspects of the program. To do so is unethical and may lead ultimately to discontinuation of the program once the facts are known. Ethical conduct is a crucial component of the evaluation process.[4]

Program planners incorporate a continuous evaluation process in the program plan to assess developmental aspects of the program. **Formative** evaluation is done during the planning and implementing processes to improve or refine the program. Determining the validity and reliability of the risk and needs assessment and pilot testing the program plan are forms of formative evaluation. **Summative** evaluation is performed at the completion of the program to determine the impact of the program on the target population. The first step is to develop the goals and objectives. Measurement of program outcomes against goals and objectives provides the answer to the question stated at the beginning of this section. How well has the program met the individual and community needs or reduced the risks for oral disease and injury? This is the foundation for summative evaluation. Once implementation is completed, summative evaluation is conducted.[7] The crucial aspect of both formative and summative evaluation is the development of an evaluation plan. The plan should include the person accountable for conducting both types of evaluations; the types of data that are to be collected; the person who is to collect, analyze, and report the data; the person who is accountable for implementing change based on the evaluation results; and the time frame for conducting the evaluation process.

Using Media in Program Planning and Promotion

It is useful to examine the use of media by health promotion professionals in delivering messages to communities with the purpose of changing health behavior. Media have been found to be the *most* effective at raising *awareness* and *interest* of health issues[6] but also effective at the remaining stages of the adoption process (i.e., *appraisal, trial, and adoption*).[52] Health promotion research has shown that media are powerful partners in shaping community opinions, values, and norms.[7] The best results occur when planners carefully match the media, the message, and the target group. For example, it serves no purpose to use English in the media approach when the target population is a group of Russian-speaking immigrants. **Figure 17-7** lists the various mass media methodologies from which to select when determining which will meet the needs of the target group and the message.[4] Careful consideration of these options should increase the likelihood of a successful media effort. An example of careful planning was reported by Black[53] regarding the 1989 *Partnership For A Drug-Free America* media campaign (involving television, newspaper, magazine, and radio) that used the *frying egg* analogy to demonstrate "your brain on drugs." The result was a 33% decline in marijuana use and a 15% decrease in cocaine use between 1988 and 1989 in markets thoroughly covered by the media campaign. Compared with similar areas without the campaign, the results were 15% and 2%, respectively, thus demonstrating that the campaign created a substantial reduction in the use of both types of drugs. The use of media can also have a negative impact on the audience, which was evidenced by the Joe Camel campaign. Using print media, billboards, clothing advertisements, and various product promotions, R. J. Reynolds increased the Camels market share among youth from about 3% in 1988 to 13% in 1993. This increase in the youth market was attributed to adolescents being about three times more sensitive/susceptible to advertising than were adults.[54]

The goals of media-based oral health initiatives are to educate the public about oral health prevention measures, to reduce individual and community risk factors, and present new community oral health initiatives. To accomplish these goals, it is suggested that the campaigns continue over long periods of time, appeal to multiple motives (*personal and public*), be combined with social support, and provide training in requisite skills.[55] Broadening the approach provides multiple stimuli to encourage participation in the program. In addition, the use of multiple approaches utilizes the principle of **synergy**; that is, the *effect of the whole is greater than the sum of the effects of the parts.* When strategies are combined, they can be more powerful in accomplishing behavioral change than if these strategies were used alone.[56] This means that for a campaign to succeed, mass media must be teamed with some form of individual interaction such as a classroom educational activity and other strategies. This allows the program to utilize the strengths of as many strategies as are reasonable. Repetition is also an important consideration in developing the plan. The impact of mass media is through a cumulative effect and is not caused by a single exposure.[56]

Multidimensional approaches are important for another reason. Unidimensional media approaches are unsuccessful because not all or even a significant part of the target group will see or hear the message. The important principle to follow *is to get the message to where the people are.* Planners must identify the locations where the greatest number of the target population congregate, reside, recreate, or work. Messages should be delivered to a variety of these locations. Even when the target population does receive the message, it is important to recognize that not all people will receive it at the same time. The rate of message reception varies by socioeconomic status of the individual or general community and the size of the community. The lower the socioeconomic status and the larger and more complex the community, the slower will be the transmission of the message. Large communities tend to have more complex communication systems; therefore, it takes longer for the message to work through the systems.[56] Consideration of these issues when planning media strategies will allow for the oral health message to be received by all socioeconomic groups, thus expanding the impact of the campaign.

Within the planning process, the committee must determine whether the message should be delivered either through face-to-face communication or through mass media communication. Breckon[4] recommends that the following criteria should be applied:

Method	Advantages	Disadvantages
Computer—Internet	Easy access, downloading, access to related information.	Must be sought out, competition, complex Web connections.
Television/Radio Public service announcements News coverage Feature presentations Consultations	Reaches the broadest segment of the population; can direct audience to other sources.	Information may be insufficiently detailed for particular target groups.
Newspapers Feature stories News coverage Advertisements	Provides greater detail than radio or TV.	Does not reach as many people in each group.
Posters Billboards Buses and trucks Public facilities	Can reach specific populations; can direct audience to additional sources of information and complement other methodologies by reinforcing various other messages.	Provides only limited amounts.
Brochures/Flyers Inserts in utility bills Health care facilities Workplace	Messages can be appropriately individualized.	May be less effective for some target groups.
Newsletters/Journals Organization newsletters Health problems updates	Messages can be appropriately individualized, detailed, and complex messages sent to segments of the population.	The longer and more complex the document, the less likely it is to be read.
Resource materials Guidelines School curriculum materials Reprints and resource directories	Provides technical information to specific target groups.	The longer and more complex the document, the less likely it is to be read.
Presentations Community groups Health care facilities	Specific information tailored to the group addressed; can be interactive.	Labor intensive; primarily information transfer only.
Workshops Drug treatment centers HIV workshops Smoking cessation	Provides detailed information and emphasizes skill development.	Labor intensive.
Counseling and testing	One-on-one counseling to individuals attempting to adopt or sustain positive health behaviors.	Very labor intensive.

Figure 17-7. Mass media methodologies. (From Breckon D, Harvey J, Lancaster R: Community Health Education, 4th ed. Gaithersburg, MD, Aspen, 1998, p 267.)

1. **Face-to-face**
   a. When the message is complex
   b. When the behavior change is extensive
   c. When the target group has low educational levels
   d. When long-term attitude and behavior change is desired

2. **Mass Media**
   a. When the message is simple and factual
   b. When change is similar to present practice or directed to those already motivated to change
   c. When the target group has high educational levels
   d. When desired decisions are short term

Once the decision is made to use mass media, what options exist to planners who are determining which mass media channels to use to deliver the oral health promotion message? Figure 17-7 outlines various media methodologies from which planners may select. Next to visits to dental offices and clinics where treatment is provided, public service announcements (PSAs) on television are the most important source of health information.[4] This is partly due to repeated

Keep messages short and simple—just one or two key points.

Repeat the subject as many times as possible.

Superimpose your main point on the screen to reinforce the verbal message.

Recommend performing specific behaviors.

Demonstrate the health problem, behavior, or skills (if appropriate).

Provide new, accurate, and complete information.

Use a slogan or theme.

Be sure that the message presenter is seen as a credible source of information, whether authority figure, target audience member, or celebrity.

Use only a few characters.

Select a testimonial, demonstration, or slice-of-life format.

Present the facts in a straightforward manner.

Use positive rather than negative appeals.

Use humor, if appropriate, but pretest to be sure it does not offend the intended audience.

Be sure the message is relevant to the target audience.

Figure 17-8. Guidelines for public service announcements. (From Breckon D, Harvey J, Lancaster R: Community Health Education, 4th ed. Gaithersburg, MD, Aspen, 1998, p 274.)

appearances and partly because PSAs combine sight, sound, motion, and color to maximize the impact of the message. As a program director develops the content of a public service announcement, the guidelines in **Figure 17-8** should be used to strategize the best approaches. Two additional considerations in the development of the PSA are to incorporate the most significant information in the beginning and use an attention-getting introduction. By placing the most important information first, you may ensure that the pertinent information will be shared with the audience. For space purposes, editors may eliminate part of the information, and generally they begin cutting at the end. Because most PSAs use emotional appeal, the PSA designer should use an attention-getting introduction to stimulate interest in the message.

Media selection should be done only after the target group is selected and the campaign objectives are developed. Once this is done, the media decisions are made and the message is developed to match the media and target group. The campaign should be pilot tested before it is fully implemented to determine how effective both the message and the media are in getting the information to the target group. The results of the pilot test will be used to revise the media plan.

SPECIAL POPULATIONS PROGRAMS

Community programs are delivered in various settings, such as nursing homes with patients who are medically compro-

mised; group homes for people with mental and physical disabilities; homeless populations within the community; schools for fluoride rinsing, sealant, and treatment programs; Hispanic neighborhood centers; smoking cessation programs in health care settings; nursing bottle syndrome in prenatal classes; cerebral palsy centers; programs for people with hearing impairments; and low income communities. Programs that address the specific prevention and treatment needs of any special needs community require the oral health professional to learn the specifics of the community. What makes the community special? What common characteristics do the members of the community possess? What medical conditions exist in the communities with special medical needs? In communities with special medical needs, whether they consist of homebound individuals, group homes, nursing or convalescent homebound individuals, or hospitalized individuals, the primary focus is the same. Oral health professionals will obtain the best results for individuals with special medical needs when their care is integrated with the medical, nursing, and allied health care plans. This requires significant coordination among the various health professionals, but the results will be much more significant than if oral health care is provided in isolation.

Sources

1. Knutson J: What is public health? In Pelton W, Wisan J (eds): Dentistry in Public Health. Philadelphia, WB Saunders, 1955, pp 20-29.
2. Block L: Dental public health: An overview. In Gluck G, Morganstein W (eds): Jong's Community Dental Health. St. Louis, CV Mosby, 1998, pp 3-24.
3. Bell C, Newby H: An Introduction to the Sociology of the Local Community. New York, Praeger, 1971, pp 27-53.
4. Breckon D, Harvey J, Lancaster R: Community Health Education, 4th ed. Gaithersburg, MD, Aspen, 1998, pp 56, 153, 154, 265-282.
5. Winslow C-EA: The untilled field of public health. Mo Med 2:183, 1920.
6. Pickett G, Hanlon J: Public Health: Administration and Practice, 9th ed. St. Louis, Times Mirror/Mosby, 1990, pp 6, 43, 222-228.
7. McKenzie J, Pinger R: An Introduction to Community Health, 2nd ed. Sudbury, MA, Jones and Bartlett, 1997, pp 4, 125-130.
8. Burt B, Eklund S: Dentistry, Dental Practice, and the Community, 4th ed. Philadelphia, WB Saunders, 1992, pp 29-37.
9. Harris N, Christen A: Primary Preventive Dentistry, 4th ed. Stamford, CT, Appleton & Lange, 1995, pp 414, 416.
10. Dunning J: Principles of Dental Public Health, 4th ed. Cambridge, MA, Harvard University Press, 1986, pp 50-54, 188-190.
11. Corbin S: National oral health objectives for the year 2000. J Public Health Dent 50:128-132, 1990.
12. United States Department of Health and Human Services: Healthy People 2000: National Health Promotion and Disease Prevention Objectives. DHHS Publication Number (Public Health Service) 91-50212. Washington, DC, United States Printing Office, 1990.
13. Gift H et al: The state of the nation's oral health: Mid-decade assessment of Healthy People 2000. J Public Health Dent 56:84-91, 1996.
14. United States Department of Health and Human Services: Healthy People 2010 (Conference Edition, Vols 1 and 2). Washington, DC, United States Printing Office, 2000.
15. United States Department of Health and Human Services: Oral Health in America: A Report of the Surgeon General-Executive Summary. Rockville, MD, US Department of Health and Human Services, National Institute of Dental and Craniofacial Research, National Institutes of Health, 2000.

16. Rogers E: Diffusion of Innovations, 3rd ed. New York, Free Press, 1983, pp 5, 11, 245-263.
17. Havelock R: Planning for Innovation. Ann Arbor, MI, University of Michigan, Institute for Social Research, 1969, pp 10-43.
18. Berlo D: The Process of Communication: An Introduction to Theory and Research. San Francisco, Rinehart Press, 1960, pp 40-71.
19. Oldenburg B, Hardcastle D, Kok G: Diffusion of innovations. In Glanz K, Lewis F, Rimers B (eds): Health Behavior and Health Education: Theory, Research, and Practice, 2nd ed. San Francisco, Jossey-Bass, 1997, pp 270-286.
20. Green L, Ottoson J: Community Health, 7th ed. St. Louis, CV Mosby, 1994, pp 54-57.
21. Green L, Gottlieb N, Parcel G: Diffusion theory extended and applied. In Ward WB (ed): Advances in Health Education and Promotion. Greenwich, CT, JAI Press, 1987.
22. Zaltman G, Duncan R: Strategies for Planned Change. New York, Wiley 1977, pp 12-16.
23. Green L: Diffusion and adoption of innovations related to cardiovascular risk behavior in the public. In Enelow A, Henderson J (eds): Applying Behavioral Sciences to CV Risk. New York, American Heart Association, 1975.
24. Minkler M, Wallerstein N: Improving health through community organization and community building. In Glanz K, Lewis F, Rimers B (eds): Health Behavior and Health Education: Theory, Research, and Practice, 2nd ed. San Francisco, Jossey-Bass, 1997, pp 241-269.
25. Cottrell L Jr: The competent community. In Warren R, Lyon L (eds): New Perspectives on the American Community. Florence, KY, Dorsey Press, 1983.
26. MacMahon B, Trichopoulos D: Epidemiology: Principles and Methods, 2nd ed. Boston, Little, Brown, 1996, pp 1-15.
27. DeBiase C: Dental Health Education Theory and Practice. Malvern, PA, Lea & Febiger, 1991.
28. Pendrys D: The epidemiology of oral diseases. In Gluck G, Morganstein W (eds): Jong's Community Dental Health. St. Louis, CV Mosby, 1998, pp 121-143.
29. Klein H, Palmer C, Knutson J: Studies on dental caries. I: Dental status and dental needs of elementary school children. Public Health Rep 53:751-765, 1938.
30. Katz R: Assessing root caries in populations: The evolution of the root caries index. J Public Health Dent 40:7-16, 1980.
31. Loe H, Silness J: Periodontal disease in pregnancy. I: Prevalence and severity. Acta Odontol Scand 21:533-551, 1963.
32. Woodall I: Comprehensive Dental Hygiene Care, 4th ed. St. Louis, CV Mosby, 1993, p 292.
33. Muhelmann H, Son S: Gingival sulcus bleeding: A leading symptom in initial gingivitis. Helvetica Odontol Acta 15:107, 1971.
34. Scarff A, Walsh M, Darby M: Periodontal and oral hygiene assessment. In Darby M, Walsh M: Dental Hygiene Theory and Practice. Philadelphia, WB Saunders, 1995, pp 359-398.
35. Polson A, Caton J: Current status of bleeding in the diagnosis of periodontal diseases. J Periodontol 56 (Special Issue):1-3, 1985.
36. Lobene R et al: Correlation among gingival indices: A methodology study. J Periodontol 60:159-162, 1989.
37. Lang N et al: Bleeding on probing: A predictor for the progression of periodontal disease? J Clin Periodontol 13:590-596, 1986.
38. Russell A: A system of scoring for prevalence surveys of periodontal disease. J Dent Res 35:350-359, 1956.
39. Ramfjord S: Indices for prevalence and incidence of periodontal disease. J Periodontol 30:51-59, 1959.
40. Ainamo J et al: Development of the World Health Organization (WHO) Community Periodontal Index of Treatment Needs. Int Dent J 32:281-291, 1982.
41. Lewis J, Morgan M, Wright F: The validity of the CPITN scoring and presentation method for measuring periodontal conditions. J Clin Periodontol 21:1-6, 1994.
42. World Health Organization: Oral Health Surveys Basic Methods, 3rd ed. Geneva, World Health Organization, 1987.
43. Loe H: The gingival index, the plaque index, and the retention index systems. J Periodontol 38 (Suppl):610-616, 1967.
44. Green L, Krueter M: Health Promotion Planning: An Educational and Environmental Approach, 2nd ed. Mountain View, CA, Mayfield, 1991, p 24.
45. Gielen A, McDonald E: The PRECEDE-PROCEED Planning Model. In K Glanz, Lewis F, Rimers B (eds): Health Behavior and Health Education: Theory, Research, and Practice, 2nd ed. San Francisco, Jossey-Bass, 1997, pp 359-371.
46. Braden C, Herban N: Community Health: A Systems Approach. New York, Appleton-Century-Crofts, 1976, pp 40-55, 58-131.
47. Mann M: Planning for community dental programs. In Gluck G, Morganstein W (eds): Jong's Community Dental Health. St. Louis, CV Mosby, 1998, pp 217-236.
48. Milgrom P: Oral hygiene Instruction and health risk assessment in dental practice. J Public Health Dent 49:24-31, 1989.
49. Siegal M, Kuthy R: Assessing Oral Health Needs: ASTDD Seven-Step Model. The Association of State and Territorial Dental Directors, funded by Maternal and Child Health, Arlington, Virginia, 1995.
50. United States Department of Health and Human Services: Healthy People 2010 Objectives: Draft for Public Comment. DHHS Publication (Public Health Service). Washington, DC, United States Printing Office, 1998.
51. McKenzie J, Smeltzer J: Planning, Implementing, and Evaluating Health Promotion Programs: A Primer. Boston, Allyn and Bacon, 1997, p 210.
52. Havelock R: The Change Agent's Guide to Innovation in Education. Englewood Cliffs, NJ, Educational Technology, 1973, p 170.
53. Black G: Changing Attitudes Toward Drug Use: The First Year Effort of the Media-Advertising Partnership for a Drug-Free America, Inc. Rochester, NY, Gordon S. Black, 1989.
54. DeSouza M, Kressin N: Dental health education. In Gluck G, Morganstein W (eds): Jong's Community Dental Health. St. Louis, CV Mosby, 1998, pp 177-216.
55. Silversin J, Kornacki M: Acceptance of preventive measures by individuals, institutions, and communities. Int Dent J 34:170, 1984.
56. Finnegan J Jr, Viswanath K: Communication theory and health behavior change: The media studies framework. In Glanz K, Lewis F, Rimer B (eds): Health Behavior and Health Education: Theory, Research, and Practice, 2nd ed. San Francisco, Jossey-Bass, 1997, pp 313-341.

Questions and Answers

Questions

You are employed by the local health department. The department just received a small federal grant to provide oral health services to the local homeless population. Your job is to manage the development of the project. Please use this information to answer questions 1 to 10.

1. All of the following areas need to be examined when performing a needs assessment EXCEPT one. The EXCEPTION is _____.
   A. demographics
   B. oral health status
   C. dental behaviors
   D. hereditary characteristics
   E. local transportation options

2. If funding is a problem, what strategy is the most effective in obtaining needed financial support?
   A. Partnering with other community agencies to develop a collaborative request to local foundations
   B. Approaching local business and industries requesting program funds
   C. Engaging community churches to conduct fundraising efforts
   D. Sending high school students door-to-door in the affluent parts of the community to solicit funds

3. To generate interest in the program, the program director should use which of the following communication strategies?
   A. Church bulletins announcements
   B. Radio and television PSAs
   C. Face-to-face exchanges
   D. Telemarketing
   E. Mass mailings

4. During the planning process, the planning committee desires to assess the caries status of a sample of homeless preschool children. Which of the following indices would be applied to this population?
   A. defs
   B. DMF
   C. RCI
   D. GI

5. Which community organization principle will provide the greatest success in developing the homeless oral health program?
   A. Funding can be sought from the state oral health department.
   B. Community members are able to use segments of the program without being required to participate in the full program.

C. Community members are able to determine that they have a personal role for making change in their health.
D. Members of the homeless community can participate in the planning process.

6. Which of the following is an EXCEPTION to a list of potential constraints to the success of the program?
   A. Local dental society position that existing dental community is serving the needs of the population
   B. Mobility of the population
   C. Increase in the community Free-Food Store donations
   D. Funding agency policy change on community programming
   E. Previous community needs assessment that was not followed through

7. What objective data might be obtained on the homeless population during the needs assessment?
   A. One-to-one interviews
   B. Existing survey results
   C. Telephone surveys
   D. CPITN
   E. Focus groups

8. Throughout the implementation phase of the program, evaluations are routinely conducted to determine if the program was implemented according to the plan procedures. Which of the following terms identifies this type of evaluation?
   A. Formative
   B. Impact
   C. Outcomes
   D. Summative

9. When seeking the ideal community member to serve on the planning committee, from which "innovation-adoption category" should the individual be a member?
   A. Innovator
   B. Early adopter
   C. Early majority
   D. Late majority

10. During an oral examination of a 25-year-old white man, the following data were collected: 26 teeth are present; Numbers 1, 16, 17, and 32 were extracted due to crowding; Number 9 is missing due to a hockey accident; Number 3 is missing due to decay. Eleven teeth have amalgam restorations, two of which are three-surface restorations. Three teeth have composite restorations. Four teeth were identified with active caries. One of the active caries is recurrent caries at the margin of an existing amalgam restoration. What is the DMFT score for this client?
    A. 16
    B. 18
    C. 24
    D. 28

11. Which sequence of the adoption process must an individual undergo to successfully move from smoking to smoking cessation?
    A. Awareness, interest, appraisal, and trial
    B. Awareness, interest, trial, and appraisal
    C. Interest, awareness, appraisal, and trial
    D. Interest, awareness, trial, and appraisal

12. Which of the following describes the role of risk assessment during the community program planning stage?
    A. Identifying the aspects of the individual(s) or community that put the individuals within the community at risk for dental disease
    B. Identifying areas within the community where oral/facial injuries may occur
    C. Identifying subgroups within the community for mini-program development
    D. Identifying where funds are used less effectively within the community to reduce dental disease

13. Including an opinion leader within the target population in developing the oral health program will result in which of the following?
    A. Increased confusion with regard to the needs of the group
    B. Focus on the agenda of the individual during the planning process
    C. Increased success in meeting program goals
    D. Increased interest of other community members

14. All of the following areas, EXCEPT one, are environmental factors that should be considered when conducting a caries epidemiologic study of a given population. The EXCEPTION is _____.
    A. fluoride intake
    B. place of residence during tooth formation
    C. oral hygiene habits
    D. emotional status
    E. nutrition status

15. Which of the following epidemiologic methods would best determine the amount and extent of oral cancer within a given community?
    A. Mail questionnaire to all community residents
    B. Age-adjusted annual incidence rates by gender and race
    C. Random sample telephone interviews
    D. Prevalence rates of oral candidiasis
    E. Root Caries Index rates

You are an oral health consultant to a nursing home community of 220 residents. One of the administrator's goals is to improve the oral health status of the residents. She asks you to develop a program to achieve this goal. Please use this information to answer questions 16 and 17.

16. Which of the following indices provides plaque and calculus information that will best demonstrate the oral health status of this population?
    A. Modified Gingival Index
    B. Sulcular Bleeding Index
    C. Loss of Periodontal Attachment
    D. Periodontal Disease Index
    E. Silness and Loe Plaque Index

17. The group score for the 220 residents using the index identified in question 16 is 2.3. Which of the following identifies the interpretation of the group score?
    A. Excellent plaque levels
    B. Good plaque levels
    C. Fair plaque levels
    D. Poor plaque levels
    E. Emergency care required

18. All of the following outcomes, EXCEPT one, are derived from the document **Healthy People 2010: Understanding and Improving Health.** Which of the following outcomes is the EXCEPTION?
    A. Dictates curricula for dental and dental hygiene education programs
    B. Establishes oral health goals and objectives
    C. Provides the basis for governmental funding
    D. Establishes the foundation for federal, state, and local oral health policy development

ANSWERS

1. **D.** Hereditary characteristics are insignificant in determining the oral needs of a community. All other factors are crucial in assessing the needs of the community group.

2. **A.** Merging the funding request with other agencies seeking support for initiatives strengthens all requests with community foundations. This strategy increases the likelihood of receiving additional funding.

3. **C.** The media strategy is to "go where the people are." The target group is a homeless population that has no mailing address or telephone number and moves regularly; therefore, church bulletins and PSAs are ineffective at reaching the population. The assessment group or workers in homeless shelters must locate the members of the population and speak directly to them regarding the program and its benefits.

4. **A.** The defs surveys the decayed, exfoliated, and filled surfaces of primary teeth. Similarly, any caries index using lower case letters addresses the caries experience of primary teeth.

5. **D.** Choices B and D are community organization principles. The other options are not. The foundation for success in any community health program is the inclusion of members of the target population in all phases of the planning process.

6. **C.** All other options are potential constraints at varying degrees of concern for community oral health program planners. Choice A, if strong enough, can prevent program implementation. The homeless population can be very mobile, and the tracking of participants is resource consuming. If the funding agency withdraws funds, the program will cease until other funding is secured. If a community participates in a needs assessment and the identified needs are not met through programming, future needs assessments will be met with significant resistance.

7. **D.** The only true *objective* data technique among the options is the CPITN Index. All others collect data using *subjective* methods.

8. **A.** Formative evaluations examine the process used in developing and implementing the program.

9. **B.** The types of individuals within the early adopters' category include opinion leaders and well-respected community members whose opinions are highly regarded. Early adopters generally know the community and can provide information that is invaluable in the planning process.

10. **B.** Teeth are counted only once regardless of the different surfaces involved in the caries and restorations. Teeth extracted for orthodontic purposes, which were lost due to injury, and teeth that are questionable regarding the existence of decay are not counted in the DMFT.

11. **A.** The innovation adoption process stages occur in this sequence. Adoption of new behaviors, attitudes, and values occurs most strongly when the individual goes through each stage and does so in the correct sequence. The adoption will be more long lasting as well.

12. **A.** Choices B, C, and D are useful data to collect, but the primary role of the risk assessment is to determine where risks occur and determine where the appropriate areas are for risk reduction to prevent oral disease and injury from occurring.

13. **C.** The inclusion of community opinion leaders is the most effective strategy when developing a community oral health program that meets the needs and thus the goals of a community program.

14. **D.** Emotional status is a *host* factor; that is, emotional status is part of the epidemiologic study of the *individual* presenting with the disease or condition.

15. **B.** Mailing questionnaires results in incomplete information due to a lack of accurate reporting and insufficient response rates. Random sampling telephone interviews fail to consider the entire population. Prevalence rates of oral candidiasis are *best* used to identify the prevalence of HIV. Use of the Root Caries Index would only indicate the amount of root caries within a given population.

16. **E.** The Silness and Loe Plaque Index is recommended as the best index for use to determine the oral health status of groups of people.

17. **D.** The interpretation scale for the Silness and Loe Plaque Index identifies a score of 2.3 as demonstrating *poor* levels of plaque accumulation.

18. **A.** All other options are intended outcomes of the *Healthy People 2010: Understanding and Improving Health: Oral Health Goal and Objectives* for the residents within the United States. Curricular changes *may* occur, but curricula are not *dictated* by the document.

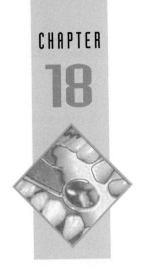

CHAPTER 18

Analyzing Scientific Information and Applying Research Results

JOAN I. GLUCH, RDH, PhD

Dental hygienists who are practicing at the start of the new millennium face many challenges from the rapidly changing health care environment and explosion of scientific information. Dental hygienists face the major challenge of assessing new information and technology to ensure that they can continue to provide dental hygiene care that is safe, effective, and appropriate for their clients' needs. These challenges are heightened in light of the increasing level of consumer expectations for high-quality practice.

In order to critically review new developments in the field, dental hygienists must have a strong knowledge base and good understanding of the role of research and the research process. Emphasis on research in dental hygiene has only occurred during the last 20 years, while the field of dental hygiene has matured to identify the need to develop a professional "body of knowledge" and a cadre of experienced researchers to expand the knowledge base.

 ## KNOWLEDGE BASE IN DENTAL HYGIENE

Dental hygiene has a strong tradition of comprehensive educational programs and has relied on traditional beliefs, expert authority, and personal experience as the major ways to develop, gather, and store knowledge about dental hygiene. Traditional beliefs shared among dentistry and dental hygiene guide many of the current dental hygiene practices, even in light of conflicting research findings. For example, the current practice of scheduling appointments for continuing dental hygiene care every 6 months is not based on research and is often inappropriate for patients who need supportive periodontal therapy on a continuing basis that is based more often on the health of their tissue. Despite re-

search evidence supporting a change in clinical practice, many dental offices continue to follow the traditional recommendation, which is based on historical practices and influenced by third party reimbursement policies. Dental hygienists have not been able to use their knowledge of the research literature to provoke a universal change in these historical practices.

The knowledge base for dental hygiene is in an early developmental phase and has borrowed extensively from the fields of dentistry, periodontics, education, and psychology. Only within the past 10 years have dental hygiene scholars developed theories and begun to build a knowledge base that is unique to dental hygiene. This is a sign of a young, developing profession, and many positive signs indicate continued expansion of dental hygiene knowledge by dental hygiene researchers.

 ## ROLE OF RESEARCH IN DENTAL HYGIENE PRACTICE

The American Dental Hygienists' Association (ADHA) has developed six roles for dental hygiene to highlight the multiple dimensions that are integral to dental hygiene practice. These six roles include **administrator/manager, clinician, educator/oral health promoter, client advocate, change agent, and researcher.** Rather than limit dental hygienists to one role, these roles were developed to display the numerous activities that are integral to the practice of dental hygiene and to help dental hygienists identify which role components are emphasized in their practices. The publication of the six roles helped to highlight the integral part of research for all dental hygienists and to encourage more dental hygienists to increase their involvement in research.

537

The six roles of dental hygiene help to place research activities on a continuum. The premise is that all dental hygienists have a role as consumers of research as an integral part of practice. For example, all dental hygienists are held increasingly accountable to critically analyze claims about new oral care products in light of research findings. Clients often ask dental hygienists to evaluate claims made for oral hygiene products, and dental hygienists need the knowledge and skills to provide clear and credible answers. Dental hygienists can cultivate their role as researchers in clinical practice by **reading and critiquing professional journals** that contain scientific articles, reviews of the literature, and case presentations of clinical techniques. These articles can provide the basis for a more scientific rationale behind recommendations for oral home care products.

DEVELOPING SKILLS IN DENTAL HYGIENE RESEARCH

Dental hygienists can attend research presentations and continuing education courses in order to discover the most recent information regarding a research perspective on practice. Unfortunately, many popular speakers in continuing education often cite their own personal experiences rather than include a careful analysis of the current research supporting the topic. Dental hygienists should carefully review information provided at continuing education courses and promotional information provided by sales representatives and should request information on the scientific literature that supports the product claims rather than depend on expert authority or broad assurances from charismatic speakers or sales personnel.

Participation in a **journal club** can be a more formal way for dental hygienists to develop more skill in analyzing scientific information. Many local dental hygiene and dental associations or academic institutions sponsor study clubs that may focus on a particular topic (e.g., implants or periodontics) or provide general topics based on the study group members' interests. For example, dental hygienists who participate in study groups have analyzed the research base for dental hygiene procedures and debated clinical topics based on published research, such as routine coronal polishing, or dÈbridement versus scaling and root planing.

A dental hygienist can also gain more experience in research activities by serving as a **clinical examiner** in a study that is conducted at an academic research center or in a clinical practice. In addition, dental hygienists who are returning to complete their bachelor's or master's degree often have the opportunity to **develop and complete a research project as part of their educational activities** and to collaborate with faculty members in portions of their research projects. These early activities provide a wonderful experience and should be viewed as a positive way to help create new knowledge for dental hygiene as part of the research process.

At the end of the continuum are those dental hygienists whose primary career activities involve **designing and conducting original research.** Research dental hygienists have training at the master's and doctoral level and are usually associated with academic health centers. The number of doctorally prepared dental hygienists has also been increasing; these experienced researchers will continue to expand the body of knowledge for dental hygiene.

SCIENTIFIC METHOD AND THE RESEARCH PROCESS

Many dental hygienists use the word "research" informally as a verb to describe the process of investigating new information and as a noun to describe the materials gathered during their search for knowledge on a particular topic. Darby and Walsh provide a broad definition of dental hygiene research, which "**develops knowledge about oral health behaviors and the promotion of oral health over the lifespan.**"

However, since the mid-1980s, this broad definition of dental hygiene research has been refined to include considerable detail and clarification from a series of four national workshops sponsored by the ADHA. Each of these workshops fostered the development of different phases of dental hygiene scholarship and research, including **theory development and theory building, mentoring programs, establishing priorities for dental hygiene research, and expanding funding and collaborative research opportunities for dental hygienists.** In 1993, the ADHA Board of Trustees approved the national research agenda to focus and direct research efforts to further develop a knowledge base for dental hygiene. Five broad categories comprise the research agenda: **(1) health promotion/disease prevention, (2) education, (3) clinical/primary care, (4) individuals/populations, and (5) basic/applied science.**

The five broad categories of the dental hygiene research agenda were further clarified by Forrest as part of the activities of the National Center for Dental Hygiene Research. Forrest and associates completed a **Delphi study** with dental hygiene experts in order to refine and gain consensus on the most important research topics for each priority area. A total of 37 dental hygiene research topics from the five research agenda categories were established and are included in **Box 18-1.**

Characteristics of Scientific Research

Burns and Grove define **research** as "diligent, systematic inquiry or study to validate and refine existing knowledge and develop new knowledge." Their definition emphasizes the research process as a logical, organized plan of action at every phase of the research project. The level of organization and systematic nature of thinking has been an important characteristic of research, which emphasizes the empirical or objective nature of observations used as data.

BOX 18-1 • Dental Hygiene Research Agenda

A. Health promotion/Disease prevention

1. Assess the effectiveness of the communication process between the client and dental hygienist that leads to oral wellness.
2. Assess the effectiveness of dental hygienists in counseling patients regarding prevention and cessation of tobacco use.
3. Explore public policy issues related to oral healthcare.
4. Identify, describe, and explain ways to promote equitable access to oral healthcare.
5. Assess the cost-effectiveness of various oral health interventions (fluorides, sealants) in promoting oral health.
6. Develop and test easy-to-use self-assessment instruments to assist individuals of all ages in learning the signs and symptoms of oral diseases.
7. Investigate ethnic/cultural group differences as they relate to the promotion of oral health and preventive behaviors.
8. Investigate legislative initiatives on issues such as those that promote autonomy and decision making by dental hygienists.
9. Investigate the concept of oral health self-care among all age, social, and cultural groups.
10. Describe, explain, or predict the relationship between environmental factors (culture, society, income, education) and oral health behaviors.
11. Explain or predict client oral health attitudes, knowledge, and behavior.
12. Assess the impact of third parties on access to and utilization of oral healthcare services.
13. Identify ways in which the unique role of the dental hygienist in the healthcare delivery system can be effectively communicated.

B. Education

1. Develop a predictive model for future needs/demands for dental hygiene personnel.
2. Identify the factors leading to curriculum modification and reform in dental hygiene academic programs.
3. Investigate the extent to which new research findings are incorporated into the dental hygiene curriculum.
4. Investigate the extent to which students are taught critical thinking and decision making skills.
5. Investigate the extent to which students are taught self-assessment and evaluation skills.

C. Clinical and primary care

1. Investigate the impact and effectiveness of alternative dental hygiene practice settings.
2. Assess methods of evaluating competency in dental hygiene.
3. Develop valid and reliable measures to be used in oral health research.
4. Assess the impact of emerging technology used by dental hygienists on the health outcomes of clients.
5. Design and evaluate alternative models for the delivery of oral healthcare.
6. Assess client compliance with recommended oral healthcare regimens.
7. Examine the extent to which knowledge derived from basic science and clinical research is used in clinical reasoning.
8. Assess compliance with established standards of practice by dental hygiene practitioners.

D. Individuals/Populations

1. Develop and test methods of primary prevention in adult populations at risk for primary and secondary enamel and root caries, with special attention to compromised, handicapped, and institutional groups.
2. Develop and test methods for early diagnosis and screening of oral diseases for individuals at high risk for dental caries, periodontal diseases, and oral cancer.
3. Evaluate the efficacy of various oral hygiene regimens with institutionalized, handicapped, or otherwise compromised patients.
4. Develop and test preventive measures to reduce the incidence of oral disease in special at-risk populations.
5. Examine the prevention, diagnosis, and treatment of oral disease in underserved and at-risk populations.

E. Basic/Applied sciences

1. Explore the effects of dental hygiene therapy on pathogenesis, wound healing, and tissue repair.
2. Test new products for use in dental hygiene practice.
3. Develop valid and reliable measures of quality dental hygiene care.
4. Test theoretical concepts in dental hygiene.
5. Assess the outcomes of client oral health self-care behaviors.
6. Develop assessment tools that provide indicators of dental hygiene care outcomes.

The **scientific method**, also called **quantitative research**, is the traditional method of inquiry that has been used most often in biomedical research. The scientific method proceeds in a controlled, orderly manner from the design and planning phase to the collection of numeric data to the analytical phase of the study. Investigators use **deductive reasoning** (i.e., the process of questioning theory and the specific expected consequences of the theory are considered) to limit the factors and the relationships important for the study. Most quantitative research studies include **hypotheses**, which are statements that predict or indicate a relationship among the variables, and factors, called variables, identified for inquiry in the study. A hallmark of quantitative research is the degree of control that the researcher exerts in the design and measurement of the study in order to provide a more objective understanding of the hypotheses and relationships among the variables.

Although most biomedical research questions are best addressed by quantitative research methods, the level of control exerted in quantitative studies often restricts the type of questions and knowledge that can be pursued, especially in light of the numerous complexities involved when studying humans. Quantitative studies have been criticized as being too controlled and too focused on reducing human experiences to readily measured scales for easy observation, which may oversimplify and limit the type of information that the researchers receive. For example, a study of clients' adherence to flossing behavior may reveal a high frequency of flossing in one group but may not explain why and how the knowledge from this group can be applied to help other clients. Many researchers have been combining or pairing quantitative and qualitative research to help provide greater depth and breadth to their scientific studies.

QUALITATIVE RESEARCH

Naturalistic methods, also called **qualitative research**, offer an intriguing alternative to the scientific method in the health sciences and are commonly used in the social sciences in order to study the nature of human complexities more directly and completely. Qualitative research takes place in the "field setting," where the behavior naturally occurs and researchers can observe and participate in the activities of their subjects. Qualitative research relies on personal methods of data collection, such as **interviews, audiotapes, videotapes, subjects' personal writings, and journals and documents from the site.** The researcher uses an **inductive process** to discover the dimensions of the problem under study by participating and recording behavior through multiple methods and then reflecting and categorizing the data systematically in order to understand more fully the dimensions or relationships. Researchers often repeat this process of observation and reflection several times in order to understand the phenomena that are being studied. This inductive method is also called the constant comparative method and distinguishes

qualitative research because of the flexible, yet disciplined nature of the research process.

Dental hygiene research has included both quantitative and qualitative studies. Most of the published research studies in dental hygiene and dentistry have followed the quantitative biomedical model and can be described in one of the following three categories: **experimental, quasi-experimental, and non-experimental** research. Polit and Hungler describe a true experimental research project as one that must include all three of the following characteristics: manipulation, control, and randomization. In order to qualify as a true experiment, the investigator must introduce an intervention or treatment (**manipulation**) to at least some of the subjects and withhold the intervention from other subjects, thus identifying a **control group.** The investigator may invoke additional levels of control by limiting the study population based on specific variables. However, the most important qualification of a true experiment is the introduction of **randomization**, which means that subjects have an equal chance of being assigned to the control group or the experimental group.

Although there are many advantages of conducting true experimental research, there are research problems and situations in which true experimental designs cannot be used. The requirement for random selection of groups is often difficult in health care situations when some characteristics cannot be controlled (e.g., health behaviors and gender) or when ethical considerations prohibit withholding treatment and make randomization difficult when known risks are present. In addition, health care research with clients cannot be as easily controlled as laboratory situations, thus quasi-experimental designs are employed in the research process.

QUASI-EXPERIMENTAL RESEARCH

Quasi-experimental research involves investigations in which the researchers introduce an intervention but are unable to design or select an appropriate control group or are unable to randomize subject selection into the study groups. Although these designs are practical and very readily conducted in health care situations, quasi-experimental research is unable to identify the causes and effects of the research problem and can only clarify the strength and direction of relationships among variables.

NON-EXPERIMENTAL RESEARCH

Non-experimental research includes a broad range of appropriate investigations in client care that are not amenable to the level of experimental manipulation and control of variables described earlier. **Descriptive research**, which is the most common type of non-experimental research, forms the core of dental hygiene research, which seeks to describe the four central concepts of **dental hygiene's paradigm: client, environment, health/oral health, and dental hygiene actions.** Because dental hygiene is a developing profession, descriptive research is critical to identify and determine the dimensions of the central concepts for further study and use in clinical practice. **Correlational studies,** another type of non-experimental research, examine the relationship of two variables from either a **retrospective** (i.e., look back in time) or **prospective** (i.e., track for a future time) dimension. By definition, all qualitative research studies are non-experimental.

Relevance to Dental Hygienists

A careful review of the research literature can be useful for dental hygienists from both a conceptual and a practical perspective. Dental hygienists may find the description of a new clinical problem intriguing and may wish to reflect on their clinical practice and review the literature to learn more about the problem. Research articles can provide a more detailed explanation about why a particular phenomenon is present and cause dental hygienists to reconsider their approach to practice. In addition, a careful review of the research literature can help dental hygienists to understand factors correlated with other health problems and to predict which clients may best respond to selected interventions. Research articles can also provoke a change in clinical care with clients in order to increase effectiveness or efficiency of practice. Dental hygienists can discover new clinical approaches to care and evaluate the differential benefits of alternative treatment approaches through consistent and systematic literature reviews.

However, dental hygienists need to develop their abilities to critique research articles thoroughly and analytically in order to determine the quality of the study and the applicability of the study results for a particular client or population. Critical analyses of articles should identify the positive and negative aspects of a study in a systematic manner in order to understand the limitations and appropriate clinical applications. Although most published articles adhere to accepted methodologic standards, few articles in the research literature are perfect. Dental hygienists should understand whether the design flaws have a minimal or fatal effect on the research results.

 CRITICAL ANALYSIS OF THE SCIENTIFIC LITERATURE

Dental hygienists should have a good understanding of the process, methods, and appropriate designs for research studies in order to complete a thorough, critical analysis of the literature. In addition to a critique of the study's methods, dental hygienists should review both the theoretical framework and the discussion of ethical principles within the study. In order to provide a framework for systematic and critical analysis of scientific literature, five phases of the scientific method are described in this section: **(1) problem formulation, (2) hypothesis formulation, (3) study design, (4) data collection,** and **(5) analysis/interpretation and conclusions.** Although these five phases are most reflective of the quantitative research tradition, application of the research process and a critique of qualitative studies are also addressed within each section.

Within the discussion of each phase of the research process, suggestions and application for critiquing literature on dentistry and dental hygiene are included. At the end of each section, sample questions are included for dental hygienists to use to critique a scientific article.

Problem Formulation

All clinicians are notoriously curious professionals, and the questions that clinicians ask frequently regarding the effectiveness and appropriateness of clinical care form the basis for investigation of new knowledge. Many researchers maintain close communication with clinicians and often continue clinical practice in order to ensure that the research problems they formulate are the most relevant and interesting ones for clinicians. For example, the following questions from clinicians are good examples of inquiries that have been studied very successfully in the dental literature. "Is this the best treatment for my client with mild to moderate periodontal disease?"; "What factors are causing my client to be so susceptible to periodontal disease?" These questions provoke a directed search into a more limited area of inquiry.

However, a broader question such as, "Is endodontic therapy or tooth extraction better for a tooth with pulpal involvement?" is a more difficult question to develop into a controlled research project. This question is too broad and laden with personal values regarding the patient's economic and personal viewpoint on tooth extraction in addition to the subjective clinical prognosis for each tooth. Research problems should be stated in realistic and practical terms in relation to the time, materials, and staff and clients available as resources for the project. The researcher should avoid making personal value judgements that are difficult to objectify and quantify.

When critically analyzing the literature, dental hygienists should consider the scope of the research questions in relation to their importance, feasibility, and relevance for application to the clinical setting. In qualitative studies, authors describe their research questions explicitly in detail and discuss how the questions changed during the course of the study; however, in quantitative studies, most authors state the purposes of their research as a way to discuss the questions posed to the researchers.

Literature Review

In quantitative research, studies are generally conducted within the context of existing knowledge, thus the critical reader should evaluate whether the research is based on a solid framework and expands the existing knowledge base sufficiently. The critical reader should expect a thorough review of the literature in both qualitative and quantitative research reports. The **literature review** should provide both a summary and an analytical critique that evaluates the adequacy of the previous research conducted on the problem. Literature reviews should not be merely reports but should describe the current state of knowledge on the subject and identify gaps in knowledge for further research.

The development and easy access to electronic databases for efficient search and retrieval of relevant literature have greatly facilitated the literature review process. The most common professional database for dentistry and dental hygiene is Medical Literature On-Line (**MEDLINE**), which can be accessed through CD-ROM or on-line search through academic libraries or Internet service providers. However, Cumulative Index to Nursing and Allied Health Literature (**CINAHL**), Psychology Literature (**PsychLIT**), and Educational Resources Information Center (**ERIC**) can also yield important sources of references for dental hygienists. Dental hygienists should be familiar with the techniques of on-line searching, which begin most commonly with a subject search using specific terminology, which can be further restricted by limiting the search to specific journals, specific languages, certain time spans, and types of research reports.

Research journals often publish articles that provide an exhaustive review of the literature on a particular topic, such as the Gutmann's literature review on air polishing. These articles can provide clinicians and researchers with a current summary of knowledge on a particular topic, and the articles are generally completed in preparation for a research project or thesis on that topic. However, literature review articles are considered to be secondary sources, because they report and review original studies. When evaluating the review of the literature section in research articles, the critical reader should look for evidence of **citation of original studies** rather than the author's sole reliance on literature review articles.

Specific questions for dental hygienists to use when evaluating both the research questions and the literature review in the first component of the research process problem formulation are included in **Box 18-2.**

Hypothesis Formulation and Study Design

In quantitative studies, researchers transform the research questions into specific statements and predictions about the relationships and outcomes of the concepts described in the research problem. The **predictive statement is called an hypothesis** (plural is hypotheses), and the **concepts to be studied are called variables.** In quantitative studies, hypotheses should always predict an outcome in specific terms in order to guide the researcher to more critically examine the data in relation to the initial prediction. Researchers for-

---

BOX 18-2 • Guidelines for Critically Analyzing the Scientific Literature

PROBLEM FORMULATION
Research Questions
- Are the research questions significant and important for dental hygiene?
- Are the research questions relevant for clinical practice?
- Are the research questions feasible and practical for study?

Literature Review
- Is the search thorough?
- Does the author cite both classic and current literature?
- Does the author report and summarize the current state of knowledge in this area?
- Does the author analyze the strengths and limitations of current knowledge in this area?

---

mulate the hypothesis by thoroughly reviewing the literature and also by reflecting on their subjective experience gained from previous research and clinical practice. When statistical tests are applied to the data, researchers use a restated hypothesis, the **null hypothesis**, which claims that no relationship exists between the variables. The null hypothesis places the burden of proof on the researcher to prove that there is a specific directional difference between the variables through statistical analysis of the data.

Variables

Variables are categorized as dependent or independent based on their relationship as stated in the hypothesis. In the example of the following hypothesis, "Systemic water fluoridation will reduce caries in school children by 30%," the independent variable is systemic water fluoridation, because it causes the expected outcome. The dependent variable is caries in school children, because it is the result. In other words, the **dependent variable** "depends" on the manipulation of the **independent variable.**

Most studies have more than one independent and dependent variable. In the hypothesis listed earlier, the researchers subdivided the dependent variable to examine the differences in rates of caries based on gender, children's ages, and socioeconomic status as multiple dependent variables. The decision to label a variable either independent or dependent is based on the context of the hypothesis and study design. No variables are inherently independent or dependent; their designation is always relative based on the study.

Extraneous variables are concepts that are inherently present in the population and may affect the study but are not included as dependent or independent variables. Researchers should provide a discussion of these extraneous variables in their report and should control them as much as

TABLE 18–1 Sample Factorial Design Using Hypothetical Data

METHOD OF APPLICATION (X_2)	TYPE OF SEALANT (X_1)		TOTAL
	PIT AND FISSURE SEALANT A	PIT AND FISSURE SEALANT B	
Applied with a bristle brush	Group I $\bar{X}_1 = 36$ months	Group II $\bar{X}_2 = 15$ months	$\bar{X} = 51$ months
Applied with a premeasured applicator	Group III $\bar{X}_3 = 20$ months	Group IV $\bar{X}_4 = 40$ months	$\bar{X} = 60$ months
TOTAL	$\bar{X} = 56$ months	$\bar{X} = 55$ months	

(From Darby ML, Bowen DM: Research Methods for Oral Health Professionals. Pocatello, JT McCann Company, 1990, p 71.)

possible based on the research design. Researchers can purposefully select individuals in order to produce a more homogenous study sample and reduce the number of extraneous variables. In addition, investigators can also match their subjects on specific variables in order to provide more control over extraneous variables. However, the best method to control extraneous variables is to use the random assignment of subjects to the control and experimental groups. **Randomization** means that subjects have an equal chance of being assigned to either group, thus the researcher can assume that the groups are comparable based on the distribution of extraneous variables.

Research Design

In the early stages of research planning, the investigator must make strategic decisions about how the project will be conducted in order to investigate the problem in the best way. The **research design** is the investigator's comprehensive plan for completing activities in order to determine the answers to the research questions and hypotheses.

Experimental Studies

The research design depends on the amount of control that the investigator has over the manipulation of the independent variable in the study. **Experimental studies** are defined by the use of randomization in assigning subjects to either a **test group**, which receives the treatment, or to a **control group**, which receives no intervention. The simplest and most powerful experimental research design is the **pre-test/post-test design** in which subjects in both groups are measured at two time points: (1) at the initial assignment to groups, and (2) at a time point after the manipulation of the independent variable. Some studies use a post-test only design, which still allows comparison between the groups but is not as powerful because baseline measurements cannot be identified to show the differences within each group.

In some true experimental studies, researchers often manipulate two or more independent variables in the same study in order to determine if there is any benefit from combining treatment methods or if there are any effects in providing treatment methods in a particular sequence. Studies that employ multiple independent variables are called **factorial designs**, which permit researchers to identify the main effects of the independent variables and the interaction effects of the combinations of independent variables, called factors. In factorial designs, subjects are assigned randomly to various combinations of independent variables, and a pretest/post-test measurement is completed in order to determine the effects of each factor both individually and in combination. Generally, two or three factors can be examined in one study; use of more than three factors expands the number of groups required and often poses problems both in recruiting a sufficient number of subjects and in managing a complex study **(Table 18-1)**.

Both the pre-test/post-test design and factorial design provide for comparisons between subjects, because different people are randomly assigned to the different groups. A **repeated measures design** involves comparisons of different treatments in the same subjects and is characterized as a within-subjects or **cross-over design (Table 18-2)**. This type of design has been used in periodontal therapy in order to minimize extraneous variables and has been also called **"split mouth design,"** because only several teeth and the associated periodontal structures are used for each treatment. A repeated measures design has several powerful advantages because of the level of control possible and because equivalence between subjects is ensured. However, carryover effects from one treatment to the other are often in-

TABLE 18–2 Hypothetical Factorial Design Demonstrating an Interaction Between Variables

	ORAL HEALTH INSTRUCTION	
	VIDEOTAPE	PERSONALIZED
Adults (21–35 years old)	Group I $\bar{X}_1 = 21$	Group II $\bar{X}_2 = 80$
Adolescents (12–19 years old)	Group III $\bar{X}_3 = 79$	Group IV $\bar{X}_4 = 22$

(From Darby ML, Bowen DM: Research Methods for Oral Health Professionals. Pocatello, JT McCann Company, 1990, p 71.)

evitable, and the sequence of experimental treatments may affect the results. In order to minimize the carry-over effects, a **"wash-out" time period** with no treatment is scheduled; however, the wash-out time may be insufficient to reduce the effect of the first treatment. Readers should carefully evaluate whether the wash-out time period and the nature of the experimental treatments can appropriately control any threats in the repeated measures design.

Quasi-experimental Studies

Quasi-experimental designs are often based on clinical situations where true random assignment is not possible, yet there is still a significant opportunity to systematically conduct research in a very realistic setting. The pre-test/post-test design can be applied in quasi-experimental situations and is called the **non-equivalent comparison group design.** This is a particularly strong strategy when randomization cannot be used, because differences both between and within groups can be measured and analyzed. An experimental group and a control group are designated in quasi-experimental studies, yet the control group is often called a **comparison group** because without randomization, inferences about the homogeneity of the groups cannot be made.

A common opportunity to implement a quasi-experimental research design occurs when a change is made in organizational procedures or when a new educational program is implemented. This research design, called the **time series design**, considers the new program to be the independent variable. The dependent variables can include test scores, productivity levels, and satisfaction levels of professionals and clients that may possibly be affected by the new intervention. Pre-test measures are taken before the new program is implemented and are compared with post-test measures of the same group after the program is implemented. In time series' designs, the same individuals serve as a comparison group, thus a level of homogeneity is ensured among the subjects. Time series' designs lack predictive power and generalizability, because many intervening factors may influence the post-test performance in addition to the implementation of the new program. However, time series' designs can be strengthened by increasing the number of post-test measurements and by lengthening the time span of the post-test evaluation. Time series' designs are quite popular and extremely useful in evaluating the implementation of new programs and in determining the outcomes of a new program in a systematic way.

Placebo Effect

A limitation of both experimental and quasi-experimental studies is the placebo effect, which may alter the responses of individuals in both the control and experimental groups. Ethical regulations mandate that individuals give voluntary consent and understand the basic study design as a condition for participation in the study; however, individuals who know that they are participating in a study-especially those who know that they are in an experimental group-may change their behavior. The **placebo effect** was first documented at the Hawthorne plant of the Western Electric Corporation, where workers in a productivity study showed increased results even when no intervention was made. Now also called the **Hawthorne effect**, the placebo effect can be controlled by keeping the group assignments secret for either the participants or examiners (**single blind study**) or for both groups (**double blind study**). However, it is often not feasible to provide a placebo medication that mimics the active drug, and it is often very difficult to mask a health promotional or educational intervention, thus investigators must be cautious when interpreting results unless they carefully consider the placebo effect.

Non-Experimental Research

Two types of non-experimental research can be described in this section: **correlational** and **descriptive** research. Correlational research seeks to describe the relationship of two variables, neither of which can be manipulated. Correlational research designs capitalize on the fact that medical records provide a wealth of information regarding clients' disease states and the conditions that may have preceded or occurred at the same time as the initiation of disease. **Retrospective studies** look back for the presence of factors that may be related to the disease and attempt to identify relationships between these factors and the specific disease condition. **Prospective studies** identify study participants and track their experience with disease states in relation to the presence of factors that may affect the initiation and progression of the disease.

A common error that is made in correlational research is the assumption that the presence of both the conditions and the disease indicate a **cause-and-effect relationship.** Correlation cannot prove causation, because there is no randomization and control over the groups and because the independent variable is not manipulated. Researchers sometimes combine correlation research with a matching technique called the **case control design.** In this research design, individuals with a certain disease are matched with subjects who do not have the disease but are alike in many background characteristics in order to control extraneous variables. Case control design then helps the researcher to track the matched individuals (cases) to determine differences that may signify an important level of relationship. Although correlational research cannot identify causation, it can be very useful when identifying important trends for further experimental research and can also provide clients with an understanding of risk factors that may be associated with disease states.

Descriptive Research

Descriptive research is also considered non-experimental research and can be conducted in both the quantitative and qualitative tradition. Quantitative descriptive research in dental hygiene and dentistry is commonly used to document and describe any number of characteristics and distribution of conditions in a population, ranging from disease states in children to the attitudes and perceptions of dental hygienists regarding practice.

Epidemiology, which can be descriptive or analytical by design, is the study of the presence and distribution of diseases in a specific group of individuals. **Epidemiologic studies** can examine the **incidence** of disease (i.e., the number of new cases over a period of time) or the **prevalence** of disease (i.e., the number of individuals in a group who have the disease at a given point in time when the measurement occurs). Researchers measure either the **morbidity rate,** which identifies the ratio of the presence of disease in individuals in proportion to the number of individuals in the group, or the **mortality rate,** which identifies the proportion of deaths due to the disease in relation to the population.

Survey research is commonly used in dental hygiene and dentistry in order to obtain descriptive information from individuals in a population regarding specific variables. Survey research is obtained by an individual's self-report, either by a written survey that is mailed or sent electronically to the subject and then returned to the researcher or by telephone or personal interview. Although surveys may be used in experimental and quasi-experimental research, they are best suited for descriptive research purposes because of the lack of control and reliance on the individual's self-report of the research data.

Other quantitative research activities include a **needs assessment** and **program evaluation research**, which are often used in community oral health programs in order to identify needs and best design appropriate programming in a community setting. Another quantitative research study is **meta-analysis,** which extends a thorough review of the literature and applies statistical techniques to analyze a group of studies together. Meta-analysis helps to summarize a number of research studies and identifies findings and trends that may not be apparent from reading the individual reports. Meta-analysis research is particularly helpful to guide clinicians in practice decisions based on the best available scientific evidence.

Qualitative Research

Qualitative studies are always descriptive and non-experimental by design, because they are situated in real life field situations and seek to explain and expand the understanding of a particular phenomenon. Researchers plan strategies for qualitative research by scheduling sessions to observe, participate in the activities of the subjects, and interview individuals and groups. However, qualitative studies do not have a formal research design imposed on the study in order to allow for flexibility to listen and discover the phenomena from the perspective of the individuals. Different types of qualitative research traditions have been described in the literature and include **grounded theory, phenomenology, and ethnography.**

For example, ethnography is a type of qualitative research common to anthropology. Ethnographers use a subjective data gathering technique called participant observation, in which they join the subjects in the study and participate in their daily activities in order to investigate the phenomena being studied. Ethnographic researchers develop a close relationship with the study participants, also called informants, who provide a detailed description about the study phenomena through both structured and unstructured interviews and meetings. Ethnographers record their observations both in writing and in audio or video recordings and always keep a journal that describes the research process and their findings.

Evaluating Internal and External Validity

When evaluating the research design of experimental and quasi-experimental studies, dental hygienists need to carefully consider the quality and appropriateness of the research design in light of the systematic control of the issues surrounding the research topic. The term **validity** has been used to refer to the overall quality of the study dependent on the amount of control that the investigators can maintain within the implementation and design of the study. Campbell and Stanley differentiate two types of validity: internal validity and external validity. **Internal validity** refers to the assurance that the independent variable is the factor influencing the change in the dependent variable, and **external validity** describes the generalizability of the results of the study to other settings.

Sample Selection

Researchers can ensure internal and external validity by selecting a **sample** that is **homogenous** and **representative** of the larger population. In a true experimental study, subjects are directed **randomly** to participate in the test or control group. Differences between the groups are minimized, because each subject has an equal chance of being assigned to either group. However, when subjects are selected randomly from the population, the researcher can be assured that the sample represents the population and that the results can be generalized to other groups in the population. Random selection of subjects from the population provides a stronger claim to a more homogenous and representative sample.

Researchers can select samples randomly from a population in three ways. The first method, **simple random sampling,** is completed by using a **table of random numbers** to select subjects from the population. The second method, **stratified random sampling**, is completed by randomly selecting several individuals from specific categories that are selected by the researcher. The third method, **systematic random sampling,** involves the systematic selection of subjects (e.g., the selection of every 10th dental hygienist named on the state licensing listing for the sample).

However, in quasi-experimental and non-experimental research, randomization is not possible, and differences among the groups may influence the change in the dependent variables. Quasi-experimental studies often use pre-existing groups, called **convenience samples**, which are more open to variation within the subjects in the sample. Although convenience samples are relatively easy to recruit, researchers have no assurances that these samples are representative of the population and that the sample is homogenous. Researchers can reduce potential bias and differences in the samples by identifying and controlling for extraneous variables and by using matching techniques; however, **bias** in sample selection remains a problematic threat to internal and external validity when convenience samples are chosen in quasi-experimental studies.

Mortality as a Threat to Internal Validity

Campbell and Stanley describe three other threats to internal validity that occur in a study: **mortality, history,** and **maturation.** All investigators face the challenge of keeping subjects active and interested in the research project, especially when members in a control group perceive that there is little personal benefit for their continued participation. **Mortality** refers to the loss of subjects, and although researchers should always expect a minimal loss of subjects, the differential loss of one group will threaten the internal validity of the study. In addition, mortality is a special threat in a study involving survey research, which depends on the cooperation of subjects to return completed questionnaires or keep scheduled interview appointments. For example, those subjects who return the questionnaires tend to be more enthusiastic and motivated about the subject and may not be representative of the sample selected and the entire population. Dental hygienists should carefully scrutinize the percentage of returned surveys that the researchers describe in the scientific report, because a low response rate means a high loss of potential subjects and a potential threat to internal validity. Kerlinger recommends that researchers strive to achieve at least an 80% response rate. If this type of return rate is not possible, researchers should include data that describe and compare the non-responders in relation to the responders in order to ensure that no bias is evident among the non-responders.

History as a Threat to Internal Validity

During the time period of the research activity, intervening **historical events** may interfere with the results of the study and threaten internal validity. For example, it is not prudent to evaluate an educational program with children to reduce their intake of refined carbohydrates and dietary sucrose in October, because children have easy access to sweet snacks at Halloween. In the true experiment, the threat of any historical event is distributed evenly between the test group and the control group; however, in quasi-experimental and non-experimental studies, historical events may be limited to one group with no possible control for the researcher.

Maturation as a Threat to Internal Validity

In a research study, subjects will change as a function of normal **growth and maturation**, which will affect the subjects as much as manipulation of the independent variable. For example, a 4-year project researching an oral hygiene program with preschool children must consider the children's level of motor skill and cognitive development in relation to the educational program, which is manipulated as the independent variable. With these children, the researchers must clarify the influence of their developing skills as a major change in the dependent variables in addition to the educational program. The maturation threat to interval validity is minimized when randomization is used; however, inflated results in true experimental research can also be achieved when the researchers do not identify and control maturation, such as normal tissue healing, postoperative recovery, or aging as a threat to internal validity.

Sample Size

When dental hygienists critically evaluate a research study, they should careful scrutinize the way that the researchers selected and maintained their research sample. A common question that many researchers ponder is the appropriate number of subjects for a research study. Although quasi-experimental studies are often limited to the convenience sample, the sample size should be based on the **research questions posed by the investigation, the size and characteristics of the population at large, and the expected differences between the test group and the control group on the post-test measures.** Quantitative researchers are generally advised to choose the largest sample size that they can manage within their budget, because a **larger sample size produces a smaller degree of sampling error.**

A formal technique called **power analysis** has been developed to help the researcher determine the optimum number of subjects for a study. Investigators are asked to determine how large a difference they expect between the experimental and control groups. When expected differences are small, a larger sample size is needed in order to ensure that the data adequately reflect the performance of the hypotheses. When small differences are expected, a small sample may not adequately reflect mathematically the true differences in the hypotheses. However, the most important criterion for sample size in a quantitative study is the ability of the sample to adequately reflect the population. Dental hygienists who critically review the research should use their judgement regarding the appropriateness of the number of subjects chosen for the sample.

It is within the second component of the research process, **hypotheses formulation and study design**, that the investigators make critical planning decisions about the organization and structure for the research project. When dental hygienists critique a scientific article, they should carefully analyze the following four subcomponents: **hypotheses, variables, research design,** and **sample selection.** Specific questions for dental hygienists to use when evaluating these subcomponents are included in **Box 18-3.**

Data Collection

When dental hygienists review the scientific literature, they should critically evaluate both the types of measures that the researchers selected for the study and the way in which these measures were used to collect the data. Researchers may choose to work with data that have already been recorded in clients' charts (e.g., records review), or they can use and re-analyze data from another research project (i.e., secondary sources); however, most researchers collect new data in order to evaluate the hypotheses.

Range of Data Collection Measures

In the research report, investigators should provide a clear rationale regarding their choice of **investigational measures.** Data collection instruments must be consistent with the research purposes and hypotheses and should ensure that the researchers have the appropriate quality and sufficient quantity of data from which to form conclusions at the end of the study. Qualitative and quantitative studies vary greatly in their choice of data collection measures and can range along a continuum from **unstructured discussions** and **subjective observations** to more **structured** forms of **interview** and **observation.** In addition, **self-report methods,** such as **surveys, social psychological scales, semantic differentials,** and **biophysiologic methods,** such as measurement of blood levels and evidence of disease symptoms, can also be found as data collection measures in both qualitative and quantitative research studies **(Table 18-3).**

Instrume nt Validity

When dental hygienists review the scientific literature, they should ensure that the researchers have thoroughly described and justified their selection of data collection measures. In quantitative investigations that employ surveys, psychological scales, or measures of disease, the researchers should identify and explain the particular data collection instruments that were selected. Critical readers should look for information regarding **instrument validity,** in which the investigators describe how realistically and appropriately the instrument measures the condition under investigation. **Content validity** measures the extent to which the instrument thoroughly represents knowledge in the selected content area. **Criterion validity** compares the newly developed instrument with a pre-existing valid and reliable instrument in order to evaluate the accuracy and appropriateness of the new instrument.

Instrument Reliability

The researchers should also describe the **reliability** of the instrument, which describes how consistently the measure identifies conditions in the same way. A data collection measure that represents a disease condition is called an **index** (the plural is indices), and dental hygiene textbooks provide several references for valid and reliable measures of caries, periodontal diseases, and associated conditions such as plaque and calculus (see Chapters 14 and 17). Sometimes, a valid and reliable measure is not available for a specific condition, and a researcher may develop an instrument unique for the study. The researcher should provide evidence that the data collection measure has been **standardized** and, when possible, provide reliability and validity scores for the instruments. The absence of a standardized instrument should not necessarily pose a threat to internal validity or detract from the generalizability of a study, especially when qualitative and quantitative designs are combined. However, valid and reliable instruments should be used whenever possible to ensure standardized collection of data.

BOX 18-3 • Guidelines for Critically Analyzing the Scientific Literature

HYPOTHESES FORMULATION AND STUDY DESIGN

Hypotheses
- Are the hypotheses stated clearly in measurable terms?
- Are the hypotheses supported by the literature review?
- Do the hypotheses predict a specific action or direction for the study?

Variables
- Are the independent and dependent variables clearly identified?
- How well are the extraneous variables discussed and controlled?

Research Design
- Is the categorization of the type of study (experimental, quasi-experimental, non-experimental) identified and rationalized?
- Is the study categorized appropriately?
- Is the study design clearly described?
- How is the placebo effect controlled?

Sample Selection
- How are the subjects in the sample chosen?
- Is the sample representative of the population?
- Is the sample size sufficient?
- How are subjects assigned to the experimental and control groups?
- How are the threats to internal validity minimized?

TABLE 18-3　Data Collection Instruments and Applications

DATA COLLECTION METHODOLOGY	INSTRUMENT	INDICATIONS	ADVANTAGES	LIMITATIONS
Direct observation of events, objects, people	Checklist, content analysis, evaluation forms, camera, tape recorder, videotape, thermometer, sphygmomanometer, rating and ranking scales	1. Used when subject recall may affect accuracy of data collection 2. Used to study behavior 3. Used to study psychomotor 4. Used in experimental research	1. Observations can be made as they occur in the "natural" setting 2. Observations can be made of behaviors that might not be reported by respondents	1. Time consuming 2. Difficulty in recording 3. Factors that may interfere with the situation 4. Difficulty in quantification of observations 5. Expensive 6. Observer-respondent interaction
Interview	Interview guide or interview schedule	1. Used for obtaining information on attitudes, beliefs, and opinions 2. Used in a survey 3. Used to gain information on past or present events	1. Flexibility 2. Questions can be clarified and explained 3. Complete data can be collected 4. Subjects do not have to read or write	1. Respondents may be inhibited to respond accurately and truthfully 2. Time consuming 3. Expensive 4. Interviewer may affect the responses
Asking questions	Questionnaire, opinionnaire	1. Used for obtaining information on attitudes, beliefs, and opinions 2. Used to gain information on past events 3. Used when impersonal interactions between researcher and respondent is required	1. Ease of administration 2. Relatively inexpensive 3. Standardization of instructions and questions 4. Economy of time 5. Data can be gathered over a wide geographic area	1. Misinterpretation of questions by respondents 2. Low return may bias results 3. Superficiality of responses 4. Incomplete data collection 5. Honesty of respondent
Survey	Questionnaire, interview, schedule, case study	1. Used for obtaining a broad range of information on the status quo 2. Used to study present conditions 3. Used in planning	1. Data can be gathered to reflect public opinion 2. Vast amount of data can be collected 3. Cross-sectional, generalized statistics can be obtained	1. Superficiality of responses 2. Control of extraneous variables is lacking
Epidemiological survey	Dental indices	1. Used to study disease patterns in a population 2. Used to evaluate the effectiveness of therapeutic or preventive treatments in a specific geographical area	1. Vast amount of data can be collected 2. Cross-sectional, generalized statistics can be obtained 3. Data are quantifiable	1. Difficulty in determining causation due to complexity of variables 2. Time consuming
Records, documents	Reports of legislative bodies and state or city officials, deeds, wills, appointment records, dental charts, report cards	1. Used to study posted events	1. Unbiased in terms of the investigator 2. Inexpensive 3. No subject-investigator interaction 4. Convenience and economy of time	1. Incomplete records 2. Accuracy of records may be unknown

(From Darby ML, Bowen DM: Research Methods for Oral Health Professionals. Pocatello, JT McCann Company, 1990, p 89.)

Examiner Training

A well-written scientific report should include specific, detailed information regarding the data collection procedures. For example, the researchers should provide information regarding the number of examiners, their training, and calibration measures that were completed to ensure that each examiner consistently completes the appropriate procedures (**intra-rater reliability**) in the same manner as the other examiners (**inter-rater reliability**). Dental hygienists should carefully review this information, because sloppy data collection procedures can spoil a good design and can be considered a threat to internal validity.

The third component of the research process, **data collection**, represents the phase in which the investigators implement their research design and gather the information that they will use to evaluate their research questions and hypotheses. When dental hygienists critique a scientific article, they should evaluate how closely the investigators monitored the study and how well they selected and designed the data collection methods. Specific questions for dental hygienists to use when evaluating these data collection methods and procedures are included in **Box 18-4.**

Data Analysis/Interpretation

Dental hygienists who are new to research often express concern regarding a critique of data analysis and statistical portions of research reports. Simply stated, statistics can be intimidating to even experienced practitioners, particularly as advanced multivariate statistical analysis has been used with more frequency in the professional literature. However, with an understanding of some of the basic principles of statistical design, dental hygienists can more readily comprehend and evaluate the investigator's use of statistical analysis to determine the significance and applicability of the research results.

Level of Measurement

The statistical analysis that is appropriate for a particular study depends on the type and level of measurement that has been completed during data collection. Polit and Hungler describe four levels of measurement: nominal, ordinal, interval, and ratio measurement. **Nominal data** involve use of numbers to represent categories of data. For example, gender is usually coded as Males = 1 and Females = 2 and is considered nominal data. This type of data is useful for basic description but is not appropriate for more advanced mathematical computation. **Ordinal measurement** involves numeric ranking of categories based on their relationship to each other and can be useful in order to quantify attributes, such as a client's perception of pain during care or a dental hygienist's ranking of her client's ability to use dental floss. However, the numeric rankings are only based in relationship to each other and do not tell us that a client's score of 2

BOX 18-4 • Guidelines for Critically Analyzing the Scientific Literature

Data Collection
- Are the measures selected by the researchers appropriate based on the research questions and hypotheses?
- Are the instruments reliable and valid?
- Are the study data collected in a systematic and standardized manner?
- How are the examiners trained and standardized?
- How is the management of the study monitored?

---

is twice as good as the other client's score of 1. Like nominal data, ordinal data restrict the type of statistical manipulation that can be completed.

Interval Scales

Interval measurement involves numeric data about an attribute that provides both rank ordering of objects and a meaningful measure of the distance between the adjacent scores. The Dental Aptitude Test (DAT) provides an example of interval data.

The scores on each portion of the DAT are ordered in meaningful units, thus a score of 8 is higher than a score of 6. In addition, the difference between the scores of 6 and 8 is equivalent to the difference between a score of 8 and 10. Most psychological and educational tests are considered interval data, and because of their assumed relationships, many sophisticated statistical analyses can be completed. However, interval measurements do not have a meaningful zero point (the lowest score that you can get is a 4, and there is not a null DAT), thus interval scores cannot provide absolute quantification of an attribute.

Ratio Scales

An example of an index that does provide an example of a scale with an absolute zero is Loe's Plaque Index, because this index uses the classification of 0 = no plaque, and the scores of 1 to 3 represent plaque measurements within each third of the tooth. This type of measurement is called a **ratio scale**, because it has a rational zero and the numbers represent a meaningful measure of the distance between the other scores. Interval and ratio scales are considered to be the highest level of measurement and are preferred because of their abilities to represent differences in an attribute for detailed statistical analysis.

Once the data have been collected, the researchers must organize it in a meaningful way and thus begin with descriptive statistics, which provide the basis for clarifying and synthesizing the data. A **frequency distribution** is a descriptive list or a graphic picture of the range and frequency of the scores in the data set. An ungrouped frequency distribution is used to organize small amounts of data (<30)

TABLE 18–4 Ungrouped Frequency Distribution of National Board Scores of 45 Dental Hygiene Students

X	F	X	F	X	F	X	F
100		90		80		70	
99	2	89	4	79	1	69	1
98	1	88	2	78	3	68	
97	1	87	2	77	1	67	
96		86		76	4	66	
95	1	85		75	1	65	
94	3	84	3	74	2	64	1
93	1	83	4	73		63	
92	1	82	2	72		62	
91	1	81	1	71		61	

(From Darby ML, Bowen DM: Research Methods for Oral Health Professionals. Pocatello, JT McCann Company, 1990, p 107.)

TABLE 18–5 Grouped Frequency Distribution and Cumulative Frequency Distribution of National Board Scores of 45 Dental Hygiene Students

CLASS INTERVAL	F	CUMULATIVE F
99–95	5	45
90–94	6	40
85–89	8	34
80–84	12	26
75–79	10	14
70–74	2	4
65–69	1	2
60–64	1	1

(From Darby ML, Bowen DM: Research Methods for Oral Health Professionals. Pocatello, JT McCann Company, 1990, p 107.)

when the distance between the scores is large **(Table 18-4).** Larger samples (>30) with scores closer together are organized using a grouped frequency distribution **(Table 18-5).** A **normal distribution,** also called the **bell curve,** is a frequently encountered distribution that is symmetric, **unimodal** (with one peak), and generally centered in distribution **(Figure 18-1).** Asymmetric distributions are referred to as **skewed. Skew** denotes the location of the tail of the distribution. A **negatively skewed distribution** means that the tail is pulled to the **left** by a few very low scores. A tail on the **right** is a **positively skewed distribution** due to the mean score being greater than the median. This is the result of several extremely high scores **(Figure 18-2).**

Measures of Central Tendency

In order to categorize the data, a summary of the scores in the data set is often helpful, and the informal term "**average**" refers to measures of **central tendency,** which can include the mean, mode, and median. The **mean,** often informally described as the average score, is the sum of the scores divided by the total number of scores. The **mode** is the most frequently occurring number; the **median score** is the central point within the distribution that divides the frequency in half. In the following set of 10 scores-1, 1, 1, 4, 5, 7, 7, 8, 9, and 9-the mean is 5.2; the mode is 1; and the median is 6.

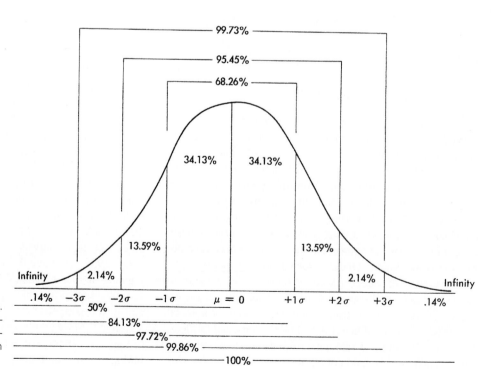

Figure 18-1. The normal curve. (From Darby ML, Bowen DM: Research Methods for Oral Health Professionals. Pocatello, JT McCann Company, 1990, p 121.)

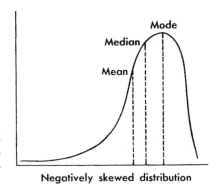 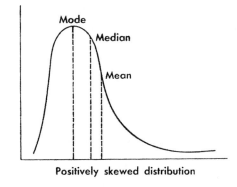

Negatively skewed distribution   Positively skewed distribution

Figure 18-2. Asymmetric distributions. (From Darby ML, Bowen DM: Research Methods for Oral Health Professionals. Pocatello, JT McCann Company, 1990, p 122.)

Measures of Variability

In addition to measures of central tendency, researchers also describe the **variability** of the data set and calculate the **range** of scores as the difference between the highest score and the lowest score. However, the most commonly used measure of variability is the **standard deviation**, which represents the average amount of deviation of the scores from the mean. In the example data set reported in the previous paragraph, the mean is 5.2; the range is 8; and the standard deviation is 3.29. Standard deviations are most often reported with the mean and place in perspective the variation of the individual scores in relation to the mean. For example, the variability of scores in this sample data set would be reported as M = 5.2 (3.29) or M = 5.2 ± 3.29, where M signifies the mean score and 3.29 signifies the standard deviation. **(See examples of the mean and standard deviation in Figures 18-3 and 18-4.)**

Bivariate Descriptive Statistics

Contingency tables provide a clear way to display differences in nominal and ordinal data in multiple dimensions. Contingency tables are frequency distributions that illustrate the relationships between variables through a tabular format. The fictitious example in **Table 18-6** provides data pre-

sented in a contingency table regarding the relationship between men and women's frequency of preventive dental hygiene visits.

In Table 18-6, gender is a nominal measurement and frequency of visits for preventive care is an ordinal measurement. The data are displayed in a cross-tabulated manner in this contingency table in order to allow the reader to quickly determine any patterns. In this example, the contingency table reveals that although 50% of clients adhere to the high-frequency interval for preventive care, 70% of the women are found in this category (or cell of the table). In addition, only 10% of the women are categorized in the low frequency of visits, yet 40% of the men are found in this low-frequency category. A contingency table provides an example of **bivariate** (i.e., with at least two variables) **descriptive statistics**.

Another example of bivariate descriptive statistics is the test for **correlation**, which describes the relationship between two measures. Test for correlation help to answer the question; for example, what is the relationship between students' scores on the DAT and their performance in dental school? Mathematical calculations are computed on the scores of both the DAT and dental school grades, and the correlation coefficient is obtained. The **correlation coefficient**, which is a number that ranges from -1 to +1, describes both the intensity and the direction of the relationship. Zero

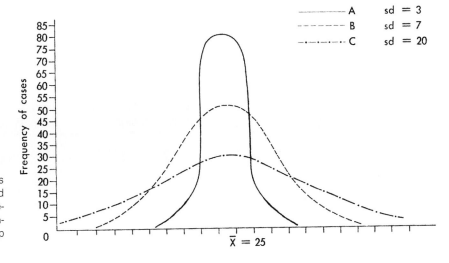

Figure 18-3. Three symmetric distributions with the same mean but different standard deviations. (From Darby ML, Bowen DM: Research Methods for Oral Health Professionals. Pocatello, JT McCann Company, 1990, p 116.)

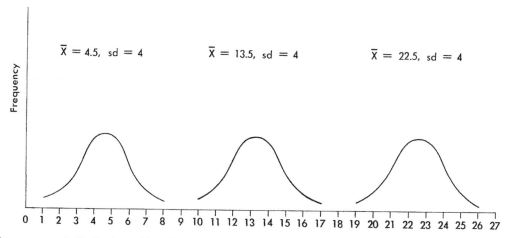

Figure 18-4. Three symmetric distributions with different means and the same standard deviations. (From Darby ML, Bowen DM: Research Methods for Oral Health Professionals. Pocatello, JT McCann Company, 1990, p 117.)

indicates that there is no relationship; a +1 is the highest positive correlation; and a -1 is the highest negative correlation. In this example, the correlation coefficient was .4, which indicates a moderate positive correlation, thus as DAT scores increase, students' dental school grades increase **(Figure 18-5).**

When working with either interval or ratio data as in the example earlier, the **product moment correlation coefficient**, also called the **Pearson's r**, is the most commonly used statistical test. When the data represent ordinal level measurement, the **Spearman's rank-order correlation**, also called **Spearman's rho,** is employed.

Inferential Statistical Tests

Although descriptive statistical testing can help to identify patterns and highlight trends, most quantitative studies contain research questions that require more analytic measures to compare and identify differences between groups. Inferential statistical tests provide the researcher with powerful data management and analysis tools to objectively test the relationships and performance of the study groups in relation to the research hypothesis.

Hypothesis Testing

In order to use statistics to test a hypothesis, the researcher must restate the research hypothesis to a **null hypothesis**, which states that there is no relationship between the independent and dependent variables and that any relationship is only a function of error. The following is an example of a research study hypothesis: "Adolescent boys who attended an educational program on the importance of wearing athletic mouthguards would wear the mouthguards for longer periods compared with boys who did not attend the educational program." The following statement formulates the hypothesis into the null hypothesis: "There is no difference in time wearing an athletic mouthguard for adolescent boys based on attendance at an educational program." **Inferential statistical tests** are designed to help the researcher decide whether to accept or reject the null hypothesis based on mathematical computations.

TABLE 18–6 Contingency Table: The Relationship Between Gender and Frequency of Preventive Dental Hygiene Visits

GENDER	HIGH FREQUENCY OF VISITS (EVERY 3–6 MONTHS)	MODERATE FREQUENCY OF VISITS (EVERY 7–15 MONTHS)	LOW FREQUENCY OF VISITS (EVERY 16–36 MONTHS)	TOTAL
Male	15 (30% of men)	15 (30% of men)	20 (40% of men)	50 (50% of sample)
Female	35 (70% of women)	10 (20% of women)	5 (10% of women)	50 (50% of sample)
TOTAL	50 (50% of sample)	25 (25% of sample)	25 (25% of sample)	100 (100% of sample)

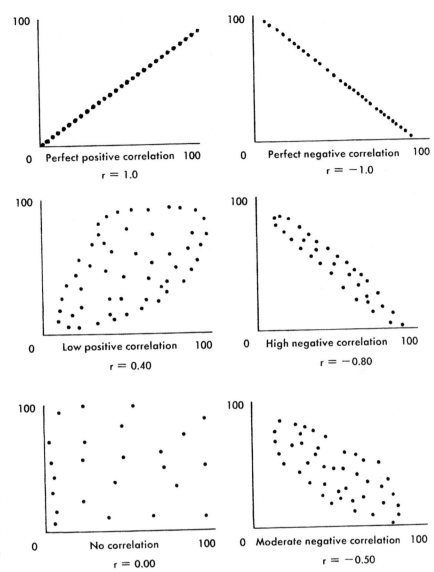

Figure 18-5. Scattergrams illustrating various relationships between two variables. (From Darby ML, Bowen DM: Research Methods for Oral Health Professionals. Pocatello, JT McCann Company, 1990, p 118.)

Type I and Type II Errors

Inferential statistics are open to two types of errors: Types I and II. **Type I errors** are errors in which the researcher rejects the null hypothesis when it really is true. **Type II errors** occur when the researcher accepts the null hypothesis when it really is false. Type I and II errors can be controlled by the researcher by adjusting the level of significance selected in the research study. The **level of significance**, also called **alpha**, is defined as the probability of rejecting a true null hypothesis, which is a type I error.

P **(probability) levels** are set at either .05 or .01, so that when researchers select a .05 significance level, they are accepting the risk that out of every 100 samples, a true null hypothesis would be rejected five times. Selection of a *P* of **.01** lowers the risk of type I errors, but it raises the risk of type II errors, because the stricter that the guidelines are set for rejecting the null hypothesis, the greater is the chance that a false null hypothesis will be accepted.

In dental and dental hygiene research, a *P* value of .05 is selected most often.

Scope of Bivariate Statistical Tests

Bivariate statistical tests can be classified as **parametric** and **nonparametric** tests and are classified based on the research design and the type of measurement employed in the study. **Parametric tests** require measurement on the interval or ratio scale; they must include at least one population parameter and mandate that the distribution of the data approximate a normal distribution. **Nonparametric tests** have less restrictive requirements and are often used with data or a nominal or ordinal scale; these tests do not require that the data resemble a normal distribution and also they do not require that the data are based on an estimation of parameters. A summary chart reprinted from Polit and Hungler is presented as **Table 18-7** and provides a summary guide to the most widely used bi-

TABLE 18–7 Summary Guide to Widely Used Bivariate Inferential Statistical Tests

NAME	TEST STATISTIC	PURPOSE	MEASUREMENT LEVEL* IV	MEASUREMENT LEVEL* DV
Parametric Tests				
t-test for independent groups	t	To test the difference between two independent group means	Nominal	Interval, Ratio
t-test for dependent groups	t	To test the difference between two dependent group means	Nominal	Interval, Ratio
Analysis of variance—ANOVA	F	To test the difference among the means of 3+ independent groups, or of more than one independent variable	Nominal	Interval, Ratio
Repeated measures ANOVA	F	To test the difference among means of 3+ related groups or sets of scores	Nominal	Interval, Ratio
Pearson's r	r	To test the existence of a relationship between two variables	Interval, Ratio	Interval, Ratio
Nonparametric Tests				
Chi-squared test	χ^2	To test the difference in proportions in 2+ independent groups	Nominal	Nominal
Mann-Whitney U-test	U	To test the difference in ranks of scores on two independent groups	Nominal	Ordinal
Kruskal-Wallis test	H	To test the difference in ranks of scores of 3+ independent groups	Nominal	Ordinal
Wilcoxon signed ranks test	$T(Z)$	To test the difference in ranks of scores of two related groups	Nominal	Ordinal
Friedman test	χ^2	To test the difference in ranks of scores of 3+ related groups	Nominal	Ordinal
Phi coefficient	ϕ	To test the magnitude of a relationship between two dichotomous variables	Nominal	Nominal
Spearman's rank order correlation	r_s	To test the existence of a relationship between two variables	Ordinal	Ordinal

*Measurement level of the independent variable (IV) and dependent variable (DV).
From Polit DF, Hungler BP: Essentials of Nursing Research. Philadelphia, JB Lippincott, 1997, p 352.

variate inferential statistical tests. This chart is subdivided into parametric and nonparametric statistical tests.

T Tests

T tests are often used in experimental and quasi-experimental research designs in order to test the statistical significance of differences in the means of the experimental and control groups. Researchers compute the **t statistic** by calculating data regarding the group means, the variability around the means, and the size of the sample. Once a t value is computed, the researchers determine the **degrees of freedom**, which are usually based on the sample size minus a specific number, and the researchers select a level of significance. After the t statistic, degrees of freedom, and P level are acquired, the researchers compare these values with the *t test table* values to determine the upper limit of the t statistic in order to accept the null hypothesis. If the computed value is higher than the table value, the null hypothesis can be rejected. If the computed value is lower, the null hypothesis cannot be rejected.

Analysis of Variance

Although t tests are limited to comparisons between two groups, **analysis of variance (ANOVA)** is a parametric test that measures the significance of differences in the means of three or more groups. The **F ratio** is calculated for ANOVA and represents the variation between the groups compared with the variation within the groups. In addition to the F ratio, two types of degrees of freedom are calculated-one for

between groups and one for within groups. After the computation is completed and the researchers select a level of significance, the values are compared with the **F distribution** table. When the computed value exceeds the value in the F distribution table, the null hypothesis that the population means are equal can be rejected.

Nonparametric Tests

Although parametric tests are powerful statistical tools to help investigators employ objective and standard ways to determine the meaning and significance of their research findings, parametric tests cannot be used in all research designs with all research data. **Nonparametric tests**, most notably the **chi-square test** and **Spearman's rank order correlation**, are helpful when categorical data are present and investigators wish to determine the level of significance of the differences among measurements for different groups.

The chi-square test is used with nominal or ordinal data to test for significance when differences are discovered in the contingency table format. The chi-squared statistic is developed by computing the expected frequencies in each portion (cell) of the table based on the assumption that there were no differences among the variables. Next, investigators subtract the differences in the computed and expected values and add all of these values together for a total chi-squared statistic. Investigators select the level of significance and compute the degrees of freedom, which are calculated by multiplying the number of rows minus 1 by the number of columns minus 1. The investigator can then consult a **chi-square table** to determine if the computed value exceeds the published table value. When the computed value exceeds the table value, the investigator can reject the null hypothesis because the values are larger than what would be expected by chance.

The bivariate parametric and nonparametric statistical tests provide a good, basic introduction to statistical analysis of research literature. Dental hygienists should understand the basic principles of selecting a test based on the type of data measurement included in the research design and should scrutinize research reports to ensure that investigators provide a strong rationale for the statistical tests that they select. In addition, dental hygienists should scrutinize the research for reports on the controls for type I and type II errors and be alert to the author's rationale for rejecting the null hypothesis and accepting the study hypothesis.

Dental and dental hygiene investigators have begun to include more powerful **multivariate statistical analysis**, which allows investigators to analyze three or more variables simultaneously. Examples of **multivariate statistical tests** include **multiple regression, analysis of covariance (ANCOVA), and factor analysis.** For example, multiple regression allow researchers to use more than one independent variable to explain and predict one dependent variable, and ANCOVA combines multiple regression with analysis of variance to provide statistical control for several troublesome extraneous variables. Although these statistical tests are more advanced than the scope of this chapter, dental hygienists should be aware of the current trend to expanded and more advanced use of statistical packages for dental and dental hygiene research.

The fourth component of the research process, **analysis/interpretation**, represents the phase in which the investigators evaluate their research questions and hypotheses through various descriptive and inferential statistical tests. **Statistical analyses** provide an objective measure for researchers to test their hypotheses and to determine if the results differed significantly from what would have been expected by chance. Statistical analyses also help the researcher to determine the strength and level of relationships of the variables in the research questions. Specific questions for dental hygienists to use when evaluating statistical methods and procedures are included in **Box 18-5.**

Results and Conclusions

As the last component of the research process, the investigators report **the results (raw data)** and provide their **interpretation of the results in the discussion and the conclusion sections** of a scientific article. These sections provide insight to the meaning that the investigators have placed on the results of the statistical tests in relation to the original research questions and hypothesis. Within these sections of the report, critical readers evaluate the investigators' findings in order to determine the appropriateness and

> **BOX 18-5 • Guidelines for Critically Analyzing the Scientific Literature**
>
> **Analysis and Interpretation**
> - Are the statistical tests described in the study?
> - Is the rationale for the selection of the statistical tests provided by the authors?
> - Are the results of the statistical tests illustrated in tables or graphs and also described in the text?
> - Are the appropriate statistical tests used in relation to the research design and the measures used in the study?

applicability of the results for clinical practice. Critical readers should address the following two issues when evaluating the results and conclusions in a research report: (1) Are the conclusions appropriate based on the research design and statistical tests used? (2) Are the conclusions realistic and relevant for clinical practice?

Conclusions must be appropriate in relation to the research design. Unfortunately, many readers skim quickly through the initial portions of a research article in order to spend most of their time reading the discussion and conclusion sections. This habit is an unfortunate choice, because it does not provide the reader with sufficient background to understand and verify the conclusions that the investigators have made. Many readers justify their complacency because of the peer review system before publication, in which professional journals such as the *Journal of Dental Hygiene* and the *Journal of Periodontology* have a strict and systematic process for accepting articles for publication. **Peer review** involves the process of review and critique by several researchers and editors before an article is accepted for publication. However, the peer review process is neither a guarantee nor a substitute for careful review and critique by the reader. In addition, some professional publications lack extensive peer review procedures, which may not be readily apparent when reviewing the publication.

Dental hygienists should read the investigators' conclusions critically and look for the evidence that the author uses to support the conclusions. Authors should be very clear when presenting this supporting evidence from the statistical analysis in tables or graphs. In addition, critical readers should look for more in-depth discussion of the evidence to support the conclusions in the results and discussion sections of the scientific article. If this information is unavailable, discriminating readers should question the conclusions, search the data presented in the article, and consider if there are any competing explanations for the results presented.

Inferential statistical analysis is built on the concept of **probability**, thus the critical reader must always consider if the null hypothesis was rejected improperly or if non-significant findings are in error. Although *P* values can be set to minimize these type I and type II errors, other sources of error, such as deviations in selecting a representative sample, insufficient sample size, or use of invalid and unreliable measurement tools can also raise the probability of error. Dental hygienists should carefully review the study methods and procedures to identify possible sources of error that may influence the hypotheses testing process and outcomes and affect the credibility of the conclusions.

Dental hygienists should evaluate carefully the type of statistical tests that are used in relation to the conclusions that are presented in the study. For example, when tests for correlation, such as Pearson's r, are used in a research study, the research conclusions are limited to descriptions of the associated relationships, and the authors cannot conclude that there is a cause-and-effect relationship. For example, in a research study about dental hygiene practice, age and hours of practice are found to be negatively correlated. The authors can conclude that these two variables are related, but they cannot present the conclusion that aging causes dental hygienists to work fewer hours. The weaker claim of association is based on the descriptive research design and limited power of the descriptive statistical test that was selected for the study.

Conclusions should be realistic and relevant for clinical practice. Dental hygienists should carefully review the researcher's conclusions in light of their experiences and current methods of practice. Are the conclusions and results believable in relation to prior clinical experiences? Often, clinical research studies provide objective analysis of accepted clinical practices but may also disprove popular clinical practices. For example, many dental hygienists were recommending that clients should use a mixture of hydrogen peroxide and baking soda as a dentifrice to reduce gingivitis; however, controlled clinical research identified the oral hygiene as the main therapeutic agent. No additional differences were seen in the treatment group with oral hygiene and experimental dentifrice compared with the group that used oral hygiene only.

Dental hygienists should also review the practicality of the methods related to research conclusions. For example, when investigators demonstrated that essential oil mouthwashes, which were readily available to consumers, could control and prevent gingivitis, the subjects in the study rinsed with 0.5 oz of the full-strength product for 30 seconds twice daily. Many clients have difficulty in rinsing with the essential oil mouthwash in a full-strength formulation for 30 seconds due to the high alcohol content of the mouthwash, which may produce burning and tissue sloughing in some clients. Although many clinicians advise patients to use a smaller amount of the product or to dilute the product, dental hygienists cannot be certain that this adapted clinical protocol will also produce the same results in terms of reduction in gingivitis that were found in the original study.

Within the last component of the research process, involving results and conclusions, the authors provide the specific detail regarding the degree to which the statistical tests supported the study hypotheses. Critical readers should expect a clear description of the results and should look for credible ex-

---

> ### BOX 18-6 • **Guidelines for Critically Analyzing the Scientific Literature**
>
> **Conclusions**
> - Are the conclusions appropriate in relation to the research design?
> - Have the authors submitted their research to a peer review journal for publication?
> - Is the evidence presented to support the conclusions made by the authors?
> - Are the potential threats to type I and type II errors discussed and controlled by the authors?
> - Are the research results practical and relevant for clinical practice?
> - Do the authors have the academic credentials, resources, and research support to the complete the type of study presented?

---

planations from the researchers that justify the results and conclusions. Readers can evaluate the credibility and validity of the results by carefully reading the way in which the results, discussion, and conclusion sections are written and presented. Specific questions for dental hygienists to use when evaluating the results and conclusions are included in **Box 18-6.**

 ETHICS

Any discussion of research principles must include a thorough review of the accepted practices and ethical principles as related to the research process. Unfortunate previous incidents have uncovered lapses in ethical behavior that have resulted in mandated procedures for the ethical review of research and required protection for human subjects involved in research. This section reviews the procedures and functions of the **Institutional Review Boards (IRB)** and includes a discussion of the rights that must be guaranteed for individuals who consent to be subjects in research projects. The current protection for human subjects and standards for the ethical conduct of research arise from three historical developments: (1) the Nuremberg Code, (2) the Declaration of Helsinki, and (3) the National Commission for the Protection of Human Subjects of Biomedical and Behavioral Research.

Nuremberg Code

Current discussion of ethical research practices arose after the discovery of multiple unethical medical experiments conducted by the Nazi regime in Germany from 1933 to 1945. Under the guise of political ambition and racial purity, several poorly designed medical experiments were conducted using disabled children and concentration camp residents of Jewish ancestry. These experiments were conducted without the subjects' consent and had little potential to benefit society. In the trials of the Nazi officials after the war, these unethical medical practices were exposed and condemned, and in 1949 the **Nuremberg code** was developed to ensure that human subjects were treated appropriately and fairly. The Nuremberg code describes procedures for ensuring both the initial voluntary consent and the continuing agreement of subjects to participate in research and includes a discussion of the general ethical practices and procedures for conducting research.

Declaration of Helsinki

As research activity began to flourish and expand throughout the world in the 1950s and 1960s, the World Medical Association developed the **Declaration of Helsinki**, which expanded the Nuremberg Code to include more formalized definitions and procedures for the conduct of research and protection of human subjects. The Declaration of Helsinki, which was originally developed in 1964 and revised in 1975, provided further differentiation of research that would provide therapeutic benefits to the individual and the riskier nontherapeutic research, which adds knowledge to the profession and future patients but no benefit for the individual. The Declaration of Helsinki strengthened the protection that healthy volunteers receive in research and placed the burden on investigators to inform and protect subjects and to justify investigations in light of the potential benefit to both subjects and society.

National Commission for the Protection of Human Subjects

Although the Nuremberg Code and the Declaration of Helsinki were adopted by most scientists and institutions, unfortunate ethical lapses in research activity were uncovered in the United States during the early 1970s. One of the most publicized infractions of ethical procedures involved the **Tuskegee study**, which was conducted to determine the natural course of syphilis in African-American men from 1932 to 1972 in Tuskegee, Alabama. Even though penicillin was discovered as an effective treatment for syphilis in the 1940s, some study subjects were not informed either of their diagnosis or of the available treatment until the study ended in 1972. Public outrage over the unethical treatment of subjects in this study and of several other studies inspired the passage of the **National Research Act** in 1974, which established the **National Commission for the Protection of Human Subjects of Biomedical and Behavioral Research.** The National Commission produced an influential document, *The Belmont Report*, which provided further clarification of scientists' rights and responsibilities regarding ethical scientific conduct.

Belmont Report

The *Belmont Report* identified three ethical principles that ensure the preservation of individuals' rights: **respect for persons, beneficence,** and **justice.** Respect for people means that all individuals make an educated choice whether or not they want to participate and continue in the study without coercion or fear of mistreatment. The ethical principles of justice and beneficence mandate that the researchers conduct the research fairly with the goal of improving the patient's condition; this has often been interpreted as "do no harm" when questions of therapeutic benefit arise for the subjects.

Current Regulations for the Protection of Human Subjects

In 1983, the US federal government's Department of Health and Human Services issued specific regulations for scientists regarding the protection of human subjects and peer review of all research projects. These guidelines come directly from the deliberations of the National Commission and the Belmont Report and draw upon the historical precedents from the Nuremberg Code and the Declaration of Helsinki.

Human subjects are protected by the requirement for written informed consent forms to be discussed and signed with all subjects participating in research. **Informed consent** means that the study has been explained to all subjects and that they understand the essential components of the study and agree to participate in the study voluntarily. Procedures and forms for informed consent must include information on the study design, how the subjects were selected, and the risks and benefits associated with the study.

Although informed consent is the major way that subjects are informed about the scope of their participation in the research study, the federal regulations mandate that peer scientists at an institution review of the research project through the establishment of the **Institutional Review Board (IRB).** The IRB reviews scientific research projects based on three levels of review: exempt, expedited, and complete (quorum) review. The assigned category and scope of the review is based on the potential risks of the study and the level of protection for human subjects. For example, educational research and projects that evaluate demonstration projects and existing programs are generally considered **exempt** because of the low potential for risk for subjects. Research projects that include survey or interview procedures are exempt unless the data collection involves the loss of confidentiality for the subject. **Expedited review** is reserved for projects that involve minimal risk for subjects, especially when confidentiality may be compromised or when blood or tissue samples are collected and protection of human subjects must be ensured. When more than minimal risk to subjects is possible, the IRB requires a **complete review** of the project. In expedited and full reviews, the study investigators must submit the research protocol, including informed consent forms and procedures, in order to minimize and justify the risks to the subjects in relation to the potential benefits. In addition, investigators must demonstrate that subjects are selected in a standard and fair manner and that all subjects complete appropriate informed consent procedures and forms.

Relevance to Dental Hygienists

All clinicians and scientists must remain vigilant to ensure that research is conducted ethically and that research subjects receive complete protection. A common way that dental hygienists begin research activity in their career is through participation as a research assistant or clinical examiner, when they may have major responsibility for completing informed consent procedures with clients. In addition, dental hygienists may participate in **clinical trials** in dental practices for a multi-site study, and they must ensure that compliance with all proper procedures, including IRB review and protection of human subjects, is maintained. Some dental hygienists may serve as members of an IRB, and they may play a major role in the review and approval of studies to ensure the highest ethical standards. All dental hygienists should be fully aware of the ethical issues in research and should serve as consumer advocates for their clients when they choose to participate in research. Specific questions for dental hygienists to use when evaluating ethical issues in scientific articles are included in **Box 18-7.**

 CONCLUSION

The scientific literature offers great opportunities for dental hygienists to advance their level of scientific knowledge and to increase the quality and efficiency of the dental hygiene care that they provide to clients. Unfortunately, many dental hygiene students and clinicians are easily intimidated by complicated or irrelevant research articles; thus, they may often report negative attitudes about their interest or involvement in research. These negative attitudes can readily be neutralized when dental hygienists learn about the exciting and dynamic qualities when they include a research perspective within their practice. Dental hygienists can begin independently to read the scientific literature, join a study club, and take academic and continuing education courses in order to expand their knowledge of the research process and increase their skills in critically reviewing the scientific literature. As scientific research continues to expand the knowledge in dental hygiene and dentistry, dental hygienists must develop their skills in evaluating scientific literature in order to provide the highest level of care for their clients.

Sources

ADHA Research Agenda: White paper by the 1993-1994 ADHA Council on Research. J Dent Hygiene 68:26-29, 1994.

Bowen D: Overview of ADHA Research Programs. Paper presented at the special session: Building alliances through dental hygiene research. J Dent Hygiene 65:13-16, 1991.

Bulman JS, Osborn JF: Statistics in Dentistry. London, BDJ, 1989.

Burns N, Grove SK: Understanding Nursing Research. Philadelphia, WB Saunders, 1995, p 3.

Campbell DT, Stanley JC: Experimental and Quasi-experimental Designs for Research. Chicago, Rand McNally, 1963.

Code of Federal Regulations: 45CFR. Washington, DC, Department of Health and Human Services, 1983.

Cohen J: Statistical Power Analysis for the Behavioral Sciences. New York, Academic Press, 1977.

Curriculum Guidelines on Research for Dental Hygiene Education. J Dent Educ 58:250-255, 1994.

Darby ML, Bowen DM: Research Methods for Oral Health Professionals. Pocatello, JT McCann Company, 1990.

Darby ML, Walsh MM: A proposed human needs conceptual model for dental hygiene, Part I. J Dent Hygiene 67:326, 1993.

Darby ML, Walsh MM: Dental Hygiene Theory and Practice. Philadelphia, WB Saunders, 1995, p 1111.

DePoy E, Gitlin LN: Introduction to Research: Multiple Strategies for Health and Human Sciences. St. Louis, CV Mosby, 1993.

Faust CC: A qualitative study of male dental hygienists' experiences after graduation. J Dent Hygiene 73:141-143, 1999.

Forrest JL, Lyons KJ, Bross TM, et al: Reaching consensus on the national dental hygiene research agenda: A Delphi study. J Dent Hygiene 69:261-269, 1995.

Gadbury-Amyot CC, Williams KB, Bray KK, et al: Validity and reliability of oral health related quality of life instrument for dental hygiene. J Dent Hygiene 73:126-133, 1999.

Glaser B, Strauss T: The Discovery of Grounded Theory: Strategies for Qualitative Research. Chicago, Aldine, 1967.

Gutmann ME: Air polishing: A comprehensive review of the literature. J Dent Hygiene 72:47-56, 1998.

Kerlinger FN: Foundation of Behavioral Research, 3rd ed. New York, Holt, Rinehart & Winston, 1986.

Leininger MM: Qualitative Research Methods in Nursing. New York, Grune & Stratton, 1985.

Lincoln YS, Guba EG: Naturalistic Inquiry. Newbury Park, CA, Sage Publications, 1985.

Loe H: The gingival index, the plaque index, and the retention index systems. J Periodontol 38(Suppl):610-621, 1967.

Mankodi S, Ross NM, Mostler C: Clinical efficacy of Listerine in inhibiting and reducing plaque and experimental gingivitis. J Clin Periodontol 14:285-291, 1987.

Morse JM, Field PA: Qualitative Research Methods for Health Professionals, 3rd ed. Thousand Oaks, CA, Sage Publications, 1995.

National Commission for the Protection of Human Subjects (1978): The Belmont Report: Ethical principles and guidelines for research involving human subjects. In Spradley JF: The Ethnographic Interview. New York, Holt, Rinehart and Winston, 1979.

Newbrun E: The use of sodium bicarbonate in oral hygiene products and practice. Compend Cont Educ Dent 18:21, 1996.

BOX 18-7 • Guidelines for Critically Analyzing the Scientific Literature

Ethics

- Was the review of the study made by the Institutional Review Board described?
- Were ethical considerations in the recruitment and selection of subjects discussed?
- How were the informed consent procedures explained to subjects?
- If vulnerable subjects were selected for the study, how were their rights protected?
- What were the risks in this study?
- What benefits outweighed the risks?
- Was there any coercion or deception involved in the study?

Polit DF, Hungler BP: Essentials of Nursing Research. Philadelphia, Lippincott Williams & Wilkins, 1997.

Spradley JF: The Ethnographic Interview. New York, Holt, Rinehart and Winston, 1979.

Walsh MM, Darby ML: Application of the human needs conceptual model of dental hygiene to the role of clinician, Part II. J Dent Hygiene 67:334-341, 1993.

Wilkins E: Clinical Practice of the Dental Hygienist, 8th ed. Philadelphia, Lea & Febiger, 1999.

Williams KB, Gadbury-Amyot CC, Bray KK, et al: Oral health related quality of life: A model for dental hygiene. J Dent Hygiene 72:19-26, 1998.

Questions and Answers

Questions

1. Which of the following best describes the differences in the quantitative and qualitative research traditions? Quantitative research
   A. provides the opportunity for in-depth exploration of a phenomenon
   B. allows the researcher to use a smaller sample size
   C. uses controlled situations to study the effects of certain variables
   D. is characterized by intensive relationships between participants and researchers

2. Which of the following is an essential part of a true experimental research study?
   A. Randomization of subjects
   B. Inclusion of at least four groups of subjects
   C. Use of laboratory facilities
   D. Introduction of an intervention to at least two groups

3. Which of the following best defines the term random selection?
   A. Asking for volunteer subjects
   B. Selecting subjects based on pre-set criteria
   C. Purposefully selecting subjects from certain subgroups
   D. Ensuring that all members of a population have an equal chance of being selected

4. All of the following represents appropriate examples of problem/question formulation in the quantitative tradition except one. Which one is this exception?
   A. Is triclosan more effective in reducing gingivitis than the pyrophosphates?
   B. Are powered toothbrushes more effective than toothbrushes for removing stains?
   C. How can we increase patient's flossing behavior?
   D. Is waxed floss more effective in proximal plaque removal than unwaxed floss?

5. Which of the following represents appropriate criteria for critiquing the literature review section of the paper?
   A. Most recent references are used; older references are avoided.
   B. The focus is on describing the range of research completed.
   C. Careful analysis of the adequacy of the literature is provided.
   D. Other review articles and secondary sources are most credible citations.

6. Which of the following is true regarding study hypothesis? Hypotheses are
   A. statements that predict relationships and outcomes of the variables.
   B. statements that claim there is no relationship between variables.
   C. questions that identify and specify the concepts to be studied.
   D. questions that provide general direction for the study design.

7. In a study with the following hypothesis, "Powered toothbrushes will remove more extrinsic stain than a manual toothbrush," what is the dependent variable?
   A. Powered toothbrush
   B. Manual toothbrush
   C. Extrinsic stain removal

8. Which of the following could be considered an extraneous variable in the study with the hypothesis described in #7?
   A. Client's ability to brush
   B. Specific brand of powered toothbrush
   C. Specific brand of manual toothbrush
   D. All of the above

9. All of the following are ways that researchers can control extraneous variables except one. Which one is this exception?
   A. Use a large convenience sample size.
   B. Use random assignment of subjects to groups.
   C. Purposefully select subjects for a more homogeneous group.
   D. Control the study design to reduce variation.

10. A true experimental study that employs multiple independent variables is called
    A. correlational study.
    B. factorial design.

C. retrospective study.

D. prospective study.

11. Which of the following best describes the placebo effect?

    A. Carry-over effects from one treatment to the other in a repeated measure design

    B. Positive results identified in a group where no intervention was made

    C. Factors inherently present in subjects that affect the outcome of the study

    D. Bias induced by beliefs of researchers

12. Research, which seeks to describe the relationship between two variables that cannot be manipulated in a study, is called

    A. true experimental.

    B. quasi-experimental.

    C. correlational.

    D. descriptive.

13. A correlational study was completed which identified a positive correlation of +.4 between advanced periodontal disease and specific types of heart disease. Can the authors state that the periodontal disease caused heart disease?

    A. Yes, that is the purpose of correlational research.

    B. Yes, because the correlation coefficient was positive

    C. No, because there is no manipulation of dependent variables.

    D. No, because there is no randomization and control in correlational studies.

14. In a correlational study regarding patterns of chocolate consumption and decay rates, the researchers found a +.2 correlation between frequency of chocolate ingestion and DMF rates. Which of the following can the authors conclude?

    A. Eating chocolate causes caries.

    B. There is a weak positive relationship between the frequency of eating chocolate and caries.

    C. There is a strong positive relationship between the frequency of eating chocolate and caries.

    D. There is no relationship between the frequency of eating chocolate and caries.

15. Which of the following describes internal validity?

    A. Amount of control researchers maintain over the study

    B. Generalizability of the results to other settings

    C. Confidence that the change in the dependent variable is due to the independent variable

    D. Subjects compliance with the study protocol

16. All of the following are considered threats to internal validity except one. Which one is this exception?

    A. Loss of subjects

    B. Intervening historical events

    C. Normal maturation of subjects

    D. Limitations in sample selection

17. Which of the following defines the reliability of an instrument? A reliable instrument

    A. consistently measures the same way in multiple attempts.

    B. thoroughly measures the content area.

    C. accurately measures the content in relation to an existing instrument.

    D. all of the above.

Questions 18-20 relate to the following data set: 1, 3, 5, 5, 5, 5, 8, 9, 9, 10.

18. What is the mode for this data set?

    A. 1

    B. 5

    C. 6

    D. 9

19. Which of the following defines the mean score?

    A. Sum of scores

    B. Sum of scores divided by the total number

    C. Most frequently occurring number

    D. Central point within the distribution

20. What is the mean for this data set?

    A. 1

    B. 5

    C. 6

    D. 9

ANSWERS

1. **C.** Qualitative research deals with data for which individual quantitative measurements (e.g., height, weight, blood pressure) are not available but that relate to the presence or absence of some characteristic (i.e., smoking, alcohol consumption).

2. **A.** A true experimental study includes at least two subgroups; the study can be accomplished in various settings (e.g., school, clinic, community) and does not require an intervention.

3. **D.** A random sample is a sample that consists of subjects who are chosen independently of each other and who have an equal chance of being included in the study.

4. **C.** Flossing behavior is not being compared with any other variable.

5. **C.** When conducting a review of the literature, all related sources should be reviewed to obtain a thorough analysis of the topic studied so that gaps in knowledge can be identified and a theoretical basis for the research can be provided. Older references may lack current knowledge; after analysis, older references may not be useful, but in some cases they provide an historical basis of understanding.

6. **A.** The hypothesis is an educated guess; a tentative answer to a problem that will be accepted or rejected by use of the scientific method.

7. **C.** The dependent variable is the measure that is believed to change as a result of manipulating the independent variable (e.g., powered and manual toothbrushes).

8. **D.** Extraneous variables are uncontrolled variables that are not related to the purpose of the study but may influence the outcome. These variables should be eliminated, if at all possible.

9. **A.** A convenience sample is easier to obtain, but randomization of this sample would help to control the extraneous variables.

10. **B.** Factorial designs allow the researcher to study the effects of several independent variables or multiple levels of the

same independent variable simultaneously in the same experiment.

11. **B.** A placebo (sugar pill), for example, is given to a group of subjects and elicits a response, even though it is not considered to be a form of treatment. Factors inherently present in subjects that affect the outcome of a study are referred to as subject relevant variables.

12. **C.** Correlational studies identify consistent relationships among variables.

13. **D.** A correlation coefficient does not indicate a cause-and-effect relationship between variables. A + .40 is a low positive correlation.

14. **B.** A correlation coefficient of + .20 is a weak positive correlation, because correlations close to 0 indicate little or no relationship between variables.

15. **C.** Answer B refers to reliability or the consistency of measurement.

16. **D.** Limitation in sample selection is a threat to external validity.

17. **A.** Reliability is the degree to which an instrument will yield the same results with the same population group in the same setting, and so forth, each time that the same information is measured.

18. **B.** The mode is the most frequently occurring score.

19. **B.** The mean is the average score.

20. **C.** Total of score (60) ÷ # of score (10) = $\bar{x}$(6)

Case Studies

SYNOPSIS OF PATIENT HISTORY	Age	14	VITAL SIGNS	
	Sex	F	Blood Pressure	102/68
	Height	4'11"	Pulse Rate	78
			Respiration Rate	18

CASE A-
Pediatric, Medically Compromised

Weight   95   lb
             43.1   kg

1. Under Care of Physician
   Yes ☑   No ☐
   Condition: Lower jaw pain

2. Hospitalized within the last 5 years
   Yes ☑   No ☐
   Reason: Cancer

3. Has or had the following conditions
   Rhabdomyosarcoma—base of the tongue

4. Current medications
   Augmentin

5. Smokes or uses tobacco products
   Yes ☐   No ☑

6. Is pregnant
   Yes ☐   No ☑   N/A ☐

MEDICAL HISTORY: Diagnosed at age 9 with rhabdomyosarcoma. Treated with radiation therapy (5000 rads) and chemotherapy. Saw physician recently for lower jaw pain, and M.D. referred child to dentist for evaluation; prescribed Augmentin.

DENTAL HISTORY: Referred to dentist after radiation and chemotherapy. After receiving hyperboric oxygen therapy, root canals and limited amalgam restorations were performed. Flouride trays were fabricated and chlorhexidine rinsing was prescribed. Trismus noted several weeks after radiation, but subsided within 3 months. Has not seen a dentist in 2 years. Did not use flouride or chlorhexidine with any regularity.

SOCIAL HISTORY: Enrolled in the 8th grade. Has missed several weeks of school due to oral pain. Diet was good until sore mouth forced her to eat only soft foods.

CHIEF COMPLAINT: "My teeth in my lower jaw hurt, and my mouth is so dry. I cannot eat."

CASE A

Current oral hygiene status
Poor oral hygiene
Rinses with old prescription of 0.12% chlorhexidine occasionally

Supplemental oral examination findings
Moderate gingivitis
Extreme tenderness—could not perform periodontal probing
Halitosis
Xerostomia

☐ Clinically visible carious lesion

✕ Clinically missing tooth

△ Furcation

▲ Through-and-through furcation

Probe 1: initial probing depth

Probe 2: probing depth 1 month after scaling and root planing

ADULT CLINICAL EXAMINATION

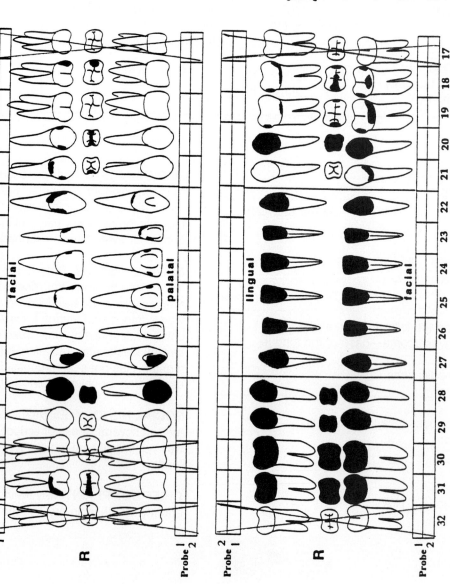

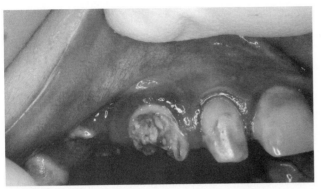

Figure A1.

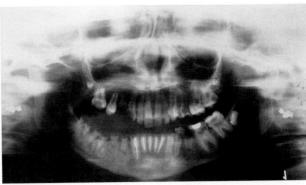

Figure A3.

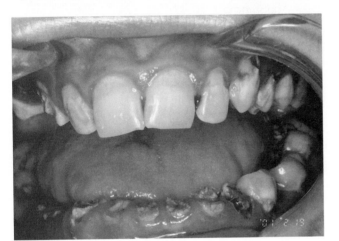

Figure A2.

CASE A — The Pediatric Medically Compromised Patient

1. Hyperbaric oxygen treatments are prescribed to reduce the risk of which of the following conditions?

   A. Xerostomia
   B. Radiation caries
   C. Osteoradionecrosis
   D. Periodontal disease

2. Which of the following conditions is most likely to be the cause of this patient's mandibular pain?

   A. Trismus
   B. Periapical infection
   C. Gingival inflammation
   D. Recurrence of the cancer

3. What dental material has been placed in the canals of the mandibular anterior teeth?

   A. Amalgam
   B. Gutta-percha
   C. Paper points
   D. Silver points

4. All of the following measures would be included in a treatment plan for this patient except one. Which one is the exception?

   A. Daily fluoride
   B. Annual recalls
   C. Extraction of severely decayed teeth
   D. Personalized oral hygiene instructions

5. The radiolucencies found at the apices of most of the mandibular teeth are indicative of which of the following conditions?

   A. Abscess
   B. Nutrient canals
   C. Incomplete root formation
   D. Normal bony trabecular patterns

6. Augmentin is found in which of the following drug classifications?

   A. Analgesic
   B. Antibiotic
   C. Anticholinergic
   D. Anti-inflammatory
   E. Nonsteroidal anti-inflammatory

7. The structure noted between tooth no. 4 and no. 6 on the panoramic radiograph is a(n) _____.

   A. odontoma.
   B. impacted tooth.
   C. dentigerous cyst.
   D. retained root tip.

8. What are the small spherical structures medial to the coronoid process?

   A. Exostoses
   B. Enamel pearls
   C. Radiographic artifacts
   D. Developing third molars

9. Which of the following teeth are most likely to be congenitally missing?

   A. No. 1
   B. No. 3
   C. No. 16
   D. No. 20
   E. No. 32

10. The severity of tooth decay noted in this young patient is **primarily** the result of which of the following factors?

    A. Soft diet
    B. Poor oral hygiene
    C. Infrequent dental visits
    D. Radiation to the salivary glands

CASE B

SYNOPSIS OF PATIENT HISTORY			
	Age	60	
	Sex	F	
	Height	5'5"	

VITAL SIGNS
Blood Pressure   135/85
Pulse Rate   85
Respiration Rate   20

CASE B -
Adult, Medically Compromised

Weight   150 lb
68.2 kg

1. Under Care of Physician
   Yes ☑   No ☐
   Condition: Sinus infection and chemotherapy

2. Hospitalized within the last 5 years
   Yes ☑   No ☐
   Reason: Mastectomy (bilateral)

3. Has or had the following conditions
   Rheumatic heart disease, Breast cancer, hyper-tension, and insulin-dependant diabetes mellitus

4. Current medications
   Tamoxifen, cyclophosphamide, clonidine, insulin, ciprofloxacin

5. Smokes or uses tobacco products
   Yes ☐   No ☑

6. Is pregnant
   Yes ☐   No ☑   N/A ☐

MEDICAL HISTORY: Sinus infection, treated with Cipro. Had rheumatic fever as a child; diagnosed with mitral valve prolapse with regurgitation 15 years ago. Bilateral mastectomy; currently undergoing chemotherapy. Allergic to penicillin. Hypertension and diabetes are usually stable.

DENTAL HISTORY: Has not had routine dental care. Several teeth extracted as a young adult. Had teeth cleaned 6 months ago at dentist of a family friend, and he referred the patient to a periodontist.

SOCIAL HISTORY: Had 3 large babies before the age of 30 years. Patient's diet is usually good but she loves candy occasionally and adjusts her insulin to compensate.

CHIEF COMPLAINT: "My mouth is sore and dry. I have a toothache somewhere in the back upper right area of my mouth. I think some of my front teeth may be decayed."

ADULT CLINICAL EXAMINATION

CASE B

Current oral hygiene status
Fair; moderate plaque; bleeding upon probing

Supplemental oral examination findings
Pt. has several maxillary anterior composites, but additional carious lesions are noted.
Generalized 2–5 mm recession
Minimal calculus
Generalized class II mobility
Xerostomia
3 2 × 3 mm = ulcerations on lining mucosa
Suppuration from No. 5

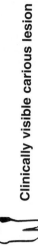 Clinically visible carious lesion

 Clinically missing tooth

△ Furcation

▲ Through-and-through furcation

Probe 1: initial probing depth

Probe 2: probing depth 1 month after scaling and root planing

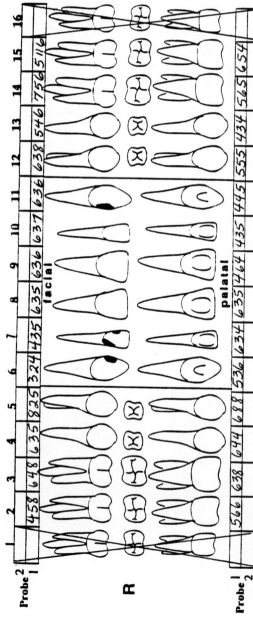

Maxillary — facial

Probe	2 / 1															
Tooth	1	2	3	4	5	6	7	8	9	10	11	12	13	14	15	16
		458	648	635	825	324	435	635	636	637	636	638	546	775	651	16

Maxillary — palatal

	566	638	644	688	536	634	635	464	435	445	555	434	565	654

Mandibular — lingual

Probe	2 / 1															
	945	565	434	736	433	332	322	424	423	324	424	444	555	
Tooth	17	18	19	20	21	22	23	24	25	26	27	28	29	30	31	32

Mandibular — facial

Probe	1 / 2															
	574	466	524	424	324	424	423	324	425	524	323	535		

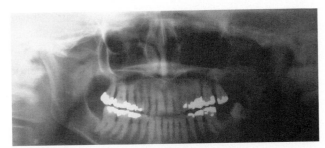

Figure B1.

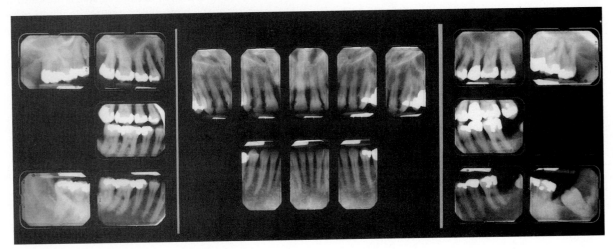

Figure B2.

CASE B —
The Adult, Medically
Compromised Patient

1. Which of the following scenerios would be recommended for this patient before treatment?

   A. The patient should be premedicated with amoxicillin.
   B. The patient should be premedicated with clindamycin.
   C. The patient's current medications are sufficient coverage for premedication.
   D. No conditions exist that warrant premedication.

2. The oral ulcerations noted on the lining mucosa are most likely the result of taking which of the following medications?

   A. Insulin
   B. Clonidine
   C. Tamoxifen
   D. Cyclophosphamide

3. The radiolucency noted between the roots of tooth no. 30 indicates which of the following?

   A. Erosion
   B. Recurrent caries
   C. Cervical burnout
   D. Furcation involvement

4. Which of the following medications is most likely to be responsible for the patient's oral xerostomia?

   A. Clonidine
   B. Tamoxifen
   C. Ciprofloxacin
   D. Cyclophosphamide

5. During periodontal débridement, this patient demonstrates flushed, dry skin, abdominal pain, and nausea. Administration of which of the following represents the best course of action?

   A. CPR
   B. Sugar Glucose
   C. Insulin
   D. Oxygen

6. The dental hygienist detects an acetone breath odor in this patient. Which of the following is the most likely cause of this condition?

   A. Hyperglycemia
   B. Insulin overdose
   C. Poor oral hygiene
   D. Medications that she is taking

7. All of the following factors have contributed to this patient's history of interproximal and occlusal caries except one. Which one is the exception?

   A. Diet
   B. Oral hygiene status
   C. Drug-induced xerostomia
   D. Diseases experienced by the patient

8. What is the status of tooth no. 17?

   A. Extracted
   B. Unerupted
   C. Congenitally missing
   9. Periodontally involved

9. Although the patient demonstrates proper brushing and flossing technique, moderate plaque deposits are noted on the teeth. Which of the following is best indicated to assist the patient in thorough plaque removal?

   A. Floss holder
   B. Rubber tip
   C. Interdental brush
   D. Listerine mouthrinse

10. According to the American Academy of Periodontology, how would this patient's periodontal status be classified?

    A. Type I
    B. Type II
    C. Type III
    D. Type IV

11. The radiolucency present at the apex of tooth no. 5 indicates which of the following?

    A. Sinus
    B. Abscess
    C. Foramen
    D. Artifact

12. If the recession measurement for the facial of tooth no. 9 is 2 mm, what is the level of attachment loss on the mesiofacial location of this tooth?

    A. 4 mm
    B. 6 mm
    C. 8 mm
    D. 10 mm

13. Instrumentation for root débridement on the mesial of tooth no. 2 can best be accomplished by using which of the following Gracey curet instruments?

    A. 11-12 Regular shank
    B. 13-14 Regular shank
    C. 11-12 After-five
    D. 13-14 After-five

14. This patient's plaque removal can be accomplished by all of the following except one. Which one is the exception?

    A. Floss
    B. Toothbrush
    C. Rubber cup polish
    D. Air-powder abrasive system

15. All of the following procedures would be recommended before periodontal débridement except one. Which one is the exception?

    A. Periodontal charting
    B. Microbiologic testing
    C. Medical history review
    D. Antimicrobial irrigation

CASE C — Community Dental Health Care

McDaniel was once a booming farming community, but now that the young people have begun seeking their fortunes in the city, there are barely 2500 residents. Through the years, the community has been unable to attract industry, and wells remain the community's primary source of water. Other than the local nursing home, the nearest health care services are located in the city 30 miles away. Declining school enrollment has resulted in the few remaining children being bused 25 miles to a consolidated school. The old schoolhouse is now a senior citizens' center.

Because there is no public dental health center in the county, the public health department has been awarded a modest grant to assess the dental health needs of youth residing in this rural area and to develop a low-cost primary preventive program.

1. The dental hygienist's initial responsibility is to determine the oral health needs of the children in this rural community. Which of the following represents the best approach?

   A. Perform a **defs** index on the schoolchildren.
   B. Survey the schoolchildren.
   C. Interview the parents.
   D. Consult with the school nurse.

2. Which resource would best contribute to the manpower needed to implement this assessment?

   A. Local service organizations
   B. Local dental/dental hygiene association
   C. County board of education
   D. Parent-teacher association

3. During analysis of the assessment data, the dental hygienist notes that the correlation between residence and the presence of dental caries is +0.88. Which of the following represents the relationship between distance that children live from the city and tooth decay?

   A. No correlation
   B. Weak correlation
   C. Moderate correlation
   D. Strong correlation

4. Which of the following objectives of the dental health program designed for these rural school-children should be implemented first?

   A. Ensure that the rural community water supply is fluoridated.
   B. Attract dental services to the rural community.
   C. Demonstrate proper oral hygiene techniques to parents.
   D. Develop a tooth brushing program in the schools.

5. The sample to be studied consists of children from all rural households in McDaniel. Although numerous households in the rural community contain more than one child, an assessment was performed on one child from each family to ensure a representative sample. This type of sampling is referred to as

   A. convenience sampling.
   B. random sampling.
   C. stratified sampling.
   D. systematic sampling.

6-9. An O'Leary's Plaque Index was completed on seven children. Their scores were as follows: 25%, 45%, 60%, 60%, 75%, 55%, and 100%.

6. Which of the following percentages represents the mean plaque score for this group?

   A. 50%
   B. 60%
   C. 65%
   D. 70%

7. Which of the following percentages represents the mode for this group?

   A. 25%
   B. 45%
   C. 55%
   D. 60%

8. Which of the following percentages represents the median score for this group?

   A. 25%
   B. 55%
   C. 60%
   D. 100%

9. Which of the following percentages represents the range of scores for this group?

   A. 55%
   B. 60%
   C. 75%
   D. 100%

10. Which of the following activities designed to improve the diet of these schoolchildren would be least effective?

    A. List appropriate snacks on the board.
    B. Chart the students' sugar exposures daily.
    C. Require students to take turns bringing in a snack for the class.
    D. Conduct a workshop with parents on proper diet and meal planning.

SYNOPSIS OF PATIENT HISTORY	Age	4	VITAL SIGNS		**CASE D**

SYNOPSIS OF PATIENT HISTORY

Age _____4_____
Sex _____M_____
Height ___34″___

VITAL SIGNS

Blood Pressure ___85/60___
Pulse Rate ___102___
Respiration Rate ___23___

CASE D -
Pediatric, Medically Compromised

Weight ___30___ lb
___13.6___ kg

CASE D

1. Under Care of Physician
   Yes ☑   No ☐   Condition: ___Neuroblastoma___

2. Hospitalized within the last 5 years
   Yes ☑   No ☐   Reason: ___Chemotherapy___
                              ___Bone marrow transplant___

3. Has or had the following conditions
   ___Neuroblastoma, Bone marrow transplant, blocked___
   ___ureter → ↓ Ⓛ kidney function___

4. Current medications
   ___Cyclosporine___

5. Smokes or uses tobacco products
   Yes ☐   No ☑

6. Is pregnant
   Yes ☐   No ☐   N/A ☑

MEDICAL HISTORY: Diagnosed with neuroblastoma at $1\frac{1}{2}$ years of age. Treated with chemotherapy. Underwent bone marrow transplant 1 year later. No complications other than small stature. Currently seen by oncologist once/month.

DENTAL HISTORY: Took bottle to bed with milk/juice until age 3. This is first dental visit, other than cursory exam prior to transplant. Child not compliant with mother brushing teeth.

SOCIAL HISTORY: Child lives with parents and infant brother in a rural town. Mom is a homemaker. Dad is a car salesman. The municipal water supply is fluoridated.

CHIEF COMPLAINT: Teeth are getting dark, and Mom is concerned that her child may have cavities.

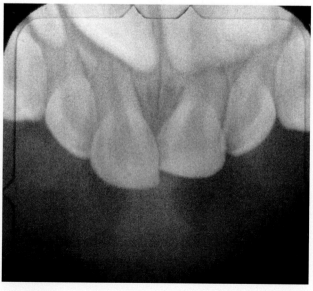

Figure D1.

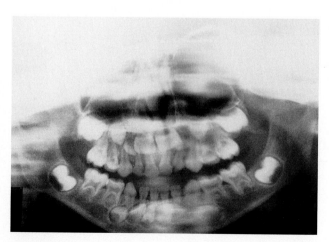

Figure D2.

CASE D

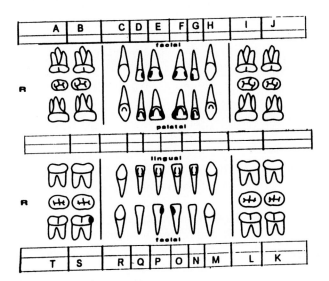

Current oral hygiene status
Fair
Generalized mild to moderate plaque

Supplemental oral examination findings
Obvious dental caries
Mild marginal gingival inflammation

 Clinically visible carious lesion

 Clinically missing tooth

△ **Furcation**

▲ **Through-and-through furcation**

Probe 1: initial probing depth

Probe 2: probing depth 1 month after scaling and root planing

CASE 4 D PEDIATRIC, Medically Compromised

1. What is the mechanism of action of the drug cyclosporine in preventing the rejection of tissue/organ transplants?

   A. Produces immunosuppression by increasing the production of lymphocytes
   B. Activates the immune response by increasing the production of lymphocytes
   C. Produces immunosuppression by decreasing the production of lymphocytes
   D. Activates the immune response by decreasing the production of lymphocytes

2. The child's small stature is most likely the result of

   A. heredity.
   B. chemotherapy.
   C. neuroblastoma.
   D. decreased kidney function.

3. Which of the following assessments would be advisable to obtain before the child receives dental treatment?

   A. White blood cell count
   B. Red blood cell count
   C. Platelet count
   D. Hematocrit

4. The dental caries experienced by this child are primarily attributed to

   A. poor oral hygiene.
   B. the administration of cyclosporine.
   C. taking a bottle to bed with milk or juice.
   D. receiving chemotherapy during eruption of the primary teeth.

5. All of the following fluoride history questions would be important to ask the patient's mother except one. The EXCEPTION is _____.

   A. Do you have a well, or do you drink the municipal water?
   B. Do you brush your child's teeth with a fluoride dentifrice?
   C. Did you have fluoride in your water when you were growing up?
   D. Was your child given a prescription for any fluoride supplements by his pediatrician?

6. Which of the following permanent teeth appear to be congenitally missing?

   A. No. 2
   B. No. 10
   C. No. 20
   D. No. 28

7. The lateral radiopaque lines found on the left side of the panoramic radiograph are indicative of

   A. lint on the intensifying screen.
   B. the normal anatomy of the spinal column.
   C. leaving one of the intensifying screens out of the cassette.
   D. static electricity resulting from pulling the film out of the cassette too rapidly.

8. Which of the following types of restorations are advised for teeth D, E, F, and G?

   A. Gold
   B. Amalgam
   C. Composite
   D. No restorations are necessary at this time.

9. What is the initial information or recommendation needed to improve this child's oral hygiene?

   A. Let the child brush his own teeth.
   B. Floss the child's teeth twice daily due to tight contacts.
   C. Determine why the child is not compliant with toothbrushing.
   D. Determine why this is the first visit, and schedule frequent recall appointments.

10. Overlap of the maxillary anterior teeth on the occlusal radiograph is indicative of

    A. improper horizontal cone placement.
    B. inadequate anterior spacing/crowding.
    C. the child moving during exposure of the film.
    D. prolonged illness during tooth development.

SYNOPSIS OF PATIENT HISTORY	Age	47	VITAL SIGNS	
	Sex	M	Blood Pressure	150/95
	Height	5'10"	Pulse Rate	80
			Respiration Rate	20

CASE E

CASE E-
Adult, Medically Compromised

Weight ___150___ lb
___67.3___ kg

1. Under Care of Physician
   Yes No
   ☑   ☐
   Condition Diabetes, End-Stage Renal Disease (ESRD)

2. Hospitalized within the last 5 years
   Yes No
   ☑   ☐
   Reason Renal Dialysis

3. Has or had the following conditions
   Arteriovenous graft for dialysis, cataracts, hypertension

4. Current medications
   Procardia, Inderal
   Insulin
   Ferrous sulfate, renal vitamin, Calcium

5. Smokes or uses tobacco products
   Yes No
   ☑   ☐

6. Is pregnant
   Yes No N/A
   ☐   ☐   ☑

MEDICAL HISTORY: Diagnosed with diabetes at age 23. Currently awaiting a kidney transplant. Smoked cigars and cigarettes since age 16. Sees physician 3 times/week for dialysis.

DENTAL HISTORY: Has only sought dental care for pain. Recently came to dentist for a pre-transplant oral evaluation.

SOCIAL HISTORY: Has been unemployed for last four years due to complications associated with diabetes. Had several toes amputated last year and was declared legally blind 2 years ago.

CHIEF COMPLAINT: "Tired of being sick; take teeth out if treating them will hold up getting kidney transplant."

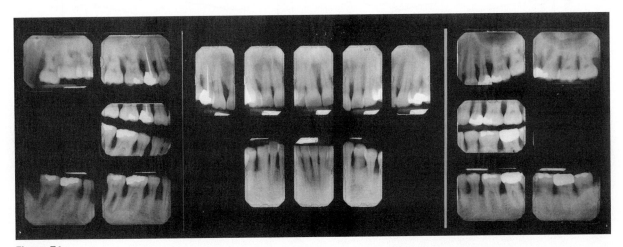

Figure E1

CASE E

Current oral hygiene status
Poor oral hygiene

Supplemental oral examination findings

Generalized 2-3 mm recession,

Bleeding upon probing, and tooth mobility

Moderate brown stain

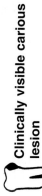 Clinically visible carious lesion

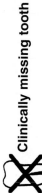 Clinically missing tooth

△ Furcation

▲ Through-and-through furcation

Probe 1: initial probing depth

Probe 2: probing depth 1 month after scaling and root planing

ADULT CLINICAL EXAMINATION

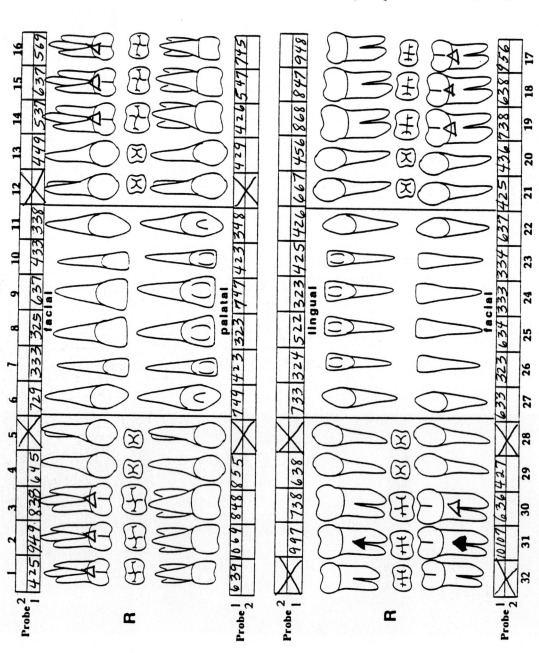

CASE E ADULT, Medically Compromised

1. Due to this patient's diagnosis of hypertension, his blood pressure should be assessed at each dental visit regardless if the visits are 1 day or 1 week apart. The patient's blood pressure should be taken in the same arm as the atrioventricular graft (shunt) to ensure an accurate reading.

    A. Statement 1 is true; statement 2 is false.
    B. Statement 1 is false; statement 2 is true.
    C. Both statements are true.
    D. Both statements are false.

2. The most suitable time to schedule a patient on renal dialysis is

    A. 2 hours before the dialysis appointment.
    B. the day between dialysis appointments.
    C. 1 hour after the dialysis appointment.
    D. after all dialysis treatments have been completed for that week.

3. Which of the following behaviors would have the most significant impact on controlling this patient's periodontal disease status?

    A. Monitoring blood pressure daily
    B. Reducing the dosage of nifedipine (Procardia) taken daily
    C. Taking oral hypoglycemic agents instead of insulin
    D. Quitting smoking or the use of tobacco products

4. Which of the following medications currently taken by this patient is responsible for staining the teeth?

    A. Insulin
    B. Inderal
    C. Procardia
    D. Ferrous sulfate

5. What is the primary reason for the supereruption of tooth no. 1?

    A. Tooth no. 1 is a microdont.
    B. The maxillary molars are crowded.
    C. There is no opposing tooth in the mandibular arch.
    D. The tooth is too far posterior and cannot be cleaned effectively.

6. Which of the following interproximal cleaning devices would be best suited for this patient?

    A. Proxabrush
    B. Fine waxed floss
    C. Wooden stimudent
    D. Rubber tip stimulators

7. What is the major contributing factor to the bone loss observed on the distal of tooth no. 30?

    A. Calculus
    B. Interproximal caries
    C. A mucogingival defect
    D. An overhanging restoration

8. Which of the following ADA and AAP classifications for periodontal disease is descriptive of this patient?

    A. Case type I
    B. Case type II
    C. Case type III
    D. Case type IV
    E. Case type V

9. Which of the following types of bitewing radiographs is best suited to the diagnosis of this patient's needs?

    A. Horizontal bitewings
    B. Vertical bitewings
    C. Reverse bitewings

10. All of the following periodontal pathogens would be elevated in this patient with one exception. The EXCEPTION is _____.

    A. *Bacteroides forsythus*
    B. *Prevotella intermedia*
    C. *Porphyromonas gingivalis*
    D. *Actinobacillus actinomycetemcomitans*

11. Antibiotic prophylaxis would be recommended for this patient prior to dental treatment. A-V shunts for hemodialysis are vulnerable to infection.

    A. Statement 1 is true; statement 2 is false.
    B. Statement 1 is false; statement 2 is true.
    C. Both statements are true.
    D. Both statements are false.

SYNOPSIS OF PATIENT HISTORY	Age	31	VITAL SIGNS			CASE F

SYNOPSIS OF PATIENT HISTORY

Age _____31_____
Sex _____M_____
Height __5'1"__

VITAL SIGNS
Blood Pressure __140/85__
Pulse Rate ____78____
Respiration Rate ____18____

CASE F

CASE F - Special Needs

Weight ____160____ lb
____72.8____ kg

1. Under Care of Physician
   Yes ☑   No ☐
   Condition _Congestive heart failure (CHF)_

2. Hospitalized within the last 5 years
   Yes ☑   No ☐
   Reason _Cardiac arrest_

3. Has or had the following conditions
   Leukemia, Down syndrome, CHF, hypertension

4. Current medications
   Lanoxin, Lasix, Vasotec, Coumadin, potassium

5. Smokes or uses tobacco products
   Yes ☐   No ☑

6. Is pregnant
   Yes ☐   No ☐   N/A ☑

MEDICAL HISTORY: Diagnosed with leukemia at age 5. Treated with chemotherapy. In remission since age 14. Diagnosed with CHF age 29. Recent loss of 25 lbs. Allergic to penicillin. IQ = 48. No hearing in right ear.

DENTAL HISTORY: Has regular dental visits, but home care is poor. Nutrition is normally good, but cannot bite down on food with front teeth due to bleeding and mobility.

SOCIAL HISTORY: Lives with mother (age 73). Works part-time in a video store. Has one older sibling of normal IQ. Father is deceased.

CHIEF COMPLAINT: Mouth is dry, and some of his teeth feel loose.

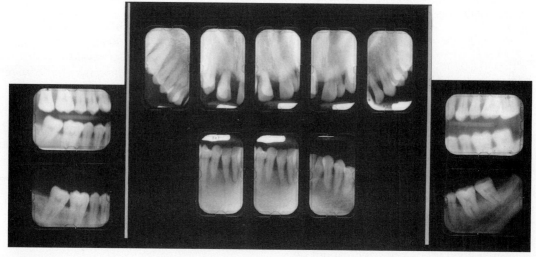

Figure F1

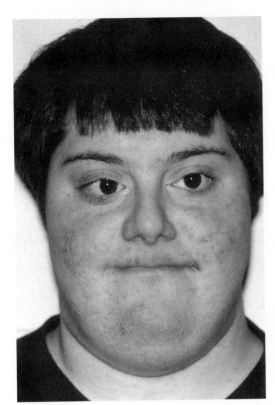

Figure F2

CASE F

Current oral hygiene status

Fair

Moderate plaque　accumulation

Supplemental oral examination findings

Bleeding upon probing (generalized)

#8–11 mobile

#22–25 mobile

Localized furcation involvement

Mild xerostomia

Crossbite-right

Clinically visible carious lesion

Clinically missing tooth

△ Furcation

▲ Through-and-through furcation

Probe 1: initial probing depth

Probe 2: probing depth 1 month after scaling and root planing

ADULT CLINICAL EXAMINATION

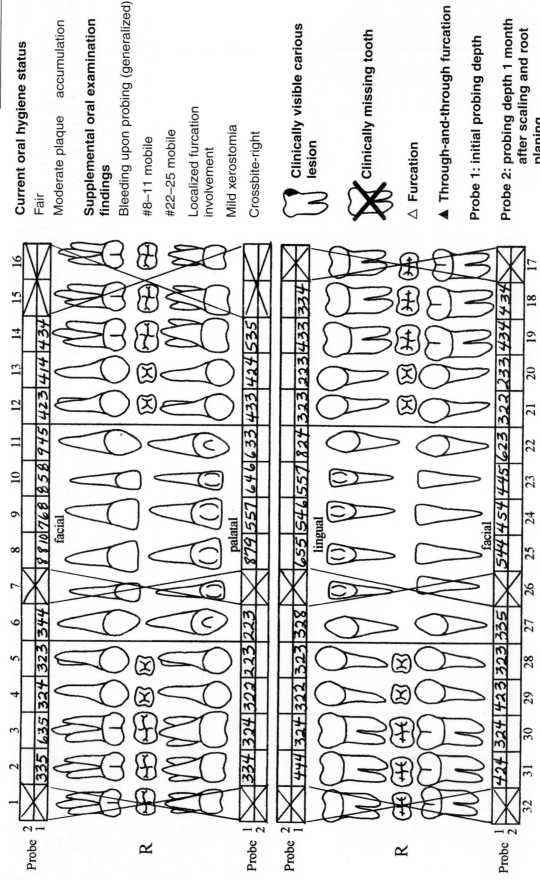

CASE 5 F SPECIAL NEEDS

1. Which of the following types of malocclusion is found most commonly in persons with Down syndrome owing to the short mid-third of the face?

   A. Class I
   B. Class II
   C. Class II, division 2
   D. Class III

2. Which of the following conditions would be contraindications for treating this patient?

   A. An international normalized ratio (INR) of 3.5
   B. A history of leukemia
   C. A history of myocardial infarction
   D. Neutrophil chemotaxis associated with Down syndrome

3. An individual with an intelligence quotient of 48 can also be called _____ mentally retarded.

   A. educable
   B. trainable
   C. severely
   D. profoundly

4. Which of the following errors may have caused the left bitewing radiograph to be too light?

   A. Excessive exposure
   B. Excessive fixation
   C. Developing solution too warm
   D. Accidental exposure to white light

5. Which of the following conditions warrant antibiotic premedication before the patient receives dental treatment?

   A. Hypertension
   B. Down syndrome
   C. History of leukemia
   D. Congestive heart failure
   E. History of myocardial infarction
   F. None of the above

6. The most likely treatment for teeth no. 8-11 is

   A. extraction.
   B. splinting.
   C. scaling and root débridement.
   D. application of a local antibiotic delivery system.

7. The most likely reason for the absence of teeth nos. 7 and 26 is

   A. trauma.
   B. dental caries.
   C. congenitally missing.
   D. periodontal involvement.

8. Which of the following medications would most likely result in xerostomia?

   A. Potassium
   B. Vasotec
   C. Coumadin
   D. Lanoxin

9. If tooth no. 22 has 2 mm of recession on the facial aspect, what would be the level of attachment loss on the mesial-facial of that tooth?

   A. 4 mm
   B. 6 mm
   C. 8 mm
   D. 10 mm

10. The best management plan for controlling periodontal disease in this patient would involve working with the patient and his mother on oral hygiene measures during biannual visits. In addition, a trial period of chlorhexidine mouthrinse brushed on the teeth and gingiva at bedtime is advised.

    A. Statement 1 is true; statement 2 is false.
    B. Statement 1 is false; statement 2 is true.
    C. Both statements are true.
    D. Both statements are false.

ANSWERS

CASE A

1. **C.** Radiation therapy used in the treatment of cancer compromises circulation to the area irradiated. The result is a change in the growth potential of bone in the affected area and a lowered resistance to infection. Osteoradionecrosis (ORN) refers to bone that has become infected as a result of radiation. Hyperbaric oxygen treatments flood the body tissues with oxygen, particularly at the time of extractions, to reduce the risk of ORN.

2. **B.** The patient's pain is caused by the obvious multiple abscessed teeth. Although trismus is a potential side effect of radiation therapy to the head and neck, no evidence of trismus exists now and no recurrence of the oral cancer has been discussed. She does have gingivitis and moderate plaque accumulation, but pain associated with periodontal disease at this stage would be much less than that experienced from the periapical infection.

3. **B.** The root canals noted on teeth no. 23 to 27 are filled with a gutta-percha. This softer material appears slightly less radiopaque radiographically than silver points. Gutta-percha has less density and a more irregular shape filling the canal. Silver points are rarely used in current endodontic treatment.

4. **B.** Annual recalls are much too infrequent for a patient with such significant decay and such a complicated medical history. A 1- to 3-month recall is advised.

5. **A.** The radiolucencies are indicative of periapical abscesses. An abscess is a localized infection or collection of pus in a circumscribed area formed by the disintegration of tissues.

6. **B.** Augmentin is a form of amoxicillin.

7. **D.** An odontoma is usually seen as a well-defined radiolucent area within bone that contains varying amounts of calcified material. A dentigerous cyst is also radiolucent. It develops from the enamel organ; therefore, it is usually associated with the crown of a tooth. Common teeth affected are third molars, canines, and embedded teeth.

8. **D.** The developing third molars are medial to the coronoid process. They appear to be microdonts.

9. **E.** Tooth no. 32 is most likely to be a congenitally missing tooth because although the other three third molars are in the early stages of development, they are visible radiographically.

10. **D.** The primary reason for a patient this young to be experiencing advanced caries of the permanent dentition is due to xerostomia induced by radiation to the salivary glands. Each of the other factors has contributed to her dental status by exacerbating the effects of a dry mouth on the teeth.

CASE B

1. **B.** The diagnosis of mitral valve prolapse with regurgitation warrants antibiotic premedication before dental treatment. Because the patient is allergic to penicillin, clindamycin is the drug of choice. In addition, ciprofloxacin is not one of the antibiotics recommended by the American Heart Association for the prevention of bacterial endocarditis. In this case, Cipro has been prescribed for a sinus infection and does not provide sufficient coverage for dental procedures.

2. **D.** Cyclophosphamide (Cytoxan) is an antineoplastic alkylating agent that often causes oral ulcerations/stomatitis as an oral side effect. Tamoxifen is also an antineoplastic drug used for advanced stages of breast cancer; the oral side effect is hypogeusia (altered taste). Clonidine is an antihypertensive drug that is known to produce xerostomia as an oral complication. Insulin rarely produces oral side effects.

3. **D.** Moderate bone loss and gingival recession have resulted in sufficient attachment loss to expose the furcation of the facial and lingual of tooth no. 30. Because the bone is missing between the mesial and distal roots, the area appears radiolucent on a radiograph.

4. **A.** Clonidine, an antihypertensive agent, causes dry mouth as a side effect.

5. **C.** A known diabetic who presents with flushed dry skin, abdominal pain, and nausea is experiencing the signs and symptoms of diabetic coma. The treatment for this medical emergency is insulin. Questioning the patient about the disease and treatment is critical when preventing or assessing and managing a medical emergency.

6. **A.** Acetone breath is one of the key signs of diabetic coma. Hyperglycemia is an elevation of the blood glucose level beyond normal limits and is the reason why the patient experiences diabetic coma. The patient's hyperglycemia may be caused by her occasional desire to indulge in candy, or she may have forgotten to take her insulin. Her obvious periodontal condition, sinus infection, or stress associated with seeing a new dentist may have contributed to this condition.

7. **D.** Caries are not initiated by the systemic diseases (e.g., rheumatic heart disease, breast cancer, hypertension, and insulin-dependent diabetes mellitus) experienced by the patient described. Caries primarily result from three factors-plaque, diet, and the susceptible host (a patient with impaired oral self-cleansing owing to drug-induced xerostomia).

8. **B.** Tooth no. 17 is unerupted. It is not visible clinically, but it can be viewed radiographically.

9. **C.** Owing to the significant amount of recession and overall attachment loss, an interdental brush is advocated as an adjunct to brushing and flossing. Listerine is contraindicated, because its high alcohol content contributes to oral dryness.

10. **D.** The patient's probing depths range from 2 to 11 mm. There is recession from 2 to 5 mm, generalized class II mobility, and furcation involvement of tooth no. 19 and no. 30. This translates to a periodontal classification of case type IV.

11. **B.** The radiolucency surrounding the apex of tooth no. 5 is indicative of an abscess. The severe attachment loss and exudate coming from this tooth, combined with the patient's report of pain in the maxillary right posterior region, are characteristics signs of infection.

12. **C.** Attachment loss is determined by combining the recession reading (2 mm) with the probing depth (6 mm) equaling a total of 8 mm.

13. **C.** Gracey 11-12 instruments are used to débride the mesial surfaces of teeth. After-five curets have elongated shanks to adapt to deeper pocket depths.

14. **D.** Air-powder abrasives contain ingestible sodium bicarbonate and may cause a drug interaction with ciprofloxacin. At least 2 hours should elapse between taking the drug and use of the Prophy Jet. Sodium is also contraindicated for this patient, because she is hypertensive.

15. **D.** An antimicrobial rinse before débridement is suggested, but irrigation is accomplished after instrumentation. Microbiologic testing must always be done before débridement to determine the types of periodontal pathogens residing in the sulcus. Treatment can be determined more definitively by the results of this testing.

CASE C

1. **A.** To determine the needs of any group, the initial procedure is to conduct an assessment of that group. A survey of schoolchildren would provide some information, but not the specific information needed to determine oral need. Looking in the mouths of these children and conducting a defs index gives the investigator a total of the number of children affected by dental caries, the number of teeth that need treatment, and the proportion of teeth that have been treated.

2. **B.** The best resource to obtain the personnel required to conduct a defs index is the local dental/dental hygiene association. These professionals are educated to conduct assessments of this type. The other groups, although often willing to lend support, would have to be trained to perform this task and they do not have the educational background to make professional judgments. These groups should be called upon to provide supplies, financial support, and so forth.

3. **D.** The strength of a correlation is determined by its proximity to 1.0. The sign (+ or -) denotes the relationship as (+) directly or (-) indirectly proportional. Therefore, a +.88 shows that a strong direct relationship exists between caries and the distance that children live from the city. As distance increases, tooth decay increases.

4. **A.** The first objective to be implemented is to reach the largest population with the least amount of compliance. Water fluoridation is the most cost-effective method to reduce dental caries, particularly because many of the children residing in rural areas drink well water that may contain little or no fluoride.

5. **C.** Stratified random sampling divides the population (i.e., children in a rural community) into subgroups (i.e., families) before selection to ensure that all families are represented.

6. **B.** The mean is the average score. You obtain the mean by adding the scores and dividing by the total number of scores. 420 (7 = 60

7. **D.** The mode is the value that occurs most frequently.

8. **C.** The median is the point that divides a score distribution into equal parts; half of the scores fall above the median and half fall below.

9. **C.** The range is the difference between the highest and the lowest scores. 100% - 25% = 75%.

10. **A.** If a change in health behavior is desired, activities must be performed that are meaningful for the person involved. Schoolchildren can change their frequency of fermentable carbohydrate intake by actively charting their daily exposures to sugar. Charting behavior influences behavior through behavior modification. Bringing in good snacks and working with the parents who are responsible for food choices and meal planning at home are activities that require active participation and have a greater chance of invoking change. A child might be able to list good snacks but may not have access to those appropriate foods at home.

CASE D

1. **C.** Cyclosporine is a drug that prevents the recipient of a transplant from rejecting the donor's organ/tissue. This is accomplished by producing immunosuppression through the inhibition of lymphocyte production.

2. **B.** The child's small stature is most likely to be the result of chemotherapy interfering with growth and development. Because chemotherapy drugs destroy cancer cells that divide in a haphazard manner, they also kill normal cells that divide rapidly, such as hair follicles and cells of the gastrointestinal and genitourinary tracts. Consequently, side effects result, particularly in children, because their cells are rapidly dividing during growth and development.

3. **A.** A white blood cell count would provide information regarding the existence and extent of immunosuppression and the need for antibiotic premedication before dental procedures.

4. **C.** Although poor oral hygiene contributes to caries, the substrate-milk or juice in the bottle at bedtime is the primary etiology for caries formation.

5. **C.** The mother's fluoride history is less relevant than the current fluoride exposures that the child is receiving. The child's past dietary habits and fair oral hygiene practices require optimal fluoride protection to prevent further decay.

6. **B.** Tooth no. 10 is the only tooth that appears to be congenitally missing at this time. The child is too young for you to see any of the remaining choices on a radiograph.

7. **B.** The lateral opaque lines represent the spinal column.

8. **C.** The interproximal decay noted on the maxillary incisors should be restored with a tooth-colored restoration despite the patient's age. Restoring the primary teeth is essential to eliminate the infection. Restoring the teeth is suggested as opposed to extracting them for reasons of aesthetics, mastication, speech and to maintain adequate spacing for the permanent teeth. Tooth G may need a polycarbonate (i.e., tooth-colored) crown, because the decay appears to have entered the pulp.

9. **C.** Initially, it is important to assess why a child is not compliant with oral hygiene. The parent(s) may need to perform daily oral hygiene on the child or at the very least supervise the child. It is usually futile to make recommendations without determining the source of the problem.

10. **B.** The overlap is anatomic and can be observed in both the occlusal and panoramic radiographs.

CASE E

1. **A.** The patient's blood pressure should always be assessed at recall appointments, and the blood pressure should be checked more often if the patient has a history of hypertension. The blood pressure should always be taken in the opposite arm of an individual who has an arteriovenous fistula for renal dialysis.

2. **B.** Most dialysis appointments are made on Monday, Wednesday, and Friday or on Tuesday and Thursday. Ideally, the patient should be seen on a day between dialysis appointments to minimize fatigue and the effects of coumadin, which was flushed through the graft site.

3. **D.** Smoking is a major risk factor in developing periodontal disease. Studies suggest that smoking may affect neutrophil function, stop serum antibody response to periodontal pathogens, and affect fibroblast function. Although diabetes is also a major risk factor in the development of periodontal disease, changing the patient's medications from insulin to an oral hypoglycemic agent would not have a significant effect on the disease. This change could actually exacerbate the periodontal condition if the oral drug was unable to control the patient's diabetes.

4. **D.** Ferrous sulfate is iron and will result in extrinsic staining of the teeth. If this medication is taken through a straw or as a tablet or capsule, staining may be eliminated.

5. **C.** Tooth no. 1 is supererupted because there is no opposing tooth in the opposite arch (i.e., no. 32 is missing) to prevent the tooth from further erupting. Teeth continue to erupt until they meet resistance.

6. **A.** Due to the significant attachment loss experienced by this patient, the interdental brush would adapt well in furcations and between open embrasures where interdental papillae have been lost.

7. **D.** In the periapical radiographs, it appears that an amalgam overhang exists on the distal of tooth no. 30. No calculus or caries is evident.

8. **D.** Case type IV refers to advanced periodontitis. Major loss of alveolar bone support and tooth mobility exist. Many probing depths exceed 6 mm, and furcation involvement is noted on several multi-rooted teeth.

9. **B.** Vertical bitewings provide a greater surface area on the film so that areas of reduced bone height are not missed (which has occurred utilizing the horizontal bitewing). Reverse bitewings are placed against the facial surfaces and are usually used for patients who have special needs and who cannot control their tongue movements or hold a bitewing on the lingual surfaces in the traditional manner.

10. **D.** *Actinobacillus actinomycetemcomitans* is usually found in juvenile or refractory forms of periodontitis.

11. **C.** Both statements are true. There is evidence that arteriovenous (A-V) shunts have a low risk for endocarditis, but are none-the-less vulnerable to infection. Peritoneal dialysis on the other hand, does not require antibiotic premedication.

CASE F

1. **D.** The short mid-facial defect commonly associated with Down syndrome results in a short constricted palate and an underdeveloped maxilla. Prognathism or a protruded mandible manifests, thus increasing the tendency for a class III malocclusion.

2. **A.** The only condition that would alter treatment is an international normalized ratio (INR) of 3.5 associated with coumadin therapy. Typically, if the level of anticoagulation (expressed in the INR) is more than 3.0, the dosage of coumadin may need to be reduced.

3. **B.** The term *trainable* is given to those individuals who have an intelligence quotient of 25-49. Trainable means that a person is capable of learning a skill or trade as opposed to being mainstreamed in the regular school system (i.e., educable).

4. **B.** Excessive exposure to fixer solution causes additional silver halide crystals to be removed from the emulsion, thus resulting in a lighter film. Insufficient development or reduced exposure of the film to the radiation source may also result in a low-density radiograph. Cool or outdated processing solutions and use of film that has expired may also produce a light radiograph.

5. **F.** None of these conditions warrants premedication prior to dental procedures.

6. **A.** Teeth no. 8-11 are severely periodontally involved (increased probing depths and mobility); therefore, extraction is recommended.

7. D. Assessment of the remaining maxillary and mandibular anterior teeth leads one to believe that periodontal involvement is the reason for the loss of teeth nos. 7 and 26.

8. **B.** Vasotec is an antihypertensive drug and is known to produce xerostomia as a side effect.

9. **C.** The facial of 22 has a 2-mm recession, and the probing depth on the mesial is 6 mm. Attachment loss equals recession plus probing depth.

10. B. Statement 1 is false, because biannual recalls (twice per year) are insufficient to manage a patient who has special needs and also moderate to severe periodontal disease.

References in *italics* indicate figures; those followed by "t" denote tables